GERONTOLOGICAL NURSING

COMPETENCIES FOR CARE

FOURTH EDITION

The Pedagogy

Gerontological Nursing: Competencies for Care, Fourth Edition drives comprehension through various strategies that meet the learning needs of students, while also generating enthusiasm about the topic. This interactive approach addresses different learning styles, making this the ideal text to ensure mastery of key concepts. The pedagogical aids that appear in most chapters include the following:

Learning Objectives These objectives provide a snapshot of information in each chapter. They serve as a checklist to guide and focus study.

Key Terms Found in a list at the beginning of each chapter, these terms will create an expanded vocabulary.

CHAPTER 10

Nursing Management of Dementia

Prudence Twigg
Christine E. Schwartzkopf

(Competencies 9, 15, 16)

LEARNING OBJECTIVES

At the end of this chapter, the reader will be able to:

> Differentiate among dementia, depression, and delirium.
> Identify the stages and clinical features of dementia.
> Describe procedures for diagnosing dementia.
> Recognize and address the common causes of delirium.
> Discuss the theoretical foundations of nursing care for persons with dementia.
> Contrast pharmacological and nonpharmacological interventions for dementia, delirium, and depression.
> Apply basic principles to provide safe and effective care for persons with dementia.
> List specific nursing interventions for behavioral and psychological symptoms of dementia.
> Recognize the role of adult day services in the care of persons with dementia.
> Identify the role that palliative care and hospice care play for individuals with dementia and their families.

KEY TERMS

Acetylcholine
Agnosia
Alzheimer's disease
Anticholinergic
Aphasia
Apolipoprotein E-e4
Apraxia

Beta-amyloid plaques
Cholinesterase
Cholinesterase inhibitor
Delirium
Dementia
Depression
Executive function

Case Studies Case studies encourage active learning and promote critical thinking. Read about real-life scenarios and analyze the situation presented.

582   Chapter 17   *Dysphagia and Malnutrition*

Case Study 17–1

Mr. C., an 81-year-old widower, is admitted for stroke rehabilitation. He underwent a cystoscopy and transurethral resection of the prostate (TURP) for benign prostatic hypertrophy (BPH) 1 week ago. After the procedure he experienced a hypotensive episode and mental status changes. A workup revealed a large left middle-cerebral artery stroke. His stroke deficits include expressive aphasia, left neglect, dysphagia, and left hemiplegia. Concurrent health problems include coronary artery disease, hypertension, and hyperlipidemia under good control prior to surgery. Prior to transfer, Mr. C. had a low hematocrit level and Hemoccult-positive stool and received a blood transfusion. He was also suspected to have pneumonia and was started on an antibiotic.

On examination, Mr. C. is noted to be thin, pale, and lethargic. He has a weak cough, facial weakness, and a mild case of thrush. An indwelling urinary catheter is draining amber urine. Nonpitting edema is noted in his right hand; his arms have multiple bruises and dry, flaky skin. The transfer report indicates he requires minimal assistance with bed mobility and moderate assistance with transfers, including toilet transfers; his sitting balance is fair; and he can self-propel his wheelchair 150 ft. with standby assistance. His son and daughter live out of town and have had to return home. They were not able to accompany him at transfer and will not be able to visit until the weekend (4 days from now).

Orders on admission include a pureed texture diet with moderate thick liquids, Isosource 1.5 cans at 0800 and 1600 and 1 can at 1200 and 2000 with 325 cc free water flush every shift via PEG tube. One scoop of Benefiber is added to tube feeding three times a day. His medication orders

include Tenormin, 25 mg once a day; Lipitor, 20 mg at bedtime; Prevacid, 30 mg once a day; ASA, 81 mg once a day; Plavix, 75 mg once a day; amiodarone, 200 mg once a day; and clindamycin, 600 mg 3 times a day.

Questions:

1. Mr. C. presents multiple challenges. Which of the common health problems discussed in this chapter are relevant to his nursing care?
2. What are the priorities for Mr. C.'s care plan during his first week of rehabilitation?
3. What are key interventions to promote recovery and prevent complications?

After 3 days, the physician orders discontinuing his indwelling catheter. He experiences frequency, urgency, and incontinence. He has developed symptoms of an allergy—he is suffering from runny nose and dry cough. His tube feeding is being dermaced as his dietary intake increases. When his family arrives, they ask about putting him on that medicine advertised on TV for overactive bladder and bring his over-the-counter (OTC) allergy medicine (Sudafed) for his cold. They also bring him his favorite soda.

Questions:

4. How would you respond to the family?
5. What actions would you take to address the problems and concerns raised?
6. How would your goals for care evolve over the next weeks of his stay?
7. What interventions would you institute to prevent the development of common health problems during his hospitalization and upon return to the community?

Clinical Reasoning Exercises

1. Delirium may manifest as hypoactive or hyperactive. Which type of delirium do you think is more likely to be identified by nurses in the clinical setting and why?
2. Why do individuals with delirium tend to be unable to communicate appropriately? What are the characteristic features associated with delirium? What are the primary risk factors for the development of delirium? Is delirium a reversible disorder?
3. Evaluate the medication list of one of your clinical clients with dementia or delirium in

relation to the Beers Criteria for potentially inappropriate medications for older adults.
4. Given the modest benefits of cholinesterase inhibitors and memantine in the treatment of dementia, debate the pros and cons of administering these medications for persons with dementia.
5. Choose a client in your clinical setting who has dementia. Practice communication strategies.

Clinical Reasoning Exercises Review key concepts from each chapter with these exercises at the end of each chapter.

Personal Reflections

1. Have you ever cared for a patient or family member with dementia? How did you feel about this experience? What did you find most frustrating? How did you handle specific symptoms that caused changes in behavior?
2. What risk factors do you personally have for AD? Are there any activities that you can do to decrease your personal risk?
3. What do you consider the difference between chronic and acute illness?
4. This chapter focused on the nurse's role, but what challenges do you think family members face in caring for loved ones with AD?

Personal Reflections Reflect critically on chapter content by exploring these questions and activities at the end of each chapter.

Clinical Tip These notes cover essential information and tactics for applicaiton to practice.

Research Highlight These boxes share important research studies for further exploration of chapter topics.

Recommended Reading, Resource List, and Web Exploration These lists point to additional resources for more in-depth learning.

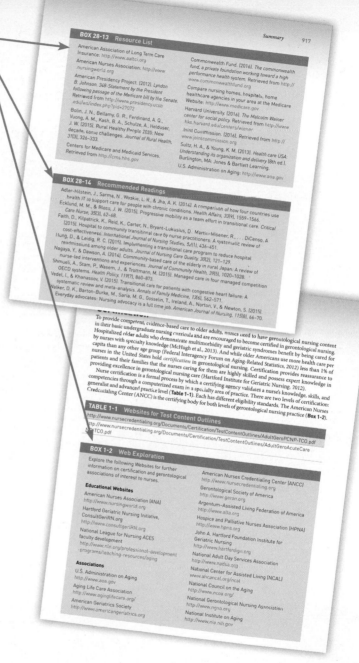

GERONTOLOGICAL NURSING

COMPETENCIES FOR CARE

FOURTH EDITION

Edited by

Kristen L. Mauk, PhD, DNP, RN, CRRN, GCNS-BC, GNP-BC, ACHPN, FAAN

Professor of Nursing
Colorado Christian University
President
Senior Care Central/International Rehabilitation Consultants, LLC
Ridgway, Colorado

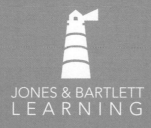

JONES & BARTLETT
L E A R N I N G

World Headquarters
Jones & Bartlett Learning
5 Wall Street
Burlington, MA 01803
978-443-5000
info@jblearning.com
www.jblearning.com

Jones & Bartlett Learning books and products are available through most bookstores and online booksellers. To contact Jones & Bartlett Learning directly, call 800-832-0034, fax 978-443-8000, or visit our website, www.jblearning.com.

13116-1

Production Credits

VP, Executive Publisher: David D. Cella
Executive Editor: Amanda Martin
Editorial Assistant: Emma Huggard
Production Manager: Carolyn Rogers Pershouse
Director of Vendor Management: Amy Rose
Vendor Manager: Juna Abrams
Senior Marketing Manager: Jennifer Scherzay
Product Fulfillment Manager: Wendy Kilborn
Composition: S4Carlisle Publishing Services

Project Management: S4Carlisle Publishing Services
Cover Design: Kristin E. Parker
Director of Rights & Media: Joanna Gallant
Rights & Media Specialist: Wes DeShano
Media Development Editor: Shannon Sheehan
Cover Image: © thinair28/Vetta/Getty
Printing and Binding: LSC Communications
Cover Printing: LSC Communications

Library of Congress Cataloging-in-Publication Data
Names: Mauk, Kristen L., editor.
Title: Gerontological nursing : competencies for care / [edited by] Kristen Mauk.
Other titles: Gerontological nursing (Mauk)
Description: 4th edition. | Burlington, MA : Jones & Bartlett Learning,
    [2018] | Includes bibliographical references and index.
Identifiers: LCCN 2016056996 | ISBN 9781284104479 (pbk. : alk. paper)
Subjects: | MESH: Geriatric Nursing—methods | Clinical Competence |
    Aging—physiology | Aging—psychology
Classification: LCC RC954 | NLM WY 152 | DDC 618.97/0231--dc23 LC record available at https://lccn.loc.gov/2016056996

6048

Printed in the United States of America
22 21 20 19 18   10 9 8 7 6 5 4 3

Dedication and Acknowledgments

Dedication

To Deanne, Cody, Amelia, Luke, and JJ

my wonderful grandchildren who make it fun to get older

Acknowledgments

Thanks to the parents and grandparents who have been a part of my life and the lives of my children:

Pete and Kay Gibson
Larry and Gracie Mauk
Phyllis Hays
Pat and Marvin Bell

Your legacies are a great gift to all the people in your lives, and you have each been influential in shaping mine.

I would also like to thank the excellent staff at Jones & Bartlett Learning for all their help, especially Emma Huggard and Amanda Martin, and to Wes and Pal for their assistance.

Contents

CHAPTER 4

Review of the Aging of Physiological Systems   67

Janice Heineman

Jennifer Hamrick-King

Beth Scaglione Sewell

(Competencies 9, 19)

UNIT III   **Health Promotion, Risk Reduction, and Disease Prevention**   **239**
(Competencies 3–6, 9, 17, 18)

CHAPTER 7   **Promoting Healthy Aging, Independence, and Quality of Life**   **241**
David Haber
(Competencies 4, 5, 9, 17, 18)

CHAPTER 8

**Identifying and Preventing Common Risk Factors
in the Elderly   271**
Joan M. Nelson
(Competencies 3, 4, 6, 9, 17)

UNIT IV   Illness and Disease Management   303
(Competencies 9, 15–18)

CHAPTER 9   Management of Common Illnesses, Diseases, and Health Conditions   305

Kristen L. Mauk

Amy Silva-Smith

(Competencies 9, 15, 17, 18)

CHAPTER 10

Nursing Management of Dementia   387
Prudence Twigg

Christine E. Schwartzkopf

(Competencies 9, 15, 16)

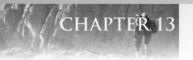

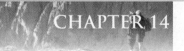

CHAPTER 15

Urinary Incontinence   517
B. Renee Dugger

(Competencies 7, 17)

CHAPTER 16

Sleep Disorders   543
Carol Enderlin

Melodee Harris

Karen M. Rose

Lisa Hutchison

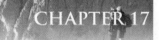

CHAPTER 17

Dysphagia and Malnutrition   577
Neva L. Crogan

(Competency 7)

CHAPTER 20

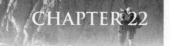

CHAPTER 25 **Pain Management and Alternative Health
Modalities** **797**
Carole A. Pepa
(Competencies 8, 9, 12, 15, 18)

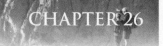

CHAPTER 26

Disaster Preparation, Response, and Recovery   829
Elaine Miller

Sharon Farra

(Competencies 14, 17)

Preface

Although numerous excellent gerontological nursing texts are available on the market today, the approach to this book is unique in that the first and second editions were based on an essential document from the American Association of Colleges of Nursing (AACN) and the John A. Hartford Foundation Institute for Geriatric Nursing (July 2000), entitled *Older Adults: Recommended Baccalaureate Competencies and Curricular Guidelines for Geriatric Nursing Care*. The third edition used the updated document, *Recommended Baccalaureate Competencies and Curricular Guidelines for the Nursing Care of Older Adults* (September 2010), published by the same two organizations. This fourth edition continues that tradition. This book is intended to be a basic baccalaureate-level gerontological nursing text, although much of the new edition is also appropriate for graduate-level coursework, and it is structured to ensure that students will obtain the recommended competencies and knowledge necessary to provide excellent care to older adults. It can be used for a stand-alone course or in sections to be integrated throughout a nursing curriculum.

Using the recommended competencies as a guide, each chapter is written to assist students of gerontological nursing to acquire the essential knowledge and skills to provide excellent care for older adults. Competencies as set forth in the AACN and Hartford Foundation document are listed at the beginning of each chapter to help direct students' learning.

This book has several outstanding features. First, the framework, as described, is unique. In addition, the text is an edited work with a diverse authorship of 50 contributors and numerous reviewers who represent all areas of gerontological nursing, including management, education, quality assurance, clinical practice in a variety of settings, advanced practice roles, research, business, consulting, and academia. This fourth edition adds several new authors, with the vast majority of authors from the last edition continuing their work in the new edition. All chapters have been updated to include current resources and evidence-based clinical practice. Interdisciplinary collaboration of many chapters was accomplished by including nurse authors' writing with colleagues whose backgrounds are in psychology, social work, pharmacy, gerontology, rehabilitation, biology, and sociology.

For this edition, comments and recommendations of instructors and reviewers who have used the text were carefully considered. In answer to requests, an entirely new chapter—Disaster Preparedness—was added. Additional practical content was added on communication, teaching, and care transitions. Many original photos and content portray older adults as actively aging.

The text has a user-friendly and comprehensive format. Several features were designed to appeal to students. Clinical tips appear as a new item throughout the text. The following pedagogical features are used:

> Learning Objectives
> Key Terms (with terms highlighted in chapter)
> Clinical Tips
> Tables that summarize key points
> Boxes to highlight interesting information and key practice points

> Web exploration and links
> Pictures, diagrams, and drawings
> Original photographs
> Research Highlights with application to practice
> Evidence-Based Practice boxes and guidelines
> Clinical Reasoning exercises
> Personal Reflection exercises
> Case Studies with Questions
> Resource Lists
> References (including websites)
> Recommended Readings
> Glossary

Students will be delighted to have a glossary at the end of the text, as well as definitions of key terms within the chapters. The competencies recommended by the AACN and Hartford Foundation are threaded throughout the book. Students will also benefit from new online resources and educational materials available from the publisher.

Instructors will find the accompanying online instructor's manual to be a time-saving tool. It is designed to provide a complete curriculum for instructors and students, even for those who may lack a strong geriatric background. The instructor's manual suggests activities for learning and in-class exercises and provides Power-Point slides for lectures that coincide with student readings in the main text. A test bank is also provided. Most of the work for development of a gerontological nursing course or integration in portions into the curriculum has already been done for instructors.

This book is divided into sections that directly follow the AACN and Hartford Foundation Institute's Competencies *Recommended Baccalaureate Competencies and Curricular Guidelines for the Nursing Care of Older Adults* (September 2010, pp. 12–13). The 19 gerontological nursing competency statements shown here, with the corresponding Essential from the AACN Baccalaureate Competencies, are those necessary to provide high-quality care to older adults and their families:

1. Incorporate professional attitudes, values, and expectations about physical and mental aging in the provision of patient-centered care for older adults and their families.
   Corresponding to Essential VIII

2. Assess barriers for older adults in receiving, understanding, and giving of information.
   Corresponding to Essentials IV and IX

3. Use valid and reliable assessment tools to guide nursing practice for older adults.
   Corresponding to Essential IX

4. Assess the living environment as it relates to functional, physical, cognitive, psychological, and social needs of older adults.
   Corresponding to Essential IX

5. Intervene to assist older adults and their support network to achieve personal goals, based on the analysis of the living environment and availability of community resources.
   Corresponding to Essential VII

6. Identify actual or potential mistreatment (physical, mental, or financial abuse; and/or self-neglect) in older adults and refer appropriately.
   Corresponding to Essential V

7. Implement strategies and use online guidelines to prevent and/or identify and manage geriatric syndromes.
   Corresponding to Essentials IV and IX

8. Recognize and respect the variations of care, the increased complexity, and the increased use of healthcare resources inherent in caring for older adults.
Corresponding to Essentials IV and IX

9. Recognize the complex interaction of acute and chronic comorbid physical and mental conditions and associated treatments common to older adults.
Corresponding to Essential IX

10. Compare models of care that promote safe, quality physical and mental health care for older adults, such as PACE, NICHE, Guided Care, Culture Change, and Transitional Care Models.
Corresponding to Essential II

11. Facilitate ethical, noncoercive decision making by older adults and/or families/caregivers for maintaining everyday living, receiving treatment, initiating advance directives, and implementing end-of-life care.
Corresponding to Essential VIII

12. Promote adherence to the evidence-based practice of providing restraint-free care (both physical and chemical restraints).
Corresponding to Essential II

13. Integrate leadership and communication techniques that foster discussion and reflection on the extent to which diversity (among nurses, nurse assistive personnel, therapists, physicians, and patients) has the potential to impact the care of older adults.
Corresponding to Essential VI

14. Facilitate safe and effective transitions across levels of care, including acute, community-based, and long-term care (e.g., home, assisted living, hospice, nursing homes) for older adults and their families.
Corresponding to Essentials IV and IX

15. Plan patient-centered care with consideration for mental and physical health and well-being of informal and formal caregivers of older adults.
Corresponding to Essential IX

16. Advocate for timely and appropriate palliative and hospice care for older adults with physical and cognitive impairments.
Corresponding to Essential IX

17. Implement and monitor strategies to prevent risk and promote quality and safety (e.g., falls, medication mismanagement, pressure ulcers) in the nursing care of older adults with physical and cognitive needs.
Corresponding to Essentials II and IV

18. Utilize resources/programs to promote functional, physical, and mental wellness in older adults.
Corresponding to Essential VII

19. Integrate relevant theories and concepts included in a liberal education into the delivery of patient-centered care for older adults.
Corresponding to Essential I

By using this text and the instructor's manual as a curricular guide, instructors should be able to ensure that nursing students will meet the essential competencies recommended for excellent care of older adults.

Reference

American Association of Colleges of Nursing and the John A. Hartford Institute for Geriatric Nursing. (2010). *Recommended baccalaureate competencies and curricular guidelines for the nursing care of older adults: A supplement to the Essentials of Baccalaureate Education for Professional Nursing Practice* (pp. 12–13). Washington, DC: Author.

Foreword

The Fourth Edition of *Gerontological Nursing: Competencies for Care* is an essential textbook for baccalaureate nursing students who seek a contemporary nursing education that is in alignment with the needs and the professional roles that follow graduation in today's society. Each day, 10,000 people in our country reach the age of 65 years, and the fastest-growing segment of the older population is the group 85 years and older. Never has the need for highly qualified registered nurses been greater or more important. Medicare expenditures in the United States account for over 18% of the federal budget, and currently our nation spends over $1 trillion annually for hospital care alone. In an era in which there is an urgent need to contain healthcare costs and deliver value in our care systems, nurses are in an optimal position to be a major part of the solutions so dramatically needed at this point in history. As the largest professional work force, the nursing profession has the greatest opportunity to implement best practices that improve care for older people and address the triple aim of better care, better health outcomes, and lower costs. The competencies in this book are those our profession's leading experts in gerontological nursing deem as crucial to the well-being and positive health outcomes for older adults.

Dr. Mauk is to be congratulated for structuring this textbook around the American Association of Colleges of Nursing gerontological nursing core competencies in a way that reflects the essence of best practice for older adults. She has carefully recruited some of our nation's leading experts to author this work and underscores the content through interesting and novel pedagogical approaches that make the learning objectives clear, concise, and meaningful. Nothing is more helpful than providing case studies that bring the content to life, and there is the wonderful opportunity to conduct self-reflections—something every nurse should do on a daily basis.

Nurses are central and essential to the care and outcomes of care for older adults across all care settings and need to claim their place as team leaders in the co-construction of thoughtful, patient-centered, patient-directed care plans that address what matters to the older person. Thoughtful partnership with family caregivers in this nursing care planning further ensures the most personalized and respectful care that older persons want and deserve.

The John A. Hartford Foundation has dedicated the last three decades to creating a well-prepared gerontological nursing workforce that has transformed the way we think about nursing care for older adults. Our Gerontological Nursing Centers of Excellence have done much to generate new knowledge that informs this textbook. We are proud to have funded the Hartford Institute for Gerontological Nursing at New York University along with the American Association of Colleges of Nursing, as the competencies first were published. We are extremely pleased that they live on in this important textbook and are not simply gathering dust on the shelf. We are excited that such a dynamic learning platform has once again been updated for the benefit of nurses everywhere and, more importantly, for the benefit of older adults.

Terry Fulmer, PhD, RN, FAAN
President, The John A. Hartford Foundation
New York City, 2017

Contributors

Demetra Antimisiaris, PharmD, CGP, FASCP
Associate Professor
University of Louisville Department of Family and
    Geriatric Medicine
Louisville, Kentucky

Stefanie E. Benton
Former Assistant Professor of Nursing
Colorado Christian University

**Terrie Black, DNP, MBA, BSN, RN, CRRN,
    FAHA, FAAN**
Clinical Assistant Professor
College of Nursing
University of Massachusetts, Amherst
Amherst, Massachusetts

Lisa Byrd, PhD, FNP-BC, GNP-BC
Gerontologist
Assistant Professor
University of Mississippi Medical Center
Jackson, Mississippi
University of South Alabama
Mobile, Alabama

Michelle Camicia, MSN, CRRN, CCM, FAHA
Director, Rehabilitation Operations
Kaiser Foundation Rehabilitation Center
Vallejo, California

Teresa Cervantez Thompson, PhD, RN, CRRN-A
Dean and Professor
College of Nursing and Health
Madonna University
Livonia, Michigan

Dennis J. Cheek, RN, PhD, FAHA
Professor
Texas Christian University
Harris College of Nursing and Health Sciences
Fort Worth, Texas

**Deborah Marks Conley, MSN, APRN-CNS-BC,
    FNGNA**
Gerontological Clinical Nurse Specialist
Nebraska Methodist Hospital
Assistant Professor of Nursing
Nebraska Methodist College
Omaha, Nebraska

**Neva L. Crogan, PhD, GNP-BC, GCNS-BC,
    FNGNA, FAAN**
Research Associate Professor
University of Arizona
College of Nursing
Tucson, Arizona

B. Renee Dugger, DNP, RN, GCNS-BC
Assistant Professor, Nursing
University of South Carolina, Beaufort
Bluffton, South Carolina

**Deborah Dunn, EdD(c), MSN, GNP-BC,
    ACNS-BC**
Associate Professor
College of Nursing and Health
Madonna University
Livonia, Michigan

Janice A. Edelstein, RN, EdD PHCNS-BC
Associate Professor
Marian University
School of Nursing and Health Professions
Fond du Lac, WI

Carol Enderlin, PhD, RN
Clinical Assistant Professor
College of Nursing
University of Arkansas for Medical Sciences
Little Rock, Arkansas

Sharon Farra, PhD, RN, CNE
Associate Professor
NDHC Co-Director, Curriculum
Wright State University
Dayton, Ohio

Dawna S. Fish, RN, BSN, COS-C
Quality Assurance Supervisor
Great Lakes Home Health and Hospice
Jackson, Michigan

Sheila Grossman, PhD, FNP, APRN-BC
Professor and Director
Family Nurse Practitioner Program
School of Nursing
Fairfield University
Fairfield, Connecticut

Lorna Guse, PhD, RN
Associate Professor
Faculty of Nursing
University of Manitoba
Winnipeg, Manitoba, Canada

David Haber, PhD
Professor
Ball State University
Muncie, Indiana

Jennifer Hamrick-King, PhD
Graduate Center for Gerontology
College of Public Health
University of Kentucky
Lexington, Kentucky

Melodee Harris, PhD, APN, GNP-BC
Associate Professor
Carr College of Nursing
Harding University
Searcy, Arizona

Linda J. Hassler, RN, MS, GCNS-BC, FNGNA
Geriatric Program Manager
Cultural Ambassador Coordinator
Meridian Health Ann May Center for Nursing and
    Allied Health
Neptune, New Jersey
Adjunct Faculty, Georgian Court University
Lakewood, New Jersey

Janice M. Heineman, PhD
Senior Research Associate
Institute for the Future of Aging Services
American Association of Homes and Services
    for the Aging
Washington, D.C.

Sandra J. Higelin, MSN, RN, CNS, CWCN, CLNC
Sandra Higelin Nursing Consulting Services
Palm Springs, California

Lisa Hutchison, PharmD, MPH, BCPS, FCCP
Associate Professor of Pharmacy Practice
University of Arkansas for Medical Sciences
Little Rock, Arkansas

Cynthia S. Jacelon, PhD, RN-BC, CRRN,
    FGSA, FAAN
Professor
Principal Investigator
UManage Center P20NR016599
Director, PhD Program
College of Nursing
University of Massachusetts, Amherst
Amherst, Massachusetts

Donald D. Kautz, PhD, RN, CNRN, CRRN-A
Assistant Professor of Nursing
University of North Carolina, Greensboro
Greensboro, North Carolina

Luana S. Krieger-Blake, MSW, LCSW
Social Worker
Pines Village Retirement Community
Valparaiso, Indiana

Carolyn A. Laabs, PhD, MA, FNP-BC
Nurse Practitioner and Supervisor
Ascension St. Ben's Clinic
Milwaukee, Wisconsin

Jean Lange, PhD, RN, CNL
Associate Professor
Fairfield University School of Nursing
Fairfield, Connecticut

Cindy Luther, PhD, FNP-BC, AGPCNP-BC,
    FAANP
Director of AGNP and PMHNP Tracks
University of Mississippi Medical Center
Jackson, Mississippi

Kristen L. Mauk, PhD, DNP, RN, CRRN,
    GCNS-BC, GNP-BC, ACHPN, FAAN
Professor of Nursing
Director, RN-BSN and MSN programs
Colorado Christian University
President
Senior Care Central/
International Rehabilitation Consultants LLC
Ridgway, Colorado

Ellyn E. Matthews, PhD, RN, AOCNS, CBSM
Associate Professor
College of Nursing
University of Arkansas for Medical Sciences
Little Rock, Arkansas

Elaine Miller, PhD, RN, CRRN, FAAN, FAHA
Professor of Nursing
Editor, *Pain Management Nursing*
University of Cincinnati, College of Nursing
Cincinnati, Ohio

Joan M. Nelson, RN, MS, DNP
Assistant Professor
University of Colorado Denver
College of Nursing
Denver, Colorado

Dennis Ondrejka, PhD, RN, CNS
Adjunct Faculty
Colorado Christian University

Carole A. Pepa, PhD, RN
Professor of Nursing
Valparaiso University
Valparaiso, Indiana

Linda L. Pierce, PhD, RN, CNS, CRRN, FAHA
Professor
College of Nursing
Medical University of Ohio, Toledo
Toledo, Ohio

Karen M. Rose, PhD, RN
Assistant Professor of Nursing
University of Virginia
Charlottesville, Virginia

Susan Saboe Rose, PhD, PMHNP-BC,
    GCNS-BC, ARNP
Legacy Medical Group
Portland, Oregon

Christine E. Schwartzkopf, MSN, RN, CRRN
Nursing Instructor
Dayton VAMC
Dayton, Ohio
Associate Professor
Valparaiso University
Valparaiso, Indiana

Beth Scaglione Sewell, PhD
Associate Professor
Valparaiso University
Valparaiso, Indiana

MaryAnne Pietraniec Shannon, PhD, RN, GCNS-BC
Professor of Nursing
Sault College BScN Collaborative with Laurentian University
Sault Ste. Marie, Ontario, Canada

Amy Silva-Smith, PhD, ANP-BC
Associate Professor
Nursing Department Chair
Helen and Arthur E. Johnson Beth-El College of Nursing and Health Sciences
University of Colorado
Colorado Springs, Colorado

Jeanne St. Pierre, MN, RN, GCNS-BC
Gerontological Clinical Nurse Specialist
Ball Memorial Hospital
Muncie, Indiana

Victoria Steiner, PhD
Assistant Professor
College of Medicine
Medical University of Ohio, Toledo
Toledo, Ohio

Prudence Twigg, PhDc, RN, ANP-BC, GNP-BC
Visiting Lecturer
Department of Family Health
Indiana University School of Nursing, Indianapolis
Gerontological Nurse Practitioner
Advanced Healthcare Associates
Indianapolis, Indiana

Brenda Tyczkowski, RN, DNP
Professional Program in Nursing
Lecturer
University of Wisconsin, Green Bay
Academic Director HIMT

Elizabeth Van Horn, PhD, RN, CNE
Assistant Professor
UNCG School of Nursing
Greensboro, North Carolina

Patricia Warring, RN, MSN, ACHPN
Clinical Nurse Specialist
Visiting Nurse Association of Porter County
Valparaiso, Indiana

DeAnne Zwicker, DrNP, ANP/GNP-BC
Assistant Professor
George Mason University School of Nursing
Manassas, Virginia

Reviewers

Susan Beck, MSN, CNS, RN
Assistant Professor
Bloomsburg University
Bloomsburg, Pennsylvania

Laura J. Blank, PhDc
Associate Clinical Professor
Northern Arizona University
Flagstaff, Arizona

Tamara Brown, MSN, RN-BC, PCCN,
    CNE, MSCRN
Professor
Georgian Court University
Lakewood, New Jersey

Lisa Byrd, PhD, FNP-BC, GNP-BC
Gerontologist
Assistant Professor
University of Mississippi Medical Center
Jackson, Mississippi
University of South Alabama
Mobile, Alabama

Maureen P. Cardoza, PhD, RN,
    CADDCT, CDP
Assistant Professor
New York Institute of Technology
Old Westbury, New York

Teresa Carnevale, PhD, MSN, RN
Assistant Professor
Department of Nursing
Appalachian State University
Boone, North Carolina

Lynn B. Clutter, PhD, APRN-CNS, CNE
Assistant Professor
The University of Tulsa
Tulsa, Oklahoma

Teresa Darnall, PhD, MSN, RN, CNE
Assistant Professor,
Director RN-BSN Program
Lees-McRae College
Banner Elk, North Carolina

Arneta Finney, MSN, FNP-C, WOCN,
    WCC, PHN
Program Manager
National University
Los Angeles, California

Jason Garbarino, DNP, RN-BC, CNL
Professor
University of Vermont
Burlington, Vermont

Marcia Gay, MSN, FNP
Adjunct Professor
California Baptist University
Riverside, California

Mary Ann Glendon, PhD RN
Associate Professor
Southern Connecticut State University
New Haven, Connecticut

Joan Harvey, DNP RN BC CCRN
Clinical Instructor
Georgian Court University
Geriatric Program Manager
Meridian Health Ann May Center
Neptune, New Jersey

Debra L. Sanders, PhD, RN, GCNS-BC, CNE, FNGNA
Assistant Professor
Bloomsburg University
Co-Founder and Co-Director
Center for Healthy Aging
Bloomsburg, Pennsylvania

Jennifer J Yeager, PhD, RN, AGNP
Assistant Professor
Director of the Graduate Nursing Program
Tarleton State University
Stephenville, Texas

Unit I
Foundations for Gerontological Nursing

(COMPETENCIES 1, 8, 9, 19)

CHAPTER 1

Introduction to Gerontological Nursing

Jeanne St. Pierre
Deborah Marks Conley

(Competencies 1, 9, 19)

LEARNING OBJECTIVES

At the end of this chapter, the reader will be able to:

> Define important terms related to nursing and the aging process.
> Outline significant landmarks that have influenced the development of gerontological nursing as a specialty.
> Identify several subfields of gerontology.
> Develop the beginnings of a personal philosophy of aging.
> Describe the unique roles of the gerontological nurse.
> Discuss the scope and standards of gerontological nursing practice.
> Examine core competencies in gerontological nursing.
> Compare the nine essentials of baccalaureate nursing education with the core competencies in gerontological nursing.
> Distinguish among the educational preparation, practice roles, and certification requirements of the various levels of gerontological nursing practice.

KEY TERMS

Ageism
Attitudes
Certification
Core competencies
Elder law
Geriatrics
Geriatric resource nurse
Gerocompetencies

Gerontological nursing
Gerontological rehabilitation nursing
Gerontology
Home care
Landmarks in gerontological nursing
Stereotype
Veterans Administration

The history and development of gerontological nursing is rich in diversity and experiences, as is the population it serves. There has never been a more opportune time than now to be a gerontological nurse (see **Figure 1-1**)! No matter where nurses practice, they will at some time in their career care for older adults. Nurses must recognize gerontological nursing as a specialty and use the science within this specialty to guide their practice. The healthcare movement is constantly increasing life expectancy; therefore, nurses should expect to care for relatively larger numbers of older people over the next decades. With the increasing numbers of acute, chronic, and terminal health conditions experienced by older adults, nurses are in key positions to provide disease prevention and health promotion, promote positive aging, and assist this growing population in end-of-life decision making.

The National Gerontological Nursing Association (NGNA), the *American Journal of Nursing,* the American Nurses Association (ANA), Sigma Theta Tau International (STTI), and the John A. Hartford Foundation Institute for Geriatric Nursing at New York University (NYU) contributed significantly to the development of the specialty of gerontological nursing. The specialty was formally recognized in the early 1960s when the ANA recommended a specialty group for geriatric nurses and the formation of a geriatric nursing division, and convened the first national nursing meeting on geriatric nursing practice. The growth of the specialty soared over the next three decades. The ANA *Standards for Geriatric Practice* and the *Journal of Gerontological Nursing* were first published (in 1970 and 1975, respectively). Following the enactment of Medicare and Medicaid, rapid growth in the healthcare industry for elders occurred. The *Veterans Administration* (VA) funded a number of Geriatric Research Education and Clinical Centers (GRECCs) at VA medical centers across the United States. Nurses were provided substantial educational opportunities to learn about the care of older veterans through the development of GRECCs. The Kellogg Foundation funded numerous certificate nurse practitioner (NP) programs at colleges of nursing for nurses to become geriatric NPs.

In 1976, the ANA Geriatric Nursing Division changed its name to the Gerontological Nursing Division and published the *Standards of Gerontological Nursing* (Ebersole & Touhy, 2006; Meiner, 2011).

The decade of the 1980s saw a substantial growth in gerontological nursing when the NGNA was established, along with the release of the revised ANA statement on the *Scope and Standards of Gerontological Nursing Practice.* Increased numbers of nurses began to obtain masters and doctoral preparation in gerontological nursing, and higher education established programs to prepare nurses as advanced practice nurses in the field (geriatric NPs and gerontological clinical nurse specialists). Thus, interest in theory to build nursing as a science grew and nurses were beginning to consider gerontological nursing research as an area of study (**Box 1-1**).

In the 1990s, the John A. Hartford Foundation Institute for Geriatric Nursing was established at the NYU Division of Nursing. It provided unprecedented momentum to improve nursing education and practice and increase nursing research in the care of older adults. Nurses Improving Care for Healthsystem Elders (NICHE) program gained a national reputation as the model of acute care for older adults and has since expanded into long-term care.

The 21st century has seen unprecedented growth in gerontological nursing care, as well as preparation of nursing faculty to teach in this specialty. As the baby boomers, who began turning sixty five years of age in 2011, continue to age, this cadre of individuals will not only expect but demand excellence in geriatric care.

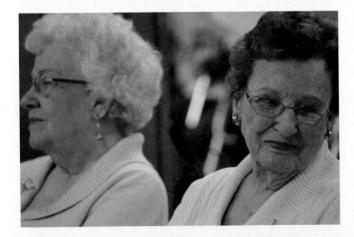

Figure 1-1 More nurses educated in gerontological nursing are needed to care for the growing number of older adults.

BOX 1-1   Research Highlight

Aim: To gain an understanding of the perspectives of minimally health literate older females and their healthcare professionals as they navigate the healthcare system.

Method/Sample: A qualitative case study approach was used to illicit and explore these perspectives through the use of guided interviews. There were two samples, which included healthcare professionals (n = 4) and older female patients (n = 8). All participants met the inclusion criteria outlined by the investigators.

Intervention: Participants were interviewed using audio-recording during a 1-hour single interview session. All interviews were conducted by the primarily investigator over a 6-month period. A semi-structured interview guide was used. Healthcare providers were interviewed at their site of employment or a destination of their choice. Patient respondents were interviewed at a place of their choice and most preferred their home. Participants were engaged in unspecific dialogue before starting the audio-recorder in order to facilitate relaxation and to encourage a steady transition to questioning. Field notes were taken, but were limited to allow undivided attention to the participant.

Audio recordings were transcribed with both electronic and hardcopy files for each interview. Transcripts were reviewed by hand and notes made to sort and organize the data. The data were entered into the computer program NVivo for analysis, categories were clustered for similarity. Word frequency criteria were limited to the categories of communication, education, relationships, listening, empowerment, and time. Relationships were ranked number one.

Findings: Demographic finds revealed the healthcare professional sample included three females (NPs) and one male (physician). Average years of experience was 13. Patient participants' age ranged from 65–89 with a mean age 71. All lived independently, five were married and three were widowed. All had graduated from high school, two had some college, and one had a Master's degree in Education.

Each of the primary categories provided development of the emerging themes. Themes included time challenges; relationships of trust, respect and empathy; patient-centered communication; and patient education, which paved the road to empowerment. Active listening was identified as the key to meeting patient needs.

Application to practice: Five primary areas were identified as impacting health care for minimally health literate older women and their professional caregivers in navigating the health system. The areas of communication and relationships were identified as critically important. A quality-patient relationship was noted to serve as a foundation for patient-centered care and communication. This quality-patient relationship promotes partnering and encourages open communication. Patients are more likely to ask questions if they do not understand what is being said, when there is honesty, openness, and trust. There were limitations to the study, which included lack of cultural diversity, age (all over 65), female gender, geography in the northwest United States, and ethnicity as all were Caucasian.

Collaborative efforts of the John A. Hartford Institute for Geriatric Nursing, the American Academy of Nursing, and the American Association of Colleges of Nursing (AACN) led to the development of the Hartford Geriatric Nursing Initiative (HGNI). This initiative substantially increased the number of gerontological nurse scientists and the development of evidence-based gerontological nursing practice. Today, there are multiple professional journals, books, Websites, and organizations dedicated to the nursing care of older adults.

In 2008, the Honor Society of Nursing, STTI, recognized the ability of nurses to influence practice and patient outcomes in geriatric health care and developed the Geriatric Nursing Leadership Academy (GNLA). This 18-month mentored leadership experience for nurses is funded by the John A. Hartford Foundation and developed in partnership with the Hartford Foundation's Centers of Geriatric Nursing Excellence. GNLA is a premier opportunity for nurses dedicated to influencing policy and geriatric health outcomes. Fellows of the GNLA become active participants in the national network of gerontological nursing leaders.

Two important gerontological nursing faculty development programs were initiated in 2009 to 2010. The Geriatric Nursing Education Consortium (GNEC) was established by the AACN and funded by the John A. Hartford Foundation to enhance gerontological nursing content in senior-level undergraduate nursing courses.

Advancing Care Excellence for Seniors (ACES) was developed through a partnership between the National League for Nursing (NLN) and Community College of Philadelphia with funding from the John A. Hartford Foundation, Laerdal Medical, and the Independence Foundation. These programs provide nursing faculty resources to prepare nurses to care for older adults (NLN, 2012). In 2015, the NGNA published a position paper on essential gerontological nursing education in registered nursing and continuing education programs. The intent of this position statement was to affirm the need for essential gerontological education for all pre-licensure registered nurse programs to build gerontological nurse competence. In addition, it recommended all registered nurses who provide care to older adults participate in ongoing gerontological nursing continuing education. The position paper can be found at http://www.ngna.org/_resources/documentation/position_papers/NGNA-Position Paper-EssentialGerontologicalNursingEducation.pdf.

A national Geropalliative Care nurse residency called AgeWISE was spearheaded in 2010 by Massachusetts General Hospital and funded in part by The Center to Champion Nursing in America, an initiative of the American Association of Retired Persons (AARP), the AARP Foundation, and the Robert Wood Johnson Foundation. Massachusetts General Hospital's Yvonne L. Munn Center for Nursing Research provided direction and oversight for the AgeWISE residency, which has been implemented in various acute care settings. More information about the AgeWISE residency may be found at http://www.mghpcs.org/eed_portal/Documents/PI_EBP/AgeWISE%20 booklet.pdf

The development of gerontological nursing as a specialty is attributed to a host of nursing pioneers. The majority of these nurses were from the United States; however, two key trailblazers were from England. Florence Nightingale and Doreen Norton provided early insights into the "care of the aged." Nightingale was truly the first gerontological nurse, because she accepted the nurse superintendent position in an English institution comparable to our current nursing homes. She cared for wealthy women's maids and helpers in an institution called the Care of Sick Gentlewomen in Distressed Circumstances (Ebersole & Touhy, 2006). Doreen Norton summarized her thoughts on geriatric nursing in a 1956 speech at the annual conference of the Student Nurses Association in London. She later focused her career on care of the aged and wrote often about the unique and specific needs of elders and the nurses caring for them. She identified the advantages of including geriatric care in basic nursing education as: (1) learning patience, tolerance, understanding, and basic nursing skills; (2) witnessing the terminal stages of disease and the importance of skilled nursing care at this time; (3) preparing for the future, because no matter where one works in nursing, older adults will be a large part of the care; (4) recognizing the importance of appropriate rehabilitation, which calls upon all the skill that nurses possess; and (5) being aware of the need to undertake research in geriatric nursing (Norton, 1956).

Landmarks in the Development of Gerontological Nursing

Nurse scientists, educators, authors, and clinicians forged the way for the overall development of gerontological nursing as we know it today. The following is a summary of significant *landmarks in the development of gerontological nursing* as a specialty:

1904 American Journal of Nursing (*AJN*) publishes first geriatric article

1925 *AJN* considers geriatric nursing as a specialty; anonymous column entitled "Care of the Aged" appears in *AJN*

1950 First geriatric nursing textbook, *Geriatric Nursing* (Newton), published First master's thesis in geriatric nursing completed by Eleanor Pingrey Geriatrics becomes a specialization in nursing

1952 First geriatric nursing study published in *Nursing Research*

1961 American Nurses Association (ANA) recommends specialty group for geriatric nurses

1962 ANA holds first National Nursing Meeting on Geriatric Nursing Practice

1966 ANA forms a Geriatric Nursing Division

First Gerontological Clinical Nurse Specialist master's program begins at Duke University

1968 First RN (L. Gunter) presents at the International Congress of Gerontology

1970 ANA creates the *Standards of Practice for Geriatric Nursing*

1973 ANA offers the first generalist certification in gerontological nursing (74 nurses certified)

1975 First gerontological nursing journal published: *Journal of Gerontological Nursing (JGN)*

First nursing conference held at the International Congress of Gerontology

1976 ANA Geriatric Nursing Division changes name to Gerontological Nursing Division

ANA publishes *Standards of Gerontological Nursing*

1977 Kellogg Foundation funds Geriatric Nurse Practitioner certificate education

First gerontological nursing track funded by the Division of Nursing at the University of Kansas

1979 First national conference on gerontological nursing sponsored by the *Journal of Gerontological Nursing*

1980 *AJN* publishes *Geriatric Nursing* journal

Education for Gerontic Nurses by Gunter and Estes suggests curricula for all levels of nursing education

ANA establishes Council of Long-Term Care Nurses

1981 First International Conference on Gerontological Nursing

ANA Division of Gerontological Nursing publishes *Statement on Scope of Practice*

John A. Hartford Foundations Hospital Outcomes Program for the Elderly (HOPE) uses a *Geriatric Resource Nurse* (GRN) model developed at Yale University under the direction of Terry Fulmer

1982 Development of Robert Wood Johnson Foundation Teaching-Nursing Home Program

1983 Florence Cellar Endowed Gerontological Nursing Chair established at Case Western Reserve University

1984 National Gerontological Nursing Association (NGNA) established ANA Division on Gerontological Nursing Practice becomes Council on Gerontological Nursing

1986 National Association for Directors of Nursing Administration in Long-Term Care established

1987 ANA revises *Standards and Scope of Gerontological Nursing Practice*

1988 First PhD program in gerontological nursing established (Case Western Reserve University)

1989 ANA certification established for Clinical Specialist in Gerontological Nursing

1990 ANA establishes Division of Long-Term Care within the Council of Gerontological Nursing

1992 Nurses Improving Care for Healthsystem Elders (NICHE) established at New York University (NYU) Division of Nursing, based on the HOPE programs

1996 John A. Hartford Foundation Institute for Geriatric Nursing established at NYU Division of Nursing; NICHE administered through the John A. Hartford Foundation Institute for Geriatric Nursing

1998 ANA certification available for advanced practice nurses as geriatric NPs or gerontological clinical nurse specialists

2000 American Academy of Nursing, the John A. Hartford Foundation, and the NYU Division of Nursing develop the Building Academic Geriatric Nursing Capacity program

2003 John A. Hartford Foundation Institute for Geriatric Nursing, the American Academy of Nursing, and the American Association of Colleges of Nursing (AACN) combine efforts to develop the Hartford Geriatric Nursing Initiative (HGNI); John A. Hartford Foundation Institute for Geriatric Nursing at NYU awards Specialty Nursing Association Partners in Geriatrics (SNAP-G) grants

2008 *Journal of Gerontological Nursing Research* emerges

2009 Geriatric Nursing Education Consortium (GNEC) (AACN, 2012) faculty development initiative of AACN established: Sigma Theta Tau International (STTI) Geriatric Nursing Leadership Academy (GNLA) launches

2010 NLN's Advancing Care Excellence for Seniors (ACES), AgeWISE Geropalliative Care Nurse Residency established

Attitudes Toward Aging and Older Adults

As a nursing student, you may have preconceived ideas about caring for older adults. Such ideas are influenced by your observations of family members, friends, neighbors, and the media, as well as your own experience with older adults. Perhaps you have a close relationship with your grandparents or you have noticed the aging of your own parents. For some of you, the aging process may have become noticeable when you look at yourself in the mirror. But for all of us, this universal phenomenon we call aging has some type of meaning, whether or not we have taken the time to consciously think about it.

The way you view aging and older adults is often a product of your environment and the experiences to which you have been exposed. Negative *attitudes* toward aging or older adults (*ageism*) often arise in the same way—from negative past experiences. Many of our attitudes and ideas about older adults may not be grounded in fact. Some of you may have already been exposed to ageism, which is often displayed in much the same way as sexism or racism—via attitudes and actions. This is one reason for studying the aging process—to examine the myths and realities, to separate fact from fiction, and to gain an appreciation for what older adults have to offer. As a nurse you will have the opportunity to influence in a positive way the lives of older adults and their families.

Population statistics show that the majority of your careers as nurses will include caring for older adults. Providing best practice in gerontological nursing requires knowledge of the intricacies of the aging process as well as the unique syndromes and disease conditions that can accompany growing older.

As you read and study this text, you are encouraged to examine your own thoughts, values, feelings, and attitudes about growing older. Perhaps you already have a positive attitude toward caring for older adults—build on that value, and consider devoting your time and efforts to the practice of gerontological nursing.

Advocates for older adults, such as Nobel laureate Elie Wiesel, feel that older adults, as repositories of our collective memories, should be appreciated and respected. Because of the rapid growth in the numbers of older adults worldwide (see Chapter 2), gerontological nursing is the place to be! Caring for the largest number of older adults in history presents enormous opportunities. With the over-85 age group being the fastest growing portion of the population, the complexity of caring for so many people with multiple physical and psychosocial changes will present a challenge for even the most experienced nurses. New graduates of nursing programs must be competent in caring for older adults across multiple health settings (Institute of Medicine, 2008), and it is vital that nursing students understand how coordinating care during significant life transitions for older adults is fundamental to ensuring culturally sensitive, individualized, holistic care for the older adult and their caregivers (see **Figure 1-2**).

The purpose of this text is to provide the essential information needed by students of gerontological nursing to provide evidence-based care to older adults. In your study of this text, you will be presented with knowledge and insights from experienced professionals with expertise in various areas of gerontological nursing. Each chapter contains thought-provoking activities and questions for personal reflection. Case studies will help you to think about and apply the information. A glossary, divided by chapter, is included at the end of this text to help you master key terms, and plenty of tables and figures summarize key information. Websites are included as a means of expanding your knowledge. Use this text as a guidebook for your study. Use all the resources available, including your instructors, to immerse yourself in the study of gerontological nursing. By the end of this text, you will have learned about the essential competencies needed to provide quality evidence-based care to older adults and their families.

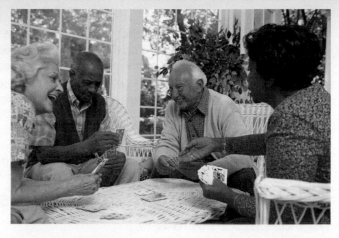

Figure 1-2 Assisted living facilities aid older people with activities of daily living (ADL).
Comstock Images/Alamy Images

Definitions

Gerontology is the broad term used to define the study of aging and/or the aged. This includes the biopsychosocial aspects of aging. Under the umbrella of gerontology are several subfields, including geriatrics, social gerontology, geropsychology, geropharmacology, gerontological nursing, and gerontological rehabilitation nursing.

What is old and who defines old age? Interestingly, although "old" is often defined as over 65 years of age, this is an arbitrary number set by the Social Security Administration. Today, the older age group is often divided into the young old (ages 65–74), the middle old (ages 75–84), and the old old, or frail elders (ages 85 and up). However, these numbers merely provide a guideline and do not actually define the various strata of the aging population. Among individuals, vast differences exist between biological and chronological aging, and between the physical, emotional, and social aspects of aging. How and at what rate a person ages depends upon a host of factors that will be discussed throughout this book. The aging population as well as theories and concepts related to aging are discussed further in Chapters 2 and 3.

Geriatrics is often used as a generic term relating to older adults, but specifically refers to the medical care of older adults. Geriatricians are physicians trained in geriatric medicine.

CLINICAL TIP

Geriatrics refers to medical care of the aged, while gerontological nursing is the preferred term for this nursing specialty.

Social gerontology is concerned with the social aspects of aging versus the biological or psychological. Geropsychology is a branch of psychology concerned with helping older persons and their families maintain well-being, overcome problems, and achieve maximum potential during later life. Geropharmacology is the study of pharmacology as it relates to older adults. Financial gerontology is another emerging subfield that combines knowledge of financial planning and services with a special expertise in the needs of older adults. *Elder law* is another area of specialty, which focuses on legal and ethical issues associated with aging.

Gerontological rehabilitation nursing combines expertise in gerontological nursing with rehabilitation concepts and practice. Nurses working in gerontological rehabilitation often care for older adults with chronic illnesses and long term functional limitations such as stroke, head injury, multiple sclerosis, Parkinson's disease, spinal cord injury, arthritis, joint replacements, and amputations. The goal of gerontological rehabilitation nursing is to assist older adults to regain and maintain the highest level of function and independence possible while preventing complications and enhancing quality of life.

Gerontological nursing falls within the discipline of nursing and the scope of nursing practice. It involves nurses advocating for the holistic care of older adults. The health status of older adults is diverse and complex. A key focus of health promotion and disease prevention in gerontological nursing is to minimize the loss of independence associated with functional decline and illness. Gerontological nurses work with healthy older adults in their communities, acutely ill elders requiring hospitalization and treatment, and chronically ill or disabled elders in long-term care facilities, skilled care, *home care*, and palliative and hospice care. The scope of practice for gerontological nursing includes all older adults from 65 years of age until death. Gerontological nursing is guided by standards of practice that will be discussed later in this chapter.

Roles of the Gerontological Nurse
Direct-Care Provider

In the role of caregiver or provider of care, the gerontological nurse gives direct, hands-on care to older adults in a variety of settings. Older adults often present with atypical symptoms that complicate diagnosis and treatment. Thus, the nurse as a direct-care provider should be educated about disease processes and syndromes commonly seen in the older population (see **Case Study 1-1**). This may include knowledge of risk factors, signs and symptoms, usual medical treatment, rehabilitation, and end-of-life care. Chapters 9, 10, and 27 review the management of common illnesses, diseases, and health conditions, imparting essential information for providing quality care. An entire unit (Chapters 11–18) of this book is devoted to the discussion of geriatric syndromes to better prepare the nurse to be a care provider.

Case Study 1–1

Rose is a 52-year-old nursing student who has returned to school for her BSN after raising a family. She is the divorced mother of two grown children and has one young grandson. In addition to being a full-time student in an accelerated program, Rose also cares for her 85-year-old mother in her own home and occasionally helps provide childcare for her grandson while his parents work. Rose's mother has diabetes and is legally blind. Rose is taking a gerontology course this semester and finds herself going home quite upset after the first week of classes when attitudes toward aging were discussed. While sharing with the course instructor her feelings and surprising emotional discomfort, Rose is helped to identify that she is afraid of getting older and being unable to care for her ailing mother and herself. As a single woman, she is unsure that she can handle what lies ahead for her.

Questions:

1. What can Rose do to become more comfortable with facing her own advancing age?
2. What factors may have influenced her discomfort with the course material?
3. Is there anything the instructor of the course might do to help Rose cope with the feelings she is having as she completes the required coursework?
4. There may be some activities that Rose can do in order to understand her feelings about aging better. Can you think of some such activities?
5. What is Rose's role as the caregiver in this situation? How may the role change over time?
6. How much does Rose's present home and living situation contribute to her fears and perceptions of aging?

Teacher

An essential part of all nursing is teaching. Gerontological nurses focus their teaching on modifiable risk factors and health promotion (see Chapters 6, 7, and 8). Many diseases and debilitating conditions of aging can be prevented through lifestyle modifications in the areas of diet, smoking cessation, weight management, physical activity, and stress management, as well as routine healthcare screenings (see Chapter 8). Nurses have a responsibility to educate the older adult population about ways to decrease their risk of certain disorders such as heart disease, cancer, and stroke, the leading causes of death for this age group. Nurses may develop expertise in specialized areas and teach skills to other nurses in order to promote evidence-based care among older adults.

CLINICAL TIP

Nurses who teach older adults should be familiar with andragogy or adult learning theory principles.

Leader

Gerontological nurses act as leaders during everyday practice as they balance the concerns of the patient, family, nursing, and the rest of the interprofessional team. All nurses must be skilled in leadership, time management, building relationships, communication, and managing change. Nurse leaders who are in management positions may supervise other nursing personnel including licensed practical nurses (LPNs), certified nursing assistants (CNAs), technicians, nursing students, and other unlicensed assistive personnel. The role of the gerontological nurse as manager and leader is further discussed in Chapter 19.

Advocate

As an advocate, the gerontological nurse acts on behalf of older adults to promote their best interests and strengthen their autonomy and decision making. Advocacy may take many forms, including active involvement at the political level or helping to explain medical or nursing procedures to family members on a unit level. Nurses may also advocate for patients through other activities such as helping family members choose the best nursing home for their loved one or supporting family members who are in a caregiving role. Whatever the situation, gerontological nurses must remember that being an advocate does not mean making decisions for older adults, but empowering them to remain independent and retain dignity, even in difficult situations.

Evidence-Based Clinician

The appropriate level of involvement for nurses at the baccalaureate level is implementation of evidence-based practice (EBP) principles. Gerontological nurses must remain abreast of current research literature, reading and translating into practice the results of reliable and valid studies. Using EBP, gerontological nurses can improve the quality of patient care in all settings. Although nurses with undergraduate degrees may be involved in research in some facilities, such as posing a clinical inquiry or assisting with data collection, their basic preparation is aimed primarily at using research in practice. All nurses should read professional journals specific to their specialty and continue their education by attending seminars and workshops, participating in professional organizations, pursuing additional formal education or degrees, and obtaining certification. By implementing EBP, gerontological nurses can improve the quality of patient care in all settings.

Expanded roles of the gerontological nurse may also include counselor, consultant, coordinator of services, administrator, collaborator, geriatric care manager, and others. Several of these roles are discussed in Chapters 19, 27, and 28.

Certification

To provide competent, evidence-based care to older adults, nurses need to have gerontological nursing content in their basic undergraduate nursing curricula and are encouraged to become certified in gerontological nursing. Hospitalized older adults who demonstrate multimorbidity and geriatric syndromes benefit by being cared for by nurses with specialty knowledge (McHugh et al., 2013). And while older Americans use more health care per capita than any other age group (Federal Interagency Forum on Aging-Related Statistics, 2012) less than 1% of nurses in the United States hold *certification* in gerontological nursing. Certification provides reassurance to patients and their families that the nurses caring for them are highly skilled and possess expert knowledge in providing excellence in gerontological nursing care (Hartford Institute for Geriatric Nursing, 2012).

Nurse certification is a formal process by which a certifying agency validates a nurse's knowledge, skills, and competencies through a computerized exam in a specialty area of practice. There are two levels of certification: generalist and advanced practice level (**Table 1-1**). Each has different eligibility standards. The American Nurses Credentialing Center (ANCC) is the certifying body for both levels of gerontological nursing practice (**Box 1-2**).

TABLE 1-1   Websites for Test Content Outlines

http://www.nursecredentialing.org/Documents/Certification/TestContentOutlines/AdultGeroPCNP-TCO.pdf

http://www.nursecredentialing.org/Documents/Certification/TestContentOutlines/AdultGeroAcuteCareNP-TCO.pdf

---

BOX 1-2   Web Exploration

Explore the following Websites for further information on certification and gerontological associations of interest to nurses.

Educational Websites

American Nurses Association (ANA)
http://www.nursingworld.org

Hartford Geriatric Nursing Initiative,
ConsultGeriRN.org
http://www.consultgeriRN.org

National League for Nursing ACES
faculty development
http://www.nln.org/professional-development
-programs/teaching-resources/aging

Associations

U.S. Administration on Aging
http://www.aoa.gov

Aging Life Care Association
http://www.aginglifecare.org/

American Geriatrics Society
http://www.americangeriatrics.org

American Nurses Credentialing Center (ANCC)
http://www.nursecredentialing.org

Gerontological Society of America
http://www.geron.org

Argentum–Assisted Living Federation of America
http://www.alfa.org

Hospice and Palliative Nurses Association (HPNA)
http://www.hpna.org

John A. Hartford Foundation Institute for
Geriatric Nursing
http://www.hartfordign.org

National Adult Day Services Association
http://www.nadsa.org

National Center for Assisted Living (NCAL)
www.ahcancal.org/ncal

National Council on the Aging
http://www.ncoa.org/

National Gerontological Nursing Association
http://www.ngna.org

National Institute on Aging
http://www.nia.nih.gov

Gerontology Certification—Entry Level

The ANCC offers a competency-based examination for certification in Gerontological Nursing that provides a valid and reliable assessment of the entry-level clinical knowledge and skills of registered nurses in the gerontological specialty. The credential awarded is Registered Nurse-Board Certified (RN-BC) (ANCC, 2016a).

In addition to holding a current, active RN license, eligibility for certification includes:

> Having practiced the equivalent of 2 years full-time as a registered nurse.
> Having a minimum of 2,000 hours of clinical practice in the specialty area of gerontological nursing within the last 3 years.
> Having completed 30 hours of continuing education in gerontological nursing within the last 3 years.

ANCC offers the generalist computerized exam in gerontological nursing at exam test sites across the country that can be located at www.prometri.com/ANCC.

Certification has been associated with improved patient outcomes and increased job satisfaction. Piazza, Donahue, Dykes, Griffin, and Fitzpatrick (2006) noted that nurse managers have reported that certification validates a nurse's specialized knowledge and demonstrates clinical competence and credibility. Additionally, by meeting national standards, certification empowers nurses as professionals and aligns them with an organizational goal of promoting positive work experiences for nurses. Certification creates an intrinsic sense of professional pride and accomplishment and validates competence in a specialized area to colleagues, peers, and the public.

Certified gerontological nurses utilize principles of gerontological nursing and gerontological competencies as they implement the nursing process with patients (AACN, 2016). Gerontological certified nurses:

> Assess, manage, and deliver health care that meets the needs of older adults
> Evaluate the effectiveness of their care
> Identify the strengths and limitations of their patients
> Maximize patient independence
> Involve patients and family members (ANCC, 2016a)

There are a number of compelling reasons for nurses to pursue gerontological nurse certification. Certified gerontological nurses:

> Experience a high degree of professional accomplishment and satisfaction
> Demonstrate a commitment to their profession
> Provide higher quality of care to older adults
> Act as resources for other nurses and interprofessional team members
> Demonstrate evidence-based gerontological nursing care
> Are recognized as national leaders in gerontological nursing care
> Create the potential for higher salaries and benefits
> Are actively recruited for employment as nursing faculty, in Magnet and NICHE designated hospitals, in long-term care facilities, in acute rehab, and in community health agencies (ANCC, 2016a; Hartford Institute for Geriatric Nursing, 2012)

See the ANCC Website (http://www.nursecredentialing.org/certification.aspx#specialty) for eligibility requirements and information about gerontological nurse certification and recertification.

Advanced Practice Certification

Many states require advanced practice registered nurses (APRNs) to hold a separate license as an APRN. The advanced practice role encompasses education, consultation, research, case management, administration, and advocacy in the care of older adults. In addition, APRNs develop advanced knowledge of nursing theory, research, and clinical practice. The APRN is an expert in providing care for older adults, families, and groups in a variety of settings

Nurse Practitioner (NP)

NPs are educated and practice at an advanced level to provide care, independently, in a range of setting and in one of six described patient populations. NPs are responsible and accountable for health promotion, disease prevention, health education and counseling, as well as the diagnosis and management of acute and chronic diseases. They provide initial, ongoing, and comprehensive care to patients in family practice, pediatrics, internal medicine, geriatrics, and women's health. NPs are prepared to practice as primary care NPs or acute care NPs, which have separate national competencies and unique certifications.

Clinical Nurse Specialist (CNS)

The CNS is educated at an advanced level to care for patients in one of the six described populations and across the continuum of care. The role of the CNS encompasses the patient, the nurse, and nursing practice, as well as the healthcare organization and system. The CNS is responsible and accountable for diagnosis and treatment of health/illness states, disease management, health promotion, and prevention of illness and risk behaviors among individuals, families, groups, and communities.

The ANCC currently offers three separate advanced practice certification exams in gerontological nursing: the Adult-Gerontology Acute Care NP, the Adult-Gerontology Primary Care NP, and the Adult-Gerontology CNS. There are different eligibility requirements for each exam and nurses must be prepared at the graduate degree level to apply. The ANCC Website has eligibility requirements and information on certification and recertification: http://nursecredentialing.org/certification.aspx.

Eligibility requirements for gerontological NP certification are the same as for the CNS with the addition of graduate coursework in health promotion and disease prevention, and differential diagnosis and disease management.

The adult-gerontology clinical nurse specialist (AGCNS-BC) focuses on three spheres of influence: patient/family care, developing nurses, and impacting organizations and systems. CNSs play important roles in acute care by developing and implementing gerontological nursing EBP. In addition, some roles involve a collaborative practice or consultative role with hospitals or long-term care facilities and interprofessional teams. In some states, the adult-gerontology CNS may obtain prescriptive authority and practice independently, following the scope of practice in the state in which she/he is practicing. While most CNSs practice in acute care, some practice in ambulatory care, nursing administration, and academia.

The Adult-Gerontology Acute Care Nurse Practitioner (ACNPC-AG) or the Adult-Gerontology Primary Care NP are the NP certifications through ANCC for adult-gerontology (ANCC, 2016b). NP who specialize in gerontology may practice in hospitals, primary care, or long-term care settings diagnosing and treating geriatric syndromes. Nurse practitioners may practice in collaboration with physicians or may practice independently, depending on the rules of the state board under which they practice. NPs can be found in diverse settings, such as rehabilitation facilities, making home visits as part of a Medical Home program, or in academic settings. Per the American Association of Nurse Practitioners (2015), about 80% of NPs are prepared in primary care, of which 22% focus on adult and geriatric patients.

Scope and Standards of Practice

The scope of nursing practice is defined by state regulation, but is also influenced by the unique needs of the population being served. The needs of older adults are complex and multifaceted, and the focus of nursing care depends on the setting in which the nurse practices.

Gerontological nursing is practiced in accordance with standards developed by the profession of nursing. In 2010, the ANA Division of Gerontological Nursing Practice published the third edition of the *Scope and Standards of Gerontological Nursing Practice,* in collaboration with the NGNA, the National Association of Directors of Nursing Administrators in Long-Term Care, and the National Conference of Gerontological Nurse Practitioners. These standards are divided into clinical care and the role of the professional nurse, both at the generalist and advanced practice nurse level of practice. There are six standards, which include assessment, diagnosis, outcome identification, planning, implementation, and evaluation. The eight standards of professional gerontological nursing performance include quality of care, performance appraisals, education, collegiality, ethics, collaboration, research, resource utilization, and transitions of care. Students should note that these are the basic standards for professional nursing, but they are specifically developed for the care of older adults. Core competencies, discussed in the next section, provide specific guidelines for gerontological nursing care. A full description and copy of the scope and standards is available at http://www.ngna.org or http://www.nursesbooks .org/Main-Menu/Specialties/Gerontology/Gerontological-Nursing-Practice.aspx.

Core Competencies

Specific *core competencies* have been identified for gerontological nursing in addition to general professional nursing preparation. These competencies are influenced by the level at which the nurse will function and the role expectations of the nurse. Core competencies provide a foundation of added knowledge and skills necessary for the nurse to implement in daily practice. Common bodies of assumptions, knowledge, skills, and attitudes that are essential for excellent clinical nursing practice with older adults have been developed and provide the basic foundation for all levels of gerontological nursing practice.

The AACN and the John A. Hartford Foundation Institute for Geriatric Nursing at NYU College of Nursing assembled input from qualified gerontological nursing experts to publish *Recommended Baccalaureate Competencies and Curricular Guidelines for Geriatric Nursing Care* in 2008. These gerocompetency statements were updated in 2010 and are a supplement to *The Essentials of Baccalaureate Education for Professional Nursing Practice* (AACN, 2008). The gerocompetency statements provide the framework for this text. There are 19 gerocompetency statements, which are divided into the 9 *Essentials* identified in the AACN document, with associated rationale, suggestions for content, teaching strategies, resources, and glossary of terms (see **Table 1-2).** The purpose of this document specific to gerontological nursing was to use the AACN's *Essentials of Baccalaureate Education for*

TABLE 1-2 **Gerontological Nursing Competency Statements**
1. Incorporate professional attitudes, values, and expectations about physical and mental aging in the provision of patient-centered care for older adults and their families. *Corresponding to Essential VIII*
2. Assess barriers for older adults in receiving, understanding, and giving of information. *Corresponding to Essentials IV & IX*
3. Use valid and reliable assessment tools to guide nursing practice for older adults. *Corresponding to Essentials IX*
4. Assess the living environment as it relates to functional, physical, cognitive, psychological, and social needs of older adults. *Corresponding to Essential IX*
5. Intervene to assist older adults and their support network to achieve personal goals, based on the analysis of the living environment and availability of community resources. *Corresponding to Essential VII*
6. Identify actual or potential mistreatment (physical, mental, or financial abuse, and/or self-neglect) in older adults and refer appropriately. *Corresponding to Essential V*

(continues)

TABLE 1-2 Gerontological Nursing Competency Statements (*continued*)

7. Implement strategies and use online guidelines to prevent and/or identify and manage geriatric syndromes.
Corresponding to Essentials IV & IX

8. Recognize and respect the variations of care, the increased complexity, and the increased use of healthcare resources inherent in caring for older adults.
Corresponding to Essentials IV & IX

9. Recognize the complex interaction of acute and chronic comorbid physical and mental conditions and associated treatments common to older adults.
Corresponding to Essential IX

10. Compare models of care that promote safe, quality physical and mental health care for older adults such as PACE, NICHE, Guided Care, Culture Change, and Transitional Care Models.
Corresponding to Essential II

11. Facilitate ethical, noncoercive decision making by older adults and/or families/caregivers for maintaining everyday living, receiving treatment, initiating advance directives, and implementing end-of-life care.
Corresponding to Essential VIII

12. Promote adherence to the EBP of providing restraint-free care (both physical and chemical restraints).
Corresponding to Essential II

13. Integrate leadership and communication techniques that foster discussion and reflection on the extent to which diversity (among nurses, nurse assistive personnel, therapists, physicians, and patients) has the potential to impact the care of older adults.
Corresponding to Essential VI

14. Facilitate safe and effective transitions across levels of care, including acute, community-based, and long-term care (e.g., home, assisted living, hospice, nursing homes) for older adults and their families.
Corresponding to Essentials IV & IX

15. Plan patient-centered care with consideration for mental and physical health and well-being of informal and formal caregivers of older adults.
Corresponding to Essential IX

16. Advocate for timely and appropriate palliative and hospice care for older adults with physical and cognitive impairments.
Corresponding to Essentials IX

17. Implement and monitor strategies to prevent risk and promote quality and safety (e.g., falls, medication mismanagement, pressure ulcers) in the nursing care of older adults with physical and cognitive needs.
Corresponding to Essentials II & IV

18. Utilize resources/programs to promote functional, physical, and mental wellness in older adults.
Corresponding to Essential VII

19. Integrate relevant theories and concepts included in a liberal education into the delivery of patient-centered care for older adults.
Corresponding to Essential I

TABLE 1-3   The Nine Essentials of Baccalaureate Education for Professional Nursing Practice

Essential I: Liberal Education for Baccalaureate Generalist Nursing Practice

Essential II: Basic Organizational and Systems Leadership for Quality Care and Patient Safety

Essential III: Scholarship for Evidence-Based Practice

Essential IV: Information Management and Application of Patient Care Technology

Essential V: Healthcare Policy, Finance, and Regulatory Environments

Essential VI: Interprofessional Communication and Collaboration for Improving Patient Health Outcomes

Essential VII: Clinical Prevention and Population Health

Essential VIII: Professionalism and Professional Values

Essential IX: Baccalaureate Generalist Nursing Practice

Reproduced from American Association of Colleges of Nursing. (2008). *The essentials of baccalaureate education for professional nursing practice.* Washington, DC: Author.

BOX 1-3   Additional Resources

American Nurses Credentialing Center (ANCC)
8515 Georgia Ave, Suite 400
Silver Spring, MD 20910

800-284-2378
http://www.nursecredentialing.org

John A. Hartford Foundation

55 East 59th Street

16th Floor

New York, NY 10022-1178

212-832-7788

Email: mail@jhartfound.org
http://www.hartfordign.org

Professional Nursing Practice (2008) as a framework to help nurse educators integrate specific nursing content into their programs. These appear in **Table 1-3.** The *gerocompetencies* in Table 1-2 correlate with and were derived from the suggestions in the more general AACN document in Table 1-3. By using these published documents as guides, nursing faculty and others who educate in the area of gerontological nursing will be able to prepare students to be competent in providing gerontological best practices to older adults and their families (**Box 1-3**). As students, we want you to understand the rationale for including gerocompetency content in your nursing education. It is essential for you to become competent in gerontological nursing concepts and principles as you move forward in your education and nursing practice, in order to be prepared for the tsunami of older adults you will be caring for (Stierle et al., 2006).

Research in Gerontological Nursing

Nursing research can be defined as the "diligent, systematic inquiry or investigation to validate and refine existing knowledge and generate new knowledge" (Burns & Grove, 2011, p. 2). Research in gerontological nursing is robust as evidenced by the growth in recent years of gerontological nursing journals, books, and other medical and nursing publications. Many colleges and universities support research in gerontological nursing, particularly the nine academic centers that host Hartford Centers for Geriatric Nursing Excellence in Arizona, Arkansas, California, Iowa, Minnesota, Oregon, Pennsylvania, and Utah.

Using nursing research in practice is called EBP, defined as "the conscientious use of best research evidence in combination with a clinician's expertise, as well as patient preferences and values, to make decisions about the type of care that is provided" (Sackett, Straus, Richardson, Rosenberg, & Haynes, 2000, p. 1). Nursing practice based on the best available evidence ensures that optimal quality of care is provided by helping nurses to know what works and how evaluate outcomes.

Gerontological nursing research has made contributions to nursing science in many areas. Examples include delirium superimposed on dementia, medication issues at discharge for patients with heart failure, and older adult *stereotypes* among care providers (see **Boxes 1-4** and **1-5**).

BOX 1-4   Research Highlight

Aim: Development of a tool to assess variables that may be related to professional caregivers' perceptions regarding the appropriateness of elderspeak.

Lombardi, Buchanan, Afflerback, Campana, Sattler, and Lai have studied caregivers' use of patronizing language when speaking to older adults and the impacts of that method of interaction. In an attempt to understand the reasons why a caregiver may employ this method of communication, the researchers created a resource to assess the variables that may lead to use of elderspeak. Sign into your database of nursing literature (CINAHL or PubMed, for example) and use the citation below to perform a search for this article. Summarize the results of this research study.

Lombardi, N. J., Buchanan J. A., Afflerbach, B. A., Campana, K., Sattler, A., & Lai, D. (2014). Is elderspeak appropriate? A survey of certified nursing assistants. *Journal of Gerontological Nursing, 40*(11), 44–52.

BOX 1-5   Research Highlight

Aim: To test the efficacy of a web-based version of a dementia feeding skills educational intervention for nursing home (NH) staff.

Methods: Two U.S. nursing homes with similar characteristics participated in the study. In the control NH staff provided usual care. In the intervention NH staff received web-based training and coaching in feeding elders with dementia. Meal observations were conducted in both NHs by trained research assistants blind to the study outcomes. In addition, staff were tested on their knowledge and self-efficacy related to items such as dementia, signs of swallowing difficulty, and feeding skills.

Findings: While aversive behaviors increased in both NH resident groups, the intervention NH staff spent more time providing assistance and meal intake doubled. In the control group, meal intake decreased. This study demonstrated the effectiveness of using an evidence-based training program to improve meal intake in NH residents with dementia.

Application to practice: For persons with dementia who have poor meal intake, staff feeding skills training can improve outcomes.

Data from Batchelor-Murphy, M., Amella, E. J., Zapka, J., Maueller, M., & Beck, C. (2015). Feasibility of a web-based dementia feeding skills training program for nursing home staff. *Geriatric Nursing, 36*, 212–218.

Summary

Gerontological nursing is a specialty practice that focuses on the unique needs of older adults and their families. It builds on the theories and foundations of nursing practice with application of a growing body of literature generated by gerontological nursing scientists. It requires specialized knowledge in the art and science of nursing, coupled with gerontological nursing best practices, to manage the complex needs of this population. Caring for older adults is influenced by many factors, one of which is recognizing one's own attitude about aging. It is imperative, with the aging of today's population, that all nurses have basic gerontological nursing concepts and principles taught in their undergraduate program. With the growth of the older population, more nurses certified and specializing in gerontological nursing will be needed. Gerontological nurses practice in almost all settings and there are emerging subfields of this specialty that offer promise of future roles for nurses who care for older adults. Focusing on the individualization of the aging person, nurses should explore the multiple career options in this rewarding, exciting, creative, and uniquely innovative field of gerontological nursing.

Clinical Reasoning Exercises

1. Go to a local card shop and browse. Look at the birthday cards that persons might buy for someone getting older. What do they say about society's attitudes toward aging? Do the cards you read point out any areas that we stereotype as problems with advancing age? What positive attributes are seen?

2. Complete this sentence: Older people are _____. List as many adjectives as you can think of. After making your list, identify how many are negative and how many are positive descriptors. Think about where your ideas came from as you did this exercise.

3. Check out the Website at http://www .consultgerirn.org. How would you use this Website to enhance your knowledge about the care of older adults? What services are available through the Website?

4. Look at the list of competencies for gerontological nurses in Table 1-2. How many of these competencies do you feel you meet at this point? Make a conscious effort to develop these skills as you go through your career.

Personal Reflections

1. How do you feel about aging? Draw a picture of yourself aging and describe the details of what you anticipate will occur as you age. Do you see advanced age as an opportunity to grow old gracefully or something to fear? What are your views about cosmetic procedures (Botox injections, face lifts, body sculpting) that are designed to make people look younger?

2. When was the last time you cared for an older adult? What was that experience like? How do you feel about caring for older adults in your nursing practice? The majority of your nursing practice will entail caring for elders and their families. Did you anticipate this when you entered nursing school?

3. What do you think about nurses who work in nursing homes? Have you ever considered a career in gerontological nursing? Describe the positives you can see about developing expertise in this field of nursing.

4. Have you ever seen ageism in practice? If so, think about that situation and how it could

have been turned into a positive scenario. If not, how have the situations you have been in avoided discrimination against older adults?

5. Which of the settings in gerontological nursing practice appeal to you most at this time in your professional career? Is there any one setting that you can see yourself working in more than another? Do you think this will change as you progress in your career?

References

American Association of Colleges of Nursing. (2008). *The essentials of baccalaureate education for professional nursing practice.* Washington, DC: Author.

American Association of Colleges of Nursing. (2012). *GNEC.* Retrieved from http://www.aacn.nche.edu/geriatric-nursing/gnec

American Association of Colleges of Nursing. (2016). Select your certificate program. Retrieved from http://www.aacn.org/wd/certifications/content/selectcert.pcms?menu=certification&lastmenu=divheader_select_your_program

American Association of Colleges of Nursing and the John A. Hartford Institute for Geriatric Nursing. (2010). *Recommended baccalaureate competencies and curricular guidelines for the nursing care of older adults: A supplement to The Essentials of Baccalaureate Education for Professional Nursing Practice.* Washington, DC: Author. Retrieved from http://www.aacn.nche.edu/geriatric-nursing/AACN_Gerocompetencies.pdf

American Nurses Association. (2010). *Scope and standards of gerontological nursing practice.* Washington, DC: Author.

American Nurses Credentialing Center. (2016a). *Gerontological nursing.* Retrieved from http://nursecredentialing.org/Certification/NurseSpecialties/Gerontological

American Nurses Credentialing Center. (2016b). *Adult gerontology CNS.* Retrieved from http://nursecredentialing.org/AdultGerontologyCNS

Batchelor-Murphy, M., Amella, E. J., Zapka, J., Maueller, M., & Beck, C. (2015). Feasibility of a web-based dementia feeding skills training program for nursing home staff. *Geriatric Nursing, 36,* 212–218.

Burns, N., & Grove, S. K. (2011). *Understanding nursing research: Building an evidence-based practice* (4th ed.). St. Louis, MO: Elsevier Saunders.

Carollo, S. (2015). Low health literacy in older women: The in influence of patient-clinician relationships. *Geriatric Nursing, 36,* 38–42.

Ebersole, P., & Touhy, T. (2006). *Geriatric nursing: Growth of a specialty.* New York, NY: Springer.

Federal Interagency Forum on Aging-Related Statistics. (2012). *Older Americans 2012: Key Indicators of Well-Being.* Washington, DC: U.S. Government Printing Office. Retrieved from https://agingstats.gov/docs/PastReports/2012/OA2012.pdf

Hartford Institute for Geriatric Nursing. (2012). Retrieved from http://www.consultgerirn.org

Institute of Medicine. (2008). *Retooling for an aging America: Building the health care workforce.* Washington, DC: The National Academies Press.

Lombardi, N. J., Buchanan J. A., Afflerbach, B. A., Campana, K., Sattler, A., & Lai, D. (2014). Is elderspeak appropriate? A survey of certified nursing assistants. *Journal of Gerontological Nursing, 40*(11): 44.

McHugh, M. D., Kelly L. A., Smith H. L., Wu, E. S., Vanak, J. M., & Aiken, L. H. (2013). Lower mortality in magnet hospitals. *Medical Care, 5,* 382–388.

Meiner, S. (2011). *Gerontologic nursing* (3rd ed.). St. Louis, MO: Mosby.

National Gerontological Nursing Association. (2015). *Position paper on essential gerontological nursing education in Registered Nursing and continuing education programs.* Retrieved from http://www.ngna.org/_resources /documentation/position_papers/NGNA-PositionPaper-EssentialGerontologicalNursingEducation.pdf

National League of Nursing. (2012). *Faculty resources.* Retrieved from http://www.nln.org/facultyprograms /facultyresources/aces/index.htm

Norton, D. (1956, July 6). The place of geriatric nursing in training. *Nursing Times, 264.*

Piazza, I. M., Donahue, M., Dykes, P. C., Griffin, M. Q., & Fitzpatrick, J. J. (2006). Differences in perceptions of empowerment among nationally certified and non-certified nurses. *Journal of Nursing Administration, 36*(5), 277–283.

Sackett, D. L., Straus, S. E., Richardson, W. S., Rosenberg, W., & Haynes, R. B. (2000). *Evidence-based medicine: How to practice and teach EBM* (2nd ed.). Edinburgh, UK: Churchill Livingstone.

Stierle, L. J., Mezey, M., Schumann, M. J., Esterson, J., Smolenski, M. C., Horsley, K. D., . . . Gould, E. (2006). Professional development. The Nurse Competence in Aging initiative: Encouraging expertise in the care of older adults. *American Journal of Nursing, 106*(9), 93–96.

For a full suite of assignments and additional learning activities, see the access code at the front of your book.

CHAPTER 2

The Aging Population

Cynthia S. Jacelon

(Competencies 1, 8, 19)

LEARNING OBJECTIVES

At the end of this chapter, the reader will be able to:

> Identify trends in aging across the globe.
> Describe social and economic issues related to aging.
> Discuss aging across cultures and countries.
> Consider challenges for aging in the 21st century.

KEY TERMS

Aging in place	Genetics
Baby boomers	Genomics
Centenarian	Health disparities
Chronic disease	Independent living
Cohorts	Indian Health Service
Elders	Oldest old
Foreign-born	Senior citizen

Individuals around the world are living longer. The increase in the actual number of older adults, those people over the age of 65, and the percentage of society comprised of older adults is affecting social policy, societal resources, business, communities, and healthcare systems in the United States and across the globe. While longer life is a resource, in order to realize the potential of a longer life span the ideas about development must be adjusted so that the extra years are not just tacked on to retirement, but expand an individual's years of productivity. Health is a key determinant for not just adding more years to life, but adding more life to years.

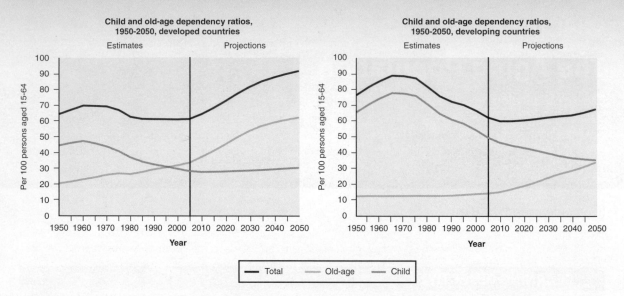

Figure 2-1 Developed and developing dependency ratios.

At the same time people are living longer, the number of babies being born is dropping (World Health Organization, 2015). Fertility of the population affects the number and percentage of older adults. The birth rate in the United States and across the globe is falling. In 1800, the average woman in the United States had 7 children; by the end of World War II, this had decreased to 2.4 children. During the baby boom the fertility rate increased, but has declined since then to 1.9 children per women (Harris-Kojetin, Sengupta, Park-Lee, & Valverde, 2013). **Figure 2-1** depicts the dependency rations for developed and developing countries, and demonstrates when the number of older individuals will exceed the number of children in the world.

Patterns of aging have changed throughout the years. In 1900, life expectancy in industrialized countries ranged from 45 to 50 years, and less for poorer countries. In 2000, life expectancy was about 65 years for the world as a whole and it is expected to increase to 75 years by 2050. In developed countries, life expectancy averages 78 years and will increase to about 85 by 2050; in developing countries, it is expected to increase from 63 to 74 years between 2005 and 2050 (United Nations, 2007).

Demographics

The global share of older people (aged 60 years or over) increased from 9.2% in 1990 to 11.7% in 2013 and will continue to grow as a proportion of the world population reaching 21.1% by 2050 (United Nations, 2013). The percentage of individuals at least 65 years old, varies by country from 3.5/100 people in the least developed countries to 17.8/100 in the most developed countries (United Nations, 2013). The variation in the percentage of older individuals is related to the birth rate. The birth rate tends to be higher in developing countries, and life span tends to be shorter than for more developed countries.

Currently, in the United States more than one out of every seven citizens (14/100) is age 65 or older. However, the distribution of older individuals is not even across the country. For example, in Alaska (9/100) and Utah (9.8/100) there are fewer than 10 seniors out of every 100 people. These states can be contrasted with Florida (18.7/100), Maine (17.7/100), West Virginia (17.3/100), and Pennsylvania, Puerto Rico, and Vermont (16.4/100) (Administration for Community Living, 2015).

In 1935, when Social Security was enacted in the United States, the life expectancy for someone who was 65 years old was 12 additional years for males (77 years total) and 13 additional years for females (78 years total). This has risen to 17.9 and 20.3 additional years, respectively. By 2080, the additional life expectancy for a 65-year-old in the United States is expected to have increased to 20 years and 23 years, respectively (Centers for Disease Control and Prevention [CDC], 2009). In 2006, life expectancy at birth was 5 years higher for Whites than for Blacks, but at age 65, Whites could expect to live only 1.5 years longer than Blacks. For those people who live to age 85, the life expectancy for Black people is slightly higher than for Whites (Federal Interagency Forum, 2010).

After World War II, between the late 1940s and the mid 1960s the birth rate surged. This period is known as the baby boom, and individuals belonging to this cohort are known as *Baby Boomers*. The baby boom ended in the mid 1960s and the birth rate across the globe began to decline. At the same time, the death rate from infectious disease also declined dramatically, leading to a steady rise in the number of individuals living into old age.

Because people are living longer, the segment of the population known as the *oldest old* (85+ years) is the fastest growing segment of the population. More people than ever before are living into the 80s or 90s and beyond. The size of this segment of the population in the United States is projected to increase from 5.5 million in 2010 to 6.6 million in 2020 (a 19% increase for the decade) (Administration on Aging, 2011a). It is anticipated that by 2018, older adults will outnumber children under the age of 5 in the world for the first time in history (Kinsella & He, 2009).

One out of seven Americans are over age 65. This represents over 14% of the current population (Administration on Aging, 2015). After 2030, the population of oldest old (those over 85 years) will grow the fastest. In fact, this oldest age group is projected to triple to 14.6 million in 2040 (Administration on Aging, 2015). In order for the promise of a long life to be realized, individuals must make healthy lifestyle choices such as avoiding smoking and controlling obesity throughout life.

Centenarians

The fastest growing segment of the population of the United States is comprised of *Centenarians*, individuals who are over 100 years old. The second fastest growing segment is comprised of individuals over 85 years. The U.S. Census Bureau (2011) estimates that there were 71,991 centenarians in the United States on December 1, 2010 and it is expected that there will be at least 601,000 centenarians in the United States by 2050, but may reach 850,000 people depending on changes in life expectancy over these years. The U.S. Census of 1990 found that four in five centenarians are women, and 78% of this age group are non-Hispanic White. African Americans make up the second largest group of centenarians at 16%.

The population of centenarians is overwhelmingly female (84%), lower educated, more impoverished, widowed, and more disabled as compared to other older cohorts (Kincel, 2014). The lower education level of this cohort is not surprising considering the increase in levels of education noted over the span of the past century. The majority of centenarians were widowed, with 84% of 100-year-old women widowed as compared to 58% of men. Women generally were more likely to live in poverty in this age group. White and Asian and Pacific Islanders centenarians were less likely than other races to live in poverty. Disability, identified as having mobility and self-care limitations is common. The increased likelihood of living in a nursing home at this age was noted in all race categories.

Genetics and Genomics

Genomics is the identification of gene sequences in the DNA, while *genetics* is the study of heredity and the transmission of certain genes through generations. Both genomics and genetics play a role in health and longevity for older adults. Research exploring genetics and genomics in relation to aging include identifying the genes that affect the aging process, the genetic origins of specific diseases such as Alzheimer's Disease and cancer, and the effect of genetics on drug metabolism. Other researchers are examining the complex interactions between environment, genes, and aging.

One interesting line of investigation is in exploring the genetic determinants of well-being in older age (O'Hara, 2014). Some researchers have suggested a genetic link for positive traits that are important for reducing the individual's response to stress. While the researchers did not identify a single gene or gene sequences, there is evidence that psychological constructs such as resilience and optimism be related to several clusters of genes on the genome (Rana et al., 2014) and contribute to longer life.

Gender and Older Age

The older population is predominantly female (See **Figure 2-2**). Because women tend to live longer than men, older women outnumber older men almost everywhere. In 2013, globally, there were 85 men per 100 women in the age group 60 years or over and 61 men per 100 women in the age group 80 years or over. These sex ratios are expected to increase moderately during the next several decades, reflecting a slightly faster projected improvement in old-age mortality among males than among females (United Nations, 2013). The difference between the number of women and the number of men increases as age increases. For the age group 65–69 in the United States, it is 112 women for every 100 men; for those 85+ the ratio is 206:100 (with more than two females for every male).In 2009, a 65-year-old female could be expected to live an additional 20 years; for males, it was 17.3 years (Administration on Aging, 2011a).

In 2010, 72% of older men were married, compared to 42% of women. Only 37% of women ages 75–84 were married; this dropped to 15% in the 85 or older age group, while 55% of men 85 years and older were married. Four times as many women as men were widowed (8.7 million women; 2.1 million men). Most older people were married at some point in their lives. The most common reason for being single is widowhood; divorce is

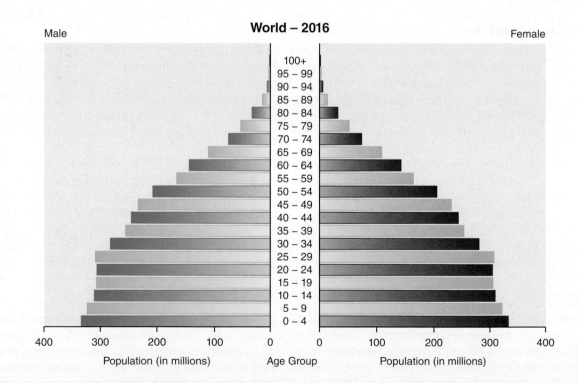

Figure 2-2 World Population Pyramid.

more unusual in this age group, and the number of individuals who have never been married is small. In 2010, 12% of older men and 13% of older women were divorced (Administration on Aging, 2015; Federal Interagency Forum, 2010).

Race and Ethnicity and Older Adults

The growing aging population consists of a significantly increased proportion of minorities. Minority elders will make up 42% of the older population over the next 40 years (Vincent & Velkoff, 2010). An understanding of cultural diversity and the unique challenges it poses is needed to address health issues and promote wellness for all older individuals. Additional information on culture and spirituality can be obtained in Chapter 22.

The older population in the United States is growing more racially and ethnically diverse as it ages. In 2010, 80% of U.S. older adults were non-Hispanic Whites, 8.4% were Black, 6.9% Hispanic, and 3.4% Asian. By 2050, the composition of the older population will be 59.4% non-Hispanic White, 19.8% Hispanic, 11% Black, 8.6% Asian, and 1% Native American and Native Alaskan (Administration on Aging, 2010; Federal Interagency Forum, 2010). In the United States health is often thought to vary based on race and ethnicity. While it is true that various ethnic and racial populations experience different disease burdens, there is growing evidence that this is not a function of genetics but of socioeconomics (Louie & Ward, 2011).

Health Disparities

Health disparities have been defined as "preventable differences in the burden of disease, injury, violence, or in opportunities to achieve optimal health experienced by socially disadvantaged racial, ethnic, and other population groups and communities" (CDC, 2013, p. 1). Not all older adults in the United States have benefited from recent advances in health care because of factors such as age, gender, race, and economic circumstances.

Substantial health disparities among race, ethnicity, and gender exist in many disease prevention and management strategies such as vaccine administration, colorectal cancer screening, coronary heart disease and stroke, preventable hospitalizations, hypertension, and hypertension control (CDC, 2010). While funding (i.e., Medicare) expands healthcare access for the older adults, it does not address older adults who do not meet criteria for Medicare funding, or lack of services available.

Even when care is available, all individuals may not receive the same services. For example, researchers in one study found that older women saw their healthcare provider as often as men did, but did not receive flu vaccinations and cholesterol screening as frequently as older males (Cameron, Song, Manheim, & Dunlop, 2010). Males in that study also tended to be admitted to the hospital more frequently. While there may be social reasons for the healthcare discrepancies between genders, it is disturbing to think that older women as a group may not receive needed preventive services because of gender rather than lack of need. Although racial and ethnic disparities in health care have also been documented for the older adult population, the core of this issue is likely complex and multifaceted, with caregiver bias, poverty level, language, literacy, and other as-yet-unidentified factors playing a role.

African American Older Adults

The number of African American older adults is projected to increase from 3.2 million in 2008 to over 9.9 million by 2050. In 2008, African Americans comprised 8.3% of the older population. By 2050, this is expected to increase to 11%. The poverty rate for older African Americans was 20% in 2008, compared to 9.7% for the total older population. Households containing families headed by African Americans age 65 years or older reported a median income of $35,025 in 2008, compared to $44,188 for all older households. The median personal income for African American men was $19,161, and $12,499 for African American women, compared to $25,503 for all older men and $14,599 for all elderly women (Administration on Aging, 2010). There is also a great disparity in

Case Study 2-1

Mrs. Johnson is an 87-year-old African American female admitted to the hospital from her home. She is widowed and has no children. Her neighbors watch out for her, bringing her groceries and making sure that she's okay each day. Mrs. Johnson's neighbor, Mrs. Edwards, accompanies her to the hospital.

Mrs. Johnson is admitted for shortness of breath, attributed to poor self-management of her medication regimen for congestive heart failure. She is alert, oriented, and very pleasant.

Mrs. Edwards takes you aside and tells you that she is concerned about Mrs. Johnson's home situation.

Questions:

1. What questions would you ask about Mrs. Johnson's financial situation? Why?
2. What questions would you ask about Mrs. Johnson's living situation? Why?
3. How might these factors contribute to her hospital admission?
4. What issues might you be thinking about as you admit Mrs. Johnson to the inpatient unit?

net worth between Black and White households headed by older Americans. In 2007, net worth among older Black households was estimated to be $46,000, compared to $280,000 among older White households (Federal Interagency Forum, 2010). The lack of economic resources and poor access to health care add to the incidence of disease and disease complications in this subgroup (see **Case Study 2-1**).

African Americans experience higher rates of diabetes, hypertension, and chronic kidney disease than other Americans (CDC, 2011). African American men have higher incidences of lung and prostate cancer as compared to Whites, and African Americans' overall risk to develop kidney disease is highest of when examined by ethnic and racial groups. However, a growing body of evidence suggests that this difference in prevalence is a function of socioeconomics, not genetics (LaViest, Thorpe, Galarrage, Bower, & Gary-Webb, 2009).

Among the most frequently occurring chronic conditions in the older African American population are hypertension (84%), arthritis (53%), heart disease (27%), diabetes (29%), sinusitis (15%), and cancer (13%). **Table 2-1** compares prevalence for several chronic diseases across race and ethnicity (Administration on Aging, 2010).

Hispanic Older Adults

The Hispanic population is now the largest ethnic minority in the United States (Porter, 2011). The over 65 year old Hispanic population is the fastest growing segment of the total U.S. population; by 2019, the Hispanic population age 65 or older is projected to be the largest racial/ethnic minority in this age group (Administration on Aging, 2010). By 2050, Hispanic elders will comprise 19.8% of all older Americans, adding up to 17 million Hispanics over the age of 65 (Administration on Aging, 2010). The Hispanic population in the United States is composed of several subgroups from Mexico, Cuba, Puerto Rico, the Dominican Republic, and other countries of Central and South America. The poverty rate in 2008 for Hispanic elders in the United States was nearly twice that of the total older population, 19.3% compared to 7.6% (Administration on Aging, 2010).

The chronic diseases including cardiovascular disease, diabetes, cancer, and cerebrovascular disease are seen in significant numbers in the Hispanic population. CDC data show Hispanics less likely to obtain preventive services such as flu and pneumonia vaccines and mammograms as compared to Whites. The top five causes of death among Hispanics are heart disease, cancer, unintentional injuries, stroke, and diabetes (CDC, 2010).

In 2008, 70% of Hispanics age 65 or over lived in four states: California, Florida, New York, and Texas (Administration on Aging, 2010). Family members frequently act as their caregivers, and multigenerational families under one roof are common. Overall, the percentage of Hispanic elders living alone is lower than that

TABLE 2-1   Comparison of the Prevalence of Chronic Disease in Older Adults by Race and Ethnicity

Disease	African American	Hispanic	Native American/ Alaskan Native	White
Hypertension	84%	75%	58%	71%
Arthritis	53%	45%	51%	49%
Heart Disease	27%	25%	*	31%
Diabetes	29%	27%	42%	18%
Cancer	13%	12%	*	22%
Three or more chronic conditions	13.7%	6.6%	15.3%	12.7%

of the general population (Administration on Aging, 2010). Older Hispanics are more likely to be married and to rely on family over friends when compared to non-Hispanic White elders.

Asians and Pacific Islander Older Adults

This ethnic group actually is composed of 40 different ethnic groups with varying economic, educational, and health profiles. National data do not usually discern between ethnicities, which complicates identifying patterns of aging for each culture. According to the U.S. Census Bureau, projections for the years 2010–2050 include population increases for Asian Americans and Pacific Islanders from 3.4% to 8.6% of the U.S. population (Administration on Aging, 2010).

Life expectancy data have historically shown an advantage for the Asian American and Pacific Islander population. Census data from 1995 showed life expectancy at birth of Asian Americans and Pacific Islanders to be 79.3 years for males and 84.9 years for females, as compared to 73.6 and 80.1 for non-Asian White males and females, respectively. Discrepancies are seen in mortality causes depending on whether persons are U.S. or foreign-born, pointing to the impact of acculturation in U.S. society. The top five causes of death among Asian Americans or Pacific Islanders are heart disease, cancer, stroke, unintentional injuries, and diabetes (CDC, 2011).

Members of this ethnic minority as the Hispanic group described above are less likely than U.S. whites to live in nursing homes. Dependence on familial and informal ethnic resources is seen more often than use of traditional health resources. Length of the family's time in this country (recent arrival vs. present for a century) affects comfort and ease of resource use.

Native American and Alaskan Native Older Adults

The census group Native American and Alaskan Natives (NA/ANs) is comprised of 566 nations, tribes, bands, and native villages in which 150 languages are used (National Council of American Indians, 2016). Overall, the 2005–2007 Current Population Survey found that the NA/AN population has larger families, less health insurance, and twice the level of poverty as other American groups (*Indian Health Service* [IHS], 2012). The 2000 Census found that the NA/AN population is younger than all other groups of the United States, with a median age of 25 years, compared to the U.S. populations median of 35 years. Although life expectancy for this group lags behind the national average, it is increasing. In 1972–1974, the life expectancy at birth for NA/ANs was 63.6 years; it is now 72.6 years, 5.2 years less than the general U.S population. Leading causes of death in this population are heart disease, cancer, unintentional injuries, diabetes, and cerebrovascular disease (Administration on Aging, 2011b).

In 2009, 50% of NA/AN elders lived in six states: California, Oklahoma, Arizona, New Mexico, Texas, and North Carolina (Administration on Aging, 2011b). Traditionally this population has lived in rural areas, although currently slighty more than half (57%) of the population resides in urban areas (IHS, 2012). Chronic disease prevalence in NA/AN increased significantly in the 20th century (see **Case Study 2-2**). Researchers have found that older NA/ANs have higher rates of hypertension, diabetes, back pain, and vision loss than the general U.S population. Nationally, more than two in five NA/AN elders has diabetes (see Table 2-1). Goins and Pilkerton (2010) found evidence that at age 55 were experiencing disease states such as cataracts more frequently found in the 70-year-old general population.

CLINICAL TIP

When caring for a person with Native American heritage, be aware of the high risk and incidence of diabetes.

NAs/ANs have the highest rates of diabetes in the United States (IHS, 2012). The NA/AN population also has higher rates of obesity, substance abuse, and mental health problems. According to the IHS, geographic isolation, economic factors, and suspicion toward traditional spiritual beliefs are some of the reasons why health among NA/ANs is poorer than other groups.

In the 2000 Census, American Indian/Alaskan Natives (AI/ANs) reported the highest rates of functional limitation, particularly in the age 55–64 years group. Disability is one of the strongest predictors of the need for nursing home admission in the older adult. This trend is "becoming increasingly important because the number of AI/ANs aged 75 years or older who will need long-term care will double in the next 25 years" (Goins, Moss, Buchwald, & Guralnik, 2007, p. 690) and Congress has a history of providing poorer funding to the healthcare services for AI/ANs compared to other U.S. populations.

The Older Foreign-Born Population in the United States

The *foreign-born* are those people who are living in the United States who were not U.S. citizens at birth. Approximately 13.1% of the total U.S. population is foreign-born. The age of newly arrived immigrants has not significantly changed since 1970. The majority of new arrivals are 18 to 44 years old, with only 5% of new immigrants 65 years old or older (Pew Research Center, 2015). Although the number of new immigrants who are 65 years old or older is small, in 2010, 11.9% of the older U. S. population were foreign-born (Population Reference

Case Study 2-2

Mr. Andrew Crow is a 67-year-old American Indian. He has been unemployed for the past 5 years.
He lives on a reservation in Oklahoma with his wife and three teenage children. Mr. Crow came to the health clinic for a routine checkup. You note that he is overweight.

Questions:

1. How should you focus your physical assessment?
2. What chronic diseases might Mr. Crow be at high risk for?
3. What are the implications for his family?
4. Develop a plan of care for Mr. Crow and his family members.

Bureau, 2013). The pattern of immigration is changing. Before 1980, over half of U.S. foreign-born individuals were from Europe and Canada. The percentage of immigrants from those countries had dropped to just over 14% in 2013 (Pew Research Center, 2015). Currently most immigrants come from Mexico (28%), other Latin American countries (24%), and Asian countries (25.8%). The changes in immigration are reflected in the aging of the portion of the U.S. population who are European-born. More than 28% of this population is now over 65 years old. (Grieco et al., 2010). Foreign-born persons comprised 12.4% of the over-65 population at the time of the 2010 Census.

CLINICAL TIP

Ask patients and families their generation of immigration (i.e., are they first, second, third generation Americans?).

Education

Level of education attained can affect the socioeconomic status of an older adult. Those with more education tend to have more money, higher standards of living, and above-average health. In 1965, 24% of the older adults in the United States had graduated from high school and 5% had at least a bachelor's degree. In 2010, 79.5% of older adults had graduated from high school, while 22.5% of older adults had at least a bachelor's degree. This increase in average education has not been universal. Differences exist in education between ethnic groups in the United States. In 2010, most older non-Hispanic Whites (84.3%), older Asians (73.6%), and older Blacks (64.8%) had completed high school. However fewer than half of older Hispanics (47%) had completed high school (Administration on Aging, 2010; Federal Interagency Forum, 2010). This could be related to a higher proportion of first-generation older individuals having fewer opportunities in their country of origin when they were children.

Living Arrangements

Before the 19th century, few individuals lived to old age. Those that did were likely to come from the upper classes, and were highly respected. If a poor person lived into later years, he or she was often seen as a burden on society, and may have lived out his or her years in a "poor-house" (Fleming, Evans, & Chutka, 2003). The poor-house was an early attempt to provide for individuals who could not provide for themselves. The conditions were often marginal at best. In the 1800s, youth came to be increasingly valued and older adults declined in status. This trend continued until, by the end of the 19th century, age stratification was prevalent in America and other western countries. Activities like school attendance, marriage, and retirement became based on age. By the start of the 1900s the number of older adults began to increase. Cultural focus shifted to business, medicine, and scientific advances. Older adults were devalued (Fleming et al., 2003), and left without means of taking care of themselves. Many were moved to poor-houses without consideration for their preferences or needs.

In the early 1900s, poor-houses in the United States had changed into old-age homes. With this change in focus the conditions gradually improved and became focused on care of older adults. When elders couldn't afford the cost of the old-age home they were transferred to state-funded mental institutions. Charitable homes came into being, run by religious organizations, benevolent societies, and ethnic organizations. For-profit homes also developed, serving the chronically ill or disabled. Standards and oversight on all of these facilities were minimal (Fleming et al., 2003).

Globally, 40% of older persons aged 60 years or over live independently, that is to say, alone or with their spouse only. *Independent living* is far more common in the developed countries, where about three quarters of older persons live independently, compared with only a quarter in developing countries and one eighth in the least developed countries. As countries develop and their populations continue to age, living alone or with a spouse

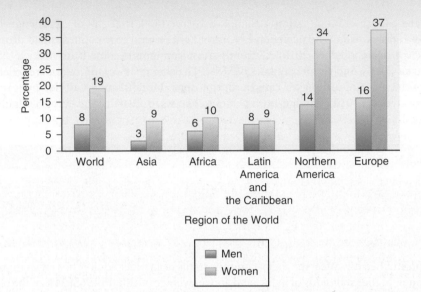

Figure 2-3 Proportion of aging population aged 60 years or older, living alone, by region and sex, 2005.

Reproduced from United Nations. (2007). *World economic and social survey 2007: Development in an ageing world.* United Nations publication, Sales No. E.07.II.C.1. Retrieved from http://www.un.org/en/development/desa/policy/wess/wess_archive/2007wess.pdf. Reprinted with permission of the United Nations.

only will likely become much more common among older people in the future (Harris-Kojetin et al., 2013). Living arrangements of older adults are linked to income, health status, culture, and the availability of caregivers. Older people who live alone are more likely than their married counterparts to live in poverty. Over one-half (55.1%) of noninstitutionalized older adults lived with their spouse in 2010. In that year, older men were more likely to be living with a spouse than were older women (69.9% compared to 41.3%). Older women were twice as likely as older men to be living alone (37.3% compared to 19.1%). The likelihood of living alone increases with age: among women age 75 or older, 47% lived alone in 2010 (see **Figure 2-3**).

A total of about 1.94 million older adults lived in households with a child present in the house in 2010. About 536,000 of these were grandparents over 65 years of age with the primary responsibility for their grandchildren who lived with them (Administration on Aging, 2015).

CLINICAL TIP

Ask patients if they are helping to care for grandchildren (in their home or elsewhere). Be ready to answer common questions related to healthcare of children, such as immunization schedules and common childhood illnesses.

Although only a small percentage (4.1%) of older adults resided in nursing homes in 2009, the percentage increases with age. This ranges from 1.1% for persons ages 65–74, to 3.5% for persons ages 75–84, and to 13.2% for persons ages 85+. Another 2.4% of older adults lived in "senior housing" in 2009, which often offers supportive services to residents (Administration on Aging, 2011a).

Elders are less likely to change residence than other age groups. From 2009 to 2010, only 5.8% of older persons moved, as opposed to 16.9% of the under-65 population. Most older movers (58.7%) stayed in the same county and 78.2% remained in the same state. Only 21.8% of the movers moved out of state or abroad (Administration on Aging, 2011a).

By 1997, approximately 4% of the older U.S. population was being cared for in nursing homes. Currently, fewer than 3% of older adults are residents in a nursing home on any given day (Harris-Kojetin et al., 2013; Administration for Community Living, 2015). Living arrangements, like education, also vary by race, ethnicity, and region of the world. Individuals in developed countries are more likely to live alone than those in developing countries and women are more likely than men to live alone. The chance of living alone increases as age increases. Older individuals who lived alone in the United States had higher poverty rates than those who lived with their spouse. In 2010, 16% of older persons who lived alone lived in poverty, but only 5% of older married men and women lived in poverty (Federal Interagency Forum, 2010).

U.S. Veterans

In 2015, one out of every two men over 65 years old were veterans. There are currently three *cohorts* of older veterans: those who served in World War II, those who served in the Korean War, and those who served in Vietnam. Changes in the population of older Americans who are veterans of the armed services are expected to continue as the Vietnam-era cohort ages and the World War II and Korean War veteran continue to die. In 2000, there were 9.8 million veterans age 65 or older in the United States. More than 95% of these veterans were male. Between 1990 and 2000, the number of male veterans age 85 or older increased from 142,000 to 400,000. There is a projected increase after 2010 as the Vietnam-era cohort ages. The number of veterans 85 or older was 1.4 million in 2015 (http://www.agingstats.gov/).

Some older veterans begin to experience symptoms of Post Traumatic Stress Disorder (PTSD) as they age. This Late Onset Stress Symptomology (LOSS) can be a result of retirement and having more time to dwell on war experiences, or other common changes occurring with age (http://www.ptsd .va.gov/public/types/war/ptsd-older-vets.asp). LOSS is different from PTSD in that LOSS is often triggered by the aging process.

Changes in military healthcare systems are a direct result of the Iraq and Afghanistan wars. It is unknown how the numbers of wounded military personnel from these wars will affect the U.S. Department of Veterans Affairs in the short or in the long term. It can be anticipated, however, that the number of veterans with significant physical and emotional disabilities will increase and that their needs for health care will also increase as this newest cohort ages. The greater incidence of those with polytraumatic injuries and multiple limb amputation who have survived the advanced weapons of war will pose an additional challenge to the healthcare system as they age. Over the last few years, there has been a shift in the age of soldiers who are deployed in Iraq and Afghanistan. Older soldiers are being re-deployed in conflict areas and soldiers are serving multiple tours. These soldiers will turn 65 in advance of the average veteran and will likely have an impact on veterans' services of older adults sooner than otherwise anticipated.

The Disabled Older Population

Advances in health care have increased the life span of persons with disabilities including individuals with acquired or congenital disabilities. This means that individuals who were anticipated to have a shortened life span are now living into old age. The success of saving lives of individuals with disabilities either at birth or at the time of the trauma has led to the unintended consequence of increasing the demands on the healthcare system later in life. Like soldiers, traumatically injured persons are now more likely to receive expert emergency services at the time of their accident thereby surviving with injuries that previously would have been fatal. Advances in intensive care services, surgical services, diagnostic services, and the knowledge and skills of healthcare workers have combined to prolong the lives of persons who previously may have died within days or months of their traumatic injuries. For the first time in history, the life span of persons with spinal cord injuries and brain injuries is similar to the average lifespan. As these individuals age, they are truly entering a time in their lives that is unpredictable, because they are the first to reach these advanced ages.

Developmentally disabled individuals are another special aging group. Technological advances and improvements in health care are prolonging the lives of those with disabilities such as mental retardation. Twelve percent of persons with developmental disabilities are now 65 or older; this translates to between 200,000 and 500,000 people. There are major implications for the U.S. healthcare system as this population continues to age, grow, and outlive their parents. These individuals are aging younger, with an increased susceptibility to chronic diseases at younger ages that the general population (Administration of Intellectual and Developmental Disabilities [AIDD], 2012).

Older Adult Prisoners

One oft-forgotten segment of the older population in the United States is prisoners. As of 2010, there were 26,100 inmates over the age of 65 in federal and state prisons, a 63% increase from 2007 (Human Rights Watch, 2012). There are two older populations in our prisons: those serving long and/or life sentences who committed crimes when young and those who are older when the crime was committed. The length of incarceration is therefore different between these two groups, and the effects of incarceration on the aging process may be different as well. There is often little motivation and power to release aged and infirm prisoners before their sentence is completed, adding to the increasing numbers of older and disabled inmates in prisons in the United States (Human Rights Watch 2012).

Older has a different connotation in prisons. Due to the stressors related to incarceration, as well as the increased likelihood of an unhealthy lifestyle preceding incarceration, prisoners aged 50–55 experience physical and mental changes normally associated with free-world citizens at least 10 years older. Substandard environment, nutrition, exercise, and medical care during incarceration likely helps to accelerate the aging process, as does the violence, anxiety, and stress associated with prison life (see **Case Study 2-3**).

CLINICAL TIP

Elderly prisoners may look considerably older than their biological age.

Older prisoners cost, on average, 8% more to incarcerate than younger prisoners because they have more health needs. Bureau of Prisons (BOP) institutions with the highest percentages of aging inmates in their population spent 5 times more per inmate on medical care than institutions with the lowest percentage of aging inmates. BOP institutions with the highest percentages of aging inmates also spent 14 times more per inmate on medication than institutions with the lowest percentage (Office of the Inspector General, 2016).

Case Study 2-3

Mr. Everett is a 62-year-old inmate in a federal penitentiary, admitted to your unit for hypertension, heart failure, and chest pain. He is accompanied by a prison guard, who watches your every move. The guard has handcuffed Mr. Everett to the bed.

This is the first prisoner that you've ever cared for. You are surprised at how old Mr. Everett looks. You complete your admission assessment and talk to him about the plans for his care.

Questions:

1. Why might this patient appear to be older than his stated age?
2. How could his social situation affect his plan of care, hospital stay, and recovery?
3. What are the implications for his ability to self-manage his chronic conditions?

In order to care for the aging prisoner population, some states, like Texas, have developed separate facilities for their geriatric prisoners. Other states have integrated telemedicine into their facilities or developed chronic care clinics. Some, recognizing the likelihood of inmates not only *aging in place* in prison but also dying of chronic disease while in prison, have implemented hospice programs for their dying, elderly prisoners.

Mortality and Morbidity

Changes in life expectancy throughout the 20th century were related to improved sanitation, advances in medical care, and the implementation of preventive health services. In the early 1900s, infectious diseases and acute illnesses were the cause of most deaths. Today, most deaths occur from *chronic disease* such as cardiovascular disease. More individuals are surviving acute events such as myocardial infarction (heart attack) and stroke, and modern medicine has made replacement of organs through transplant possible. These medical advances have contributed to the increased longevity. Healthcare costs, including medication costs, have become a primary issue for many *senior citizens* in the United States. In other developed countries, national health care alleviates this expense for elders. In developing countries, healthcare services and medicines for chronic diseases simply may not exist. The repercussions of rising healthcare costs have been felt within the state and federal governments, as they seek to help support their senior citizens' health. Nearly 95% of healthcare expenditures for older Americans are for chronic diseases (Centers for Medicare and Medicaid Services [CMS], 2012).

Chronic Diseases

The incidence of chronic diseases increases with age. Across the globe noncommunicable diseases are replacing infectious diseases as the major cause of morbidity and mortality. Six of the seven leading causes of death among older Americans are chronic diseases such as heart disease, stroke, cancer, and diabetes. There is a gender component to the incidence of chronic disease; older women report higher incidence of chronic diseases such as hypertension and arthritis, whereas men report more heart disease and cancer.

Obesity is a chronic condition that is increasing in prevalence in the United States. According to the Center for Disease Control, more than one-third of older adults aged 65 and over were obese in 2010, the most recent year for which statistics are available. Obesity prevalence was higher among those aged 65–74 as compared with those aged 75 and over in both men and women. These rates suggest that the effects of obesity will increase with age.

Sensory impairments and oral health problems become more frequent with aging. Early detection can prevent or postpone the physical, social, and emotional effects that these changes have on a senior's life. Nearly 25% of those aged 65–74 and 50% of those who are 75 and older have disabling hearing loss (National Institutes of Health, 2016b). Men are more likely to report hearing loss than women. Alterations in vision affects about one in five of older adults. Common eye conditions resulting in vision loss include glaucoma, macular degeneration, and cataracts. These changes in sensory function can lead to decreased function, independence, and social isolation.

Thirty-four percent of persons 85 years of age or older reported edentulism (lack of teeth). Poorer older adults were less likely to have teeth than those above the poverty threshold (42% compared to 23%) (Federal Interagency Forum, 2010). Glasses, hearing aids, and dentures can be difficult to obtain for financial reasons: They are expensive and they are not covered services under Medicare. Thus, many older adults may not possess these assistive devices, or may have out-of-date or ill-fitting devices, which can affect cognitive status (hearing aids and glasses), nutritional intake (dentures), and likelihood of falling (glasses).

Decline in memory, particularly short term memory, is another chronic problem that can affect older individuals. However sudden memory loss or confusion is a sign of acute illness. Approximately 30–40% of individuals over 65 years old report normal, age-related memory change. An additional 10% of people over 65 years develop mild cognitive impairment, a precursor to Alzheimer's Disease (National Institutes of Health, 2016a). These percentages increase as age increases. As the elderly U.S. population grows, the number of individuals with dementia will also increase, making planning for the long-term care needs of those individuals increasingly important.

The trend toward increasing chronic disease is global, however when compared to European elders, older individuals in the United States report worse health than their European counterparts (World Health Organization, 2015). The age-adjusted proportion of people in the United States age 65 or older with chronic disabilities actually declined from 1984 to 1999. Older women reported more difficulties in physical functioning than older men. In 2007, 32% of older women reported that they were unable to perform at least one of five activities, compared to 19% of men. Those aged 85 years or older had more physical limitations than those between 65 and 74 years. (Federal Interagency Forum, 2010).

Causes of Death

The leading cause of death for older adults in the United States in 2013 was diseases of the heart, followed by malignant neoplasms, chronic lower respiratory diseases (CLRD), accidents, cerebrovascular diseases, Alzheimer's disease, diabetes, and influenza and pneumonia (Xu, Murphy, Kochanek, & Bastian, 2016). In 2014, age-adjusted death rates among older males were higher than among older females for heart disease, cancer, CLRD, diabetes, stroke, and unintentional injuries. Age-adjusted death rates for Alzheimer's disease were lower among older males than females (CDC, 2016). Globally, heart disease is followed by a cause of death by stroke, pulmonary disease, HIV/AIDS, diabetes mellitus, Alzheimer's disease, diarrheal diseases, tuberculosis, and injury. (World Health Organization, 2017).

Healthy Aging

Although the statistics can sound grim, in actuality, the vast majority of elders report adequate health. Seventy-five percent of adults younger than 64 years old report having three or fewer chronic conditions such as high blood pressure or high cholesterol. This is compared with 71% of individuals aged 65–74 years old. That means that the youngest group of elders is experiencing health comparable to younger adults. The middle old and oldest old report more chronic illness, with 45% of middle old and more than half of the oldest old with more than 4 chronic conditions (CMS, 2012). The secret to good health in old age is good health during an individual's younger years. Lifestyle is a major contributor to how people age. Avoiding smoking and obesity and engaging in regular exercise can make a substantial difference to health in old age (Ortman & Velkoff, 2014).

Summary

This chapter has reviewed important facts and statistics about the aging population. The aging of the world population will affect society as the baby boomers enter the old age. The challenge for successful aging will be to reduce the incidence of chronic disease across the lifespan, and to optimize the additional years of life. Finally, successful aging is thought to be possible with wise lifestyle choices and avoidance of risk factors. These are further discussed throughout this text.

Resource List

Aging Statistics

  Administration on Aging:
  http://www.aoa.gov/

  American Association of Retired Persons:
  http://www.aarp.org

  American Geriatrics Society:
  http://www.americangeriatrics.org

  Centers for Disease Control and Prevention:
  http://www.cdc.gov/aging/

  Federal Interagency Forum on Aging-Related
  Statistics:
  http://www.agingstats.gov

  Gray Panthers:
  http://www.graypanthers.org

  Merck Manual of Health and Aging:
  http://www.merck.com/pubs/mmanual_ha
  /sec1/ch03/ch03a.html

  National Institute on Aging:
  http://www.nia.nih.gov/

Online Journals

  BMC Geriatrics:
  http://www.biomedcentral.com/bmcgeriatr

  Geriatrics:
  http://www.geri.com/geriatrics/

  Geriatrics and Aging:
  http://www.geriatricsandaging.com

Longevity

  Estimate your longevity potential by accessing
  the Life Expectancy Calculator at:
  http://www.livingto100.com

  CDC/National Center for Health Statistics:
  http://www.cdc.gov/nchs/fastats/lifexpec.htm

Clinical Reasoning Exercises

1. **You will be one of the nurses caring for the baby boomers as they age**. How will the prevalence of aged patients affect your nursing practice? What are the implications for your ongoing nursing education?

2. **Healthful living becomes ever more important to prevent the chronic diseases of the aged.** Fewer chronic diseases in the aged could mean that more healthcare services are available for those without chronic diseases. What is healthful living? What will your role be in promoting healthful living to your patients? Should nurses be responsible for promoting healthful living when they could be caring for sick patients?

3. **The health care of the baby boomers will likely be affected by changes in Social Security, Medicare, and Medicaid.** What implications does this have for your nursing practice? How might you address this issue as a nurse? How might you address this issue as a citizen?

4. **The population of the United States is becoming ever more ethnically and culturally diverse.** What healthcare issues can you foresee as this ethnically diverse population ages?

5. **Think about older celebrities in the United States and abroad,** and compare your thoughts about them to your thoughts about older people in general. Do you have different thoughts and feelings about Bill Clinton and George W. Bush (former presidents, both age 69 in 2016) than you do about a nursing home patient? How about those celebrities who are growing older—Cher (singer), Barbra Streisand (singer), Colin Powell (general), Clint Eastwood (actor)? Compare and contrast a well-known senior celebrity with an aged patient you have recently met.

Personal Reflection

The aging of America will affect you both personally and professionally. Government resources will become more and more strained as the baby boomers become elders and begin to use these resources. Medicare, Medicaid, and Social Security may not continue to exist as we know them. There will be fewer beds available in both acute and chronic care facilities to care for the growing aged population. There may not be enough geriatric specialty physicians and nurses to care for the vast numbers of older adults. How could these circumstances affect you and your family? What are your personal plans for your own aging? Have you started to save money for retirement? Are you living a healthy lifestyle, eating "right," and exercising? Are you or your children overweight? Do you smoke or drink excessive alcohol? Are you ready to become involved in the political process so that your opinion is heard?

References

Administration for Community Living. (2015). *Administration on aging: Geographic distribution.* Retrieved from http://www.agid.acl.gov/

Administration of Intellectual and Developmental Disabilities (AIDD). (2012). *Bridging aging and developmental disabilities service networks.* Retrieved from http://www.acl.gov/programs/aidd/Program_Resource_Search/Resources/Bridging Aging_DD Srvc Networks.aspx

Administration on Aging, Department of Health and Human Services. (2010). A profile of older Americans: 2010. Retrieved from https://aoa.acl.gov/Aging_Statistics/Profile/2010/2.aspx

Administration on Aging, Department of Health and Human Services. (2011a). *A profile of older Americans: 2011.* Retrieved from http://www.aoa.gov/AoARoot/Aging_Statistics/Profile/2011/docs/2011profile.pdf

Administration on Aging, Department of Health and Human Services. (2011b). *A statistical profile of American Indian and Native Alaskan elderly.* Retrieved from https://aoa.acl.gov/Aging_Statistics/Minority_Aging/Facts-on-AINA-Elderly2008-plain_format.aspx

Administration on Aging, Department of Health and Human Services. (2015). *A profile of older Americans: 2015.* Retrieved from http://www.aoa.acl.gov/aging_statistics/profile/2014/2.aspx

Cameron, K. A., Song, J., Manheim, L. M., & Dunlop, D. D. (2010). *Gender disparities in health and healthcare among older adults.* Retrieved from http://www.ncbi.nlm.nih.gov/pmc/articles/PMC2965695/

Centers for Disease Control and Prevention. (2009). *Fast stats: Life expectancy.* Retrieved from http://www.cdc.gov/nchs/fastats/older_americans.htm

Centers for Disease Control and Prevention. (2011). *Office of minority health and health disparities.* Retrieved from http://www.cdc.gov/omhd/Populations/HL/HL.htm#Ten

Centers for Disease Control and Prevention. (2013). *Fact sheet: CDC health disparities and inequalities report.* Retrieved from https://www.cdc.gov/mmwr/pdf/other/su6203.pdf

Centers for Disease Control and Prevention. (2016). *Fast stats on older persons' health.* Retrieved from http://www.cdc.gov/nchs/fastats/older-american-health.htm

Centers for Medicare and Medicaid Services. (2012). *Chronic conditions among medicare beneficiaries, chartbook, 2012 edition.* Baltimore, MD: Centers for Medicare and Medicaid Services.

Federal Interagency Forum on Aging-Related Statistics. (November 2010). *Older Americans 2010: Key indicators of well-being.* Washington, DC: U.S. Government Printing Office. Retrieved from https://agingstats.gov/docs/PastReports/2010/OA2010.pdf

Fleming, K., Evans, J. M., & Chutka, D. S. (2003). A cultural and economic history of old age in America. *Mayo Clinic Proceedings, 78*(7), 914–921.

Goins, R. T., Moss, M., Buchwald, D., & Guralnik, J. M. (2007). Disability among older American Indians and Alaska Natives: An analysis of the 2000 Census public use microdata sample. *Gerontologist, 47*(5), 690–696.

Goins, R. T., & Pilkerton, C. S. (2010). Comorbidity among older American Indians: The Native Elder Care Study. *Journal of Cross-Cultural Gerontology, 25*(4), 343–354.

Grieco, M., Acosta, Y. D., de la Cruz, G. P., Gambino, C., Gryn, T., Larsen, L. J., et al. (2010). *The foreign-born population in the United States*; 2010 (American Community Survey Reports). Retrieved from http://www.census.gov/prod/2012pubs/acs-19.pdf

Harris-Kojetin, L., Sengupta, M., Park-Lee, E., & Valverde, R. (2013). *Long-term care services in the United States: 2013 overview.* Hyattsville, MD: National Center for Health Statistics.

Human Rights Watch. (2012). *Old behind bars: The aging prison population in the United States.* Retrieved from http://www.hrw.org/sites/default/files/reports/usprisons0112webwcover_0.pdf

Indian Health Service. (2012). *Fact sheets.* Retrieved from http://www.ihs.gov/PublicAffairs/IHSBrochure/

Kincel, B. (2014). *The centenarian population: 2007–2011.* U.S. Census Bureau. Retrieved from https://www.census.gov/prod/2014pubs/acsbr12-18.pdf

Kinsella, G., & He, W. (2009). *An aging world, 2008.* U.S. Census Bureau, International Population Reports, P95/09-1. Washington, DC: U.S. Government Printing Office.

LaViest, T., Thorpe, R., Galarrage, J., Bower, K., & Gary-Webb, T. (2009). Environmental and socio-economic factors as contributors to racial disparities in diabetes prevalence. *Journal of General Internal Medicine, 24*(10), 1144–1148.

Louie, G., & Ward, M. (2011). Socioeconomic and ethnic differences in disease burden and disparities in physical function in older adults. *American Journal of Public Health, 101*(7), 1322–1329.

National Institutes of Health. (2016a). *Age page: Forgetfulness: Knowing when to ask for help.* Retrieved from https://www.nia.nih.gov/health/publication/forgetfulness

National Institutes of Health. (2016b). *Quick statistics on hearing.* Retrieved from https://www.nidcd.nih.gov/health/statistics/quick-statistics-hearing

National Council of American Indians. (2016). *Indians 101.* Retrieved from http://www.ncai.org/about-tribes

Office of the Inspector General, U.S. Department of Justice. (2016). *The Impact of an Aging Inmate Population on the Federal Bureau of Prisons.*

O'Hara, R. (2014). Commentary on "Individual and societal wisdom: explaining the paradox of human aging and high well-being" by Dilip V. Jeste and Andrew J. Oswald: Uncovering the genetic basis of well-being in older adults. *Psychiatry: Interpersonal & Biological Processes, 77*(4), 440–443.

Ortman, J., & Velkoff, V. (2014). *An aging nation: The older population in the United States.* Washington, DC: U.S. Census Bureau.

Pew Research Center. (2015, September 28). *U.S. foreign-born-populaion trends.* Retrieved from http://www.pewhispanic.org/2015/09/28/chapter-5-u-s-foreign-born-population-trends/

Population Reference Bureau. (2013). *Today's research on aging.* Washington, DC: Population Reference Bureau.

Porter, C. (2011). *Hispanics are largest minority group in United States.* Embassy of the United States, Brussels, Belgium. Retrieved from http://iipdigital.usembassy.gov/st/english/article/2011/03/20110328152807enelrahc0.5275232.html#axzz4YOlreuV3

Rana, B., Darst, B., Bloss, C., Shih, P., Depp, C., Nievergelt, C., et al. (2014). Candidate SNP associations of optimism and resilience in older adults: Exploratory study in 935 community-dwelling adults. *American Journal of Geriatric Psychiatry, 22*(10), 997–1006.

United Nations. (2007). *World economic and social survey2007: Development in an ageing world.* Retrieved from http://www.un.org/en/development/desa/policy/wess/wess_archive/2007wess.pdf

United Nations, Department of Economic and Social Affairs, Population Division. (2013). *World population ageing 2013*.

U. S. Census Bureau. (2011). *Older Americans month: May, 2011*. Retrieved from http://www.census.gov /newsroom/releases/archives/facts_for_features_special_editions/cb11-ff08.html

Vincent, G. K., & Velkoff, V. A. (2010). *The next four decades: The older population in the United States: 2010–2050*. Retrieved from http://www.census.gov/prod/2010pubs/p25-1138.pdf

World Health Organization (2015). *World report on ageing and health*. Luxembourg: World Health Organization.

World Health Organization. (2017). The top 10 causes of death. Retrieved from http://www.who.int/mediacentre /factsheets/fs310/en/

World population: The world in 2100. (2011, May 13). *The Economist*. Retrieved from http://www.economist .com/blogs/dailychart/2011/05/world_population

Xu, J., Murphy, S., Kochanek, K., & Bastian, B. (2016). *Deaths, final data for 2013*. Hyattsville, MD: National Center for Health Statistics.

For a full suite of assignments and additional learning activities, see the access code at the front of your book.

CHAPTER 3

Theories of Aging

Jean Lange
Sheila Grossman

(Competencies 1, 19)

LEARNING OBJECTIVES

At the end of this chapter, the reader will be able to:

> Identify the major theories of aging.
> Compare the similarities and differences between biological and psychosocial theories.
> Describe the process of aging using a biological and a psychosocial perspective.
> Analyze the rationale for using multiple theories of aging to describe the complex phenomenon of aging.
> Describe a general theoretical framework, taken from all of the aging theories that will assist nurses in making clinical decisions in gerontology.

KEY TERMS

Apoptosis	Mitochondria
Capacity	Nonstochastic theories of aging
Free radicals	Reactive oxygen species
Human needs theory	Senescence
Immunomodulation	Stochastic theories of aging
Lipofuscin	Telomerase
Maslow	Telomere
Melatonin	

From the beginning of time, preserving youth has been a topic of discussion in science, health care, technology, and everyday life. Is there anyone who would not be interested in knowing how the human organism ages? Doesn't everyone want to live a long and healthy life? There are few who would not want to see what the future holds for our bodies and minds; even more curiosity surrounds what advances have been made or will possibly be made to alter and slow the aging process. Understanding what knowledge theories of aging may contribute to answering these questions is a first step toward understanding the mystery of aging.

Complex physiological, social, economic, and psychological challenges often present themselves as we age. Declining health and cognitive or physical functioning may necessitate moving to supportive care environments that drain financial resources. Losing friends or loved ones, grappling with the meaning of life, maintaining quality of life in the face of increasing disability, adapting to retirement and contemplating death are just a few of the challenges that aging adults face.

Theories that are validated through research can guide nurses in helping elderly patients navigate the changes they experience. Cultural, spiritual, regional, socioeconomic, educational, and environmental factors as well as health status impact older adults' perceptions and choices about their healthcare needs. According to Haight and colleagues, "a good gerontological theory integrates knowledge, tells how and why phenomena are related, leads to prediction, and provides process and understanding. In addition, a good theory must be holistic and take into account all that impacts a person throughout a lifetime of aging" (Haight, Barba, Tesh, & Courts, 2002, p. 14).

Sociologists, psychologists, biologists, and more recently nurses have proposed varying theories about the aging process. The purpose of this chapter is to review the chronological development of aging theories, describe

TABLE 3-1   Psychosocial Theories of Aging

Theory	Description
Sociological Theories	Changing roles, relationships, status, and generational cohort impact the older adult's ability to adapt.
Activity	Remaining occupied and involved is necessary to a satisfying late life.
Disengagement	Gradual withdrawal from society and relationships serves to maintain social equilibrium and promote internal reflection.
Subculture	The elderly prefer to segregate from society in an aging subculture sharing loss of status and societal negativity regarding the aged. Health and mobility are key determinants of social status.
Continuity	Personality influences roles and life satisfaction and remains consistent throughout life. Past coping patterns recur as older adults adjust to physical, financial, and social decline and contemplate death. Identifying with one's age group, finding a residence compatible with one's limitations, and learning new roles postretirement are major tasks.
Age stratification	Society is stratified by age groups that are the basis for acquiring resources, roles, status, and deference from others. Age cohorts are influenced by their historical context and share similar experiences, beliefs, attitudes, and expectations of life-course transitions.
Person-Environment-Fit	Function is affected by ego strength, mobility, health, cognition, sensory perception, and the environment. Competency changes one's ability to adapt to environmental demands.
Gerotranscendence	The elderly transform from a materialistic/rational perspective toward oneness with the universe. Successful transformation includes an outward focus, accepting impending death, substantive relationships, intergenerational connectedness, and unity with the universe.

what evidence supports or refutes these theories and discuss their application to nursing practice. CINAHL, the National Library of Medicine, the Web of Science, PsycINFO, Science in Context, and Sociological Abstracts databases were reviewed to assess the support for and clinical application of these theories.

Psychosocial Theories of Aging

The earliest theories on aging came from the psychosocial disciplines (see **Table 3-1**). These theories focus on changes in behavior, personality, and attitude as we age. The authors propose that aging is a lifelong process characterized by transitions. Psychological theories relate these transitions to personality or ego development and the accompanying challenges associated with various life stages. They speak to how mental processes, emotions, attitudes, motivation, and personality influence adaptation to physical and social demands.

Sociological theorists consider how changing roles, relationships, and status within a culture or society impact an older adult's ability to adapt. They assert that societal norms can affect how individuals perceive and enact their role within a community. How living through key events such as the Vietnam War or civil rights eras affects aging is an important component of sociological theories of aging.

Theory	Description
Psychological Theories	Explain aging in terms of mental processes, emotions, attitudes, motivation, and personality development that is characterized by life stage transitions.
Human needs	Five basic needs motivate human behavior in a lifelong process toward need fulfillment.
Individualism	Personality consists of an ego and personal and collective unconsciousness that views life from a personal or external perspective. Older adults search for life meaning and adapt to functional and social losses.
Stages of personality	Personality develops in eight sequential stages with corresponding life development tasks. The eighth phase, integrity versus despair, is characterized by evaluating life accomplishments; struggles include letting go, accepting care, detachment, and physical and mental decline.
Life-course/life span	Life stages are predictable and structured by roles, relationships, values, development, and goals. Persons adapt to changing roles and relationships. Age-group norms and characteristics are an important part of the life course.
Selective optimization	Individuals cope with aging losses through activity/role selection, optimization, and compensation. Critical life points are morbidity, mortality, and quality of life. Selective optimization with compensation facilitates successful aging.

Sociological Theories of Aging

Activity Theory

Havighurst and Albrecht (1953) proposed one of the first aging theories by studying a group of adults. They concluded that society expects retirees to remain active in their communities. Havighurst and Albrecht published the Activity Theory in 1963, which states that staying occupied and involved is necessary to having a satisfying late-life (Havighurst, Neugarten, & Tobin, 1963; see **Figure 3-1**). Havighurst and Albrecht (1953) did not, however explain what sorts of activity are linked to life satisfaction but clearly believed that activity was associated with psychological health. They suggested that being active helps to prolong middle age and thus delay the adverse effects of old age.

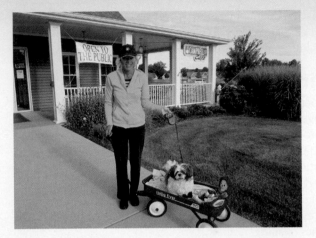

Figure 3-1 Activity theory suggests that remaining involved and engaged is a needed ingredient to a satisfying late life.

Others disagree with Havighurst and Albrecht's perspective, arguing that Activity Theory fails to consider that choices are often limited by physical capabilities, finances, and access to social resources (Birren & Schroots, 2001). Maddox (1963) suggests a more optimistic view; that leisure time in retirement presents new opportunities for community service that may be more consistent with physical, economic, and resource limitations. A second criticism of Activity Theory is the unproven assertion that staying active necessarily delays the onset of the negative effects of aging. Furthermore, Birren and Schroots assert that roles assumed by older adults are highly influenced by societal expectations so that older adults may be limited in what activities they can choose.

Despite these criticisms, Activity Theory's central theme—that remaining active in old age is desirable—is supported by most researchers. Lemon and colleagues found a direct relationship between being active and life satisfaction among older adults (Lemon, Bengston, & Peterson, 1972). They also observed that older adults viewed the quality of activity to be more important than the quantity.

Other investigators suggested that the type of activity matters. Activities that connected people socially, such as meeting friends for lunch or pursuing hobbies through group activities were more likely to improve life satisfaction than formal or solitary activities (Longino & Kart, 1982). Harlow and Cantor (1996) agreed that the social component was important. In their study, sharing tasks was an important predictor of life satisfaction, particularly among retirees. Schroots (1996) proposed that successful aging means being able to do things despite limitations. These studies suggest that the type of activity may be an important consideration rather than merely the frequency of engagement.

Disengagement Theory

In stark contrast to activity theorists, sociologists Cumming and Henry (1961) asserted that aging is characterized by gradual disengagement from society and relationships. The authors contended that this separation is desired by society and older adults, and that it serves to maintain social equilibrium. Cumming and Henry proposed that by disengaging, older adults are freed from social responsibilities and gain time for internal reflection, while the transition of responsibility from old to young maintains a continuously functioning society unaffected by lost members. The outcome of disengagement is a new equilibrium that is ideally satisfying to both the individual and society.

Challengers of Disengagement Theory argue that the emphasis on social withdrawal is inconsistent with what appears to be a key element of life satisfaction: being engaged in meaningful relationships and activities

(Baltes, 1987; Lemon et al., 1972; Neumann, 2000; Schroots, 1996). Others contend that the decision to withdraw varies across individuals and that disengagement theory fails to account for differences in sociocultural settings and environmental opportunities (Achenbaum & Bengtson, 1994; Marshall, 1996). Rapkin and Fischer (1992) reported that demographic disadvantages and age-related transitions were related to a greater desire for disengagement, support, and stability. Elders who were married and healthy were more likely to report a desire for an energetic lifestyle.

In support of Disengagement Theory, Adams developed an instrument to measure change in activity among older adults (Adams, 2004). The author reported, "In almost all instances, the group 75 years old and older reported a higher proportion of disengaged responses; they were particularly less invested than their younger counterparts in keeping up with hobbies, making plans for the future, making and creating things, and taking care of others" (p. 102). Several authors also agree with Cumming and Henry's assertion that a fit between societal needs and older adult activity is necessary (Back, 1980; Birren & Schroots, 2001; Riley, Johnson, & Foner, 1972). One example of the restrictions society can pose on older adult activity is the Social Security laws that reduce payment to older adults who make more than a set income. As life expectancy increases however, society is reframing its notions about the capability of older adults to make valuable contributions (Uhlenberg, 1992). Many adults are working past retirement age or begin to work part-time in a new field. Others are actively engaged in a variety of volunteer projects that benefit their communities. The many examples of what is now termed "successful aging" are challenging the common association of aging with disease.

Subculture Theory

Unlike activity theorists, Rose (1965) theorized that older adults form a unique subculture within society to defend against society's negative attitude toward aging and the accompanying loss of status. As in disengagement theory, Rose contended that older adults prefer to interact among themselves. He suggested that social status is determined more by health and mobility than occupation, education, or income; therefore older adults have a social disadvantage regarding status and associated respect because of the functional decline that accompanies aging.

Research to support or refute Rose's Subculture Theory is lacking. The growing number of older adults in developed countries around the world however necessitates greater attention to the needs of this age group and challenge the sociological theorists' view of aging as negative, undesirable, burdensome, and lacking status. Questions are beginning to be asked about whether society should be more supportive of older adults in terms of their environment, health care, work opportunities, and societal resources. The emphasis on whether society's or older adults' needs take precedence is beginning to shift in favor of older adults. In summary, McMullin (2000) argued that sociological theories need to more clearly address the diversity among older adults as well as the disparity versus younger age groups.

Continuity Theory

In the late 1960s, Havighurst and colleagues recognized that neither activity, subculture nor disengagement theories fully explained successful aging (Havighurst, Neugarten, & Tobin, 1968). Borrowing from psychology, they created Continuity Theory, which hypothesizes that personality influences the roles we choose and how we enact them. This in turn influences satisfaction with living. Continuity Theory suggests that personality is well developed by the time we reach old age and tends to remain consistent throughout our lives.

Havighurst and associates (1963) identified four personality types from observations of older adults: integrated, armored-defended, passive-dependent, and unintegrated. Integrated personality types have adjusted well to aging, as evidenced by activity engagement that may be broad (reorganizers), more selective (focused), or disengaged. Armored-defended individuals tend to continue the activities and roles held during middle age, whereas passive-dependent persons are either highly dependent or exhibit disinterest in the external world. Least well-adjusted are unintegrated personality types who fail to cope with aging successfully.

BOX 3-1   Research Highlight

Aim: This study investigated the relationship between social support and psychological distress in older adults over an 8-year period.

Methods: Canadian National Population Health Survey telephone survey data from 1998 and 2007 regarding residents' health, sociodemographic status, health services utilization, predictors of health, chronic conditions, and activity restrictions were analyzed. Respondents included 2,564 adults aged 55–89 years (mean age 64 years). Bivariate autoregressive cross-lagged models were used to analyze the data. Four dimensions of social support (emotional/informational support, tangible support, positive social interactions, and affectionate support) were examined in relationship to psychological distress, defined as a nonspecific negative psychological state that includes feelings of depression and anxiety. Structural equation modeling was used to analyze relationships among the variables.

Findings: Emotional/informational support, positive social interactions, and affectionate support were directly related to psychological distress. Higher psychological distress was related to subsequently higher levels of positive social interaction and emotional/informational support. Prior affectionate support predicted later support, and prior psychological distress predicted later levels of distress.

Application to practice: Psychological distress among older adults may predict subsequent levels of social support. Implications for these findings include the need for a greater awareness of the bidirectional nature of the relationship between social support and psychological distress among those who develop programs targeting older adults.

Robitaille, A., Orpana, H., & McIntosh, C. N. (2012). Reciprocal relationship between social support and psychological distress among a national sample of older adults: An autoregressive cross-lagged model. *Canadian Journal on Aging—La Revue Canadienne Du Vieillissement, 31*(1), 13.

Havighurst (1972) later defined adjusting to physical, financial, and social decline; contemplating death; and developing a personal and meaningful perspective on the end of life as the tasks of older adulthood (**Box 3-1**). Successful accomplishment of these tasks, he proposed is evidenced by identifying with one's age group, finding a living environment that is compatible with physical functioning, and learning new societal roles postretirement. The authors suggest that identifying a person's personality type provides clues as to an older adult will adjust to changes in health, environment, or socioeconomic conditions, and in what activities he or she will engage. Continuity Theory was the first sociological theory to acknowledge that responses to aging differ among individuals.

Several studies support Continuity Theory. Troll and Skaff (1997) asked older adults how they thought they had changed over the years. Almost all respondents thought they were still essentially the same person. Responders who believed they had stable personalities over time tended to have a more positive affect. In another study, Efklides, Kalaitzidou, and Chankin, (2003) investigated the effects of demographics, health status, attitude, and adaptation to old age on perceived quality of life. A positive attitude about adaptation to old age were associated with better perceptions about quality of life in this Greek sample (Efklides et al., 2003). Agahi, Ahacic, and Parker (2006) used continuity theory to examine patterns of change in older adults' participation in leisure activities over time. Consistent with continuity as well as activity and disengagement theories, the authors found that active participation tends to decline over time, and lifelong participation patterns predict involvement later in life. Critics of continuity theory, however, caution that the social context within which one ages may be more important than personality in determining what and how roles are played (Birren & Schroots, 2001).

Age Stratification Theory

In the 1970s, sociologists began to examine the interdependence between older adults and society (Riley et al., 1972). Riley and colleagues observed that society is stratified into different age categories that are the basis for acquiring resources, roles, status, and deference from others in society. In addition, they observed that age cohorts are influenced by the historical context in which they live and can vary across generations. People born in the same cohort have similar experiences, ideologies, orientations, attitudes, and values as well as expectations regarding the timing of life transitions such as retirement and life expectancy (Riley, 1994). Age Stratification Theory highlighted the importance of cohorts and the associated socioeconomic and political impact on how individuals age (Marshall, 1996).

Several authors support the Age Stratification Theory. Uhlenburg (1996) used Age Stratification Theory to define the societal needs of specific aging cohorts. Yin and Lai (1983) explained the varied status among older adults based on cohort differences. Cohorts were also found to affect outcomes in residential settings with mixed versus homogenous groups (Hagestad & Dannefer, 2002; Uhlenberg, 2000).

Person-Environment-Fit Theory

Following the broader view of aging that emerged in the 1970s, another shift occurred in the early 1980s that blended existing theories from different disciplines. Lawton's (1982) Person-Environment-Fit Theory proposed that *capacity* to function in one's environment is an important aspect of successful aging, and that function is affected by ego strength, motor skills, biologic health, cognitive capacity, and sensori-perceptual capacity, as well as external conditions imposed by the environment. Functional capacity influences an older adult's ability to adapt to his or her environment. Those individuals functioning at lower levels can tolerate fewer environmental demands.

Lawton's (1982) theory helps us think about the fit between the environment and an older adult's ability to function. It can help nurses identify needed modifications in their homes or in residential settings. Several authors lend support to this theory. Wahl (2001) developed six models to explain relationships between aging and the environment, home, institution, and relocation decision making using Lawton's theory. O'Connor and Vallerand (1994) used Lawton's theory to examine the relationship between long-term care residents' adjustment and their motivational style and environment. Older adults with self-determined motivational styles were better adjusted when they lived in homes that provided opportunities for freedom and choice, whereas residents with less self-determined motivational styles were better adjusted when they lived in high-constraint environments. The authors concluded that their findings supported the person-environment-fit theory of adjustment in old age.

Gerotranscendence Theory

One of the newest sociological aging theories is Tornstam's (1994) theory of gerotranscendence. This theory proposes that aging individuals undergo a cognitive transformation from a materialistic, rational perspective toward "oneness" with the universe. Characteristics of successful transformation include a more outward or external focus, accepting impending death without fear, an emphasis on substantive relationships, a sense of connectedness with preceding and future generations and spiritual unity with the universe. Gerotranscendence borrows from disengagement theory but does not accept its idea that social disengagement is a necessary and natural development. Rather, Tornstam asserted that activity and participation must be the result of one's own choices and that control over one's life in all situations is essential for successful adaptation to aging.

Gerotranscendence has been tested in several studies. Schroots (2003) used this theory to investigate how people manage their lives, cope with transformations and react to affective-positive and negative life events. Wadensten

(2002) used the Theory of Gerotranscendence to develop guidelines for the care of older adults living in a nursing home. Her results suggest that the guidelines may be useful for facilitating the process of gerotranscendence among nursing home residents.

Psychological Theories of Aging

Human Needs Theory

At the same time that activity theory was being developed, *Maslow* (1954), a psychologist, published the *human needs theory*. In this theory, Maslow surmised that a hierarchy of five needs motivates human behavior: physiologic, safety and security, love and belonging, self-esteem, and self-actualization. These needs are prioritized such that more basic needs like physiological functioning or safety take precedence over personal growth needs (love and belonging, self-esteem, and self-actualization). Movement is multidirectional and dynamic in a lifelong process toward need fulfillment. Self-actualization requires the freedom to express and pursue personal goals and be creative in an environment that is stimulating and challenging.

Maslow asserted that failure to grow leads to feelings of failure, depression, and the perception that life is meaningless.

Since its inception, Maslow's theory has been applied to varied age groups in many disciplines. Ebersole, Hess, and Luggen (2004) suggested that the tasks of aging described by several theorists (Havighurst, 1972; Peck, 1968) are linked to the basic needs described in Maslow's model. Jones and Miesen (1992) used Maslow's hierarchy to present a model for the nursing care of elderly persons in residential settings.

Theory of Individualism

Jung's Theory of Individualism, like Maslow's theory is not specific to aging. Jung (1960) proposed that our personality develops over a lifetime and is composed of an ego or self-identity that has a personal and collective unconsciousness. Personal unconsciousness is the private feelings and perceptions surrounding important persons or life events. The collective unconscious is shared by all persons. It contains latent memories about human origin. The collective unconscious is the foundation of personality on which the personal unconsciousness and ego are built. Jung's theory says that people tend to view life through either their own "lens" (introverts) or the lens of others (extroverts).

As individuals age, they begin to reflect on their beliefs and life accomplishments. According to Jung, one ages successfully when he or she accepts the past, adapts to physical decline, and copes with the loss of significant others. Neugarten (1968) supported Jung's theory by asserting that introspection promotes positive inner growth. Subsequent theorists also describe introspection as a part of healthy aging (Erikson, 1963; Havighurst et al., 1968).

Stages of Personality Development Theory

Similar to his colleagues Erikson's theory, Stages of Personality Development focuses on personality development. According to Erikson (1963), personality develops in eight sequential stages. Each stage has a life task at which we may succeed at or fail. During the final stage, "ego integrity versus despair" individuals search for the meaning of their lives and evaluate their accomplishments. Satisfaction leads to integrity, while dissatisfaction creates a sense of despair. In later years, Erikson and colleagues suggested that older adults face additional challenges or life tasks including physical and mental decline, accepting the care of others and detaching from life (Erikson, Erikson, & Kivnick, 1986). Peck (1968) expanded Erikson's definition of "integrity versus despair" to include three other challenges: creating a meaningful life after retirement, dealing with an "empty nest" as children move away, and contemplating the inevitability of death.

Erikson's theory is widely employed in the behavioral sciences. In nursing, Erikson's model is often used as a framework to examine the challenges faced by different age groups. In a study of frail elderly men and women, Neumann (2000) used Erikson's theoretical framework when asking participants to discuss their perceptions about the meaning of their lives. She found that older adults who expressed higher levels of meaning and energy described a sense of connectedness, self-worth, love, and respect that was absent among participants who felt unfulfilled. This finding is consistent with the positive or negative outcome that may result from Erikson's developmental stage, "integrity versus despair." In another study, Holm and colleagues examined the value of storytelling among dementia patients. Investigators told stories linked to Erikson's developmental stages to stimulate sharing among the participants. The authors reported that these stages were clearly evident in the experiences related by the participants (Holm, Lepp, & Ringsberg, 2005).

CLINICAL TIP

Nurses can help older adults identify meaningful experiences in their lives and thereby help prevent feelings of despair that may arise with advanced age.

Life-Course (Life Span Development) Theory

In the 1980s, behavioral psychology theorists shifted from personality development as the basis for understanding aging to the concept "life course," in which life, although unique to each individual, is divided into stages with predictable patterns (Back, 1980). Most theorists up to this point had focused primarily on childhood; for example Erikson's devotes only one of eight stages to adults over 65 years (1963). An emphasis on adulthood corresponded to an aging demographic, the emergence of gerontology as a specialty, and the availability of data from longitudinal studies that began during the 1920s and 1930s (Baltes, 1987). Life-course Theory is concerned with understanding age group norms and their characteristics.

Life-course theories encompass aspects of psychological theories such as tasks during different stages of personality development with sociological tenets regarding the interconnectedness of individuals and society. The central theme of life course is that life occurs in stages that are structured according to one's roles, relationships, internal values, and goals. Goal achievement is linked to life satisfaction but people's goals are limited by external factors. Individuals adapt to changing roles and relationships that occur throughout life, such as getting married, finishing school, completing military service, getting a job, and retiring (Cunningham & Brookbank, 1988). Successful adaptation to life changes may require revising one's beliefs to be consistent with society's expectations.

The life-course perspective remains a dominant theme in the psychology literature today. Selective optimization with compensation, discussed in the following section, is one example of a theory that emerged from the life-course perspective.

Selective Optimization with Compensation Theory

Baltes's (1987) theory of successful aging emerged from his study of psychological processes across the lifespan. He asserted that individuals learn to cope with the functional losses of aging through the processes of selection, optimization, and compensation. Aging individuals adjust activities and roles as limitations present themselves; at the same time, they choose those activities and roles that are most satisfying (optimization). Coping with illness and functional decline may lead to greater or lesser risk of mortality. Ideally, selective optimization with compensation is a positive coping process that facilitates successful aging (Baltes & Baltes, 1990).

Much of the research testing psychosocial theories centers on the more recent life-course paradigm (Baltes, 1987; Caspi, 1987; Caspi & Elder, 1986; Quick & Moen, 1998; Schroots, 2003). In an ongoing longitudinal study called "Life-Course Dynamics," Schroots' examined behavior in a longitudinal study about behavior across the life course. He observed that life structure tended to be consistent over time but influenced by life events and experiences. He further proposed that aging and development are ongoing, lifelong processes that are intertwined (Schroots, 2012). To further explain the interaction of structure and experiences, other theorists use life-course theory to explain how historical events and retirement conditions influence behavior as we age. They argued that the influence of social change on life course is intertwined with individual factors (Caspi, 1987; Quick & Moen, 1988).

Biological Theories of Aging

The biological theories explain the physiologic processes that change with aging. In other words, how is aging manifested on the molecular level in the cells, tissues, and body systems; how does the body-mind interaction affect aging; what biochemical processes impact aging; and how do one's chromosomes impact the overall aging process? Does each system age at the same rate? Does each cell in a system age at the same rate? How does chronological age influence an individual who is experiencing a pathophysiological disease process—how does the actual disease, as well as the treatment, which might include drugs, *immunomodulation*, surgery, or radiation, influence the organism? Several theories purport to explain aging at the molecular, cellular, organ, and system levels; however, no one predominant theory has evolved. Both genetics and environment influence the multifaceted phenomenon of aging.

Some aging theorists divide the biological theories into two categories:

1. A stochastic or statistical perspective, which identifies episodic events that happen throughout one's life that cause random cell damage and accumulate over time, thus causing aging.
2. The nonstochastic theories, which view aging as a series of predetermined events happening to all organisms in a timed framework.

Others believe aging is more likely the result of both programmed and stochastic concepts as well as allostasis, which is the process of achieving homeostasis via both behavioral and physiological change (Carlson & Chamberlain, 2005; Miquel, 1998). For example, there are specific programmed events in the life of a cell, but cells also accumulate genetic damage to the *mitochondria* due to free radicals and the loss of self-replication as they age. The following discussion presents descriptions of the different theories in the stochastic and nonstochastic theory categories, and also provides studies that support the various theoretical explanations.

Stochastic Theories

Studies of animals reflect that the effects of aging are primarily due to genetic defects, development, environment, and the inborn aging process (Harman, 2006; Goldsmith, 2011). There is no set of statistics to validate that these same findings are true with human organisms. The following *stochastic theories of aging* are discussed in this section: free radical theory, Orgel/error theory, wear and tear theory, and connective tissue theory.

Free Radical Theory

Oxidative free radical theory postulates that aging is due to oxidative metabolism and the effects of *free radicals*, which are the end products of oxidative metabolism. Free radicals are produced when the body uses oxygen, such as with exercise. This theory emphasizes the significance of how cells use oxygen (Hayflick, 1985). Also known as superoxides, free radicals are thought to react with proteins, lipids, deoxyribonucleic acid (DNA), and ribonucleic acid (RNA), causing cellular damage. This damage accumulates over time and is thought to accelerate aging.

Free radicals are chemical species that arise from atoms as single, unpaired electrons. Because a free radical molecule is unpaired, it is able to enter reactions with other molecules, especially along membranes and with nucleic acids. Free radicals cause:

> Extensive cellular damage to DNA, which can cause malignancy and accelerated aging due to oxidative modification of proteins that impact cell metabolism
> Lipid oxidation that damages phospholipids in cell membranes, thus affecting membrane permeability
> DNA strand breaks and base modifications that cause gene modulation

This cellular membrane damage causes other chemicals to be blocked from their regularly friendly receptor sites, thus mitigating other processes that may be crucial to cell metabolism. Mitochondrial deterioration due to oxidants causes a significant loss of cell energy and greatly decreases metabolism. Ames (2004) and Harman (1994) suggested some strategies to assist in delaying the mitochondrial decay, such as:

> Decrease calories in order to lower weight
> Maintain a diet high in nutrients, including antioxidants
> Avoid inflammation
> Minimize accumulation of metals in the body that can trigger free radical reactions

Additionally, studies have demonstrated that mitochondrially targeted antioxidant treatments may decrease the adverse effects of Parkinson's Disease, Alzheimer's disease, and cardiovascular disease (Smith & Murphy, 2011).

With the destruction of membrane integrity comes fluid and electrolyte loss or excess, depending on how the membrane was affected. Little by little there is more tissue deterioration. The older adult is more vulnerable to free radical damage because free radicals are attracted to cells that have transient or interrupted perfusion. Many older adults have decreased circulation because they have peripheral vascular, as well as coronary artery, disease. These diseases tend to cause heart failure that can be potentially worsened with fluid overload and electrolyte imbalance.

The majority of the evidence to support this theory is correlative in that oxidative damage increases with age. It is thought that people who limit calories, fat, and specific proteins in their diet may decrease the formation of free radicals. Roles of *reactive oxygen species* (ROS) are being researched in a variety of diseases such as atherosclerosis, vasospasms, cancers, trauma, stroke, asthma, arthritis, heart attack, dermatitis, retinal damage, hepatitis, and periodontitis (Gans, Putney, Bengtson, & Silverstein, 2009). Lee, Koo, and Min (2004) reported that antioxidant nutraceuticals are assisting in managing and, in some cases, delaying some of the manifestations of these diseases. Poon and colleagues described how two antioxidant systems (glutathione and heat shock proteins) are decreased in age-related degenerative neurological disorders (Poon, Calabrese, Scapagnini, & Butterfield, 2004). They also cited that free radical-mediated lipid peroxidation and protein oxidation affect central nervous system function.

Examples of some sources of free radicals are listed in **Box 3-2**. In some instances, free radicals reacting with other molecules can form more free radicals, mutations, and malignancies. The free radical theory supports that as one lives, an accumulation of damage has been done to cells and, therefore, the organism ages. Grune and Davies (2001) go so far as to describe the free radical theory of aging as "the only aging theory to have stood the test of time" (p. 41). They further described how free radicals can generate cellular debris rich in lipids and proteins called lipofuscin, which older adults have more of when compared to younger adults. It is thought that *lipofuscin*, or age pigment, is a nondegradable material that decreases lysosomal function, which in turn impacts already disabled mitochondria (Brunk & Terman, 2002). Additionally, lipofuscin is considered a threat to multiple cellular systems including the ubiquitin/proteasome pathway, which leads to cellular death (Gray & Woulfe, 2005).

Orgel/Error Theory

This theory suggests that, over time, cells accumulate errors in their DNA and RNA protein synthesis that cause the cells to die (Orgel, 1970). Environmental agents and randomly induced events can cause error, with ultimate cellular changes. It is well known that large amounts of X-ray radiation cause chromosomal abnormalities. Thus,

BOX 3-2	Exogenous Sources of Free Radicals	
Tobacco smoke	Organic solvents	Ozone
Pesticides	Radiation	Selected medications

this theory proposes that aging would not occur if destructive factors such as radiation did not exist and cause "errors" such as mutations and regulatory disorders.

Hayflick (1996) did not support this theory, and explained that all aged cells do not have errant proteins, nor are all cells found with errant proteins old.

Wear and Tear Theory

Over time, cumulative changes occurring in cells age and damage cellular metabolism. An example is the cell's inability to repair damaged DNA, as in the aging cell. It is known that cells in heart muscle, neurons, striated muscle, and the brain cannot replace themselves after they are destroyed by wear and tear. Researchers cite gender-specific effects of aging on adrenocorticotropic activity that are consistent with the wear and tear hypothesis of the ramifications of lifelong exposure to stress (Van Cauter, Leproult, & Kupfer, 1996). There is some speculation that excessive wear and tear caused by exercising may accelerate aging by increasing free radical production, which supports the idea that no one theory of aging incorporates all the causes of aging, but rather that a combination of factors is responsible.

Studies of people with osteoarthritis suggest that cartilage cells age over time, and this degeneration is not due solely to strenuous exercise but also to general wear and tear. The studies point out that aged cells have lost the ability to counteract mechanical, inflammatory, and other injuries due to their *senescence* (Aigner, Rose, Martin, & Buckwalter, 2004).

Connective Tissue Theory

This theory is also referred to as cross-link theory, and it proposes that, over time, biochemical processes create connections between structures not normally connected. Several cross-linkages occur rapidly between 30 and 50 years of age. However, no research has identified anything that could stop these cross-links from occurring. Elastin dries up and cracks with age; hence, skin with less elastin (as with the older adult) tends to be drier and wrinkled. Over time, because of decreased extracellular fluid, numerous deposits of sodium, chloride, and calcium build up in the cardiovascular system. No clinical application studies were found to support this theory.

Nonstochastic Theories

The *nonstochastic theories of aging* are founded on a programmed perspective that is related to genetics or one's biological clock. Goldsmith (2004) suggests that aging is more likely to be an evolved beneficial characteristic and results from a complex structured process and not a series of random events. The following nonstochastic theories are discussed in this section: programmed theory, gene/biological clock theory, neuroendocrine theory, and immunologic/autoimmune theory.

Programmed Theory

As people age, more of their cells start to decide to commit suicide or stop dividing. The Hayflick phenomenon, or human fibroblast replicative senescence model, suggests that cells divide until they can no longer divide, whereupon the cell's infrastructure recognizes this inability to further divide and triggers the *apoptosis* sequence or death of the cell (Gonidakis & Longo, 2009; Sozou & Kirkwood, 2001). Therefore, it is thought that cells have a finite doubling potential and become unable to replicate after they have done so a number of times. Human cells age each time they replicate because of the shortening of the telomere. *Telomeres* are the most distal appendages of the chromosome arms. This theory of programmed cell death is often alluded to when the aging process is discussed. The enzyme *telomerase*, also called a "cellular fountain of youth," allows human cells grown in the laboratory to continue to replicate long past the time they normally stop dividing. Normal human cells do not have telomerase.

It is hypothesized that some cancer, reproductive, and virus cells are not restricted, having a seemingly infinite doubling potential, and are thus immortal cell lines. This is because they have telomerase, which adds back DNA to the ends of the chromosomes. One reason for the Hayflick phenomenon may be that chromosome telomeres become reduced in length with every cell division and eventually become too short to allow further division. When telomeres are too short, the gene notes this and causes the cell to die or apoptosize. Shay and Wright (2001) suggest that telomerase-induced manipulations of telomere length are important to study to define the underlying genetic diseases and those genetic pathways that lead to cancer.

Although it is unknown what initial event triggers apoptosis, it is generally acknowledged that apoptosis is the mechanism of cell death (Thompson, 1995). Henderson (2006) reviewed how fibroblast senescence is connected to wound healing and discussed the implications of this theory for chronic wound healing. Increased cell apoptosis rates do cause organ dysfunction, and this is hypothesized to be the underlying basis of the pathophysiology of multiple organ dysfunction syndrome (MODS) (Papathanassoglou, Moynihan, & Ackerman, 2000).

Gene/Biological Clock Theory

This theory explains that each cell, or perhaps the entire organism, has a genetically programmed aging code that is stored in the organism's DNA. Slagboom and associates describe this theory as comprising genetic influences that predict physical condition, occurrence of disease, cause and age of death, and other factors that contribute to longevity (Slagboom, Bastian, Beekman, Wendendorf, & Meulenbelt, 2000).

A significant amount of research has been done on circadian rhythms and their influence on sleep, *melatonin*, and aging (Ahrendt, 2000; Moore, 1997; Richardson & Tate, 2000). These rhythms are defined as patterns of wakefulness and sleep that are integrated into the 24-hour solar day (Porth, 2009). The everyday rhythm of this cycle of sleep–wake intervals is part of a time-keeping framework created by an internal clock. Research has demonstrated that people who do not have exposure to time cues such as sunlight and clocks will automatically have sleep and wake cycles that include approximately 23.5 to 26.5 hours (Moore, Czeisler, & Richardson, 1983). This clock seems to be controlled by an area in the hypothalamus called the suprachiasmatic nucleus (SCN), which is located near the third ventricle and the optic chiasm. The SCN, given its anatomic location, does receive light and dark input from the retina, and demonstrates high neuronal firing during the day and low firing at night. The SCN is connected to the pituitary gland, explaining the diurnal regulation of growth hormone and cortisol. Also because of the linkage with the hypothalamus, autonomic nervous system, and brain stem reticular formation, diurnal changes in metabolism, body temperature, and heart rate and blood pressure are explained (Porth, 2009). It is thought that biological rhythms lose some rhythmicity with aging.

Melatonin is secreted by the pineal gland and is considered to be the hormone linked to sleep and wake cycles because there are large numbers of melatonin receptors in the SCN. Researchers have studied the administration of melatonin to humans and found a shift in humans' circadian rhythm similar to that caused by light (Ahrendt, 2000). The sleep–wake cycle changes with aging, producing more fragmented sleep, which is thought to be due to decreased levels of melatonin.

This theory indicates that there may be genes that trigger youth and general well-being as well as other genes that accelerate cell deterioration. Why do some people have gray hair in their late 20s and others live to be 60 or beyond before graying occurs? It is known that melanin is damaged with ultraviolet light and is the ingredient that keeps human skin resilient and unwrinkled. People who have extensive sun exposure have wrinkles earlier in life due to damage to collagen and elastin. But why, if we know that people have a programmed gene or genes that trigger aging, wouldn't we prevent the gene(s) from causing the problems they are intending to promote?

For example, hypertension, arthritis, hearing loss, and heart disease are among the most common chronic illnesses in older adults (Cobbs, Duthie, & Murphy, 1999). Each of these diseases has a genetic component to it. So if the healthcare profession can screen people when they are younger before they develop symptoms of target organ disease due to hypertension, loss of cartilage and hearing, and aspects of systolic and diastolic dysfunction, it is possible for people to live longer without experiencing the problems connected to these chronic illnesses.

The knowledge being acquired from the genome theory is greatly impacting the possibility of being able to ward off aging and disease. Studies of tumor suppressor gene replacement, prevention of angiogenesis with tumor growth, and regulation of programmed cell death are in process (Daniel & Smythe, 2003). Parr (1997) and Haq (2003) cited that caloric restriction extends mammalian life. By restricting calories there is a decreased need for insulin exposure, which consequently decreases growth factor exposure. Both insulin and growth factor are related to mammals' genetically determined clock, controlling their life span, so there is more evidence supportive of aging being influenced by key pathways such as the insulin-like growth factor path (Haq, 2003). More and more genetic findings are being related to aging and disease, such as the significance of the apolipoprotein E gene and correlations of more or less inflammation and DNA repair to aging (Stessman et al., 2005; Christenson, Johnson, & Vaupel, 2006).

Neuroendocrine Theory

This theory describes a change in hormone secretion, such as with the releasing hormones of the hypothalamus and the stimulating hormones of the pituitary gland, which manage the thyroid, parathyroid, and adrenal glands, and how it influences the aging process. The following major hormones are involved with aging:

> Estrogen decreases the thinning of bones, and when women age, less estrogen is produced by the ovaries. As women grow older and experience menopause, adipose tissue becomes the major source of estrogen.
> Growth hormone is part of the process that increases bone and muscle strength. Growth hormone stimulates the release of insulin-like growth factor produced by the liver.
> Melatonin is produced by the pineal gland and is thought to be responsible for coordinating seasonal adaptations in the body.

There is a higher chance of excess or loss of glucocorticoids, aldosterone, androgens, triiodothyronine, thyroxine, and parathyroid hormone when the hypothalamus-pituitary-endocrine gland feedback system is altered. When the stimulating and releasing hormones of the pituitary and the hypothalamus are out of synch with the endocrine glands, an increase in disease is expected in multiple organs and systems. Of significance are the findings of Rodenbeck and Hajak (2001), who cited that, with physiological aging and also with certain psychiatric disorders, there is increased activation of the hypothalamus-pituitary-adrenal axis, which causes increased plasma cortisol levels. The increased cortisol levels can be linked with several diseases.

Holzenberger, Kappeler, and De Magalhaes Filho (2004) stated that by inactivating insulin receptors in the adipose tissue of mice, the life span of the mice increases because less insulin exposure occurs. This further supports the idea that the neuroendocrine system is connected to life span regulation. Grossman and Porth (2014) suggest that as one ages, there is a loss of neuroendocrine transmitter function that is related to the cessation of reproductive cycles as well as the development of reproductive organ tumors. This would correspond well with Zuevo's (2015) research that the neuroendocrine system impacts aging by decreasing heart rate variability and other physiological processes that would impact the "normal" regulatory feedback mechanisms. Additionally, Takahashi and colleagues (2012) describe the concept of neuroplasticity, which refers to changes in neural connections in the brain that may increase as humans age. Thus, neurological changes occurring secondary to trauma, inflammation, and other neurological events may be reversible with the aging brain given that the brain has the ability to restructure itself.

Immunologic/Autoimmune Theory

This theory was proposed almost 50 years ago and describes the normal aging process of humans and animals as being related to faulty immunological function (Effros, 2004). There is a decreased immune function in the elderly due to the thymus gland shrinking to 15% of its capacity, altered lymphocyte function, and decreased cell mediated and humoral immune response (Grossman & Porth, 2014). The elderly are more susceptible to infections as well as cancers. There is a loss of T-cell differentiation, so the body incorrectly perceives old, irregular cells as foreign bodies and attacks them, hence, increased autoimmune disorders are diagnosed in old age.

There is also an increase in certain autoantibodies such as rheumatoid factor and a loss of interleukins. Some think that this change increases the chance of the older adult developing an autoimmune disease such as

TABLE 3-2 Biological Theories of Aging	
Theory	**Description**
Stochastic Theories	Based on random events that cause cellular damage that accumulates as the organism ages.
Free radical theory	Membranes, nucleic acids, and proteins are damaged by free radicals, which causes cellular injury and aging.
Orgel/error theory	Errors in DNA and RNA synthesis occur with aging.
Wear and tear theory	Cells wear out and cannot function with aging.
Connective tissue/cross-link theory	With aging, proteins impede metabolic processes and cause trouble with getting nutrients to cells and removing cellular waste products.
Nonstochastic Theories	Based on genetically programmed events that cause cellular damage that accelerates aging of the organism.
Programmed theory	Cells divide until they are no longer able to, and this triggers apoptosis or cell death.
Gene/biological clock theory	Cells have a genetically programmed aging code.
Neuroendocrine theory	Problems with the hypothalamus-pituitary-endocrine gland feedback system cause disease; increased insulin growth factor accelerates aging.
Immunological theory	Aging is due to faulty immunological function, which is linked to general well-being.

rheumatoid arthritis. Older adults are more prone to infection such as wound and respiratory infections, as well as to infections if they are hospitalized.

Venjatraman and Fernandes (1997) cite that active and healthy older adults who participated in endurance exercises had a significantly increased natural killer cell function that, in turn, caused increased cytokine production and enhanced T-cell function. In contrast, those not exercising see a loss of immunological function as they age. The idea that increased exercise causes new growth of muscle fibers is not new, but that it also causes an increased immunological function is significant. Also important to note is that there should be a balance of exercising and resting because overdoing exercise can lead to injuries, and this would support the wear and tear theory of aging.

Table 3-2 summarizes the major theories of aging originating from a biological perspective. It seems that no one theory fully describes the etiology of aging. Kirkwood (2000) cited the impact that single gene mutations and various environmental interventions such as diet and stress have on aging. Of all the theories discussed in this section, it appears that the gene theory and free radical theory seem to have the most support.

Implications for Nursing

Nursing has incorporated psychosocial theories such as Erikson's personality development theory into its practice (Erikson, 1963). Psychological theories enlighten us about the developmental tasks and challenges faced by older adults and the importance of finding and accepting meaning in one's life. From sociologists, nursing has learned how support systems, functionality, activity and role engagement, cohorts, and societal expectations can influence adjustment to aging and life satisfaction. Nurses can learn from these theories to help minimize the challenges of aging by connecting older adults to resources. These may include an occupational therapist that can help families adapt a home environment to that it is safe for an older adult to "age in place," suggesting visiting nurse or physical therapy visits to help manage chronic illnesses such as heart failure or diabetes, or to optimize physical functioning, or to enlist a pharmacist to evaluate how medication regimens may be causing side effects that adversely affect functioning. Dealing with loss of friends, spouse, and other important relationships can lead to isolation and depression. Connecting older adults to their communities through senior centers, online groups like "Meetup" or "Road Scholar," adult education programs, or volunteer groups can help them explore new passions and develop new relationships. Others may benefit from counseling with a mental health provider or religious leader (see **Case Study 3-1**).

Biological and psychosocial theories however, lack the specificity and holistic perspective needed to fully guide the nursing care of older adults. Nurse theorists have attempted to address this gap by building upon past theories of

Case Study 3-1

Mr. Ronald Dea, 64 years old, had been planning for many years to retire from his position as an accountant at a software company at his 65th birthday. Then his wife of 40 years died of lymphoma last year. He now finds that he only gets out of his house to work. He has let his racquetball membership, swimming club, and night out with his neighborhood friends slide. He finds he does not go out socially at all anymore except for visiting his two children and their families, who live out of town, when invited. He is no longer active in the Lions Club nor does he regularly attend his church where he and his wife used to be very involved.

Now he is deliberating whether to retire or not because he is aware that his work has become the only thing in his life. He is finding he does not have the energy he used to and that he is not excited about the weekend time he used to enjoy so much. He also has found he does not enjoy food shopping, so Mr. Dea generally buys his main meal at work and then snacks on crackers and cheese at night. He generally eats a donut or a bagel for breakfast. On the weekends, Mr. Dea stays in bed until noon and does not eat anything until night when he goes to the nearby fast food drive-in window to pick up fried chicken or has a pizza delivered.

He has not changed anything in his bedroom since his wife died nor removed any of his wife's belongings from the home. Mr. Dea has been delaying his regularly scheduled visits to his hematologist for management of his hemochromatosis. He has been gaining weight, approximately 14 pounds, since his wife was first diagnosed with cancer about 2.5 years ago. He has also started smoking a cigar just about every evening. It was after his nightly smoke, when he was walking up the hill in his backyard one evening, that he fell and fractured his hip.

Mr. Dea has just been discharged home from the rehabilitation center, and you are the visiting nurse assigned to him. He has planned judiciously for his retirement but has been afraid to prepare the paperwork. Mr. Dea confides in you that he wants to remain independent as long as possible. He shares his concerns with you and inquires what your opinion is of how he should proceed. One of his daughters is at his home for the next 2 weeks to assist him and is pushing him to retire and move in with her and her family.

Drawing from aging theory, what are some of the challenges you believe Mr. Dea is dealing with? What would you, given the knowledge you have learned regarding aging theories, recommend to Mr. Dea regarding retirement? Would you recommend he sell his house and move out of the town he has lived in for so many years? What other living arrangements might be conducive for Mr. Dea? Who would you suggest he and his daughter talk with regarding his everyday needs if he chooses to stay in his house during his convalescence? What are his priority needs for promoting his health? How would these be best managed? Use aging theory to support your responses.

aging. In a quest for a theoretical framework to guide caregiving in nursing homes, Wadensten (2002) and Wadensten and Carlsson (2003) studied 17 nursing theories that were generated from the 1960s to the 1990s and found that none of the theorists discussed what aging is, nor did the theorists offer advice on how to apply their theory to caring for older adults. Wadensten wrote that existing "nursing theories do not provide guidance on how to care for older people or on how to support them in the developmental process of aging. There is a need to develop a nursing care model that, more than contemporary theories, takes human aging into consideration" (p. 119). Others concur that nursing needed to develop more situation-specific theories of aging to guide practice (Bergland & Kirkevold, 2001; Haight et al., 2002; Miller, 1990; Putnam, 2002). Two newer theories, Functional Consequences (Miller, 1990) and the Theory of Thriving (Haight et al., 2002), are nurse-authored and attempt to address this need.

Nursing Theories of Aging

Functional Consequences Theory

Functional Consequences Theory (see **Table 3-3**) was developed to provide a guiding framework for older adults with physical impairment and disability (Miller, 1990). Miller asserted that aging adults experience environmental and biopsychosocial consequences that impact their functioning. The nurse's role is to assess age-related changes and accompanying risk factors, and to design interventions that minimize age-associated disability. The goal is to maximize functioning in ways that improve patient safety and quality of life (Miller, 1990).

Functional Consequences Theory assumes that quality of life, functional capacity and dependency are connected and that positive consequences are possible despite age-related limitations. Miller's theory (1990) applies to high as well as low functioning older adults. Her theory defines the focus of nursing interventions in varied settings (inpatient, outpatient, acute, or long-term care); thus, her theory can be used in many contexts. The interventions include other healthcare providers, older adults and significant others, so this theory is patient centered as well as interprofessional in scope. Miller's theory has been used to create an assessment tool for the early detection of hospitalized elderly patients experiencing acute confusion and to prevent further complications (Kozak-Campbell & Hughes, 1996). Additional testing is needed however to determine the utility of the functional consequences theory in other settings.

Theory of Thriving

The theory of thriving (Haight et al., 2002) was developed to explain the experience of nursing home residents. Failure to thrive first appeared in the aging literature as a diagnosis for older adults with vague symptoms such as fatigue, cachexia, and generalized weakness (Campia, Berkman, & Fulmer, 1986). Other disciplines later added malnutrition, physical and cognitive dysfunction, and depression as major attributes (Braun, Wykle, & Cowling, 1988). Newbern and Krowchuk (1994) suggested that difficulty with social relationships (disconnectedness and inability to find meaning in life, give of oneself, or attach to others) and physical/cognitive dysfunction (consistent unplanned weight loss, signs of depression, and cognitive decline) were related to a failure to thrive. Haight and colleagues (2002) proposed

TABLE 3-3	Nursing Theories of Aging
Theory	**Description**
Functional consequences theory	Environmental and biopsychosocial consequences impact functioning. Nursing's role is risk reduction to minimize age-associated disability in order to enhance safety and quality of living.
Theory of thriving	Failure to thrive results from a discord between the individual and his or her environment or relationships. Nurses identify and modify factors that contribute to disharmony among these elements.

that the environment is an important contributor to how people age. They asserted that people thrive when they are in harmony with their environment and personal relationships and fail to thrive when there is discord. This theory has helped bring together elements of earlier aging theorists in ways that make it accessible for nursing practice.

> **CLINICAL TIP**
>
> The theory of thriving in older adults living in nursing homes is often compared to failure to thrive seen in neglected infants.

Theory of Successful Aging

Twenty-first century literature has focused on what it means to age well. Flood (2006) proposed that aging well is defined by the extent to which older adults adapt to the cumulative physical and functional changes they experience. Moreover, a person's perception about how well he or she has aged is fundamentally connected to believing that one's life has meaning and purpose; thus, spirituality is a central ingredient of Floods theory. Flood proposed that:

> aging is a progressive process adaptation,
> aging may be successful or unsuccessful, depending upon a person's ability to cope,
> successful aging is influenced by a person's choices, and
> aging people experience changes, which uniquely characterize their beliefs and perspectives in ways that differ from those of younger adults (Flood, 2006).

According to this theory, aging successfully means remaining physically, psychologically, and socially engaged in meaningful ways that are individually defined. Achieving a comfortable acceptance of impending death is also a hallmark of successful aging.

Ji, Ling, and McCarthy (2014) have used Flood's Theory of Successful Aging in several studies. They concluded that transcendence or finding a sense of meaning and well-being was the main predictor of life satisfaction. Relationships, creativity, contemplation, introspection, and spirituality are all important elements of transcendence.

> **CLINICAL TIP**
>
> One theory of aging does not explain all that is observed in the aging process. This is why using a variety of theories is often preferred.

Summary

Nursing theories of thriving and functionality contribute to our understanding of aging; however, neither encompass all of the holistic elements (cultural, spiritual, geographic, psychosocioeconomic, educational, environmental, and physical) of concern to nursing. Flood's theory of successful aging provides a more comprehensive framework to guide nursing practice and has been validated by some authors; however additional studies are needed to confirm this theory.

Given the diversity of older adults living in independent, assisted, and residential care settings, much can be learned from the theories of other disciplines. From the stochastic and programmed biological theories of aging, nurses can better manage nutrition, incontinence, sleep rhythms, immunological response, catecholamine surges, hormonal and electrolyte balance, and drug efficacy for older adults with chronic illnesses. Using psychosocial aging theories, nurses can assist both the older adult and his or her family in recognizing that the life they have lived has been one of integrity and meaning and facilitate peaceful death with dignity. Ego integrity contributes to older adults' well-being and reduces the negative psychological consequences that are often linked to chronic illness and older age. Finally, being cognizant of older adults' socioeconomic resources will assist the nurse and older adult in planning cost-effective best practices to improve symptom management and treatment outcomes.

Using knowledge gained from aging theories, nurses can:

> Help people to use their genetic makeup to prevent comorbidities
> Facilitate best practices for managing chronic illnesses
> Maximize individuals' strengths relative to maintaining independence
> Facilitate creative ways to overcome individuals' challenges
> Assist in cultivating and maintaining older adults' cognitive status and mental health

In conclusion, aging has many dimensions that have been explained by multiple theoretical perspectives. Collectively, these theories reveal that aging is a complex phenomenon still in need of research. How one ages is a result of biopsychosocial factors. Nurses can use this knowledge as they plan and implement ways to promote health care to all age groups. As in other disciplines, the state of the science on aging is rapidly improving within the nursing profession. Nursing is developing a rich body of knowledge regarding the care of older adults. Programs and materials developed by the Hartford Institute for Geriatric Nursing, the End of Life Nursing Education Consortium, the American Association of Colleges of Nursing and the Mather Institute provide a strong foundation for developing and disseminating our current knowledge (see **Boxes 3-3** and **3-4**). Nursing research must continue to view aging holistically and contribute to the literature in ways that help confirm, develop or refute these theories. Ultimately theories that can predict patient outcomes hold the greatest promise for guiding nursing practice in ways that help each individual patient age successfully.

BOX 3-3　Web Exploration

End-of-Life Nursing Education Consortium
(http://www.aacn.nche.edu/elnec)

The core curriculum in end-of-life consists of nine content modules with a syllabus, objectives, student note-taking outlines, detailed faculty content outlines, slide copies, reference lists, and supplemental teaching materials.

The Geriatric Nursing Education Project
(www.aacn.nche.edu/Education/Hartford)

Offers faculty development institutes, online interactive case studies, a guide for integrating gerontology into nursing curricula, and a complimentary catalog of geriatric nursing photos that may be used free of charge for print or Web-based media by schools of nursing.

Consult GeriRN
(http://consultgerirn.org/)

An evidence-based online resource for nurses in clinical and educational settings. Includes many resources on a wide variety of topics related to aging including evidence-based geriatric protocols, hospital competencies for older adults, continuing education contact hours, the "Try This" series of assessment tools, information related to common geriatric problems, and links to additional age-related agencies and references.

The John A. Hartford Foundation Institute for Geriatric Nursing
(www.hartfordign.org)

A wealth of resources including core curriculum content for educators in academic and practice settings, consisting of detailed content outlines, case studies, activities, resources, PowerPoint slides, an online gerontological nursing certification review course, research support programs, best practice guidelines, consultation services, and geriatric nursing awards.

(continues)

BOX 3-3   Web Exploration (*continued*)

Mather LifeWays Institute on Aging
(http://www.matherlifeways.com/re
_researchandeducation.asp)

Offers programs for faculty development
(web-based), long-term care staff, and family
caregivers.

National Institute on Aging
(http://newcart.niapublications.org)

Free publications about older adults for health
professionals and patients.

**Toolkit for Nurturing Excellence at End-of-Life
Transition**
(www.tneel.uic.edu/tneel.asp)

A package for palliative care education on
CD-ROM that includes audio, video, graphics,
PowerPoint slides, photographs, and animations
of individuals and families experiencing end-of-
life transitions. An evidence-based self-study
course on palliative care will soon be available
for the national and international nursing
community.

BOX 3-4   Recommended Reading

Azinet. (2003–2014). Resources on aging
  information: How do we age? Retrieved from
  http://www.azinet.com/aging/
Bragg, E. J., Warshaw, G. A., van der Willik, O.,
  Meganathan, K., Weber, D. Cornwall, D. et al.

(2011). Paul B. Beeson career development
awards in aging research and United States
medical schools aging and geriatric medicine
programs. *Journal of American Geriatric Society*,
59(9), 1730–1738.

Clinical Reasoning Exercises

1. **Mrs. Smith, 72 years old and recently
   diagnosed with a myocardial infarction**, asks
   why she should take a cholesterol-lowering
   drug for her hyperlipidemia at her age. Why
   should she engage in the lifestyle changes
   (increased exercise, low fat & low sodium
   diet, and low stress living) her nurse is
   recommending?

2. **Your 82-year-old patient, Rodney Whitishing,
   has been healthy most of his life** and now is
   experiencing, for the second winter in a row,
   an extremely severe case of influenza. He
   has never received a flu shot as a preventive
   measure because he felt he was very strong

and healthy. Explain how you would describe
the older adult's weakened immune system
and why older adults seem to be more
vulnerable to influenza.

3. **John, an 85-year-old man with emphysema**,
   is brought to your clinic by his family because
   of increasing complaints about shortness of
   breath. John uses oxygen at home, but states
   that he is afraid to walk more than a few steps
   or show any emotion because he will become
   unable to get enough air. John tells you that
   he feels his life is not worth living. Using the
   theories of aging, how might you respond to
   this situation?

Personal Reflections

1. Develop a philosophy of how theories of aging can support or refute the idea of categorizing people in the young-old, middle-old, and old-old classifications according to chronological age. What other characteristics could be used to categorize people as they age? Give an example of how you would perceive a relative or friend of yours who is in the seventh or eighth decade of life.

2. Comparable to infant–child development stages, generate five or six stages of development for older adults to accomplish as they complete their work stage and begin their retirement era.

3. Using theories of aging with biological, psychological, and sociological perspectives, hypothesize how these frameworks influence the older adult's development.

References

Achenbaum, W. A., & Bengtson, B. L. (1994). Re-engaging the disengagement theory of aging: On the history and assessment of theory development in gerontology. *Gerontologist, 34,* 756–763.

Adams, K. B. (2004). Changing investment in activities and interests in elders' lives: Theory and measurement. *International Journal of Aging & Human Development, 58*(2), 87–108.

Agahi, N., Ahacic, K., & Parker, M. G. (2006). Continuity of leisure participation from middle age to old age. *The Journals of Gerontology, 61B*(6), S340–S346.

Ahrendt, J. (2000). Melatonin, circadian rhythms, and sleep. *New England Journal of Medicine, 343,* 1114–1115.

Aigner, T., Rose, J., Martin, J., & Buckwalter, J. (2004). Aging theories of primary osteoarthritis: From epidemiology to molecular biology. *Rejuvenation Research, 7*(2), 134–145.

Ames, B. (2004). Mitochondrial decay, a major cause of aging, can be delayed. *Journal of Alzheimer's Disease, 6*(2), 117–121.

Back, K. (1980). *Life course: Integrated theories and exemplary populations.* Boulder, CO: Westview Press.

Baltes, P. B. (1987). Theoretical propositions of life-span developmental psychology: On the dynamics between growth and decline. *Developmental Psychology, 23,* 611–626.

Baltes, P. B., & Baltes, M. M. (1990). Psychological perspectives on successful aging: The model of selective optimization with compensation. In P. B. Baltes & M. M. Baltes (Eds.), *Successful aging: Perspectives from the behavioral sciences* (pp. 1–34). New York, NY: Cambridge University Press.

Bergland, A., & Kirkevold, M. (2001). Thriving: A useful theoretical perspective to capture the experience of well-being among frail elderly in nursing homes? *Journal of Advanced Nursing, 36,*426.

Birren, J. E., & Schroots, J. J. F. (2001). History of gero-psychology. In J. E. Birren (Ed.), *Handbook of the psychology of aging* (5th ed., pp. 3–28). San Diego, CA: Academic Press.

Braun, J. V., Wykle, M. N., & Cowling, W. R. (1988). Failure to thrive in older persons: A concept derived. *Gerontologist, 28,* 809–812.

Brunk, U., & Terman, A. (2002). The mitochondrial-lysosomal axis theory of aging—Accumulation of damaged mitochondria as a result of imperfect autophagocytosis. *European Journal of Biochemistry, 269*(8), 1996–2002.

Campia, E., Berkman, B., & Fulmer, T. (1986). Failure to thrive for older adults. *Gerontologist, 26*(2), 192–197.

Carlson, E., & Chamberlain, R. (2005). Allostatic load and health disparities: A theoretical orientation. *Research in Nursing & Health, 28*(4), 306–315.

Caspi, A. (1987). Personality in the life course. *Journal of Personality and Social Psychology, 53,* 1203–1213.

Caspi, A., & Elder, G. H. (1986). Life satisfaction in old age: Linking social psychology and history. *Psychology and Aging, 1,* 18–26.

Christensen, K., Johnson, R. E. & Vaupel, J. W. (2006). The quest for genetic determinants of human longevity: Challenges and insights. *National Review of Genetics. 7,* 436–448.

Cobbs, E., Duthie, E., & Murphy, J. (Eds.). (1999). *Geriatric review syllabus: A core curriculum in geriatric medicine* (4th ed.). Dubuque, IA: Kendall/Hunt for the American Geriatric Society.

Cumming, E., & Henry, W. (1961). *Growing old.* New York, NY: Basic Books.

Cunningham, W., & Brookbank, J. (1988). *Gerontology: The physiology, biology and sociology of aging.* New York, NY: Harper & Row.

Daniel, J., & Smythe, W. (2003). Gene therapy of cancer. *Seminars of Surgical Oncology, 21*(3), 196–204.

Ebersole, P., Hess, P., & Luggen, A. S. (2004). *Toward healthy aging: Human needs and nursing response* (3rd ed.). St. Louis, MO: Mosby.

Effros, R. (2004). From Hayflick to Walford: The role of T cell replicative senescence in human aging. *Experimental Gerontology, 39*(6), 885–890.

Efklides, A., Kalaitzidou, M., & Chankin, G. (2003). Subjective quality of life in old age in Greece: The effect of demographic factors, emotional state, and adaptation to aging. *European Psychologist, 8,* 178–191.

Erikson, E. (1963). *Childhood and society.* New York, NY: W. W. Norton.

Erikson, E. H., Erikson, J. M., & Kivnick, H. Q. (1986). *Vital involvement in old age: The experience of old age in our time.* New York, NY: W. W. Norton.

Flood, M. (2006). A mid-range theory of successful aging. *Journal of Theory Construction and Testing, 9*(2), 35–39.

Gans, D., Putney, N. M., Bengtson, V. L., & Silverstein, M. (2009). The future of theories of aging. In V. Bengtson, M. Silverstein, N. Putney, & D. Gans (Eds.), *Handbook of theories of aging* (pp. 723–738). New York, NY: Springer,

Goldsmith, T. (2004). Aging as an evolved characteristic—Weismann's theory reconsidered. *Medical Hypotheses, 62*(2), 304–308.

Goldsmith, T. C. (2011). *Theories of aging and implications for public health.* Crownsville, MD: Azinet.

Gonidakis, S., & Longo, V. D. (2009). Programmed longevity and programmed aging theories. In V. Bengtson, M. Silverstein, N. Putney, & D. Gans (Eds.), *Handbook of theories of aging* (pp. 215–228). New York, NY: Springer.

Gray, D., & Woulfe, J. (2005). Lipofuscin and aging: A matter of toxic waste. *Science of Aging Knowledge Environment, 5,* 1.

Grossman, S. & Porth, C. (2014). *Porth's pathophysiology: Concepts of altered health states* (9th ed.). Philadelphia, PA: Wolters Kluwer Lippincott Williams & Wilkins.

Grune, T., & Davies, K. (2001). Oxidative processes in aging. In E. Masoro & S. Austad (Eds.), *Handbook of the biology of aging* (5th ed., pp. 25–58). San Diego, CA: Academic Press.

Hagestad, G. O., & Dannefer, D. (2002). Concepts and theories of aging: Beyond microfication in social sciences approaches. In R. H. Binstock & L. K. George (Eds.), *Handbook of aging and the social sciences* (5th ed., pp. 3–21). San Diego: Academic Press.

Haight, B. K., Barba, B. E., Tesh, A. S., & Courts, N. F. (2002). Thriving: A life span theory. *Journal of Gerontological Nursing, 28*(3), 14–22.

Haq, R. (2003). Age-old theories die hard. *Clinical Investigative Medicine, 26*(3), 116–120.

Harlow, R. E., & Cantor, N. (1996). Still participating after all these years: A study of life task participation in later life. *Journal of Personality and Social Psychology, 71,* 1235–1249.

Harman, D. (1994). Aging: Prospects for further increases in the functional life-span. *Age, 17*(4), 119–146.

Harman, D. (2006). Understanding and modulating aging: An update. *Annals of the New York Academy of Sciences, 1067,* 10–21.

Havighurst, R. (1972). *Developmental tasks and education.* New York, NY: David McKay.

Havighurst, R. J., & Albrecht, R. (1953). *Older people.* Oxford, England: Longmans, Green.

Havighurst, R. J., Neugarten, B. L., & Tobin, S. S. (1963). Disengagement, personality and life satisfaction in the later years. In P. Hansen (Ed.), *Age with a future* (pp. 419–425). Copenhagen, Denmark: Munksgoasrd.

Havighurst, R. J., Neugarten, B. L., & Tobin, S. S. (1968). Disengagement and patterns of aging. In B. L. Neugarten (Ed.), *Middle age and aging* (pp. 67–71). Chicago, IL: University of Chicago Press.

Hayflick, L. (1985). Theories of biologic aging. *Experimental Gerontology, 10,* 145–159.

Hayflick, L. (1996). *How and why we age.* New York, NY: Ballantine Books.

Henderson, E. (2006). The potential effect of fibroblast senescence on wound healing and the chronic wound environment. *Journal of Wound Care, 15*(7), 315–318.

Holm, A. K., Lepp, M., & Ringsberg, K. C. (2005). Dementia: Involving patients in storytelling—A caring intervention. A pilot study. *Journal of Clinical Nursing, 14*(2), 256–263.

Holzenberger, M., Kappeler, L., & De Magalhaes Filho, C. (2004). IGF-1 signaling and aging. *Experimental Gerontology, 39*(11–12), 1761–1764.

Ji, H., Ling, J., & McCarthy, V. L. (2014). Successful aging in the United States and China: A theoretical basis to guide nursing research, practice, and policy. *Journal of Transcultural Nursing.* doi:10.1177/1043659614526257

Jones, G. M., & Miesen, B. L. (Eds.). (1992). *Care-giving in dementia: Research and applications.* New York, NY: Tavistock/Routledge.

Jung, C. G. (1960). *The structure and dynamics of the psyche. Collected works (Vol. VIII).* Oxford, England: Pantheon.

Kirkwood, T. (2000). Molecular gerontology: Bridging the simple and complex. *Annals of the New York Academy of Sciences, 908,* 14–20.

Kozak-Campbell, C., & Hughes, A. M. (1996). The use of functional consequences theory in acutely confused hospitalized elderly. *Journal of Gerontological Nursing, 22*(1), 27–36.

Lawton, M. P. (1982). Competence, environmental press, and the adaptation of older people. In M. P. Lawton, P. G. Windley, & T. O. Byerts (Eds.), *Aging and the environment: Theoretical approaches* (pp. 33–59). New York, NY: Springer.

Lee, J., Koo, N., & Min, D. (2004). Reactive oxygen species, aging, and antioxidative nutraceuticals. *Comprehensive Reviews in Food Science and Food Safety, 3*(1), 21–33.

Lemon, B. W., Bengston, V. L., & Peterson, J. A. (1972). An exploration of the activity theory of aging: Activity types and life satisfaction among in-movers to a retirement community. *Journal of Gerontology, 27,* 511–523.

Longino, C. F., & Kart, C. S. (1982). Explicating activity theory: A formal replication. *Journal of Gerontology, 35,* 713–722.

Maddox, G. L. (1963). Activity and morale: A longitudinal study of selected elderly subjects. *Social Forces, 42,* 195–204.

Marshall, V. W. (1996). The stage of theory in aging and the social sciences. In R. H. Binstock & L. K. George (Eds.), *Handbook of aging and the social sciences* (4th ed., pp. 12–26). San Diego, CA: Academic Press.

Maslow, A. H. (1954). *Motivation and personality.* New York, NY: Harper & Row.

McMullin, J. A. (2000). Diversity and the state of sociological aging theory. *Gerontologist, 40,* 517–530.

Miller, C. A. (1990). *Nursing care of older adults: Theory and practice.* Glenview, IL: Scott, Foresman/Little, Brown Higher Education.

Miquel, J. (1998). An update on the oxygen stress-mitochondrial mutation theory of aging: Genetic and evolutionary implications. *Experimental Gerontology, 33*(1–2), 113–126.

Moore, M., Czeisler, C., & Richardson, G. (1983). Circadian time-keeping in health and disease. *New England Journal of Medicine, 309,* 469–473.

Moore, R. (1997). Circadian rhythms: Basic neurobiology and clinical application. *Annual Review of Medicine, 48,* 253–266.

Neugarten, B. L. (1968). Adult personality: Toward a psychology of the life cycle. In B. L. Neugarten (Ed.), *Middle age and aging: A reader in social psychology* (pp. 137–147). Chicago, IL: University of Chicago Press.

Neumann, C. V. (2000). *Sources of meaning and energy in the chronically ill frail elder.* Unpublished paper prepared for the Ronald E. Mcnair Research Program, University of Wisconsin-Milwaukee.

Newbern, V. B., & Krowchuk, H. V. (1994). Failure to thrive in elderly people: A conceptual analysis. *Journal of Advanced Nursing, 19,* 840–849.

O'Connor, B. P., & Vallerand, R. J. (1994). Motivation, self-determination, and person-environment fit as predictors of psychological adjustment among nursing home residents. *Psychology and Aging 9*(2), 189–194.

Orgel, L. (1970). The maintenance of the accuracy of protein synthesis and its relevance to aging: A correction. *Proceedings of the National Academy of Sciences, 67,* 1476.

Papathanassoglou, E., Moynihan, J., & Ackerman, M. (2000). Does programmed cell death (apoptosis) play a role in the development of multiple organ dysfunction in critically ill patients? A review and a theoretical framework. *Critical Care Medicine, 28*(2), 537–549.

Parr, T. (1997). Insulin exposure and aging theory. *Gerontology, 43*(3), 182–200.

Peck, R. C. (1968). Psychological development in the second half of life. In B. L. Neugarten (Ed.), *Middle age and aging: A reader in social psychology* (pp. 88–92). Chicago, IL: University of Chicago Press.

Poon, H., Calabrese, V., Scapagnini, G., & Butterfield, D. (2004). Free radicals in brain aging. *Clinics in Geriatric Medicine, 20*(2), 329–359.

Porth, C. (2009). Pathophysiology: *Concepts of altered health states* (8th ed.). Philadelphia, PA: Lippincott Williams & Wilkins.

Putnam, M. (2002). Linking aging theory and disability models: Increasing the potential to explore aging with physical impairment. *Gerontologist, 42,* 799–806.

Quick, H. E., & Moen, P. (1998). Gender, employment, and retirement quality: A life course approach to the differential experiences of men and women. *Journal of Occupational Health Psychology, 3,* 44–64.

Rapkin, B. D., & Fischer, K. (1992). Personal goals of older adults: Issues in assessment and prediction. *Psychology and Aging, 7,* 127–137.

Richardson, G., & Tate, B. (2000). Hormonal and pharmacological manipulation of the circadian clock: Recent developments and future strategies. *Sleep, 23*(Suppl. 3), S77–S88.

Riley, M. W. (1994). Age integration and the lives of older people. *Gerontologist, 34,* 110–115.

Riley, M. W., Johnson, M., & Foner, A. (1972). *Aging and society: A sociology of age stratification (Vol. 3).* New York, NY: Russell Sage Foundation.

Robitaille, A., Orpana, H., & McIntosh, C. N. (2012). Reciprocal relationship between social support and psychological distress among a national sample of older adults: An autoregressive cross-lagged model. *Canadian Journal on Aging—La Revue Canadienne Du Vieillissement, 31*(1), 13.

Rodenbeck, A., & Hajak, G. (2001). Neuroendocrine dysregulation in primary insomnia. *Reviews of Neurology, 157*(11 Pt 2), S57–S61.

Rose, A. M. (1965). The subculture of the aging: A framework for research in social gerontology. In A. M. Rose & W. Peterson (Eds.), *Older people and their social worlds* (pp. 3–16). Philadelphia, PA: F. A. Davis.

Schroots, J. J. F. (1996). Theoretical developments in the psychology of aging. *Gerontologist, 36,* 742–748.

Schroots, J. J. F. (2003). Life-course dynamics: A research program in progress from the Netherlands. *European Psychologist, 8,* 192–199.

Schroots, J. J. F. (2012) On the dynamics of active aging. *Current Gerontology and Geriatrics Research,* Retrieved from http://dx.doi.org/10.1155/2012/818564

Shay, J., & Wright, W. (2001). Telomeres and telomerase: Implications for cancer and aging. *Radiation Research, 155*(1), 188–193.

Slagboom, P., Bastian, T., Beekman, M., Wendendorf, R., & Meulenbelt, I. (2000). Genetics of human aging. *Annals of the New York Academy of Science, 908,* 50–61.

Smith, R. A. & Murphy, M. P. (2011). Mitochondria-targeted antioxidants as therapies. *Discovery Medicine, 11*(57), 106–114.

Sozou, P., & Kirkwood, T. (2001). A stochastic model of cell replicative senescence based on telomere shortening, oxidative stress, and somatic mutations in nuclear and mitochondrial DNA. *Journal of Theoretical Biology, 213*(4), 573–586.

Stessman, J., Maaravi, Y., Hammerman-Rozenberg, R., Cohen, A., Nemanov, L., . . . Ebstein, R. P. (2005). Candidate genes associated with ageing and life expectancy in the Jerusalem longitudinal study. *Mechanisms of Ageing Development. 126*, 333–339.

Takahashi, A. C., Porta, A., Melo, R. C., Quitério, R. J., da Silva, E., Borghi-Silva, A., . . . Catai, A. M. (2012). Aging reduces complexity of heart rate variability assessed by conditional entropy and symbolic analysis. *Journal of Internal and Emergency Medicine. 7*, 229–235.

Thompson, C. (1995). Apoptosis in the pathogenesis and treatment of disease. *Science, 267*, 1456–1462.

Troll, L. E. & Skaff, M. M. (1997). Perceived continuity of self in very old age. *Psychology and Aging, 12*(1), 162–169. doi:10.1037/0882-7974.12.1.162

Tornstam, L. (1994). Gerotranscendence: A theoretical and empirical exploration. In L. E. Thomas & S. A. Eisenhandler (Eds.), *Aging and the religious dimension* (pp. 203–226). Westport, CT: Greenwood.

Uhlenberg, P. (1992). Population aging and social policy. *Annual Review of Sociology, 18*, 449–474.

Uhlenberg, P. (1996). The burden of aging: A theoretical framework for understanding the shifting balance of care giving and care receiving as cohorts age. *Gerontologist, 36*, 761–767.

Uhlenberg, P. (2000). Why study age integration? *Gerontologist, 40*, 261–266.

Van Cauter, E., Leproult, R., & Kupfer, D. (1996). Effects of gender and age on the levels and circadian rhythmicity of plasma cortisol. *Journal of Clinical Endocrinology Metabolism, 81*(7), 2468–2473.

Venjatraman, F., & Fernandes, G. (1997). Exercise, immunity and aging. *Aging, 9*(1–2), 42–56.

Wadensten, B. (2002). *Gerotranscendence from a nursing perspective: From theory to implementation.* Uppsala University. Retrieved from http://www.samfak.uu.se/Disputationer/Wadensten.htm

Wadensten, B., & Carlsson, M. (2003). Nursing theory views on how to support the process of ageing. *Journal of Advanced Nursing, 42*(2), 118–124.

Wahl, H. W. (2001). Environmental influences on aging and behavior. In J. E. Birren & K. W. Schaie (Eds.), *Handbook of the psychology of aging* (5th ed., pp. 215–237). San Diego, CA: Academic Press.

Yin, P., & Lai, K. H. (1983). A reconceptualization of age stratification in China. *Journal of Gerontology, 38*, 608–613.

Zuevo, M.V. (2015). Fractality of sensations and the brain health: The theory linking neurodegenerative disorders with distortion of spatial and temporal scale invariance supports and fractal complexity of visible world. *Frontiers in Aging Neuroscience, 7*(135), 1–24.

For a full suite of assignments and additional learning activities, see the access code at the front of your book.

CHAPTER 4

Review of the Aging of Physiological Systems

Janice Heineman
Jennifer Hamrick-King
Beth Scaglione Sewell

(Competencies 9, 19)

LEARNING OBJECTIVES

At the end of this chapter, the reader will be able to:

> Describe the aging process of each physiological system.
> Distinguish between intrinsic aging and age-related disease.
> Describe how the aging process of each physiological system correlates with the functional ability of the older adult.
> Explain how the aging process of one system interacts with and/or affects other physiological systems.
> Acknowledge that not every aspect of every physiological system changes with age.
> Recognize that aging changes are partially dependent upon an individual's health behaviors and preventive health measures.

KEY TERMS

Alpha-adrenoceptors	Andropause
Acquired immunity	Anemia
Actin	Anorexia of aging
Adrenal cortex	Antibodies
Adrenal glands	Antigen
Adrenal medulla	Apoptosis
Adrenocorticotropic hormone	Arteries
Aldosterone	Atria
Alveoli	Autoimmunity
Amino acid neurotransmitters	Autonomic nervous system

B cells

Beta-adrenoceptors

Baroreceptors

Baroreflex

Basic multicellular units

Calcitonin

Cancer

Cardiac output

Cartilaginous joints

Catecholamines

CD34$^+$ cells

Cell-mediated immunity

Chemoreceptors

Cholinergic neurons

Chronological aging

Clonal expansion

Colon

Complement system

Cortical bone

Corticotropin-releasing hormone

Cortisol

Cytokines

Dehydroepiandrosterone

Dermis

Detrusor

Diaphragm

Diastole

Dopaminergic system

Elastic recoil

Epidermis

Epinephrine

Erythrocytes

Esophagus

Extrinsic aging

Fast-twitch fibers

Follicle-stimulating hormone

Forced expiratory volume

Free radical

Gallbladder

Gastrointestinal immunity

Glomerular filtration rate

Glomeruli

Glucagon

Glucocorticoids

Glucose tolerance

GLUT4

Gonadotropin-releasing hormone

Growth hormone

Hematopoiesis

Homeostasis

Hormones

Humoral immunity

Hypogeusia

Hypophysiotropic

Hypothalamic-pituitary-adrenal (HPA) axis

Immovable joints

Immunosenescence

Inflammatory response

Inhibin B

Innate immunity

Insulin

Insulin resistance

Islets of Langerhans

Keratinocytes

Killer T cells

Langerhans cells

Leukocytes

Lipofuscin

Liver

Luteinizing hormone

Macrophages

Mechanoreceptors

Melanin

Melanocytes

Melatonin

Menopause

Mineralocorticoids

Monoaminergic system

Motor unit	Reproductive axis
Muscle quality	Sarcomeres
Muscle strength	Sarcopenia
Myocardial cells	Sarcoplasmic reticulum
Myofibrils	Skeletal muscles
Myosin	Slow-twitch fibers
Natural killer (NK) cells	Somatic
Nephrons	Stem cell progenitors
Nerve cells	Subcutaneous layer
Neurogenesis	Suppressor T cells
Neurotransmitter	Synapses
Nocturia	Synaptogenesis
Norepinephrine	Synovial fluid
Olfaction	Synovial joint
Osteoblasts	Synovium
Osteoclasts	Systole
Osteocytes	T cells
Pain	Tangles
Pancreas	T-helper cells
Parathyroid gland	Thrombocytes
Parathyroid hormone	Thyroid
Pathophysiology	Thyroid-stimulating hormone
Pharynx	Thyroxine
Photoaging	Total lung capacity
Pineal gland	Trabecular bone
Plaques	Triiodothyronine
Plasma cells	Ureters
Plasticity	Urethra
Pluripotent stem cells	Vasopressin
Presbycusis	Ventilatory rate
Presbyopia	Ventricles
Replicative senescence	Vital capacity

Without the physiological changes of aging, we might never say that a person ages. The general population's concept of aging is generally, and almost instinctively, characterized by changes in physical appearance, functional decline, and chronic disease. All of these characteristics are the result of physiological change. Even the psychological and social changes associated with aging, such as depression and social withdrawal, are often rooted in changes in the structure and function of the body's physiological systems. Thus, it could be argued that the physiology of aging is true aging.

Aging processes that occur in one physiological system can directly or indirectly influence other physiological systems. Thus, although it is relatively easy to focus on changes in only one physiological system, a broader scope is necessary to truly understand the influences and consequences of aging on physiological structure and function. This is especially true given that people are now living longer and for longer periods of time in the stage of life that is currently considered to be old age. Although each cohort ages differently, general aging changes tend to remain stable. In this chapter we will review the aging process of each of the body's major physiological systems. We ask, however, that the reader remain mindful that physiological aging is an extremely individual process and that how the body ages is greatly affected by a person's genetic makeup, health behaviors, and availability of resources.

The Cardiovascular System

The cardiovascular system consists of the heart, associated vasculature, and blood. The heart and vasculature deliver the blood to every organ system in the body, maintaining oxygen levels, supplying nutrients, and carrying toxins away to be filtered by the spleen and liver. The structural and functional abilities of the cardiovascular system are crucial to sustaining the human body. Age-related changes to the cardiovascular structure and function will be evaluated in this section.

Overview of the Cardiovascular Structure and Function

The heart contains four chambers, consisting of the two upper atria and the two lower ventricles (Digiovanna, 2000). Blood from the venous system enters the two *atria*. Oxygen-rich blood from the lungs enters the left atrium, proceeds to the left *ventricles*, and is expelled into the aorta for delivery to the entire body, excluding the lungs. Oxygen-poor blood returns from the body's venous system to the right atrium. The right ventricle expels oxygen-poor blood into pulmonary arteries that carry the blood to the lungs for reoxygenation (Digiovanna, 2000; Moore, Mangoni, Lyons, & Jackson, 2003). When ventricles contract during *systole* or peak blood pressure, blood fills the arteries. Once the ventricles relax during *diastole*, or low pressure, blood is propelled into the capillaries (Digiovanna, 2000; Moore et al., 2003; Pugh & Wei, 2001).

Larger *arteries* are associated with the structure and function of the heart, whereas smaller arteries and arterioles are associated with systemic structure and function. The arterial system as a whole is responsible for the qualities of pressure and resistance that are characteristic of the cardiovascular system (Moore et al., 2003). The veins carry over half of the total blood in the cardiovascular system and are associated with the qualities of volume and conformity (Moore et al., 2003). **Figure 4-1** illustrates the arterial and venous systems within the body and organ systems, and **Figure 4-2** demonstrates the structural overview of the heart and the path of blood flow into and out of the heart.

The main function of the cardiovascular system is to maintain homeostasis by transferring oxygen, nutrients, and hormones to other organ systems. The cardiovascular system also provides defense mechanisms through white blood cells (WBCs). In addition, this physiological system regulates body temperature and contributes to acid–base balance within the range of pH 7.35 to 7.45 (Digiovanna, 2000). **Figure 4-3** illustrates the pathway of oxygen-rich and oxygen-depleted blood circulation to corresponding organs and body areas.

Aging Changes in Cardiovascular Structure

Cardiac Aging

Enlargement of heart chambers and coronary cells occurs with age, as does increased thickening of heart walls, especially in the left ventricle (Maruyama, 2012; Priebe, 2000; Pugh & Wei, 2001). This enlargement and thickening cause a decline in ventricle flexibility (Pugh & Wei, 2001) and an overall increase in heart weight of about

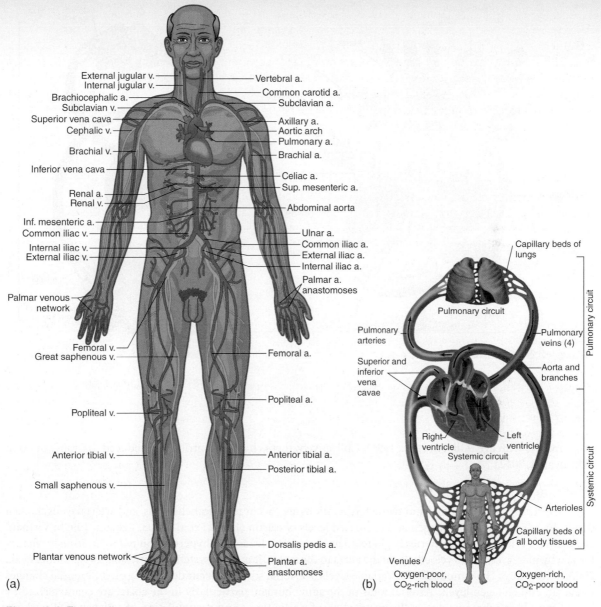

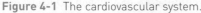

Figure 4-1 The cardiovascular system.

1.5 grams/year in women and 1.0 gram/year in men, measured from age 30 to age 90 years (Ferrari, Radaelli, & Centola, 2003; Lakatta, 1996). Ventricles in the heart also begin to thicken and stiffen in correlation with continued steady production of collagen. In addition, there is a decline in the number of *myocardial cells* and a subsequent enlargement of the remaining cells (Ferrari et al., 2003; Olivetti, Melessari, Capasso, & Anversa, 1991; Pugh & Wei, 2001). Early studies found that the total number of myocardial cells declines by approximately 40–50% between the ages of 20 and 90, but more recent investigations have concluded that women maintain myocardial

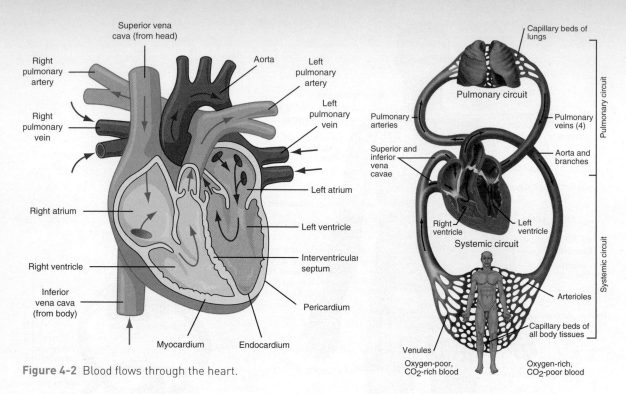

Figure 4-2 Blood flows through the heart.

Figure 4-3 The circulatory system.

cell numbers with age (Olivetti et al., 1991). Collectively, these changes contribute to reduced diastolic function (Maruyama, 2012)

Vascular Aging

Aged arteries become extended and twisted. Alterations also occur in endothelial cells, and arterial walls thicken due to increased levels of collagen and decreased levels of elastin (Ferrari et al., 2003; Lakatta, 1999b; Virmani et al., 1991). With age, large arteries begin to dilate and stiffen, leading to hypertension *pathophysiology* characterized by increased blood velocity from the aorta to the systemic arterial system (Maruyama, 2012; Moore et al., 2003; O'Rourke & Hashimoto, 2007). Variable levels of arterial stiffness occur depending on differential changes in elastin and collagen levels. Arterial walls of the aging human, particularly in the aorta, are characterized by loss of muscle attachments due to disorganization of elastic tissue and accumulation of collagen (O'Rourke & Hashimoto, 2007). The level of arterial stiffness also depends on whether the affected arteries are central elastic arteries or peripheral muscular arteries (Pugh & Wei, 2001; Robert, 1999). Peripheral arteries can show increased stiffness due to accumulating mineral (calcium), lipid, and collagen residues (Lakatta, 1993a; Richardson, 1994; Robert, 1999). Whereas arteries stiffen due to alterations in elastin and collagen, arterioles undergo atrophy, affecting their ability to expand with pressure alterations (Richardson, 1994).

Although the aorta and other arteries begin to stiffen with age, the left ventricle pumps the same amount of blood. This combination of arterial stiffening and stable blood flow results in increased wave velocity of blood traveling toward the arterial system and increased pressure in late systole (Carroll, Shroff, Wirth, Halsted, &

Rajfer, 1991; Lakatta, 1993a; Maruyama, 2012; O'Rourke & Hashimoto, 2007; Schulman, 1999). The aorta and proximal elastic arteries are able to stretch by 10% during systole in youth; however, this dilation is reduced to 2–3% in aged subjects (O'Rourke & Hashimoto, 2007). The flexibility of the aorta remains greater in women than in men until menopause, at which time aortic flexibility declines. However, estrogen replacement recovers some of the lost aortic expandability (Hayward, Kelly, & Collins, 2000; Rajkumar et al., 1997).

Overall vascular tone tends to decline with age due to deterioration in endothelium regulation of vascular relaxation (Pugh & Wei, 2001; Quyyumi, 1998). All four cardiac valves increase in circumference in older adults, with the greatest increase occurring in the aortic valve. In addition, calcium deposits accrue in the valves and may lead to stenosis (Pugh & Wei, 2001; Roffe, 1998; Tresch & Jamali, 1998).

In the cardiac conduction system, the sinoatrial (SA) node demonstrates some fibrosis as well as loss of pacemaker cells, down to approximately 10% of those observed at age 20 (Lakatta, 1993a; Wei, 1992). Also with age, the atroventricular (AV) node may be affected by nearby calcification of cardiac muscle (Pugh & Wei, 2001). In contrast to those of the arterial system, age-related changes to the venous system have not been well described in the literature (Moore et al., 2003). **Table 4-1** summarizes cardiovascular age-related structural changes.

Cardiovascular Aging Mechanisms

Finding the mechanism responsible for the aging of the cardiovascular system could lead to interventions and therapies aimed at reducing the age-associated physiological factors that alter cardiovascular structure and functioning. Some potential mechanisms include free radicals, apoptosis, inflammatory processes, advanced glycation end products, and gene expression (Pugh & Wei, 2001; Nilsson, 2012). Free radicals have been implicated in the overall aging process of the body, as described in Chapter 3 and also mentioned later in this chapter under "The Aging Brain." The presence of *lipofuscin*, a brown pigment found in aging cells, relates to oxidative mechanisms. In combination with mitochondrial dysfunction, lipofuscin may result in the increased production of free radicals (Roffe, 1998; Wei, 1992).

Increased levels of free radicals can foster *apoptosis*, or cell death. Due to the very limited regenerative properties of cardiomyocytes, or heart cells, apoptosis can have detrimental effects on cardiovascular structure and functioning (Pugh & Wei, 2001). The proposed triggers for induction of apoptosis include elevated levels of noradrenaline and initiation of the renin-angiotensin system with age (Sabbah, 2000). Another possible trigger for apoptosis is gene expression, which causes changes in the messenger RNA (mRNA) associated with

TABLE 4-1   Summarization of Cardiovascular Structural and Functional Changes That Occur with Age

Type of change	Change with age
Structural	Decreased myocardial cells, decreased aortic distensibility, decreased vascular tone Increased heart weight, increased myocardial cell size, increased left ventricle wall thickness, increased artery stiffness, increased elastin levels, increased collagen levels, increased left atrium size
Functional	Decreased diastolic pressure (during initial filling), decreased diastolic filling, decreased reaction to beta-adrenergic stimulus Increased systolic pressure, increased arterial pressure, increased wave velocity, increased left ventricular end-diastolic pressure, elongation of muscle contraction phase, elongation of muscle relaxation phase, elongation of ventricle relaxation
No change	Ejection fraction, stroke volume, overall systolic function

the *sarcoplasmic reticulum* and the related enzyme ATPase (Lakatta, 1993a). These mRNA changes lead to both qualitative and quantitative alterations in the sarcoplasmic reticulum and ATPase. These alterations, in turn, lead to functional changes in relaxation of the heart and diastolic filling (Lakatta, 1993a; Lompre, 1998; Pugh & Wei, 2001). Aging mechanisms associated with the heart continue to be researched in depth, hopefully leading to new insights in the near future.

Aging Changes in Cardiovascular Function

Cardiac Aging

According to several studies, the ability of the heart to exert force or to contract does not change with age (Colcombe et al. 2004; Gerstenblith et al., 1977; Maruyama, 2012; Rodeheffer et al., 1984). At rest, the aging heart adapts and maintains necessary functioning quite efficiently (Pugh & Wei, 2001). Although the ability of the cardiac muscle to exert force does not change with age, the actual muscle contraction as well as the relaxation phase does elongate (Lakatta, 1993a; Lakatta, Gerstenblith, Angell, Shock, & Weisfeldt, 1975; Roffe, 1998; Schulman, 1999). The prolonged contraction and relaxation phases with age correlate with extended release of calcium as well as decline in calcium reuptake (Roffe, 1998).

Ventricles also experience prolonged relaxation due to age-related declines in the sarcoplasmic reticulum pump and the associated enzyme ATPase, which produces energy for the cardiovascular system (Lompre, 1998; Pugh & Wei, 2001). The left atrium in the heart enlarges, contributing to functional changes in its filling. Furthermore, research has demonstrated that increased arterial stiffness along with the extended relaxation period leads to increased left ventricular end-diastolic pressure. This is demonstrated by a decline in pressure at the beginning of diastolic filling and an increase in pressure during late diastolic filling (Kane, Ouslander, Abrass, & Resnick, 2013; Lakatta, 1993a; Miller et al., 1986; Pugh & Wei, 2001; Roffe, 1998). With age, diastolic filling declines at a rate of approximately 6–7% each decade both during exercise and at rest, but diastolic heart failure rarely occurs (Schulman, 1999). Increased pressure during ventricular systole due to increased aortic stiffening has been correlated with left ventricle hypertrophy (O'Rourke & Hashimoto, 2007). In turn, increased left ventricle mass has been correlated with age-related declines in initial diastolic filling (Salmasi, Alimo, Jepson, & Dancy, 2003). The increase in left ventricular mass correlates with increased total blood flow and elevated systolic blood pressure (Maruyama, 2012). Although no age-related change occurs in ejection fracture or stroke volume (Ferrari et al., 2003; Gerstenblith et al., 1977; Rodeheffer et al., 1984), the increase in left ventricular mass and concomitant increase in left ventricle oxygen requirements predisposes the development of left ventricular failure (Levy, Larsen, Vasan, Kannel, & Ho, 1996).

Vascular Aging

Aging does not appear to change the overall maximum capacity, maximum vasodilation, or perfusion of coronary vessels (Maruyama, 2012). However, resistance increases with age in the aorta, arterial wall, and vascular periphery. In addition, blood viscosity increases between the ages of 20 and 70 years (Lakatta & Levy, 2003; Morley & Reese, 1989). Cardiovascular symptoms of hypertension parallel the usual aging changes seen in older adults. Such symptoms, however, are exhibited at younger ages as well and are sometimes exaggerated. These differences have led to use of the term *muted hypertension* to describe cardiovascular aging changes (Lakatta, 1999b). Other changes such as moderate accumulation of cardiac amyloid and lipofuscin do not appear to alter functional abilities, but they are present in approximately half of individuals over age 70, and elevated levels could produce degenerative changes (Pugh & Wei, 2001). Small arteries (< 400 mm), arterioles (< 100 mm), and the capillaries comprise the microcirculation. Specific structural changes of the microcirculation are generally unnotable with aging (O'Rourke & Hashimoto, 2007). No age-related changes occur in blood–tissue exchange via the capillaries, suggesting a possible compensatory mechanism such as capillary thickening (Richardson, 1994).

Autonomic Nervous System Aging Effects

A few of the age-related changes in the cardiovascular system occur due to the autonomic nervous system. Orthostatic hypotension has a prevalence as high as 30% in individuals over 75 years of age (Gupta & Lipsitz, 2007). Changes related to orthostatic hypotension include decreased reaction of the entire system, both myocardial and vascular, to beta-adrenergic stimulus as well as reduced *baroreflex* activity relating to an imbalance in neuroendocrine control (Lakatta, 1999b; Maruyama, 2012; Phillips, Hodsman, & Johnston, 1991; Pugh & Wei, 2001). *Norepinephrine* concentrations increase with age, causing overactivation of the sympathetic nervous system. This overactivation subsequently leads to overstimulation of *beta-adrenoceptors*, even to the point of desensitization (Esler et al., 1995; Lakatta, 1993a, 1999a; Moore et al., 2003). With usual functional abilities, however, stimulation of the beta-adrenoceptors triggers vessel dilation. In contrast, *alpha-adrenoceptors* that control vessel constriction remain stable with age (Maruyama, 2012; Priebe, 2000). Reduced arterial baroreflex activity, which controls peripheral vessels, has been correlated with several changes, including arterial stiffening, neural modifications, and decreased stimulation of *baroreceptors* (Hunt, Farquar, & Taylor, 2001). These changes in baroreflex activity can lead to impaired sympathetic nerve response and resistance in peripheral vessels. As a result, blood pressure becomes unstable and hypotension may result (Ferrari et al., 2003). Table 4-1 summarizes age-associated changes in the functional abilities of the cardiovascular system.

Exercise and Aging

When older adults exercise, the cardiovascular response is different from the response of younger individuals. Cardiovascular condition during exercise is usually measured using maximum oxygen consumption (VO_{2max}), which equals the sum of cardiac output and systemic oxygen reserve. VO_{2max} shows age-related declines of around 10% per decade beginning in the second decade of life and reductions of around 50% by age 80 (Aronow, 1998; Maharam, Bauman, Kalman, Skolnick, & Perle, 1999). Furthermore, declines are accelerated as aging progresses, from 3% to 6% per decade in the 20s and 30s to more than 20% per decade in the 70s and beyond (Bearden, 2006; Fleg et al., 2005). Cardiovascular reserve is best measured using maximum *cardiac output*, which is equal to heart rate multiplied by stroke volume during exercise (Fleg, 1986). With age, the increased heart rate and contractility usually associated with exercise become less pronounced; however, opposition to blood flow increases (Maruyama, 2012). With these changes, an overall decline in cardiac function and cardiac output is observed with initiation of exercise (Maruyama, 2012; Pugh & Wei, 2001).

A number of individuals from the Baltimore Longitudinal Study, aged 20–80 years and without heart disease, participated in an exercise program so that their cardiovascular functioning could be assessed (Rodeheffer et al., 1984). The researchers conducting this study observed and concluded that when older adults began to exercise, their heart rate did not respond as well, a greater end-systolic volume existed, and heart contractility declined. However, as these older adults continued to exercise, the end-diastolic volume increased, producing greater stroke volume and ending with an unchanged cardiac output. Other research has shown similar conclusions with exercise, including decreased heart rate and contractility, decreased peak heart rate and ejection fraction, decreased end-systolic volume, increased end-diastolic volume, and preserved stroke volume, further supporting the findings of increased left ventricle end-diastolic volume and maintained cardiac output during exercise (Fleg et al., 1995; Lakatta, 1993a, 1999a; Roffe, 1998; Wei, 1992). Exercise also increases vascular resistance and elevates both systolic and diastolic pressure (Lind & McNicol, 1986). Salmasi et al. (2003) conducted a research study involving 55 patients younger than 50 years of age and 45 patients older than 50 years of age, and evaluated them for left ventricle diastolic function at rest and during isometric exercise. These researchers concluded that degeneration in left ventricle diastolic functioning occurred in the group 50 years and older, both at rest and during isometric exercise, due to ventricle stiffening leading to decreased diastolic filling initially (Salmasi et al., 2003). Conclusions on cardiovascular change with exercise must be evaluated carefully to discern age associated alterations across time and across individuals (see **Table 4-2**).

TABLE 4-2   Lifestyle Interventions to Maintain or Improve Physiological Functioning in Aging

Physical activity	1. Do some type of exercise at least 30 minutes per day and more involved exercise 3–5 days per week. 2. Include cardiovascular training, weight-bearing exercise, resistance, balance training, and flexibility exercise.
Nutrition	1. Low-calorie diet 2. Low-fat diet 3. Low-cholesterol diet 4. Low-sodium diet 5. At least five fruits and vegetables per day 6. Plenty of whole grains 7. Eight glasses of water a day
Vitamins and minerals	1. Vitamins: B_6, B_{12}, D, K, A, C, E, beta-carotene, and folic acid 2. Minerals: Selenium, calcium, and iron
Examples of self-report assessment measures of physical activity and nutrition status	1. The Physical Activity Scale for the Elderly (PASE) (Washburn et al., 1993) 2. Nutritional Risk Index (Wolinsky et al., 1990) 3. The DETERMINE Screen (Nutrition Screening Initiative, 1992)

Prevalence rates of weight, dietary intake, and physical activity in individuals age 65 and over	1. Obese: Men—27%, Women—32%
	    Age 65–74: Men—32%, Women—39%
	    Age 75 and over: Men—18%, Women—24%
	    Overweight: Men—73%, Women—66%
	    Underweight: Men—1%, Women—3%
	2. Diet (Healthy Eating Index):
	    19% good diet, 67% needed improvement, 14% poor diet
	      *Low score on daily fruit and dairy servings
	      *High score on variety of food and cholesterol intake
	3. Nonstrenuous physical activity: 21% total for 65 and over; regular strenuous physical activity:
	    Age 65–74: 26%
	    Age 75–84: 18%
	    Age 85 and over: 9%

Data from Drewnowski, A., & Evans, W. (2001). Nutrition, physical activity, and quality of life in older adults: Summary. *Journals of Gerontology Series A: Biological Sciences and Medical Sciences, 56A* (Special Issue II), 89–94; Federal Interagency Forum on Aging-Related Statistics. (2004). *Older Americans 2004: Key indicators of well-being.* Washington, DC: U.S. Government Printing Office; McReynolds, J., & Rossen, E. (2004). Importance of physical activity, nutrition, and social support for optimal aging. *Clinical Nurse Specialist, 18*(4), 200–206; Topp, R., Fahlman, M., & Boardley, D. (2004). Healthy aging: Health promotion and disease prevention. *Nursing Clinics of North America, 39*(2), 411–422.

Although structural and functional changes occur in the cardiovascular system with age, some changes remain variable across time and across individuals. Some research studies comparing cardiovascular function across different age cohorts do not take into account nutrition practices, exercise regimens or lack thereof, and other effects such as the lifestyle of older adults across time and space compared to younger individuals (Lakatta, 1999b; Mohanlal, Parsa, & Weir, 2012). For example, older adults today often will say they grew up on a farm with large meals and a lack of concern for fat content; however, younger individuals today are very health conscious, with tremendous focus on fat and calories. Nutrition and exercise habits as well as other health-related practices continually change over time, which brings up the question of how comparable younger individuals are to older individuals in terms of cardiovascular functioning (McReynolds & Rossen, 2004).

The Respiratory System

The respiratory system refers to the parts of the body involved in breathing. This system works in close collaboration with the cardiovascular system to provide the body with a continuous supply of oxygen necessary to produce energy and to eliminate unwanted carbon dioxide. This gaseous exchange is vital to life, and, hence, proper functioning of the respiratory system and its constituent parts is critical to human survival.

Structure and Function of the Respiratory System

The respiratory system is composed of the mouth, nose, pharynx, trachea (or windpipe), and lungs, as well as the diaphragm and rib muscles. During respiration (**Figure 4-4a**), oxygen first passes through the mouth and nasal passages, where it is filtered of any large contaminants. It then enters the *pharynx*, where it absorbs water vapor and is warmed. Next, the oxygen flows through the trachea, a tube extending into the chest cavity, and into two smaller tubes called the bronchi, each of which splits into tubes called the bronchioles. Oxygen flows through the bronchi into the bronchioles and then into the lungs through many smaller tubes called alveolar ducts.

From the alveolar ducts, oxygen travels into tiny, spongy air sacs called *alveoli* (**Figure 4-4b**), of which there are approximately 600 million in the average, healthy adult lung (Krauss Whitbourne, 2002). The alveoli

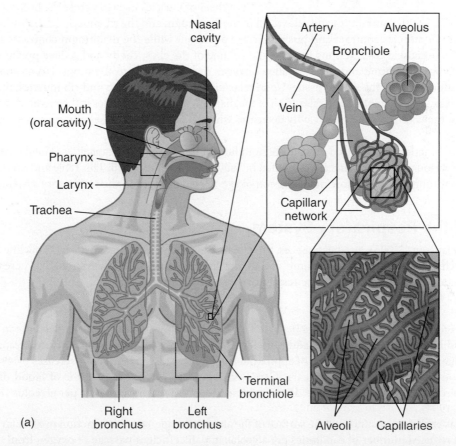

Figure 4-4a The respiratory system.

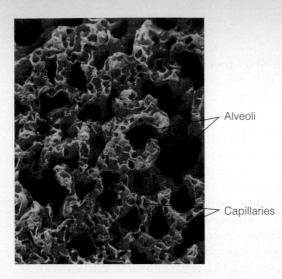

Alveoli

Capillaries

Figure 4-4b Alveolar structure.

are the functional units of the lungs and the site of gas exchange. Once in the alveoli, oxygen is diffused through the capillaries into the blood. The blood then carries the oxygen to the cells of the body. Carbon dioxide exits the body through the same, albeit reverse, pathway through which oxygen entered.

The lungs, more specifically the alveoli, are composed of elastic tissue that allows them to expand and recoil during inhalation and exhalation, respectively. The more the alveoli can expand and recoil, the more oxygen they can bring in and the more carbon dioxide they can expel. The alveoli also secrete a substance known as surfactant, which reduces the surface tension within the lungs. This reduction in surface tension helps keep the lungs from collapsing after each breath. Hence, surfactant aids in maintaining lung stability.

Respiration is highly controlled by respiratory muscles, including the diaphragm and rib muscles. The *diaphragm* is a sheet of muscles located across the bottom of the chest. Respiration occurs with contraction and relaxation of the diaphragm and the rib muscles. To allow for the intake of oxygen, the rib muscles contract and push the ribs up and out while the diaphragm contracts and is pulled downward. These muscle contractions increase the volume of the chest cavity and reduce pressure within the cavity. The change in volume and pressure allows oxygen to be sucked into the lungs. Expansion of the lung during inhalation expands the elastic tissue. Upon relaxation of the diaphragm and rib muscles, the lung tissue and the ribs relax. Supplementing the relaxation of the diaphragm and rib muscles is the recoil of the lung tissue. Consequently, the volume of the chest cavity decreases while its pressure increases and carbon dioxide is forced out of the lungs.

Respiratory function is measured in terms of both lung volumes and lung capacities. The names and definitions of these various measurements are presented in **Table 4-3** and **Figure 4-5**. This table and this figure should be referred to throughout the following discussion of age-related changes in the respiratory system.

Aging of the Respiratory System

According to Janssens (2005), as a person ages, three main physiological changes occur: (1) decline in chest wall ability, (2) decline in elastic recoil of the lung, and (3) decline in respiratory muscle strength. These three factors contribute to the functional decline of the respiratory system.

Alveoli

As a person ages, the alveoli of the lungs become flatter and shallower, and there is a decrease in the amount of tissue dividing individual alveoli. In addition, there is a decrease in the alveolar surface area. A person 30 years of age has an alveolar surface area of approximately 75 m². This surface area decreases by 4% per decade thereafter to around 60 m² by age 70 years (Carpo & Campbell, 1998). The volume of blood distributed to pulmonary circulation declines with age due to a decreasing number of capillaries per alveolus (Meyer, 2005; Nitzan et al., 1994).

Because gas exchange occurs over the surface of the alveoli, the age-related reduction in alveolar surface area as well as the reduced number of capillaries per alveolus impairs efficient passage of oxygen from the alveoli to the blood (De Martinis & Timiras, 2007; Meyer, 2005).

TABLE 4-3   Respiratory Volumes and Capacities

Volumes	Definition	Age-related
Tidal volume (TV)	Amount of air inspired and expired during a normal breath	Decrease
Inspiratory reserve volume (IRV)	Amount of air that can be inspired after maximum inspiration	Decrease
Expiratory reserve volume (ERV)	Amount of air that can be expired after maximum expiration	Decrease
Residual volume (RV)	Amount of air remaining in the lungs following maximum expiration	Increase
Forced expiratory volume (FEV)	Amount of air that can be forcefully expelled in 1 second	Decrease
Capacity	**Definition**	**Age-related**
Total lung capacity (TLC)	Maximum capacity to which the lungs can expand during maximum inspiratory effort	No change
Vital capacity (VC)	Amount of air that can be expelled following maximum inspiration	Decrease
Inspiratory capacity (IC)	Maximum amount of air that can be inspired after reaching the end of a normal expiration	Decrease
Functional residual capacity (FRC)	Amount of air remaining in the lungs following a normal expiration	Increase

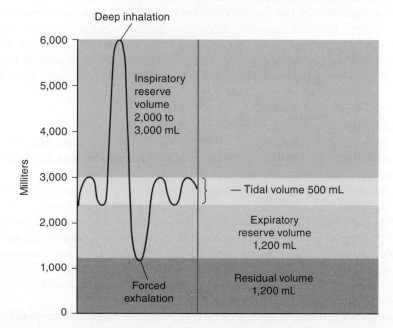

Figure 4-5 Measuring lung capacity.

Reproduced from Moffett, D., Moffett, S., & Schauff, C.L. (1993). *Human physiology: Foundations and frontiers* (2nd ed.). St. Louis, MO: Mosby.

Lung Elasticity

With age there is a decrease in the lungs' elasticity, which in turn causes a change in the elastic recoil properties of the lungs. During expiration, *elastic recoil* helps to keep the lungs open until all air is expelled and the lungs are forced to collapse due to the action of the respiratory muscles. Loss of elastic recoil causes the lungs to close prematurely, trapping air inside and preventing the lungs from emptying completely. As a result, unexpired air remains in the lungs and, consequently, during the next inhalation less air can be inspired (Krauss Whitbourne, 2002). Despite the reduced inspiratory capacity, *total lung capacity*—the maximum volume to which the lungs can expand during greatest inspiratory effort—remains virtually unchanged with age. After adjustment for age-related decreases in height, total lung capacity of both men and women decreases by less than 10% between the ages of 20 and 60 years (De Martinis & Timiras, 2007).

Changes in lung elasticity can decrease the efficiency of oxygen delivery. Due to the effects of gravity, more blood flows through the lower than the upper portion of the lungs. However, because of the reduced ability of the aging lungs to expand during inhalation, less air reaches the lower portion of the lungs. As a result, air is more likely to flow through the upper portion of the lungs, yet it is the lower lung that has a greater capillary network and blood supply for oxygen delivery. Thus, the decrease of airflow through the lower lung results in less efficient delivery of oxygen to the body. Consequently, as individuals age they must breathe in more air to achieve the same amount of gas exchange, a task that is difficult to accomplish with a loss of lung elasticity. This same upper–lower lung disparity is seen in young people. However, because of their greater lung elasticity, younger individuals are better able to compensate for the disparity by bringing more air into the lungs (Krauss Whitbourne, 2002).

The Chest Wall

The chest wall becomes stiffer with advancing age, decreasing the ease with which the thoracic cavity can expand. The increase in stiffness is largely due to a loss of rib elasticity as well as age-related calcification of the cartilage that attaches the ribs to the breastbone. The stiffness of the chest reduces its ability to expand during inhalation and contract during exhalation. Age-related vertebral kyphosis, arthritis of the costovertebral joints, as well as the increased rigidity of the thoracic cavity lead to increased anteroposterior diameter, which results in flattening of the diaphragm (El Solh & Ramadan, 2006). Older persons rely heavily on the diaphragm for expansion and contraction of the chest cavity when they breathe (Digiovanna, 1994). However, the diaphragm may weaken by up to 25–31% (Beers & Berkow, 2000; Janssens, 2005) with age. This weakening, combined with an age-associated loss of overall muscle mass, reduces the contractual abilities of the diaphragm, limiting respiration.

Changes in Respiratory Measures

As a result of the age-related changes in lung tissue and the chest wall, the respiratory system of older adults is less able to provide sufficient gas exchange to meet the body's demand for oxygen, particularly at times of maximum physical exertion (Arking, 1998). This insufficiency is demonstrated by age-related changes in respiratory measures (see Table 4-3).

Research has shown that *vital capacity*—the maximum amount of air that can be expelled following a maximum inspiration—decreases with advancing age. Between the ages of 20 and 70 years, vital capacity is reduced by approximately 40% (Krauss Whitbourne, 2002), and in some cases vital capacity in the seventh decade may decrease to almost 75% of its value at 17 years of age (De Martinis & Timiras, 2007). Residual volume, however, increases nearly 50% with age (De Martinis & Timiras, 2007). This increase, in combination with reduced vital capacity, leads to a reduction in the amount of air that can be inspired. In addition, any fresh air that is inhaled is mixed with stale, residual air. This mixing, together with diminished inhalation, contributes to the lungs' reduced ability to deliver sufficient oxygen to the body (Krauss Whitbourne, 2002).

Residual volume is inversely related to *forced expiratory volume* (FEV), the amount of air that can be forcefully expelled in 1 second. As residual volume increases, FEV decreases. Thus, evidence supporting a marked decrease in FEV with age is congruent with the age-related increase in residual volume (Arking, 1998; Hollenberg, Yang, Haight, & Tager, 2006).

Another respiratory measure known to change with age is the *ventilatory rate*, or the minute respiratory rate. Ventilatory rate is defined as the volume of air inspired in a normal breath (i.e., tidal volume) multiplied by the frequency of breaths per minute. At low levels of exertion, age does not appear to have any effect on ventilatory rate. However, at maximal exertion levels the ventilatory rate shows an age-related decline. Young adult males have a maximum capacity for inspiration of about 125–170 liters of air per minute, but this rate can be sustained for only approximately 15 seconds, while a ventilatory rate of 100–120 liters of air per minute can be maintained for prolonged periods of time. However, by the age of 85 years, the ventilatory rate has decreased to approximately 75 liters per minute (Arking, 1998).

Age-Related Pathologies of the Respiratory System

The proportion of deaths due to respiratory disease is at its highest, approximately 30%, in the first year of life. By late adolescence and early adulthood, only about 5% of deaths are attributed to respiratory disease. However, from the fifth decade of life on, there is a steady increase in the incidence of respiratory disease, and among persons over 85 years of age, respiratory disease accounts for 25% of all deaths (De Martinis & Timiras, 2007). Two of the most prevalent respiratory diseases among older adults are chronic obstructive pulmonary disease (COPD) and pneumonia.

Chronic Obstructive Pulmonary Disease

COPD is characterized by limited airflow and impaired gas exchange. It encompasses chronic bronchitis, chronic obstructive bronchitis, emphysema, or a combination of these disorders (Barnes, 2000). The pathology of COPD is characterized by a decreased ability of the lungs to respire properly. Environmental irritants such as cigarette smoke promote the production of excessive amounts of mucus within the airways. As this mucus builds up, the airways become restricted. The result is inefficient respiration in which excessive air accumulates in the alveoli, causing them to remain perpetually inflated. This constant inflation damages the alveolar walls, and the body repairs this damage by replacing the normally elastic tissue with fibrous tissues that are much less permeable to gas exchange. In addition, the fibrous tissue decreases elastic recoil, further contributing to inefficient and difficult respiration (Arking, 1998). Individuals with COPD often experience excessive cardiac workload as the heart tries to compensate for impaired airflow by pumping more blood to the lungs (Arking, 1998).

Pneumonia

Pneumonia is characterized by lung inflammation generally brought on by infection. The impaired immune response with age (see "The Immune System" later in this chapter) is thought to play a significant role in the high prevalence of pneumonia seen among elderly persons. Older individuals are more susceptible to severe pneumonia and complications of pneumonia than are younger persons. In addition, mortality from pneumonia is known to be significantly higher in those age 60 years or older (Naughton, Mylotte, & Tayara, 2000).

The Gastrointestinal System
Aging in Key Components of the Gastrointestinal Tract

Overall, the gastrointestinal (GI) system (see **Figure 4-6**) appears to be relatively preserved in aging, with only minor changes. The two GI areas most affected by age are the upper tract (the pharynx and *esophagus*) and the *colon*, also referred to as the large intestine (Hall, 2002; Salles, 2007). Changes in the GI system can have multiple and varied effects, including effects upon consumption and absorption of nutrients and waste secretion.

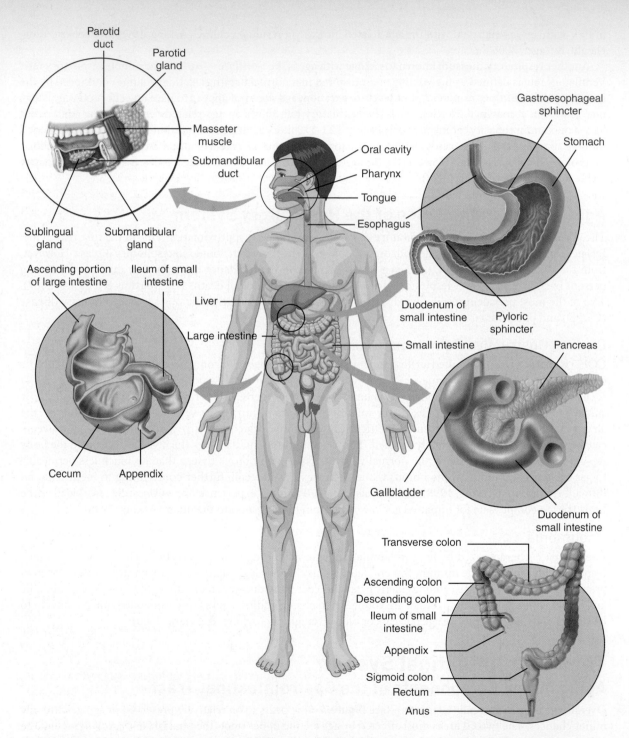

Figure 4-6 The gastrointestinal system.

In this section, age-related changes of the GI system, from the mouth to the large intestine and the accompanying glands and organs, will be evaluated.

The Mouth

The GI system begins at the mouth, which shows some signs of age-related changes that affect the ability to chew. Changes in taste also occur, as described in this chapter's "The Nervous System" section. The mouth is utilized for mastication, or chewing, and for moistening food with saliva. The chewing and moistening of food allows for easier passage of the processed content to the pharynx and esophagus (Arking, 1998; Hall & Wiley, 1999).

Dental decay and tooth loss affect many older individuals today, making it more difficult to chew and prepare food to be swallowed (Hall, 2009). Age-related changes in teeth cause them to be less sensitive and more brittle (Devlin & Ferguson, 1998). However, in the near future, tooth decay and loss may decline due to increased health awareness, improved dentistry practices, and higher availability of fluoride toothpaste and floss that were not available when today's generation of older adults was maturing.

With age, there is atrophy of those muscles and bones of the jaw and mouth that control mastication. Consequently, it is more difficult for older adults to chew their food (Devlin & Ferguson, 1998; Digiovanna, 2000; Karlsson, Persson, & Carlsson, 1991; Newton, Yemm, Abel, & Menhinick, 1993). Along with changes in the skeletal muscle, changes occur in the nerves that innervate the oral region. As a result, there is some change in the ability of the nerves and muscles to coordinate functioning (Digiovanna, 2000). Refer to "The Muscle" later in this chapter for additional information regarding aging changes in skeletal muscle.

Saliva produced and secreted by salivary glands and the oral mucosa assists in removing food from teeth, neutralizing acid, replacing minerals in enamel, inhibiting bacteria and fungi growth, and breaking down starch molecules (Devlin & Ferguson, 1998; Digiovanna, 2000). Salivary flow is controlled by the autonomic nervous system and is influenced by food touching the mouth, by jaw movement, and by olfaction and gustation input (Bourdiol, Mioche, & Monier, 2004; Digiovanna, 2000). Although almost 40% of older adults complain of dry mouth, salivary gland function remains stable with age due to the large secretory reserve in the main salivary glands (Bourdiol et al., 2004; Devlin & Ferguson, 1998; Ghezzi & Ship, 2003; Tepper & Katz, 1998). Dry mouth can be attributed to prescription and over-the-counter medications, nutritional deficiencies, disease, and treatment therapies such as chemotherapy (Devlin & Ferguson, 1998; Ghezzi & Ship, 2003; Ship, Pillemer, & Baum, 2002).

The Esophagus

A study in 1964 showing impaired esophageal motility function in older individuals led to the development of the term *presbyesophagus*; however, the study included many individuals with diseases such as diabetes and neuropathy that confounded the findings (Soergel, Zboralske, & Amberg, 1964). Studies have since demonstrated preservation of esophageal functioning in aging until around age 80, when some changes occur. These changes include decline in upper esophageal sphincter pressure, increased time for the upper esophageal sphincter to relax, and decreased intensity of esophageal contractions, potentially caused by loss of muscle abilities and nerve innervations (Fulp, Dalton, Castell, & Castell, 1990; Hall, 2009; Orr & Chen, 2002; Schroeder & Richter, 1994). The lower esophageal sphincter was once thought to demonstrate age-related declines in contractions and impaired relaxation; however, recent work has shown that no real changes occur to the lower sphincter (Hall, 2009).

Swallowing is controlled by the brain through cortical input to the medulla oblongata swallowing centers, which have nerve endings in the skeletal muscle controlling the pharynx and esophagus (Hall, 2009). The esophagus also contains smooth muscle that is controlled by nerve endings from the intestines and by the vagus nerve in the brain (Hall, 2009). Rao, Mudipalli, Mujica, Patel, and Zimmerman (2003) conducted a study evaluating sensory and mechanical changes in both skeletal and smooth muscle located in the esophagus and found that older adults demonstrated stiffening of the esophageal wall and less sensitivity to discomfort and *pain* in the esophagus. These changes affect the older patient's ability to swallow. The gag reflex also appears to be absent in around 40% of healthy older adults (Davies, Kidd, Stone, & MacMahon, 1995). Dysphagia (difficulty swallowing), reflux, heartburn, and chest pain are common complaints that relate to changes in the pharynx and esophagus; approximately 35% of older individuals report such complaints (Bhutto & Morley, 2008; Hall 2009; Orr & Chen, 2002; Reinus & Brandt, 1998; Shaker, Dua, & Koch, 1998). Although frequency of reflux episodes does not appear to vary with age, the duration of gastroesophageal episodes appears to be more prolonged in older adults (Ferriolli, Oliveira, Matsuda, Braga, & Dantos, 1998).

The Stomach

Several studies have determined that age-related declines in peristaltic contractions and stomach emptying do not appear to be clinically significant (Brogna, Ferrara, Bucceri, Lanteri, & Catalano, 1999; O'Mahony, O'Leary, & Quigley, 2002). A study by Madsen and Graff (2004) assessing gastrointestinal motility in aging concluded that no changes in gastric emptying occurred with age. Furthermore, enteric nerves or nerves innervating the intestinal system that control gastric motility do not change with age (Madsen & Graff, 2004). Other studies have shown that peristalsis and gastric contractile force are mildly reduced in the elderly and that the reduction reaches significance in less active elderly subjects rather than in those who maintain an active lifestyle (O'Donovan et al., 2005; Shimamoto, Hirata, & Hiraike, 2002). Gastric acid secretions do not appear to change with age, but pepsin, bicarbonate, and sodium ion secretions and prostaglandin content do show age-related decline (Hall, 2009). These secretion changes cause a decline in gastric defense mechanisms and create an increased potential for mucosal injury in the stomach (Hall, 2009).

The Small Intestine

Small intestine motility needed for digestion and absorption of nutrients has been reported to show no change or only minor changes in contraction intensity with age (Brogna et al., 1999; O'Mahony et al., 2002; Orr & Chen, 2002; Shaker et al., 1998). Madsen and Graff (2004) also discovered no age-related change in small intestine transit rate (the time needed for digested material to move through the length of the small intestine). This finding supports results from other studies. The endocrine and nervous system aid in motility functioning in the intestines, and any changes in these specific systems could potentially cause changes in intestinal abilities (Shaker et al., 1998). However, no clinically significant motility changes appear to occur in the small intestine with age.

A common consequence of prolonged gastric emptying is a decrease in gastric acid secretion in approximately 32% of elderly people (Saffrey, 2004). This decreased acid production, along with motility disturbances in the small intestine, can lead to bacterial overgrowth in the small intestine, a common clinical finding in the older population, causing malabsorption and malnutrition (Madsen & Graff, 2004; O'Mahony et al., 2002; Orr & Chen, 2002; Salles, 2007). Absorption of nutrients generally does not change with age, though changes in vitamin absorption are seen with particular vitamins but not others (Hall, 2009). For instance, vitamin A absorption increases in older adults whereas vitamin D, zinc, and calcium absorption decreases. Absorption of vitamins B_1, B_{12}, and C and iron does not change with age (Baik & Russell, 1999; Hall, 2009; Simon, Leboff, Wright, & Glowacki, 2002; Tepper & Katz, 1998).

The Large Intestine

The large intestine, also referred to as the colon, measures approximately 5 feet long when stretched out and covers the area from the small intestine to the anus (Digiovanna, 2000). In aging, a loss of enteric, or intestinal, neurons and nerve connections to the smooth muscle in the colon occurs (Gomes, deSouza, & Liberti, 1997; Shaker et al., 1998). Madsen and Graff (2004) concluded that older adults experience longer colonic transit time (the amount of time needed for fluid and excrement to travel the length of the colon). This change again relates to age-related loss of neurons and receptors in the enteric nervous system. Increased colonic transit time also correlates with increased fibrosis in the colon (Hall, 2002). Colonic pressure in the intralumen also increases with age, but can be lowered with fiber supplementation (Hall, 2002).

The rectum, a colonic structure that is located before the anus, shows an age-related increase in fibrous tissue. This increase reduces the rectum's ability to stretch as feces pass through (Digiovanna, 2000). In the anus, the external anal sphincter shows an age-related decrease in motor neurons responsible for sphincter control. This sphincter also thins with age; however, the internal anal sphincter thickens with age, possibly as a compensatory mechanism. Nonetheless, it shows a decline in contractile abilities (Digiovanna, 2000; Nielson & Pedersen, 1996; O'Mahony et al., 2002; Rociu, Stoker, Eijkemans, & Lameris, 2000). Aging women experience a greater risk of anal sphincter changes due to laxity of the pelvic floor, decreased pressure in the rectum, and even menopause (Hall, 2002).

Aging in Accessory Glands and Organs

As people age, relatively no changes occur in the secretions of the liver, pancreas, and gallbladder (Hall, 2002). However, these accessory glands and organs, which work in close association with the GI system, remain crucial for intestinal stability.

The Liver

The *liver* is the largest gland in the body and contributes to the conversion of food by secreting bile into the small intestine and by screening blood from the stomach and small intestine for toxic substances, excess nutrients, and ammonia (Digiovanna, 2000). With age, the liver's size as well as its blood flow and perfusion can decrease by 30–40%. In addition, hepatocytes, or liver cells, can undergo structural alterations. However, due to the liver's large reserve capacity and the hepatocytes' ability to regenerate after damage, no functional changes result from these changes in structure (Digiovanna, 2000; Hall, 2009; James, 1998; Marchesini et al., 1988; Schmucker, 1998; Wynne et al., 1989). Decreased drug clearance in the older population can occur due to the declines in liver size and blood flow as well as age-related changes in the kidneys, but this is highly variable among individuals (Bhutto & Morley, 2008; James, 1998; Le Couteur & McLean, 1998; McLean & Le Couteur, 2004).

The Gallbladder

The *gallbladder* is a small sac located below the liver that stores the bile sent from the liver until it receives intestinal and pancreatic signaling via the hormone cholecystokinin. This signaling indicates a readiness for digestion and, in response, bile is released into the ducts of the small intestine (Digiovanna, 2000; MacIntosh et al., 2001). Refer to Figure 4-6 for the location and anatomical structure of the gallbladder. With age, no overall structural changes occur in the gallbladder with the exception of the bile ducts (Digiovanna, 2000). However, in older adults the gallbladder appears to demonstrate declines in emptying rates so that less bile is secreted when food is digested (Hall, 2009). Increased bile volume in the gallbladder has been correlated with gallstones in older adults. This increase in bile volume is more common in older women than men (Bates, Harrison, Lowe, Lawson, & Padley, 1992; Hall, 2009). The bile ducts tend to widen with age, allowing potential gallstones to pass through more easily; however, the duct near the opening of the small intestine becomes narrower, trapping the gallstones and leading to abnormal changes (Digiovanna, 2000).

The Pancreas

The *pancreas* is a gland located below the stomach and above the small intestine. Refer to Figure 4-6 for pancreatic location and structure. The pancreas secretes pancreatic fluid, which neutralizes stomach acid and accelerates the transport of large nutrients into ducts that eventually converge with the bile duct leading into the small intestine (Digiovanna, 2000; Hall, 2009). The pancreas decreases in weight with age and shows some histological changes such as fibrosis and cell atrophy (Hall, 2009). However, due to the large reserve capacity of the pancreas, the small changes that occur, including changes in the enzymes that aid in stomach acid neutralization and nutrient breakdown, do not affect overall pancreatic function as a person ages (Digiovanna, 2000; Hall, 2009).

Gastrointestinal Immunity

The GI tract, with a mucosal lining containing immunological properties, is the largest organ (Hall, 2009). The immune response in the GI system depends on the congruent work of lymphoid and epithelial cells (Schmucker, Thoreux, & Owen, 2001). Secretion of antibodies into the intestinal mucosa works to neutralize toxins, block bacteria from adhering to surfaces, and block antigens from crossing the mucosa (Holt, 1992; Schmucker et al., 2001). Research has suggested a decline in immunological function in the aging GI system. This decline can increase rates of infections that occur via the GI system. Infection may, in turn, lead to mortality and morbidity (Arranz, O'Mahony, Barton, & Ferguson, 1992; Schmucker et al., 2001; Schmucker, Heyworth, Owen, & Daniels, 1996; Schmucker, Owen, Outenreath, & Thoreux, 2003). A decline in *gastrointestinal immunity* can be attributed to a change in lymphoid cells or epithelial cells or possibly both cell types (Schmucker et al., 2001).

Although relatively few changes occur in the aging GI system, changes that do occur increase the risk of diseases and disorders. Age-related changes, compounded by other influential factors such as comorbidity and medication use, place older individuals at increased risk of gallstones, constipation, fecal incontinence, and infection.

The Genitourinary System
Overview of the Genitourinary System

The genitourinary system (**Figure 4-7**) in both males and females contains the kidneys and associated renal arteries and veins, the ureters, the bladder, and the urethra running through the genitalia (Digiovanna, 2000; Lindeman, 1995). The urinary system provides many functions that help the body to maintain *homeostasis*, or balance of the organ systems. For instance, the urinary system (1) removes wastes and toxins such as ammonia, uric acid, and some medications from the blood; (2) regulates osmotic pressure in the blood and interstitial fluid; (3) regulates concentration levels of calcium, sodium, potassium, magnesium, and phosphorus; (4) controls the acid–base balance by making necessary adjustments; (5) regulates blood pressure; (6) activates vitamin D in order to maintain calcium levels; and (7) regulates oxygen level through stimulation of erythropoietin, the hormone responsible for increased red blood cell (RBC) production in the bone marrow (Digiovanna, 2000; Lye, 1998). The kidneys form urine through a process of filtration, reabsorption, and secretion with constant homeostasis maintained throughout the process (Digiovanna, 2000). Under usual living conditions the kidneys can be maintained on as little as 30% capacity, but under stressful conditions, such as high temperatures, kidney reserves are needed to maintain proper functioning (Digiovanna, 2000). In this section, aging structural and functional changes in the urinary system will be evaluated. For age-related changes in genitalia, refer to the section "The Reproductive System."

Urinary Structural Changes with Age

The Kidneys

With age, the kidneys shrink in length and weight. At 30 years of age, the average kidney weighs 150 to 200 grams. By age 90, weight has declined to between 110 and 150 grams (Beck, 1998a, 1999b; Jassal, Fillit, & Oreopoulos, 1998; Lindeman, 1995; Martin & Sheaff, 2007; Minaker, 2011; Pannarale et al., 2010). The number of *glomeruli* decreases by as much as 30–40% by age 90 due to glomerulosclerosis. Remaining glomeruli decrease in size but increase in basement membrane thickness (Beck, 1999a; Lindeman, 1995; Musso, Ghezzi, & Ferraris, 2004). The size and number of *nephrons*, the combination of the Bowman's capsule and renal tubule with the glomerulus, also decrease with age (Jassal & Oreopoulos, 1998; Jassal et al., 1998; Minaker, 2011). On average, renal blood flow declines 10% per decade beginning as early as 20 years of age. Young adults (20 years) average a renal blood flow of 600 mL/minute, whereas average blood flow in older adults (80 years) averages only 300 mL/minute (Beck, 1999b; Digiovanna, 2000; Jassal et al., 1998; Lindeman, 1995; Minaker, 2011). Furthermore, blood flow declines with age due to changes in the arteries and capillaries in the kidneys (Digiovanna, 2000; Jassal et al., 1998;

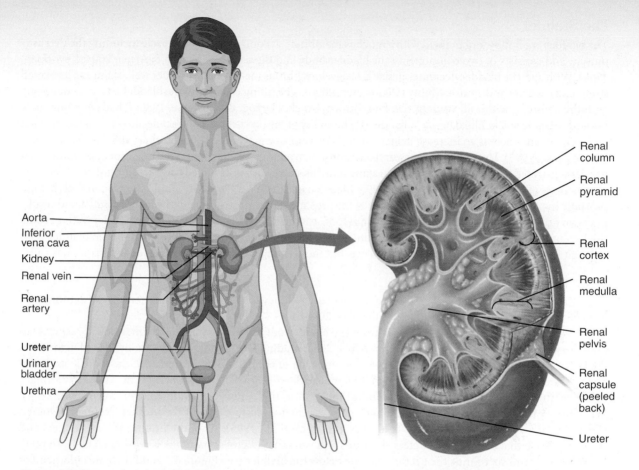

Figure 4-7 The genitourinary system.

McLean & Le Couteur, 2004). Renal blood flow in the cortical section of the kidneys declines at a much quicker rate compared to the average renal blood flow rate; this indicates that cortical nephrons are severely affected by age (Lindeman, 1995). Changes in blood flow and glomerular filtration rate (GFR) account for the majority of functional disability in the kidneys with age. With disease and some medications, blood flow and GFR can be further compromised (Beck, 1999b; Digiovanna, 2000; Lindeman, 1995; Martin & Sheaff, 2007). The GFR variably declines with age. This decline is measured by creatinine or insulin clearance and usually begins in the third decade as a result of changes in glomeruli, clustering of capillaries, and renal blood flow rate (Digiovanna, 2000; Jassal et al., 1998; McLean & Le Couteur, 2004; Rowe, Andres, Tobin, Norris, & Shock, 1976). A decline in GFR becomes significant as people age because elimination of waste and toxins declines, causing an accumulation of harmful substances such as uric acid and medications in the body (Digiovanna, 2000; McLean & Le Couteur, 2004). Renal tubules also show age-related changes, including decreased number and length. There is also evidence of age-related interstitial fibrosis and thickening of renal tubule basement membranes, which can affect reabsorption and excretion (Beck, 1999b; Jassal & Oreopoulos, 1998; Jassal et al., 1998). Despite age-related structural changes, the kidneys contain a large reserve capacity and functional abilities remain relatively stable unless stressed (Beck, 1999b; Jassal et al., 1998; Minaker, 2011).

The Bladder

The bladder is a hollow organ lined with a mucous membrane; it contains smooth muscle including the detrusor muscle, and consists of two components, the bladder body and the base (Andersson & Arner, 2004; Kevorkian, 2004). With age, the bladder decreases in size and develops fibrous matter in the bladder wall, changing its overall stretching capacity and contractibility (Digiovanna, 2000). The filling capacity of the bladder also declines along with the ability to withhold voiding (Diokno, Brown, Brock, Herzog, & Normolle, 1988; Elbadawi, Diokno, & Millard, 1998; Resnick, Elbadawi, & Yalla, 1995). The ability of the *detrusor* to contract declines in both aging men and women, and there is an increase in incidence of detrusor overactivation (Diokno et al., 1988; Minaker, 2011; Resnick et al., 1995). However, other research has not shown any age-related changes in detrusor contractility, but has demonstrated that the detrusor in usual aging remains stable with unchanged contractility and no observable obstructions (Elbadawi, Yalla, & Resnick, 1993; Madersbacher et al., 1998). In around 50% of men with benign prostatic hyperplasia (BPH), the enlargement of the prostate causes obstruction of the bladder outlet and results in urinary dysfunction (Resnick et al., 1995). In response to bladder outlet obstruction, the bladder walls become thicker and stronger to recompense for declining function (Elbadawi et al., 1998). Overall, the bladder goes through few variable structural changes with age, but these changes can have an impact on a person physically.

Ureters and the Urethra

The urinary system contains two *ureters* that connect each kidney to the bladder, but ureters do not demonstrate any age-specific changes (Cutler, 2006; Digiovanna, 2000).

The *urethra* forms the canal that leads from the bladder out of the body and also functions in response to excitatory or inhibitory stimuli (Andersson & Arner, 2004; Brading, Teramoto, Dass, & McCoy, 2001; Digiovanna, 2000). In males, the sphincter elevates from the prostate, encompassing the urethra (Strasser, Tiefenthaler, Steinlechner, Bartsch, & Konwalinka, 1996). In females, the urethra extends about 3–4 cm. Males have longer urethras; this is due to the urethra's anatomical location in the penis (Digiovanna, 2000; Kevorkian, 2004). With age, both the length of the urethra and the pressure needed to close off the urethra decline in women (Elbadawi et al., 1998; Madersbacher et al., 1998; Resnick et al., 1995). Also, the urethra thins with age, and striated muscle that controls sphincters also thins and weakens (Digiovanna, 2000; Kevorkian, 2004). In men, the prostate gland surrounds the urethra directly below the bladder (see Figure 4-7) and prostate enlargement around the bladder and urethra can cause urinary dysfunction (Digiovanna, 2000; Hollander & Diokno, 2007; Resnick et al., 1995).

Urinary Functional Changes with Age

Urination

Urination involves both the central and peripheral nervous systems and requires that bladder contraction and urethral relaxation occur simultaneously (Andersson & Arner, 2004; Kevorkian, 2004). The amount of urine expelled from the body decreases with age, correlating with increases of around 50–100 mL in postvoid residual (Cutler, 2006; Madersbacher et al., 1998; Minaker, 2011). Renal changes affect the ability to concentrate and dilute the urine, causing electrolyte imbalance (Jassal & Oreopoulos, 1998). Urine osmolality in the older adult only reaches about half of that in a younger adult, leading to increased water loss in the aged (Beck, 1999c). Older individuals also experience an increase in *nocturia* or an increased number of fluid voids occurring at night, which can disturb sleep patterns (Asplund, 2004; Kirkland, Lye, Levy, & Banerjee, 1983; Lubran, 1995; Mühlberg & Platt, 1999).

Prostate volume increases in aging males, and it is possible that, with longevity, every male will experience BPH (Madersbacher et al., 1998). BPH can lead to prostatic changes that influence lower urinary tract function as well as erectile and ejaculatory disorders (Cutler, 2006; Hafez & Hafez, 2004; Hollander & Diokno, 2007; Paick, Meehan, Lee, Penson, & Wessells, 2005; Rosen et al., 2003). More specifically, in BPH the prostate enlarges enough to encroach on the urethra and bladder, causing urinary retention, difficulty voiding, urinary tract infections, and, in advanced stages, renal failure (Hollander & Diokno, 2007; Resnick et al., 1995). Nerve stimulations to the smooth muscle of the prostate, bladder, and urethra occur in BPH, causing voiding difficulty. However, blocking the stimulus allows the muscle to relax, improving voiding abilities in BPH (Hollander & Diokno, 2007).

Glomerular Filtration Rate

The *glomerular filtration rate* (GFR), usually measured by creatinine clearance, declines in older individuals, but there is no resultant increase in blood creatinine concentration (Beck, 1999b; Minaker, 2011). Creatinine clearance is measured by the Cockcroft–Gault equation (Cockcroft & Gault, 1976):

$$\frac{140 - \text{age (years)} \times \text{IBW (ideal body weight) (kg)}}{72 \times \text{serum creatinine (mg/dL)}}$$

*Note: Multiply by 0.85 for females.

Measuring creatinine does not yield an accurate concentration rate because (1) the creatinine production rate is variable, (2) the tubules also secrete creatinine, and (3) elders have decreased muscle mass. Inaccuracy in measurement generally results in an overestimation of creatinine level of about 20–30% (Fliser et al., 1997; Lindeman, 1995; McLean & Le Couteur, 2004). The Cockcroft–Gault equation can be used to predict renal disease but may not reflect the usual aging process. As a result, use of the equation can lead to medication underdosing in healthy older adults and overdosing in compromised older adults (Fliser et al., 1997; Lubran, 1995; McLean & Le Couteur, 2004; Rule et al., 2004). A closer estimation of actual GFR comes from inulin clearance or non–radio-labeled iothalamate (Lubran, 1995; Mühlberg & Platt, 1999; Rule et al., 2004).

Adverse drug reactions occur approximately 3–10 times more often in the older population compared to in younger cohorts (Mühlberg & Platt, 1999). Adverse drug reactions in the older population occur as a result of changes in the kidneys, more specifically changes in GFR and renal clearance. Adverse drug reactions also can occur due to changes in tubular filtration (Abernathy, 1999; Mühlberg & Platt, 1999). Estimates of GFR among older adults correlate with aging tubular filtration and are often used to determine the amount of a drug to use in the older population (Lindeman, 1990). The key phrase in geriatric pharmacy remains "start low and go slow" because of renal changes that affect pharmacokinetics and pharmacodynamics with age (Abernathy, 1999; Mühlberg & Platt, 1999). Furthermore, polypharmacy and medication compliance are also associated with increased adverse events in the older population (Abernathy, 1999).

Homeostasis Changes

Overall, the aging kidneys function relatively well in maintaining fluid levels and electrolyte concentration balance; however, age-related changes are more readily observed under conditions of stress such as dehydration and high temperatures (Arking, 1998; Minaker, 2011). Age-related structural changes in the kidneys lead to some functional declines such as a decrease in the ability to regulate sodium concentrations under usual conditions. In addition, there is a decline in the ability to maintain sodium and potassium homeostasis and conserve water during times of stress (e.g., dehydration; Jassal & Oreopoulos, 1998; Minaker, 2011). The inability to properly regulate sodium can be attributed to malfunctioning of the ascending loop of Henle in addition to increases in prostaglandin levels and tubular unresponsiveness to aldosterone (Musso et al., 2004). A decline in overall potassium level in the body also occurs with age due to low potassium secretion resulting from the decline in tubular reaction to aldosterone (Jassal & Oreopoulos, 1998; Mühlberg & Platt, 1999; Musso et al, 2004). Older adults also experience changes in their ability to reabsorb water and, in conjunction with decreased thirst in older adults, the body can become dehydrated more quickly (Lye, 1998; Musso et al., 2004). Acid–base homeostasis appears to be relatively stable (pH 6.9 to 7.7) in older adults under usual conditions; however, under conditions of acid overload, older adults cannot excrete acid as quickly as younger adults (Lindeman, 1998; Mühlberg &

Platt, 1999; Sorribas et al., 1995). The nephron functionally serves the kidneys by balancing sodium and water and eliminating waste from the bloodstream (Arking, 1998). With age, nephrons shrink in size and decrease in number. This is partly caused by decreased blood flow in the glomeruli, which causes an increase in solute levels and eventually renders the nephron nonfunctional (Arking, 1998; Jassal et al., 1998; Minaker, 2011). Changes in homeostasis can negatively affect both the structural and functional capacity of the renal system.

Hormone Changes

Plasma renin and aldosterone concentration levels gradually decline with age, beginning around 40 years of age (Mühlberg & Platt, 1999). With age, the renin-angiotensin system undergoes a decline in its ability to maintain salt levels following salt deprivation (Corman et al., 1995; Mimran, Ribstein, & Jover, 1992). In addition, the renin-angiotensin-aldosterone (RAA) axis fails to adequately respond to hormone volume changes in healthy older adults without deprivation; therefore, maximum sodium levels cannot be attained (Beck, 1999b; Mühlberg & Platt, 1999; Weinstein & Anderson, 2010). During normal renal functioning, antidiuretic hormone release is responsible for reabsorption of fluid in the tubules and production of concentrated urine to maintain blood osmolarity. Studies concerning changes in the basal levels of antidiuretic hormone in the elderly have been inconclusive. Several studies, however, have indicated that changes in reabsorption are related to loss of responsiveness of antidiuretic hormone receptors in the tubules, leading to nocturnal polyuria with frequent nighttime voiding (Jassal & Oreopoulos, 1998; Johnson, Miller, Pillin, & Auslander, 2003; Musso, Liakopoulos, Ioannidis, Eleftheriadias, & Stefandis, 2006). Aging changes also occur in the calcium-parathormone-vitamin D_3 axis, as exhibited by decreased serum calcium levels, increased parathyroid hormone levels resulting from GFR decline, and declines in vitamin D metabolism by the aging kidneys (Chapuy, Durr, & Chapuy, 1983; Marcus, Masdirg, & Young, 1984; Massry et al., 1991; Mühlberg & Platt, 1999; Vieth, Ladak, & Walfish, 2003). Due to the decline in vitamin D metabolism by the kidneys, vitamin D supplementation is usually recommended in the older population (Vieth et al., 2003).

Age-related changes in the genitourinary system lead to alterations in genital structures, voiding behaviors, toxin and medication clearance, hormone levels, and overall physiological homeostasis of the body. Overall structural and functional changes can vary with age, but these changes can have an impact on a person physically, emotionally, psychologically, and socially, especially when urinary function declines and becomes abnormal, as seen with incontinence. Although aging changes in the kidneys can vary among older adults, as seen with GFR, as a whole these changes are quite common and should be considered when evaluating and treating an older population.

The Reproductive System

Female changes in the reproductive system are most notably associated with the onset of menopause and subsequent declines in estrogen. Menopause and symptoms associated with menopause serve as the physical reminder of reproductive aging, but underlying neuroendocrine and ovarian changes occur years earlier (Randolph et al., 2004). Male changes in the reproductive system are mostly associated with androgen deficiency and physical syndromes such as impotency. However, changes in reproductive hormones affect not only the reproductive system, but also other physiological systems. This section will provide an overview of all of the changes associated with reproductive aging in both women and men. The reader should refer to **Figures 4-8** and **4-9** for illustrations of the female and male reproductive systems.

Female Reproductive Aging

Neuroendocrine Function

The *reproductive axis* refers to the integration of the hypothalamus, pituitary gland, and gonads (ovaries for women). This axis controls reproductive hormones and ovulatory cycles (Chakraborty & Gore, 2004; Hall, 2004). The hypothalamus releases *gonadotropin-releasing hormone* (GnRH), which binds to corresponding

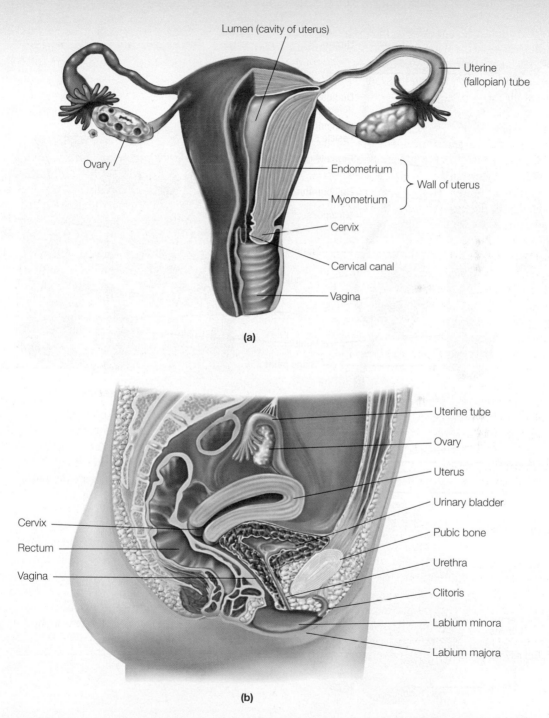

Figure 4-8 The female reproductive system. (a) Cross-section front view; (b) Cross-section side view.

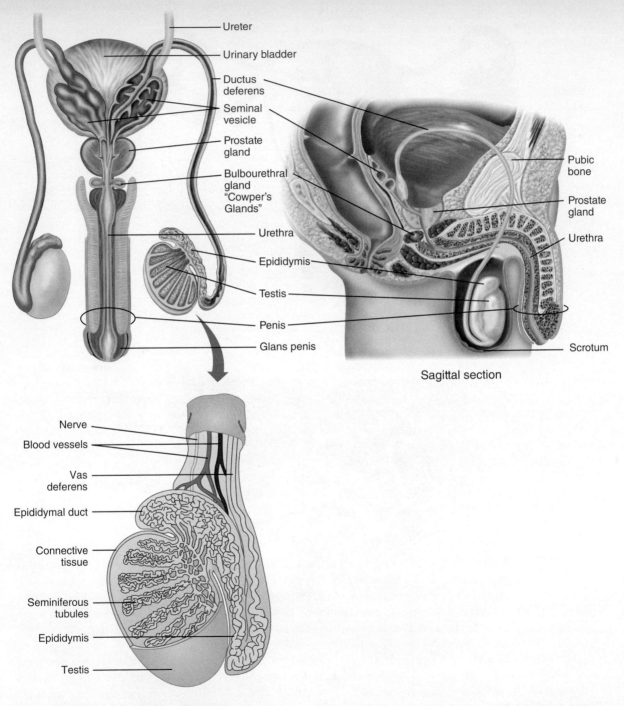

Ureter

Urinary bladder

Ductus deferens

Seminal vesicle

Prostate gland

Bulbourethral gland "Cowper's Glands"

Urethra

Epididymis

Testis

Penis

Glans penis

Pubic bone

Prostate gland

Urethra

Scrotum

Sagittal section

Nerve

Blood vessels

Vas deferens

Epididymal duct

Connective tissue

Seminiferous tubules

Epididymis

Testis

Figure 4-9 The male reproductive system.

gonadotropin receptors in the pituitary, stimulating the synthesis and release of *follicle-stimulating hormone* (FSH) and *luteinizing hormone* (LH) (Hall, 2004, 2007). FSH regulates ovarian follicle development and the conversion of androstenedione to estrogen, while LH regulates ovulation, supports the corpus luteum, and helps synthesize androgens (Hall, 2004, 2007; Yialamas & Hayes, 2003). Reproductive function relies heavily on hormone signaling from the ovaries to the hypothalamus and pituitary, as demonstrated by FSH secretion in the development of mature oocytes (Hall, 2004, 2007). The menstrual cycle functions on a negative feedback system, but also relies on positive feedback with estrogen to produce the LH surge for ovulation (Hall, 2004, 2007). **Figure 4-10** demonstrates the menstruation cycle along with corresponding changes in ovarian hormone levels throughout the cycle.

Age-related changes in neuroendocrine function include a change in gonadotropin levels. This change occurs before ovarian age–related changes, implicating involvement of the hypothalamus. With age, FSH levels begin increasing before menopause occurs and continue to increase throughout and after menopause. Estradiol levels tend to increase right before and while transitioning into menopause and then drastically decrease during menopause (Joffe, Soares, & Cohen, 2003; White, 2014). *Inhibin B*, a glycoprotein synthesized in the ovaries that usually suppresses FSH, also decreases in older women, explaining the observed increase in FSH (Hansen et al., 2005; Klein et al., 1996; Santoro, Adel, & Skurnick, 1999). Age-related changes in circulating hormones (estrogen and progesterone) strongly affect hypothalamic and pituitary responses to positive and negative hormone feedback systems. Finally, age-related changes occur in estrogen and progestin receptors located in the brain. These changes occur independently of changes in circulating hormone levels in the body (Chakraborty & Gore, 2004; Gill, Sharpless, Rado, & Hall, 2002; Hall, Lavoie, Marsh, & Martin, 2000; Rossmanith, Handke-Vesel, Wirth, & Scherbaum, 1994).

Age-related decline in estrogen affects the brain, resulting in some cognitive changes, insomnia, or even depression. Estrogen decline also affects other areas of the body that contain estrogen receptors and estrogen-dependent tissue (Smith, 1998; Wise, Dubal, Wilson, Rau, & Bottner, 2001; Wise, Krajnak, & Kashon, 1996). For example, with decreased estrogen levels the skin contains less collagen and becomes thin, sweat and sebaceous glands become dry, hair follicles begin to dry, bones lose calcium and undergo increased bone resorption, breasts lose connective tissue but gain adipose tissue, lipoproteins increase, bladder function decreases, cardiovascular function and blood pressure change, and the absorption and metabolism of nutrients become less efficient (Smith, 1998; Wise et al., 1996). A majority of the emphasis concerning estrogen has been on neuroprotective effects, including delay of onset in Alzheimer's disease (AD) and Parkinson's disease (PD) as well as protection against nerve cell death and brain injury (Roof & Hall, 2000; Wise et al., 2001; Wise, Dubal, Wilson, Rau, & Liu, 2001).

Female System Changes

The Ovaries

With age, the ovaries atrophy to such a small size that they can become impalpable during an examination (Smith, 1998). The number of ovarian follicles decreases with age, leading to a decline in fertility. This decline usually begins in the 30s or 40s, and more rapid declines occur after age 35 (Digiovanna, 2000; Hall, 2004; Smith, 1998). The ovarian follicles that remain through these declining years tend to be underdeveloped, and only a few follicles ovulate and form a corpus luteum. Eventually, by the age of 50–65 years, a woman will have no remaining viable follicles (Digiovanna, 2000; Smith, 1998; Wise et al., 1996).

In the late reproductive years, around age 45, when fertility declines, FSH levels tend to increase earlier in the follicular phase due to age-related decline in inhibin B. The earlier decline in FSH occurs even before increases in levels of LH or decreases in levels of estradiol (Hall, 2004; White, 2014; Wise et al., 1996). The increase in FSH levels is attributed to the drastic age-related decline in inhibin B (Hall, 2004; Wise et al., 1996). Decline in inhibin B along with the increase in FSH establishes the earliest age-related changes in the ovaries (Hall, 2004). In the clinical setting, FSH values are determined at day 3 of the menstrual cycle in order to indicate the stage

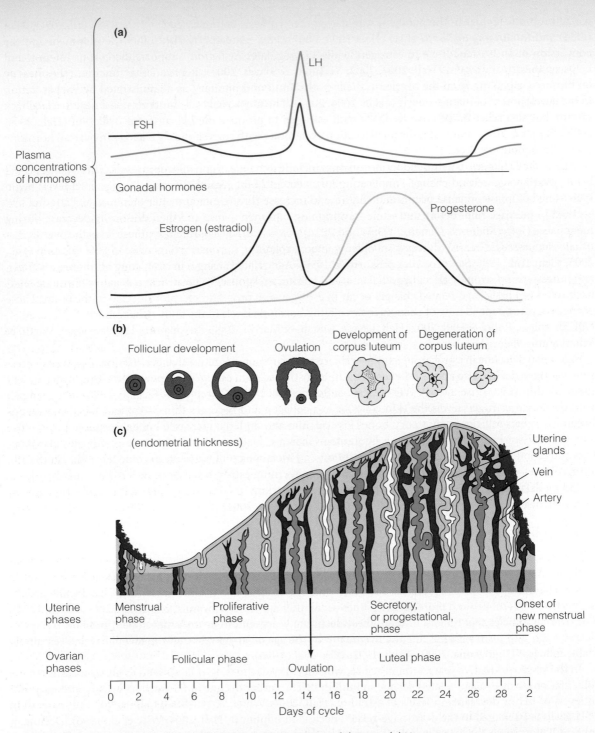

Figure 4-10 The menstrual cycle. (a) Gonadotrophic hormones; (b) Ovary; (c) Uterus.

of reproductive age (Hall, 2004). Reproductive aging causes a decline in estrogen due to a decrease in ovarian follicles. A decline in progesterone also occurs (Chakraborty & Gore, 2004; Smith, 1998). The ovaries produce about 25% of the testosterone in women, with the rest being supplied by the adrenal glands and conversion of androstenedione, a testosterone precursor (Horton & Tait, 1966; Yialamas & Hayes, 2003). However, testosterone levels in women are only about one tenth of those found in men (Judd & Yen, 1973; Yialamas & Hayes, 2003). These changes in the ovaries, including ovarian failure and oocyte depletion, are causally linked to the triggering of menopause (Hall, 2004; Wise et al., 1996).

The Uterus

Age-related decreases in uterine endometrial thickening during menstrual cycles occur as the result of decreased estrogen and progesterone levels (Digiovanna, 2000). This thickening leads to a decline in menstrual flow, eventually causing missed menstrual cycles and permanent cessation of ovulation and menstruation (Digiovanna, 2000; White, 2014). The supporting ligaments attached to the uterus are weakened with age, causing the uterus to tilt backward or fall out of position (prolapse) (Digiovanna, 2000; White, 2014). Over the postmenopausal period the uterus decreases in size by as much as 50% and may become so small as to be impalpable in women over the age of 75 (Digiovanna, 2000; Smith, 1998). As a result of stenosis and possible retraction, the cervix, the structure at the opening of the uterus, also may be unidentifiable upon physical examination in postmenopausal women (Smith, 1998).

The Vagina

With age, the vagina becomes shorter and narrower and the vaginal walls tend to thin and weaken (Smith, 1998; White, 2014). These structural changes, especially thinning of the vaginal walls and loss of elasticity, increase the chances for vaginal injury in the older female (Digiovanna, 2000). A loss of mucosal layers in the vagina as well as a large decrease in discharge causes a loss of lubrication. As a result, the vagina can become very dry, causing sexual intercourse to be painful (Digiovanna, 2000; Smith, 1998). With age, vaginal pH levels also shift from an acidic environment (3.8–4.2) toward an alkaline environment (6.5–7.5). The shift occurs because of decreased glycogen levels in vaginal tissue, which results in an environment in which microbes flourish (Digiovanna, 2000; Smith, 1998). With all of these changes, vaginal infections tend to increase with age (Digiovanna, 2000). The increased rate of infection also may be due in part to shrinkage of the labia majora, part of the external genitalia. As a result of this shrinkage, the labia become separated, which exposes a greater surface area upon which microbes and infectious agents can nest (Digiovanna, 2000; White, 2014).

Menopause

On average, *menopause* occurs around 51 years of age, but the reproductive changes described in this section begin years earlier (Digiovanna, 2000; Hall, 2004; Joffe et al., 2003). The late reproductive stage begins around 35 years of age with a decrease in fertility marked by a decrease in inhibin B, a decrease in progesterone, a slight increase in estradiol, and an increase in FSH (Hall, 2004, 2007; Joffe et al., 2003; Soules et al., 2001; White, 2014). The menopausal transition is defined by declines in estradiol along with the onset of variable menstrual cycles in both early and late stages. Periods of amenorrhea trigger the move into the late stage (Hall, 2004; Soules et al., 2001). Menopause is said to have occurred 1 year after the final menstrual period (Digiovanna, 2000; Hall, 2004, 2007; Soules et al., 2001). The postmenopausal period is characterized by drastic decreases in ovarian hormone functioning and changes in corresponding hormone-related systems such as bone formation and resorption (Hall, 2004, 2007; Soules et al., 2001). **Table 4-4** classifies the stages of menopause along with corresponding changes that occur within each stage.

Menopause is usually causally linked with ovarian failure and complete oocyte depletion, but research also implicates the hypothalamus and pituitary via a decline in estrogen negative feedback on LH release (Soules et al.,

TABLE 4-4   Classification of the Stages of Menopause and the Characteristics Associated with Each Stage as Defined by STRAW

Reproductive Late	Menopausal Transition Early/Late	Menopause	Postmenopause Early/Late
Variable symptoms: Vasomotor (hot flashes), breast tenderness, insomnia, migraines, premenstrual anxiety, and/or depression	Early: Menstrual cycle lengths vary Late: Two or more skipped cycles and some amenorrhea	Begins 12 months after the final menstrual period	Early: 5 years after the final menstrual period; ovarian hormone function decreases; increased bone loss Late: 5 years after the final menstrual period until death
Begin FSH elevation, decreased inhibin B, slight increase in estradiol, decreased progesterone	FSH elevation, LH elevation, decreased inhibin B, decreased estradiol	FSH elevation, LH elevation, decreased inhibin B, decreased estradiol	FSH elevation, LH elevation, decreased inhibin B, decreased estradiol, increased GnRH

Data from Soules, M., Sherman, S., Parrott, E., Rebar, R., Santoro, N., Utian, W., . . . STRAW + 10 Collaborative Group. (2001). Executive summary: Stages of reproductive aging workshop (STRAW). *Fertility and Sterility, 76*(5), 874–878; Hall, J. (2004). Neuroendocrine physiology of the early and late menopause. *Endocrinology and Metabolism Clinics of North America, 33*(4), 637–659.

2001; Weiss, Skurnick, Goldsmith, Santoro, & Park, 2004). Estrogen and progesterone are still present in small amounts during early postmenopausal years, but ovarian production of these hormones eventually declines and ceases completely during late postmenopausal years (Chakraborty & Gore, 2004; Digiovanna, 2000). Estrogen levels decrease by 80% by the postmenopausal years and progesterone decreases by 60% (Smith, 1998).

During menopause, the ovaries decrease production of androstenedione by 50%. This decline could help explain loss of libido and energy in the older female (Yialamas & Hayes, 2003). Although some studies have shown that there are slight declines in testosterone levels during and after menopause, others have shown no change in testosterone levels (see **Case Study 4-1**). Thus, the question of whether androgen deficiency occurs in older women remains unanswered (Laughlin, Barrett-Connor, Kritz-Silverstein, & von Muhlen, 2000; Yialamas & Hayes, 2003; Zumoff, Strain, Miller, & Rosner, 1995).

Physical symptoms that are often described by menopausal women include hot flashes, mood disturbance, weight gain, vaginal dryness, bladder infections, loss of sex drive, fatigue, insomnia, cognitive decline, hair loss, backaches, and joint pain (Hafez & Hafez, 2004; Joffe et al., 2003). Aging effects on the entire reproductive axis contribute to reproductive aging and eventual menopause in women.

Male Reproductive Aging

Neuroendocrine Changes

The male reproductive axis also involves the integration of the hypothalamus and pituitary, but for males the gonads involved are the testes (Sampson, Untegassan, Plas, & Berger, 2007; Schlegel & Hardy, 2002; Yialamas & Hayes, 2003). Similar to the female reproductive axis, the hypothalamus secretes gonadotropin-reducing hormone (GnRH) into the blood. GnRH then travels to the pituitary, where it stimulates the secretion of the gonadotropins FSH and LH (Schlegel & Hardy, 2002; Seidman, 2003). The gonadotropins travel to the testes, where LH stimulates the Leydig cells to produce testosterone while FSH stimulates the Sertoli cells to initiate and maintain sperm production (Schlegel & Hardy, 2002; Seidman, 2003; Yialamas & Hayes, 2003). Sertoli cells, however, have the ability

Case Study 4–1

H. M. is a 72-year-old white woman with a history of osteopenia for the past 4 years and shortness of breath related to 42 years of smoking. She presents today with complaints of painful sexual intercourse and a constant feeling of being cold. Upon questioning, she reports sometimes experiencing dizziness and light-headedness upon standing from a chair; however, she never loses consciousness when standing. She also reports a few episodes of forgetting her two grandchildren's names in the past several months. On evaluation of mental status using the Mini Mental State Exam (MMSE) she scores a 26. On physical examination, she has a blood pressure of 140/89, a weight loss of 6 pounds, and a loss of a 1/2 inch from her height from the previous visit 8 months ago. She reports no discomfort in her back or neck regions. She has no history of stroke, seizure, heart disease, or thyroid disease.

H. M. did not begin hormone therapy at any point during or after menopause by her own choosing. She did begin taking calcium supplements during menopause and within the past 5 years began taking over-the-counter herbal estrogen to self-treat some of her noted symptoms.

Questions:

1. What steps would you take to address H.M.'s chief complaints for today's visit?
2. List possible laboratory tests, therapeutic options, and recommendations for the patient during this visit.
3. Would you address other existing issues or would you reevaluate at the next visit?
4. List potential areas that will be noted for continuing evaluation and possible future treatment.

to suppress FSH secretion via inhibin B (Schlegel & Hardy, 2002). In males, a negative feedback system among the testes, the hypothalamus, and the pituitary controls the rate of sperm production and testosterone release. This is demonstrated by the relationship between FSH and Sertoli cells as well as by the effect of testosterone on GnRH and gonadotropin secretion (Schlegel & Hardy, 2002; Seidman, 2003; Yialamas & Hayes, 2003). Testosterone is the most available androgen in the male reproductive system, with secretory bursts occurring around six times per day (Partin & Rodriguez, 2002; Seidman, 2003). Testosterone binds to androgen receptors located in the brain and spinal cord, activating cellular mechanisms that influence androgen-dependent tissues (Seidman, 2003).

Age-related changes to the male reproductive axis include increases in FSH and LH levels, decreases in both serum and bioavailable testosterone levels, and a decline in Leydig cell function (Kandeel, Koussa, & Swerdloff, 2001; Morley et al., 1997; Sampson et al., 2007; Schlegel & Hardy, 2002). Testosterone levels in men decline with age, but can show variability from small decreases to major decreases depending on health status (Seidman, 2003). As testosterone levels decline in older males, the amount of estrogen remains stable, leading to a decline in the testosterone-to-estrogen ratio (Kandeel et al., 2001). A decline in testosterone is often associated with decreases in libido, spontaneous erections, sexual desire, and sexual thoughts (Seidman, 2003).

Male System Changes

The Testes

In aging, the testes decrease in both size and weight, but with high variability among men (Digiovanna, 2000; Hurd, 2014). The Leydig cells decrease in number but not in structure. In addition, these cells decrease their production of testosterone (Digiovanna, 2000; Hurd, 2014); Yialamas & Hayes, 2003). In contrast, the small amount of estrogen secreted by the testes does not decline with age, nor does the estrogen that is aromatized from androstenedione. As a result, the ratio of estrogen to testosterone increases in older males (Partin & Rodriguez, 2002). In stages over time, the seminiferous tubules show thinning of the walls and narrowing of lumen, known as sclerosis (Hurd, 2014). The lumen can become so narrow that the tubules become blocked (Digiovanna, 2000). Other dynamics that may contribute to or enhance the aging of the structure and function of the seminiferous tubules include decreased blood flow and changes in testosterone production (Digiovanna, 2000). Although a decline in sperm production occurs in aging males, the production never ceases, so the older male remains fertile (Digiovanna, 2000; Hurd, 2014).

Glands

The seminal vesicles and the bulbourethral glands demonstrate no age-related changes (Digiovanna, 2000). However, the biggest concern in older males is changes in the prostate gland. The lining and muscle layer of the prostate gland become thinner with age, probably due to the reduced blood flow to the area (Digiovanna, 2000). BPH, which is dependent on age and androgen production, remains very common in aging males, with approximately 50% of men experiencing nodules by age 60 and around 90% by age 85 (Hollander & Diokno, 2007; Hurd, 2014; Letran & Brawer, 1999). By age 60, approximately 13% of males will be diagnosed with clinical BPH that requires medical attention. By age 85, this percentage has increased to 23% (Letran & Brawer, 1999). BPH causes the prostate to grow very large, which may result in urethral blockages (Hafez & Hafez, 2004; Hollander & Diokno, 2007). Common complaints with BPH include increased frequency and discomfort with urination, bladder and kidney infections, and erectile and ejaculatory dysfunction (Hafez & Hafez, 2004; Hollander & Diokno, 2007; Paick et al., 2005; Rosen et al., 2003).

The Penis

The penis begins to show fibrous changes in erectile tissue around the urethra starting in the 30s and 40s. By ages 55–60 years, increased fibrosis occurs in all erectile tissues (Digiovanna, 2000). This fibrosis in erectile tissue causes an increase in the amount of time it takes to achieve an erection in the older male; however, the ability to have an erection is maintained with age and is usually most affected by medication or disease (Digiovanna, 2000; Kandeel et al., 2001). In addition to the increase in time to obtain an erection, older males also require more stimulation to maintain the erection, experience less intense orgasms and ejaculation, have decreased ejaculatory volume, and undergo a longer refractory period following ejaculation (Kandeel et al., 2001; Schlegel & Hardy, 2002).

Andropause

Andropause is classified as a decline and eventual deficiency in testosterone levels significant enough to cause clinical symptoms (American Society for Reproductive Medicine [ASRM] Practice Committee, 2004; Hafez & Hafez, 2004; Yialamas & Hayes, 2003). Unlike menopause, andropause occurs gradually over time and does not occur in all aging males (Hafez & Hafez, 2004). A decline in the functional ability of the entire reproductive axis causes decreased production of testosterone in aging males (Yialamas & Hayes, 2003). When testosterone is produced in the adult male it stimulates negative feedback of GnRH, FSH, and LH secretion. In the older adult male this negative feedback is enhanced (Yialamas & Hayes, 2003). During andropause, when testosterone becomes extremely low, a recovery mechanism triggers increases in FSH and LH in an attempt to elevate testosterone levels (Hafez & Hafez, 2004). Androgen deficiency in the aging male (ADAM) includes symptoms of low libido; decreased energy, strength, and stamina; increased irritability; and cognitive changes (ASRM Practice Committee, 2004; Janowsky, Oviatt, & Orwoll, 1994; Korenman et al., 1990; Sternbach, 1998; van den Beld, de Jong, Grobbee, Pols, & Lamberts, 2000; Yialamas & Hayes, 2003). Physiological symptoms of ADAM include erectile dysfunction, osteopenia, osteoporosis, breast enlargement, decreased muscle mass, shrinkage of the testes, and increased fat deposition (ASRM Practice Committee, 2004; Greendale, Edelstein, & Barrett-Connor, 1997; Hafez & Hafez, 2004; Turner & Wass, 1997; Vermeulen, Goemaere, & Kaufman, 1999; Yialamas & Hayes, 2003). Diagnosis of andropause generally occurs via measurement of total serum testosterone levels; however, measures of the true testosterone level should be based on total testosterone and testosterone metabolites as well as androgen receptor activity (Yialamas & Hayes, 2003).

Although the hypothalamus-pituitary-gonadal axis controls both male and female reproductive systems, the age-related changes in the axis and the physiological effects are very diverse. All males and females experience age-related changes in the reproductive system; however, these changes occur with tremendous variability among individuals.

The Nervous System

Introduction to the Nervous System

The two components of the nervous system, central and peripheral, have the potential to affect the entire body through continual communication via nerve innervations and signals. As a person ages, natural changes occur in the nervous systems that can have direct or indirect effects on the rest of the body. The central nervous system (CNS) consists of the brain and the spinal cord; the peripheral nervous system encompasses the motor and sensory neurons located in the sensory-somatic system and the autonomic system (see **Figure 4-11**). The *autonomic nervous system* consists of the motor and sensory neurons that maintain homeostasis within the body. It can be further divided into the parasympathetic and sympathetic systems. Communication among the brain, spinal cord, and peripheral nerves is responsible for maintenance of homeostasis. This communication process within the nervous system and between organ systems and the nervous system is demonstrated in **Figure 4-12**.

The process of aging in the nervous system could lead to profound effects on other organ systems, considering the constant communication that occurs. Any change in the nervous system has the potential to influence the stability of the entire body, even if minimally. In this section, the age-related changes that occur in the brain, spinal cord, and peripheral nerves will be discussed.

The Aging Brain

The human brain goes through many developmental changes throughout a person's lifespan. Aging should still be considered on a developmental scale, not a decrement scale. Although brain changes do occur as humans grow older, one should not assume that cognitive function will automatically decline. Memory changes can be observed by the fifth decade, but changes remain variable among individuals (**Box 4-1**). There is also great variation in the type of memory affected (Erickson & Barnes, 2003).

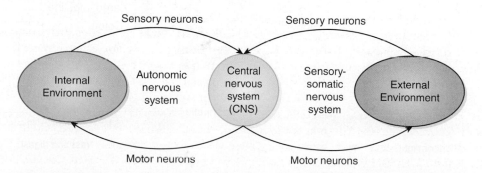

Figure 4-11 The central nervous system and the peripheral nervous system have a constant feedback loop between each system as well as the external and internal environments.

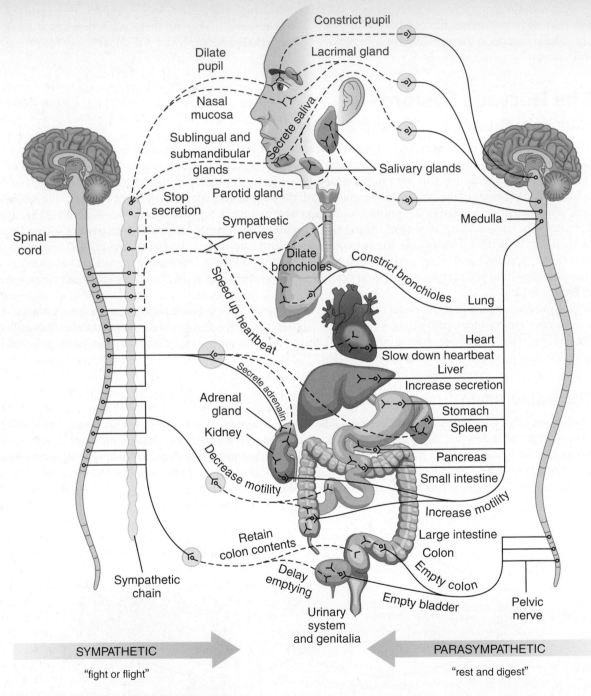

Figure 4-12 The autonomic nervous system.

BOX 4-1   Research Highlight

Hötting, Reich, Holzschneider, Kauschke, Schmidt, Reer, Braumann, and Röder have studied the impact of exercise, namely cardiovascular exercise, on brain function and cognition in older adults. Observing exercise patterns at a baseline and over a 6-month period of exercising two times per week, they arrived at an interesting finding. Sign into your database of nursing literature (CINAHL or PubMed, for example) and use the citation below to perform a search for this article. What were the results of this study? Why is this important in the care of older adults?

Hötting, K., Reich, B., Holzschneider, K., Kauschke, K., Schmidt, T., Reer, R., Braumann, K. M., & Röder, B. (2012). Differential cognitive effects of cycling versus stretching/coordination training in middle-aged adults. *Health Psychology, 31*(2), 145–155.

Overall Structural Changes

The brain decreases in size and weight as men and women age (Arking, 1998; Digiovanna, 1994; Minaker, 2011). At birth, the brain weighs approximately 357 grams; brain weight peaks at about 1,300 grams around the age of 20 years. This weight is maintained until 55 years of age, after which the brain weight begins to decline (Arking, 1998). This decline can result in a brain weight that is 11% smaller than that observed in the young adult brain (Arking, 1998); however, measurements of brain weight may show bias due to individual differences in head size and body weight. Measuring changes in individual brain volume helps diffuse this inherent bias. Brain volume appears to be stable from ages 20–60, followed by a significant decline of between 5% and 10% (Arking, 1998; Minaker, 2011). Magnetic resonance imaging (MRI) studies have demonstrated that, compared to women, men demonstrate greater age-related volume loss in the brain as a whole as well as in the temporal and frontal lobes specifically (Leon-Carrion, Salgado, Sierra, Marquez-Rivas, & Dominguez-Morales, 2001; Murphy, DeCarli, Schapiro, Rapoport, & Horwitz, 1992). In the same MRI study, researchers showed that women had a greater loss of volume in the hippocampus and parietal lobes than that observed in men. From ages 30–90 years both men and women experience a volume loss of 14% in the cerebral cortex, 35% in the hippocampus, and 26% in the cerebral white matter (Anderton, 2002; Raz et al., 2005). Ventricles within the brain enlarge throughout the aging process, such that ventricle size at age 90 may be as much as three to four times ventricle size at age 20. Ventricle enlargement may help explain some loss of brain volume (Arking, 1998; Beers & Berkow, n.d.; Digiovanna, 1994). Although the ventricles on the inside of the brain enlarge, the gyri—raised ridges on the surface of the brain—shrink, and the sulci—grooves between the gyri—become wider (Digiovanna, 1994).

Neuron Changes

The brain is composed of gray matter and white matter. The gray matter is located on the surface of the brain, known as the cerebral cortex, and contains the nerve cell bodies. The white matter contains no cell bodies or dendrites, but is strictly myelinated nerve fibers (Arking, 1998). **Figure 4-13** demonstrates the composition of a nerve cell and fibers. The average number of neocortical neurons is 19 billion in female brains and 23 billion in male brains, a 16% difference. A study by Pakkenberg and Gundersen (1997) that focused on neuron numbers in 20- to 90-year-old individuals showed that approximately 10% of all neocortical neurons are lost over the lifespan in both sexes. Cell loss remains minimal in some parts of the brain, whereas other areas show tremendous neuron

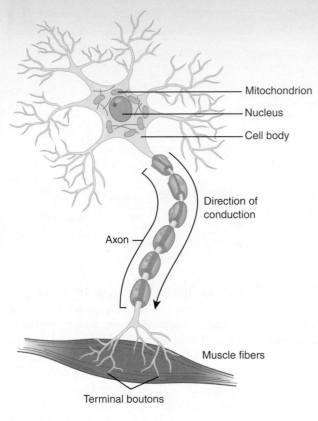

Mitochondrion

Nucleus

Cell body

Direction of
conduction

Axon

Muscle fibers

Terminal boutons

Figure 4-13 A neuron.

decrease (Katzman, 1995). According to Beers and Berkow (n.d.), neuronal cell loss remains minimal in the brainstem nuclei, paraventricular nuclei, and supraoptic nuclei, whereas losses in other areas can be great: 10–60% in the hippocampus, 55% in the superior temporal gyrus, and 10–35% in the temporal lobe. However, anatomical studies have not shown any statistically significant age-related change in neuron numbers in the hippocampus, the primary center for learning and memory (Erickson & Barnes, 2003). Unlike previous studies, these more recent anatomical studies have taken into account age-related tissue shrinkage and have utilized better-controlled stereological methods in making the determination that no neuronal decreases occur (Anderton, 2002; Peters, 2002).

Other sources describe a significant decline of neurons in the cerebrum, which controls voluntary movement, vision, hearing, and other senses. Only a minimal neuronal loss is seen in the cerebellar cortex and the basal ganglia, which are responsible for muscle movement and control (Digiovanna, 1994, 2000). The brainstem demonstrates some loss of neurons in the nucleus of Meynert (acetylcholine production) and the locus coeruleus (norepinephrine production), which aids in sleep regulation (Digiovanna, 1994, 2000).

Early reports of neuron loss should be considered carefully because more recent studies have used more carefully controlled human tissue samples, study design, and neuron counting techniques (Peters, 2002). A loss of neurons in the aging brain occurs, but not to the extent that researchers have reported in the past (Morrison & Hof, 1997; Peters, 2002; Peters, Morrison, Rosene, & Hyman, 1998). The myelin sheath, which surrounds the axon on every neuron and promotes faster electrical signaling along each neuron, breaks down in aging (Bartzokis et al., 2004; Dickson, 1997; Peters, 2002). Myelination of the axon appears to continue until middle age, followed by a breakdown in the structural integrity of the myelin (Bartzokis et al., 2004; Dickson, 1997). This degradation of myelin may cause neuronal disruption by slowing the nerve impulses as they travel through the nervous system. This may help to explain mild age-related declines in cognition and motor control (Dickson, 1997).

The loss of a neuron or a decrease in neuron participation causes disruption of neural circuits and hence neural signaling. Dendrites serve as the system through which nerve impulses are relayed to the neuron. The synapse serves as the messenger system between dendrites. **Figure 4-14** demonstrates how a synapse works to relay chemical messages between neurons. The number of dendrites and dendritic spines decreases with age, but this change is not uniformly distributed in the brain (Arking, 1998). Several human studies focusing on synapse change in different areas of the brain throughout the lifespan have shown no significant changes (Scheff, Price, & Sparks, 2001). However, synapse loss has been shown in multiple brain areas in postmortem AD tissue when compared to control tissue (Lippa, Hamos, Pulaski, Degennaro, & Drachman, 1992; Scheff & Price, 1998, 2001; Scheff, Sparks, & Price, 1996).

The brain demonstrates remarkable compensatory mechanisms to recover from loss, even in old age. *Plasticity*, or the ability to lengthen and/or form new neuronal connections onto available existing neurons, is one of these compensatory mechanisms (Beers & Berkow, n.d.; Digiovanna, 1994, 2000). Plasticity can occur through many avenues, including *neurogenesis*, *synaptogenesis*, synaptic alteration, synaptic efficacy, long-term potentiation, axon sprouting, and dendrite transformation (Teter & Ashford, 2002). An example of synaptic alteration is the ability of the *synapses* to broaden and cover more surface area, possibly compensating for synapse loss in some brain regions (Digiovanna, 1994, 2000; Terry, DeTeresa, & Hansen, 1987). In aging or injury, new neuronal connections specifically compensate for the loss of neurons in certain brain areas to aid in preservation of function (Beers & Berkow, n.d.). Plasticity does diminish with age, but is not completely lost. Aging effects include a decrease in long-term potentiation and synaptogenesis in addition to delays in axon sprouting, which in turn affect the formation of new connections (Teter & Ashford, 2002).

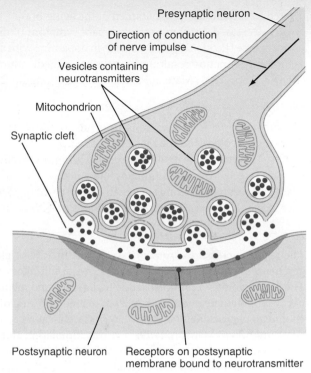

Figure 4-14 A synapse and synaptic transmission.

Neurotransmitter Changes

A *neurotransmitter* is a chemical messenger encapsulated in synaptic vesicles that is released from the axon into the synaptic space and onto corresponding receptors on the postsynaptic neuron. Neurotransmitter changes during the aging process can influence memory and cognition as well as behavior and motor function.

Cholinergic

Cholinergic neurons, which release the neurotransmitter acetylcholine, play a significant role in learning and memory in humans and animals (Arking, 1998; Mattson, 1999). Acetylcholine induces learning and memory via cholinergic input to the hippocampus and neocortex in the brain (Kelly & Roth, 1997; Mattson, 1999). With age, acetylcholine synthesis and release from synaptic vesicles begin to decline. The postsynaptic acetylcholine receptors, known as nicotinic and muscarinic receptors, and transport of choline also demonstrate age-related deficits (Beers & Berkow, n.d.; Kelly & Roth, 1997; Mattson, 1999). In AD these cholinergic deficits are more pronounced, which led to the development of acetylcholinesterase inhibitor medications now on the market to treat the disease. The objective of the medication is to decrease the degradation of acetylcholine in the synaptic space, thereby increasing the amount of acetylcholine available to bind with postsynaptic receptors.

Dopaminergic

The *dopaminergic system* involves the neurotransmitter dopamine, mainly in the substantia nigra and striatum (Arking, 1998). In aging, dopamine levels decrease by around 10% per decade, and dopamine transport in the neuron also diminishes (Katzman, 1995; Mattson, 1999; Peters, 2006). Age-related changes are also found in dopamine receptors, and the ability of dopamine to bind to postsynaptic receptors also decreases (Katzman, 1995; Mattson, 1999). Positron emission tomography (PET) studies have shown a decline in dopamine receptors located in the caudate and putamen of the aging brain (Mozaz & Monguio, 2001). In PD, dopamine levels are greatly decreased, leading to the hallmark symptom of diminished motor control and compromised cognitive performance (Peters, 2006). Decreases in dopamine with age may explain some age-related motor deficits as well as motor dysfunction resulting from the use of medications targeting the dopaminergic neurotransmitter system (Kelly & Roth, 1997; Mattson, 1999; Mozaz & Monguio, 2001; Volkow et al., 1998).

Monoaminergic

The *monoaminergic system* consists mainly of the neurotransmitters norepinephrine and serotonin located in the locus coeruleus and the raphe nucleus (brainstem), respectively (Arking, 1998; Kelly & Roth, 1997; Mattson, 1999). Norepinephrine tends to increase with age in certain brain regions, but corresponding receptors have been shown to decrease in both humans and animals (Gruenewald & Matsumoto, 1999; Mattson, 1999). Serotonin levels and receptor binding sites both decrease with age, which may play a role in depression and sleep changes later in life (Mattson, 1999; Mattson, Maudsley, & Martin, 2004; Ramos-Platon & Beneto-Pascual, 2001).

Amino Acid Transmitters

The *amino acid neurotransmitters* consist mainly of glutamate, the major excitatory neurotransmitter, and gamma-aminobutyric acid (GABA), the major inhibitory neurotransmitter (Kelly & Roth, 1997; Mattson, 1999). The hippocampus, a central location for learning and memory, contains high levels of glutamate. This relationship between glutamate and memory leads to a questioning of the idea that memory decline is tied solely to acetyl-choline depletion (Kelly & Roth, 1997). Glutamate receptors decline with age, but the change in glutamate with age is unknown (Mattson, 1999). The overstimulation and release of glutamate may be significant in AD, PD, and Huntington's disease, as well as stroke (Mattson, 1999). GABA concentrates in the brain areas of the substantia nigra and the globus pallidus (Kelly & Roth, 1997). Age-related changes in the GABA neurotransmitter are unknown; however, decreases in GABA have been correlated with aggressive behavior (Jimenez, Cuartero, & Moreno, 2001; Mattson, 1999). GABA can synthesize glutamate, which can convert to GABA via the enzyme glutamic acid decarboxylase (Gluck, Thomas, Davis, & Haroutunian, 2002). So, changes in glutamate could have a direct or indirect effect on GABA in the aging brain and vice versa.

Neuroendocrine Changes

Age-related changes to neuroendocrine functioning affect many other systems in the body. **Figure 4-15** demonstrates body systems that are controlled and/or affected by changes in neuroendocrine functioning, with an emphasis on the pituitary gland. Aging changes in secretion of hypothalamic-releasing hormone are studied indirectly by observing changes in pituitary secretion response to hypothalamic-releasing hormone, to chemicals that block feedback mechanisms, and to chemicals that stimulate the release of hypothalamic-pituitary hormone (Gruenewald & Matsumoto, 2009). One example of a neuroendocrine age-related change is in the reproductive axis, or the hypothalamic-pituitary-gonadal axis, that controls the regulation of male and female hormones (Chakraborty & Gore, 2004; Hall, 2004). (Refer to "The Reproductive System" earlier in this chapter for further discussion of age-related neuroendocrine function of gonadal hormones.)

Another example is the *hypothalamic-pituitary-adrenal (HPA) axis* that integrates the endocrine, immune, and nervous systems. This integration allows for great adaptability (Ferrari et al., 2001). The HPA axis regulates glucocorticoid levels in the body and allows the body to respond to stressful conditions (Ferrari et al., 2001; Gruenewald & Matsumoto, 2009). Age changes in the negative feedback system of glucocorticoids on the HPA axis may cause glucocorticoids to circulate for longer periods. Consequently, damage may occur to hippocampal neurons needed for cognitive function (Gruenewald & Matsumoto, 1999).

In the CNS, the neurotransmitters dopamine and norepinephrine affect hypothalamic and pituitary hormone release, and with age these neurotransmitters cause changes in hormone secretions (Gruenewald & Matsumoto, 2009). Hypothalamic neurons release dopamine, which inhibits prolactin release from the pituitary. Prolactin

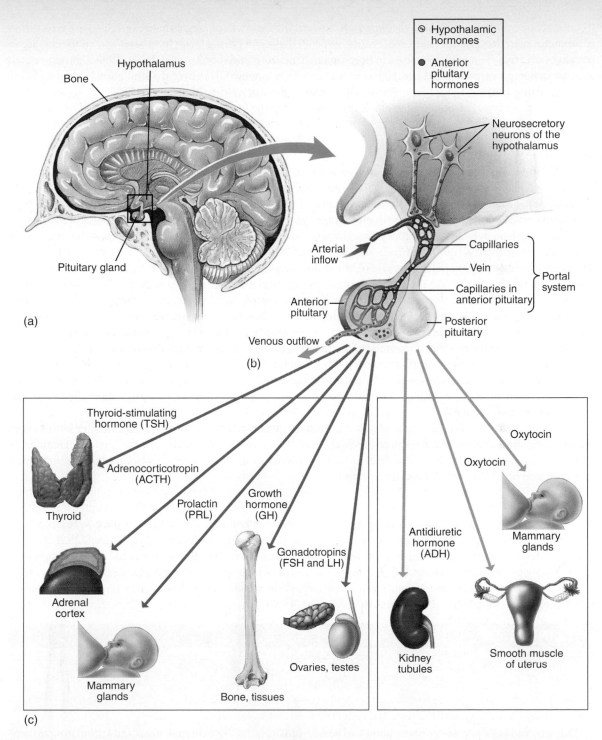

Hypothalamic hormones
Anterior pituitary hormones

Hypothalamus
Bone
Neurosecretory neurons of the hypothalamus

Arterial inflow
Capillaries
Vein
Capillaries in anterior pituitary
Portal system
Anterior pituitary
Posterior pituitary
Pituitary gland
Venous outflow

(a)
(b)

Thyroid-stimulating hormone (TSH)
Oxytocin
Adrenocorticotropin (ACTH)
Oxytocin
Thyroid
Prolactin (PRL)
Growth hormone (GH)
Mammary glands
Antidiuretic hormone (ADH)
Gonadotropins (FSH and LH)
Adrenal cortex
Mammary glands
Bone, tissues
Ovaries, testes
Kidney tubules
Smooth muscle of uterus

(c)

Figure 4-15 The pituitary gland.

stimulates dopaminergic neurons in the hypothalamus, but with age dopaminergic changes can lead to deregulation of prolactin secretion (Gruenewald & Matsumoto, 2009). Norepinephrine levels have been shown to increase in certain brain areas even with a decrease in noradrenergic neurons and receptors (Mattson, 1999). An age-related increase in norepinephrine could affect the release of growth hormone (GH), thyroid-stimulating hormone (TSH), and luteinizing hormone (LH) from the pituitary gland (Gruenewald & Matsumoto, 2009). Neuroendocrine changes with age have the potential to affect many systems in the body via hormone alterations. These changes are an example of how the nervous system plays an integral role in every aspect of the human body.

Vascular Changes

Cerebral blood flow decreases with age, reportedly by an average of 20%. Decreased blood flow is accompanied by decreased glucose utilization and metabolic rate of oxygen in the brain (Arking, 1998; Beers & Berkow, n.d.; Dickson, 1997; Mattson, 1999). According to Katzman (1995), the National Institute of Mental Health longitudinal study revealed that individuals with an average age of 70 years were comparable in cerebral blood flow to individuals with an average age of 20.8 years. However, an 11-year follow-up showed that the older cognitively intact participants had a significant reduction in cerebral blood flow, leading to the conclusion that the eighth decade of life was a turning point. The rate of blood flow in women decreases slightly more rapidly than in men; however, blood flow is usually greater in women than in men until age 60 (Beers & Berkow, n.d.). Potential explanations for decreased cerebral blood flow include cerebrovascular disease, structural changes in cerebral blood vessels, and neuron loss accompanied by a reduction in blood flow need (de la Torre, 1997). Cerebral blood vessels display less elasticity and increased fibrosis, which may lead to increased vascular resistance (Mattson, 1999).

The blood–brain barrier shows age-related degradation of capillary walls. This degradation affects the ability of nutrients such as glucose and oxygen to nourish the brain (Arking, 1998; de la Torre, 1997; Mattson, 1999). In conjunction with the inability to effectively nourish the brain, changes in capillaries could also prevent waste by-products from effectively exiting the blood–brain barrier, in turn causing a build-up of potentially neurotoxic substances (de la Torre, 1997).

A number of studies have associated increased lesions in myelinated areas, known as white matter lesions, with increased cerebrovascular risk, a reduced cerebral blood flow, and loss of vascular density (Artero, Tiemeier, & Prins, 2004; Atwood et al., 2004; Moody et al., 2004). It remains unclear, however, whether these lesions are a causative step or a result of the vascular compromise.

Plaques and Tangles

Neurofibrillary tangles and beta-amyloid plaques are considered hallmarks of AD (see **Figure 4-16**), but both also can be found in older individuals without evidence of dementia (Anderton, 2002; Beers & Berkow, n.d.; Dickson, 1997; Schmitt et al., 2000) (see **Box 4-2**). *Plaques* occur outside of the neuronal cell and consist of gray matter with a protein core surrounded by abnormal neurites (Anderton, 2002). Each plaque consists of a core of protein, with the dominant protein being amyloid beta-peptide, which is formulated from a larger protein known as amyloid precursor protein (Anderton, 2002; Dickson, 1997).

CLINICAL TIP

The Nun Study suggested that the phenomenon of idea density was a factor in whether the nuns in the study manifested the signs and symptoms of AD, even in those whose brains showed the characteristic plaques and tangles.

This amyloid beta-peptide has been shown to be neurotoxic, inducing oxidative stress and stimulating inflammatory processes (Mattson, 1999). However, in the aging brain, plaques are disseminated, unlike in the AD brain, where plaques are very numerous and dense (Dickson, 1997).

Normal   **Alzheimer's**

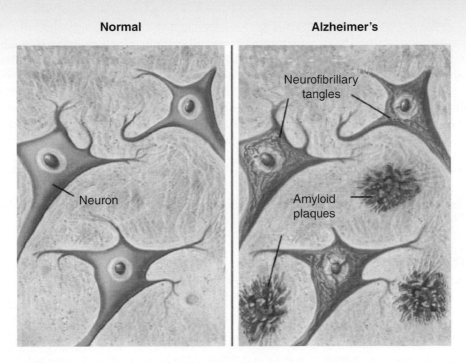

Figure 4-16 The difference between control and AD tissue in relation to amyloid plaques and neurofibrillary tangles. Plaques and tangles can be present in control tissue with no signs of memory problems.
Image courtesy of: Alzheimer's Disease Research, a program of BrightFocus Foundation. www.brightfocus.org/alzheimers

---

BOX 4-2   Web Exploration

Explore the findings from the Nun Study, which provide some unique insight into the development and manifestations of AD. Go to http://www.mc .uky.edu/nunnet/ and follow the links, or visit

http://www.mc.uky.edu/nunnet/AWGExcerpt.htm to read an excerpt from *Aging with Grace*, a book about the Nun Study by David Snowdon (2001).

Neurofibrillary *tangles* occur in the neuronal cell body and consist of paired helical filaments and a few straight filaments (Anderton, 2002; Dickson, 1997). The main protein associated with neurofibrillary tangles is known as tau, a phosphoprotein that supports microtubule stability (Binder, Guillozet-Bongaarts, Garcia-Sierra, & Berry, 2005; Dickson, 1997). In neurofibrillary tangles, tau protein undergoes abnormal phosphorylation and increases in density (Dickson, 1997). In aging, tangles are found in very low numbers and usually concentrate in areas of the entorhinal cortex, hippocampus, and amygdala (Anderton, 2002; Dickson, 1997; Mattson, 1999). In the aged brain, the greatest density of tangles appears in the entorhinal cortex, whereas in the AD brain plaques spread throughout the entire cortex (Dickson, 1997).

Free Radicals

A *free radical* is a molecule with an unpaired electron in the outer shell of electrons that remains unstable until paired with another molecule (Mattson, 1999). In humans, oxygen is the major molecule in the generation of free radicals. Although the brain makes up only 2% of total body weight, it consumes around 20% of the total oxygen uptake (Benzi & Moretti, 1997; Tortora & Derrickson, 2014). In the cell, mitochondria continuously emit oxygen free radicals during the electron transport process, which manifests oxidative stress and can cause oxidative damage (Benzi & Moretti, 1997; Mattson, 1999; Sohal, Mockett, & Orr, 2002). Antioxidants and repair mechanisms for oxidative stress in biological systems are covered under the oxidative stress hypothesis (see Chapter 3). Oxygen free radicals, or oxyradicals, continually increase and accumulate with age, causing oxidative damage to lipids, proteins, and DNA in human tissue, including the brain (Mattson, 1999; Sohal et al., 2002). Oxidative damage to proteins, such as cell membrane proteins, could be highly significant in brain aging. Such damage can result in loss of structural integrity and subsequent cell dysfunction and neuron degeneration (Mattson, 1999; Sohal et al., 2002). Nuclear DNA in the nervous system does not incur much oxidative damage in aging; however, oxidative damage is tremendous in mitochondrial DNA because mitochondria are the main source of free radical production (Mattson, 1999). A decrease in available cell energy and impairment in cell metabolism could be mechanisms in promoting free radical production with age (Mattson, 1999; Sohal et al., 2002).

The Aging Spinal Cord

Cells

Overall, the number of spinal cord cells remains stable until around age 60 and then declines thereafter (Beers & Berkow, n.d.; Digiovanna, 1994). Interneuron loss in the lower spinal cord has been reported. Neuron decrements of up to 25% to 45% are observed in those neurons of the spinal layer that correlate to the cerebral cortex (Arking, 1998).

Nerve Conduction

According to Abrams, Beers, and Berkow (1995), the aging spine may narrow due to pressure on the spinal cord resulting from bone overgrowth. Because of this narrowing, spinal cord axons decrease and can eventually cause changes in sensation. However, these effects may be correlated not only with age, but also with degenerative disease processes or compression of spinal disks that clamp nerves (Beers & Berkow, n.d.). An MRI study by Ishikawa, Matsumoto, Fujimura, Chiba, and Toyama (2003) focused on age-associated changes of the cervical spinal cord and spinal canal. These researchers concluded that the transverse area of the cervical spinal cord decreased with age and the spinal canal narrowed with age. These aging changes may directly or indirectly affect motor control and/or sensory systems in the body.

The Aging Peripheral Nervous System

The peripheral nervous system contains approximately 100 billion *nerve cells*. These cells form nerve fibers that cascade throughout the body, connecting the CNS to the rest of the body. Hence, these cells work as a relay messenger system (Abrams et al., 1995). The *somatic* nervous system connects the brain and spinal cord to skeletal muscles and sensory receptors. The autonomic nervous system regulates organ function through activation of nervous system response and inhibition of parasympathetic response (Abrams et al., 1995). See Figure 4-12 for a diagram of the autonomic pathway of the peripheral nervous system. Nerve conduction speed slows with age as a result of the degradation of the myelin sheaths that coat axons (Bartzokis et al., 2004; Beers & Berkow, n.d.; Mozaz & Monguio, 2001; Peters, 2002). In addition, calcium modulation appears to be functionally compromised with advancing age. Calcium is a key regulator of nervous signaling, from excitability to neurotransmitter release. Calcium's dysregulation also has been implicated in loss of cell viability in nervous tissue (Buchholz, Behringer, Pottorf, Pearce, & Vanterpool, 2007). Changes in motor speed, such as reaction times to stimuli, and changes in sensory abilities, such as changes in taste or smell, may be explained by these age-related changes in the peripheral nervous system.

Sensory Neurons

Sensory neuron function declines with age, leading to alterations in reflexes and voluntary actions and influencing certain quality of life areas such as memories, thoughts, and emotion (Digiovanna, 1994, 2000). The sense of touch changes with age due to changes in the touch receptors, or Meissner's corpuscles, and the pressure receptors, or Pacinian corpuscles. However, only small changes in sensory neurons related to touch are observed (Digiovanna, 1994, 2000). Sensory neurons for smell, or olfactory neurons, decrease with age, causing a lessened ability to detect and identify certain smells. This dampened ability could affect eating habits and, due to the inability to detect toxic fumes, also may place older adults in potentially dangerous situations (Digiovanna, 1994, 2000). The sense of taste involves the flavors of salty, sweet, sour, bitter, and umami. Aging changes occur on an individual basis, usually affecting salty and bitter flavors, with salty flavors declining the most (Digiovanna, 1994, 2000). However, the sense of smell also may play a significant role in the age-related changes in taste. This may occur because of the strong link between certain food aromas and taste expectations. The sense of taste has a rapid compensatory response to injury, such as burning the tongue with hot food, and even aging. This compensatory response is characterized by replacement of taste receptors and sensory neurons (Digiovanna, 1994, 2000). Other sensory neurons that decline with age affect the monitoring of blood pressure, thirst, urine in the bladder, and fecal matter in the intestine and rectum. Bone, joint, and muscle position and function are also affected by age-related changes in sensory neurons (Digiovanna, 1994, 2000).

Somatic Motor Neurons

With age, there is a decrease in the number of motor neurons. As a result, there is a reduction in the number of muscle cells and consequent muscle degeneration and weakness (Digiovanna, 1994, 2000). Age changes in the remaining motor neurons include myelin breakdown and cell membrane damage. These changes lead to a slower relay of messages, which in turn alters the ability of the muscle to contract and relax (Bartzokis et al., 2004; Digiovanna, 1994, 2000). Changes in both sensory and motor peripheral nerve pathways cause voluntary movements to become slower, less accurate, and less coordinated with age (Digiovanna, 1994). These aging changes that affect muscle strength and movement abilities can be lessened with daily exercise aimed at increasing and retaining the performance of remaining muscle.

Autonomic Motor Neurons

Aging causes changes to both the sympathetic and parasympathetic pathways to organ systems. One example of these changes is seen in the body's response to changes in blood pressure. When blood pressure drops too low, sympathetic neurons usually help to increase blood pressure by stimulating the heart and constricting blood vessels. However, with age the sympathetic response is delayed, causing low blood pressure and subsequent orthostatic hypotension. When blood pressure rises, the parasympathetic pathway helps slow the heart rate, but this function declines with age, resulting in elevated blood pressure as well as a decrease in the time required to return to homeostasis (Digiovanna, 1994, 2000). Autonomic neuron age-related changes also can affect thermoregulation. The sympathetic pathway normally acts to constrict blood vessels, thereby preventing heat loss in cold conditions. However, with age there is a decline in this action and this decline, together with age-related changes in blood vessels, results in increased risk of hypothermia (Digiovanna, 1994, 2000). Other age-related changes in the autonomic pathway that affect vision, swallowing, and sexual arousal will be covered in other sections of this chapter.

Injury Responsiveness

Throughout life, peripheral nerve injury is usually repaired through new axon growth and nerve reinnervation of the damaged area, but age decreases these reparative properties (Beers & Berkow, n.d.). These changes in the peripheral nervous system cause older individuals to become slower in detecting and recognizing stimuli, thereby making actions and reactions more difficult (Digiovanna, 1994).

The nervous system remains the most integral organ system in the body due to its influence on every other organ system. Age-related changes that occur at the central and peripheral nerve levels can directly and indirectly influence the homeostasis of the entire body. When observing an age-related change in the older adult, professionals need to broaden their scope of observation to integrate other body systems so that they may better understand the aging changes in the person as a whole.

The Endocrine System

The endocrine system consists of various glands, groups of cells that produce and secrete chemical messengers known as hormones. *Hormones* transfer information from one set of cells to another as they work to maintain overall homeostasis and regulate the body's growth, metabolism, and sexual development and function. The major glands comprising the endocrine system are the hypothalamus, pituitary gland, thyroid, parathyroids, pineal gland, adrenal glands, and the reproductive glands (ovaries and testes). The pancreas, together with its hormones, is also considered part of the endocrine system. Age-related changes to the endocrine system as a whole are best presented through individual discussion of the glands, their hormones, and the functions they perform.

The Hypothalamus and Pituitary Gland

The hypothalamus is a collection of cells located in the lower, central portion of the brain, and it provides a link between the nervous system and endocrine system. Nerves within the hypothalamus produce *hypophysiotropic* hormones that either stimulate or suppress the secretion of hormones from the pituitary gland. Thus, the hypothalamus acts primarily as a mechanism of control for pituitary hormone secretion. The hypothalamus provides hormonal messages to the pituitary, which in turn produces and secretes its own hormones.

The pituitary gland, only the size of a pea, is located just below the hypothalamus at the base of the brain. It is often termed the "master gland" because it produces hormones that regulate numerous other endocrine glands. These regulatory hormones include GH, *vasopressin*, thyrotropin, and corticotropin. GH and vasopressin will be discussed here, and thyrotropin and corticotropin will be discussed with the thyroid and adrenal glands, respectively.

Growth Hormone

Growth hormone (GH) is released from the pituitary gland in response to GH-releasing hormone (GRH) secreted by the hypothalamus. GH stimulates the uptake of amino acids into cells and the synthesis of proteins from these amino acids. In so doing, it promotes the growth of bone, muscle, and other body tissues. GH also plays a role in the body's handling of nutrients because it causes increased breakdown of fat for energy. In addition, GH is known to act antagonistically to insulin and increase blood sugar levels. (See the discussion of the pancreas and its function later in this chapter.)

Evidence suggests that with advancing age there is a decline in the level of GH. The reason for this observed decline has not been well defined, but may involve changes in the diurnal rhythm of GH secretion or decreases in GRH output from the hypothalamus (Russell-Aulet, Jaffe, Mott-Friberg, & Barkans, 1999). In young adults, GH secretion and blood levels of GH rise during the night, reaching a nocturnal peak during the first 4 hours of sleep (Gersten, 2007), and taper off toward morning, with GH levels reaching a minimum during the day. Results from studies examining age-related changes in GH show an overall decrease in nightly GH secretion as well as a damping of the hormone's nocturnal peak (Prinz, Weitzman, Cunningham, & Karacan, 1983). It is thought that over time the nightly increase in GH secretion may cease completely and become constant at all times (Digiovanna, 1994). Whatever the mechanisms behind it, the age-related decline in GH is of great importance because it contributes to age-associated loss of muscle mass, decreased bone formation, reduced protein synthesis, reduced tissue repair, and decline in immune function (Chahal & Drake, 2007; Gersten, 2007).

Vasopressin

Vasopressin, also known as antidiuretic hormone (ADH), is secreted by neurons that originate in the hypothalamus and extend into the pituitary gland. Vasopressin works to regulate homeostatic levels of osmotic pressure and blood pressure. The release of vasopressin is stimulated by either a decrease in blood pressure or an increase in osmotic pressure. Once secreted, vasopressin promotes water reabsorption by the kidneys. This reabsorption of water prevents increases in the body's osmotic pressure and helps maintain a substantial blood volume, thereby preventing blood pressure from becoming too low. Vasopressin secretion also helps maintain blood pressure by stimulating the constriction of blood vessels. The release of vasopressin is inhibited by increased blood pressure or decreased osmotic pressure, as well as by alcohol. Decreased levels of vasopressin result in the loss of water through the urine, which leads to increases in osmotic pressure as well as decreases in blood volume and blood pressure.

With age there is an average increase in levels of circulating vasopressin. However, this age-related increase does not produce a subsequent rise in water reabsorption as would be expected, possibly due to the loss of vasopressin receptor responsiveness noted in the genitourinary section (Johnson et al., 2003; Gersten, 2007). The reason for this is unclear, but most research suggests that the failure to respond to increased vasopressin levels with increased water reabsorption occurs primarily in individuals with kidney infections or hypertension and, thus, should not be viewed as a usual characteristic of the aging process (Gersten, 2007). In general, age-related changes in vasopressin levels are not known to have significant effects on body homeostasis. Furthermore, the ability of vasopressin to respond appropriately to low blood pressure remains unchanged with age.

The Thyroid Gland

T4 and T3

The *thyroid* is a small, butterfly-shaped gland located in the lower front portion of the neck. The secretion of the thyroid hormones, *thyroxine* (T_4) and *triiodothyronine* (T_3), occurs through collaboration with the hypothalamus and pituitary glands. The hypothalamus produces and secretes thyrotropin-releasing hormone (TRH), which in turn stimulates the secretion of *thyroid-stimulating hormone* (TSH) from the pituitary gland. Finally, TSH stimulates the synthesis and secretion of T_4 and T_3. Utilizing a negative feedback loop, T_4 and T_3 inhibit TSH secretion. Thus, with higher levels of T_4 and T_3, levels of TSH are lower and vice versa. In addition to its role of regulating the T_4 and T_3 levels, TSH acts to maintain the growth and structural integrity of the thyroid gland. An absence or deficit of TSH results in atrophy of the thyroid (P. S. Timiras, 2007).

During the early years of life, the thyroid gland is essential for growth of the whole body and its organs as well as development and maturation of the central nervous system. In adulthood, however, the thyroid functions mainly to regulate the body's metabolic rate. T_4 and T_3 both promote an increase in metabolic rate. Heat is a by-product of the metabolic process and, hence, increased metabolic rate leads to an increase in heat production; this means that the thyroid hormones also act to regulate body temperature. The thyroid gland is not essential for life (P. S. Timiras, 2007); however, without this gland there is a slowing of the metabolic rate, general lethargy, and poor resistance to cold. In contrast, abnormally high levels of the thyroid hormones result in a potentially dangerous elevation of metabolic rate.

As the body ages, thyroid hormone levels decrease slightly yet remain in the lower range of normal. Because there is less negative feedback because of lower T_3 and T_4 levels, the level of TSH increases with age (Tortora & Derrickson, 2014). Borderline abnormal values of T_4, T_3, and TSH are more common in women than men (P. S. Timiras, 2007). However, there is a large degree of variability in these hormone levels among older adults and hormone levels may depend on age, general health, and gender. Yet, in general, the ability of the thyroid and its hormones to provide metabolic and thermal regulation is not impaired with age.

Calcitonin

Most thyroid cells produce T_4 and T_3, but some cells—known as c cells—produce a hormone called calcitonin. *Calcitonin* promotes a decrease in blood calcium by stimulating increased uptake of calcium by bone-forming cells. Conversely, calcitonin inhibits the action of cells involved in the breakdown of bone. Unlike secretion of T_4 and T_3, calcitonin secretion does not involve the hypothalamus or pituitary; instead, its release is regulated by blood calcium levels. High levels of calcium trigger the secretion of calcitonin, which then causes calcium to be removed from the blood, thereby lowering blood calcium levels. The lower calcium levels then feed back and inhibit calcitonin secretion.

Little is known about age-related changes in calcitonin; however, there have been some reports of decreased calcitonin levels with age. Such a decrease would have profound effects on older persons' risk of osteoporosis given the effects of calcitonin on bone formation and breakdown.

The Parathyroid Gland

The *parathyroid gland* consists of groups of cells located on the back of the thyroid gland, and it secretes a hormone known as *parathyroid hormone* (PTH). Parathyroid hormone acts antagonistically to calcitonin, and homeostasis of blood calcium depends heavily on a proper balance between PTH and calcitonin. Parathyroid hormone release is stimulated by low blood calcium levels, whereas elevated calcium levels inhibit PTH secretion. Thus, PTH works to raise blood calcium levels, which it does through a variety of mechanisms including the removal of calcium from bone, the decline of calcium release into the urine by the kidneys, and the activation of vitamin D by the kidneys, which in turn stimulates calcium absorption by the small intestine. Blood levels of PTH increase with aging, possibly due to decreases in calcium intake (Tortora & Derrickson, 2014).

In children and young adults, calcium levels are maintained through the consumption and subsequent intestinal absorption of dietary calcium. At these ages maintenance of blood calcium levels has no effect on bone (P. S. Timiras, 2007). However, in older persons, calcium levels are maintained primarily through calcium reabsorption from bone. The reason for this shift in mechanisms of calcium level regulation is not fully understood. However, it is thought that with age, PTH may have a decreased ability to stimulate production of active vitamin D by the kidneys and/or that active vitamin D may be impaired in its ability to stimulate intestinal absorption of calcium.

The Pineal Gland

The *pineal gland*, a tiny gland located deep within the brain, secretes the hormone melatonin. Secretion of *melatonin* is highly influenced by light properties, including light intensity, length of light exposure, and light wavelength (i.e., color; Digiovanna, 1994). Detection of increased light exposure (day) inhibits melatonin secretion, whereas detection of decreased light exposure (night) stimulates hormone secretion. Hence, blood levels of melatonin follow a diurnal rhythm with hormone levels highest at night and lowest during the day. It is melatonin that synchronizes internal body functions with a day–night cycle that shifts in response to seasonal changes in the length of said day–night cycle (P. S. Timiras, 2007; Tortora & Derrickson, 2014).

Age is accompanied by a decline in melatonin levels. This decline can have a negative impact on other diurnal rhythms such as sleep patterns. Melatonin is known to reach peak concentrations during sleep, and administration of doses of melatonin equivalent to nighttime levels have been shown to promote and sustain sleep (P. S. Timiras, 2007). Thus, age-related declines in melatonin may be linked to the poor sleep quality and insomnia of some elderly persons.

The Adrenal Glands

The *adrenal glands* are paired glands located above the kidneys. Each gland is composed of an outer region known as the adrenal cortex and an inner region known as the adrenal medulla.

The Adrenal Cortex

The *adrenal cortex* secretes three types of hormones: glucocorticoids, mineralocorticoids, and sex hormones. Secretion of both glucocorticoids and sex hormones from the adrenal cortex is stimulated by pituitary *adrenocorticotropic hormone* (ACTH). The secretion of ACTH follows a diurnal rhythm and is itself stimulated by *corticotropin-releasing hormone* (CRH) from the hypothalamus. Thus, release of glucocorticoids and sex hormones from the adrenal cortex relies on the HPA pathway or axis.

Glucocorticoids

Glucocorticoids have several metabolic functions, including increased amino acid uptake and glucose production by the liver, decreased amino acid uptake and protein synthesis in muscle, inhibition of somatic (non-reproductive) cell growth, suppression of GH secretion from the pituitary gland, and mobilization of lipids and cholesterol. Glucocorticoids also have antiinflammatory actions, including the inhibition of inflammatory and allergic reactions.

The primary glucocorticoid in humans is cortisol. *Cortisol* is synthesized from cholesterol, and its synthesis follows the diurnal rhythm of ACTH release. Cortisol levels are highest in the early morning hours and lowest in the evening. However, both ACTH and cortisol can be secreted independently of this diurnal rhythm under periods of physical or psychological stress (Aeron Biotechnology, 2005). Cortisol is, in fact, often referred to as the stress hormone because it promotes the production of increased energy necessary for dealing with stress.

When cortisol is secreted it stimulates a breakdown of muscle protein, releasing amino acids that can in turn be used by the liver to produce glucose for energy. Cortisol also makes fatty acids, an energy source from fat cells, available for use.

The net effect is an increase in energy supply that allows the brain to more effectively coordinate the body's response to a stressor. The increased energy supply also helps the muscles respond quickly and efficiently to a stressor or threat that requires a physical response.

Early research suggested that cortisol secretion decreases slightly with advancing age, but that this decreased secretion is compensated for by a simultaneous decrease in cortisol excretion from the body. As a result, normal cortisol levels would be maintained as a person ages. More recent studies, however, suggest that as long as individuals are healthy, cortisol secretion remains unchanged with age (Gersten, 2007, P. S. Timiras, 2007).

Studies conducted in animals have provided evidence that under stressful conditions, corticosterone (equivalent to the human cortisol) is more elevated among old than young animals. In addition, this elevated level persists for a longer period in some older animals. It has been hypothesized that the high levels of corticosterone following a stressor represent a loss of resiliency of the HPA axis such that the axis fails to decrease ACTH in response to elevated corticosterone levels and, consequently, fails to stop corticosterone release once the stress has passed. In rats, there is evidence that the elevated levels of corticosterone may be toxic to the brain, particularly the hippocampus. To date, there is little evidence to support an age-related decline in the competence of the HPA axis among humans. However, given the age-associated changes found in animal models, further study of the changes in the HPA axis among older humans is warranted (Gersten, 2007).

Clearly, glucocorticoids stimulate a beneficial response during times of stress. However, glucocorticoids also have some undesirable effects, including suppression of cartilage and bone formation, stimulation of bone demineralization, inhibition of portions of the immune response, and promotion of GI tract bleeding and ulcer formation (Digiovanna, 1994). When glucocorticoids are administered therapeutically for their antiinflammatory effects, their concentration in the blood can rise to extremely high levels. Excessively high levels of glucocorticoids exacerbate their aforementioned negative physiological effects. Given that older persons are generally at greater risk for osteoporosis and infection, as well as high blood pressure, therapeutic administration of glucocorticoids in this population should be carefully monitored.

Mineralocorticoids

The *mineralocorticoids* derive their name from their critical role in regulating extracellular concentrations of minerals, principally sodium and potassium. The primary mineralocorticoid is *aldosterone*, which targets the kidneys. Aldosterone has three major physiological effects: increased renal reabsorption of sodium or decreased urinary secretion of sodium, increased renal reabsorption of water and consequent expansion of extracellular fluid volume, and increased renal excretion of potassium. These physiological effects of aldosterone aid in the maintenance of fluid–electrolyte balance within the body. In addition, aldosterone helps to maintain blood pressure through its effects on sodium and water retention and increased fluid (i.e., blood) volume (Gersten, 2007).

Secretion of aldosterone is stimulated primarily through the release of the enzyme renin from the kidneys and activation of the RAA system. Renin is released in response to low blood pressure, increased osmotic pressure, and adverse changes in sodium concentrations. Once released, renin promotes the production of angiotensin, a peptide that then stimulates secretion of aldosterone (Gersten, 2007). Conversely, high blood pressure, decreased osmotic pressure, and favorable changes in sodium concentrations will inhibit the release of renin and activation of the renin-angiotensin system. As a result, the production and release of aldosterone is suppressed (Digiovanna, 1994).

The stimulation and suppression of aldosterone also have secondary regulatory mechanisms. The release of aldosterone is secondarily stimulated by pituitary ACTH. Suppression of aldosterone release is secondarily controlled by high sodium concentrations, potassium deficiency, and the release of atrial natriuretic factor, a hormone released by the heart in response to increased blood volume (Digiovanna, 1994).

Aldosterone levels decrease with age. The primary reason for this decrease is thought to be a decline in renin activity and subsequent decline in the activity of the RAA system. The release of aldosterone in response to ACTH does not appear to undergo age-related changes (University of California Academic Geriatric Resource Program, 2004). Because aldosterone stimulates sodium retention, decreased levels of aldosterone predispose older persons to sodium loss and possible hyponatremia, a condition characterized by water–mineral imbalance.

In addition to the overall decrease in aldosterone levels, older persons have an impaired ability to increase aldosterone secretion and aldosterone blood levels when necessary. Thus, there is a decline in aldosterone reserve capacity. This decline is not due to age-related changes in the adrenal cortex; rather, it is thought to be the result of decreased ability of the kidneys to secrete renin when needed (Digiovanna, 1994).

Adrenal Sex Hormones

The primary adrenal sex hormone of interest among aging persons is *dehydroepiandrosterone* (DHEA). DHEA is, in fact, the most abundant hormone in the human body (Chahal & Drake, 2007; Shealy, 1995; Yen & Laughlin, 1998). As a neurosteroid, it is thought that DHEA may have antidiabetic, antiobesity, cardioprotective, and immune-enhancing properties (Chahal & Drake, 2007; Yen & Laughlin, 1998). The exact physiological function of DHEA is not well understood; however, it is known to convert to a multitude of other hormones, mainly the sex hormones testosterone and estrogen. The major effects of DHEA are largely the result of the actions of those hormones to which it is converted (Dhatariya & Nair, 2003).

DHEA levels are high at birth but then undergo a precipitous drop until between the 6th and 10th year of life, at which time DHEA levels begin to steadily increase, achieving maximal concentrations during the third decade (Arlt, 2004). By age 70–80 years, DHEA levels are only 5–10% of peak values achieved in early adulthood (Hinson & Raven, 1999). Very low levels of DHEA are also observed in a variety of often age-related disease states, including diabetes, cardiovascular disease, AD, and various *cancers*. Thus, DHEA appears to be one of the most critical hormones in predicting disease. It has been hypothesized that low DHEA levels may be a marker of poor health status and, as a result, are associated with not only increased risk of disease, but also increased mortality (Arlt, 2004). As a result of DHEA's association with aging and disease, DHEA replacement has been touted as a means of slowing, if not reversing, the aging process, as well as the chronic disease and disability with which it is often accompanied.

DHEA replacement studies in humans have produced equivocal results. For example, research has shown positive effects of DHEA replacement on muscle strength and body composition, including increased muscle strength and decreased fat mass. Positive effects on bone, including increased bone mineral density, also have been demonstrated. However, numerous other studies have found no change in muscle strength, body composition, or bone density with DHEA replacement (Dhatariya & Nair, 2003). Overall, there is no consensus regarding the benefits of DHEA replacement. Although low levels of DHEA may predispose an individual to disease, there is no evidence that these low levels of DHEA cause disease. In addition, most studies of DHEA replacement have been short term and, thus, there is a paucity of information regarding the benefits (or risks) of DHEA use over long periods (Hinson & Raven, 1999). DHEA is currently available without a prescription, but given the relative lack of information regarding the risks and benefits of its use, especially in the long term, caution should be taken in self-administration of the hormone without medical supervision.

Adrenal Medulla

The *adrenal medulla* is part of the sympathetic division of the autonomic nervous system. Hormones called *catecholamines*, mainly epinephrine (adrenaline) and norepinephrine (noradrenaline), are produced in the adrenal medulla and released in response to sympathetic nervous system activity. Much like cortisol, *epinephrine* and norepinephrine play a critical role in the body's stress response, and their release is greatly increased under stressful conditions. Major physiological effects mediated by epinephrine and norepinephrine hormones include increased heart rate and blood pressure, increased metabolic rate, and increased blood glucose levels, which lead to increased energy. There is also an inhibition of nonessential activities such as GI secretion. This preparing of the body to respond to stress or threat is often termed the "fight or flight" response. Activation of adrenal medullary hormones is stimulated through a variety of means, including low blood sugar, hemorrhage, threat of bodily harm, emotional distress, and even exercise.

With aging there is a decrease in epinephrine secretion from the adrenal medulla. One study has reported that, under resting conditions, epinephrine secretion is 40% less in older men compared to younger men; however, there is a 20% simultaneous age-related decrease in epinephrine clearance from the circulation (Esler et al., 1995). As a result, levels of epinephrine concentration do not change significantly with age (Seals & Esler, 2000). Mechanisms for the age-related decline in epinephrine secretion have not been well investigated. Hypothesized mechanisms include (1) age-related attenuation in the adrenal medulla's response to nervous system activity, and (2) an overall age-associated decrease in nervous system activity to the adrenal medulla. It also has been hypothesized that reduced epinephrine secretion with age may be the result of decreased synthesis and storage of epinephrine in the adrenal medulla (Seals & Esler, 2000).

Under stressful conditions there is a characteristic increase in epinephrine secretion. This increase is markedly attenuated in older persons. Research has found that the increase in epinephrine secretion in response to a stressor is reduced by 33–44% in older men compared to that in their younger counterparts (Seals & Esler, 2000). Thus, the ability of the adrenal medulla to effectively respond to stressful situations is greatly impaired, even in healthy older adults.

Reproductive Hormones

Please refer to the previous discussion of the reproductive system for a review of age-related changes in the reproductive axis and female and male reproductive hormones.

The Pancreas

The hormone-secreting cells of the pancreas occur in tiny clusters known as the *islets of Langerhans*. Four islet cell types have been identified: the alpha (A), beta (B), delta (D), and pancreatic polypeptide (PP) cells. These cells secrete, respectively, glucagon, insulin, somatostatin, and pancreatic polypeptide. Of these hormones, only insulin is secreted exclusively by its particular cell type (B cells). The other hormones are also secreted by the GI mucosa, and somatostatin can be found in the brain. The function of PP cells has not been well identified, and therefore will not be discussed here.

Both *insulin* and *glucagon* are integral parts of metabolism regulation, and their secretion is regulated principally by blood glucose levels. High blood glucose levels stimulate the release of insulin and inhibit glucagon secretion. The released insulin then stimulates the cells of the body to absorb an amount of glucose from the blood that is sufficient to meet the body's energy needs. It also acts to promote storage of excess glucose in the liver, muscle, and fat cells and to suppress the release of this stored glucose. The result is a lowering of blood glucose levels. Conversely, low blood glucose levels stimulate glucagon release and inhibit insulin secretion. Secreted glucagon then promotes the release of stored glucose, and the result is a rise in blood glucose level. Somatostatin can inhibit the release of both insulin and glucagon, but the overall role of this hormone in regulation of blood glucose levels has not been firmly established.

Blood Glucose Levels

Blood glucose level is generally expressed as the amount (in milligrams) of glucose per deciliter (100 mL) of blood. According to the guidelines of the American Diabetes Association (ADA, 2016), normal fasting plasma glucose (FPG) level is below 100 mg/dL. When the FPG level lies between 100 and 125 mg/dL, an individual is said to have impaired fasting glucose, or impaired *glucose tolerance*, meaning that he or she is unable to reverse a dramatic rise in blood glucose levels and restore glucose homeostasis. An FPG of 126 mg/dL indicates a diagnosis of diabetes (ADA, 2016).

In addition to the FPG, a person's ability to respond to increased blood glucose levels also can be measured by the oral glucose tolerance test (OGTT). The OGTT involves drinking a solution of concentrated glucose after having fasted for at least 10 hours. Blood glucose levels are measured at the beginning of the test and then periodically thereafter for 3 hours. Individuals with normal glucose tolerance will exhibit a rise in glucose levels following consumption of the glucose solution, but glucose levels will return to normal within 2 hours. In persons with impaired glucose tolerance, blood glucose levels will remain high for longer than 2 hours. According to ADA guidelines, a person whose blood glucose level is 140 mg/dL or less after 2 hours is considered to have a normal glucose response. A person whose blood glucose level falls to between 140 and 199 mg/dL after 2 hours is said to be glucose intolerant. When, after 2 hours, blood glucose levels are elevated to 200 mg/dL or above, a person has diabetes (ADA, 2005).

Age-Related Glucose Intolerance

First documented by Spence (1921) and since confirmed by numerous others, biological aging is associated with a decline in glucose tolerance. This decline is generally associated with impaired response to a glucose challenge such as the OGTT rather than with fasting glucose levels. Although a small rise in fasting glucose of 1–2 mg/dL per decade has been observed by some, it is postprandial (following a meal) glucose levels that show the greatest increase, up to 15 mg/dL per decade (Morrow & Halter, 1994). Thus, the glucose intolerance of aging is associated primarily with response to glucose challenge or oral glucose load (Jackson, 1990). Approximately 40% of individuals ages 65–74 years have some degree of impairment in glucose homeostasis. This percentage rises to 50% in those over the age of 80 years (Harris, 1990; Minaker, 1990). The altered glucose metabolism that comes with increased age has potentially important pathophysiological consequences, because these age-related changes have been associated with an accumulation of advanced glycosylation end products (AGEs) that are believed to contribute to varying age-related pathologies as well as long-term complications in those who have diabetes (Chang & Halter, 2004). Mechanisms proposed as contributing to age-related glucose intolerance include impaired insulin secretion, insulin resistance, and alterations in glucose counterregulation.

Insulin Secretion

Studies of the effects of aging on insulin secretion provide some evidence that aging may be associated with subtle impairment in insulin release (Chen, Halter, & Porte, 1987). Other research, however, has found no alteration in insulin secretion with age (Peters & Davidson, 1997), and, overall, results from various studies have provided equivocal results regarding the role of insulin secretion in the impaired glucose tolerance of aging. Although the inability to secrete sufficient amounts of insulin to overcome the heightened blood glucose levels and insulin resistance associated with aging may contribute to the phenomenon, impaired insulin secretion is generally not regarded as the primary cause of age-related glucose intolerance.

Insulin Resistance

A defect in insulin action is generally presented as the greatest contributing factor in impaired glucose tolerance among elderly persons. Evidence suggests that the primary effect of the aging process on glucose homeostasis is the development of a resistance to the actions of insulin—that is, *insulin resistance* (Peters & Davidson, 1997). This resistance leads to an impaired ability to suppress glucose release from the liver as well as an impaired glucose uptake, with the latter defect predominating. Skeletal muscle is considered the primary site of the impaired glucose uptake (Jackson, 1990). The mechanism(s) through which this impairment develops is still poorly understood. However, because insulin receptors on cell membranes appear to be unchanged with age (Fink, Kolterman, Griffin, & Olefsky, 1983; Rowe, Minaker, Pallotta, & Flier, 1983), the principal cause of resistance to insulin uptake is assumed to be a postreceptor defect. It is hypothesized this defect may involve the transportation of glucose from the membrane receptor into the cell. Glucose uptake in virtually all cells is mediated by transporter proteins. *GLUT4* is an insulin-mediated transporter located within vesicles in the cells' cytoplasm. Upon stimulation by insulin, these vesicles travel to the cell membrane and release the GLUT4 transporters, which in turn serve as a port of cell entry for glucose. In the absence of insulin stimulation, GLUT4 is transferred back to vesicles and the entry of glucose is slowed (Czech, Erwin, & Sleeman, 2004). Thus, GLUT4 plays a central role in the maintenance of glucose homeostasis, and it is hypothesized that impaired GLUT4 synthesis, transfer, and activity may lead to insulin resistance (Chang & Halter, 2004).

Glucose Counterregulation

Research has reported that glucose counterregulation by glucagon, as well as other hormones—such as epinephrine, cortisol, and GH—that tend to raise blood glucose levels, is impaired in healthy elderly individuals (Marker, Cryer, & Clutter, 1992; Meneilly, Cheung, & Tuokko, 1994b). Rather than contributing to an elevation of plasma glucose levels, such a defect in glucose counterregulation results in delayed recovery from the hypoglycemic (low blood sugar) state. Thus, the impaired glucose homeostasis that characterizes aging is marked not only by elevated fasting plasma glucose but also by periods of prolonged hypoglycemia. The latter gains even greater importance when it is recognized that in comparison to younger subjects, elders demonstrate reduced awareness of the autonomic warning signs of hypoglycemia (Meneilly, Cheung, & Tuokko, 1994a). Furthermore, they exhibit impaired psychomotor performance during hypoglycemic episodes and thus are less likely to take the action necessary to return glucose levels to normal even if they are aware of the existing hypoglycemia (Meneilly, 2001).

Confounding Factors of the Glucose Intolerance of Aging

A general consensus exists that the processes of biological and physiological aging are themselves the most important contributors to impaired glucose homeostasis among elders (Meneilly, 2001). However, other factors exist that may contribute to the severity of the impairment. These include genetic predisposition (Chang & Halter, 2004) as well as various lifestyle and environmental factors.

Adiposity

Aging is associated with a decrease in lean body mass (Peters & Davidson, 1997) and an overall increase in adiposity as well as a redistribution of adipose tissue to the intraabdominal region (Kotz, Billington, & Levine, 1999). This tissue redistribution places the elderly population at increased risk of development of insulin resistance and glucose intolerance because clinical studies have shown that persons with this adipose distribution pattern exhibit greater insulin resistance as well as increased risk of diabetes (Despres & Marette, 1999; Garg, 1999). Research shows that adipose tissue in the abdominal region is metabolically more active than that in other regions of the body because of elevated fatty acid concentrations in this area (Bjorntorp, 1997; Garg, 1999). It is hypothesized that this increased metabolic activity may be the cause of the increased insulin resistance associated with overweight and obesity (Despres & Marette, 1999). Indeed, it has been shown that older people who are classified as having normal glucose tolerance have less adiposity, particularly less intraabdominal or central adiposity, and they do not experience a detectable difference in sensitivity to insulin (Chang & Halter, 2004).

Physical Activity

Physical activity is known to increase insulin action through heightened insulin sensitivity (Dela, Mikines, & Galbo, 1999; Jackson, 1990). Thus, decreased levels of physical activity may contribute to the development of insulin resistance. Aging is generally associated with declines in functional mobility and a decrease in physical activity, thereby placing elders at greater risk of impaired glucose tolerance. Older individuals with greater degrees of physical activity exhibit better glucose tolerance and less evidence of insulin resistance than do less active older people (Chang & Halter, 2004). It has been shown that glucose uptake is high in elderly athletes and low in bedridden elders compared with elderly controls (Dela et al., 1999). Furthermore, among elders, endurance training has been shown to produce improvements in insulin-mediated glucose uptake similar to those observed in young subjects (Dela et al., 1999). It must be noted, however, that elders who are more physically active are also more likely to have less body fat and less central adiposity, so it is most likely the combined effects of reduced abdominal adiposity and increased levels of physical activity that give rise to greater insulin sensitivity and glucose tolerance (Chang & Halter, 2004).

Diet

There is some evidence that impaired glucose tolerance in aging may be due at least in part to the diminished dietary carbohydrate intake often observed in elderly persons (Peters & Davidson, 1997). It has been shown that increased carbohydrate intake improves glucose tolerance in both young and old subjects. However, the older subjects exhibit decreased glucose tolerance at each level of matched carbohydrate intake when compared to the younger population (Chen et al., 1987). This idea is supported by studies showing that when old and young subjects are fed diets comparable in carbohydrate levels, age differences in glucose tolerance, insulin secretion, and insulin action are diminished but still persistent (Chang & Halter, 2004). Thus, age itself appears to be correlated with decreased glucose tolerance. However, poor levels of dietary carbohydrate intake are likely to exacerbate the age-related impairments in glucose metabolism.

Polypharmacy

Several pharmacological agents are known to affect glucose metabolism, and older adults are frequent users of such agents. Therefore, when evaluating alterations in blood glucose levels among elders, their medication regimens must be considered and attention must be paid to potential drug interactions (Minaker, 1990; Morley & Perry, 1991). Drugs known to affect glucose metabolism include, but are not limited to, beta-blockers, calcium channel blockers, glucocorticoids, and other nonpharmacological agents such as alcohol, caffeine, and nicotine (Bressler & DeFronzo, 1997). Furthermore, in treating the elderly patient with diabetes, sulfonylureas should be used with caution. These pharmacological agents stimulate insulin secretion and can contribute to the development of hypoglycemia (Graal & Wolffenbuttel, 1999). In addition, the interaction of sulfonylureas with some drugs can increase the hypoglycemic effect of the sulfonylureas (Peters & Davidson, 1997). Thus, elderly persons are at increased risk of the development of prolonged hypoglycemia when treated with sulfonylureas.

The Muscle

The body's muscular system is composed of three types of muscle—skeletal muscle, smooth muscle, and cardiac muscle. *Skeletal muscles*, examples of which include the bicep, tricep, quadricep, hamstring, and gastrocnemius (calf) muscle, make up the majority of the body's overall muscle mass. Skeletal muscle is also the muscle type in which most age-related changes occur. Thus, skeletal muscle and its changes with age will be the focus of our discussion about the aging muscle.

Skeletal Muscle: Structure and Function

Skeletal muscles are composed of several thin muscle bundles (see **Figure 4-17**). These bundles are held together with connective tissue but are able to move independently of one another (Arking, 1998). The muscle bundles are composed of several muscle fibers, each of which is formed from the fusion of numerous individual myofibrils.

Myofibrils contain two types of protein molecules: actins and myosins. *Actin* and *myosin* molecules are arranged in a parallel, overlapping manner within compartments called *sarcomeres*. The overlap of actin and myosin within the sarcomere results in a pattern of alternating light and dark bands, which accounts for the striated, or striped, appearance of skeletal muscle. In a state of rest, actin molecules overlap both ends of the myosin molecules, which are centered within the sarcomere. Muscle contraction results when actin molecules are pulled toward the center of the sarcomere in a ratcheting motion. This contraction of skeletal muscle is controlled by an individual's own volition; hence, skeletal muscle has also been termed voluntary muscle.

Although muscle fibers have a common basic structure, they can be divided into two distinct physiological types, *fast-twitch fibers* and *slow-twitch fibers*. These two fiber types produce the same amount of force per contraction; however, they produce this force at different rates. White fast-twitch fibers contract quickly and provide short bursts of energy, but they fatigue quickly. As a result of these contractile properties, fast-twitch fibers are generally used for high-intensity, low-endurance, generally anaerobic activities such as sprinting and weight lifting. Red slow-twitch fibers contract slowly but steadily and are not easily fatigued. Therefore, these fibers are best suited for use in aerobic activities of low intensity but high endurance, such as long-distance running. Slow-twitch fibers are also used for postural activities, such as the supporting of the head by the neck.

Every person is born with a fixed ratio of fast-twitch to slow-twitch muscle fibers. However, the ratio may vary from one body location to another, and one person may have a greater ratio of fast-twitch to slow-twitch fibers in a particular location than does another person. This phenomenon is part of what can result in one individual being, for example, a better sprinter or better long-distance runner than another.

Aging of the Skeletal Muscle

Sarcopenia

A reduction in muscle mass occurs to at least some degree in all elderly persons as compared to young, healthy, physically active young adults (Roubenoff, 2001; Tortora & Derrickson, 2014). This reduction in muscle mass is known as *sarcopenia* (from the Greek meaning poverty of flesh) and is distinct from muscle loss due to disease or starvation. One population-based study estimated that the prevalence of sarcopenia rises from 13–24% in

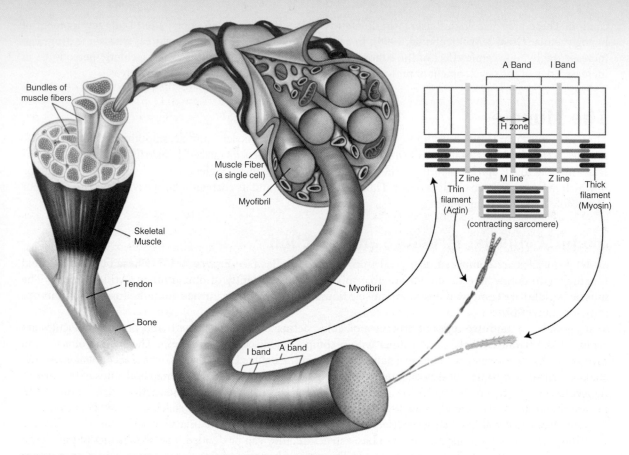

Figure 4-17 Structure of the skeletal muscle fiber, myofibril and sarcomere.

individuals under the age of 70 years to greater than 50% in persons over the age of 80 years (Baumgartner et al., 1998). Sarcopenia is of great consequence to older persons because it is associated with tremendous increases in functional disability and frailty. Older sarcopenic men are reported to have 4.1 times higher rates and women 3.6 times higher rates of disability than their gender-specific counterparts with normal muscle mass (Baumgartner et al., 1998).

The total cross-sectional area of skeletal muscle is reported to decrease by as much as 40% between the ages of 20 and 60 years (Doherty, 2003), with the greatest loss occurring in the lower limbs (Doherty, 2003; Vandervoot & Symons, 2001). Men are known to have greater total muscle mass than women; however, men experience greater relative muscle loss with age than do their female counterparts (Janssen, Heymsfield, Wang, & Ross, 2000). The reason for this gender difference has not been clearly defined, but it is postulated to relate to hormonal factors (Janssen et al., 2000). Although men experience greater relative muscle loss, it has been noted that sarcopenia may be of greater concern for older women given their longer life expectancy and higher rates of disability in old age (Roubenoff & Hughes, 2000).

Gender is not the only factor contributing to differences in the rate of sarcopenia. The loss of muscle mass is highly individualized and greatly dependent upon genetics, lifestyle, and other factors that influence the varied mechanisms proposed to underlie sarcopenia. The most commonly proposed mechanisms include a decline in the number and size of muscle fibers, loss of motor units, hormonal influences, altered protein synthesis, nutritional factors, and lack of physical activity, all of which are discussed later.

Changes in Muscle Fibers

With age, there is an overall loss in the number of both fast-twitch and slow-twitch muscle fibers. By the ninth decade, approximately 50% fewer muscle fibers are present in the vastus lateralis muscle (the lateral portion of the quadriceps) than are observed in the same muscle of a 20-year-old (Lexell, Taylor, & Sjöström, 1988). In addition, a reduction in the size of muscle fibers has been observed, with the greatest reduction seen in fast-twitch muscle fibers. Reduction in the size of fast-twitch fibers ranges from 20–50% with age, whereas slow-twitch fibers have been shown to reduce in size by only 1–25% as a person ages (Doherty, 2003).

Loss of Motor Units

Muscle fibers are innervated by motor nerves, which extend from the spinal cord. Each nerve innervates several muscle fibers. The combination of a single nerve and all the fibers it innervates is known as a *motor unit*, and it is this motor unit that allows muscles to contract. Beginning about the seventh decade of an individual's life, the number of functional motor units begins to decline precipitously (Vandervoot & Symons, 2001). One group of researchers found that the estimated number of motor units in the bicep-brachialis muscle declined by nearly half, from an average of 911 motor units in subjects younger than 60 years of age to 479 in subjects older than 60 years of age (Brown, Strong, & Snow, 1988). A similar degree of motor unit loss was shown in a group of subjects ages 60–80 years compared with a group of subjects ages 20 to 40 years (Doherty & Brown, 1993).

The loss of motor units with age is due to an age-related loss of muscle innervation (Deschenes, 2004). As motor units are lost, surviving motor nerves adopt muscle fibers that have been abandoned due to their loss of innervation (Roubenoff, 2001). This results in an increase in the size of the adopting motor unit. Thus, older persons generally have larger, yet less efficient, motor units than do younger persons (Roubenoff, 2001). Because these enlarged motor units are now responsible for the contraction of a greater number of muscles, they are generally less efficient; this inefficiency can lead to tremors and weakness (Enoka, 1997) and, together with the atrophy of fast-twitch muscle fibers, can result in a decline in coordinated muscle action (Morley, Baumgartner, Roubenoff, Mayer, & Nair, 2001). Furthermore, abandoned muscle fibers that are not adopted by surviving motor units begin to atrophy as a result of disuse secondary to their loss of innervation. This atrophy contributes to an overall loss of muscle mass. Muscle atrophy secondary to nerve cell death is clearly demonstrated through the loss of muscle mass observed in persons who have had a stroke (Roubenoff, 2001).

Hormonal Influences

Estrogen and testosterone are anabolic hormones—hormones that promote the build-up of muscle. With age, levels of these hormones decline, thereby contributing to muscle atrophy and sarcopenia. Accelerated loss of muscle around the time of menopause lends support to the idea that estrogen may play a role in the maintenance of muscle mass (Poehlman, Toth, & Gardner, 1995). There is evidence supporting estrogen replacement therapy as a means of attenuating the loss of muscle mass among older women (Dionne, Kinaman, & Poehlman, 2000; Phillips, Rook, Siddle, Bruce, & Woledge, 1993). However, some research suggests that the beneficial effects of estrogen replacement are most pronounced in the perimenopausal period and may have little to no effect on the loss of muscle mass among postmenopausal women (Doherty, 2003). Among older men, testosterone supplementation has been shown to increase muscle mass; however, studies performed to date have been conducted among healthy older men, so it is not known whether testosterone supplementation would have the same beneficial effects on muscle mass in older men with physical impairments, chronic disease, or frailty (Bhasin, 2003). Testosterone supplementation also has been shown to increase muscle strength among elderly women (Davis, McCloud, Strauss, & Burger, 1995).

GH (see "The Endocrine System" earlier in this chapter) is another anabolic hormone that declines with age. The decline in GH begins during the fourth decade of life and parallels the decline in muscle mass (Roubenoff, 2001). Because of the strong association between GH and muscle mass, administration of GH has been suggested as a potential method by which age-related loss of muscle mass might be attenuated. However, research investigating the effects of GH on muscle mass has produced equivocal results, and there is no evidence that GH administration results in any increase in muscle strength (Borst, 2004). In addition, the use of GH is accompanied by numerous side effects, including fluid retention, hypotension, and carpal tunnel syndrome, and these side effects are reported to be more severe among older persons (Borst, 2004). Given the equivocal results regarding its efficacy as well as the side effects associated with its use, GH is not recommended as an intervention for sarcopenia (Doherty, 2003).

Protein Synthesis

Excluding water, protein is the primary component of skeletal muscle and accounts for approximately 20% of its weight (Proctor, Balagopal, & Nair, 1998). Furthermore, muscle is the body's largest repository for protein (Balagopal, Rooyackers, Adey, Ades, & Nair, 1997; Proctor et al., 1998). When protein breakdown within the body exceeds protein synthesis, muscle atrophy occurs. Some research findings suggest that aging is associated with a reduced capacity of skeletal muscle to synthesize protein. Such a reduction is likely to lead to a decrease in muscle mass among elderly persons. However, other research (Volpi, Sheffield-Moore, Rasmussen, & Wolfe, 2001) has found no difference in the synthesis rate of muscle protein with age. Thus, further studies are needed to elucidate the role that protein synthesis plays in sarcopenia.

Nutritional Factors

Food intake declines with age, with greater decline occurring among men than women (Morley et al., 2001). This decline is often referred to as the *anorexia of aging*, and it is hypothesized to be associated with a decrease in the senses of smell and taste as well as an earlier rate of satiation with age (Morley et al., 2001). It is thought that the anorexia of aging may result in protein intake below the level necessary to maintain muscle mass and consequently contribute to sarcopenia (Morley et al., 2001; Drewnowski & Evans, 2001); however, the degree to which alterations in protein intake with age may play a role in age-related loss of muscle mass is unknown and requires further study.

Muscle Strength

Loss of *muscle strength*, the muscle's capacity to generate force, is thought to be secondary to declines in muscle mass (Ivey et al., 2000), and decreases in muscle strength are seen with advancing age. Data from one study demonstrated that 71% of men between the ages of 40 and 59 and 85% of men age 60 or older had declines in muscle strength over a 9-year period (Kallman, Plato, & Tobin, 1990). Age-related decreases in strength are reported to range from 20 to 40%, with even greater decreases of 50% or more occurring in persons in their ninth decade or beyond (Doherty, 2003). Older men experience greater absolute declines in muscle strength than women; however, because men have greater total muscle mass than women, relative losses in strength are similar between males and females (Doherty, 2003). The rate at which the decline in muscle strength occurs has not been well defined, but longitudinal studies have shown rates of strength loss of about 1–3% per year (Doherty, 2003).

Muscle Quality

In addition to declines in muscle mass and strength, advancing age is also associated with a loss of *muscle quality*, strength generated per unit of muscle mass. However, research shows that age-related declines in muscle quality differ by both gender and muscle group. Studies (Lynch et al., 1999; Ostchega, Dillon, Lindle, Carroll, & Hurley, 2004) of arm and leg muscle quality in men and women found that age-related differences in arm muscle quality declined more among males than females, yet leg muscle quality declined at similar rates among both genders. In addition, among men the rates of decline of leg and arm muscle quality were similar, but among women there was a greater rate of decline of leg muscle quality than arm muscle quality. Lower limb weakness is of particular concern because it results in an inability to perform most daily tasks, such as standing up from a chair, walking, or stair climbing (Olivetti et al., 2007; Ostchega et al., 2004).

Resistance Training and Aging Muscle

Older persons who are less physically active have less muscle mass and greater rates of disability and debilitating falls than persons who remain physically active as they age (Evans, 2002; Moreland, Richardson, Goldsmith, & Clase, 2004). There is a large body of evidence demonstrating that exercise can not only slow or prevent muscle loss with age, but also increase muscle mass as well as muscle strength among older persons. Resistance exercise, exercise aimed at increasing the force generated by muscle, has been shown to have the most beneficial effects on aging muscle. One study of 66-year-old men found that a 12-week program of resistance training resulted in significant increases in the cross-sectional area of both fast-twitch and slow-twitch muscle fibers (Frontera, Meredith, O'Reilly, Knuttgen, & Evans, 1988). In addition, muscle strength improved significantly. Even among very elderly persons, resistance exercise has shown benefits for age-related changes in muscle. An 8-week resistance training program conducted among men and women in their 90s resulted in a 15% increase in muscle cross-sectional area and a nearly 175% increase in the amount of weight subjects were capable of lifting (Fiatarone et al., 1990). Numerous other studies have shown that resistance training programs of 10–12 weeks' duration, with training 2–3 days per week, result in significant increases in muscle strength among older persons (Doherty, 2003). It has been reported that resistance training may restore approximately 75% of lost muscle mass and 40% of lost muscle strength (Roubenoff, 2003). Significant increases in muscle strength are also achieved using weight-bearing exercise regimes (Olivetti et al., 2007).

Resistance training has also been shown to improve muscle quality. Following a 9-week training program, older men and women showed statistically significant increases in muscle quality. Furthermore, subsequent to the initial 9-week program there was a 31-week detraining period after which levels of muscle quality remained significantly greater than levels measured before the start of the 9-week program (Ivey et al., 2000).

Finally, there is also evidence to support an increase in protein synthesis with resistance exercise. One study reported an approximately 50% increase in protein synthesis among 65- to 75-year-old men following a 16-week progressive resistance training program (Yarasheski, Zackwieja, Campbell, & Bier, 1995). Improvements in protein synthesis have also been demonstrated among frail elderly men and women ages 76–92 years (Yarasheski et al., 1999). Other research has reported increases in protein synthesis of over 100% following resistance training (Hasten, Pak-Loduca, Obert, & Yarasheski, 2000).

The plethora of benefits to muscle that result from resistance training demonstrate the extreme importance of regular physical activity, especially of the resistance type, among aging men and women (Vincent, Raiser, & Vincent, 2012). It is no wonder that many have cited resistance training as the most important factor in preventing and even reversing the losses in muscle mass, strength, and power that come with advancing age.

The Skeletal System

The skeletal system is composed of the 206 bones of the body as well as the joints that connect them. The skeleton, extremely strong yet relatively lightweight, gives shape and support to the human body. It also acts to protect the body; for example, the skull protects the brain and eyes, the ribs protect the heart, and the vertebrae protect the spinal cord. The skeleton also provides a structure to which muscles can attach by tendons, enabling the body to move. Furthermore, it acts as a set of levers to modify movement provided by the muscles, increasing or decreasing the distance, speed, and force obtained from muscle contraction (Digiovanna, 1994; Marieb & Hoehn, 2015; Tortora & Derrickson, 2014). When one considers the importance of the functions performed by the skeletal system, it becomes apparent that any alteration or destruction of the skeletal system would have potentially serious consequences for the overall health and physical functioning of the human body.

Bone

In addition to the aforementioned functions of the skeletal system, each component of bone has its own unique function(s). A principal function of bone is mineral storage and the maintenance of free mineral homeostasis. The predominant mineral stored within bone is calcium, which is necessary for, among other things, muscle contraction and nerve impulse conduction. If it is to aid in these functions, calcium must be readily and continuously available in a free form. However, too much free calcium may be toxic and too little calcium may impair or prevent cell functioning. Thus, there must be a means of maintaining mineral homeostasis, and bone cells assist in this maintenance.

Bone cells are of four types: osteogenic cells, osteoblasts, osteocytes, and osteoclasts. Osteogenic cells are unspecialized stem cells capable of cell division. The resulting cells develop into osteoblasts. *Osteoblasts* secrete collagen and minerals to produce a bone matrix; hence, these cells are responsible for the construction of new bone and the repair of damaged or broken bone. They mature into *osteocytes*, the main cells in bone tissue that maintain daily activities of the bone such as exchange of nutrients and wastes with the blood (Tortora & Derrickson, 2014). The fourth bone cell type is the *osteoclasts*, which break down or resorb existing bone, dissolving minerals of the bone matrix so that these minerals can be used by the body.

The formation and resorption of bone are not separately regulated processes. Osteoblasts and osteoclasts occur together in temporary anatomic structures known as *basic multicellular units* (BMUs). A mature BMU is composed of osteoblasts, osteoclasts, a vascular supply, a nerve supply, and connective tissue (Manolagas, 2000). A BMU has a lifespan of approximately 6–9 months, longer than the lifespan of osteoblasts and osteoclasts. Thus, the BMU must be continually supplied with new cells.

During development and growth, BMUs mold bone to achieve proper size and shape by osteoclastic removal of bone from one site and osteoblastic deposition at a different one. This process is known as modeling. By adulthood, the skeleton has reached maturity and modeling no longer occurs. However, in adulthood there is periodic replacement of old bone with new bone, a process known as bone remodeling. Through bone remodeling, the human skeleton is completely regenerated every 10 years (Manolagas, 2000). The purpose of bone remodeling is not well understood; however, it is hypothesized that remodeling occurs to repair fatigue and damage and to prevent excessive aging. Thus, the primary purpose of bone remodeling may be to attenuate if not prevent the accumulation of old bone (Manolagas, 2000).

Bone remodeling by the osteoblasts and osteoclasts is principally controlled through hormonal regulation. As previously noted in the discussion of the endocrine system, thyroid calcitonin inhibits bone resorption, lowering blood calcium levels. Parathyroid hormone from the parathyroid gland has the opposite effect—it increases bone resorption and mobilizes calcium, thereby increasing blood calcium levels. Other hormones are also involved in bone remodeling, yet often indirectly. Glucocorticoids promote bone resorption, and GH and insulin work to increase bone formation.

Bone Types

There are two types of bone—cortical, or compact bone, and trabecular, or spongy bone. *Cortical bone* comprises the outer layer of bone and is composed of numerous osteons—long, narrow cylinders of bone matrix. The osteons are tightly fused to one another and possess a complex system of blood vessels and nerves. Osteons are continually dissolved and replaced anew. Cortical bone surrounds and protects trabecular bone and provides the majority of skeletal strength.

Trabecular bone makes up the inner portion of bone and is composed of small pieces of bone matrix known as trabeculae. The trabeculae are arranged in very irregular patterns. Compared to cortical bone, trabecular bone provides only minimal skeletal strength. The ratio of cortical bone to trabecular bone varies throughout the body; cortical bone is predominant in the limbs, whereas trabecular bone is predominant in bones of the axial skeleton, such as the ribs, vertebrae, and skull.

Aging of the Bone

Bone Loss

In order to ensure that there is no net loss of bone, the amount of bone resorbed by the BMU must not exceed the amount formed. As the body ages, it loses the ability to maintain this balance between bone resorption and formation (Tortora & Derrickson, 2014). The BMU is said to be in a negative balance and bone loss occurs. Negative BMU balance begins as early as the third decade, long before menopause in women (Seeman, 2003b). After several decades have passed, skeletal mass may be reduced to half of what it was at 30 years of age (Timiras & Navasio, 2007).

Estrogen promotes apoptosis or programmed cell death of osteoclasts. Thus, the osteoclast lifespan is increased by estrogen deficiency whereas the lifespan of osteoblasts declines with such a deficiency (Tortora & Derrickson, 2014). Consequently, BMU balance becomes more negative. Thus, estrogen deficiency is a key contributor to bone loss, and bone loss accelerates in women after menopause due to a decline in estrogen levels (Seeman, 2003b). Simultaneously, as osteoclast activity increases and more bone is resorbed, the remaining bone becomes more porous. The result of this increased porosity is a decline in bone mineral density. Unfortunately, bone loss continues from the lower density bone and at a higher rate than before menopause. The increased rapidity of bone loss is explained by (1) the increasingly negative BMU, (2) a higher remodeling rate, and (3) reduction in the mineral content of bone due to the replacement of older, more densely mineralized bone with younger, less densely mineralized bone (Seeman, 2003c).

Estrogen deficiency also plays a role in bone loss among men. Although men do not undergo the midlife acceleration in bone resorption characteristically seen in women, decreased bone mineral density among men is due to a decline in levels of estrogen, not testosterone (Seeman, 2003b). It has been suggested that estrogen may regulate bone resorption whereas both estrogen and testosterone may regulate bone formation (Falahati-Nini et al., 2000). At any given age, bone mass is greater in men than in women, but the rate of bone loss is generally accelerated among women (Arking, 1998). However, the overall loss of bone is quantitatively similar in persons of both genders, suggesting that bone loss may occur over a longer period in men than in women (Seeman, 2003c).

Bone Type

The majority of bone resorption occurs within trabecular bone, and in both men and women bone loss occurs at least a decade earlier in trabecular bone than in cortical bone (Arking, 1998). As the body ages, trabeculae become thinner and weaker. In addition, some may disappear entirely and cannot be replaced. As a result of these changes the bone becomes permanently weaker at the site of trabeculae thinning or loss. Furthermore, some trabeculae may become disconnected from the others, resulting in a decline in bone strength (Digiovanna, 1994).

Corticol bone loss is not detected until about 40 years of age, at which time the rate of loss begins to increase. However, the loss of cortical bone still occurs at only half the rate of trabecular bone loss (Digiovanna, 1994). Loss of trabecular bone occurs from the inside of the bone outward. Normally, old osteons shrink and are dissolved while new osteons form next to them and eventually fill the space left by the old ones. With age, however, new osteons are unable to fill this space completely, leaving increasingly larger gaps between existing osteons. The result is a weakening of the bone.

Bone Strength

With age there is not only a loss of bone, but also a loss of bone strength. This loss of strength has been attributed to at least two different processes. The first is the increased porosity of bone that occurs due to continuous bone remodeling. Greater porosity reduces the structural strength of bone. The second is an age-related loss of collagen due to decreased protein synthesis, which increases the ratio of bone minerals to collagen, leading to increased brittleness of bone (Arking, 1998; Tortora & Derrickson, 2014). Reduction in collagen fiber strength may be related to decreases in GH production, which was noted earlier in the endocrine section. In childhood, approximately two thirds of bone is composed of collagen and connective tissues, whereas in aged individuals minerals make up two thirds of bone structure (Timiras & Navasio, 2007).

Bone tensile strength is a property that allows bone to withstand forces applied to the skeleton during movements such as bending and stretching. Strong, young bones will respond to force with flexibility and resilience, bending as needed; however, aged bones are more likely to snap when subjected to force. Consequently, the age-associated decline in bone strength increases older persons' risk of bone fracture (Arking, 1998). See the following section for further discussion of bone fractures among older persons.

Age-Related Disease and Injury of the Bone

Osteoporosis

Osteoporosis is a disease that results from reductions in bone quantity and strength that are greater than the usual age-related reductions. Bones of those with osteoporosis are generally very porous, containing numerous holes or empty pockets. In addition, they are thin and fragile and, consequently, extremely prone to fracture (discussed in the following section). An estimated 10 million Americans suffer from osteoporosis and another 34 million have low bone mass that puts them at increased risk of the disease. The majority of osteoporosis cases, 8 million (80%), occur in women whereas only 2 million (20%) occur in men (National Osteoporosis Foundation, 2015).

Bone Fracture

Osteoporosis and the general progressive loss of bone mass with age leads to increased risk of fracture among older persons. Fifty percent of women and 25% of men over the age of 50 years will experience an osteoporosis-related fracture in their lifetime. Fractures in elderly persons often occur as the result of only minimal or moderate trauma, whereas in younger persons considerable force is required to fracture a bone. In addition, the fractures that occur in old age generally occur at different sites than those that occur at younger ages. Among younger persons the most common site of fracture is the bone shaft, whereas in older persons fractures generally occur next to a joint (Timiras & Navasio 2007). Regardless of the site of fracture, fractures among older adults are generally more difficult to prevent or repair, and recovery from fracture occurs much more slowly in older persons than in young individuals.

In young adults, fractures occur more frequently among males than females. This is hypothesized to be the result of males' generally more frequent engagement in physical activity and exposure to accidental falls (Timiras & Navasio, 2007). In older adults, however, women generally experience greater fracture rates than men. This gender difference may be due, at least in part, to the fact that women begin life with a smaller skeleton that adapts less well to aging than that of men (Seeman, 2002a). This gender difference in fracture incidence with age is most evident in fractures of the vertebrae, forearm, and hip (Timiras & Navasio, 2007).

There are also racial differences in the rate of fracture. The rates of fracture associated with old age are significantly lower among African Americans than whites, specifically three times lower among African American women and five times lower among African American men. These racial differences may be explained by the 10–20% greater bone mass and density of adult bone among African Americans. In addition, bone remodeling occurs more slowly among African Americans than whites (Timiras & Navasio, 2007).

Joints

Joints or articulations are junctions between two or more bones. Three types of joints comprise the body's articular system. *Immovable joints*, or fibrous joints, consist of collagen fibers that bind bones tightly together.

The toughness of collagen allows minimal, if any, shifting of bones, and thus the joints are immovable. Skull bones are examples of immovable joints. These joints keep the skull in place, allowing support and protection of the brain.

Cartilaginous joints have a layer of cartilage that separates the two connected bones. These joints also may have ligaments to aid in holding bones together. Cartilaginous joints allow for slight movement. Examples of this type of joint include the joints between vertebrae. These cartilaginous joints are known as intervertebral disks, and together with strong ligaments they hold the vertebrae together and aid the vertebrae in supporting the weight of the body. They also allow the vertebral column to bend and twist slightly.

The third and most common type of joint is the *synovial joint*. The bones that this type of joint connects contain smooth cartilage on their opposing ends. This cartilage minimizes friction when the joint moves. A sleeve of connective tissue encapsulates the ends of the two bones that have been joined. The joint capsule is lined with the *synovium*, a membrane that secretes *synovial fluid*. The fluid is thick and slippery, allowing easy movements of the bones. In addition, it absorbs part of the shock sustained by the joint. Although synovial joints, together with reinforcing ligaments, bind two bones tightly together, they are characterized by free range of motion. Nearly all the joints in the arms, legs, shoulders, and hips are synovial joints.

Aging of the Joints

Immovable Joints

With increasing age the collagen between the bones of immovable joints becomes coated with bone matrix. As a result, the space between bones gets even narrower and the bones may eventually fuse together completely. Consequently, the joints become stronger; therefore, with age immovable joints actually improve.

Cartilaginous Joints

The aging process is associated with a stiffening of the cartilage comprising cartilaginous joints. Ligaments also become stiffer and less elastic. The result of these changes is a reduction in the amount of movement allowed by the cartilaginous joints. Vertebral movement is decreased, and there is a decline in the ability of intervertebral disks to support the body and cushion the spinal cord. With age the vertebrae weaken and, as a result, the weight of the body forces the intervertebral disk to expand into the vertebrae, forming a concave region. This change appears to force more of the weight of the body onto the outer edge of the intervertebral disk, compressing the disk (Digiovanna, 1994). The result is a shortening of the spinal column and a decrease in body height.

Synovial Joints

The functional ability of synovial joints begins to decline around 20 years of age (Digiovanna, 1994). As a person ages, both the joint capsule and the ligaments become shorter, stiffer, and less able to stretch. In addition, the cartilage lining the bones becomes calcified, thinner, and less resilient (Arking, 1998; Tortora & Derrickson, 2014). Consequently, it becomes more difficult to move, and range of motion and efficiency of the joint are reduced. As a result, both the initiation and speed of movement begin to slow with age. This leads to a lessened ability to maintain balance and makes it difficult to act quickly to minimize the force of impact resulting from a fall or other physically harmful event.

With age the synovial membrane also becomes stiffer and less elastic. In addition, it loses some of its vasculature, which in turn reduces its ability to produce synovial fluid. The fluid that is produced is thinner and less viscous (Arking, 1998). As a result of these changes in the synovial membrane and fluid, there is a decline in the ease and comfort with which the joints move within the joint capsule as a person ages.

The net result of the aging of synovial joints is often increased injury and decreased activity performance. However, there is evidence to demonstrate that this net result can be slowed or minimized through continual physical activity. Exercise can increase flexibility of the joint components and also appears to increase circulation to the joints (Digiovanna, 1994; Tortora & Derrickson, 2014).

It should be noted here that at least some, if not many, of the changes in joints with age may be due not to the aging process but to repeated injuries the joints experience over time due to the performance of regular daily activities. It is often difficult to distinguish these latter effects from true biological aging (Digiovanna, 1994).

Diseases of the Joints
Osteoarthritis

Age-related changes in the joints often result in or are compounded by arthritis, a disease characterized by inflammation of the joints and accompanied by joint pain and injury. There are more than 100 different types of arthritis, but the two most common forms are osteoarthritis and rheumatoid arthritis.

Osteoarthritis is by far the most common form of arthritis, accounting for more than half of all arthritis cases (Digiovanna, 1994). More than 20 million people in the United States have osteoarthritis, and the disease is much more common among older persons. More than half of people 65 years of age or older would show radiographic evidence of osteoarthritis in at least one joint. Before age 45, osteoarthritis is more common among men, but after age 45 it becomes more common in women (National Institute of Arthritis and Musculoskeletal and Skin Diseases, 2016).

Osteoarthritis frequently affects the weight-bearing joints, such as the hips, knees, and lower spine. Finger joints also are common sites of osteoarthritis. This form of arthritis causes a breakdown and weakening of cartilage, which results in a decreased ability to cushion the ends of the bones. If enough cartilage is lost, the bones will begin to rub against each other. The bones then respond by producing more bone matrix, which builds up and can lead to an enlargement of the joints and difficulty in joint movement. In addition, the bone matrix produced may be rough and jagged and, when it rubs against soft tissues, can cause pain. Furthermore, with age there is a decrease in synovial fluid concentration and viscosity. This decrease may lower the lubricating and cushioning properties of the joints, making movement of the joint difficult and painful (Moskowitz, Kelly, & Lewallen, 2004).

The Sensory System

The sensory system provides constant stimulation to the body and relays important messages to the mind and body. The sensory system can evoke emotion and memories and when disrupted can influence quality of life (Arking, 1998; Digiovanna, 1994; Weiffenbach, 1991). Age-related changes to touch, smell, taste, vision, and hearing lead older individuals to interact with the environment differently than they did at a younger age.

Touch

The ability to touch and distinguish texture and sensation tends to decline with age due to a decrease in the number and alteration in the structural integrity of touch receptors, or Meissner's corpuscles, and pressure receptors, or Pacinian corpuscles (Arking, 1998; Digiovanna, 1994, 2000). Receptors related to the sense of touch are also known as *mechanoreceptors*. See **Figure 4-18** for an illustration and location of mechanoreceptors in the integumentary system. Changes to these touch and pressure receptors lead to a decrease in the ability to acknowledge that an object is touching or applying pressure to the skin, a decrease in the ability to identify where the touch or pressure is occurring, an inability to distinguish how many objects are touching the skin, and a decreased ability to identify objects just by touch (Digiovanna, 1994, 2000). Aging changes to the skin as well as changes in surface hair may also play a role in diminished touch. (See the following section, "The Integumentary System.") Arking (1998) suggests that the skin on the hands, the most sensitive to touch, undergoes the most age-related change in touch. In addition to the hands, Stevens and Choo (1996) found that the feet undergo major declines in touch sensitivity with age. This conclusion may be explained by a higher concentration of receptors in the hands and feet whereas the rest of the body has a larger surface area over which receptors are dispersed.

Stevens and Patterson (1995) conducted a spatial acuity study of touch that involved changes in stimuli related to discontinuity, skin location, and area on the skin as well as changes in the orientation of stimuli in older versus younger adults. Conclusions from this study showed that all four acuity measures declined with age at a rate of 1% per year between the ages of 20 and 80. Furthermore, these researchers demonstrated that acuity at sites such as the forearm and lip declined less quickly than acuity in the fingertips. These changes to touch can be related to a decline in the number of sensory neurons and a decreased ability of the remaining sensory neurons to efficiently relay signals critical to the detection, location, and identification of touch or pressure on the skin (Digiovanna, 1994, 2000).

Of particular concern for the elderly is loss of sensation and proprioception, or reception of information regarding body movements and position (Shaffer & Harrison, 2007). Recent data suggest that aging results in loss of lower limb sensory fibers and receptors for vibration and discriminative touch as well as impaired lower extremity proprioception. These compromises along with declines in ability to initiate corrective movements leave elderly adults more prone to imbalances and falls (Maki & McIlroy, 2006; Shaffer & Harrison, 2007).

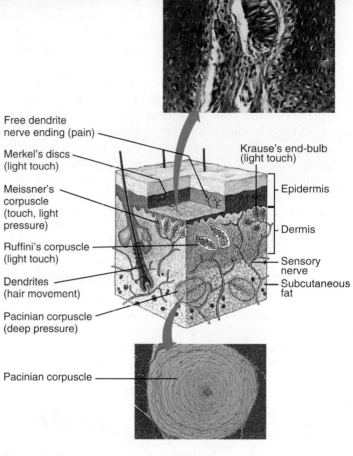

Figure 4-18 General sense receptors.

Smell

Olfactory System Anatomy

The chemical senses of smell and taste work together and influence each other as a functional entity (Weiffenbach, 1991). The olfactory system contains supporting cells for mucus production, olfactory receptors, and basal cells that replenish every 2 months and eventually transform into new olfactory receptors (Sherwood, 2014). When basal cells transform into receptors, the entire neuron, including the axon that projects into the brain, is completely replaced (Sherwood, 2014). The olfactory axons connect to the olfactory bulb and the olfactory nerve layer. The nerve layer synapses into the glomerulus, sending messages to the primary olfactory cortex of the brain (Kovacs, 2004). Approximately 5 million olfactory receptors of about 1,000 different types are located in the nose. Each receptor type detects one miniscule component of an odor instead of the odor as a whole (Sherwood, 2014).

Age-Related Olfactory Changes

Olfaction, or the sense of smell, appears to be reduced with age, as demonstrated by threshold studies of stimulus strength. A decrease in smell is also referred to as hyposmia (Seiberling & Conley, 2004). Evidence shows peaks in the senses of smell and taste during the 20s and 40s, but by the 60s and 70s there is a decline in olfaction. This decline includes reduced ability for both odor detection and identification, especially among males. Over 50% of people age 65 years or older have significant olfactory dysfunction (Arking, 1998; Kovacs, 2004; Marieb & Hoehn, 2015; Seiberling & Conley, 2004). A decrease in the number of olfactory neurons and the weakening of olfactory neural pathways to the brain lead to a reduction in the ability to identify and distinguish aromas (Digiovanna, 1994, 2000; Seiberling & Conley, 2004). At the age of 25 years, the olfactory bulb contains approximately 60,000 mitral cells. By the age of 95 years, there are only 14,500 mitral cells. This decline in cell numbers decreases the functional ability of the olfactory neural system (Bhatnagar, Kennedy, Baron, & Greenberg, 1987). As discussed in "The Nervous System" section, neurofibrillary tangles and amyloid plaques can be observed in the aging brain and have been documented in the olfactory bulb (Kovacs, 1999, 2004). See **Figure 4-19** to identify olfaction pathways and neural correlates. Age-related gender differences include that males show greater declines in detection and identification of odors than do females (Arking, 1998; Kovacs, 2004).

Concerns associated with the declining sense of smell in older populations include the inability to smell harmful odors such as gas or smoke in the home and the inability to smell pleasurable, memory-invoking aromas such as flowers (Digiovanna, 1994, 2000; Kovacs, 2004; Stevens, Cain, & Weinstein, 1987). A decline in the ability to smell also can influence the sense of taste, often causing older individuals to change their eating habits and to receive less enjoyment from food (Cowart, 1989; Marieb & Hoehn, 2015; White & Ham, 1997). The decline in

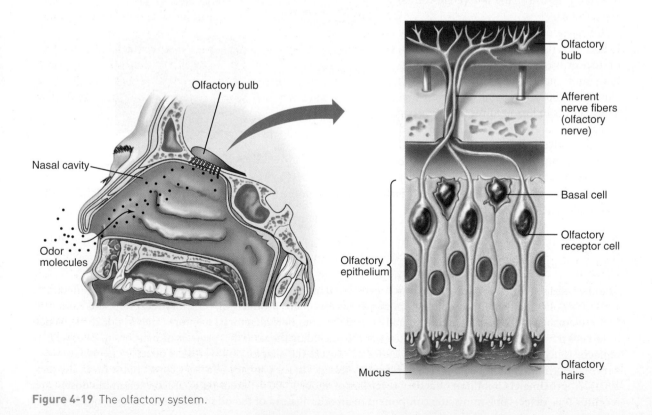

Figure 4-19 The olfactory system.

smell is much more predominant than the decline in taste, but individuals often say that the sense of taste has changed when actually it is the sense of smell that is impaired (Seiberling & Conley, 2004).

Taste

Anatomy of Gustation

Taste, or gustation, and the *chemoreceptors* for taste are located in approximately 10,000 taste buds found mostly on the tongue, but also in the rest of the oral cavity and throat (Sherwood, 2014). Taste receptors renew about every 10 days through generation of new receptor cells (Sherwood, 2014). The four primary tastes are sweet, salty, bitter, and sour; a fifth primary taste known as umami, a sensation related to the presence of the amino acid glutamate, also has been discovered (Digiovanna, 1994, 2000; Lindemann, 2000; Sherwood, 2014).

Age-Related Gustation Changes

Aging causes a decrease in taste, also known as *hypogeusia*, usually more noticeable around the age of 60 and with more severe declines occurring after the age of 70 (Seiberling & Conley, 2004). However, the sense of taste seems to decrease only slightly with age and can be variable among individuals (Digiovanna, 1994, 2000). Threshold studies, or studies that evaluate the lowest level of stimulus needed to reach threshold to invoke a response, are often used to measure taste (Digiovanna, 1994, 2000). Threshold studies have demonstrated some age-related, quality-specific changes in taste. The ability to detect salt changes the most with age, whereas detection of sugar appears to remain steady (Bartoshuk & Duffy, 1995; Cowart, 1989; Digiovanna, 1994, 2000; Weiffenbach, 1991; Weiffenbach, Baum, & Burghauser, 1982). Taste changes with age are not as well understood as changes in smell, but it has been hypothesized that there is a decrease in the number of taste buds as well as a change in taste receptors and cell membrane ion channels with age (Mistretta, 1984; Seiberling & Conley, 2004). Because taste buds have the ability to regenerate every 10 days, any changes in taste are most likely correlated with disruptions in taste receptors and cell membranes. Of course, taste sensation can be disrupted for other reasons, including medication use, smoking, disease, infections, and poor oral health (Schiffman, 1997; Seiberling & Conley, 2004; Wilson et al., 2005). The most common concerns related to changes in taste, which are strongly tied to changes in smell, are food poisoning and malnutrition (Marieb & Hoehn, 2015; Schiffman, 1997; Wilson et al., 2005).

Vision

The eyes monitor objects and conditions around the body, continually sending sensory messages to the brain such that the body can elicit appropriate responses to the outside environment (Digiovanna, 2000).

Anatomy and Age-Related Changes in Eye Structure

Many older adults experience dry eyes and/or a feeling of irritation, as if an object is in the eye. This condition is known as dry eye syndrome (Kollarits, 1998). Dry eye syndrome may be explained by age-related decline in the amount of tears produced by the lacrimal glands. The conjunctiva, which also normally helps lubricate the eye and eyelid with a mucous secretion, may have functional declines (Digiovanna, 1994, 2000; Kalina, 1999). The cornea, a transparent structure behind the conjunctiva, refracts or bends light rays traveling through the eye; with age the cornea tends to decrease in transparency. This decrease can cause a reduction in the amount of light entering the eye as well as an increase in light scattering (Digiovanna, 1994, 2000). The scattered light still reaches the retina, albeit in incorrect areas, causing bright areas in the field of view. This phenomenon is known as glare (Digiovanna, 1994, 2000). See **Figure 4-20** for an overview of the physiology of the eye. Behind the cornea lies the iris, which contains a hole called the pupil. The pupil allows light to pass into the eye (Digiovanna, 1994, 2000).

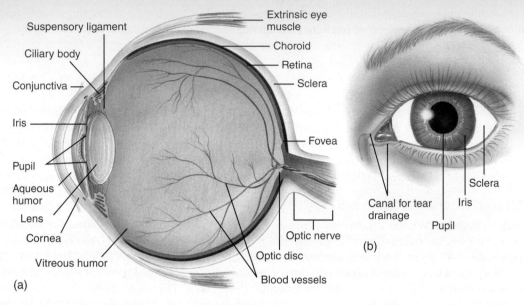

Figure 4-20 Anatomy of the human eye.

Collagen fibers in the eye begin to thicken and muscle cell numbers decrease with age. These changes reduce the ability of the pupil and iris to work together to constrict and dilate. As a result, the eye is unable to appropriately adapt to changing light intensities (Digiovanna, 1994, 2000; Kalina, 1999). The lens of the eye demonstrates an age-related loss of elasticity that also has been attributed to changes in collagen fibers. With age, the lens of the eye becomes less curved and more flat. In addition, there is a decreased transparency to colors of light, especially blue, and formation of opaque spots that block and scatter light (Digiovanna, 1994, 2000; Marieb & Hoehn, 2015). Retinal rods of the eye that are responsible for low-light vision demonstrate age-related changes, whereas retinal cones remain relatively stable (Kalina, 1999). The center of the eye contains vitreous humor, a gel containing collagen fibrils. With age, the vitreous humor loses transparency and there is an increase in the scattering of light, which may potentially cause floaters (Digiovanna, 2000; Kalina, 1999; Kollarits, 1998). The amount of aqueous humor, or fluid between the cornea and lens, produced declines with age, resulting in structural corneal changes such as flattening (Digiovanna, 2000; Kalina, 1999). All of these age-related structural changes in the eye explain many of the age-associated changes in vision.

Age-Related Changes in Visual Function

One of the most common visual concerns in aging that occurs over time but becomes most notable around 40 years of age and older, is *presbyopia*, or the inability to focus on nearby objects, such as newsprint. This inability is also known as farsightedness (Digiovanna, 1994; Jackson & Owsley, 2003). Presbyopia is generally corrected using bifocals and trifocals in lenses (Jackson & Owsley, 2003). Several studies have shown a decline in visual acuity, or the smallest object or detail that can be seen, even in individuals wearing corrective lenses. This decline may be correlated with a decrease in the neurons along the visual pathway as well as changes in the actual lens of the eye (Jackson & Owsley, 2003). Sensitivity to contrast, or the ability to observe a pattern in different light and intensity, also declines with age as a result of changes in the optics of the eye. Contrast sensitivity further declines under conditions of low light. Such a decline is likely due to changes in the neural pathways (Jackson & Owsley, 2003; Owsley, Sekular, & Siemsen, 1983; Sloane, Owsley, & Alzarez, 1988). Decline in contrast sensitivity is demonstrated by older individuals' complaints that driving and seeing road signs at night is very difficult, prompting them to drive only in daylight. All of these changes can be associated with aging of the cornea. Corneal aging is characterized by decreased transparency, greater scattering of light, and a flattening effect that results in reduced refraction, as previously described (Digiovanna, 1994). Another common complaint among older individuals pertains to changes in the visual field. Studies have demonstrated a narrowing of both the central and peripheral visual fields in older adults as compared to those of young adults. Narrowing is greater in peripheral fields as a result of disruption in the visual neural pathway (Haas, Flammer, & Schneider, 1986; Jackson & Owsley, 2003; Johnson, Adams, & Lewis, 1989). This decrease in the visual field area causes a lessened ability to visually search environmental surroundings, making it difficult to identify and discriminate objects and moving targets (Jackson & Owsley, 2003). Other consequences of aging changes in the visual neural pathway are demonstrated by decreased detection and awareness of moving objects as well as a diminished ability to distinguish one motion from another very similar motion (Ball & Sekuler, 1986; Gilmore, Wenk, Naylor, & Stuve, 1992; Jackson & Owsley, 2003). For instance, a police officer directs traffic around an accident scene on a two-lane highway by motioning one lane to slow and stop while motioning a car in the opposite lane to proceed slowly around. From a distance the older driver may not be able to clearly distinguish the hand movements of the officer until he or she is much closer to the scene. The speed with which individuals can visually process information also tends to slow in the older adult. As a result, older adults need to focus on an object for a longer time to identify and describe it (Jackson & Owsley, 2003; Salthouse, 1993).

Visual attention, divided attention, and selective attention also decrease with aging, with more pronounced deficits occurring when objects or information are shown very quickly (Jackson & Owsley, 2003). Impaired divided attention can be observed when an older adult is given two simultaneous tasks to complete, such as viewing a series of two pictures side by side on a computer screen for 5 seconds. If the older adult is instructed to learn the name on a building in one picture and to count how many animals are in the other picture, he or she will eventually begin to focus on only one picture.

Age-related changes in color vision lead to impaired color discrimination, especially along the blue–yellow color continuum. This indicates increased absorption of short wavelengths and a deficiency in those cones associated specifically with short wavelengths (Jackson & Owsley, 2003). The photoreceptors—rods and cones—also demonstrate age-related changes. The rod photoreceptors aid vision in the dark and in other low-light situations and demonstrate a greater age-related decline in density than do cone photoreceptors. Cone photoreceptors aid vision in regular and bright light situations and are involved in color vision. These photoreceptors maintain relative stability in density with age (Curcio, Millican, Allen, & Kalina, 1993; Jackson & Owsley, 2003). The decline in rod photoreceptors also provides evidence to support the common complaint of older individuals that they do not see as well at night, especially when driving.

Age-Related Eye Diseases

The most common causes of vision loss in the older adult population are cataracts, glaucoma, macular degeneration, and diabetic retinopathy (Heine & Browning, 2002; Jackson & Owsley, 2003; Kollarits, 1998; Marieb & Hoehn, 2015). These are all eye diseases or conditions that manifest more frequently in the aging population, but should not be considered a part of usual aging (National Eye Institute, 2004). The presence of cataracts, or a decrease in the transparency of the lens in the eye, is fairly common in the older population, and everyone who lives long enough will experience some degree of cataracts (Digiovanna, 1994; Kollarits, 1998). By the age of 75, approximately 50% of older adults will show signs of cataracts and about 25% of these cases will be advanced cataracts, with more instances occurring in women than men (Klein, Klein, & Linton, 1992a). Risk of glaucoma, increased intraocular pressure, is partly genetic but is also subject to environmental influences. Glaucoma causes loss in the peripheral visual field (Duggal et al., 2005; Kollarits, 1998). In general, intraocular pressure increases with age (Kalina, 1999). Around 2% of individuals in the United States over the age of 40 experience glaucoma, with a higher prevalence in African Americans (Kollarits, 1998). Adults age 75 or older also demonstrate a high incidence of macular degeneration (Klein et al., 1992b), which is a major cause of irreversible vision impairment and blindness. It accounts for 22% of cases of blindness in one eye and 75% of cases of legal blindness in adults 50 years of age or older (Klein, Wang, Klein, Moss, & Meuer, 1995). Diabetic retinopathy relates directly to the presence of diabetes. Diabetes is a disease state and not a part of usual aging; therefore, this topic will not be covered in this section (National Eye Institute, 2004).

Hearing

The External Canal

The external canal of the ear consists of the visible external ear opening, known as the pinna or auricle, and the canal that extends to the eardrum or tympanic membrane (Digiovanna, 2000; Patt, 1998; Tortora & Derrickson, 2014). Small vellus hairs cover the entire ear canal, and larger tragus hairs concentrate only in the most external portion of the canal (Patt, 1998). Cerumen glands situated in the ear canal open into hair follicles and onto skin, producing the odor associated with cerumen, or earwax (Patt, 1998). Age-related shrinkage of cerumen glands causes cerumen to become dryer. In turn, there is often blockage of the external canal and a decreased ability to hear (Digiovanna, 2000; Patt, 1998; Rees, Duckert, & Carey, 1999). In aging, the outer ear loses elasticity, the external ear canal narrows, and the tympanic membrane stiffens (Heine & Browning, 2002; Schuknecht, 2010). The skin on the ear becomes thinner and more susceptible to tears and infection (Rees et al., 1999), and hair on the external ear becomes longer and denser (Digiovanna, 2000; Patt, 1998).

The Middle Ear

The middle ear consists of three small bones called the auditory ossicles. These bones are the malleus, incus, and stapes (Digiovanna, 2000; Tortora & Derrickson, 2014). The ossicles amplify the vibrations sent from the external ear so as to maintain intensity of the sound wave traveling to the cochlea of the inner ear (Digiovanna, 2000; Tortora & Derrickson, 2014). The middle ear also loses elasticity and the ossicles tend to shrink with age (Heine & Browning, 2002; Patt, 1998; Schuknecht, 2010). Narrowing of the joint space between ossicles occurs as a result of age-related calcification of the joint capsule and deterioration of the cartilage; however, this narrowing does not seem to cause loss of sound waves in the middle ear (Jerger, Chmiel, Wilson, & Luchi, 1995; Patt, 1998; Rees et al., 1999).

The Inner Ear

The cochlea of the inner ear, also called the hearing organ, is spiral in shape and is filled with perilymph liquid (Digiovanna, 2000; Patt, 1998; Tortora & Derrickson, 2014). Within the cochlea, vibrations pass from the perilymph through the vestibular membrane into endolymph, another cochlear liquid, and finally to the basilar membrane (Digiovanna, 2000). **Figure 4-21** for representation of ear anatomy as well as changes to the ear and hearing process.

Age-related hearing loss occurs as a result of changes in the inner ear (Digiovanna, 2000; Rees et al., 1999; Tortora & Derrickson, 2014). The inner ear shows a loss of elasticity in the basilar membrane as well as degeneration of the organ of Corti, manifested as increased shrinkage and loss of hair cells (Heine & Browning, 2002; Schuknecht, 2010). Degeneration of small blood vessels in the cochlea leads to a reduction in endolymph production and a diminished ability of vibrations to travel through the ear (Digiovanna, 2000; Tortora & Derrickson, 2014). In the auditory portion of the brain, the cortex displays shrinkage, loss of neurons, and decreased blood flow (Heine & Browning, 2002; Schuknecht, 2010).

The Vestibular System

The inner ear encompasses the cochlea as well as the vestibule and balance organs (Patt, 1998). In the vestibular system, age-related decline occurs in hair cells, ganglion cells, and sensory nerve fibers (Patt, 1998; Rees et al.,

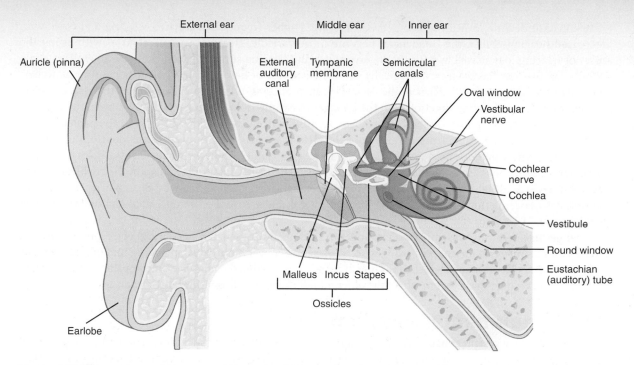

Figure 4-21 The anatomy of the ear and the parts of the ear that show changes with age.

1999). The vestibular system, together with the eye and proprioceptors, helps to maintain the body's physical balance or equilibrium (Rees et al., 1999). Compromises in vestibular balance occur with more frequency in the elderly and may lead to one of the most common complaints among older adults: dizziness. Among those age 65 or older, 90% of reports of vertigo or other imbalance result in physician office visits (Patt, 1998; Rees et al., 1999).

Hearing Mechanism

Hearing is the result of sound waves entering the external ear and canal, traveling to the tympanic membrane, and sending vibrations according to sound wave intensity. These vibrations are relayed to the ossicles and on toward the cochlea, which is considered the hearing organ (Jerger et al., 1995). The vibrations initiate a wave motion in the cochlea, causing changes in the basilar membrane and, in turn, stimulating the hair cells in the cochlea. Eventually, signals are sent through nerve fibers to the central auditory system (Jerger et al., 1995).

Hearing Loss

Aging changes that cause hearing loss include the alteration and decline in threshold sensitivity, the ability to hear high frequency sounds, and the ability to discern speech (Rees et al., 1999). Age-related hearing loss, also known as *presbycusis*, remains the most common sensory deficit in the older population. Approximately 35% of men and women age 60–70 years and 39% of those over the age of 75 report difficulty with conversation when they are in areas with background noise (Fransen, Lemkens, Van Laer, & Van Camp, 2003; Rees et al., 1999). Ringing in the ears, or tinnitus, is also a frequent occurrence in the elderly (Tortora & Derrickson, 2014). Typically, hearing loss, observed more often among males than females, occurs in both ears. The ability to hear higher frequency sounds is generally affected the most. Hearing loss is most closely correlated with sensorineural disruption (Fransen et al., 2003; Rees et al., 1999).

A constant decline in hearing is observed in aging. Higher frequencies are affected first and then, with decreased hearing ability, the frequencies become more variable. Hearing acuteness varies with age at the onset of hearing loss as well as with progressive states and hearing severity (Fransen et al., 2003; Rees et al., 1999). Hearing loss has been physiologically correlated to loss of hair cells and cochlear neurons as well as degeneration of the stria vascularis in the ear (Fransen et al., 2003). Four categories of presbycusis correlate the deterioration in hearing function with the changes in ear physiology, particularly changes in the cochlea. High-frequency hearing loss, or sensory presbycusis, results from the loss of hair cells in the cochlea of the ear. Strial presbycusis results from shrinkage of the stria vascularis. Neural presbycusis develops as a result of cochlear neuron deterioration and can cause a loss of the ability to discriminate words. Finally, cochlear conductive presbycusis causes gradual threshold loss correlated with potential changes in the cochlear duct in the ear (Rees et al., 1999; Schuknecht & Gacek, 1993). Along with usual aging processes, intrinsic and extrinsic factors such as occupation, loud noise, nutrition, cholesterol, and arteriosclerosis also affect the auditory system (Digiovanna, 2000; Rees et al., 1999).

Changes in the sensory system include changes in the anatomy of sensory organs and corresponding neural circuits and brain areas. Age-related changes occur variably for every individual, meaning that one person may not experience noticeable changes while another experiences severe decrements or even complete loss of a sensory system. These changes have an impact on the older adult's quality of life on a variety of levels.

The Integumentary System

The integumentary system consists of the skin and its accessory structures, including hair, nails, and the sweat and sebaceous (oil) glands. The integumentary system protects the body's tissues and internal organs, serves as a barrier against injury and infection, helps regulate body temperature, and acts as a receptor for stimuli of touch, pressure, and pain. It is also the physiological system most visible to the human eye, and thus the system that most readily displays the signs of aging.

Skin: Structure and Function

The skin, the largest of all human organs, comprises three primary layers—the epidermis, the dermis, and the subcutaneous layer (see Figure 4-18 earlier in the chapter). Each layer has a unique structure and function.

The Epidermis

The *epidermis* is the thin, outermost layer of the skin. It is composed of three primary cell types—keratinocytes, melanocytes, and Langerhans cells. *Keratinocytes* produce the protein keratin. As keratin accumulates in the cells, the cells die, and eventually these dead cells are pushed outward by the production of new cells beneath them. The keratinized cells begin to form a superficial layer of the epidermis known as the stratum corneum that protects the surface of the human body. These cells are exfoliated, or shed, and replaced by new cells. This process of cell exfoliation and replacement is cyclical, with one cycle normally lasting 14 to 28 days, depending on the region of the body (Marieb & Hoehn, 2015; M. L. Timiras, 2007).

The *melanocytes* produce *melanin*, a pigment essential to protecting the body from ultraviolet (UV) rays. Exposure to UV radiation leads to damage of the DNA and other components in cells of both the epidermis and dermis. Melanin blocks and absorbs UV radiation and, in so doing, protects against cellular dysfunction and lowers the risk of tumor formation. Because of their role in protection against UV radiation, melanocytes are found in increased numbers in sun-exposed skin.

The *Langerhans cells*, although they constitute only 1–2% of epidermal cells (Fossel, 2004), play a critical role in the body's immune defense system, particularly cutaneous immune reactions. These cells recognize foreign antigens and, in response, activate immune defenses. The main functions of Langerhans cells include antigen binding, processing, and presentation to naïve T cells (see "The Immune System" later in this chapter;

Schmitt, 1999). Langerhans cells, in addition to responding to antigens, launch immune responses to tumor cells. Thus, Langerhans cells help protect the body against both infection and skin cancer.

In addition to these cellular functions, the epidermis plays a critical role in the production of vitamin D_3, which is produced when its epidermal precursor form is activated through the skin's exposure to UV radiation—that is, sunlight (Yaar & Gilchrest, 2001). Ninety percent of the body's supply of vitamin D is produced in this manner (Holick, 2003). Vitamin D_3 plays a significant role in calcium homeostasis and bone metabolism, and deficiencies in vitamin D_3 have been associated with osteoporosis and osteomalacia as well as numerous other diseases, including cardiovascular disease, multiple sclerosis, diabetes, and a variety of cancers (Holick, 2003).

The Dermis

The *dermis* is composed primarily of the connective tissue fibers of collagen and elastin. Collagen provides structure to the skin. Due to its flexibility and extreme strength, collagen offers resistance against pulling forces (Arking, 1998) and thus helps protect the skin from being torn when stretched. Elastin, woven throughout collagen, adds resilience and flexibility to skin. Elastin is responsible for maintaining skin tension while simultaneously allowing skin to stretch to permit necessary movement of muscles and joints.

In addition to its connective tissue structure, the dermis is rich in vasculature. This dense vasculature allows for the provision of nutrients to the epidermis and assists in the control of body temperature through regulation of blood flow. The dermis also contains an abundance of nerves that relay information to the brain in response to a variety of sensory stimuli. Pressure and touch stimuli are detected and responded to by nerve endings known, respectively, as Pacini's and Meissner's corpuscles (see "The Sensory System" earlier in this chapter).

The Subcutaneous Layer

The *subcutaneous layer* is made up of loose collagen and subcutaneous fat. Collagen provides structure to the skin, much as it does in the dermis. Subcutaneous fat, with its rich vasculature, acts as an insulator against extensive heat loss. Thus, this layer of the skin plays an extremely important role in thermoregulation. Fat also serves as a shock absorber to prevent injury and trauma to bone, muscle, and internal organs. In addition, subcutaneous fat acts as a storage area for caloric reserves.

The Aging Skin

Changes in skin structure and function can be classified as either chronological (intrinsic) aging or extrinsic aging. *Chronological aging* refers to those changes considered to be caused only to the passage of time (see **Table 4-5**), while *extrinsic aging* is the result of chronic exposure of the skin to external factors such as smoking, poor nutrition, and especially UV light, which induces *photoaging* (Baumann, 2007). Chronologically aged skin is characterized by thinness and a reduction in elasticity. The wrinkles caused by chronological aging are usually very fine and thus the skin appears relatively smooth. In contrast, photoaged skin is characterized by deep wrinkles, sagging, and a leathery appearance (Scharffetter-Kochanek et al., 2000). Generally, chronological aging and photoaging become superimposed upon one another and compound each other's effects. Chronological aging primarily affects skin's function rather than its appearance.

With age, there is an overall decrease in the turnover rate of epidermal keratinocytes. By the eighth decade (Fossel, 2004), turnover rate has decreased by as much as 50%. The reduced turnover rate slows the exfoliation–replacement rate of dead keratinocytes. As a result, exposure of epidermal cells to harmful carcinogens is prolonged and the risk of skin cancer increases (M. L. Timiras, 2007). Risk of infection also increases. In addition, decreased epidermal turnover rate contributes to the slower wound repair seen in elderly persons.

The number of active melanocytes also declines with age, at a rate of 10–20% per decade (Fossel, 2004). This decline weakens the body's protective barrier against UV radiation, resulting in an increased risk of UV-induced DNA damage. Such damage greatly increases the risk of tumor formation and the development of skin cancer,

TABLE 4-5 Chronological or Intrinsic Aging Changes of the Integumentary System

	Structure	Function	Consequence
Skin			
Epidermis	Decreased turnover rate of keratinocytes Decreased number of active melanocytes Reduction in pigment granules in melanocytes Grouping and increased size of melanocytes Reduction in number of Langerhans cells Decline in vitamin D_3 production	Prolonged exposure of the epidermal cells to the environment Weakening of the protective barrier against UV radiation Dampened cell-mediated immune response	Increased risk of skin cancer Slower wound repair Increased risk of tumor formation and skin cancer Reduced ability to tan Age spots Increased susceptibility to infection and tumor development Increased risk of osteoporosis, osteomalacia, and other diseases
Dermis	Loss of thickness Loss of collagen elasticity and overall loss of collagen Elastin loses resiliency and becomes more brittle Loss of vascularity Decline in number of Pacini's and Meissner's corpuscles	Reduced ability to maintain skin suppleness Reduced ability to return skin to normal tension Decline in blood flow; impaired thermoregulation Reduced response to pressure and touch	Increased likelihood of sagging and wrinkling Sagging Decrease in skin temperature; dampened ability to adapt to temperature change; reduction in sweat and oil production Increased risk of injury Impaired ability to perform fine maneuvers with hands
Subcutaneous layer	Loss of thickness	Impaired ability to insulate and protect	Increased risk of heat loss and hypothermia Increased risk of injury and bruising
Skin Derivatives			
Hair	Thinning and loss; changes in length, appearance, and site of growth; graying		
Nails	Decline in linear growth rate; change in color, texture, and shape		
Eccrine glands	Decreased number of glands	Reduced efficiency of sweat production	Impaired thermoregulation; increased risk of heat exhaustion and heat stroke
Sebaceous glands		Reduction of oil and wax production	Increased roughness, dryness, and itchiness of skin

especially among the elderly population in which the DNA repair rate is slowed (Yaar & Gilchrest, 2001). With age, the remaining melanocytes generally have fewer pigment granules, making aged skin less likely to tan (Krauss Whitbourne, 2002). In addition, the melanocytes tend to increase in size and group together, which results in the so-called age spots that appear on elderly skin.

CLINICAL TIP

The integumentary system (including skin, hair, nails) often shows the most visible signs of aging.

Langerhans cells show an age-associated numerical decline of 20–50% from early to late adulthood (Yaar & Gilchrest, 2001). As a result, cell-mediated immune response is dampened with age. In fact, both animal and human studies have found immune system abnormalities to be associated with defects in the structure and function of skin cells (Arking, 1998). A depressed immune response can increase susceptibility to skin infection as well as skin allergens. In addition, when coupled with the reduction in melanocytes' protective action, the weakened immune response only further increases older persons' risk of tumor development.

Finally, vitamin D_3 production by the epidermis declines with age. This is the result of both a decrease in epidermal vitamin D_3 precursor and a reduction in sun exposure among older adults. The lower levels of vitamin D_3 put older adults at greater risk for poor overall bone health, osteoporosis, and numerous other diseases, as mentioned earlier.

In young skin, the epidermal and dermal layers are held tightly together through a series of interdigitations called dermal papillae, and it is nearly impossible to separate this epidermal–dermal junction. With age, however, there is a flattening of the epidermal–dermal junction as its interdigitated structure is lost. This flattening of the junction allows the epidermis to more easily separate from the underlying dermis. In turn, this separation renders older persons more susceptible to bruising and tearing of the skin as well as to blister formation. Furthermore, the decreased area of surface contact between the epidermis and dermis may compromise communication and nutrient transfer between these two layers of the skin (Baumann, 2007; Yaar & Gilchrest, 2001). The rate of change in the epidermal–dermal junction differs between women and men. In women, changes occur rather sharply between 40 and 60 years of age, most likely as a result of hormonal changes with menopause. Among men, the rate of change is much more constant throughout adulthood (Yaar & Gilchrest, 2001).

The greatest changes in aging skin are seen in the dermis. There is a general thinning of the dermal layer, with loss of thickness averaging 20% in older persons (Baumann, 2007; Beers & Berkow, 2000). This thinning of the dermis is due in large part to a general loss of collagen—approximately a 1% loss per year in adulthood (M. L. Timiras, 2007)—as well as a decrease in its flexibility. In addition, elastin becomes increasingly brittle and less resilient. This change in elastin results in a loss of the ability of the dermis to return to its original tension after it is stretched by the movement of underlying muscles and joints. Consequently, skin is more likely to sag. The overall effect of these changes in the connective tissues of the dermis is the looseness, loss of suppleness, and increased fine wrinkling that is characteristic of old, chronologically aged skin. It is of interest to note that the dermal layer is generally thicker in males than females, and this may account for the apparently greater rate of deterioration of female skin, especially following menopause (Arking, 1998).

With age the dermis also undergoes a decline in vascularity and blood flow is reduced by approximately 60% (Beers & Berkow, 2000). This reduction results in a decrease in skin temperature, making the skin of older adults generally cool to the touch. Diminished vascularity also contributes to impaired thermoregulation. The avascularity characterizing older skin can give a paler appearance to the skin, and generally the bones and remaining blood vessels beneath the skin become more visually prominent.

Nerve endings in the dermis also undergo changes as a person ages. In particular, the number of Pacini's and Meissner's corpuscles decreases, leading to a decline in the sensations of pressure and touch. Consequently, older persons are more prone to injuries resulting from poor detection of sensory stimuli. In addition, sensory loss leads to a decline in the ability to perform fine maneuvers with the hands.

The skin's subcutaneous layer thins dramatically with age. This loss of thickness occurs primarily in the skin of the face and hands (Arking, 1998). There is a general redistribution of body fat to the intraabdominal region with age. Thus, subcutaneous thickness of the skin around the hips and abdomen may, in fact, increase (Fenske & Lober, 1986). The subcutaneous layer ordinarily acts as an insulator against excessive loss of body heat. Thus, as it thins, the ability to conserve heat declines, making the older person more prone to low body temperature and possible hypothermia when exposed to the cold (Krauss Whitbourne, 2002). The thinning of the subcutaneous layer also limits its ability to act as protective cushioning. Consequently, bones, major organs, arteries, and nerves receive more concentrated impacts (Fossel, 2004), in turn increasing the risk of injury and bruising.

CLINICAL TIP

Due to the changes in the skin's ability to conserve heat, older persons may have a lower baseline body temperature. This should always be noted on admission, as a later temperature reading of 99.9 degrees Fahrenheit may actually be a fever and a warning sign of infection in a person with a lower baseline temperature.

Estrogen and Aging Skin

Sex hormones greatly influence the aging process, and the skin is a target organ for these hormones. Therefore, a change in sex hormone levels with age will affect any skin functions that are under hormonal control (Sator, Schmidt, Rabe, & Zouboulis, 2004). Estrogen is a sex hormone and has been extensively studied for its influence on skin aging. Research has shown that the reduction in estrogen associated with menopause is associated with impaired structure and function of the skin (Phillips, Demircay, & Sahu, 2001; Shah & Maibach, 2001). Postmenopausal women receiving hormone replacement therapy (HRT) have been shown to have thicker, healthier skin and show statistically greater collagen content than those not receiving HRT (Phillips et al., 2001). In addition, the skin of those receiving hormonal treatment exhibits less loss of elasticity, in turn exerting a positive effect on skin sagging (Pierard, Letawe, Dowlati, & Pierard-Franchimont, 1995). One national study found that estrogen use may prevent both skin drying and skin wrinkling (Dunn, Damesyn, Moore, Reuben, & Greendale, 1997).

Aging of Skin Accessory Structures

Hair

Hair is produced by hair follicles underneath the surface of the skin. With age, the germination centers that produce hair follicles undergo changes and may, in fact, be destroyed (Baumann, 2007; Krauss Whitbourne, 2002). As a result, thinning and loss of scalp hair occur with age, in both men and women. There also may be a thinning of facial hair in men. Simultaneously, however, the hair on older men's eyebrows and inside their ears may become longer and coarser. Similarly, women may develop unwanted facial hair, especially following the hormonal changes associated with menopause.

Hair also tends to gray over time. Graying is due primarily to gradual loss of functional melanocytes from hair bulbs and a general decline in melanin production. The age of onset of graying varies somewhat based on heredity and racial background. For whites, the average age of graying onset is the mid-30s, for Asian Americans, late-30s, and for African Americans, mid-40s. Despite these variations, however, it can generally be said that by 50 years of age, 50% of people have 50% gray hair (Tobin & Paus, 2001).

Nails

The linear growth rate of nails decreases with age (M. L. Timiras, 2007). In addition, nails tend to become thinner, drier, and more brittle as a person ages. Nails also undergo a change in shape, generally becoming flat or concave instead of convex (Beers & Berkow, 2000). Longitudinal grooves or ridges may form on the nails.

Glands

Both sweat glands and sebaceous glands undergo changes with age. The number of sweat glands decreases by approximately 15% during adulthood (Beers & Berkow, 2000; Tortora & Derrickson, 2014). In addition, the glands' efficiency declines and less sweat is produced. The result is impaired thermoregulation and difficulty in staying cool; this leaves older adults at greater risk for heat exhaustion and heat stroke.

Sebaceous glands do not decrease in number with age; however, the size and activity of the glands does decrease. Soon after puberty, oil production declines at a rate of 23% per decade in men and 32% per decade in women (Jacobsen et al., 1985). Clinical manifestations associated with age-related changes of the sebaceous glands include increased dryness, roughness, and itchiness of the skin as well as, in rare cases, sebaceous gland carcinoma (Zouboulis & Boschnakow, 2001).

The Immune System

The immune system is a network of cells and biochemicals responsible for defending the body against foreign microorganisms such as bacteria, viruses, fungi, and parasites. Whenever the immune system is compromised, the body is left vulnerable to a variety of infections and infectious diseases, from the flu and common cold to tuberculosis and acquired immunodeficiency syndrome (AIDS). The numerous and, at times, life-threatening consequences of a weakened immune system illustrate the tremendous importance of the system in maintaining good health.

The crucial feature of the immune system that makes it such a remarkable system of defense is its ability to distinguish the body's own cells ("self") from any foreign cells or microorganisms ("nonself"). A foreign substance invading the body is known as an *antigen*. Antigens carry marker molecules on their surface that identify them as foreign, and it is these marker molecules that allow for the discernment of self and nonself. In cases in which this discernment process fails, the immune system will attack its own cells. This attack of self is termed *autoimmunity* and can lead to a variety of autoimmune diseases, such as rheumatoid arthritis and multiple sclerosis. Once again, these consequences of a disrupted immune system demonstrate its critical role in protecting the health of an organism.

The defense mechanisms of the immune system are divided into two primary types, innate (or nonspecific) immunity and acquired (also called specific or adaptive) immunity. Each type of immunity is characterized by its own components and method of function. However, the two must work in close collaboration, often through the use of *cytokines*, to fulfill their common responsibility: the protection of the body against infection and disease.

Innate Immunity

The innate immune system is the one with which a person is born. It is always present and is activated almost immediately upon exposure to an antigen. It is the body's initial attempt at ridding the body of foreign substances. Although *innate immunity* allows for the general discernment of self versus nonself, it does not have the ability to recognize a specific antigen. Thus, even if the body is repeatedly exposed to the same antigen, it will react each time to that particular antigen as if it had never before been encountered. Innate immunity does not adapt to or remember a specific antigen, so it is unable to improve the effectiveness of its defense against that antigen. Innate immunity, therefore, is antigen-independent and results in no immunological memory of prior encounters with an antigen.

Innate immunity operates through a variety of mechanisms. One of these mechanisms involves the use of physical barriers, in particular the skin and mucosal membranes. The skin may be the most basic and yet one of the most important mechanisms of immunity, because it is the first site most antigens encounter and the site at which many are stopped. Mucosal membranes, such as those lining the eyes, airways, and gastrointestinal and genitourinary tracts, also provide physical barriers of protection, as do mucosal secretions, such as saliva and tears, which contain enzymes that destroy potential infectious agents.

If an antigen manages to breach physical barriers such as skin and mucosa, the innate immune system continues its attack on the antigen by launching additional defense mechanisms. These include the actions of macrophages, *natural killer (NK) cells*, and the complement system, as well as the inflammatory response.

Macrophages act through a process called phagocytosis. During phagocytosis an antigen is completely engulfed and, through the use of destructive enzymes, literally consumed by the macrophage. Macrophages also secrete cytokines that stimulate the actions of NK cells. When NK cells are activated, they work to kill cells that have been altered through infection by an antigen. Destruction of these cells occurs through two mechanisms. First, NK cells literally punch holes in the membranes of the altered cells and release enzymes that promote self-induced death (or apoptosis) of the altered cells. Second, NK cells release cytokines that target macrophages and enhance their destructive action. Thus, macrophages and NK cells work synergistically to augment each other's actions and thereby provide a stronger defense against invading antigens.

The *complement system* is a collection of proteins that can kill antigens directly or help destroy antigens by attaching to and marking them for destruction by macrophages and other cells of the immune system. The complement system also initiates the *inflammatory response*, which results in the release of several chemical messengers that signal macrophages and other phagocytic cells to destroy the antigen. These chemical messengers also increase blood flow and cause blood vessels to release fluid, resulting in redness and swelling, respectively, at the site of invasion. The swelling helps isolate an antigen and prevent it from coming in further contact with body tissues. The inflammatory response also generates heat, and thus fever, in an attempt to overheat and kill antigens.

Innate immunity provides an early and strong line of defense against foreign antigens. In addition, the very occurrence of the innate immune response serves as a signal for initiation of the acquired immune response, effectively stimulating further mechanisms of defense. When they act in concert, innate and acquired immunity provide the body with its most powerful protection against infection and disease.

Acquired Immunity

Acquired immunity consists of two branches (see **Table 4-6**). The first, *humoral immunity*, is mediated by antigen-attacking proteins called *antibodies* and is responsible for defending the body against extracellular antigens found in the blood and other body fluids or "humors." The second branch, *cell-mediated immunity*, is responsible for destroying intracellular antigens. Acquired immunity involves the actions of two primary types of leukocytes— B cells and T cells. Both cell types are produced in the bone marrow; however, only *B cells* continue to mature in the marrow. *T cells* are transported to the thymus, a small organ behind the breastbone, for maturation. Once both

TABLE 4-6 Comparison of Humoral and Cell-Mediated Immunity	
Humoral	Cell-Mediated
Principal cellular agent is the B cell.	Principal cellular agent is the T cell.
B cells respond to bacteria, bacterial toxins, and some viruses.	T cells respond to cancer cells, virus-infected cells, single-cell fungi, parasites, and foreign cells in an organ transplant.
When activated, B cells form memory cells and plasma cells, which produce antibodies to these antigens.	When activated, T cells differentiate into memory cells, cytotoxic cells, suppressor cells, and helper cells; cytotoxic T cells attack the antigen directly.

cell types have reached maturity they reside mainly in the lymph nodes and spleen. B cells are involved primarily in humoral immunity and T cells principally in cell-mediated immunity. However, there is strong communication between the two cell types, reflecting the collaborative action of the two branches of acquired immunity.

Humoral Immunity

B cells are activated through encounters with antigens; however, not just any antigen will activate any B cell. Each B cell is programmed to respond to only one specific antigen. Once activated by this antigen, the B cell undergoes a process known as *clonal expansion* in which it multiplies to produce a multitude of B-cell clones. These clones then differentiate into antibody-producing B cells, or plasma cells. *Plasma cells* are capable of producing and secreting antibodies against only the specific antigen that initiated the humoral immune response. The antibodies are released into the bloodstream, where they bind with the targeted antigen. This binding action neutralizes the antigen and prompts other immune cells, such as macrophages, into action.

Following clonal expansion, not all B-cell clones will differentiate into antibody-producing cells. Some will become memory B cells. Upon formation, these memory cells do not produce antibodies; however, they effectively remember the antigen against which they were produced and retain the ability to produce antibodies in the future should the antigen be reintroduced. The memory cells survive, perhaps for years, and circulate in the bloodstream, primed to launch a rapid response if and when they again encounter their antigen. Thus, humoral immunity is characterized by immunological memory.

Cell-Mediated Immunity

T cells are of three types—T-helper cells, killer T cells, and suppressor T cells (see **Table 4-7**).

T-helper cells are the primary regulatory agents of the immune system. They identify foreign antigens and, in response, proliferate through clonal expansion and release chemical messengers that stimulate action of the killer T cells. T-helper cells also have an indirect role in humoral immunity. Only nonprotein antigens have the ability to cause direct activation of B cells. Protein antigens require that B cells first interact with and receive chemical signals from T helper cells before the B cells can be activated and an antibody-mediated humoral response launched. This T-helper cell activation of the B cells provides an excellent example of the interaction between humoral and cell-mediated immunity.

Killer T cells, also known as cytotoxic T cells, directly attack and destroy infected cells within the body. Most commonly, killer T cells operate against virally infected cells; however, they are also responsible for ridding the body of cells that have been transformed by cancer. In addition, killer T cells are the cells responsible for the rejection of organ and tissue grafts.

TABLE 4-7	Summary of T Cells
Cell Type	**Action**
Cytotoxic T cells	Destroy body cells infected by viruses, and attack and kill bacteria, fungi, parasites, and cancer cells.
Helper cells	Produce a growth factor that stimulates T cells, B-cell proliferation and differentiation, and antibody production by plasma cells; enhance activity of cytotoxic T cells
Supressor cells	May inhibit immune reaction by T cells, decreasing B- and T-cell activity and B- and T-cell division
Memory cells	Remain in the body awaiting contact with the antigen they remember, at which time they proliferate and differentiate into cytotoxic T cells, helper T cells, suppressor T cells, and additional memory cells

Suppressor T cells are the final players in an immune response. These cells counteract the actions of T-helper and killer T cells as well as B cells, bringing an end to the immune response once an infection has passed. In addition, suppressor T cells act to damp the immune response when it becomes overactive. This damping action is crucial given that overaction of the immune response can lead to both allergic reactions and autoimmune disease. Thus, the action of suppressor T cells is critical to ensuring that the overall immune response remains properly balanced.

Like humoral immunity, cell-mediated immunity is characterized by immunological memory. During proliferation T cells produce a pool of memory cells. These cells remain dormant until they again come in contact with the antigen they remember; they then unleash a faster and more powerful immune response than the first. Some memory cells are able to survive for the lifetime of an individual; this ability is what provides us with lifelong immunity to diseases such as chickenpox and measles.

Immunosenescence

The term *immunosenescence* refers to the aging of the immune system. To date, the aging process is thought to involve primarily innate immunity and the T cells of acquired immunity. B cells are less highly affected by immunosenescence; however, the majority of investigations have been performed only in animal models (Aw, Silva, & Palmer, 2007).

Innate Immunity

Clinical evidence suggests a dysfunction in the innate immune system. With aging, elevated levels of proinflammatory cytokines released from fibroblasts and macrophages are believed to be linked to age-associated diseases such as diabetes, osteoporosis, and atherosclerosis that appear to have an inflammatory pathway involved (Aw et al., 2007; Gomez, Boehmer, & Kovacs, 2005; Licastro et al., 2005). A number of studies have also indicated that phagocytosis is reduced in the aging immune system and that the destructive capacity of neutrophils and macrophages is inhibited by decreased levels of production of the superoxide anion, which is responsible for the destruction of ingested material (Aw et al., 2007, Plackett, Boehmer, Faunce, & Kovacs, 2004). Some studies have also implicated depressed NK function in some of the decline in innate immunity (Aw et al., 2007; Gruver, Hudson, & Sempowski, 2007; Mocchegiani & Malavolta, 2004; Solana & Mariani, 2000).

Thymus Involution

The most prominent morphological change characterizing immunosenescence is the involution, or atrophy, of the thymus (Aw et al., 2007). The thymus begins to atrophy around puberty and continues as an individual ages. Extrapolating from known rates of thymic involution, it has been postulated that if an individual were to live to 120 years of age, the thymus would atrophy completely (Aspinall & Andrew, 2000). Given that the thymus is responsible for T-cell maturation and differentiation, it is not surprising that the involution of this organ results in changes in the T-cell population.

Naïve-to-Memory T-Cell Ratio

At any given time, both naïve and memory T cells are present in the body. Naïve T cells are those that have not yet been exposed to an antigen; these are the cells that respond to any new antigen that might attack the body. Memory T cells, as discussed earlier, are T cells that are programmed to respond to specific and previously encountered antigens. With age there is a shift in the ratio of naïve T cells to memory T cells. In young persons, this ratio is quite high, with more naïve T cells than memory T cells. Over time, however, many more naïve cells become exposed to antigens and converted to memory T cells. In addition, as a result of thymic involution, fewer naïve T cells are produced with age. As a result of these changes, the population of naïve T cells is depleted over time, so the ratio of naïve T cells to memory T cells is very low in older persons. Consequently, elderly persons respond much less efficiently to new antigens that may threaten the body (Gruver et al., 2007; Linton & Dorshkind, 2004; Whitman, 1999), leaving them more vulnerable to infection and disease.

Replicative Senescence

The greater the number of B or T cells available to fight off infection and disease, the more likely it is that the immune response will be effective. Thus, the replication or proliferation of immune cells subsequent to stimulation by an antigen is crucial to efficient immune function. However, cells can undergo only a finite number of divisions, after which there can be no further proliferation of cells. This phenomenon is known as *replicative senescence*. Replicative senescence is the result not of the passage of time per se, but of repeated cell division (Effros & Pawelec, 1997). Nonetheless, over time older cells will have experienced more demands for cell division than younger cells. Consequently, older cells are more likely to have exhausted their ability to divide and to have reached a state of replicative senescence. This is particularly true of immune cells that repeatedly encounter their antigens (Effros, Dagarag, & Valenzuela, 2003) (e.g., antigens giving rise to the common cold). In addition to the increased number of cells that reach replicative senescence as a person ages, research has also shown that replicative senescence occurs earlier (i.e., after fewer divisions) in T cells from old individuals. This suggests that T cells may have a reduced ability to proliferate in old age (Wick & Grubeck-Loebenstein, 1997).

The primary result of replicative senescence is a decline in the overall number of immune cells available to ward off invading antigens. In addition, if immune cells reach replicative senescence during an active immune response, they will be unable to continue cell division, thereby leading to premature termination of the immune response (Effros & Pawelec, 1997). Thus, with age the immune response is greatly weakened due to the inability of immune cells to divide indefinitely. Replicative senescence appears to be of particular concern for T cells and cell-mediated immunity.

Cell Signaling

Effective cell-mediated immunity requires that when a T cell binds to its antigen, the presence of that antigen must be communicated or signaled to the interior of the cell. One of the key molecules involved in this signaling process is CD28, located on the surface of T cells. Without the presence of CD28, the cell is unable to respond to an invading antigen and thus remains inactive. With age, there is a progressive increase in the number of T cells lacking CD28, which leads to an increased likelihood of disruption to the signaling pathway and, ultimately, T cell function is impaired (Hirokawa, 1999).

Calcium, essential for numerous biochemical reactions, is also crucial for effective cell signaling. In general, calcium deficiency becomes more likely as a person ages. In addition, calcium mobilization from intracellular stores is inhibited in older subjects as compared to younger subjects (Aw et al., 2007). This deficiency contributes to impaired cell signaling within the immune system of older persons. Calcium is also a central player in the production of cytokines. Thus, calcium deficiency can inhibit production of these chemical messengers, thereby hindering immune system communication and the overall coordination of the immune response (Whitman, 1999).

Autoimmunity

Despite the age-related decrease in immune response to foreign antigens, there is an increase in autoimmunity. There is an overall increase in the percentage of T cell– and B cell–generated antibodies that are directed against many of the body's own cells. The reason for the increase in autoimmunity is not well understood; however, it has been hypothesized that although T cells directed against the body's own cells are normally destroyed in the thymus before they are fully matured, involution of the thymus with age allows these cells to persist. In turn, these T cells could also prompt B cells to produce autoantibodies—antibodies against the body's own cells. Ultimately, there is an increase in autoimmunity.

Clinical Implications of Immunosenescence

Vaccinations

Due to changes characterizing immunosenescence, older individuals are more susceptible to infection and disease than are younger individuals. One method of strengthening the immune defenses is to administer vaccines such as those against influenza and pneumonia. By introducing the body to a foreign antigen, vaccines stimulate the production of antibody-producing B cells as well as memory T cells against the antigen. However, older individuals' antibody response to vaccines is slower and weaker than that seen in younger individuals (Whitman, 1999). In addition, due to the decrease in naïve T cells with age, the T-cell response of older persons to a new antigen, such as that introduced by vaccine, may be particularly impaired (Wick & Grubeck-Loebenstein, 1997). T cells of older adults have, in fact, been shown to respond less quickly to vaccines. Overall, the age-related changes in response to vaccines generally render them less effective in older patients.

Infection and Disease

Immunosenescence is associated with increased incidence of infectious diseases such as bronchitis and influenza. It is also implicated in the increased incidence of tumors and cancer that occurs with age. In addition, immunosenescence has been associated with a number of age-related autoimmune diseases and inflammatory reactions, including diabetes, arthritis, osteoporosis, cardiovascular disease, and dementia. Inarguably, the aging of the immune system has widespread implications for disease incidence and overall health within the elderly population.

The Hematopoietic System

The hematopoietic system is responsible for the production, differentiation, and proliferation of mature blood cells from stem cells. The site of blood cell production, or *hematopoiesis*, changes with the developmental stage of an organism. In the fetus, blood cells are produced in the liver, spleen, and yolk sac. In children and adults, blood cells are produced in the bone marrow. At birth, the cavities of nearly all bones are filled with active bone marrow; however, by adulthood, active bone marrow is found only in the femur, humerus, sternum, vertebrae, and ribs as well as the pelvic bones and some skull bones.

Hematopoiesis

Hematopoiesis begins with *pluripotent stem cells*. Pluripotent describes the cells' ability to differentiate into any of several different types of progeny cells, or *stem cell progenitors*. Each type of progenitor is committed to the production of only one particular type of mature blood cell (e.g., RBCs, WBCs, and platelets, as discussed below) (see **Table 4-8**). Pluripotent stem cells and stem cell progenitors comprise the body's stem cell pool. The stem cells are capable of self-renewal and, thus, the stem cell pool is maintained throughout an individual's life. The self-renewal capacity of stem cells together with the unlimited differentiation potential of pluripotent stem cells allow for regeneration of all hematopoietic cells as needed.

Hematopoiesis is regulated by a network of several biochemical messengers known as cytokines. Any imbalance in cytokine production or decreased sensitivity to cytokines by pluripotent stem cells and/or stem cell progenitors can result in disruption of hematopoiesis. Likewise, disruption may result from a reduction in the number of pluripotent stem cells available for differentiation into mature blood cells. The hematopoietic system is responsible for a variety of functions, including oxygen delivery to cells, the immune response, and hemostasis or the control of blood loss. Given the importance of these functions, any interruption to hematopoiesis will have potentially serious consequences for efficient and proper functioning of the body.

The Blood Cells

Erythrocytes

Erythrocytes (see Table 4-8), or RBCs, are biconcave in shape and have no nuclei. They are red due to the presence of hemoglobin, an iron-containing protein pigment. Erythrocytes are responsible for the transport of oxygen, which binds to hemoglobin molecules and is then carried from the lungs to the cells where it is needed for metabolism.

TABLE 4-8 Summary of Blood Cells

Name	Light Micrograph	Description	Concentration (Number of Cells/mm³)	Lifespan	Function
Red blood cells (RBCs)		Biconcave disk; no nucleus	4–6 million	120 days	Transports oxygen and carbon dioxide
White blood cells (WBCs) Neutrophil		Approximately twice the size of RBCs; multilobed nucleus; clear-staining cytoplasm	3,000–7,000	6 hours to a few days	Phagocytizes bacteria
Eosinophil		Approximately same size as neutrophil; large pink-staining granules; bilobed nucleus	100–400	8–12 days	Phagocytizes antigen-antibody complex; attacks parasites
Basophil		Slightly smaller than neutrophil; contains large, purple cytoplasmic granules; bilobed nucleus	20–50	Few hours to a few days	Releases histamine during inflammation
Monocyte		Larger than neutrophil; cytoplasm grayish-blue; no cytoplasmic granules; U- or kidney-shaped nucleus	100–700	Lasts many months	Phagocytizes bacteria, dead cells, and cellular debris
Lymphocyte		Slightly smaller than neutrophil; large, relatively round nucleus that fills the cell	1,500–3,000	Can persist many years	Involved in immune protection, either attacking cells directly or producing antibodies
Platelets		Fragments of megakaryocytes; appear as small dark-staining granules	250,000	5–10 days	Play several key roles in blood clotting

The efficient delivery of oxygen is a key function of erythrocytes, and the production and functional activity of erythrocytes increases in response to hypoxia, or oxygen deprivation.

Once produced in the bone marrow, erythrocytes mature in 24–48 hours. They have a lifespan of approximately 120 days, after which they die and are removed from circulation. Erythrocytes, however, have the capacity for continual self-renewal, allowing for the replenishment of the RBC supply. This replenishment balances the routine destruction of erythrocytes and, thus, a relatively constant number of RBCs is maintained in the circulation.

Leukocytes

Leukocytes (see Table 4-8), or WBCs, are classified on the basis of their nuclear shape as well as the presence or absence of cytoplasmic granules. Leukocytes are of two primary types—granular and agranular—and function principally within the immune system. Granular leukocytes, or granulocytes, include the neutrophils, basophils, and eosinophils. Neutrophils are phagocytic cells that ingest and kill bacteria. Basophils and eosinophils are involved in inflammatory reactions. Agranular leukocytes, also termed mononuclear leukocytes, consist of lymphocytes and monocytes. The lymphocytes include B lymphocytes and T lymphocytes, which are involved in humoral and cell-mediated immunity, respectively. (See "The Immune System" earlier in this chapter.) Monocytes are also involved in the immune response. These cells leave the blood and enter tissues, where they mature into macrophages, the cells necessary for the destruction of infectious agents.

Thrombocytes

Thrombocytes (Table 4-8), or platelets, are responsible for hemostasis, the prevention of blood loss. Hemostasis involves the aggregation of thrombocytes to form a clot. The clot then acts to seal off and impede blood loss from wounds.

Aging of the Hematopoietic System

Changes that are most often discussed in regard to the aging hematopoietic system include the reduced proliferative and self-replicative capacity of stem cells and changes in the cytokine network. However, the degree to which these changes are the result of aging per se remains controversial. There is a great deal of evidence to suggest that functioning of the hematopoietic system, when under basal or steady-state conditions, undergoes no significant changes with aging. Many of the changes in the hematopoietic system of older individuals are evidenced only under certain circumstances, such as hemorrhaging or anemia, in which the system is under stress and experiencing an increase in functional demand.

Stem Cells and Aging

The Proliferative Capacity of Stem Cells

Some research suggests that stem cells' proliferative capacity is limited and may decrease with age, reaching a state of exhaustion (Globerson, 1999). Reduction in proliferative capacity is thought to result from continual shortening of telomeres, the terminal sections of chromosomes. Once telomeres become too short to allow for further cell replication, cell proliferation ceases. If and when stem cell proliferation is stopped, the body becomes limited in its ability to renew the supply of mature hematopoietic cells. A reduction in mature hematopoietic cells would in turn affect the efficiency with which these cells perform their respective functions, such as oxygen delivery and the immune response.

Telomerase is the enzyme that stimulates the addition of telomeric portions to the end of chromosomes, thereby maintaining the self-renewal capacity of cells. Telomerase activity is upregulated in response to chemical messages from cytokines and downregulated in response to cell proliferation. Although the action of telomerase may limit telomere shortening and subsequent reductions in proliferative capacity, it has not been shown to entirely prevent reduction in telomere length (Engelhardt et al., 1997; Kamminga & DeHaan, 2006). Thus, potential methods by which telomerase activity is increased will not lead to a cessation of the loss of proliferative capacity. Furthermore, research has suggested that indeed other factors besides the action of telomerase are involved in regulation of telomere shortening (Lansdorp et al., 1997). Thus, certainly the mechanisms influencing loss of proliferative capacity with age have yet to be clarified and will require further research.

As mentioned earlier, many of the age-related changes in the hematopoietic system are most evident not when the body is in the basal state, but when the body is under hematopoietic stress. Hematopoietic stress requires a fairly rapid increase in the number of functional blood cells, thereby necessitating an efficient process of stem cell proliferation. Hence, the reduction of stem cell proliferative capacity illustrates well how age-related changes would be most clearly evident under conditions of stress.

CD34⁺ Progenitor Stem Cells

CD34⁺ cells, the primary circulating progenitor stem cells, are believed to decrease in number with age. This decrease is evidenced by one study, which found that among normal human volunteers (ages 20–90 years) CD34⁺ cells exhibited an inverse correlation with age (Egusa, Fujiwara, Syahruddin, Isobe, & Yamakido, 1998). The decline in CD34⁺ cells witnessed among older adults ages 66 to 73 years was similar to that witnessed in centenarians. This research suggests that reduction in CD34⁺ cell counts is primarily an early age-related phenomenon. Centenarians and those with great longevity are unlikely to exhibit decreases in CD34⁺ progenitor cells beyond that which they experienced in the early stages of aging (Bagnara et al., 2000).

Age-Related Changes in the Cytokine Network

Cytokines involved in the regulation of hematopoiesis include interleukin 3 (IL-3), granulocyte-macrophage colony-stimulating factor (GM-CSF), interleukin 6 (IL-6), and tumor necrosis factor alpha (TNF-α). IL-3 and GM-CSF stimulate proliferation of hematopoietic cells; conversely, IL-6 and TNF-α act to inhibit hematopoiesis (Balducci, Hardy, & Lyman, 2000; Baraldi-Junkins, Beck, & Rothstein, 2000). These cytokines show changes in older populations, which may implicate them in many of the age-related changes in the hematopoietic system.

The peripheral blood of older individuals is reported to have a reduced capacity to produce IL-3 and GM-CSF (Bagnara et al., 2000), thereby limiting their efficiency in stimulating the production of hematopoietic cells. IL-6 and TNF-α, in contrast, show an increased concentration with age in both animals and humans (Balducci et al., 2000). This increase has the potential to disrupt homeostatic regulation of hematopoiesis and may be partially responsible for poor response to hematopoietic stress with age. Furthermore, increased IL-6 concentrations show an association with increased risk of death, anemia, and functional decline in older persons (Balducci, 2003).

Anemia and Aging

Anemia is a condition in which a deficiency in the number of erythrocytes or the amount of hemoglobin they contain limits the exchange of oxygen and carbon dioxide between the blood and tissues. Anemia is a common condition among older persons. Of the elderly population, 8% to 44% have anemia, with a higher prevalence among older men (Nilsson-Ehle, Jagenburg, Landahl, & Svanborg, 2000). These prevalence statistics are based on the World Health Organization's (WHO's) criteria for a diagnosis of anemia—hemoglobin less than 12 g/dL blood in women and less than 13 g/dL blood in men (De Martinis & Timiras, 2007).

Despite the relatively ubiquitous nature of anemia among elderly persons, it is important to note that most forms of anemia in this population are due to causes other than aging. This is demonstrated by the fact that hemoglobin and hematocrit remain essentially unchanged among healthy older persons. In addition, when anemia is diagnosed in older adults there is almost always another comorbid medical condition present and underlying the anemia (De Martinis & Timiras, 2007). Thus, anemia should not be considered an age-related disease; it is not a universal or even usual condition that develops as the body ages.

Genetics and Aging

How well a person ages is often attributed to intrinsic factors, such as genetics and hereditary factors, as well as extrinsic factors, such as diet and exercise. Scientifically, the natural process of aging has been attributed to free radical damage, a by-product of metabolism, as well as by direct genetic inheritance and genetic changes with age (Hekimi & Guarente, 2003; Lee & Wei, 2012). As mentioned previously in the "Cardiovascular Aging

Mechanisms" and the "Nervous System" sections of this chapter, free radicals cause damage to cells and proteins, leading to increased processes of aging. However, research has shown that steps can be taken to slow aging. For instance, caloric restriction studies in animals have demonstrated increased longevity in multiple species (Mair & Dillin, 2008; Stein et al., 2012). Caloric restriction slows the aging process through increased protein renewal along with declines in molecular damage (Lee, Kloop, Weindruch, & Prolla, 1999). Important to note is that caloric restriction does not mean malnutrition, which can be dangerous and lead to death.

Longevity, the ability to live a long life, has been a focus of countless studies in order to unlock the secrets of aging. Centenarians, older adults who live to 100 years are longer, are studied to research genetic components, disease states, dietary habits, exercise regimens, and other factors throughout the lifespan. Aging twin studies also offer insight into variances in environmental versus genetic factors of aging processes (Tan, Ohm, Kruse, & Christensen, 2010). More controlled laboratory studies utilize animals for genetic testing of longevity manipulation. Studies of longevity demonstrate that a strong genetic component exists with protectors against oxidative stress and cardiovascular disease (Vijg & Suh, 2005; Nair & Ren, 2012). Biological aging is commonly associated with cardiovascular aging changes (Nair & Ren, 2012). Globally, the ability to study and manipulate the aging process and utilization of antiaging products remain in high demand. One antiaging gene therapy study involving telomerase in mice demonstrated an increase in lifespan along with positive effects in other physiological areas, including osteoporosis in bone, insulin sensitivity in the pancreas, and neuromuscular function (Bernardes de Jesus et al., 2012).

Summary

As the content in this chapter has discussed, many biological and physiological changes occur with normal aging. Even in the absence of pathology, normal changes to the human body may necessitate older persons making adjustments in their activities and lifestyle to safely accommodate some of these changes. Recognizing normal changes in the various systems of the aging body will assist the nurse in identifying subtle changes that could indicate the beginning of a health problem. Readers are encouraged to refer to this chapter as needed while learning from the following chapters and to use this material for comparison in recognizing common abnormalities of aging.

Clinical Reasoning Exercises

1. Choose an age-related disease in which you have a particular interest and discuss how this disease might affect the functional ability, independence, and psychosocial well-being of an older adult.

2. Many people within and outside the field of geriatrics and gerontology use the term normal aging to refer to physiological changes that occur over the passage of time. Do you believe there is such a thing as "normal aging"? Why or why not? How do you believe the use of the term *normal aging* might affect the clinical care received by older adults?

3. Read "No Truth to the Fountain of Youth" by S. Jay Olshansky, Leonard Hayflick, and Bruce A. Carnes in *Scientific American*, Vol. 286, No. 6, pp. 92–95 (June 2002). This article can also be found online https://www.scientificamerican.com/article/no-truth-to-the-fountain-of-youth/. Do you agree with the arguments made by the authors of this article? Discuss your reactions to and thoughts on the article with your classmates. You may also want to consider reviewing the two articles on antiaging medicine listed in this chapter's Recommended Readings list (**Box 4-3**).

BOX 4-3   Recommended Readings

Bhutto, A., & Morley, J. (2008). The clinical significance of gastrointestinal changes with aging. *Current Opinion in Clinical Nutrition & Metabolic Care, 11*(5), 651–660.

de Haan, G. (2002). Hematopoietic stem cells: Self-renewing or aging? *Cells Tissues Organs, 171*(1), 27–37.

DeVault, K. (2002). Presbyesophagus: A reappraisal. *Current Gastroenterology Reports, 4*(3), 193–199.

Enoch, J., Werner, J., Haegerstrom-Portnoy, G., Lakshminarayanan, V., & Rynders, M. (1999). Forever young: Visual functions not affected or minimally affected by aging: A review. *Journal of Gerontology Series A: Biological Sciences and Medical Sciences, 54*(8), B336–B351.

Federal Interagency Forum on Aging-Related Statistics. (2004). *Older Americans 2004: Key indicators of well-being*. Washington, DC: U.S. Government Printing Office.

Finch, C. (2005). Developmental origins of aging in brain and blood vessels: An overview. *Neurobiology of Aging, 26*(3), 303–307.

Fukunaga, A., Uematsu, H., & Sugimoto, K. (2005). Influences of aging on taste perception and oral somatic sensation. *Journal of Gerontology Series A: Biological Sciences and Medical Sciences, 60A*(1), 109–113.

Greenwald, D. (2004). Aging, the gastrointestinal tract, and risk of acid-related disease. *American Journal of Medicine, 117* (Suppl. 5A), 8S–13S.

Harman, S., & Blackman, M. (2004). Use of growth hormone for prevention and treatment of effects of aging. *Journals of Gerontology Series A: Biological Sciences and Medical Sciences, 59*(7), 652–658.

Hazzard, W. R., Blass, J. P., Halter, J. B., Ouslander, J. G., & Tinetti, M. E. (Eds.). (2003). *Principles of geriatric medicine and gerontology* (5th ed.). New York, NY: McGraw-Hill Professional.

Henderson, V., Paganini-Hill, A., Miller, B., Elble, R., Reyes, P., Shoupe, D., . . . Farlow, M. R. (2000). Estrogen for Alzheimer's disease in women: Randomized, double-blind, placebo-controlled trial. *Neurology, 54*(2), 295–301.

Hötting, K., Reich, B., Holzschneider, K., Kauschke, K., Schmidt, T., Reer, R., . . . Röder, B. (2012). Differential cognitive effects of cycling versus stretching/coordination training in middle-aged adults. *Health Psychology, 31*(2), 145–155.

Hurwitz, J., & Santaro, N. (2004). Inhibins, activins, and follistatin in the aging female and male. *Seminars in Reproductive Medicine, 22*(3), 209–217.

Jackson, R. (2001). Elderly and sun-affected skin: Distinguishing between changes caused by aging and changes caused by habitual exposure to sun. *Canadian Family Physician, 47*, 1236–1243.

Janssens, J. (2005). Aging of the respiratory system: Impact on pulmonary function tests and adaptation to exertion. *Clinical Chest Medicine, 26*(3), 469–484.

Linton, P., & Thoman, M. (2001). T cell senescence. *Frontiers in Bioscience, 1*(6), D248–D261.

Marder, K., & Sano, M. (2000). Estrogen to treat Alzheimer's disease: Too little, too late? So what's a woman to do? *Neurology, 54*, 2035–2037.

Nikolaou, D., & Templeton, A. (2004). Early ovarian ageing. *European Journal of Obstetrics and Gynecology and Reproductive Biology, 113*(2), 126–133.

O'Dononvan, D., Hausken, T., Lei, Y., Russo, A., Keough, J., Horowitz, M., & Jone, K. (2005). Effects of aging on transpyloric flow, gastric emptying and intragastric distribution in healthy humans—impact on glycemia. *Digestive Diseases and Sciences, 50*(4), 671–676.

Olshansky, J., Hayflick, L., & Perls, T. T. (2004a). Anti-aging medicine: The hype and the reality, Part I. *Journals of Gerontology Series A: Biological Sciences and Medical Sciences, 59A*(6), B513–B514.

Olshansky, J., Hayflick, L., & Perls, T. T. (2004b). Anti-aging medicine: The hype and the reality, Part II. *Journals of Gerontology Series A: Biological Sciences and Medical Sciences, 59A*(7), B649–B651.

(continues)

BOX 4-3   Recommended Readings (*continued*)

Rosenzweig, E., & Barnes, C. (2003). Impact of aging on hippocampal function: Plasticity, network dynamics, and cognition. *Progress in Neurobiology, 69*, 143–179.

Salvador, J., Adams, E., Ershler, R., & Ershler, W. (2003). Future challenges in analysis and treatment of human immune senescence. *Immunology and Allergy Clinics of North America, 23*(1), 133–148.

Scharffetter-Kochanek, K., Brenneisen, P., Wenk, J., Herrmann, G., Ma, W., Kuhr, L., . . . Wlaschek, M. (2000). Photoaging of the skin from phenotype to mechanisms. *Experimental Gerontology, 35*(3), 307–316.

Sullivan, M., & Yalla, S. (2002). Physiology of female micturition. *Urology Clinics of North America, 29*, 499–514.

Timiras, P. S. (Ed.). (2007). *Physiological basis of aging and geriatrics* (4th ed.). Boca Raton, FL: CRC Press.

Topp, R., Fahlman, M., & Boardley, D. (2004). Healthy aging: Health promotion and disease prevention. *Nursing Clinics of North America, 39*(2), 411–422.

Troncale, J. (1996). The aging process: Physiologic changes and pharmacologic implications. *Postgraduate Medicine, 99*(5), 111–114, 120–122.

Uylings, H., & De Brabander, J. (2002). Neuronal changes in normal human aging and Alzheimer's disease. *Brain and Cognition, 49*(3), 268–276.

Van Zant, G., & Liang, Y. (2003). The role of stem cells in aging. *Experimental Hematology, 31*(8), 659–672.

Verdaguer, E., Junyent, F., Folch, J., Beas-Zarate, C., Auladell, C., Pallas, M., & Camins, A. (2012). Aging biology: A new frontier for drug discovery. *Expert Opinion on Drug Discovery, 7*(3), 217–219.

Vijg, J., & Suh, Y. (2005). Genetics of longevity and aging. *Annual Review of Medicine, 56*, 193–212.

Vincent, H., Raiser, S., & Vincent, K. (2012). The aging musculoskeletal system and obesity-related considerations with exercise. *Ageing Research Reviews, 11*(3), 361–373.

Wade, P., & Cowen, T. (2004). Neurodegeneration: A key factor in the ageing gut. *Neurogastroenterology and Motility, 16*(Suppl. 1), 19–23.

Wakamatsu, M. (2003). What affects bladder function more: Menopause or age? *Menopause, 10*(3), 191–192.

Weinstein, J., & Anderson, S. (2010). The aging kidney: Physiological changes. *Advances in Chronic Kidney Disease, 17*(4), 302–307.

Personal Reflections

1. Discuss with an older adult (such as a grandparent or great-grandparent) the significant physical changes that occurred as a consequence of the aging process— not involving disease—over his or her life course. Focus on changes that led to lifestyle alterations and changes that most affected him or her personally. What specific alterations stand out the most in your mind? Which ones most affect quality of life?

2. Review several Websites about aging and discuss what healthy aging means from a media perspective versus a research or personal perspective. Compare your own experiences of aging processes with those found in other arenas. How could you use these resources in your nursing practice?

3. Identify preventive techniques that may enhance the aging experience or delay aging processes throughout the life course. Discuss how these techniques work on the body for every organ system and how they might help delay aging or maintain a healthy aging status. Correlate your discussion with older individuals you know. How could you use this knowledge to make you more sensitive toward caring for the aged?

| BOX 4-4 | Resource List |

American Federation for Aging Research:
http://www.afar.org

American Society on Aging:
http://www.asaging.org

Baltimore Longitudinal Study of Aging:
https://www.blsa.nih.gov/

Centers for Disease Control and Prevention,
Healthy Aging:
http://www.cdc.gov/aging/

Geriatrics and Aging:
http://www.geriatricsandaging.com

National Council on Aging:
http://www.ncoa.org

National Institute on Aging (NIA):
http://www.nia.nih.gov

National Institute on Aging Age Pages:
https://www.nia.nih.gov/health/publication
/agepages/content/booklets/research_new_age
/page3.htm

The Nun Study:
http://www.mc.uky.edu/nunnet/

University of California at San Francisco Academic
Geriatric Resource Center Online Curriculum:
https://www.cmecalifornia.com/Activity/1920990
/Detail.aspx

References

Abernathy, D. (1999). Aging effects on drug disposition and effect. *Geriatric Nephrology and Urology, 9*(1), 15–19.

Abrams, W., Beers, M., & Berkow, R. (Eds.). (1995). *The Merck manual of geriatrics* (2nd ed.). Whitehouse Station, NJ: Merck & Company.

Aeron Biotechnology. (2005). Salivary hormone monitoring: Cortisol. Retrieved from http://www.aeron.com/new_page_27.htm

American Diabetes Association. (2016). Diagnosing diabetes and learning about prediabetes. Retrieved from http://www.diabetes.org/diabetes-basics/diagnosis/

American Society for Reproductive Medicine Practice Committee. (2004). Treatment of androgen deficiency in the aging male. *Fertility and Sterility, 82*(Suppl. 1), S46–S50.

Andersson, K., & Arner, A. (2004). Urinary bladder contraction and relaxation: Physiology and pathophysiology. *Physiological Reviews, 84*(3), 935–986.

Anderton, B. (2002). Ageing of the brain. *Mechanisms of Ageing and Development, 123*(7), 811–817.

Arking, R. (1998). *Biology of aging: Observations and principles* (2nd ed.). Sunderland, MA: Sinauer Associates.

Arlt, W. (2004). Adrenal androgens. Retrieved from http://www.thelancet.com/journals/lancet/article/PIIS0140-6736(04)16503-3/abstract

Aronow, W. (1998). Effects of aging on the heart. In R. Tallis, H. Fillit, & J. Brocklehurst (Eds.), *Brocklehurst's textbook of geriatric medicine and gerontology* (5th ed., pp. 255–262). London, England: Churchill Livingstone.

Arranz, E., O'Mahony, S., Barton, J., & Ferguson, A. (1992). Immunosenescence and mucosal immunity: Significant effects of old age on secretory IgA concentrations and intraepithelial lymphocyte counts. *Gut, 33*(7), 882–886.

Artero, S., Tiemeier, H., & Prins, N. (2004). Neuroanatomical localization and clinical correlates of white matter lesions in the elderly. *Journal of Neurology and Neurosurgery Psychiatry, 75*, 1304–1308.

Aspinall, R., & Andrew, D. (2000). Thymic involution in aging. *Journal of Clinical Immunology, 20*(4), 250–256.

Asplund, R. (2004). Nocturia, nocturnal polyuria, and sleep quality in the elderly. *Journal of Psychosomatic Research, 56*(5), 511–525.

Atwood, L., Wolf, P., Heard-Costa, N., Massaro, J., Beiser, A., D'Agostino, R., & DeCarli, C. (2004). Genetic variation in white matter hyperintensity volume in the Framingham study. *Stroke, 35*(7), 1609–1613.

Aw, D., Silva, A., & Palmer, D. (2007). Immunosenescence: Emerging challenges for an ageing population. *Immunology, 120*(4), 435–446.

Bagnara, G. P., Bonsi, L., Strippoli, P., Bonifazi, F., Tonelli, R., D'Addato, S., . . . Franceschi, C. (2000). Hemopoiesis in healthy old people and centenarians: Well-maintained responsiveness of CD34+ cells to hemopoietic growth factors and remodeling of cytokine network. *Journals of Gerontology: Biological Sciences, 55A*(2), B61–B66.

Baik, H., & Russell, R. (1999). Vitamin B_{12} deficiency in the elderly. *Annual Review of Nutrition, 19*, 357–377.

Balagopal, P., Rooyackers, O. E., Adey, D. B., Ades, P. A., & Nair, K. S. (1997). Effects of aging on in vivo synthesis of skeletal muscle myosin heavy-chain and sarcoplasmic protein in humans. *American Journal of Physiology, 273*(4 Pt 1), E790–E800.

Balducci, L. (2003). Anemia, cancer, and aging. *Cancer Control, 10*(6), 478–486.

Balducci, L., Hardy, C. L., & Lyman, G. H. (2000). Hemopoietic reserve in the older cancer patient: Clinical and economic considerations. *Cancer Control, 7*(6), 539–547.

Ball, K., & Sekuler, R. (1986). Improving visual perception in older observers. *Journal of Gerontology, 41*(2), 176–182.

Baraldi-Junkins, C., Beck, A., & Rothstein, G. (2000). Hematopoiesis and cytokines: Relevance to cancer and aging. *Hematology and Oncology Clinics of North America, 14*(1), 45–61.

Barnes, P. J. (2000). Chronic obstructive pulmonary disease. *New England Journal of Medicine, 343*(4), 269–280.

Bartoshuk, L., & Duffy, V. (1995). Taste and smell. In E. Masoro (Ed.), *Handbook of physiology: Section 11, aging* (pp. 363–376). New York, NY: Oxford Press.

Bartzokis, G., Sultzer, D., Lu, P., Nuechterlein, K., Mintz, J., & Cummings, J. (2004). Heterogeneous age-related breakdown of white matter structural integrity: Implications for cortical "disconnection" in aging and Alzheimer's disease. *Neurobiology of Aging, 25*(7), 843–851.

Bates, T., Harrison, M., Lowe, D., Lawson, C., & Padley, N. (1992). Longitudinal study of gallstone prevalence at necropsy. *Gut, 33*(1), 103–107.

Baumann, L. (2007). Skin aging and its treatment. *Journal of Pathology, 211*, 241–251.

Baumgartner, R., Koehler, K., Gallagher, D., Romero, L., Heymsfield, S., Ross, R., . . . Lindeman, R. D. (1998). Epidemiology of sarcopenia among the elderly in New Mexico. *American Journal of Epidemiology, 147*(8), 755–763.

Bearden, S. (2006). Effect of aging on the structure and function of skeletal muscle microvascular networks. *Microcirculation, 13*(4), 305–314.

Beck, L. (1998a). Changes in renal function with aging. *Clinical Geriatric Medicine, 14*(2), 199–209.

Beck, L. (1999b). Aging changes in renal function. In W. Hazzard, J. Blass, W. Ettinger Jr., J. Halter, & J. Ouslander (Eds.), *Principles of geriatric medicine and gerontology* (4th ed., pp. 767–776). New York, NY: McGraw-Hill.

Beck, L. (1999c). Fluid and electrolyte balance in the elderly. *Geriatric Nephrology and Urology*, 9, 11–14.

Beers, M., & Berkow, R. (Eds.). (n.d.). *The Merck manual of geriatrics* (3rd ed.) [Online ed.]. Kenilworth, NJ: Merck & Company, Inc. Retrieved from http://www.merck.com/mrkshared/mm_geriatrics/home.jsp

Beers, M. H., & Berkow, R. (Eds.). (2000). *The Merck manual of geriatrics* (3rd ed.). New York, NY: John Wiley & Sons.

Benzi, G., & Moretti, P. (1997). Contribution of mitochondrial alterations to brain aging. *Advances in Cell Aging & Gerontology, 2*, 129–160.

Bernardes de Jesus, B., Vera, E., Schneeberger, K., Tejera, A., Ayuso, E., Bosch, F., & Blasco, M. (2012). Telomerase gene therapy in adult and old mice delays aging and increases longevity without increasing cancer. *EMBO Molecular Medicine, 4*(8), 691–704.

Bhasin, S. (2003). Testosterone supplementation for aging-associated sarcopenia. *Journals of Gerontology: Medical Sciences, 58A*(11), 1002–1008.

Bhatnagar, K., Kennedy, R., Baron, G., & Greenberg, R. (1987). Number of mitral cells and the bulb volume in the aging human olfactory bulb: A quantitative morphological study. *Anatomical Record Part A, 218*, 73–87.

Bhutto, A., & Morley, J. (2008). The clinical significance of gastrointestinal changes with aging. *Current Opinion in Clinical Nutrition & Metabolic Care, 11*(5), 651–660.

Binder, L., Guillozet-Bongaarts, A., Garcia-Sierra, F., & Berry, R. (2005). Tau, tangles, and Alzheimer's disease. *Biochimica et Biophysica Acta (BBA)—Molecular Basis of Disease, 1739*(2–3), 216–223.

Bjorntorp, P. (1997). The relationship between obesity and diabetes. In K. Alberti, P. Zimmet, R. DeFronzo, & H. Keen (Eds.), *International textbook of diabetes mellitus* (Vol. 1, pp. 611–627). New York, NY: John Wiley & Sons.

Borst, S. E. (2004). Interventions for sarcopenia and muscle weakness in older people. *Age and Ageing, 33*(6), 548–555.

Bourdiol, P., Mioche, L., & Monier, S. (2004). Effect of age on salivary flow obtained under feeding and non-feeding conditions. *Journal of Oral Rehabilitation, 31*(4), 445–452.

Brading, A., Teramoto, N., Dass, N., & McCoy, R. (2001). Morphological and physiological characteristics of urethral circular and longitudinal smooth muscle. *Scandinavian Journal of Urology and Nephrology: Supplementum, 207*, 12–18.

Bressler, P., & DeFronzo, R. (1997). Drug effects on glucose homeostasis. In K. Alberti, P. Zimmet, R. DeFronzo, & H. Keen (Eds.), *International textbook of diabetes mellitus* (2nd ed., Vol. 1, pp. 231–254). New York, NY: John Wiley & Sons.

Brogna, A., Ferrara, R., Bucceri, A., Lanteri, E., & Catalano, F. (1999). Influence of aging on gastrointestinal transit time: An ultrasonographic and radiologic study. *Investigative Radiology, 34*(5), 357–359.

Brown, W., Strong, M., & Snow, R. (1988). Methods of estimating numbers of motor units in biceps-brachialis muscles and losses of motor units with aging. *Muscle and Nerve, 11*(5), 423–432.

Buchholz, J., Behringer, E., Pottorf, W., Pearce, W., & Vanterpool, C. (2007). Age-dependent changes in Ca^{2+} homeostasis in peripheral neurones: Implications for changes in function. *Aging Cell, 6*, 285–296.

Carpo, R., & Campbell, E. (1998). Aging of the respiratory system. In A. P. Fishmen (Ed.), *Pulmonary diseases and disorders* (pp. 251–264). New York, NY: McGraw-Hill.

Carroll, J., Shroff, S., Wirth, P., Halsted, M., & Rajfer, S. (1991). Arterial mechanical properties in dilated cardiomyopathy: Aging and the response to nitroprusside. *Journal of Clinical Investigation, 87*(3), 1002–1009.

Chahal, H., & Drake, W. (2007). The endocrine system and ageing. *Journal of Pathology, 211*(2), 173–180.

Chakraborty, T., & Gore, A. (2004). Aging-related changes in ovarian hormones, their receptors, and neuroendocrine function. *Experimental Biology and Medicine, 229*(10), 977–987.

Chang, A., & Halter, J. (2004). Effects of aging on glucose homeostasis. In D. LeRoith, S. Taylor, & J. Olefsky (Eds.), *Diabetes mellitus, a fundamental and clinical text* (3rd ed., pp. 869–877). Philadelphia, PA: Lippincott Williams & Wilkins.

Chapuy, M., Durr, F., & Chapuy, P. (1983). Age-related changes in parathyroid hormone and 25-hydroxycholecalciferol levels. *Journal of Gerontology, 38*(1), 19–22.

Chen, M., Halter, J., & Porte, D. (1987). The role of dietary carbohydrate in the decreased glucose tolerance of the elderly. *Journal of the American Geriatrics Society, 35*(5), 417–424.

Chiras, D. D. (2012). *Human biology* (7th ed.). Burlington, MA: Jones & Bartlett Learning.

Cockcroft, D., & Gault, M. (1976). Prediction of creatinine clearance from serum creatinine. *Nephron, 16*(1), 31–41.

Colcombe, S. J., Kramer, A. F., Erickson, K. I., Scalf, P., McAuley, E., Cohen, N. J., . . . Elavsky, S. (2004). Cardiovascular fitness, cortical plasticity, and aging. *Proceedings of the National Academy of Sciences of the United States of America, 101*(9), 3316–3321.

Corman, B., Barrault, M., Klingler, C., Houot, A., Michel, J., Della Bruna, R., . . . Soubrier, F. (1995). Renin gene expression in the aging kidney: Effect of sodium restriction. *Mechanisms of Ageing and Development, 84*(1), 1–13.

Cowart, B. (1989). Relationships between taste and smell across the adult life span. *Annals of the New York Academy of Science, 561*, 39–55.

Curcio, C., Millican, C., Allen, K., & Kalina, R. (1993). Aging of the human photoreceptor mosaic: Evidence for selective vulnerability of rods in central retina. *Investigative Ophthalmology & Visual Science, 34*(12), 3278–3296.

Cutler, R. (2006). Effects of aging on the urinary tract. In R. S. Porter & J. L. Kaplan (Eds.), *The Merck Manual: Home Health Handbook*. Retrieved from http://www.merckmanuals.com/home/kidney_and_urinary_tract _disorders/biology_of_the_kidneys_and_urinary_tract/effects_of_aging_on_the_urinary_tract.html

Czech, M., Erwin, J., & Sleeman, M. (2004). Insulin action on glucose transport. In D. LeRoith, S. Taylor, & J. Olefsky (Eds.), *Diabetes mellitus: A fundamental and clinical text* (pp. 335–347). Philadelphia, PA: Lippincott-Raven.

Davies, A., Kidd, D., Stone, S., & MacMahon, J. (1995). Pharyngeal sensation and gag reflex in healthy subjects. *Lancet, 345*, 487–488.

Davis, S., McCloud, P., Strauss, B., & Burger, H. (1995). Testosterone enhances estradiol's effects on postmenopausal bone density and sexuality. *Maturitas, 21*(3), 227–236.

Dela, F., Mikines, K., & Galbo, H. (1999). Physical activity and insulin resistance in man. In G. Reaven & A. Laws (Eds.), *Insulin resistance: The metabolic syndrome X* (pp. 97–120). Totowa, NJ: Humana Press.

de la Torre, J. (1997). Cerebrovascular changes in the aging brain. In P. Timiras & E. Bittar (Eds.), *Advances in cell aging and gerontology: The aging brain* (Vol. 2, pp. 707–717). Greenwich, CT: Jai Press.

De Martinis, M., & Timiras, P. S. (2007). The pulmonary respiration, hematopoiesis, and erythrocytes. In P. S. Timiras (Ed.), *Physiological basis of aging and geriatrics* (pp. 319–336). Boca Raton, FL: CRC Press.

Deschenes, M. (2004). Effects of aging on muscle fiber type and size. *Sports Medicine, 34*(12), 809–824.

Despres, J.-P., & Marette, A. (1999). Obesity and insulin resistance: Epidemiologic, metabolic, and molecular aspects. In G. Reaven & A. Laws (Eds.), *Insulin resistance: The metabolic syndrome X* (pp. 51–81). Totowa, NJ: Humana Press.

Devlin, H., & Ferguson, M. (1998). Aging and the orofacial tissues. In R. Tallis, H. Fillit, & J. Brocklehurst (Eds.), *Brocklehurst's textbook of geriatric medicine and gerontology* (5th ed., pp. 789–802). London, England: Churchill Livingstone.

Dhatariya, K. K., & Nair, K. S. (2003). Dehydro-epiandrosterone: Is there a role for replacement? *Mayo Clinic Proceedings, 78*(10), 1257–1273.

Dickson, D. (1997). Structural changes in the aging brain. In P. Timiras & E. Bittar (Eds.), *Advances in cell aging and gerontology: The aging brain* (Vol. 2, pp. 51–76). Greenwich, CT: Jai Press.

Digiovanna, A. G. (1994). *Human aging: Biological perspectives*. New York, NY: McGraw-Hill.

Digiovanna, A. G. (2000). *Human aging: Biological perspectives* (2nd ed.). Boston, MA: McGraw-Hill.

Diokno, A., Brown, M., Brock, B., Herzog, A., & Normolle, D. (1988). Clinical and cystometric characteristics of continent and incontinent noninstitutionalized elderly. *Journal of Urology, 140*, 567–571.

Dionne, I., Kinaman, K., & Poehlman, E. (2000). Sarcopenia and muscle function during menopause and hormone-replacement therapy. *Journal of Nutrition, Health, and Aging, 4*(3), 156–161.

Doherty, T., & Brown, W. (1993). The estimated numbers and relative sizes of thenar motor units selected by multiple point stimulation in young and older animals. *Muscle and Nerve, 16*(4), 355–366.

Doherty, T. J. (2003). Invited review: Aging and sarcopenia. *Journal of Applied Physiology, 95*(4), 1717–1727.

Drewnowski, A., & Evans, W. (2001). Nutrition, physical activity, and quality of life in older adults: Summary. *Journals of Gerontology Series A: Biological Sciences and Medical Sciences, 56A*(Special Issue II), 89–94.

Duggal, P., Klein, A., Lee, K., Iyengar, S., Klein R., Bailey-Wilson, J., & Klein, B. E. (2005). A genetic contribution to intraocular pressure: The Beaver Dam Eye Study. *Investigative Ophthalmology and Visual Science, 46*(2), 555–560.

Dunn, L. B., Damesyn, M., Moore, A. A., Reuben, D. B., & Greendale, G. A. (1997). Does estrogen prevent skin aging? Results from the First National Health and Nutrition Examination Survey (NHANES I). *Archives of Dermatology, 133*(3), 339–342.

Effros, R. B., & Pawelec, G. (1997). Replicative senescence of T cells: Does the Hayflick limit lead to immune exhaustion? *Immunology Today, 18*(9), 450–454.

Effros, R. B., Dagarag, M., & Valenzuela, H. F. (2003). In vitro senescence of immune cells. *Experimental Gerontology, 38*(11–12), 1243–1249.

Egusa, Y., Fujiwara, Y., Syahruddin, E., Isobe, T., & Yamakido, M. (1998). Effect of age on human peripheral blood stem cells. *Oncology Reports, 5*(2), 397–400.

Elbadawi, A., Diokno, A., & Millard, R. (1998). The aging bladder: Morphology and urodynamics. *World Journal of Urology, 16*(Suppl. 1), S10–S34.

Elbadawi, A., Yalla, S., & Resnick, N. (1993). Structural basis of geriatric voiding dysfunction, Part II. Aging detrusor: Normal vs. impaired contractility. *Journal of Urology, 150*(5 Pt 2), 1657–1667.

El Solh, A., & Ramadan, F. (2006). Overview of respiratory failure in older adults. *Journal of Intensive Care Medicine, 21*(2), 345–351.

Engelhardt, M., Kumar, R., Albanell, J., Pettengell, R., Han, W., & Moore, M. (1997). Telomerase regulation, cell cycle, and telomere stability in primitive hematopoietic cells. *Blood, 90*(1), 182–193.

Enoka, R. (1997). Neural strategies in the control of muscle force. *Muscle and Nerve, 5*(Suppl.), S66–S69.

Erickson, C., & Barnes, C. (2003). The neurobiology of memory changes in normal aging. *Experimental Gerontology, 38*(1–2), 61–69.

Esler, M., Kaye, D., Thompson, J., Jennings, G., Cox, H., Turner, A., . . . Seals, D. (1995). Effects of aging on epinephrine secretion and regional release of epinephrine from the human heart. *Journal of Clinical Endocrinology and Metabolism, 80*(2), 435–442.

Evans, W. J. (2002). Effects of exercise on senescent muscle. *Clinical Orthopaedics and Related Research, 403S*, S211–S220.

Falahati-Nini, A., Riggs, B. L., Atkinson, E. J., O'Fallon, W. M., Eastell, R., & Khosla, S. (2000). Relative contributions of testosterone and estrogen in regulating bone resorption and formation in normal elderly men. *Journal of Clinical Investigation, 106*(12), 1553–1560.

Federal Interagency Forum on Aging-Related Statistics. (2004). *Older Americans 2004: Key indicators of well-being.* Washington, DC: U.S. Government Printing Office

Fenske, N., & Lober, C. (1986). Structural and functional changes of normal aging skin. *Journal of the American Academy of Dermatology, 15*(4 Pt 1), 571–585.

Ferrari, A., Radaelli, A., & Centola, M. (2003). Invited review: Aging and the cardiovascular system. *Journal of Applied Physiology, 95*(6), 2591–2597.

Ferrari, E., Cravello, L., Muzzoni, B., Casarotti, D., Paltro, M., Solerte, S., . . . Magri, F. (2001). Age-related changes of the hypothalamic-pituitary-adrenal axis: Pathophysiological correlates. *European Journal of Endocrinology, 144*, 319–329.

Ferriolli, E., Oliveira, R., Matsuda, N., Braga, F., & Dantos, R. (1998). Aging, esophageal motility and gastroesophageal reflux disease. *Journal of the American Geriatric Association, 46*, 1534–1537.

Fiatarone, M., Marks, E., Ryan, N., Meredith, C., Lipsitz, L., & Evans, W. (1990). High-intensity strength training in nonagenarians: Effects on skeletal muscle. *Journal of the American Medical Association, 263*(22), 3029–3034.

Fink, R., Kolterman, O., Griffin, J., & Olefsky, J. (1983). Mechanisms of insulin resistance in aging. *Journal of Clinical Investigation, 71*(6), 1523–1535.

Fleg, J. (1986). Alterations in cardiovascular structure and function with advancing age. *American Journal of Cardiology, 57*, 33C–44C.

Fleg, J., Morrell, C., Bos, A., Brant, L., Talbot, L., Wright, J., & Lakatta, E. G. (2005). Accelerated longitudinal decline of aerobic capacity in healthy older adults. *Circulation, 112*(5), 674–682.

Fleg, J., O'Connor, F., Gerstenblith, G., Becker, L., Clulow, J., Schulman, S., & Lakatta, E. G. (1995). Impact of age on the cardiovascular response to dynamic upright exercise in healthy men and women. *Journal of Applied Physiology, 78*(3), 890–900.

Fliser, D., Franek, E., Joest, M., Block, S., Mutschler, E., & Ritz, E. (1997). Renal function in the elderly: Impact of hypertension and cardiac function. *Kidney International, 51*(4), 1196–1204.

Fossel, M. B. (2004). *Cells, aging, and human disease.* New York, NY: Oxford -University Press.

Fransen, E., Lemkens, N., Van Laer, L., & Van Camp, G. (2003). Age-related hearing impairment (ARHI): Environmental risk factors and genetic prospects. *Experimental Gerontology, 38*(4), 353–359.

Frontera, W., Meredith, C., O'Reilly, K., Knuttgen, H., & Evans, W. (1988). Strength conditioning in older men: Skeletal muscle hypertrophy and improved function. *Journal of Applied Physiology, 64*(3), 1038–1044.

Fulp, S., Dalton, C., Castell, J., & Castell, D. (1990). Aging-related alterations in human upper esophageal sphincter functions. *American Journal of Gastroenterology, 85*, 1569–1572.

Garg, A. (1999). The role of body fat distribution in insulin resistance. In G. Reaven & A. Laws (Eds.), *Insulin resistance: The metabolic syndrome X* (pp. 83–96). Totowa, NJ: Humana Press.

Gersten, O. (2007). The adrenals and pituitary: Stress, adaptation & longevity. In P. S. Timiras (Ed.), *Physiological basis of aging and geriatrics* (4th ed., pp. 137–157). Boca Raton, FL: CRC Press.

Gerstenblith, G., Frederiksen, J., Yin, F., Fortuin, N., Lakatta, E., & Weisfeldt, M. (1977). Echocardiographic assessment of a normal adult aging population. *Circulation, 56*(2), 273–278.

Ghezzi, E., & Ship, J. (2003). Aging and secretory reserve capacity of major salivary glands. *Journal of Dentistry Research, 82*(10), 844–848.

Gill, S., Sharpless, J., Rado, K., & Hall, J. (2002). Evidence that GnRH decreases with gonadal steroid feedback but increases with age in postmenopausal women. *Journal of Clinical Endocrinology and Metabolism, 87*(5), 2290–2296.

Gilmore, G., Wenk, H., Naylor, L., & Stuve, T. (1992). Motion perception and aging. *Psychology and Aging, 7*(4), 654–660.

Globerson, A. (1999). Hematopoietic stem cells and aging. *Experimental Gerontology, 34*(2), 137–146.

Gluck, M., Thomas, R., Davis, K., & Haroutunian, V. (2002). Implications for altered glutamate and GABA metabolism in the dorsolateral prefrontal cortex of aged schizophrenic patients. *American Journal of Psychiatry, 159*(7), 1165–1173.

Gomes, O., deSouza, R., & Liberti, E. (1997). A preliminary investigation of the effects of ageing on the nerve cell number in the myenteric ganglia of the human colon. *Gerontology, 43*, 210–217.

Gomez, C., Boehmer, E. D., & Kovacs, E. (2005). The aging innate immune system. *Current Opinion in Immunology, 17*(5), 457–462.

Graal, M., & Wolffenbuttel, B. (1999). The use of sulphonylureas in the elderly. *Drugs and Aging, 15*(6), 471–481.

Greendale, G., Edelstein, S., & Barrett-Connor, E. (1997). Endogenous sex steroid and bone mineral density in older women and men. The Rancho Bernardo Study. *Journal of Bone Mineral Research, 12*, 1833–1843.

Gruenewald, D., & Matsumoto, A. (2009). Aging of the endocrine system. In W. Hazzard, J. Blass, W. Ettinger Jr., J. Halter, & J. Ouslander (Eds.), *Principles of geriatric medicine and gerontology* (6th ed., Ch. 107). New York, NY: McGraw-Hill.

Gruver, A., Hudson, L., & Sempowski, G. (2007). Immunosenescence of ageing. *Journal of Pathology, 211*(2), 144–156.

Gupta, V., & Lipsitz, L. (2007). Orthostatic hypotension in the elderly: Diagnosis and treatment. *American Journal of Medicine, 120*(10), 841–847.

Haas, A., Flammer, J., & Schneider, U. (1986). Influence of age on the visual fields of normal subjects. *American Journal of Ophthalmology, 101*(2), 199–203.

Hafez, B., & Hafez, E. (2004). Andropause: Endocrinology, erectile dysfunction, and prostate pathophysiology. *Archives of Andrology, 50*(1), 45–68.

Hall, J. (2004). Neuroendocrine physiology of the early and late menopause. *Endocrinology and Metabolism Clinics of North America, 33*(4), 637–659.

Hall, J. (2007). Neuroendocrine changes with reproductive aging in women. *Seminars in Reproductive Medicine, 25*(5), 344–355.

Hall, J., Lavoie, H., Marsh, E., & Martin, K. (2000). Decrease in gonadotropin-releasing hormone (GnRH) pulse frequency with aging in postmenopausal women. *Journal of Clinical Endocrinology and Metabolism, 85*, 1794–1800.

Hall, K. (2002). Aging and neural control of the GI tract. Part II. Neural control of the aging gut: Can an old dog learn new tricks? *American Journal of Physiology: Gastrointestinal and Liver Physiology, 283*(4), G827–G832.

Hall, K. (2009). Effect of aging on gastrointestinal function. In W. Hazzard, J. Blass, W. Ettinger Jr., J. Halter, & J. Ouslander (Eds.), *Principles of geriatric medicine and gerontology* (6th ed.). New York, NY: McGraw-Hill.

Hansen, K., Thyer, A., Sluss, P., Bremner, W., Soules, M., & Klein, N. (2005). Reproductive ageing and ovarian function: Is the earlier follicular phase FSH rise necessary to maintain adequate secretory function in older ovulatory women? *Human Reproduction, 20*(1), 89–95.

Harris, M. (1990). Epidemiology of diabetes mellitus among the elderly in the United States. *Clinics in Geriatric Medicine, 6*(4), 703–719.

Hasten, D., Pak-Loduca, J., Obert, K., & Yarasheski, K. (2000). Resistance exercise acutely increases MHC and mixed muscle protein synthesis rate in 78–84 and 23–32 yr olds. *American Journal of Physiology, 278*(4), E620–E626.

Hayward, C., Kelly, R., & Collins, P. (2000). The role of gender, the menopause and hormone replacement on cardiovascular function. *Cardiovascular Research, 46*(1), 28–49.

Heine, C., & Browning, C. (2002). Communication and psychosocial consequences of sensory loss in older adults: Overview and rehabilitation directions. *Disability and Rehabilitation, 24*(15), 763–773.

Hekimi, S., & Guarente, L. (2003). Genetics and the specificity of the aging process. *Science, 299*(5611), 1352–1354.

Hinson, J., & Raven, P. (1999). DHEA deficiency syndrome: A new term for old age? *Journal of Endocrinology, 163*, 1–5.

Hirokawa, K. (1999). Age-related changes of signal transduction in T cells. *Experimental Gerontology, 34*(1), 7–18.

Holick, M. F. (2003). Vitamin D: A millennium perspective. *Journal of Cellular Biochemistry, 88*(2), 296–307.

Hollander, J., & Diokno, A. (2007). Prostate gland disease. In E. Duthie, P. Katz, & M. Malone (Eds.), *Practice of geriatrics* (4th ed., Ch. 43). Philadelphia, PA: W. B. Saunders.

Hollenberg, M., Yang, J., Haight, T., & Tager, I. (2006). Longitudinal changes in aerobic capacity: Implications for concepts of aging. *Journals of Gerontology, 61A*(8), 851–858.

Holt, P. (1992). Clinical significance of bacterial overgrowth in elderly people. *Age and Ageing, 21*, 1–4.

Horton, R., & Tait, J. (1966). Androstenedione production and interconversion rates measured in peripheral blood and studies on the possible site of its conversion to testosterone. *Journal of Clinical Investigation, 45*(3), 301–313.

Hunt, B., Farquar, W., & Taylor, J. (2001). Does reduced vascular stiffening fully explain preserved cardiovagal baroreflex function in older, physically active men? *Circulation, 103*, 2424–2427.

Hurd, R. (2014). Aging changes in the male reproductive system. Bethesda, MD: Medline Plus, National Library of Medicine, National Institutes of Health. Retrieved from http://www.nlm.nih.gov/medlineplus/ency/article/004017.htm

Ishikawa, M., Matsumoto, M., Fujimura, Y., Chiba, K., & Toyama, Y. (2003). Changes of cervical spinal cord and cervical spinal canal with age in asymptomatic subjects. *Spinal Cord, 41*, 159–163.

Ivey, F., Tracy, B., Lemmer, J., NessAiver, M., Metter, E., Fozard, J., & Hurley, B. F. (2000). Effects of strength training and detraining on muscle quality: Age and gender comparisons. *Journals of -Gerontology: Biological Sciences, 55A*(3), B152–B157.

Jackson, G., & Owsley, C. (2003). Visual dysfunction, neurodegenerative diseases, and aging. *Neurology Clinics of North America, 21*, 709–728.

Jackson, R. (1990). Mechanisms of age-related glucose intolerance. *Diabetes Care, 13*(Suppl. 2), 9–19.

Jacobsen, E., Billings, J., Frantz, R., Kinney, C., Stewart, M., & Downing, D. (1985). Age-related changes in sebaceous wax ester secretion rates in men and women. *Journal of Investigative Dermatology, 85*(5), 483–485.

James, O. (1998). The liver. In R. Tallis, H. Fillit, & J. Brocklehurst (Eds.), *Brocklehurst's textbook of geriatric medicine and gerontology* (5th ed., pp. 841–862). London, England: Churchill Livingstone.

Janowsky, J., Oviatt, S., & Orwoll, E. (1994). Testosterone influences spatial cognition in older men. *Behavioral Neuroscience, 108*(1), 325–332.

Janssen, I., Heymsfield, S., Wang, Z., & Ross, R. (2000). Skeletal muscle mass and distribution in 468 men and women aged 18–88 yr. *Journal of Applied Physiology, 89*(1), 81–88.

Janssens, J. (2005). Aging of the respiratory system: Impact on pulmonary function tests and adaptation to exertion. *Clinical Chest Medicine, 26*(3), 469–484.

Jassal, S., & Oreopoulos, D. (1998). The aging kidney. *Geriatric Nephrology and Urology, 8*(3), 141–147.

Jassal, V., Fillit, H., & Oreopoulos, D. (1998). Aging of the urinary tract. In R. Tallis, H. Fillit, & J. Brocklehurst (Eds.), *Brocklehurst's textbook of geriatric medicine and gerontology* (5th ed., pp. 919–924). London, England: Churchill Livingstone.

Jerger, J., Chmiel, R., Wilson, N., & Luchi, R. (1995). Hearing impairment in older adults: New concepts. *Journal of the American Geriatrics Society, 43*(8), 928–935.

Jimenez, M., Cuartero, E., & Moreno, J. (2001). Neurobehavioral syndromes in patients with cerebrovascular pathology. In J. Leon-Carrion & M. Giannini (Eds.), *Behavioral neurology in the elderly* (pp. 337–362). Boca Raton, FL: CRC Press.

Joffe, H., Soares, C., & Cohen, L. (2003). Assessment and treatment of hot flashes and menopausal mood disturbance. *Psychiatric Clinics of North America, 26*(3), 563–580.

Johnson, C., Adams, A., & Lewis, R. (1989). Evidence for a neural basis of age-related visual field loss in normal observers. *Investigative Ophthalmology and Visual Science, 30*(9), 2056–2064.

Johnson, T., Miller, M., Pillin, D., & Auslander, J. (2003). Arginine vasopressin and nocturnal polyuria in older adults with frequent nighttime voiding. *Journal of Urology, 170*(2), 480–484.

Judd, H., & Yen, S. (1973). Serum androstenedione and testosterone levels during the menstrual cycle. *Journal of Clinical Endocrinology and Metabolism, 36*(3), 475–481.

Kalina, R. (1999). Aging and visual function. In W. Hazzard, J. Blass, W. Ettinger Jr., J. Halter, & J. Ouslander (Eds.), *Principles of geriatric medicine and gerontology* (4th ed., pp. 603–616). New York, NY: McGraw-Hill.

Kallman, D., Plato, C., & Tobin, J. (1990). The role of muscle loss in the age-related decline of grip strength: Cross-sectional and longitudinal perspectives. *Journals of Gerontology, 45*(3), M82–M88.

Kamminga, L., & DeHaan, G. (2006). Cellular memory and hematopoietic stem cell aging. *Stem Cells, 24*(5), 1143–1149.

Kandeel, F., Koussa, V., & Swerdloff, R. (2001). Male sexual function and its disorders: Physiology, pathophysiology, clinical investigation, and treatment. *Endocrine Reviews, 22*(3), 342–388.

Kane, R., Ouslander, J., Abrass, I., & Resnick, B. (2013). Cardiovascular disorders. In S. Zollo & M. Navrozov (Eds.), *Essentials of clinical geriatrics* (7th ed., Ch. 11). New York, NY: McGraw-Hill.

Karlsson, S., Persson, M., & Carlsson, G. (1991). Mandibular movement and velocity in relation to state of dentition and age. *Journal of Oral Rehabilitation, 18*(1), 1–8.

Katzman, R. (1995). Human nervous system. In E. Masoro (Ed.), *Handbook of physiology: Section 11, aging* (pp. 325–344). New York, NY: Oxford University Press.

Kelly, J., & Roth, G. (1997). Changes in neurotransmitter signal transduction pathways in the aging brain. In P. Timiras & E. Bittar (Eds.), *Advances in cell aging and gerontology: The aging brain* (Vol. 2, pp. 243–278). Greenwich, CT: Jai Press.

Kevorkian, R. (2004). Physiology of incontinence. *Clinics in Geriatric Medicine, 20*(3), 409–425.

Kirkland, J., Lye, M., Levy, D., & Banerjee, A. (1983). Patterns of urine flow and electrolyte excretion in healthy elderly people. *British Medical Journal, 287,* 1665–1667.

Klein, B., Klein, R., & Linton, K. (1992a). Prevalence of age-related lens opacities in a population: The Beaver Dam Eye Study. *Ophthalmology, 99*(4), 546–552.

Klein, B., Klein, R., & Linton, K. (1992b). Prevalence of age-related maculopathy: The Beaver Dam Eye Study. *Ophthalmology, 99*(6), 933–943.

Klein, N., Illingworth, P., Groome, N., McNeilly, A., Battaglia, D., & Soules, M. (1996). Decreased inhibin B secretion is associated with the monotropic FSH rise in older, ovulatory women: A study of serum and follicular fluid levels of dimeric inhibin A and B in spontaneous menstrual cycles. *Journal of Clinical Endocrinology and Metabolism, 81,* 2742–2745.

Klein, R., Wang, Q., Klein, B., Moss, S., & Meuer, S. (1995). The relationship of age-related maculopathy cataract, and glaucoma to visual acuity. *Investigative Ophthalmology and Visual Science, 36*(1), 182–191.

Kollarits, C. (1998). Ophthalmologic disorders. In E. Duthie & P. Katz (Eds.), *Practice of geriatrics* (3rd ed., pp. 457–466). Philadelphia, PA: W. B. Saunders.

Korenman, S., Morley, J., Mooradian, A., Davis, S., Kaiser, F., Silver, A., . . . Garza, D. (1990). Secondary hypogonadism in older men: Its relation to impotence. *Journal of Clinical Endocrinology and Metabolism, 71,* 963–969.

Kotz, C., Billington, C., & Levine, A. (1999). Obesity and aging. *Clinics in Geriatric Medicine, 15*(2), 391–412.

Kovacs, T. (1999). B-amyloid deposition and neurofibrillary tangle formation in the olfactory bulb in ageing and Alzheimer's disease. *Neuropathology and Applied Neurobiology, 25*(6), 481–491.

Kovacs, T. (2004). Mechanisms of olfactory dysfunction in aging and neurodegenerative disorders. *Ageing Research Review, 3*(2), 215–232.

Krauss Whitbourne, S. (2002). *The aging individual: Physical and psychological perspectives* (2nd ed.). New York, NY: Springer.

Lakatta, E. (1993a). Cardiovascular regulatory mechanisms in advanced age. *Physiological Reviews, 73*(20), 413–467.

Lakatta, E. (1993b). Deficient neuroendocrine regulation of the cardiovascular system with advancing age in healthy humans. *Circulation, 87*(2), 631–636.

Lakatta, E. (1996). Cardiovascular aging in health. In M. Chizner (Ed.), *Classic teachings in clinical cardiology* (Vol. 2, pp. 1369–1390). Cedar Grove, NJ: Laennec.

Lakatta, E. (1999a). Cardiovascular aging research: The next horizons. *Journal of the American Geriatrics Society, 47,* 613–625.

Lakatta, E. (1999b). Circulatory function in younger and older humans in health. In W. Hazzard, J. Blass, W. Ettinger Jr., J. Halter, & J. Ouslander (Eds.), *Principles of geriatric medicine and gerontology* (4th ed., pp. 645–660). New York, NY: McGraw-Hill.

Lakatta, E., Gerstenblith, G., Angell, S., Shock, N., & Weisfeldt, M. (1975). Prolonged contraction duration in aged myocardium. *Journal of Clinical Investigation, 55*(1), 61–68.

Lakatta, E., & Levy, D. (2003). Arterial and cardiac aging: Major shareholders in cardiovascular disease enterprises, Part II. Aging arteries: A setup for vascular disease. *Circulation, 107*(1), 139–146.

Lansdorp, P., Poon, S., Chavez, E., Dragowska, V., Zijlmans, M., Bryan, T., . . . Martens, U. (1997). Telomeres in the hematopoietic system. *CIBA Foundation Symposium, 211,* 209–222.

Laughlin, G., Barrett-Connor, E., Kritz-Silverstein, D., & von Muhlen, D. (2000). Hysterectomy, oophorectomy, and endogenous sex hormone levels in older women: The Rancho Bernardo Study. *Journal of Clinical Endocrinology and Metabolism, 85,* 645–651.

Le Couteur, D., & McLean, A. (1998). The aging liver: Drug clearance and an oxygen diffusion barrier hypothesis. *Clinical Pharmacokinetics, 34*(5), 359–373.

Lee, C., Kloop, R., Weindruch, R., & Prolla, T. (1999). Gene expression profile of aging and its retardation by caloric restriction. *Science, 285*(5432), 1390–1393.

Lee, H., & Wei, Y. (2012). Mitochondria and aging. *Advances in Experimental Medicine and Biology, 942,* 311–327.

Leon-Carrion, J., Salgado, H., Sierra, M., Marquez-Rivas, J., & Dominguez-Morales, M. (2001). Neuroanatomy of the functional aging brain. In J. Leon-Carrion & M. Giannini (Eds.), *Behavioral neurology in the elderly* (pp. 67–84). Boca Raton, FL: CRC Press.

Letran, J., & Brawer, M. (1999). Disorders of the prostate. In W. Hazzard, J. Blass, W. Ettinger Jr., J. Halter, & J. Ouslander (Eds.), *Principles of geriatric medicine and gerontology* (4th ed., pp. 809–822). New York, NY: McGraw-Hill.

Levy, D., Larsen, M. G., Vasan, R. S., Kannel, W. B., & Ho, K. K. (1996). The progression from hypertension to congestive heart failure. *Journal of the American Medical Association, 275*(20), 1557–1562.

Lexell, J., Taylor, C., & Sjöström, M. (1988). What is the cause of aging atrophy? Total number, size and proportion of different fiber types studied in whole vastus lateralis muscle from 15- to 83-year-old men. *Journal of the Neurological Sciences, 84*, 275–294.

Licastro, F., Candore, G., Lio, D., Porcellini, E., Colonna-Romano, G., Franceschi, C., & Caruso, C. (2005). Innate immunity and inflammation in ageing: A key for understanding age-related diseases. *Immunity and Ageing, 2*, 8.

Lind, A., & McNicol, G. (1986). Cardiovascular response to holding and carrying weights by hand and shoulder harness. *Journal of Applied Physiology, 25*(3), 261–267.

Lindeman, R. (1990). Overview: Renal physiology and pathophysiology of aging. *American Journal of Kidney Diseases, 16*(4), 275–282.

Lindeman, R. (1995). Renal and urinary tract function. In E. Masoro (Ed.), *Handbook of physiology: Section 11, aging* (pp. 485–502). New York, NY: Oxford University Press.

Lindeman, R. (1998). Renal and electrolyte disorders. In E. Duthie & P. Katz (Eds.), *Practice of geriatrics* (3rd ed., pp. 546–562). Philadelphia, PA: W. B. Saunders.

Lindemann, B. (2000). A taste for umami. *Nature Neuroscience, 3*(2), 99–100.

Linton, P. J., & Dorshkind, K. (2004). Age-related changes in lymphocyte development and function. *Nature Immunology, 5*(2), 133–139.

Lippa, C., Hamos, J., Pulaski, S., Degennaro, L., & Drachman, D. (1992). Alzheimer's disease and aging: Effects on perforant pathway perikarya and synapses. *Neurobiology of Aging, 13*(2), 405–411.

Lompre, A. (1998). The sarco(endo)plasmic reticulum Ca^{2+}-ATPases in the cardiovascular system during growth and proliferation. *Trends in Cardiovascular Medicine, 8*(2), 75–82.

Lubran, M. (1995). Renal function in the elderly. *Annals of Clinical and Laboratory Science, 25*(1), 122–133.

Lye, M. (1998). Disturbances of homeostasis. In R. Tallis, H. Fillit, & J. Brocklehurst (Eds.), *Brocklehurst's textbook of geriatric medicine and gerontology* (5th ed., pp. 925–948). London, England: Churchill Livingstone.

Lynch, N., Metter, E., Lindle, R., Fozard, J., Tobin, J., Roy, T., . . . Hurley, B. F. (1999). Muscle quality, Part I. Age-associated differences between arm and leg muscle groups. *Journal of Applied Physiology, 86*(1), 188–194.

MacIntosh, C., Horowitz, M., Verhagen, M., Smout, A., Wishart, J., Morris, H., . . . Chapman, I. M. (2001). Effect of small intestinal nutrient infusion on appetite, gastrointestinal hormone release, and gastric myoelectrical activity in young and older men. *American Journal of Gastroenterology, 96*(4), 997–1007.

Madersbacher, S., Pycha, A., Schatzl, G., Mian, C., Klingler, C., & Marberger, M. (1998). The aging lower urinary tract: A comparative urodynamic study of men and women. *Urology, 51*(2), 206–212.

Madsen, J. L., & Graff, J. (2004). Effects of aging on gastrointestinal motor function. *Age and Ageing, 33*(2), 154–159.

Maharam, L., Bauman, P., Kalman, D., Skolnik, H., & Perle, S. (1999). Masters athletes: Factors affecting performance. *Sports Medicine, 28*(4), 273–285.

Mair, W., & Dillin, A. (2008). Aging and survival: The genetics of life span extension by dietary restriction. *Annual Review of Biochemistry, 77*, 727–754.

Maki, B., & McIlroy, W. (2006). Control of rapid limb movements for balance recovery: Age-related change and implications for fall prevention. *Age and Aging, 35*(S2), ii12–ii18.

Manolagas, S. C. (2000). Birth and death of bone cells: Basic regulatory mechanisms and implications for the pathogenesis and treatment of osteoporosis. *Endocrine Reviews, 21*(2), 115–137.

Marchesini, G., Bua, V., Brunori, A., Bianchi, G., Pisi, P., Fabbri, A., . . . Pisi, E. (1988). Galactose elimination capacity and liver volume in aging man. *Hepatology, 8*(5), 1079–1083.

Marcus, R., Masdirg, P., & Young, G. (1984). Age-related changes in parathyroid hormone and parathyroid hormone action in normal humans. *Journal of Clinical Endocrinology and Metabolism, 58*(2), 223–230.

Marieb, E., & Hoehn, K. (2015). *Human anatomy and physiology* (10th ed.). San Francisco, CA: Pearson/Benjamin Cummings.

Marker, J., Cryer, P., & Clutter, W. (1992). Attenuated glucose recovery from hypoglycemia in elderly. *Diabetes, 41*, 671–678.

Martin J., & Sheaff, M. (2007). Renal ageing. *Journal of Pathology, 211*(2), 198–205.

Maruyama, Y. (2012). Aging and arterial-cardiac interactions in the elderly. *International Journal of Cardiology 155*(1), 14–19.

Massry, S., Faddy, G., Zhou, X., Chandrasoma, P., Cheng, L., & Filburn, C. (1991). Impaired insulin secretion of aging: Role of renal failure and hyperparathyroidism. *Kidney International, 40*, 662–667.

Mattson, M. (1999). Cellular and neurochemical aspects of the aging human brain. In W. Hazzard, J. Blass, W. Ettinger Jr., J. Halter, & J. Ouslander (Eds.), *Principles of geriatric medicine and gerontology* (4th ed., pp. 1193–1208). New York, NY: McGraw-Hill.

Mattson, M., Maudsley, S., & Martin, B. (2004). BDNF and 5-HT: A dynamic duo in age-related neuronal plasticity and neurodegeneration disorders. *Trends in Neuroscience, 27*(10), 589–594.

McLean, A., & Le Couteur, D. (2004). Aging biology and geriatric clinical pharmacology. *Pharmacological Reviews, 56*(2), 163–184.

McReynolds, J., & Rossen, E. (2004). Importance of physical activity, nutrition, and social support for optimal aging. *Clinical Nurse Specialist, 18*(4), 200–206.

Meneilly, G. (2001). Pathophysiology of diabetes in the elderly. In A. Sinclair & P. Finucane (Eds.), *Diabetes in old age* (2nd ed., pp. 17–23). New York, NY: John Wiley & Sons.

Meneilly, G., Cheung, E., & Tuokko, H. (1994a). Altered responses to hypoglycemia of healthy elderly people. *Journal of Clinical Endocrinology and Metabolism, 78*(6), 1341–1348.

Meneilly, G., Cheung, E., & Tuokko, H. (1994b). Counterregulatory hormone responses to hypoglycemia in the elderly patient with diabetes. *Diabetes, 43*(3), 403–410.

Meyer, K. (2005). Aging. *Proceedings of the American Thoracic Society, 2*(5), 433–439.

Mimran, A., Ribstein, J., & Jover, B. (1992). Aging and sodium homeostasis. *Kidney International Supplement, 37*, S107–S113.

Minaker, K. (1990). What diabetologists should know about elderly patients. *Diabetes Care, 13*(Suppl. 2), 34–46.

Minaker, K. (2011). Common clinical sequelae of aging. In L. Goldman & A. Schafer (Eds.), *Cecil textbook of medicine* (24th ed.). Philadelphia, PA: Elsevier/Saunders.

Mistretta, C. (1984). Aging effects on anatomy and neurophysiology of taste and smell. *Gerodontology, 3*(2), 131–136.

Mocchegiani, E., & Malavolta, M. (2004). NK and NKT cell functions in immunosenescence. *Aging Cell, 3*(4), 177–184.

Moffett, D., Moffett, S., & Schauff, C. L. (1993). *Human physiology: Foundations and frontiers* (2nd ed., p. 458). St. Louis, MO: Mosby.

Mohanlal, V., Parsa, A., & Weir, M. (2012). Role of dietary therapies in the prevention and treatment of hypertension. *Nature Reviews: Nephrology, 8*(7), 413–422.

Moody, D., Thore, C., Anstrom, J., Challa, C., Langefield, C., & Brown, W. (2004). Quantification of afferent vessels shows reduced brain vascular density in subjects with leukoaraiosis. *Radiology, 233*(3), 883–890.

Moore, A., Mangoni, A., Lyons, D., & Jackson, S. (2003). The cardiovascular system in the ageing patient. *British Journal of Clinical Pharmacology, 56*(3), 254–260.

Moreland, J., Richardson, J., Goldsmith, C., & Clase, C. (2004). Muscle weakness and falls in older adults: A systematic review and meta-analysis. *Journal of the American Geriatrics Society, 52*(7), 1121–1129.

Morley, J., Kaiser, F., Perry, H., Patrick, P., Morley, P., Stauber, P., . . . Garry, P. J. (1997). Longitudinal changes in testosterone, luteinizing hormone, and follicle-stimulating hormone in healthy older men. *Metabolism, 46*(4), 410–413.

Morley, J., & Perry, H. (1991). The management of diabetes mellitus in older individuals. *Drugs, 41*(4), 548–565.

Morley, J., & Reese, S. (1989). Clinical implications of the aging heart. *American Journal of Medicine, 86*, 77–86.

Morley, J. E., Baumgartner, R., Roubenoff, R., Mayer, J., & Nair, K. S. (2001). Sarcopenia. *Journal of Laboratory and Clinical Medicine, 137*(4), 231–243.

Morrison, J., & Hof, P. (1997). Life and death of neurons in the aging brain. *Nature, 279*, 112–119.

Morrow, L., & Halter, J. (1994). Treatment of the elderly with diabetes. In C. Kahn & G. Weir (Eds.), *Joslin's diabetes mellitus* (13th ed., pp. 552–559). Philadelphia, PA: Lea & Febiger.

Moskowitz, R., Kelly, M., & Lewallen, D. (2004). Understanding osteoarthritis of the knee: causes and effects. *American Journal of Orthopaedics, 33*(Suppl. 2), 5–9.

Mozaz, M., & Monguio, I. (2001). Motor functions and praxis in the elderly. In J. Leon-Carrion & M. Giannini (Eds.), *Behavioral neurology in the elderly* (pp. 125–150). Boca Raton, FL: CRC Press.

Mühlberg, W., & Platt D. (1999). Age-dependent changes of the kidneys: pharmacological implications. *Gerontology, 45*(5), 243–53.

Murphy, D., DeCarli, C., Schapiro, M., Rapoport, S., & Horwitz, B. (1992). Age-related differences in volumes of subcortical nuclei, brain matter, and cerebro-spinal fluid in healthy men as measured with magnetic resonance imaging (MRI). *Archives of Neurology, 49*(8), 839–845.

Musso, C., Ghezzi, L., & Ferraris, J. (2004). Renal physiology in newborns and old people: Similar characteristics but different mechanisms. *International Urology and Nephrology, 36*, 273–276.

Musso, C., Liakopoulos, V., Ioannidis, I., Eleftheriadias, T., & Stefandis, I. (2006). Acute renal failure in the elderly: Particular characteristics. *International Journal of Urology and Nephrology, 38*, 787–793.

Nair, S., & Ren, J. (2012). Autophagy and cardiovascular aging: Lesson learned from rapamycin. *Cell Cycle, 11*(11), 2092–2099.

National Eye Institute. (2004). *Prevalence of blindness data*. Retrieved from https://nei.nih.gov/eyedata/pbd _tables

National Institute of Arthritis and Musculoskeletal and Skin Diseases. (2066). *Handout on health: Osteoarthritis*. Retrieved from https://www.niams.nih.gov/Health_Info/Osteoarthritis/default.asp#2

National Osteoporosis Foundation. (2015). What is osteoporosis? Retrieved from http://www.nof.org/articles/7

Naughton, B., Mylotte, J., & Tayara, A. (2000). Outcome of nursing home-acquired pneumonia: Derivation and application of a practical model to predict 30 day mortality. *Journal of the American Geriatrics Society, 48*(10), 1292–1299.

Newton, J., Yemm, R., Abel, R., & Menhinick, S. (1993). Changes in human jaw muscles with age and dental state. *Gerodontology, 10*(1), 16–22.

Nielson, M., & Pedersen, J. (1996). Changes in the anal sphincter with age: An endosonographic study. *Acta Radiologica, 37*(3), 357–361.

Nilsson, P. (2012). Impact of vascular aging on cardiovascular disease: The role of telomere biology. *Journal of Hypertension*, 30(Suppl.), S9–S12.

Nilsson-Ehle, H., Jagenburg, R., Landahl, S., & Svanborg, A. (2000). Blood haemoglobin declines in the elderly: Implications for reference intervals from age 70 to 88. *European Journal of Haematology, 65*(5), 297–305.

Nitzan, M., Mahler Y., Schechter, D., Yaffe, S., Bocher, M., & Chisn, R. (1994). A measurement of pulmonary blood volume increase during systole in humans. *Physiological Measures, 15*(4), 489–498.

O'Donovan, D., Hausken, T., Lei, Y., Russo, A., Keough, J., Horowitz, M., & Jones, K. L. (2005). Effects of aging on transpyloric flow, gastric emptying and intragastric distribution in healthy humans—impact on glycemia. *Digestive Diseases and Sciences, 50*(4), 671–676.

Olivetti, G., Melessari, M., Capasso, J., & Anversa, P. (1991). Cardiomyopathy of the aging human heart: Myocyte loss and reactive cellular hypertrophy. *Circulation Research, 68*(6), 1560–1568.

O'Mahony, D., O'Leary, P., & Quigley, E. (2002). Aging and intestinal motility: A review of factors that affect intestinal motility in the aged. *Drugs Aging, 19*(7), 515–527.

O'Rourke, M., & Hashimoto, J. (2007). Mechanical factors in arterial aging: A clinical perspective. *Journal of the American College of Cardiology, 50*(1), 1–13.

Orr, W., & Chen, C. (2002). Aging and neural control of the GI tract, Part IV. Clinical and physiological aspects of gastrointestinal motility and aging. *American Journal of Physiology: Gastrointestinal and Liver Physiology, 283*, G1226–G1231.

Ostchega, Y., Dillon, C., Lindle, R., Carroll, M., & Hurley, B. (2004). Isokinetic leg muscle strength in older Americans and its relationship to a standardized walk test: Data from the National Health and Nutrition Examination Survey 1999–2000. *Journal of the American Geriatric Society, 52*, 977–982.

Owsley, C., Sekular, R., & Siemsen, D. (1983). Contrast sensitivity throughout adulthood. *Vision Research, 23*(7), 689–699.

Paick, S., Meehan, A., Lee, M., Penson, D., & Wessells, H. (2005). The relationship among lower urinary tract symptoms, prostate specific antigen and erectile dysfunction in men with benign prostatic hyperplasia: Results from the Proscar Long-Term Efficacy and Safety Study. *Journal of Urology, 173*, 903–907.

Pakkenberg, B., & Gundersen, J. (1997). Neocortical neuron number in humans: Effect of sex and age. *Journal of Comparative Neurology, 384*(4), 312–320.

Pannarale, G., Carbone, R., Del Mastro, G., Gallo, C., Gattullo, V., Naalicchio, L., . . . Tedesco, A. (2010). The aging kidney: Structural changes. *Journal of Nephrology, 23*(Suppl. 15), S37–S40.

Partin, A., & Rodriguez, R. (2002). The molecular biology, endocrinology, and physiology of the prostate and seminal vesicles. In P. Walsh (Ed.), *Campbell's urology* (8th ed.). Philadelphia, PA: W. B. Saunders.

Patt, B. (1998). Otologic disorders. In E. Duthie & P. Katz (Eds.), *Practice of geriatrics* (3rd ed., pp. 449–456). Philadelphia, PA: W. B. Saunders.

Peters, A. (2002). The effects of normal aging on myelin and nerve fibers: A review. *Journal of Neurocytology, 31*, 581–593.

Peters, A., & Davidson, M. (1997). Aging and diabetes. In K. Alberti, P. Zimmet, & R. Defronzo (Eds.), *International textbook of diabetes mellitus* (2nd ed., Vol. 2, pp. 1151–1176). Chichester, England: John Wiley & Sons.

Peters, A., Morrison, J., Rosene, D., & Hyman, B. (1998). Are neurons lost from the primate cerebral cortex during aging? *Cerebral Cortex, 8*(4), 295–300.

Peters, R. (2006). Ageing and the brain. *Postgrad Medical Journal, 82*(964), 84–85.

Phillips, P., Hodsman, G., & Johnston, C. (1991). Neuroendocrine mechanisms and cardiovascular homeostasis in the elderly. *Cardiovascular Drugs and Therapy, 4*(Suppl. 6), 1209–1213.

Phillips, S., Rook, K., Siddle, N., Bruce, S., & Woledge, R. (1993). Muscle weakness in women occurs at an earlier age than in men, but strength is preserved by hormone replacement therapy. *Clinical Science, 84*(1), 95–98.

Phillips, T. J., Demircay, Z., & Sahu, M. (2001). Hormonal effects on skin aging. *Clinics in Geriatric Medicine, 17*(4), 661–672.

Pierard, G. E., Letawe, C., Dowlati, A., & Pierard-Franchimont, C. (1995). Effect of hormone replacement therapy for menopause on the mechanical properties of skin. *Journal of the American Geriatrics Society, 43*(6), 662–665.

Plackett, T., Boehmer, E., Faunce, D., & Kovacs, E. (2004). Aging and innate immune cells. *Journal of Leukocyte Biology, 76*(2), 291–299.

Poehlman, E., Toth, M., & Gardner, A. (1995). Changes in energy balance and body composition at menopause. *Annals of Internal Medicine, 123*(9), 673–675.

Priebe, H. (2000). The aged cardiovascular risk patient. *British Journal of Anaesthesia, 85*(5), 763–778.

Prinz, P., Weitzman, E., Cunningham, G., & Karacan, I. (1983). Plasma growth hormone during sleep in young and aged men. *Journals of Gerontology, 38*(5), 519–524.

Proctor, D., Balagopal, P., & Nair, K. (1998). Age-related sarcopenia in humans is associated with reduced synthetic rates of specific muscle proteins. *Journal of Nutrition, 128*(Suppl. 2), 351S–355S.

Pugh, K., & Wei, J. (2001). Clinical implications of physiological changes in the aging heart. *Drugs & Aging, 18*(4), 263–276.

Quyyumi, A. A. (1998). Endothelial function in health and disease: New insights into the genesis of cardiovascular disease. *American Journal of Medicine, 105*, 325–395.

Rajkumar, C., Kingwell, B., Cameron, J., Waddell, T., Mehra, R., Christophidis, N., . . . Dart, A. M. (1997). Hormonal therapy increases arterial compliance in postmenopausal women. *Journal of the American College of Cardiology, 30*(2), 350–356.

Ramos-Platon, M., & Beneto-Pascual, A. (2001). Aging, sleep, and neuropsychological functioning outcomes. In J. Leon-Carrion & M. Giannini (Eds.), *Behavioral neurology in the elderly* (pp. 203–242). Boca Raton, FL: CRC Press.

Randolph, J., Sowers, M., Bondarenko, I., Harlow, S., Luborsky, J., & Little, R. (2004). Change in estradiol and follicle-stimulation hormone across the early menopausal transition: Effects of ethnicity and age. *Journal of Clinical Endocrinology and Metabolism, 89*(4), 1555–1561.

Rao, S., Mudipalli, R., Mujica, V., Patel, R., & Zimmerman, B. (2003). Effects of gender and age on esophageal biomechanical properties and sensation. *American Journal of Gastroenterology, 98*(8), 1688–1695.

Raz, N., Lindenberger, U., Rodrigue, K., Kennedy, K., Head, D., Williamson, A., . . . Acker, J. D. (2005). Regional brain changes in aging healthy adults: General trends, individual differences and modifiers. *Cerebral Cortex, 15*(11), 1676–1689.

Rees, T., Duckert, L., & Carey, J. (1999). Auditory and vestibular dysfunction. In W. Hazzard, J. Blass, W. Ettinger Jr., J. Halter, & J. Ouslander (Eds.), *Principles of geriatric medicine and gerontology* (4th ed., pp. 617–632). New York, NY: McGraw-Hill.

Reinus, J., & Brandt, L. (1998). The upper gastrointestinal tract. In R. Tallis, H. Fillit, & J. Brocklehurst (Eds.), *Brocklehurst's textbook of geriatric medicine and gerontology* (5th ed., pp. 803–826). London, England: Churchill Livingstone.

Resnick, N., Elbadawi, A., & Yalla, S. (1995). Age and the lower urinary tract: What is normal? *Neurourology and Urodynamics, 14*, 577–579.

Richardson, D. (1994). Adjustments associated with the aging process. In N. Mortillaro & A. Taylor (Eds.), *The pathophysiology of the microcirculation* (pp. 200–204). Boca Raton, FL: CRC Press.

Robert, L. (1999). Aging of the vascular wall and atherosclerosis. *Experimental Gerontology, 34*(4), 491–501.

Rociu, E., Stoker, J., Eijkemans, M., & Lameris, J. (2000). Normal anal sphincter anatomy and age- and sex-related variations at high-spatial-resolution endoanal MR imaging. *Radiology, 217*(2), 395–401.

Rodeheffer, R., Gerstenblith, G., Becker, L., Fleg, J., Weisfeldt, M., & Lakatta, E. (1984). Exercise cardiac output is maintained with advancing age in healthy human subjects: Cardiac dilatation and increased stroke volume compensate for a diminished heart rate. *Circulation, 69*(2), 203–213.

Roffe, C. (1998). Ageing of the heart. *British Journal of Biomedical Science, 55*(2), 136–148.

Roof, R., & Hall, E. (2000). Gender differences in acute CNS trauma and stroke: Neuroprotective effects of estrogen and progesterone. *Journal of Neurotrauma, 17*(5), 367–388.

Rosen, R., Altwein, J., Boyle, P., Kirby, R., Lukacs, B., Meuleman, E., . . . Giuliano, F. (2003). Lower urinary tract symptoms and male sexual dysfunction: The multinational survey of the aging male (MSAM-7). *European Urology, 44*(6), 637–649.

Rossmanith, W., Handke-Vesel, A., Wirth, U., & Scherbaum, W. (1994). Does the gonadotropin pulsatility of postmenopausal women represent the unrestrained hypothalamic-pituitary activity? *European Journal of Endocrinology, 130*, 485–493.

Roubenoff, R. (2001). Origins and clinical relevance of sarcopenia. *Canadian Journal of Applied Physiology, 26*(1), 78–89.

Roubenoff, R. (2003). Sarcopenia: Effects on body composition and function. *Journals of Gerontology: Medical Sciences, 58A*(11), 1012–1017.

Roubenoff, R., & Hughes, V. A. (2000). Sarcopenia: Current concepts. *Journals of Gerontology: Medical Sciences, 55A*(12), M716–M724.

Rowe, J., Andres, A., Tobin, J., Norris, A., & Shock, N. (1976). The effect of age on creatinine clearance in men: A cross-sectional and longitudinal study. *Journal of Gerontology, 32*(2), 155–163.

Rowe, J., Minaker, K., Pallotta, J., & Flier, J. (1983). Characterization of the insulin resistance of aging. *Journal of Clinical Investigation, 71*(6), 1581–1587.

Rule, A., Gussak, H., Pond, G., Bergstralh, E., Stegall, M., Cosio, F., & Larson, T. S. (2004). Measured and estimated GFR in healthy potential kidney donors. *American Journal of Kidney Diseases, 43*(1), 112–119.

Russell-Aulet, M., Jaffe, C., Mott-Friberg, R., & Barkans, A. (1999). In vivo semiquantification of hypothalamus growth hormone releasing hormone (GHRH) output in humans: Evidence for relative GHRH deficiency in aging. *Journal of Clinical Endocrinology Metabolism, 84*(10), 3490–3497.

Sabbah, H. (2000). Apoptotic cell death in heart failure. *Cardiovascular Research, 45*, 704–712.

Saffrey, M. (2004), Aging of the enteric nervous system. *Mechanism of Ageing and Development, 125*(12), 899–906.

Salles, N. (2007). Basic mechanisms of the aging gastrointestinal tract. *Digestive Diseases, 25*(2), 112–117.

Salmasi, A., Alimo, A., Jepson, E., & Dancy, M. (2003). Age-associated changes in left ventricular diastolic function are related to increasing left ventricular mass. *American Journal of Hypertension, 16*(6), 473–477.

Salthouse, T. (1993). Speed mediation of adult age differences in cognition. *Developmental Psychology, 29*(4), 722–738.

Sampson, N., Untegassan, G., Plas, E., & Berger, P. (2007). The ageing male reproductive tract. *Journal of Pathology, 211*(1), 206–218.

Santoro, N., Adel, T., & Skurnick, J. (1999). Decreased inhibin tone and increased activin A secretion characterize reproductive aging in women. *Fertility and Sterility, 71*(4), 658–662.

Sator, P. G., Schmidt, J. B., Rabe, T., & Zouboulis, C. C. (2004). Skin aging and sex hormones in women: clinical perspectives for intervention by hormone replacement therapy. *Experimental Dermatology, 13*(Suppl. 4), 36–40.

Scharffetter-Kochanek, K., Brenneisen, P., Wenk, J., Herrmann, G., Ma, W., Kuhr, L., . . . Wlaschek, M. (2000). Photoaging of the skin from phenotype to mechanisms. *Experimental Gerontology, 35*(3), 307–316.

Scheff, S., & Price, D. (1998). Synaptic density in the inner molecular layer of the hippocampal dentate gyrus in Alzheimer disease. *Journal of Neuropathology and Experimental Neurology, 57*(12), 1146–1153.

Scheff, S., & Price, D. (2001). Alzheimer's disease-related synapse loss in the cingulate cortex. *Journal of Alzheimer's Disease, 3*(5), 495–505.

Scheff, S., Price, D., & Sparks, D. (2001). Quantitative assessment of possible age-related change in synaptic numbers in the human frontal cortex. *Neurobiology of Aging, 22*(3), 355–365.

Scheff, S., Sparks, D., & Price, D. (1996). Quantitative assessment of synaptic density in the outer molecular layer of the hippocampal dentate gyrus in Alzheimer's disease. *Dementia, 7*(4), 226–232.

Schiffman, S. (1997). Taste and smell losses in normal aging and disease. *Journal of the American Medical Association, 278*(16), 1357–1362.

Schlegel, P., & Hardy, M. (2002). Male reproductive physiology. In P. Walsh (Ed.), *Campbell's urology* (8th ed., pp. 1358–1377). Philadelphia, PA: W. B. Saunders.

Schmitt, D. (1999). Immune functions of the human skin: Models of in vivo studies using Langerhans cells. *Cell Biology and Toxicology, 15*(1), 41–45.

Schmitt, F., Davis, D., Wekstein, D., Smith, C., Ashford, J., & Markesbery, W. (2000). Preclinical AD revisited: Neuropathology of cognitively normal older adults. *Neurology, 55*(3), 370–376.

Schmucker, D. (1998). Aging and the liver: An update. *Journal of Gerontology Section A: Biological Sciences & Medical Sciences, 53*(5), B315–B320.

Schmucker, D., Heyworth, M., Owen, R., & Daniels, C. (1996). Impact of aging on gastrointestinal mucosal immunity. *Digestive Diseases and Sciences, 41*(6), 1183–1193.

Schmucker, D., Owen, R., Outenreath, R., & Thoreux, K. (2003). Basis for the age-related decline in intestinal mucosal immunity. *Clinical and Developmental Immunology, 10*, 167–172.

Schmucker, D., Thoreux, K., & Owen, R. (2001). Aging impairs intestinal immunity. *Mechanisms of Ageing and Development, 122*(13), 1397–1411.

Schroeder, P., & Richter, J. (1994). Swallowing disorders in the elderly. *Practical Gastroenterology, 18*, 19–41.

Schuknecht, H. (2010). *Pathology of the ear*. Cambridge, MA: Harvard University Press.

Schuknecht, H., & Gacek, M. (1993). Cochlear pathology in presbycusis. *Annals of Otology, Rhinology and Laryngology, 102*(1 Pt. 2), 1–16.

Schulman, S. (1999). Cardiovascular consequences of the aging process. *Cardiology Clinics, 17*(1), 35–49.

Seals, D. R., & Esler, M. D. (2000). Human ageing and the sympathoadrenal system. *Journal of Physiology, 528*(3), 407–417.

Seeman, E. (2002a). Pathogenesis of bone fragility in women and men. *Lancet, 359*, 1841–1850.

Seeman, E. (2003a). Invited review: Pathogenesis of osteoporosis. *Journal of Applied Physiology, 95*, 2142–2151.

Seeman, E. (2003b). Reduced bone formation and increased bone resorption: Rational targets for the treatment of osteoporosis. *Osteoporosis International, 14*(Suppl. 3), S2–S8.

Seiberling, K., & Conley, D. (2004). Aging and olfactory and taste function. *Otolaryngologic Clinics of North America, 37*(6), 1209–1228.

Seidman, S. (2003). The aging male: Androgens, erectile dysfunction, and depression. *Journal of Clinical Psychiatry, 64*(Suppl. 10), 31–37.

Shaffer, S., & Harrison, A. (2007). Aging of the somatosensory system: A translational perspective. *Physical Therapy, 87*(2), 193–207.

Shah, M. G., & Maibach, H. I. (2001). Estrogen and skin. An overview. *American Journal of Clinical Dermatology, 2*(3), 143–150.

Shaker, R., Dua, K., & Koch, T. (1998). Gastroenterologic disorders. In E. Duthie & P. Katz (Eds.), *Practice of geriatrics* (3rd ed., pp. 505–523). Philadelphia, PA: W. B. Saunders.

Shealy, C. N. (1995). A review of dehydroepiandrosterone (DHEA). *Integrative Physiological and Behavioral Science, 30*(4), 308–313.

Sherwood, L. (Ed.). (2014). *Human physiology: From cells to systems* (9th ed.). Boston, MA: Cengage Learning.

Shimamoto, C., Hirata, I., & Hiraike, Y. (2002). Evaluation of gastric motor activity in the elderly by electro gastrography and the 13C-acetate breath test. *Gerontology, 48*(6), 381–386.

Ship, J., Pillemer, S., & Baum, B. (2002). Xerostomia and the geriatric patient. *Journal of the American Geriatrics Society, 50*(3), 535–543.

Simon, J., Leboff, M., Wright, J., & Glowacki, J. (2002). Fractures in the elderly and vitamin D. *Journal of Nutrition, Health, and Aging, 6*(6), 406–412.

Sloane, M., Owsley, C., & Alzarez, S. (1988). Aging, senile miosis and spatial contrast sensitivity at low luminance. *Vision Research, 28*(11), 1235–1246.

Smith, M. (1998). Gynecologic disorders. In E. Duthie & P. Katz (Eds.), *Practice of geriatrics* (3rd ed., pp. 524–534). Philadelphia, PA: W. B. Saunders.

Snowdon, D. A. (2002). *Aging with Grace: What the Nun Study Teaches us about Leading Long, Healthier, and more Meaningful Lives.* New York, NY: Bantam.

Soergel, K., Zboralske, F., & Amberg, J. (1964). Presbyesophagus: Esophageal motility in nonagenarians. *Journal of Clinical Investigation, 43*, 1972–1979.

Sohal, R., Mockett, R., & Orr, W. (2002). Mechanisms of aging: An appraisal of the oxidative stress hypothesis. *Free Radical Biology & Medicine, 33*(5), 575–586.

Solana, R., & Mariani, E. (2000). NK and NK/T cells in human senescence. *Vaccine, 18*(16), 1613–1620.

Sorribas, V., Lotscher, M., Loffing, J., Biber, J., Kaissling, B., Murer, H., & Levi, M. (1995). Cellular mechanisms of the age-related decrease in renal phosphate reabsorption. *Kidney International, 50*, 855–863.

Soules, M., Sherman, S., Parrott, E., Rebar, R., Santoro, N., Utian, W., . . . STRAW + 10 Collaborative Group. (2001). Executive summary: Stages of reproductive aging workshop (STRAW). *Fertility and Sterility, 76*(5), 874–878.

Spence, J. (1921, July). Some observations on sugar tolerance with special reference to variations found at different ages. *Quarterly Journal of Medicine*, 314–326.

Stein, P., Soare, A., Meyer, T., Cangemi, R., Holloszy, J., & Fontana, L. (2012). Caloric restriction may reverse age-related autonomic decline in humans. *Aging Cell, 11*(4), 644–650.

Sternbach, H. (1998). Age-associated testosterone decline in men: Clinical issues for psychiatry. *American Journal of Psychiatry, 155*(10), 1310–1318.

Stevens, J., Cain, W., & Weinstein, D. (1987). Aging impairs the ability to detect gas odor. *Fire Technology, 23*(3), 198–204.

Stevens, J., & Choo, K. (1996). Spatial acuity of the body surface over the life span. *Somatosensory and Motor Research, 13*(2), 153–166.

Stevens, J., & Patterson, M. (1995). Dimensions of spatial acuity in the touch sense: Changes over the life span. *Somatosensory and Motor Research, 12*(1), 29–47.

Strasser, H., Tiefenthaler, M., Steinlechner, M., Bartsch, G., & Konwalinka, G. (1996). Urinary incontinence in the elderly. *Age and Ageing, 25*, 285–291.

Tan, Q., Ohm, K., Kruse, T., & Christensen, K. (2010). Dissecting complex phenotypes using the genomics of twins. *Functional and Integrative Genomics, 10*(3), 321–327.

Tepper, R., & Katz, S. (1998). Overview: Geriatric gastroenterology. In R. Tallis, H. Fillit, & J. Brocklehurst (Eds.), *Brocklehurst's textbook of geriatric medicine and gerontology* (5th ed., pp. 783–788). London, England: Churchill Livingstone.

Terry, R., DeTeresa, R., & Hansen, L. (1987). Neocortical cell counts in normal human adult aging. *Annals of Neurology, 21*(6), 530–539.

Teter, B., & Ashford, J. (2002). Neuroplasticity in Alzheimer's disease. *Journal of Neuroscience Research, 70,* 402–437.

Timiras, M. L. (2007). The skin. In P. S. Timiras (Ed.), *Physiological basis of aging and geriatrics* (3rd ed., pp. 397–404). Boca Raton, FL: CRC Press.

Timiras, P. S. (2007). The thyroid, parathyroid, and pineal glands. In P. S. Timiras (Ed.), *Physiological basis of aging and geriatrics* (4th ed., pp. 205–218). Boca Raton, FL: CRC Press.

Timiras, P. S., & Navasio, F. M. (2007). The skeleton, joints, and skeletal and cardiac muscles. In P. S. Timiras (Ed.), *Physiological basis of aging and geriatrics* (4th ed., pp. 329–344). Boca Raton, FL: CRC Press.

Tobin, D., & Paus, R. (2001). Graying: Gerontobiology of the hair follicle pigmentary unit. *Experimental Gerontology, 36,* 29–54.

Topp, R., Fahlman, M., & Boardley, D. (2004). Healthy aging: Health promotion and disease prevention. *Nursing Clinics of North America, 39*(2), 411–422.

Tortora, G., & Derrickson, B. (2014). *Principles of anatomy and physiology* (14th ed.). Hoboken, NJ: John Wiley and Sons.

Tresch, D., & Jamali, I. (1998). Cardiac disorders. In E. Duthie & P. Katz (Eds.), *Practice of geriatrics* (3rd ed., pp. 353–374). Philadelphia, PA: W. B. Saunders.

Turner, H., & Wass, J. (1997). Gonadal function in men with chronic illness. *Clinical Endocrinology, 47*(4), 379–403.

van den Beld, A., de Jong, F., Grobbee, D., Pols, H., & Lamberts, S. (2000). Measures of bioavailable serum testosterone and estradiol and their relationship with muscle strength, bone density, and body composition in elderly men. *Journal of Clinical Endocrinology and Metabolism, 85,* 3276–3282.

Vandervoot, A. A., & Symons, T. B. (2001). Functional and metabolic consequences of sarcopenia. *Canadian Journal of Applied Physiology, 26*(1), 90–101.

Vermeulen, A., Goemaere, S., & Kaufman, J. (1999). Sex hormones, body composition, and aging. *Aging Male, 2,* 8–15.

Vieth, R., Ladak, Y., & Walfish, P. (2003). Age-related changes in the 25-hydroxyvitamin D versus parathyroid hormone relationship suggest a different reason why older adults require more vitamin D. *Journal of Clinical Endocrinology and Metabolism, 88*(1), 185–191.

Vijg, J., & Suh, Y. (2005). Genetics of longevity and aging. *Annual Review of Medicine, 56,* 193–212.

Vincent, H., Raiser, S., & Vincent, K. (2012). The aging musculoskeletal system and obesity-related considerations with exercise. *Ageing Research Reviews, 11*(3), 361–373.

Virmani, R., Avolio, A., Margner, W., Robinowitz, M., Herderick, E., Cornhill, J., . . . O'Rouke, M. (1991). Effect of aging on aortic morphology in populations with high and low prevalence of hypertension and atherosclerosis: Comparison between Occidental and Chinese communities. *American Journal of Pathology, 139,* 1119–1129.

Volkow, N., Gur, R., Wang, G., Fowler, J., Moberg, P., Ding, Y., . . . Logan, J. (1998). Association between decline in brain dopamine activity with age and cognitive and motor impairment in healthy individuals. *American Journal of Psychiatry, 155*(3), 344–349.

Volpi, E., Sheffield-Moore, M., Rasmussen, B. B., & Wolfe, R. R. (2001). Basal muscle amino acid kinetics and protein synthesis in healthy young and older men. *Journal of the American Medical Association, 286*(10), 1206–1212.

Washburn, R. A., Smith, K. W., Jette, A. M., & Janney, C. A. (1993). The physical activity scale for the elderly (PASE): Development and evaluation. *Journal of Clinical Epidemiology, 46*(2), 153–62.

Wei, J. (1992). Age and the cardiovascular system. *New England Journal of Medicine, 327,* 1735–1739.

Weiffenbach, J. (1991). Chemical senses in aging. In T. Getchell, R. Doty, L. Bartoshuk, & J. Snow (Eds.), *Smell and taste in health and disease* (pp. 369–380). New York, NY: Raven Press.

Weiffenbach, J., Baum, B., & Burghauser, R. (1982). Taste threshold: Quality specific variation with aging. *Journal of Gerontology, 37*(3), 372–377.

Weinstein, J., & Anderson, S. (2010). The aging kidney: Physiological changes. *Advances in Chronic Kidney Disease, 17*(4), 302–307.

Weiss, G., Skurnick, J., Goldsmith, L., Santoro, N., & Park, S. (2004). Menopause and hypothalamic-pituitary sensitivity to estrogen. *Journal of the American Medical Association, 292*(24), 2991–2996.

White, C. (2014). Aging changes in the female reproductive system. Bethesda, MD: Medline Plus, National Library of Medicine, National Institutes of Health. Retrieved from http://www.nlm.nih.gov/medlineplus/ency/article/004016.htm

White, J., & Ham, R. (1997). Nutrition. In R. Ham & P. Sloane (Eds.), *Primary care geriatrics: A case-based approach* (3rd ed., pp. 108–127). New York, NY: Mosby.

Whitman, D. B. (1999, March). *The immunology of aging.* Retrieved from http://www.csa.com/discoveryguides/archives/immune-aging.php

Wick, G., & Grubeck-Loebenstein, B. (1997). Primary and secondary alterations of immune reactivity in the elderly: Impact of dietary factors and disease. *Immunological Reviews, 160*, 171–184.

Wilson, M., Thomas, D., Rubenstein, L., Chibnall, J., Anderson, S., Baxi, A., . . . Morley, J. E. (2005). Appetite assessment: Simple appetite questionnaire predicts weight loss in community-dwelling adults and nursing home residents. *American Journal of Clinical Nutrition, 82*(5), 1074–1081.

Wise, P., Dubal, D., Wilson, M., Rau, S., & Bottner, M. (2001). Minireview: Neuroprotective effects of estrogen— New insights into mechanisms of action. *Endocrinology, 142*(3), 969–973.

Wise, P., Dubal, D., Wilson, M., Rau, S., & Liu, Y. (2001). Estrogens: Trophic and protective factors in the adult brain. *Frontiers in Neuroendocrinology, 22*(1), 33–66.

Wise, P., Krajnak, K., & Kashon, M. (1996). Menopause: The aging of multiple pacemakers. *Science, 273*(5271), 67–70.

Wolinsky, F. D., Coe, R. M., McIntosh, W. A., Kubena, K. S., Prendergast, J. M., Chavez, M. N., Miller, D. K., . . . Landmann, W. A. (1990). Progress in the development of a nutritional risk index. *Journal of Nutrition, 120*(Suppl. 11), 1549–53.

Wynne, H., Cope, E., Mutch, E., Rawlins, M., Woodhouse, K., & James, O. (1989). The effect of age upon liver volume and apparent liver blood flow in healthy man. *Hepatology, 9*(2), 297–301.

Yaar, M., & Gilchrest, B. A. (2001). Skin aging: Postulated mechanisms and consequent changes in structure and function. *Clinics in Geriatric Medicine, 17*(4), 617–630.

Yarasheski, K., Pak-Loduca, J., Hasten, D., Obert, K., Brown, M., & Sinacore, D. (1999). Resistance exercise training increases mixed muscle protein synthesis rate in frail women and men. *American Journal of Physiology, 40*(1, Pt 1), E118–E125.

Yarasheski, K., Zackwieja, F., Campbell, J., & Bier, D. (1995). Effect of growth hormone and resistance exercise on muscle growth and strength in older men. *American Journal of Physiology, 268*(2, Pt 1), E268–E276.

Yen, S., & Laughlin, G. (1998). Aging and the adrenal cortex. *Experimental Gerontology, 33*(7–8), 897–910.

Yialamas, M., & Hayes, F. (2003). Androgens and the ageing male and female. *Best Practice and Research Clinical Endocrinology and Metabolism, 17*(2), 223–236.

Zouboulis, C. C., & Boschnakow, A. (2001). Chronological ageing and photoageing of the human sebaceous gland. *Clinical Dermatology, 26*(7), 600–607.

Zumoff, B., Strain, G., Miller, L., & Rosner, W. (1995). Twenty-four hour mean plasma testosterone concentration declines with age in normal premenopausal women. *Journal of Clinical Endocrinology and Metabolism, 80*(4), 1429–1430.

For a full suite of assignments and additional learning activities, see the access code at the front of your book.

Unit II
Communication and Assessment

(COMPETENCIES 2–6, 13, 15)

CHAPTER 5

Teaching and Communication with Older Adults and Their Families

Dennis Ondrejka

(Competencies 2, 5, 13, 15)

LEARNING OBJECTIVES

At the end of this chapter, the reader will be able to:

> State the importance of communication with older adults.
> Identify effective and ineffective communication strategies.
> Understand how normal and pathological changes of aging effect communication.
> Discuss communication strategies for older adults with common normal and pathological changes of aging.
> Describe person-centered communication.
> Apply gerogogy strategies for enhancing teaching and learning of older adults.
> Explore changing demographics for older adults as it affects the teaching–learning process.
> Adjust teaching related to the diversity in learning styles of older adults.
> Draw correlations between effective communication and teaching strategies.
> Examine teaching variations needed for those with chronic illness.
> Identify assessments for the older adult in and out of healthcare settings.

KEY TERMS

Active memory	Broca's aphasia
Activities of daily living	Cataract
Alzheimer's disease	Cognition
Andragogy	Communication Enhancement Model
Anomia	Compensatory scaffolding
Aphasia	Compensatory strategies
Apraxia	Compliance scaffolding
Background noise	Declarative memory

Dementia

Depression

Diabetic retinopathy

Dual sensory impairment

Dysarthria

Eden Alternative

Elderspeak

Episodic memory

Frequencies

Gerogogy

Glaucoma

Global aphasia

HCHAPS surveys

Hearing aids

Isolation

Language

Lexical memory

Literacy

Long-term memory

Macular degeneration

Major neurocognitive disorder

Nondeclarative memory

Nonverbal communication

Parkinson's disease

Partnering communication model

Patient-centered communication

Pay-for-performance

Pedagogy

Person-first language

Personal amplification devices

Presbycusis

Presbyopia

Relational teaching

Restorative strategies

Scaffolding Theory of Aging
     and Cognition

Semantic memory

Short-term memory

Social networks

Successful aging

Tinnitus

Wernicke's aphasia

Working memory

Communication links all of us to each other and to the environment and is a key factor in how we relate and coexist. People use communication to provide and receive information from others for a variety of reasons. For many decades, scientists have created communication models from the work of Satir (1967), in which she states, "Communication is a two-sided affair: senders are receivers, and receivers are also senders" (p. 88). Successful communication involves conveying a looping message between a sender and a receiver in which their roles continuously reverse and cycle back. However, many issues must be addressed for this communication to be effective. Effective communication is a dynamic process that includes an ongoing exchange of information with feedback, context, clarifications, language, definitions, and removal of barriers between the sender and receiver—it suggests a partnership that increases understanding going both directions. When considering how best to communicate with and to teach older adults, several key principles must be considered. Basic knowledge of communication with older adults is fundamental to effective teaching. These concepts are discussed in this chapter.

Communication Basics for Older Adults

Communication relies heavily on intact senses, such as hearing, vision, physical, and cognitive processes. Any level of distortion or failure of one or more senses can cause significant challenges for effective communication. The individual's cognitive abilities and a conducive environment must be present for effective message transmission because background noise and internal distortions can be serious barriers.

Communication is complex and encompasses verbal and nonverbal messaging that may have a cultural dynamic to its meaning. In some cases, communication is affected by the variances seen in different age groups and how these various age groups create meaning. A common example is how boomers and millennials define the word *sick*. The boomer generation thinks the word means *to be ill and not well*. Millennials define the word to mean *impressive and outstanding* (using boomer terms). We are seeing additional strategies affecting the way most people communicate with the use of symbols ($), emoji (☺), and various forms of short hand (lol).

In the past, communication tended to be more linear, with a feedback mechanism to help clarify what was being said. Today it may be dynamic and more of a constant building of beliefs and ideas that must be sorted and integrated by the reader to give it meaning. There are several methods for showing one's emotions when the individual cannot be seen in person, using emoji symbols, where in the past you would typically use bold or all capital letters. On Facebook® and Twitter®, you can see the building of what a person is thinking regarding an idea that also has pictures with multiple persons giving opinions and feelings to the threaded discussions. The language of symbols is updated regularly, and refinements are put into smartphones for current generational understanding. The following link is a place where these updates can be seen and then integrated: https://twitter .com/Emojipedia?ref_src=twsrc%5Egoogle%7Ctwcamp%5Eserp%7Ctwgr%5Eauthor (Emojipedia, n.d.). The Internet can quickly give you definitions, perspectives, and variations in meaning, but there is very little support for the older adult who has not learned this language or is having cognitive confusion.

Most new computers and electronic devices have voice-activated messaging, searching, and responses such as seen with *Siri* on an iPhone®. Television remotes allow you to speak into the remote and that channel will appear, or it will find all movies or shows on a given topic. However, many older adults have difficulty with fast-paced change and are not always willing to use all this valuable technology unless they have a chance to practice and become comfortable.

Building a Framework for Understanding Normal and Abnormal Aging

If you are the average adult and well under this age group, you probably have beliefs similar to those of other persons who might have participated in the exercise. Examine your own thinking right this minute regarding some beliefs you have regarding people ages 70 to 90. Write them on a piece of paper. Many of the stereotypes are negative and do not suggest favorable characteristics for the older adult. Having negative and significant cognitive decline of this group is a myth, and even clinicians get caught in this thinking. "Perhaps one of the most serious assumptions made by many psychologist is that of universal cognitive decline" (Shaie, 2016, p. 4). Shaie's (2013) longitudinal study of older adults suggest there is a decline in various domains (verbal, spatial, word fluency, and inductive reasoning), but it is so individualized that generalizations are not useful. It has been shown that a significant population of older adults do not show any decline until they are near death.

Normal Language and Speech

One area of *language* that has been shown to improve with age is vocabulary. The longer one lives, the more that person is exposed to a variety of words and meanings, and thus their vocabulary continues to expand. When verbal knowledge was compared between adults ages 20 and 80 years, the 80-year-old group had better scores than the 20-year-old group (Park et al., 2002). Syntax (the structure of sentences) remains intact throughout the process as well. How older adults use language to interact remains relatively strong, but people tend to be more verbose and/or drift off topic. The rate of speech slows, and word articulation becomes less clear because of the slowing rate of cognitive processing and declining strength and range of movement of the mouth, tongue, and jaw. Having missing teeth or dentures that do not fit properly are also factors that influence word articulation.

CLINICAL TIP

Older adults are not all the same, nor do they have all the same issues related to normal aging.

Complex and lengthy verbal and written information may be more difficult to understand (Lubinski, 2010) and often causes frustration on the part of listeners. It is easy to identify caregivers who think they cannot give any more time to a given conversation and may quit listening, be more directing, or even show frustration and anger to cut off the conversation. In addition, comprehension during conversation may be more challenging because of hearing, vision, or sensory loss, cognitive changes, or emotional factors.

A study by Haro and Isaki (2009) found that older adults had more cohesive and organized speech and used fewer fillers (e.g., like, um, uh) compared to younger adults. Older individuals continue to display abilities to learn and retain world knowledge as well. Appropriate content of sentences, vocabulary, and grammar remain strengths for normal-aging older adults. However, the length and complexity of sentences is reduced (Schreck, 2010). Nonspecific language (she, they, thing) becomes more prevalent, leaving the listener to guess or ask more questions to understand to whom they are referring. Although there are changes in being able to recall names of people, places, and objects, the ability to functionally communicate remains intact.

During the process of normal aging, some start to notice changes in strength, endurance, memory, vision, hearing, sensation, and taste. Body hormone levels shift, affecting libido and causing night sweats, sleep changes, energy reduction, and weight variances. Lifelong relationships are reinforced for different reasons, and staying active becomes a necessity if a person is attempting to counteract some of these normal aging changes. Changes in communication patterns and functional abilities are a part of this aging process, with some older adults becoming less interactive for various reasons. Some nonresponsive behaviors during conversations occur because the person is not sure what he or she heard or may not be clear on the topic being discussed. In some cases, the individual thinks what he or she has to say does not matter or there may be an opposite response, with the older adult thinking he or she must be heard and present *the truth* on a topic. There is a group of older adults who think that if they do not present *the truth* on a certain topic, no one will. A few older adults may invade the conversation with bold and unwavering absolutes that cannot be reasoned away or discounted through any rational reasoning. There is significant diversity in how older adults respond during conversations. This is something you may have already noticed in your own experience. The latter two responses presented are often a challenging issue for healthcare providers because there is a tendency to argue or present a *more rational way of thinking*. **Case Study 5-1** is a real example of how different older adults think. Both of these older men are in total independent living situations and both are in this author's personal life.

CLINICAL TIP

Developmental maturational paths have a significant impact on the cognitive abilities in later years.

Schaie (2008, 2016) suggests "there are four major patterns that will describe most of the observed aging trajectories" (p. 5). These are as follows:

> *Super-normal or successful aging*: This group is able to be very successful, engaged, and socially advantaged and hit a peak of their mental abilities in late midlife. They are usually doing what they enjoy right up to their death.
> *Normal aging*: This group does well and hits their social and cognitive peaks in early midlife, but can have a couple of divergent endings. One group stays very independent and the other needs significant support.

Case Study 5-1

I went to breakfast with my neighbor John, who is now 80. He was born in Poland with a German heritage and lived in Germany during World War II from ages 8 to 10. John's view of Hitler sounded like this: "Hitler was not all bad, and he did a lot of good for the German people. You know, the Jews brought much of their problems on themselves. Hitler wanted them to give more to the poor people of Germany, because most of the Jews in Germany had significant wealth, and they would not give it up." Other conversations centered around how his family hid a Jewish neighbor from the Gestapo who came looking for him, but the Jewish farmer was their friend and they risked everything to protect this man.

John does not listen to the news media in the United States and thinks everything in the U.S. news is filtered in an unacceptable way. He only listens to the foreign news media so he can, "hear the truth about what is happening in the world." John, when given the opportunity, wants to tell the "real story" about what is happening in the world, and there is no changing his opinion. It is a conspiracy story with a few unknown people running everything—elections, leader assassinations, policies, and all major money activities.

The medical system is just as corrupt, and he will see a physician for the specific purpose of getting a blood test and then uses the data to treat himself using natural vitamins and minerals. He takes more than 20 types of naturalist supplements and does not trust that any traditional medical clinicians could advise him accurately. He had self-overdosed on some of these vitamins, with significant muscle weakness, and then spent 10 months reassessing his regimen and finally recovered. There is not an invasive procedure he would undergo for any reason. After tearing one bicep tendon, he decided to let it heal on its own with more than 5 years of problems from his decision. However, after 5 years, his bicep appeared to become connected on its own.

Bert is 82 and has been involved in more than 100 men's personal growth retreats. He enjoys small groups who work closely together and worked most of his life in the railroad industry. He has pain in his hips and back, is hard of hearing, and is a man of faith and spirituality. He listens most of the time with an expressionless affect until he decides to engage and speak on a topic. He likes to tell jokes and laughs along with everyone else, or he will give a comment with some emotion. Sometimes Bert's wisdom moves others with words of encouragement, insight, or how he would address a particular issue in his own life. He cautions others not to think like him, but would like them to hear his wisdom and see if it is valuable for them. He is still being asked to give talks at various men's retreats—then he offers wisdom from all his years of living.

Bert receives traditional medical care for his back pain and functional limitations. There are times when he has difficulty maneuvering, but understands his limitations.

Both men struggle with remembering simple things: the name of a street, a place they want to have breakfast, the name of someone they met. They both drive, own a home, enjoy company, continue to engage the world in their own way, and remember historical information like it just happened.

> *Mild cognitive impairment (MCI) or unsuccessful aging*: This group has earlier than normal cognitive losses and struggles with normal functioning as they progress past their midlife years.
> *Dementia group*: This group is diagnosed with some form of dementia and is in need of constant attention. They are considered to age and progress very differently from those in the other three groups.

Developmental models provide reasons for such diverse responses to life, as seen in the vignette. Some aging deficits seem more universal, whereas other issues are very individual. As presented in Schaie's model and in the two stories of John and Bert, there may be major differences on how older adults connect to others and how they see the world.

Categories of Normal and Abnormal Barriers to Communication

Communication failures occur when barriers to communication exist in any component of the older adult, regardless of what technology is being used to assist in the process. Normal and abnormal aging barriers might be:

> *Internal* (e.g., cognition and physical deficits)
> *External* (e.g., speaking too softly, noisy room, elderspeak)
> *Language* (e.g., misunderstanding of terms, the use of a word in a different generational context, idiom, and slang)

Internal Barriers and Interventions

The older adult has a natural progression of sensory and *cognition* reduction over time, but it is not uniform or consistent from person to person. Think about how someone at the age of 70 struggles to navigate through a room or drive a car. There are others, such as Paul Newman, who raced competitively to age 70, hitting speeds of 140 m.p.h. in his 1988 Nissan race car. Here is a video of Paul Newman in action: https://youtu.be/4Szj0gCkFuk. The variations in internal decline are present; however, eventually body and cognitive functioning lose the race against time. Schaie's model (2016, 2008) suggest the four types of identifiable groups, but some general statements can be addressed with this in mind.

Maturational Variations in Cognition

Part of a people's cognitive ability is related how they functioned throughout their life. Worldviews, educational level, conspiracy beliefs, religious beliefs, political views, and how the person has related to others continue into older age. Erik Erikson's stages of development can be misleading if the reader thinks all persons mature in the same way (Schaie, 2016) and each person makes it to the eighth stage (see Erikson's Eight Stages of Psychosocial Development: http://web.cortland.edu/andersmd/ERIK/sum.HTML). This site presents a summary chart of the eight stages presented by Erikson, but there are different thoughts today as to how these stages are really played out and at what age (Schaie). Regardless of the debate, we can examine an example of a person who keeps failing at each stage of development. It is possible for an older adult to mistrust, have shame and doubt, carry guilt, feel inferior, have role confusion, become isolated and stagnant, and then fall into despair. The cognitive coping abilities of such a person would be minimal, and care partners might see a person wishing to die, even when the person is not ill. This person would fall into the maturational group called unsuccessful aging, presented earlier.

An alternative view of older adults might have a very different perspective of development. They learned to trust in others, developed autonomy, and had initiatives with successes. They may have developed skills and an identity in how they worked and lived to include fostering intimacy in relationships. These older adults might go on to become generous and giving as they maintained a sense of healthy ego identity or a sense of purpose for their creator. This older adult moves into a world equipped to manage a host of issues that come as challenges, problems, or obstacles and falls into the Schaie model under the heading of super-normal and successful aging. Developmental maturational paths have a significant impact on the cognitive abilities in later years. Despite this variance, there are still issues that have an impact on many older adults, but it may happen at different ages or their response to these difficulties can be significantly varied.

Brain Function and Cognition

As people age, there is a gradual decrease in brain mass and neuronal function that results in cognitive changes. Long-term and short-term memory declines as people age. *Short-term memory* is limited in capacity, and information remains for only a few seconds. Older adults are thought to hold approximately five to nine pieces of information, such as a phone number, in short-term memory. Some information in the short-term memory is then encoded to be stored in *long-term memory*. Long-term memory is suggested to be more expansive than short-term memory, and there is no limit as to how long information can be stored (Lustig & Lin, 2016).

Bayles and Tomoeda (2007) describe two subgroups found in long-term memory: declarative and nondeclarative. The authors present *declarative memory* as factual information that can be presented objectively and has three subtypes:

> *Episodic* (events)
> *Semantic* (concepts)
> *Lexical* (word) memory

If you thought of a specific time you went to a park, you used *episodic memory* (event) memory. If you are asked to imagine a beautiful park, you might think of swing sets, flowers, grass, barbeques, or a sunny day, all of which requires *semantic memory* (concept). *Lexical memory* is the memory of words, including meanings, spellings, and pronunciations. If you decided to write about going to the park or tell a friend what you did, then you would be using lexical memory to select and communicate the words you think have universal meaning. *Nondeclarative memory* includes the following:

> Motor skills
> Cognitive skills
> Reflex responses
> Priming
> Conditioned responses

Repetition typically strengthens nondeclarative memory. Examples of nondeclarative memory are how you might solve a math problem, how you get angry when someone cuts in front of you on the highway, or a conditioned response to loud noises.

Bayles and Tomoeda (2007) also describe *working memory*, which includes executive functions such as:

> Planning
> Attention
> Inhibition
> Encoding
> Monitoring

They define *active memory* as an immediate brain function that can describe what you are thinking at any given moment. Phelps (2004) expanded the idea of memory as being more vivid and memorable if it is tied to an emotional state created by the amygdala charging the hippocampal memory system. Unfortunately, the amygdala is also involved in symptom severity of posttraumatic stress disorder (PTSD), bringing forth memories and symptoms associated with those memories, even when they are not wanted (Shin, Rauch, & Pitman, 2006). This allows the individual to integrate positively or negatively several memories. The individual may have a sematic memory that is a reflex memory that bypasses cognitive processing and goes directly to an emotional response that is expressed as PTSD or a positive emotional feeling of love and peace. Based on your history of listening to music, it is possible to experience this effect in this moment (active memory). To engage in this experience, complete the first critical thinking exercise at the end of this chapter.

Normal Aging Changes in Cognition with Compensatory Strategies

As people age, certain types of memory are more vulnerable to decline than others. Episodic memory and working memory are the most affected in the aging processes, whereas semantic, lexical, and nondeclarative memory are more likely to be preserved (Bayles & Tomoeda, 2007). It may be difficult for these persons to recall what they did the day before or what they ate for breakfast (episodic memory). There may be difficulty with multitasking (e.g., talking and writing a check) because of a decline in working memory in which the individual is attending to information, encoding, or planning. Studies show that memories that are especially difficult to recall are often the result of not having a connection with the hippocampus (Tulving & Markowitsch, 1998). It is much easier for an older adult to recall a story that happened decades earlier because the information has already been stored in areas of long-term memory not affected by the hippocampus. Repeating new names or developing an association with the name or face of a person can help older adults create instinctive remembering, but either way this memory loss may cause frustrations for the individual. Nondeclarative memory may be slower, yet still accurate, which is seen in some sports activities (Bayles & Tomoeda, 2007). For example, an older individual who has played golf for many years can still play at the same level as at a younger age, but it may take more time to complete one round.

With normal aging, cognitive processing slows and abstract reasoning becomes more difficult. Also, new information becomes harder to remember (Lubinski, 2010). Attending to daily tasks may be mildly impaired, especially when there are distracting factors such as the phone ringing or television noise (Schreck, 2010). On a day-to-day basis, older adults may show that they have challenges with following conversations, managing money, driving, safety, and complex tasks (Schreck, 2010). Because of brain changes, individuals over 65 "are slower in perceiving, processing, and reacting especially when the situation requires rapid processing of complex information" (Bayles & Tomoeda, 2007, p. 49). The overall knowledge does not diminish. However, the time necessary to process and retrieve that information does increase. This can appear as knowledge impairment to family members and care providers, so it is important to provide adequate time for older individuals to process and respond.

Aging causes changes in the physical brain (Park & Farrell, 2016), but it is important to remember that the maturational development of individuals varies in how they adjust and compensate for losses. For some older adults, cognitive integration is as strong as it has ever been and there may be greater coping strategies compared to their younger years as they have progressed positively during maturational development. One theory on how the compensation occurs is called *compensatory scaffolding* and has been recently described in the model by Reuter-Lorenz and Park (2014) as the *Scaffolding Theory of Aging and Cognition* (STAC) (p. 90). It is described as a process in which the individual's brain recruits additional neuron connections for maintaining memory and decoding what has been observed.

Pathological Changes that Affect Cognition and Communication

Dementia is defined as memory loss accompanied by speech and language impairments and/or decline in executive functioning (Bayles & Tomoeda, 2007). It been called a *major neurocognitive disorder* as a clinical diagnostic category (American Psychological Association, [APA] 2014). Because changes in memory occur with normal aging, the symptoms have to be significant enough to interfere with social, occupational, or daily activities before it is diagnosed medically. There are different types of dementia, including Alzheimer's disease (AD), vascular dementia, dementia with amyloid deposits, mixed dementia, and frontotemporal dementia (Park & Farrell, 2016). Dementia can be seen in numerous other conditions, such as Parkinson's disease (PD), Huntington's disease, Creutzfeldt–Jakob disease, Wernicke–Korsakoff syndrome, and normal pressure hydrocephalus (NPH). *Alzheimer's disease* is the most common form of dementia and accounts for 60–80% of dementia cases (Alzheimer's Association, n.d.). AD is a progressive degenerative brain disease that first affects memory (Bayles & Tomoeda, 2007; Park & Farrell, 2016). As it progresses, physical movement, communication, cognition, personality, and emotional and mental health are affected. In the United States, 1 in 8 people over the age of 65 has AD and individuals 85 and older have a 50% chance of having AD (Alzheimer's Association, 2012). With a growing population that is older than 65, we can expect a greater need for care partners to become more competent in memory care as they work with dementia patients in need of special understanding. Strategies for caring for persons with dementia are discussed further in Chapter 10.

The Effect of Cognitive Issues on Communication

Effective communication relies heavily on an intact memory. When we are listening, we first have to attune to the speaker and then use our memory to recall what the person said in order to make an appropriate response. When speaking, we use our memory to recall stories and information as well as to select the right words to convey what we mean. As with the aging process, episodic memory is the first to be affected in individuals with AD (Bayles & Tomoeda, 2007). The difference between age-related changes and AD–related change in episodic memory is the rapidness with which one forgets the information. Individuals with AD, as well as individuals with PD plus dementia, forget within seconds. In addition to short-term memory issues, persons affected with AD experience long-term memory problems. Because of short-term memory impairments, people with dementia will repeat the same stories or repeatedly ask the same questions. If persons with a memory impairment are asked what they did yesterday, common responses include "I don't remember," "I don't know," or saying something vague such as "Oh, you know, the usual." Long-term memories from distant times, such as events that happened in childhood through young adulthood, are easier to recall and discuss with aging dementia. The aim in working with all types of dementia is to reduce the individual's frustration when communicating by minimizing the demands on memory and providing enjoyable communicative opportunities. This process can be facilitated by the use of pictures, objects, or music from the older adult's past, which allows individuals to practice communication without having to rely on memory.

CLINICAL TIP

For persons with dementia, reduce their frustration during communication by minimizing the demands on memory and focusing on enjoyable communication opportunities that do not rely on memory.

Dysarthria and *apraxia* are speech and motor impairments caused by neurological changes in the body. Speech apraxia is a speech impairment with an inability of the individual to send the correct messages to the mouth muscles for making motor planning. Dysarthria refers to muscle weakness difficulties of the mouth affecting speech movements. Some adults who have had a stroke will have brain damage that has an impact on what the person wants to say, causing the language impairment *aphasia*. These persons continue normal intellect but are unable to connect the brain to the speech motor receptors (Yorkston, Beukelman, Strand, & Hakel, 2010). Although other conditions and diseases can cause language impairments, the term *aphasia* is used if it is primarily a language deficit. If cognition, personality, or speech is impaired, it does not fit the diagnosis of aphasia. There are several types of aphasia that are categorized by fluency, comprehension, and repetition abilities. All types of aphasia share one common feature—*anomia*, which is a naming impairment (Bayles & Tomoeda, 2007).

When damage occurs to Broca's area of the brain, it is called *Broca's aphasia*. With this type of aphasia, comprehension remains intact, but spoken communication is not fluid. Speech is slow, effortful, choppy, and often lacks proper grammatical markers, such as "-ed" at the end of a verb to indicate past tense. Individuals have difficulty initiating speech, but they provide good content. Repetition is moderately to severely impaired, and most people with Broca's aphasia are aware of their impairments and try self-correcting (Bayles & Tomoeda, 2007).

Another nonfluent type of aphasia is *global aphasia*, with even greater damage to the left hemisphere than found with Broca's aphasia. The effects on communication are more devastating, causing the person to have very limited spoken language and individuals may use only single words that are not always understood. Unlike Broca's aphasia, comprehension of written and spoken information is significantly impaired. In addition, written expression is equally as impaired as the spoken form (Bayles & Tomoeda, 2007). This form of aphasia has a poor prognosis for recovery of meaningful use of language.

A common fluent type of aphasia is *Wernicke's aphasia,* which is caused by damage to the Wernicke's area of the brain. People with this aphasia have fluent speech with unintelligible content. Individuals will use real or nonsense words, but the string of words has no clear meaning. Comprehension of spoken and written information is impaired, as is repetition. Unlike Broca's aphasia, those with Wernicke's are generally unaware of their communication deficits and seem to have a cognitive filter that makes sense in their own mind but not to others, (Bayles & Tomoeda, 2007).

Individuals with *Parkinson's disease* often experience dysarthria. PD is a progressive degenerative brain condition that includes symptoms such as resting tremors, slow movements, rigidity of limbs or trunk, and unstable balance (National Parkinson's Foundation, 2012a). Research estimates there are 50,000 to 60,000 Americans diagnosed with PD each year (National Parkinson's Foundation, 2012b) and there is a higher prevalence in individuals over the age of 60 (American Parkinson Disease Association, n.d.).

Approximately 15% of individuals with PD develop dementia as the condition progresses. Slow movements and rigidity have a negative impact on producing speech. Because of rigidity of the trunk, people with Parkinson's have a reduction of air pressure needed to adequately support speech, causing a weakened voice. Other common problems include hoarse voice, monotonous voice, difficulty initiating speech, and reduced word articulation. When reduction in the word articulation occurs, listeners find it more difficult to understand what is being said. Rigidity also prevents a full range of motion of the facial and jaw muscles, contributing to reduced intonation and soft speech tones. In addition, individuals often appear to have a flat affect with minimal facial expressions, leaving some to think the Parkinson's patient is disconnected from the conversation (Yorkston et al., 2010).

In the early stages of a progressive dementia such as AD, sentences are typically grammatically correct, but fragmented and repetitious. At this point, there are signs of declining vocabulary, and words may be substituted with similar words (e.g., "look" for "took"). In addition, the person may perseverate on an idea or a topic. In the middle stages, attention, memory, speech, and language skills continue to decline. Speech becomes slower and more repetitive, and the content becomes less cohesive. At this point, comprehension of written and spoken language is typically impaired.

Interventions for Those with Cognitive and Language Barriers

To effectively communicate with patients who have speech, language, and/or cognitive impairments, it is imperative to use a multitude of modalities to aid in communication. Although oral communication is what we generally think of most when we think of communication, written information, pictures, drawings, concrete symbols (such as letters and numbers), gestures, and facial expressions all aid in effectively communicating a message. Some approaches will help patients communicate better than others. It is important to collaborate with the patient, family members, care partners, and speech–language pathologists to determine approaches that work best for that specific person.

Questions that incorporate confrontation naming should be avoided. One common example of confrontation naming involves the care partners looking at family pictures in a patient's room and then asking, "Who is this?" or "What's her name?" In early stages of dementia progression, individuals are typically aware that they should know the information but simply cannot remember. This can lead to frustration, anger, guilt, and sadness. Caregivers and care partners need to switch from a confrontational naming question to a comment about a picture or ask multiple-choice and yes/no questions. Nurses can convert a "Who is this?" to "This is a beautiful picture. Is this your daughter?" In later stages of dementia, it may be simply, "I like this picture on your wall," eliminating any expected response.

Daily factual postings may be useful for some dementia patients to know the day, what is happening today, or what is on the menu for today. Care partners can use items such as whiteboards or large wall calendars to

TABLE 5-1 Strategies for Communication with Persons with Dementia That Support Personhood

Strategy	Definition	Example
Recognition	Acknowledge the person, know the person's name, affirm uniqueness.	"Come along Mrs. Jones, your dinner is being served."
Negotiation	Consult the person regarding preferences, desires, needs.	"That was a nice bit of fresh air. I'm ready for my dinner now; would you like to join me?"
Validation	Acknowledge the person's emotions and feelings and respond.	"Mrs. Johnson, it sounds like you would like to wait for your bath."
Facilitation and collaboration	Work together, involve the person. Enable the person to do what he or she otherwise would not be able to do by providing the missing parts of the action.	"What is it you are looking for Mrs. Smith? Can I help? Tell me what it is and we can look for it together."

Modified from Ryan, E.B., Byrne, K., Spykerman, H., & Orange, J.B. (2005). Evidencing Kitwood's personhood strategies: Conversation as care in dementia. In B. Davis (Ed.), *Alzheimer talk, text and context: Enhancing communication*. New York, NY: Palgrave Macmillan.

post their names, the time for various activities, or other daily facts that the patient may ask about. Expect such care recipients to ask the same questions anyway. The ability of the care partner to respond in a calm and reassuring voice going back to the whiteboard and showing the information as if it were for the first time, is useful for reorientation to the reference board without sending a nonverbal message of frustration, guilt assigning, or contempt for the question being asked. **Table 5-1** provides guidance on how to communicate with persons who have cognitive deficits.

Normal and Abnormal Changes in Vision

Another internal barrier affected by normal and abnormal aging is vision. As people age, functioning of anatomical structures decreases, which is true in respect to vision. Age-related changes can start occurring in the 30s. Over time, the cornea becomes less sensitive and the pupils decrease to about one third of the size during young adulthood. It also takes longer for one's eyes to adjust from light to dark environments, such as walking out of a movie theater on a sunny day. The lenses become less flexible, slightly yellowed, and cloudy (Dugdale, 2011). Visual acuity also decreases with age. In the normal aging process, *presbyopia* (*aging eye*) occurs and causes difficulty seeing at close range, such as in reading (National Eye Institute, National Institutes of Health [NIH], n.d.). This change in vision can affect anyone over the age of 35. Although the age that presbyopia becomes apparent may vary from person to person, it is expected to affect everyone at some point. This type of vision impairment may be corrected by wearing glasses with bifocals or contact lenses or by various forms of surgery, such as Karma inlay, monovision Lasik, or refractive lens exchange (Boxer-Wachler, 2016). As presbyopia increases with age, care partners and family may need to set up regular annual vision assessments to determine any progressive changes affecting the older adult over time. If there is a reduction in reading, headaches, or eye fatigue, the older adult may need new glasses and lenses regardless of how they made these adjustments earlier in life.

It is common for older adults to experience an increase in sensitivity to light and glare. Too little or too much light may hinder vision. This will vary from person to person, but typically older individuals require more light to be able to see adequately. On the other hand, bright lights, such as headlights, may be temporarily blinding

Case Study 5-2

Mark is a 60-year-old active man who was driving his car down the interstate on a sunny Colorado day. He blinked his left eye and noticed the cars ahead of him shrink instantly from both sides. He then did it intentionally to see what his right eye was seeing. Everything pulled in and seemed to shrink. Not sure what was happening, he went home and looked at the TV in the same way—closing his left eye and then noticing the TV shrink in from its sides to be narrower than it was. Not only did it shrink, but there was a dark spot directly in his vision and faces on the screen disappeared. Mark moved his vision with his right eye to the left and right of faces on the television and they would reappear, and then disappear when he looked directly at the faces. Not sure of what was happening, he kept testing himself. Yes, he could make things disappear with just his right eye open. In the distance the blank spot was larger and could cover a car. As he looked at closer objects, a piece of the object would go dark and shrink at the same time. As he began to read an article in a magazine, the words would not become clear unless he looked to the right of the word, and then the letters became clear.

Mark went to see a retinal specialist and eventually was diagnosed with a macular hole. The treatment was to have a vitrectomy (removal of inner eye fluid), with argon gas put in the eye. Mark was to lie face down on his stomach or in a back massage chair for 2 weeks to aid in preventing the hole from enlarging. After the 2 weeks, it was 4 weeks of a water line slowly rising in the right eye as the fluid returned— like having a fish bowl in his right eye. The complications could be a *cataract* from the gas used. Yes, Mark had a cataract in less than 6 months and then went for cataract surgery. "OK, now I should be good to go" Mark thought. Fortunately, the left eye became increasingly more dominate and the blind spot was not as bothersome and the macular hole did stabilize. Unfortunately, there was significant loss of peripheral lower right side vision that was present after the second surgery. In addition, the right eye continued to become dominate after being in bright sunlight. As Mark goes from outside to inside a house, he has significant eye adjustment delays to see clearly indoors.

and impair the ability to drive at night (Ayalon, Feliciano, & Arean, 2006). Reading material with a glossy cover or on glossy paper may reflect light and make it more difficult to read. Changes also occur in the cones of the eyes, which affect how a person sees colors. For older adults, it is more difficult to differentiate between green and blue than between red and yellow.

There are many diseases of the eye (*diabetic retinopathy*, *macular degeneration*, retinal detachment, macular holes, vessel ruptures, *glaucoma*, herpes, and cancer) that will make seeing more difficult regardless of having just the right amount of light. All of these diseases and more affect the quality of life of older adults, with a constant reduction of activity and accurate vision. These changes in activities include the climbing of stairs, walking exercise, driving a car, and many other *activities of daily living* (ADLs). As various diseases progress, more *isolation* is likely, with activities needing guidance from family and friends. The vignette in **Case Study 5-2** describes how one older person noticed changes caused from a macular hole in one eye.

Case Study 5-2 demonstrates how a simple eye issue can have an impact on ADLs for older adults. Chronic vision changes, regardless of the cause, can affect driving, reading, watching television, working on a computer, and many sports activities.

Care Partner Strategies for Vision Barriers

Contrasting warm and cool colors should be used when creating visuals such as calendars, instructions, and signs with a contrasting dark print for reading messages. Overall eye movement and peripheral vision are reduced as well, and anything that can be a tripping point or low-level obstacle should be placed far from walking areas. The older adult may need larger print papers, books, or tablet screen print and icons. If vision is nearly gone, they may need auditory visual support, as seen in movies and books for the visually impaired, or talking computers. There is also value in being in direct line of sight while speaking, because they may be watching mouth movements and gestures to understand more clearly. Correct lighting for the task is important. Reading lamps are useful and special magnifying devices can be used to see something that has fine detail or smaller print.

Normal Aging Changes in Hearing

Hearing loss has a great impact on individuals' daily activities, relationships, socialization, psychological health, and quality of life. Work environments often rely on communication between people. Whether it is the employer and employees, therapist or doctor and patients, teacher and students, or clerk and customers, good communication is fundamental to working relationships. Some individuals who have difficulty hearing leave jobs because they feel they can no longer do their job or they become frustrated with the situation. People may feel embarrassed about having a hearing loss and do not want to address it with coworkers, family, or friends. Hearing loss also can put a strain on marital and familial relationships. If a spouse or family member continually repeats things, frustration and increased relational stress are likely to occur.

Certain levels of hearing loss are a safety risk, and attempting to guide the person by commands is significantly reduced. More visual communication with gestures and movements, and showing mouth movements, may be needed if vision is not impaired. If hearing loss is severe, there may be a need for warning lights or alarms. Some environmental noises are important for safety and need to be heard. For example, a tornado siren warning people to take cover may sound like a soft noise in the background or may not be heard and should trigger a light instead. Another example involves pedestrian safety in which the sound of an approaching car may not be heard when an individual is crossing the street. These sounds provide important information regarding the surrounding environment and influence choices people make.

Being able to understand conversation over the phone is one of the most difficult situations for individuals with hearing loss because it increases the barriers to those they had frequent contacts with in the past. When communicating over the phone, there are no visual cues to help the person fill in what he or she cannot hear as one could if the conversation took place face to face. Social situations also may be avoided. Restaurants, parties, meetings, and family celebrations are just a few social situations in which there are multiple competing sounds. If there is music or television playing in the background or multiple people talking, it makes it more difficult for the person to hear and understand conversations.

Persons with hearing loss may experience *depression*, loneliness, and decreased quality of life (Ayalon et al., 2006). In addition, hearing loss has been shown to have a negative impact on cognitive functioning and it increases the risk of dementia (Oyler, 2012).

Like vision, hearing declines as people age. Normal hearing loss in older adults begins with the inability to hear higher frequencies. Microscopic hair cells within the cochlea (inner ear) detect frequencies from sound waves and then send signals to the brain. The hair cells that detect high *frequencies* (6,000 and 8,000 hertz [Hz]) are the most vulnerable to damage. With age, these higher frequency hair cells deteriorate and lose their function. They cannot be repaired nor do new hair cells grow back; this is called *presbycusis* and is permanent (Lin, 2012). As hearing loss progresses and moves to speech frequencies from various forms of damage or very old age, the person ends up with much more serious health issues. The most common complaint from someone with progressive presbycusis is that the person can hear but does not understand what was said (Norrix & Harris, 2008). As damage begins to affect the speech frequencies of 500, 1,000, 2,000, 3,000, and 4,000 Hz, several speech consonants are not heard (p, t, k, f, s, th, sh, ch) because they are produced at 4,000 to 6,000 Hz and are a low-intensity sound. The loss of these specific tones can greatly affect the meaning of words being heard. Older adults are affected by more than not hearing a word; they do not understand what you are trying to say. When all the frequencies of a word are not present, the word does not sound like a true word. People with progressive presbycusis affecting speech frequencies often claim that the speaker is mumbling. At some point, the ability to understand speech, listen to music, and hear environmental noises is seriously impaired (Norrix & Harris, 2008).

One in three adults ages 60 years and older and one in two adults over the age of 85 are reported to have some level of hearing loss. There are estimates of 26.7 to 35 million U.S. adults with hearing impairment, but less than 15% use hearing aids to assist in their hearing (Hear-it, n.d.; Lin, 2012). Fortunately, the speech frequencies (500–4,000 Hz) are not significantly lost in normal aging until much later in life. One can expect mild losses in 28% of older adults (Dalton et al., 2002). Dalton et al. also studied the impact on ADLs in older adults who had hearing loss and found 24% of the 2,688 subjects tested had moderate to severe hearing loss that also affected speech frequencies, and this group had significantly impaired ADLs. Assuming Dalton's research can be generalized even further, one should expect to see moderate to severe hearing loss in 24% of the older adult population that will worsen over time. Such losses will need care partners and family members to assist with ADLs.

Tinnitus is also fairly common in older individuals. This is a continual, abnormal sound in one or both ears and is similar to the internal noise one hears after being exposed to loud sounds, such as at a concert. Tinnitus is generally caused by some mild hearing loss and can be extremely annoying to the person. For some individuals, the symptoms are temporary, but others may experience this long-term (Vorvick & Schwarz, 2011). In some cases, it interferes with being able to adequately hear speech or go to sleep easily. It can appear louder if persons are in a quiet place or when they turns their head into the pillow and try to sleep. Early mornings may be very problematic, as the person is in a quiet time, but the sound seems extremely loud. Other sounds may override the tinnitus, or, during very busy activities, the brain will ignore the ringing, so it appears to come and go. There are medical specialties that state they can do something for tinnitus, and others state it is best just to learn to live with it.

Hearing loss can be more progressive and more serious as a result of various factors: excessive noise, diseases such as measles, trauma, medications that are ototoxic, and genetic predispositions. Obtaining a very complete health history is key to starting the assessment process for what is causing hearing loss. Was the loss caused by a conductive process, a sensorineural issue, or both?

Care Partner Interventions for Hearing Impairments

Most care partners think of *hearing aids* to amplify the speech frequencies when considering interventions. There are many devices with varying costs, and they are effective only if used. Older adults have a host of reasons why they may not be using the devices even if they have them. Some parts may be lost, the older adult does not like the negative side effects with certain devices, and the devices require management and cleaning. If hearing aids are not a viable option due to financial constraints or noncompliance from the patient, there are *personal amplification devices* that can aid in hearing and are less expensive (**Box 5-1**). These not only amplify the speaker's message but also reduce *background noise* if they are the right type of device.

Ferguson (2012) found that persons who use clear vowel pronunciation, could be understood more easily by older adults with hearing loss. Unfortunately, it is challenging for those with moderate to severe hearing loss to understand foreign accents, strong English dialects, and those who speak rapidly. It would be important to use a second form of communication to augment the verbal speech, such as writing, using pictures, or speaking in a native language if possible. In addition, there is value in looking at these individuals directly so they can augment their hearing with some lip reading that may have been learned over time, even though these persons may not know this is a skill they were developing.

BOX 5-1   Research Highlight

Ferguson sought to study the impact of speech perceptions, namely, those associated with vowel sounds, on the interpretation of speech by older adults with hearing loss. The researcher sought to discover whether the clarity of speech that benefits those with normal hearing would also be of benefit to those with auditory limitations. Sign into your database of nursing literature (CINAHL or PubMed, for example) and use the citation below to perform a search for this article. What were the results of this study? What did Ferguson conclude? How can these findings help caregivers and the older adults they care for?

Ferguson, S. H. (2012). Talker differences in clear and conversational speech: Vowel intelligibility for older adults with hearing loss. *Journal of Speech, Language, and Hearing Research, 55*(3), 779–790.

Case Study 5-3

I went to see my mother, who was 93 and in her last stage of life: cardiac ejection fracture less than 30%, legs completely edematous and oozing with open sores, and in severe pain with every movement. I assisted her throughout the night and called the hospice nurse for more medication so she could sleep. I had my noise blocking headphones from my flight to her care center and I had music that I knew she liked on my smart phone. I put the head phones on her and played Whispering Hope by Phil Coulter (https://youtu.be/3t3_yWQH1Go), which I knew she loved to sing. Her face relaxed, and her fidgeting stopped for several minutes as she listened. Julie was exhausted and tired and then would fall asleep for short periods. As she awoke, I played another song by Phil Coulter https://youtu.be/-8MmeVhkMv8 and she continued to rest for 10 more minutes—it seemed longer as she relaxed and had peace on her face.

Later that morning she was not able to do much except struggle for pain relief, which the nurse supported with oral medication. I read from her large print Bible, and sang softly in her ear as her breathing changed and finally stopped.

When using hearing devices, place them on correctly and make sure they are working properly before having a conversation that is important or you are expecting the patient to understand. You may need access to spare batteries, ensure proper prong insertion, and adjust to the right sound level.

As the aging process progresses, many elders move to what they know and trust the most—music from their past and common sounds from their generational life experience, such as religious music and old movies. Past familiar sounds become more important, and with headphones and music, they have the opportunity to go to something they can hear and remember well. One of our best gifts could be music from their past that has enough sound quality to make up for high frequency losses. Today, we have background noise–reducing headphones, which may be excellent for the older adult or those in their end-of-life, as presented in the next vignette. **Case Study 5-3** gives an example of how special noise-reducing headphones made a dying woman comfortable during a very painful night.

Physical Limitations

Physical abilities can decrease dramatically in a short period of time. The age when such physical limitations are noticed may be different for everyone. An older adult may say, "Oh, I have been doing this for years. I can garden and keep the house clean by myself. I don't need help." The following year this individual may want to move to a place without yard work, no stairs, no snow shoveling, and no gardening. Physical ability seems to have a mind of its own, and sometimes the denial of this change can result in an injury. Take time right now to view the personal stories of some older adults and how they stay fit. These YouTube video links are listed in the resources at the end of the chapter.

Dual Sensory Impairment

Dual sensory impairment is when one experiences a loss in two or more sensory functions. Research indicates that 21% of individuals over the age of 70 experience dual sensory impairment. As age increases, the prevalence increases. This has a significant effect on functioning and overall quality of life. One system is unable to compensate for the impaired system, because both are impaired. For example, if only a hearing loss is present, then information can be given in written form to help compensate for the hearing loss, or if vision is impaired, the individual relies on auditory input for communication. When both hearing and vision are impaired, it is more difficult for the message to be received. It has been predicted that this dual impact has a greater effect on quality of life and function compared to a single impairment (Saunders & Echt, 2011), which seem to make sense on a practical level with decreased ability to experience life or communicate.

Although it is difficult to find research on multiple sensory impairment, there is research on the *vascular-depression-dementia* connection. If there is a vascular blockage, especially in the frontostriatal brain, it can cause a dementia that also brings on depression symptoms (Barry & Byers, 2016). We still have much to learn regarding complex cases having multiple sensory and cognitive losses.

External Barriers and Interventions

Environmental Noise

The environment has been called a place of healing or a place that can increase disease. Florence Nightingale's nursing model centered around creating healthy environments so patients could heal (Nightingale, [1859], 1969). Nursing and hospital architects have been concerned about the patient's environment for some time, utilizing different construction strategies aimed at healing environments (Malkin, 1992).

Power of Choice

Balchik (2002) identified many environmental strategies that could be applied to hospitals to improve patient healing. A key component is the ability of the individual to control their lighting, room temperature, privacy, visitors and visitor exposure, type and volume of music played, and the timing and types of meals provided. She states, "It has been demonstrated that in all settings—not just hospitals—feeling as if we have control over our own environment reduces our stress. When we know we have options, even in the most minimal sense, we feel better" (p. 10). Power (2010) offers a way to give choice for those suffering from dementia, by creating options of choice versus commands to eat. He suggests "Pointing to the food on a plate and asking, 'What would you like to try first?'" (p. 93). This allows for a choice that everyone can find acceptable without a *telling* approach being used.

Physical Environment

Combining personal control with the physical environment makes the environment even better. Architects are putting in water fountains, fish aquariums, soft music, garden views, and interactive works of art as a part of healthcare environment construction (Malkin, 1992). Part of the Hospital Consumer Assessment of Healthcare

Providers and Systems (HCAHPS) quality strategy for patients in hospitals is to reduce noise for patients (Zusman, 2012), which is often a major complaint by those who are trying to sleep. Living environments for the elderly are discussed in detail by authors specializing in elder care. Power (2010) provides research and guidance on lighting (ambient, targeted, and natural), glare prevention, floor space, noise control, comfort of the chairs and bed, privacy areas, and asking care partners to experience the environment exactly as the residents do. Powers presents a story in which a resident was falling repeatedly every night for days. The nurse reviewed the medications and staff talked to the resident about her need for using the rest room and pain management or if she was hungry. They could not find anything that was causing this resident to leave her bed each night, and the resident was not sure why she felt the need to get out of the bed. One of the certified nursing assistants (CNAs) working on the unit decided to lie in the place in which the resident would be sleeping. A glare came through the door and hit her directly in the eyes. After removing this glaring light, the falls stopped. Sometimes there is value in putting ourselves in the place of the older adult to see if we are affected by something they find problematic.

Most older adults think normal room temperatures are too cold as their metabolism slows with age. This is a common concern for the elderly and should be monitored closely. If the environment is not easily adjusted, care partners may need to provide sweaters or more blankets when the resident is sleeping or resting.

Cultural Shifts in Living Environment

There are programs that have changed the entire culture of an elderly living residence. One such program is the *Eden Alternative*. These facilities use a different language, the naming of living areas having street names; words are selected with positive intent, with *behavior problems* becoming *behavior expressions*; and the idea of *care partners* versus *caregiver* is supported (Powers, 2010), which has been used throughout this chapter. In Eden facilities, "words make worlds" (p. 82). The Eden Alternative Golden Rule is, "as management does unto staff, so shall staff do unto the elders" (p. 52). There is little argument against the value of healing environments, but there certainly is a resistance to making such changes.

A person's home seems to be a key place for healing without the risk of hospital-acquired infections or excessive noise found in many hospitals today. There is an attempt to keep the elderly in their homes as long as possible and to offer necessary care in their familiar surroundings. Power (2010) describes this as the "death of the nursing home—aging in community" (p. 121). There are many levels of community involvement that might be used: family members, church family, helpful neighbors, healthcare aids, and assisted living facilities. The movement for Program[s] of All-Inclusive Care for the Elderly (PACE), or Naturally Occurring Retirement Communit[ies] (NORC) is driven by community standards and not insurance or regulatory requirements (Power). The home has advantages and disadvantages. The risks associated with staying home are being unsafe with the stove or electrical devices, falling, and various injuries from utensils or home equipment. Many older adults have neighbors who can check on them daily, have *Meals-on-Wheels* food delivery, or can wear an emergency alert button around their neck if they cannot reach a phone. These are useful services for those staying at home.

The home environment has some unique issues that are both positive and very dangerous. The positive comes from the older adult being familiar with how things operate, and they often have high levels of control on what the environment is like. However, there is a serious abuse of the older adult coming from scam letters, phone calls, and easy television purchasing, if they have a credit card. Alves and Wilson (2008), identify the older adult as being much more vulnerable to scam strategies by telemarketers or phone solicitors. A high level of loneliness may exist, and these phone and mail racketeers can remember names, wish them a personal good day, chat as if they are old friends, and then ask for various forms of money or sell a host of services or products the person does not need. Some are so convincing they are able to obtain checking account access or credit card numbers (**Case Study 5-4**).

Stories like Norma's are very common. There is an entire network of scam systems in place to take advantage of the older adult living alone, and making important changes are difficult for the family members to control.

Case Study 5-4

Norma, age 82, was living alone in her home, where she would receive two to four calls per day and 20 solicitation pieces of mail per week. She purchased special journals that were cheaply copied papers full of conspiracy theories, and would donate monthly for those publishing the journal in order to have her views go toward governmental change. The organizations were fake, and the addresses were post office box numbers.

Some of the money requests were tailored to her religious views that were obtained during phone calls. She would put cash in 4 or 5 envelops per week supporting different issues. Her son, who came to stay with her after a hip surgery, was concerned she was giving away hundreds of dollars every 2 weeks and wanted to stop mailing the envelops. After he left her house, the process continued, with Norma overdrawing her checking account twice by over $400 each time. In her mind, the bank had to be taking her money, but in reality she was giving it away. This process continued until she was 91 years old and was finally told she would need assistance with her checking account and finances. In addition, her phone was changed to an unlisted number. Yes, these changes created an angry Norma, who felt a lack of control as she was spiraling into deeper debt. When talking to her about these changes, Norma was told the person writing the checks would let her know how much money she had after she paid her bills first. Then some funds were put in a safe place and other money was given to Norma each month to spend on her choice of programs and vitamins she thought were helpful. She could choose to save it or spend it. Her vitamin orders were rationed with no more overstocked inventories. Her bills were then covered and eventually paid off. All her friends were notified of the phone number change, but she really missed the calls and complained of being more alone. The family was asked to call her more often and to let her talk even if they were listening to the same stories week after week. Giving some choice, but taking away risk, is a hard balancing act and was not easy to navigate.

Language for Improving Communication with Older Adults

The diversity of issues presented by older adults, and the demands on the time for the care partner, make effective communication very challenging. However, tools are available that can assist in most cases, starting with building trust.

Building Trust and Respect

Verbal strategies that support communication include addressing the older adult by name, listening and responding on topic or guiding the conversation back to a topic, reflecting on feelings, while holding space for delusions, paranoia, repeated stories, and attacking language. Buffering oneself and learning not to take attacks as something that has to be responded to is a critical behavioral outcome for those working with some older adults. Care partners are more likely to build trust in chaotic situations if they remain calm, do not have an emotional response to an attack, and are able to smoothly move the patient back to the topic at hand. Trust and respect continue to be built as the care partner continues to address and monitor communication tools and avoid elderspeak.

Avoiding elderspeak. Nurses are typically younger than older adult patients, creating an intergenerational relationship when it comes to communication. Society has adopted negative stereotypes of aging with beliefs that older adults are less competent at communication as well as in other functional areas. Because of this, younger persons often modify their speech when they talk to older adults. Modifications include simplification in which care partners reduce the complexity of a statement or use fragmented sentences. In some cases, these healthcare partners use clarification strategies, which include adding repetitions, stressing certain words, or altering the pitch of one's speech. The end result is speech that is overly caring or controlling and less respectful than normal adult-to-adult speech. This type of speech has been called *elderspeak* and is widespread in community and elder-care settings. Elderspeak is similar to *babytalk*, which has been documented to sound the same as that used by those who work in day care and are speaking to children (Caporael, 1981). Common features of elderspeak include terms of endearment (e.g., "honey," "dearie," and "sweetie") and tag questions that prompt the older adult to respond as the younger person wishes. Examples of elderspeak include:

"You're ready for lunch now, aren't you?" (controlling and not a real question)

"Honey, you can do this, and be a good girl." (terms of endearment)

"Let's go take our bath now." (inappropriate)

The *Communication Predicament of Aging Model* describes how speech modifications occur and lead to negative outcomes for older adults (Ryan, Hummert, & Boich, 1995). Aging individuals who receive elderspeak messages may recognize they are being talked down to and respond by withdrawing from engagement in such patronizing conversations, or they may suffer increased depression or decreased self-esteem. Older adults also may respond by enacting behaviors consistent with their own negative stereotypes of a frail elder and may avoid self-care activities.

Pay attention to the nonverbal. It is important to note that healthcare providers have had a long history with effective and ineffective communication patterns with patients and residents. *Nonverbal communication* is more powerful than verbal messages (Satir, 1967). Powers (2010), continues this theme and states,

Only about 7% of the meaning we glean is communicated through the words themselves. Another 38% is paralinguistic, meaning that it is a function of how the words are spoken—the tone and inflection of the voice. The remaining 55% comes from facial expression and body language [non-verbal]. (p. 105)

Unfortunately, not all care partners are aware of the nonverbal messages they are sending.

Many messages and conversations are not really useful for the patient or resident, but are really a desire by the healthcare provider to get tasks completed and move on.

Partnering communication. Person-centered communication is an integral part of person-centered care and reflects a focus on the patients and their unique perceptions and experiences with health and illness. A key approach to this type of care is to partner with patients and meet them at eye level. Nursing interventions include providing information to promote health and healing and to engage patients in self-care or in more compliant behaviors. Person-centered care includes methods that build trust and respect. Various methods can be used; one example is the 5Ps *Partnering Communication Model* when establishing a relationship with the patient (Ondrejka, 2014). The 5Ps method provides a unique example of person-centered care that builds trust and respect in any setting, but has been built for in-patient care settings originally. Ondrejka presents this model as a partnering dialogue that states the following:

1. Tell the [patient] your name and your role as you sit at eye level.
2. Ask the patient his or her priorities for the day so you can assist him or her in meeting these goals.
3. Let the patient know what your practice needs are during your shift and look at integrating your needs and the patient's needs for the day.
4. Put your name, contact number [how to reach you], and partnered goals on the whiteboard [or other visible area].

5. Continue with the five Ps:
   a. You did **partnering** already
   b. Ask about the restroom needs—**potty**
   c. Obtain a **pain** assessment
   d. Make **positioning** adjustments.
   e. Check the **pump(s)** to reduce potential noise distractions.
6. Address pain or your first assessment of the day and do both soon.
7. Before leaving, ask if there is anything he or she needs before you leave to finish your regular rounds. (p. 42)

Partnering communication involves a person-centered approach such as the 5Ps, being respectful, and being flexible to accomplish all that is needed for the patient. It allows patients to participate in their own care as well as partnering with them for the care they must provide to the patient.

Use person-first language. When referring to the patient, regardless of whether the patient is present, use *person-first language.* This stresses the person as an individual who has some condition or disease instead the condition or disease as a defining factor of the individual. For example, say or write *person with dementia* instead of dementia or demented patient and a *person with hearing loss,* not a hearing-impaired person. This communicates respect for the individual.

Include the patient. In some situations, family members and caregivers speak as if the person being talked about is not in the room. Be sure to include the individual in the conversation. If conversations are taking place with the patient in the room, speak as though the person can understand you. Do not have conversations about the person in front the person and not include him or her, especially if you say something that might be hurtful or embarrassing to the person (e.g., *she does not remember anything anymore*).

Speak slower and pause between phrases. Slowing the rate at which you speak allows you to speak more clearly and provides distinct separation of words for better comprehension. Pause time between sentences allows for older adults whose retrieval and processing has decreased in speed to process and respond. This helps individuals with hearing loss as well.

Provide additional time for the person to respond. After asking a question or making a comment that you expect a response to, wait 5 to 10 seconds for a response. Processing time slows in adults with and without pathological conditions, so providing additional time allows the person to process what was said, plan what to say, and then provide an oral or written response.

Simplify vocabulary and avoid jargon. Try to use language that is easy to understand; refrain from using slang and medical jargon, especially. Watch to see if the person understands what you are saying. If you think the person did not understand or the person says that he or she does not understand, rephrase your sentence.

Use short, direct, clear phrases. Comprehension of complex sentences becomes more difficult as people age. Use short phrases, but remember to still use respectful language. Limit instructions to one or two steps at a time. Using short, clear phrases may help reduce the number of times you repeat the information. If the person forgets the topic being discussed, summarize what has been said to help guide the person back into the conversation

Use appropriate touch to communicate. Some individuals have difficulty with attention and alertness due to cognitive issues, medication side effects, and/or medical health problems. Gently touch the person on the hand, shoulder, arm, or leg to help gain his or her attention. If you start speaking when the person is not attending, you will likely have to repeat your message.

Speak in the direction of the person. Make sure you are in the same room and are looking at the individual. This will help the person prepare to listen. Being in the same room eliminates an environmental barrier, as talking to a person in another room or across the room leads to a reduced speech signal to the listener.

Speak into the ear with less or no hearing loss. For those who have hearing impairments, be sure look in their charts for information about their hearing. If one ear has better hearing, position yourself so that you are speaking in the direction of that ear.

Write out information. If the person does not understand you, write down key words, phrases, or sentences so the person can read the information. This will help ensure that the message is clearly communicated.

Provide written information in large, easy-to-read print. For individuals who have difficulty seeing written text, make sure that text is in an easy-to-read, large font. Stick to high-contrasting colors (e.g., black ink on white paper) and avoid using blue and green ink.

Request clarification. If you did not understand the intent of the person's message, ask questions that help to clarify. Another option is to say what you think was said and ask the person if you understood correctly.

Encourage use of clues. There are times when we all struggle with finding the word we want to say. Because this typically occurs more often in older adults, encourage them to provide clues so you can then guess the word. For example, you should suggest they describe appearance, function, and/or location.

Eliminate or minimize background noise. Additional sounds compete with the speech sounds, making it more difficult to determine what was said. Music, television, and other conversations all make it more difficult to attend to the conversation at hand.

Limit the number of speakers. Typically, group settings and social events have numerous people speaking at the same time or rapidly taking turns. This requires quick processing to be able to understand and keep up with the conversation. Because older adults are slower to process and respond to the information, it is best to limit the number of people speaking. This is less cognitively demanding for the individual.

Position yourself in the person's direct line of vision. This will let the person know that you are engaging in communication with him or her. Also, it provides visual information about what is being said. The person will be able to look at your lips and perhaps fill in what he or she does not understand simply by hearing. If understanding of nonverbal communication is still intact, positioning yourself in front of the person will allow for him or her to tune into nonverbal communication (posture, facial expressions, gestures). Another element to keep in the mind is lighting. Be sure there is adequate lighting so the person can see you. Individuals with vision impairments often require more lighting than those without vision issues.

Use gestures to aid in communication. Gestures help clarify the message when perhaps not all of it was understood. Pointing and demonstrating actions may aid understanding.

Say names. Say the person's name before providing instructions to get his or her attention. If memory is an issue, state your name as you enter the room so that the person does not have to guess who you are. When possible, use proper names instead of pronouns.

Make sure any assistive devices are on and working. This includes hearing aids and other assistive listening devices. If the person needs glasses to see, make sure the person has easy access to them. If the person has difficulty hearing, ask the person to wear his or her hearing aids or properly place hearing aids before speaking.

Using the Communication Enhancement Model

The *Communication Enhancement Model* (Ryan, Meredith, Maclean, & Orange, 1995) provides direction for effective healthcare–provider communication. This model directs the younger adult healthcare provider to make an individualized assessment of the communication abilities of each older adult and modify speech only as needed to support effective communication with that individual. For example, many younger adults assume that all older adults have hearing loss and speak loudly and slowly to all elders. For older adults with intact hearing, excessively loud and high-pitched speech can be distorted and make it harder for them to understand.

There are two types of strategies to help with communication issues: compensatory and restorative. *Compensatory strategies* focus on providing mechanisms to assist the person with the physical or neurological impairment. Several types of compensatory strategies are used with older adults, such as adapting the environment, using relational communication, and adding technological devices or memory aids. *Restorative strategies* address rebuilding the patient's skills that are currently impaired. A man with nonfluent aphasia might start to focus on saying common single words to help communicate his wants and needs. As his ability to say these words increases, more words are taught. In most cases, a person needs to be assessed by a speech–language pathologist to determine appropriate evidence-based strategies to implement during this restorative phase.

Regulatory Communication Goals for Older Adults

Communication is an integral part of quality health care, as identified by the Institute of Medicine (2001) report. A key to quality includes *patient-centered communication* as a key characteristic of quality health care. Patient-centered communication is a very complex issue with many forces at play. Healthcare providers have struggled to show any improvements in their communication scores with patients until just recently. Dimensions of patient centeredness include respect for patient values, preferences, and expressed needs, along with a focus on information, communication, and education of patients using terms they would understand. Is it possible that improving communication with older adults is only being implemented part of the time or may be ignored by healthcare providers for various reasons? Consistent and effective communication between patient and clinician has been associated with improved patient satisfaction, safety, better health outcomes, and lower healthcare costs. In contrast, communication breakdown has been implicated in healthcare disparities and medical errors. Professional standards include respectful and effective communication as key factors in informed consent and a trusting relationship (Paget et al., 2011). We must ask ourselves if there are some barriers for healthcare providers, as the outcomes that were expected did not occur until just recently and after *HCHAPS surveys* and *Pay-for-Performance* were implemented under the Affordable Health Care for America Act of 2010 (Schimpff, 2012; Zusman, 2012).

Communication is essential for the giving and receiving of information and the exchange of ideas, thoughts, and feelings. We communicate to exchange information and meet our physical, social, and emotional needs, as well as to meet the needs of others. The Joint Commission on American Hospitals has recognized and mandated attention be placed on effective communication in healthcare settings to prevent errors and safety issues (Joint Commission, 2014). Research indicates that older adults who have a positive relationship to nurses state they are also highly satisfied with their care and the nurses who work with them. In addition, this positive relationship between the patient and nurse provides higher levels of job satisfaction for the nurses (Grau, Chandler, & Saunders, 1995; Parsons, Simmons, Penn, & Furlough, 2002). It is apparent that we need to have compassionate, patient-centered communication that builds trust and mutual respect. However, it is not always that easy to accomplish with communication being so complex.

Communicating with Families and Significant Others

Care partners can support family members caring for older adults by assisting them to overcome communication barriers as they occur. Healthcare providers must be aware of the need to include the older adult in communication regarding health matters as much as possible and then include family members as appropriate. Permission to communicate about the patient's health condition with family and significant others is a key privacy issue that may be complicated. Ensure the patient is willing to have this information passed on, or encourage the patient to give this information to the family himself or herself.

Care partners also can help significant others to understand their role in caregiving as well as their need to recognize stress they may encounter. Be ready to explain what resources are available to aid the significant other in providing care. Nurses frequently counsel family caregivers, make referrals for resources such as respite care, and serve as role models for care partner communication practices. If this is not your skill set, have the name of someone who can offer such assistance.

Quick Intervention Table

The content in this chapter has focused on the importance of communication. Many older adults may have significant sensory or cognitive impairments that affect their ability to communicate, and care partners can use the techniques discussed in this chapter to facilitate appropriate communication. Health *literacy* should also be taken into account when planning teaching or providing educational materials. By choosing the most applicable strategies for information exchange, care partners can positively influence the communication process with older adults.

Table 5-2 is a quick tool describing what you can do to be an effective communicator with many older adults having significant communication barriers. Use it wisely and where it fits the patient's needs. Avoid the many traps and myths about working with older adults presented in this chapter. Greet and treat everyone like you would like them to connect to you.

TABLE 5-2 Strategies for Effective Communication with Persons with Vision, Hearing, Cognitive, and/or Speech–Language Impairments	
Impairment Type	**Communication Strategies**
Vision	• Use person-first language • Include the patient • Provide written information in large, easy to read print • Position yourself in the person's direct line of vision • Make sure glasses or contacts are worn • Use relational connections and partner with the patient
Hearing	• Use person-first language • Use slower speaking rate and pause between phrases • Include the patient and ask if you are speaking loud enough • Provide additional time for the person to respond • Summarize • Speak into the ear with less hearing loss • Write out information • Eliminate or minimize background noise • Limit the number of speakers in the room • Position yourself in the person's direct line of vision • Make sure the hearing aid(s) or assistive listening device is on and working • Say the person's name • Use touch to gain attention • Use relational connections and partner with the patient

(continues)

TABLE 5-2   Strategies for Effective Communication with Persons with Vision, Hearing, Cognitive, and/or Speech–Language Impairments (*continued*)

Impairment Type	Communication Strategies
Cognition	• Use person-first language • Use slower speaking rate and pause between phrases • Include the patient • Provide additional time for the person to respond • Simplify vocabulary and avoid jargon • Summarize • Write out information • Eliminate or minimize background noise • Limit the number of speakers in the room • Say the person's name • Encourage use of clues for word-finding difficulty • Use touch to communicate or to gain attention • Request clarification • Use relational connections and be calm and nonreactive, partner with the patient
Speech and language	• Use person-first language • Use slower speaking rate and pause between phrases • Include the patient • Provide additional time for the person to respond • Simplify vocabulary and avoid jargon • Summarize • Write out information • Eliminate or minimize background noise • Limit the number of speakers in the room • Position yourself in the person's direct line of vision • Make sure the assistive devices are on and working • Say the person's name • Encourage use of clues for word-finding • Request clarification • Use relational connections and partner with the patient

Teaching Older Adults and Their Families

Older adults may have unique physical, psychological, or cognitive limitations that affect learning ability similar to how these same limitations affect speech and communication. The American Nurses Association (ANA) in collaboration with the National Gerontological Nursing Association developed the document *Gerontological Nursing: Scope and Standards of Practice* (ANA, 2010), which identifies a standard requiring nurses working with older adults to include health education of patients and their families. This is not always an easy task as the nurses may be confronted with a host of barriers on the part of the patient, their partners, or family members.

As a quick reminder, **Box 5-2** lists some of the areas that will challenge the older adult in the effort to become educated or to learn some type of health advice from their care partners.

Care partners would need specialized training to teach older adults having many of the barriers presented. However, there is knowledge that can support best teaching strategies for various educational and health needs. These same methods also can be used for the patient's partners or family members when needed.

BOX 5-2 Physical, Psychological, and Cognition Changes Impacting Learning	
• Impaired vision, hearing, and speech • Literacy level • Multidimensional motor sequence impairment • Decreased reflexes, tremor, muscle weakness • Chronic illness or pain	• Cognitive and memory changes and losses • Fear, anxiety, and confusion • Reality disturbances and hallucinations • Depression • Culture and habitual patterns of living

Theory of Adult Learning

Knowles (1973) provided well-known principles for addressing the way adults are motivated and prefer to learn. He is attributed with coining the term *andragogy* in the early 1970s and provided six principles that distinguish it from *pedagogy* used for younger learners with these principles being refined over time. More recently they have been described as:

> Adults need to know why they need to learn something before learning it.
> The self-concept of adults is heavily dependent on a move toward self-direction.
> Prior experience of the learner provides a rich resource for learning.
> Adults typically become ready to learn when they experience a need to cope with a life situation or perform a task.
> Adults' orientation to learning is life-centered; education is a process of developing increased competency levels to achieve their full potential.
> The motivation for adult learners is internal rather than external. (Knowles, Holton, & Swanson, 2005, p. 159)

The idea that andragogy principles need to be flexible has been emphasized in more recent years, as there are many factors affecting the various learners that change the teaching methods. "It seems clear that Knowles always knew, and then confirmed through use, that andragogy could be utilized in many different ways and would have to be adapted to fit individual situations" (Knowles et al., p. 147). The patient variances could be situational or individual, and each person has different strengths and weaknesses for learning new things. Older adults are just like any other adults in that they have situational and personal attributes for learning that vary in many ways to include specific barriers to learning presented in Box 5-2.

CLINICAL TIP

The good teacher tailors each teaching session to the learner's internal abilities to learn and then integrates this with the teaching method being used.

Gerogogy in Transition

John (1988) presented some of the first ideas on what it takes to have a teaching method for the older adult. He defined *gerogogy* as "the process involved in stimulating and helping older persons to learn" (p. 12). It has more recently been described as an art and a science of using teaching strategies that lead older adults to higher levels of empowerment and emancipation (Formosa, 2002; Thomas, 2007).

CLINICAL TIP

Gerogogy is the process of stimulating and helping older persons to learn (John, 1988, p. 12).

Categorizing Diverse Learners

Hunt (2013) suggests using Felder's historical categories for teaching to the type of learner the person is: visual, sensing, inductive/deductive, active, and sequential, which may be useful for those without impairments. In reality, the care partner may need to switch the typical learner preference with an alternative when there is a specific barrier. Visual learners who cannot see well may be able to complement their learning by active learning and touching things that would be looked at only in the past. Capitalizing on the patients' most functional senses is a great resource for teaching older adults. There may be more difficulty in assessing other forms of learning styles, and it is easier to connect to broader generalizations identified by surveys of older adults (American Association for Retired Persons [AARP], 2000) and exploring more universal highly effective teaching methods. Strategies for teaching older adults appear in **Boxes 5-3** and **5-4**.

Use a Relational Approach to Teaching

Many assume that humans are persuaded by rational approaches to decision making. This assumption has been challenged for years (Pilkington, 1997). Our real challenge is to see what others think they are seeing.

Building a *relational communication* approach to patients in clinical or teaching settings means connecting to the patients and integrating their perspective in a life-giving and caring way. This approach also has been called *biogenic* (Watson, 2008) and described as a connection that is life giving and life receiving. Ondrejka (2014) describes *relational teaching* as having many levels, from a toxic to a powerfully life-sustaining relationship; the

---

BOX 5-3   Preparing a Short Educational Program for Older Adults and Families

1. Assure that the goal of the presentation is to provide information that the group is interested in. Work with the facility to be certain that the date and time of the presentation does not interfere with other regularly planned activities.

2. If the program being presented is for a regularly scheduled support group for elders with chronic disease and their families, make sure that the information is specific to the needs of the group. For example, if the session is about coping with COPD, assure that the content is specific to the needs of the elder (medications, activity, oxygen use) as well as the family in assisting them to cope with the challenges that the disease presents.

3. The information presented should be relevant to the group both in content and format. Ask older adults who may attend what topics they are interested in and want to know more about.

4. The more current research done on the subject, the more comfortable the presenter will be. If a health-related topic, assure application of the principles of health literacy.

5. For the program itself, employ strategies appropriate to teaching older adults (Box 5-4).

6. Plan at least one interactive activity to increase group participation; this can aid in overall understanding of the presented material.

7. Intersperse questions throughout the class to:
   a. Evaluate understanding by learners and allow changes in presentation.
   b. Allow learners to feel connected to the presentation by answering questions and making them feel that each question is important and will add to the material already presented.
   c. Encourage participants to share their personal stories, as this will make the presentation more realistic to those participants.

8. Be flexible. Allow extra break time if needed and plan to stay after the program to answer individual questions as necessary.

BOX 5-4   Strategies for Teaching Older Adults

Use the principles of adult learning theory.
- Assess readiness to learn
- Involve the audience in the presentation
- Draw the learners into the discussion
- Provide reasons for them to learn by pointing out the significance of the topic

Use multiple teaching modalities to keep the material interesting and maintain attention.
- PowerPoint slides
- DVDs
- Handouts, brochures, or pamphlets
- Posters
- Demonstration/samples
- Quizzes/games
- Social media, e.g., YouTube
- Internet Websites

Remember to accommodate any unusual physical needs.
- Avoid glare; control environmental temperature and noise level
- Use a microphone and speak slowly
- Face the audience as many elders lip read to fill in what they cannot hear

- Limit content to 30–40 minutes so questions can be answered
- Handouts should be in large font
- Make sure the room is large enough for the number of learners and their adaptive equipment
- If possible, have a helper to assist learners who need to leave for any reason or who come late

Make presentations elder-friendly
- Choose content that elders are interested in, such as advance directives, nutrition, heart health, medication safety, etc.
- Create a catchy title that will pique interest
- Use the principles of literacy and avoid "jargon" that may confuse the learner, but don't talk down to them. If you ask a few questions you should be able to judge the literacy level and speak at that level.
- Invite special speakers who are well known in the area to promote attendance.
- Provide a take-home item for all participants (e.g., handouts, pill organizers, etc.)

---

latter takes a deep understanding of self on the part of the instructor. Freire (1998) was one of the great Brazilian education reformers, and states, "In short it is impossible to teach without a forged invented, and well-though-out capacity to *love*" (in Darder, 2002, p. 91). A similar view is also expressed by two great American educators, Nodding (2005) and Palmer (2007). Nodding even warns teachers that having knowledge of having a caring relationship is not enough,

> Knowledge alone is unlikely to establish a caring relationship. In fact a number of studies have shown that qualities such as 'counselor relationship' or 'teacher relationship' are only slightly correlated with multi-cultural knowledge. Knowing something about the other cultures is important and useful, but it is not sufficient to produce positive relationships. (p. 113)

Palmer continues to support a deeper inner awareness as a necessary component for the teacher and states,

> Good teachers possess a capacity for *connectedness*. They are able to weave a complex web of connections among themselves, their subjects, and their students so that students can learn to weave a world for themselves. . . . . The connections made by good teachers are held not in their methods but in their hearts—meaning heart in the ancient sense, as the place where intellect and emotion and spirit will converge in the human self. (p. 11)

A *relational teaching* approach has been described in detail by Ondrejka (2014) and expanded here for older adults who need to have *choice* (Balchik, 2002). In addition, older adults are more likely to comply when they have *compliance scaffolding* (James, 2010) or there is connection from the request to something that is important for them or has personal meaning. The final step is show *care* and *acceptance* (Watson, 2008) from a *deep connectedness* of knowledge, feelings, passion, and spirit (Freire, 1998, cited in Darder, 2002; Nodding, 2005; Palmer 2007). The relational approach to teaching provides content, compassion, empathy, caring acceptance, and expresses this with a spirit of love for the older adult.

An example of a relational approach can be seen in a situation in which patients may think their medicine is poison and the care partners have been told they have no right to make the patient take this poison. The request to take medication becomes a teaching, effective communication and a challenging request for this person. A care partner who is avoiding a rationalizing approach might use this *relational* approach: "Mr. Hide *(dignity)*, I do care about you and what you think *(acceptance)*, and I know this medicine will help your heart be stronger *(teaching)* so you have energy to talk to your family when they come *(compliance scaffolding)*. That is why I think you should take the medicine *(request)*. Would you like to take it with water or juice *(choice)*?" [while holding his hand, or having a soft touch on the shoulder, *caring presence*]. Connection of these approaches can build trust and a positive relationship with patients so they are more likely to agree with you and there is a better clinical outcome.

Many care partners continue to use the rational approach. The rational approach might sound like this, "Mr. Hide, this medicine is not poison. The doctor wants you to take it so you will feel better, so please take the medicine." In this response, there is no caring acceptance, no scaffolding, and no choice imbedded in the message. It has a message that is factual but lacks a deeper connection that is needed to build to trust. It is important to remember that during times of patient frustration, delusion, or paranoia, rational conversations have very little value for compliance or teaching and in many cases can escalate to aggressive responses. James (2010) suggest, "part of our role is to try to get staff to empathize with the person's [patients] situation, to think what she might be thinking in that situation and to try to understand the reasons behind the challenging behavior" (p. 183). James thinks the deeper need for patients showing challenging behaviors is their need for respect, acceptance of feelings, and a way to sustain their dignity. Relational communication shows respect, does not argue, does not discount the patient's beliefs, builds on the relationship, and offers acceptable choices that still allow for compliance where needed. This same approach can be used for various types of teaching for the patient—especially those struggling with cognitive impairments.

Older Adults' Preferences on Teaching

The AARP Survey on Lifelong Learning (2000) provides teaching preferences desired by most older adults. They include the following:

> Methods that are easy to access, require small investments of time and money to get started, and allow learning to begin immediately
> Methods that are direct, hands-on experiences—putting hands on something, playing with it, listening to it, watching it, and thinking about it
> Newspapers, magazines, books, and journals are the most frequently used tools for gathering information (nontechnology driven).
> Methods that enable them to keep up with what's going on in the world, for their own spiritual or personal growth and/or for the simple joy of learning something new
> Subjects that will improve the quality of their lives, build on a current skill, or enable them to take better care of their health
> Ability to use what they have learned right away or in the near future

We can also examine the adult learning principles and adjust them to meet gerogogy methods as seen in building effective communication. A modified version to meet this need is as follows:

> Older adults need to know the teacher is providing information because they really care about them as a care partner.

> The self-concept of older adults is heavily dependent on a relationship that shows a partnership between them and the teacher.
> Prior experience of the learner provides a rich resource for learning.
> Older adults typically become ready to learn when they experience a need to cope with a life situation or if it supports more independence.
> Older adults' orientation to learning is life-sustaining, independence-promoting, and personal goal–oriented using resources, including technology, when needed.
> Older adults benefit by presentations that engage their functional senses using diverse and experiential learning methods in which there is engagement with objects and each other.
> Older adults need a simple reminder tool(s) for the critical content presented that does not require complex access. This is moving increasingly more to technology methods.

Technology for Older Adults' Lifelong Learning

Many think the older adult is more likely to reject technology, and this has been shown to be a myth. According to a 2008 Pew Internet Survey on older adults and use of the Internet, 70% of those ages 50–64 and 38% of adults 65 or older reported using the Internet. The fastest growing age group learning to use the Internet is those 55 and older. Madden (2010) found that social networking among Internet users 50 years of age and older nearly doubled between 2009 and 2010, so that now half of Internet users between the ages 50 and 64 and 26% of users age 65 and older use social networking sites. Older adults are more likely to use email than social networking, with 89% of adults 65 and over who use the Internet sending or receiving an email on a typical day. Additionally, "among Internet users ages 65 and older, 62% look for news online" (Madden, p. 4), with 34% doing so on a typical day. Older adults who were living with chronic disease used the Internet for blogging and participating in online health discussions. The process of aging may present challenges to older adults who wish to use computers to enhance learning, but it is clear that many older adults are embracing the use of computers and the Internet in some aspect of their lives. Advances in voice activation have led to computers that can send or receive messages verbally. Barriers to the use of computers and the Internet for older adults include the cost of computers and access to the Internet, concerns about being able to learn how to use a computer, and fears about privacy and security of computers and the Internet. Some of the challenges associated with the use of computer technology can be overcome (see **Table 5-3**). Chapter 21 provides a thorough discussion on technology and older adults.

Teaching Older Adults Using Technology

Wolfson, Cavanagh, and Kraiger (2013) offer specific strategies for older adults to promote higher levels of success with technology, as follows:

> Develop a structured and simple interface process
> Maintain feedback processes offering ways to make adjustments
> Be ready to assist the user in how he or she thinks through an issue and give guidance for decision making
> Integrate learning principles allowing for diverse ways of gaining information

The day has come when senior centers either have or will teach classes with titles such as *Getting Comfortable with Technology* as older adults are constantly being exposed to new technology. Older adults are seeing how some of their peers are staying connected to family members from a distance through technology and may want to connect in the same way. It is useful for older adults to have computer tablets with the following:

> Simple and consistent access keys
> Uncluttered screens without multiple apps
> A talking interface or problem-solving ques for a single social media platform

TABLE 5-3	Aging Alterations That Can Be Overcome Using Computer Technology	
Alteration	**Effect on Computer Use**	**Possible Solutions**
Decreased hearing	Sound from computer may not be heard	Use of external speakers and headphones to enhance sound
Decreased visual acuity	Need for bifocals or trifocals, viewing monitor size may be too small, alteration in light/color distinction due to glaucoma or cataracts	Adjust monitor tilt to decrease glare Get larger monitor Change size of font to 14 to 16 Adjust contrast to ensure clarity Adjust screen resolution to promote color contrast
Motor control or tremors Arthritis	May affect use of keyboard or control of mouse	Use "larger" mouse Use control arrows to move through text Purchase "touch screen" or voice-activated computer
Attention span	Inability to focus for extended periods and comprehend new informational subjects	Programs contain small modules of information Repetition of last concept in each new module Utilization of multimedia presentations (PowerPoint, streaming video, summary sheets)

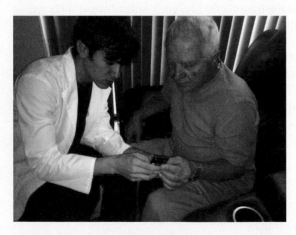

Figure 5-1 Nurse teaching older patient to program his smart phone with a medication reminder.
Courtesy of Sergio Medina.

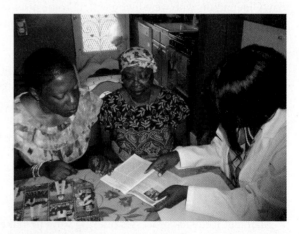

Figure 5-2 Nurse teaching older patient and her daughter about her chronic illness.
Courtesy of K. Steele.

These simple approaches could be just the right strategy, as suggested by the theories in the work of Wolfson et al. (2013). Keeping older adults from technology just because they appear confused at first may be short-sighted for care partners, family members, and the future of advancing older adult technology access (see **Figures 5-1** and **5-2**).

Additional Internet Resources for Teaching Older Adults

There are a variety of Internet resources for older adults who want to learn and stay connected (**Case Study 5-5**). **Box 5-5** provides a variety of choices.

Case Study 5-5

Marjorie Hanes is 70 years old. She always wanted to learn how to speak Spanish and enrolled in the local college, despite having a hearing impairment. She was enjoying her classes as she continued her responsibilities in her home, including caring for her husband who had hypertension. Unfortunately, her husband suffered a stroke and Ms. Hanes had to assume the responsibility of primary care partner, resulting in her withdrawing from college. She purchased some audiovisuals to help her practice Spanish. When her husband recovered from his stroke, Ms. Hanes was able to reenroll at the college; however, her hearing loss had become worse over time, which made it difficult to continue learning a language in class. Ms. Hanes decided to continue using books and audiotapes to learn Spanish, but she also had a new interest in plants and used educational programs on television to learn more about horticulture and working in her garden. These activities provided Ms. Hanes with educational activities in the home while she continued to care for her husband, who died 3 years later. After her husband's death, Ms. Hanes was feeling isolated and decided to go back to the college and continue her learning. She found a cohort of older adults who were also interested in continuing their education in a variety of ways. At this time, Ms. Hanes was enjoying art and took a class in art history—something she had always wanted to learn more about. Taking this class was not hindered by her hearing loss. She visited art galleries and was involved in group discussions that were led by class participants under supervision of the instructor. As an older adult, Ms. Hanes was engaged in a variety of learning experiences that changed over time because of circumstances in her life.

Consider the following regarding Ms. Hanes:

1. How has Ms. Hanes incorporated lifelong learning into her older years?
2. How has Ms. Hanes adapted to the challenges she has faced to overcome barriers and continue her lifelong learning?
3. How might technology have been used to help Ms. Hanes continue her learning when her husband became ill?
4. In your role as a nurse educator, what would you recommend to Ms. Hanes to enhance her education or to meet her lifelong learning needs?

BOX 5-5 Recommended Internet Resources for Teaching Older Adults

- Administration on Aging (AoA): http://www.AoA.gov
- American Association for Retired Persons (AARP): http://www.aarp.org
- American Society on Aging (ASA): http://www.asaging.org
- Association for Continuing Higher Education: http://www.acheinc.org
- Association for Gerontology in Higher Education (AGHE): http://www.aghe.org
- Gerontological Society of America (GSA): http://www.geron.org
- The John A. Hartford Foundation Institute for Geriatric Nursing: http://www.hartfordign.org
- National Council on Aging (NCOA): http://www.ncoa.org
- National Gerontological Nurses Association (NGNA): http://www.ngna.org
- National Institute on Aging (NIA): http://www.nia.nih.gov
- Osher Lifelong Learning Institute: http://www.olli.gmu.edu

Additional Web resources for health education are available for specific disease processes from focused organizations, including the American Heart Association, American Diabetes Association, and Alzheimer's Association.

Summary

What has become valuable for geriatric care partners is the significant amount of support for individually working with older adults in any setting. Assessment tools that were created for one setting work just as well in a host of other settings, including the home. The critical issue is to see the patient as a person—not just an older person. This video at the following Website allows the reader to note a potential flaw in what you are seeing: https://youtu.be/LOtNdn_GsMc. This video reflects what might be in the mind of the older adult as the care partner is focused on something different. Take a moment to *see them*, do not just do to them—this is a constant concern for older adults.

You have been asked to accept the assumption that **older adults are not the same, nor do they all have the same issues related to normal aging**. Some aging deficits seem more universal, whereas other issues are very individual. As presented in the two stories of John and Bert, **there may be major differences in how older adults connect to others and how they see the world**. However, most want to really be seen. Diversity is not just a cultural issue. It is a human phenomenon. Be ready to see all people in their diverse and unique selves.

A second assumption presented asked the readers to remember—**even when there is evidence of universal aging barriers to effective communication, continue to be open to the idea that effective communication strategies may not be age specific, but human specific**. Is it possible that everyone needs what has been offered in this chapter as valuable support for effective communication, teaching methods, and specialty assessments? Keep in mind that children, young adults, and older adults all may enjoy having care partners who are aware of what might be affecting effective communication and what they can do to address these deficits.

Care partners need to be prepared to meet the unique educational needs of the growing population of older adults who increasingly reflect a diversity of ethnicity, race, religion, gender, sexual orientation, and socioeconomic status. In addition to these factors, the older adult population also represents a wide diversity in age, ranging from 65 to 100 or more years of age. The increased longevity and diversity indicates that there will be greater needs for health teaching related to health promotion, illness and injury prevention, and chronic disease management (**Box 5-6**). Older adults need to have a reason to engage in learning activities that is relevant to their lives and situation. Older adults are becoming more comfortable with technology and are accessing health information from the Internet. Care partners will need to be flexible and adaptable to meet the needs of older adults and use flexible gerogogy to make learning appealing and interesting.

By combining knowledge of appropriate communication techniques with older adults and the principles of gerogogy, nurses can be become more effective teachers with older adults and their families.

BOX 5-6   Evidence-Based Practice Highlight

The authors examined learning theories and programs for older adults with chronic kidney disease. They concluded that "there is evidence that programs exist to address effective self-management of chronic illnesses and health literacy of the older adult. However, there are no programs in place to address health literacy specifically for the older adult with chronic kidney disease. The best way to address this issue is to have large, well-designed studies that will explore the most effective way to educate older adults with kidney disease. There is a definite need to conduct more research studies in this area of practice so the evidence can be translated to this growing population of individuals". p. 525

Elliott, R. W. (2014). Educating older adults with chronic kidney disease. *Nephrology Nursing Journal, 41*(5), 522–528. Reprinted from the *Nephrology Nursing Journal*, 2014, Volume 41, Number 5, pp. 522-528. Reprinted with permission of the American Nephrology Nurses Association, East Holly Avenue/Box 56, Pitman, NJ 08071-0056; (856) 256-2300; Fax (856) 589-7463; Website: www.anna.org; For a sample copy of the journal, please contact the publisher.

Clinical Reasoning Exercises

1. Realizing not everyone has the same past experience, but in an effort to connect the dots to what was presented in this chapter, you are being provided two music videos and are encouraged to listen to them. Play them both, and close your eyes. See where they take you in your memory. See if you touch old memory. Is it automatic? Does it bring an immediate emotional feeling and memory? Take the time now.
   - https://youtu.be/7E88RUqyjts?list=RD1SC OimBo5tg
   - https://youtu.be/7VBex8zbDRs

2. Choose one of these videos or music below from YouTube referred to in this chapter. Listen and review. What does this teach you about communication, individuality, and diversity that occurs with age?
   - https://youtu.be/4Szj0gCkFuk Paul Newman racing at 70 years of age.
   - http://web.cortland.edu/andersmd/ERIK /sum.HTML Summary of Erikson's stages of development.

- https://youtu.be/7E88RUqyjts?list=RD1SCO imBo5tg Tell me 'bout the good-ole days.
- https://youtu.be/7VBex8zbDRs Gravity
- https://youtu.be/3t3_yWQH1Go Phil Coulter
- https://youtu.be/-8MmeVhkMv8 Phil Coulter
- https://youtu.be/H6cl_RJUMqM Dave's Story on aging
- https://youtu.be/iVEiAU_F2qw How we age
- https://youtu.be/vPawWPXp5eg SPICES assessment model
- https://youtu.be/aPLt9OjwFTk KATZ assessment model
- https://youtu.be/_hRBPrfDQVI Cognition and Memory Assessment Model
- https://youtu.be/LOtNdn_GsMc Just being human

3. What older persons in your own life demonstrate diversity in the way they communicate with others?

4. Do you agree with the chapter author's assumption that older adults are not the same, nor do they have all the same issues related to normal aging? Why or why not?

Personal Reflections

1. Think about one of your older relatives. How did this person's maturational state contribute to his or her ability to learn or see the viewpoints of others?

2. What has been your experience with older adults and their use of technology? Do you think older adults are using more technology to communicate (i.e., cellphones, email, tablets, Twitter, Facebook)? What teaching strategies have you found to be most effective when teaching older adults? Does this change if teaching in a one-on-one situation versus a large group?

References

Alves, L. M., & Wilson, S. R. (2008). The effects of loneliness on telemarketing fraud vulnerability among older adults. *Journal of Elder Abuse & Neglect, 20*(1), 63–85.

Alzheimer's Association. (n.d.). *Key types of dementia.* Retrieved from http://www.alz.org/alzheimers_disease_related _diseases.asp

Alzheimer's Association. (2012). 2012 Alzheimer's disease facts and figures. *Alzheimer's and Dementia, 8,* 131–168.

American Association for Retired Persons. (2000). *Survey on lifelong learning.* Retrieved from http://assets.aarp .org/rgcenter/general/lifelong.pdf

American Nursing Association. (2010). *Gerontological nursing: Scope and standards of practice.* Silver Spring, MD: American Nursing Association Press.

American Parkinson Disease Association. (n.d.). *Basic info about PD.* Retrieved from http://www.apdaparkinson .org/publications-information/basic-info-about-pd/

American Psychological Association. (2014). *Diagnostic and statistical manual of mental disorders* (5th ed.). Washington, DC: Author.

Balchik, G. (2002). A better place to heal. *Health Forum Journal, 45*(4), 10–15.

Barry, L. C., & Byers, A. L. (2016). Risk factors and prevention strategies for late-life mood and anxiety disorders. In K. W. Schaie & S. L. Willis (Eds.), *Handbook of the psychology of aging* (8th ed., pp. 409–427). New York, NY: Academic Press.

Bayles, K. A., & Tomoeda, C. K. (2007). *Cognitive-communication disorders of dementia.* San Diego, CA: Plural.

Boxer-Wachler, B. S. (2016). Surgery for presbyopia. Retrieved from http://www.allaboutvision.com/visionsurgery /presbyopia_surgery.htm

Caporael, L. (1981). The paralanguage of caregiving: Baby talk to the institutionalized aged. *Journal of Personality and Social Psychology, 40*(5), 876–884.

Dalton, D. S., Cruickshanks, K. J., Klein, B. E. K., Klein, R., Wiley, T. L., & Nondahl, D. M. (2002). The impact of hearing loss on quality of life in older adults, *The Gerontologist, 43*(5), 661–668.

Dugdale III, D. C. (2011). Aging changes in the senses. Bethesda, MD: Medline Plus, National Library of Medicine, National Institutes of Health. Retrieved from http://www.nlm.nih.gov/medlineplus/ency/article/004013.htm

Elliott, R. W. (2014). Educating older adults with chronic kidney disease. *Nephrology Nursing Journal, 41*(5), 522–528.

Emojipedia (n.d.). Retrieved from https://twitter.com/Emojipedia?ref_src=twsrc%5Egoogle%7Ctwcamp%5Ese rp%7Ctwgr%5Eauthor

Ferguson, S. H. (2012). Talker differences in clear and conversational speech: Vowel intelligibility for older adults with hearing loss. *Journal of Speech, Language, and Hearing Research, 55,* 779–790.

Formosa, M. (2002). Critical gerogogy: Developing practical possibilities for critical educational gerontology. *Education and Ageing, 17*(1), 73–85.

Darder, A. (2002). Teaching as an act of love: The classroom and critical praxis. In: *Reinventing Paulo Freire: A pedagogy of love* (p. 91). Boulder, CO: Westview Press.

Grau, L., Chandler, B., & Saunders, C. (1995). Nursing home residents' perceptions of the quality of their care. *Journal of Psychosocial Nursing, 33*(5), 34–41.

Haro, S., & Isaki, E. (2009). Age effects on language: Differences between young and normal aging adults. Retrieved from http://www.asha.org/Events/convention/handouts/2009/2386_Isaki_Emi/

Hear-it. (n.d.). Retrieved from http://www.hear-it.org

Hunt, D. D. (2013). *The new nurse educator: Mastering academe.* New York, NY: Springer Publishing Company.

Institute of Medicine. (2001). *Crossing the quality chasm.* Washington, Dc.: National Academies Press.

James, I. A. (2010). *Cognitive Behavioral therapy with older adults.* Philadelphia, PA: Jessica Kingsley Publishing.

John, M. T. (1988). *Geragogy: A theory for teaching the elderly.* Binghamton, NY: Haworth Press.

Joint Commission. (2010). *Advancing effective communication, cultural competence, and patient-and-family-centered care: A roadmap for hospitals.* Oakbrook Terrace, IL: Author.

Joint Commission. (2014a). *Hospital accreditation standards.* Oakbrook Terrace, IL: Author

Joint Commission. (2014b). *Joint commission and CMS crosswalk: Comparing hospital standards and CoPs.* Oakbrook Terrace, IL: Author

Kiely, D. K., Simon, M. A., Jones, R. N., & Morris, J. N. (2000). The protective effect of social engagement on mortality in long-term care. *Journal of the American Geriatrics Society, 48*(12), 1367–1372.

Knowles, M. (1973). *The adult learner: A neglected species.* Houston, TX: Gulf.

Knowles, M., Holton III, E. F., & Swanson, R. A. (2005). *The adult learner: The definitive classic in adult education and human resource development* (6th ed.). New York, NY: Elsevier.

Lin, F. R. (2012). Hearing loss in older adults: Who's listening? *The Journal of the American Medical Association, 307*(11), 1147–1148.

Lubinski, R. (2010). Communicating effectively with elders and their families. *The ASHA Leader, 15,* 12–15. Retrieved from http://leader.pubs.asha.org/article.aspx?articleid=2291892.

Lustig, C., & Lin, Z. (2016). Memory: Behavior and neural basis. In K. W. Schaie & S. L. Willis (Eds.), *Handbook of the psychology of aging* (8th ed., pp. 147–163). New York, NY: Academic Press.

Madden, M. (2010). *Older adults and social media.* Washington, DC: Pew Research Center. Retrieved from http://pewinternet.org/~/media//Files/Reports/2010/Pew%20Internet%20-%20Older%20Adults%20and%20Social%20Media.pdf

Malkin, J. (1992). *Hospital interior architecture*, Hoboken, NJ: John Wiley and Sons.

National Eye Institute. (n.d.). Presbyopia. Retrieved from https://nei.nih.gov/health/presbyopia

National Parkinson's Foundation. (2012a). What are the early symptoms of Parkinson's disease? Retrieved from http://www.parkinson.org/understanding-parkinsons/10-early-warning-signs

National Parkinson's Foundation. (2012b). What is Parkinson's disease? Retrieved from http://www.parkinson.org/Parkinson-s-Disease/PD-101/What-is-Parkinson-s-disease

Nightingale, F. ([1859], 1969). *Notes on nursing: What it is and what it is not.* (A Dover Republication) Mineola, NY: Dover Publication, Inc.

Nodding, N. (2005). *The challenge to care in schools: an alternative approach to education* (2nd ed.). New York, NY: Teachers College Press.

Norrix, L., & Harris, F. P. (2008). Disorders of hearing in adults. In E. Plante & P. M. Beeson, *Communication and communication disorders: A clinical introduction* (3rd ed.). Boston, MA: Pearson Education.

Ondrejka, D. (2014). *Affective teaching in nursing: Connecting to feelings, values, and inner awareness.* New York, NY: Springer Publishing.

Oyler, A. L. (2012, January). Untreated hearing loss in adults: A growing national epidemic. Retrieved from http://www.asha.org/Articles/Untreated-Hearing-Loss-in-Adults/

Paget, L., Han, P., Nedza, S., Kurtz, P., Racine, E., Russell, S., . . . Von Kohorn, I. (2011). Patient-clinician communication: Basic principles and expectations. Washington, DC: Institute of Medicine. Retrieved from http://www.iom.edu/pcc

Palmer, P. (2007). *The courage to teach: Exploring the inner landscape of a teaching life* (10th Anniversary ed.). San Francisco, CA: Jossey-Bass.

Park, D. C., & Farrell, M. E. (2016). The aging mind in transition: Amyloid deposition and progression toward Alzheimer's disease. In K. W. Schaie & S. L. Willis (Eds.), *Handbook of the psychology of aging*, (8th ed., pp. 87–103). New York, NY: Academic Press.

Park, D. C., Lautenschlager, G., Hedden, T., Davidson, N. S., Smith, A. D., & Smith, P. K. (2002). Models of visuospatial and verbal memory across the adult life span. *Psychology and Aging, 17*(2), 299–320.

Parsons, S. K., Simmons, W. P., Penn, K., & Furlough, M. (2002). Determinants of satisfaction and turnover among nursing assistants. *Journal of Gerontological Nursing, 29*(3), 51–58.

Phelps, E. A. (2004). Human emotion and memory: Interactions of the amygdala and hippocampal complex. *Current Opinion in Neurolbiology, 14*(2), 198–202.

Pilkington, F. B. (1997). Knowledge and evidence: Do they change patterns of health? *Nursing Science Quarterly, 10*(4), 156–157.

Plante, E., & Beeson, P. M. (Eds.) (2008). *Communication and communication disorders: A clinical introduction* (3rd ed.). Needham Hcights, MA: Allyn & Bacon.

Power, G. A. (2010). *Dementia beyond drugs: Changing the culture of care.* Baltimore, MA: Health Professions Press.

Remen, N. R. (1996). *Kitchen table wisdom: Stories that heal.* New York, NY: Riverhead Books.

Reuter-Lorenz, P. A., & Park, D. C. (2014). How does it STAC up? Revisiting the Scaffolding Theory of Aging and Cognition, *Neuropsychology Review, 24*(3), 355–370.

Ryan, E. B., Byrne, K., Spykerman, H., & Orange, J. B. (2005). Evidencing Kitwood's personhood strategies: Conversation as care in dementia. In B. Davis (Ed.), *Alzheimer talk, text and context: Enhancing communication.* New York, NY: Palgrave Macmillan.

Ryan, E. B., Hummert, M. L., & Boich, L. H. (1995). Communication predicaments of aging: Patronizing behavior toward older adults. *Journal of Language and Social Psychology, 14*(1–2), 144–166.

Ryan, E. B., Meredith, S. D., Maclean, M. J., & Orange, J. B. (1995). Changing the way we talk with elders: Promoting health using the communication enhancement model. *International Journal of Aging and Human Development, 41*(2), 89–107.

Satir, V. (1967). *Conjoint family therapy.* Palo Alto, CA: Science and Behavior Books.

Saunders, G. H., & Echt, K. (2011). Dual sensory impairment in an aging population. *The ASHA Leader, 16,* 5–7. Retrieved from http://leader.pubs.asha.org/article.aspx?articleid=2279013.

Schaie, K. W. (2013). *Developmental influences on adult intellectual development: The Seattle longitudinal study* (2nd rev. ed.). New York, NY: Oxford University Press.

Schaie, K. W. (2016). Theoretical perspectives for the psychology of aging in lifespan context. In K. W. Schaie & S. L Willis (Eds.), *Handbook of the psychology of aging,* (8th ed., pp. 3–13). New York, NY: Academic Press.

Schimpff, S. C. (2012). *The future of health-care delivery.* Washington, DC: Potomac Books.

Schreck, J. (2010, November). *The impact of "normal" aging on cognitive-communication skills.* Paper presented at the ASHA Annual Convention, Philadelphia, PA.

Shelkey, M., & Wallace, M. (2002, April). Katz Index of Independence in Activities of Daily Living (ADL). *Medical Surgical Nursing.* Retrieved from http://go.galegroup.com/ps/anonymous?id=GALE%7CA84866004&sid=googleScholar&v=2.1&it=r&linkaccess=fulltext&issn=10920811&p=AONE&sw=w&authCount=1&isAnonymousEntry=true

Shin, L. M., Rauch, S. L., & Pitman, R. K. (2006). Amygdala, medical prefrontal cortex, and hippocampal function in PTSD. *Psychology of Posttraumatic Stress Disorder: A Decade of Progress, 1071,* 67–79.

Thomas, C. M. (2007). Bulletin boards: A teaching strategy for older audiences. *Journal of Gerontological Nursing, 33*(3), 45–52.

Tulving, E., & Markowitsch, H. J. (1998). Episodic and declarative memory: Role of the hippocampus. *Hippocampus (8),* 3, 198-204.

Vorvick, L. J., & Schwartz, S. (2011, May). Hearing loss. Bethesda, MD: Medline Plus, National Library of Medicine, National Institutes of Health. Retrieved from http://www.nlm.nih.gov/medlineplus/ency/article/003044.htm

Watkins, J. M., & Mohr, B. J. (2001). *Appreciative inquiry: Change at the speed of imagination.* San Francisco, CA: Jossey-Bass/Pfeiffer.

Watson, J. (2008). *Nursing: The philosophy and science of caring,* (Rev. ed). Denver, CO: University Press of Colorado.

Wolfson, N. E., Cavanagh, T. M., & Kraiger, K. (2013). Older adults and the technology-based instruction: Optimizing learning outcomes and transfer. *Academy of Management: Learning and Education, 13*(1), 26–44. Retrieved from http://amle.aom.org/content/13/1/26.short

Yorkston, K. M., Beukelman, D. R., Strand, E. A., & Hakel, M. (2010). *Management of motor speech disorders in children and adults* (3rd ed.). Austin, TX: Pro-ed.

Zusman, E. E. (2012). HCAHPS replaces Press Ganey survey as quality measure for patient hospital experience. *Neurosurgery, 71*(2), 21–24.

For a full suite of assignments and additional learning activities, see the access code at the front of your book.

CHAPTER 6

Comprehensive Assessment of the Older Adult

Lorna Guse

(Competencies 3, 4, 6)

LEARNING OBJECTIVES

At the end of this chapter, the reader will be able to:

> Identify the major components of comprehensive assessment of older adults, including functional, physical, cognitive, psychological, social, and spiritual assessments.
> Name tools that are frequently used in the assessment of older adults.
> Recognize the challenges of conducting comprehensive assessments of older adults.
> Value the role of other health professionals in the assessment of older adults.
> Describe some of the issues in relation to comprehensive assessment of older adults.

KEY TERMS

Agnosia	Osteoarthritis
Aphasia	Osteoporosis
Apraxia	Otosclerosis
Cataracts	Overflow incontinence
Cerumen	Personhood
Constipation	Polydipsia
Dysphagia	Polyphagia
Excess disability	Polyuria
Functional incontinence	Presbycusis
Glaucoma	Presbyopia
Health literacy	Stress incontinence
Ketones	Treatment options
Longevity	Urge incontinence
Macular degeneration	

The basis of an individualized plan of care for an older adult is a comprehensive assessment. Enhanced skills in comprehensive geriatric assessment can improve health outcomes, increase nursing assessment confidence, and provide a role model for healthcare teams (Stolee et al., 2003). Assessment has been described as the cornerstone of gerontological nursing, and the goal is to conduct a systematic and integrated assessment (Olenek, Skowronski, & Schmaltz, 2003). The health and healthcare needs of older adults are complex, deriving from a combination of age-related changes, age-associated and other diseases, heredity, and lifestyle. Assessment requires knowledge and an understanding of these complex factors, and a comprehensive baseline assessment is necessary in order to recognize changes that occur in relation to these complex factors. In assessing and providing care to older adults, nurses are members of a healthcare team that includes physicians, therapists, social workers, spiritual care workers, pharmacists, nutritionists, and others. Each member of the team has a contribution to make, and nurses should draw upon the knowledge of other team members to enhance the assessment process.

Comprehensive assessments can be lengthy, and this presents a challenge to nurses because depending on health status and energy level, the older adult may not be well or strong enough for an extensive physical or verbal-based assessment. If the older adult is experiencing memory problems, the reliability of question-based assessment may be suspect. The role of the family and particularly family caregivers (often spouses and adult children) adds another dimension. The literature suggests that when family members act as proxies for health information, there can be underestimates and overestimates of functional ability, cognition, and social functioning (Ostbye, Tyas, McDowell, & Koval, 1997). Assessment tools do not always identify the source of information, and even experienced nurses sometimes rely too much on secondary sources such as family members and caregivers rather than focusing on the older adult as the primary source of information (Luborsky, 1997). This is important to note, as a study compared preferences of nursing home residents with dementia with those as reported by their family members and nursing staff; the authors found that family and staff were relatively inaccurate in determining the preferences of residents (Mesman, Buchanan, Husfeldt, & Berg, 2011).

Since the early 1960s, when major tools to measure function were introduced, the number of assessment tools from which nurses can choose has increased exponentially. Part of this increase has been due to the refinement of existing tools and the testing and tailoring of tools across patient populations, as well as the creation of new tools. The current growth in the development of clinical practice guidelines has not yet reached the stage where nurses have identified a complete roster of the "best" tools to use with older adults across all settings for specific areas of assessment (see http://www.consultgerirn.org for examples). However, certain tools are used by nurses because they have been used traditionally to provide a foundation for decision-making and intervention strategies. In this chapter, we will identify these common tools and provide guidelines for assessment. In addition, several of the chapters in this text give examples of assessment tools related to specific content.

A cautionary note is needed. Comprehensive assessment is not a neutral process; the sources of information and tools used as well as the nurse's skill level have consequences for the older adult's individualized plan of care. The physical and social environment can support or suppress an older adult's abilities. Comprehensive assessment consists of objective and subjective elements, and how the assessment data are interpreted is of major importance. As Kane (1993) has suggested, interpretation is an art, and it is an art that nurses must aspire to master both as students and as practitioners.

Functional Assessment

Nurses typically conduct a functional assessment in order to identify an older adult's ability to perform self-care, self-maintenance, and physical activities, then plan appropriate nursing interventions based on the results. There are two approaches: One approach is to ask questions about ability, and the other approach is to observe ability through evaluating task completion. However, although we tend to speak of "ability," our verbal and observational tools tend to screen for "disability." Disability refers to the impact that health problems have on an individual's ability to perform tasks, roles, and activities, and it is often measured by asking questions about the performance of activities of daily living (ADLs) (such as eating and dressing) and instrumental activities of daily living (IADLs) (such as meal preparation and hobbies) (Verbrugge & Jette, 1994). The basis of our understanding of ability, disability, physical function, ADLs, and any contextual factors comes from work initiated by the World Health Organization (WHO) almost 30 years ago.

The International Classification of Impairment, Disability and Handicap (ICIDH) was first published by the WHO in 1980. It suggested relationships among impairment, disability, and handicap. In attempting to move away from a disease perspective and toward a health perspective, the WHO discontinued using the term handicap and made definitional changes, creating a new International Classification of Functioning, Disability, and Health (ICIDH-2) in 2001 (World Health Organization, 2001). The ICIDH-2 uses the term *disability* to reflect limitations in activities based on an interaction between the individual's health (including impairment, or problems in body function or structure) and the physical, social, and attitudinal environment. This broader perspective on health, activity, and environment is illustrated in the WHO definitions provided in **Box 6-1**. Kearney and Pryor (2004) have suggested that nursing has not yet integrated the ICIDH-2 framework into research, practice, and education; specifically, they suggest that the ICIDH-2 framework provides nurses with a broad structure "to address more fully, activity limitations and participation restrictions associated with impairment" (2004, p. 166). Moreover, they argue that in nursing education, students should be encouraged to develop "a healthcare plan that outlines strategies to promote maximum health, function, well-being, independence and participation in life for the individual" (2004, p. 167). Kearney and Pryor are, in fact, promoting an "ability" perspective rather than emphasizing deficits.

Taking an ability perspective on comprehensive assessment of older adults builds upon the ICIDH-2 framework and is informed by the work of Kearney and Pryor (2004) and others. Functional assessment should first emphasize an older adult's ability and the appropriate nursing interventions to support, maintain, and maximize ability; second, it should focus on an older adult's disability and the appropriate nursing interventions to compensate for and prevent further disability. Nursing interventions that create excess disability are not appropriate. *Excess disability* is defined as "functional disability greater than that warranted by actual physical and physiological impairment of the individual" (Kahn, 1964, p. 112). For example, assisting an older adult in a nursing home to get dressed in the morning when that individual is mentally and physically able to do this task creates excess disability, curbs independence, and discourages optimal wellness.

Tools to assess functional ability tend to address self-care (basic activities of daily living, or ADLs), higher-level activities necessary to live independently in the community (instrumental activities of daily living, or IADLs), or highest-level activities (advanced activities of daily living, or AADLs) (Adnan, Chang,

---

BOX 6-1 World Health Organization (2001) ICIDH-2 Definitions

In the context of health:

Body functions are the physiological functions of body systems (including psychological functions).

Body structures are anatomical parts of the body such as organs, limbs, and their components.

Impairments are problems in body function or structure such as significant deviation or loss.

Activity is the execution of a task or action by an individual.

Participation is involvement in a life situation.

Activity limitations are difficulties an individual may have in executing activities.

Participation restrictions are problems an individual may experience in involvement in life situations.

Environmental factors make up the physical, social, and attitudinal environment in which people live and conduct their lives.

Arseven, & Emanuel, 2005). AADLs include societal, family, and community roles, as well as participation in occupational and recreational activities.

In selecting or using tools to measure functional ability, the nurse must be clear on two questions. First, is performance or capacity being assessed? Some tools ask, "Do you dress without help?" (performance) whereas others ask, "Can you dress without help?" (capacity). Asking about capacity places the emphasis on ability. The second question is, "Who is the source of information on functional ability?" Is information gained verbally from the family or from the older adult? Does the nurse assess functional ability by direct observation or by relying on the observations of others?

In 1987, the Omnibus Budget Reconciliation Act (OBRA) mandated the use of the Minimum Data Set (MDS) in all Medicaid-and Medicare-funded nursing homes. This assessment tool attempted to identify a resident's strengths, preferences, and functional abilities in a systematic way in order to better address his or her needs. The MDS was revised in 1995 and a home-based version was also later developed. In this chapter, we will not be looking at this particular assessment tool. Instead, examples of tools to assess functional ability will be presented in relation to ADL, IADL, and AADL. In addition, the use of physical performance measures will be discussed in relation to functional assessment.

Activities of Daily Living

The original ADL tool was developed by Katz and his colleagues during an 8-year period at the Benjamin Rose Hospital, a geriatric hospital in Cleveland, Ohio, using observations of patients with hip fractures and their performance of activities during recovery (Katz, Ford, Moskowitz, Jackson, & Jaffee, 1963). The Katz Index of ADL (Katz, Down, Cash, & Grotz, 1970) distinguished between independence and dependence in activities and created an ordered relationship among ADLs. It addressed the need for assistance in bathing, eating, dressing, transfer, toileting, and continence.

Other similar tools followed the Katz Index of ADL and are still being developed and refined. These tools can be divided into those that are generic and those that are disease-or illness-specific. Some tools are designed to provide a more sensitive assessment of ability for older adults with cognitive limitations. Such tools attempt to separate disability stemming from cognitive limitations from those caused by physical limitations. Generally speaking, since the early work of Katz and his colleagues, there has been an emphasis on more detailed assessments of ADL. Unfortunately, the development of different tools with different foci (for example, performance vs. capacity) has tended to create confusion because these differences can lead to varying outcomes (Parker & Thorslund, 2007).

One widely used ADL tool is the Barthel Index (Mahoney & Barthel, 1965). This index was designed to measure functional levels of self-care and mobility, and it rates the ability to feed and groom oneself, bathe, go to the toilet, walk (or propel a wheelchair), climb stairs, and control bowel and bladder. Tasks typically assessed with ADL tools are listed in **Box 6-2**. In using the Barthel Index or any ADL assessment tool, it is critical that the assessment be detailed and individualized. For example, the Barthel item for "personal toilet" includes several

---

BOX 6-2 Tasks Typically Assessed with ADL Assessment Tools	
Eating	Ascending/descending stairs
Dressing	Communication
Bathing/washing	Transferring (e.g., from bed to chair)
Grooming	Toileting (bowel and bladder)
Walking/ambulation	

tasks (wash face, comb hair, shave, clean teeth), and the older adult may be independent in some but not all of them and may require an assistive device for some but not all of them. A detailed assessment will provide information for appropriate nursing interventions, that is, those designed to promote ability and compensate for and prevent further disability for that individual.

Some older adults, specifically those with cognitive limitations but with good physical abilities, can manage their ADLs with direction and support (cueing and supervising). As pointed out by Tappen (1994), most ADL assessment tools were developed for physically impaired individuals and "are not sensitive to the functional difficulties experienced by the persons with Alzheimer's disease and related dementia" (1994, p. 38). The Refined ADL Assessment Scale is composed of 14 separate tasks within 5 selected ADL areas (toileting, washing, grooming, dressing, and eating) (Tappen, 1994). This scale represents an approach to ADL assessment known as "task segmentation," which means breaking down the ADL activity into smaller steps (Morris & Morris, 1997). For example, the steps of washing one's hands or getting dressed in the morning are fairly complex for someone with cognitive limitations. However, by cueing as needed, the nurse can assess which of the steps are challenging and which are not. In getting dressed in the morning, some older adults with cognitive limitations will require help in selecting clothing, but once these clothing pieces are selected and laid out, the older adult may require limited cueing to progress through the complex task of dressing. Beck (1988) has developed a dressing assessment tool for persons with cognitive limitations that is particularly detailed. Another consideration for assessment is the use of assistive devices to support older adults and their ADLs. The development and use of assistive devices has increased among all segments of the older adult population, from those in nursing homes to those living in the community. It is important to ask about such devices and how they are used to perform ADLs.

The most common ADL scale used in rehabilitation of older adults is the Uniform Data System for Medical Rehabilitation (UDSMR) Functional Independence Measure (FIM). The FIM instrument scores a person from 1 (needing total assistance or not testable) to 7 (complete independence) and is considered a reliable and valid tool. Categories measured include self-care, bowel and bladder, transfer, locomotion, communication, and social cognition (UDSMR, 1996). This measure is done at admission, discharge, and several times in between to assess progress in rehabilitation.

Instrumental Activities of Daily Living

IADLs include a range of activities that are considered to be more complex compared with ADLs and address the older adult's ability to interact with his or her environment and community. It is readily apparent that items in IADL assessment tools are geared more for older adults living in the community; for example, items often ask about doing the laundry or shopping for groceries. It has also been suggested that IADL tools emphasize tasks traditionally associated with women's work in the home (Lawton, 1972). IADLs include the ability to use the telephone, cook, shop, do laundry and housekeeping, manage finances, take medications, and prepare meals. Missing from most IADL tools are activities that may be more associated with men, such as fixing things around the house or lawn care. One of the earliest IADL measures was developed by Lawton and Brody (1969). Tasks typically assessed with IADL tools are listed in **Box 6-3**.

Advanced Activities of Daily Living

AADLs include societal, family, and community roles, as well as participation in occupational and recreational activities. AADL assessment tools tend to be used less often by nurses and more often by occupational therapists and recreation workers to address specific areas of social tasks. One tool that seems to combine elements of ADLs, IADLs, and AADLs is the Canadian Occupational Performance Measure (COPM) (Chan & Lee, 1997). Developed by Law and colleagues (1994), this tool is designed to detect changes in self-perception of occupational performance over time.

BOX 6-3   Tasks Typically Assessed with IADL Assessment Tools

Using the telephone	Light or heavy housekeeping
Taking medications	Light or heavy yard work
Shopping	Home maintenance
Handling finances	Using transportation
Preparing meals	Leisure/recreation
Laundry	

The COPM asks older adults to identify daily activities that are difficult for them to do but, at the same time, are self-perceived as being important to do. The tool asks about self-care activities (personal care, functional mobility, and community management), productivity (paid/unpaid work, household management, and play/school), and leisure (quiet recreation, active recreation, and socialization). Consequently, interventions to enhance and support ability are planned to address those activities of importance to the older adult. The strength of the COPM is that it focuses on the older adult's functional priorities by asking about importance so that interventions can be tailored to enhance those priority activities and increase satisfaction.

Physical Performance Measures

One of the criticisms directed toward ADL and IADL assessment tools is that they are highly subjective, relying on the perspectives of older adults (and sometimes their family members) or on healthcare professionals who may tend to be more conservative in estimating ability (Guralnik, Branch, Cummings, & Curb, 1989). In contrast, physical performance measures involve direct observation of activities, such as observing the older adult prepare and eat a meal, but also include tasks related to balance, gait, and the ability to reach and bend. The Physical Performance Test (PPT) is one example of a physical performance assessment tool (Reuben & Sui, 1990). The seven-item version asks the individual to write a sentence, transfer five kidney beans from an emesis basin to a can (one at a time), put on and remove a jacket, pick up a penny from the floor, turn 360 degrees, and walk 50 feet (Reuben, Valle, Hays, & Sui, 1995).

The benefit of using physical performance measures is related to a potential relationship between physical ability and functional ability. The question is, does assessment of physical performance relate meaningfully to the ADL and IADL abilities of older adults? Does difficulty with walking and climbing stairs, for example, go hand-in-hand with ADL and IADL abilities such as toileting or grocery shopping? Findings have been inconsistent due at least in part to the several ways of measuring physical performance and functional ability. Some studies have suggested that physical performance measures provide good information to identify older adults who may be at risk for losing functional ability in ADL and becoming prone to falls (Gill, Williams, & Tinetti, 1995; Tinetti, Speechley, & Ginter, 1988).

Physical Assessment

Conducting a physical assessment of an older adult is based on technical competence in physical assessment, knowledge of the normal changes (Chapter 4) and diseases associated with aging, and good communication skills (Chapter 5). In this chapter, a basis in technical competence is taken for granted and the emphasis is on presenting physical assessment information that is particularly relevant to the older adult (see **Case Study 6-1**). Physical assessment with a "systems" approach reviews each body system by first taking a history and then conducting a physical examination. It is important to ask questions that produce an accurate description of the older adult's

Case Study 6-1

You are visiting an older couple in the community in order to assess the couple's functional ability and the potential for their needing assistance with ADLs or IADLs. Mr. and Mrs. Boyd are 72 and 67 years old, respectively, and have been married for 45 years. They have lived in the same neighborhood since Mr. Boyd retired from his bank manager job 12 years ago. Mrs. Boyd has been a housewife since her marriage. Mr. and Mrs. Boyd have one child, a son who lives in another city about 500 miles away. There are no other family members in their community.

As you sit with both of them at the kitchen table, Mrs. Boyd tells you to direct all your questions to her because Mr. Boyd has trouble understanding questions. She goes on to explain that Mr. Boyd used to garden and maintain the yard but no longer seems interested in doing anything. He sleeps a great deal, seems to be eating less, and is often uncommunicative when she speaks to him. She says that her husband is getting quite forgetful and that this worries her because he was always socially engaging and a man who could speak on several subjects.

Mrs. Boyd tells you that she makes all the decisions and spends most of her time planning meals, doing housework, and attending her ladies' church group. She says that she could really use some help with outdoor tasks because these tasks had been handled by Mr. Boyd until just recently. When you ask what she means by "recently," Mrs. Boyd replies that a change seems to have occurred within the last 6 months.

You thank Mrs. Boyd for sharing this information with you, and you indicate that most of the questions can be directed to her but that you will be asking Mr. Boyd some questions as part of the assessment. Mrs. Boyd seems concerned by this but agrees to give you an opportunity to try and ask some questions of Mr. Boyd. You begin your assessment by asking Mrs. Boyd about her functional abilities, including ADLs and IADLs, indicating that you will be asking the same questions of Mr. Boyd.

Questions:

1. Drawing from the 10 principles of comprehensive assessment (Box 6-9) and your knowledge of functional, physical, cognitive, psychological, social, and spiritual assessment of older adults, what are the areas of assessment that you think should be explored first with Mr. and Mrs. Boyd?
2. Will you be relying on self-report, proxy report, performance measures, or all of these for the assessment?
3. Mrs. Boyd seems to want to dominate the interview. How will this affect the assessment process?
4. Which other health professionals do you think should be involved directly or in consultation in relation to your assessment?

physical health status, and furthermore, explore the meaning and implications of physical health status on an individual basis. The same changes in visual acuity for two older adults may have quite different meanings and implications—for one older adult, the changes may not affect their everyday activities whereas for the other, they may mean the loss of a driver's license and accompanying distress and hardship in relation to unmet transportation needs and decreased social contact.

Physical assessment by body systems usually involves a healthcare team approach. Physicians, including specialists such as a cardiologist, and nurses are key members of the team. Nurses often do an initial assessment or act as case finders in the community and in clinics. Other members of the healthcare team include a nutritionist, respiratory therapist, social worker, kinesiologist, physical therapist, and psychologist.

Circulatory Function

Several factors play a role in older adults and their circulatory status. Age-related changes in the heart muscle and blood vessels result in overall decreased cardiac function. These changes plus lifestyle, including limited exercise and physical activity, increase the likelihood that older adults will experience diminished circulatory function. Other lifestyle factors that have an impact on circulatory function are smoking behaviors and the consumption of alcohol. When the current cohort of older adults was young, the benefits of exercise and physical activity and the detrimental effects of smoking were not common knowledge. The social context was different compared with our current one.

The cumulative effects of age-related changes, heredity, and lifestyle mean that there can be great variation among older adults in relation to their circulatory function. In addition, through the use of medications and assistive devices, diminished circulatory function may have a greater or lesser impact on their day-to-day life. Although diseases of the circulatory system can occur at all ages, these diseases are associated with people in their older years, and comprehensive assessment will include taking a cardiac history and performing a physical examination.

The circulatory health assessment should address family history; current problems with chest pain or discomfort, especially if associated with exertion; current diagnoses and associated medications as well as over-the-counter and herbal medicines; sources of stress; and adherence to current medical regimens. The assessment should also include a physical examination, assessing blood pressure, listening to chest sounds, and taking a pulse rate. Other assessment protocols may include an exercise stress test, blood and serum tests, electrocardiograms, and other tests for imaging and assessing the condition of the heart and blood vessels. These advanced laboratory assessment protocols are usually ordered by physicians and the results are shared by the healthcare team as detailed assessment information.

Respiratory Function

Age-related changes to bones, muscles, lung tissue, and respiratory fluids all contribute to the respiratory difficulties experienced by some older adults. Older adults are particularly susceptible to respiratory diseases, and the signs of infection may not be as obvious as they are in younger adults; therefore, assessment of respiratory function should occur more often, particularly with older adults who may have compromised respiratory function because of disease, injury, or previous exposure to occupational or environmental pollutants. Older adults who have restricted mobility and are on extended bed rest are especially at risk for respiratory infections and serious sequential complications.

The respiratory assessment should ask about current medications (including prescribed, over-the-counter, and herbal) and take a history of smoking behavior and exposure to environmental pollutants during the life span. Other areas for assessment include current difficulties and anxieties associated with breathing, decreased energy to complete everyday tasks, frequent coughing, and production of excessive sputum. Physical examination includes observation of posture and breathlessness, and listening to chest sounds. Other assessment protocols include blood and pulmonary function tests, chest X-rays, and sputum analysis. Information from these tests assists the nurse in a total assessment of respiratory function.

Gastrointestinal Function

Age-related changes in the gastrointestinal system are not dramatic and therefore, may not be noticed by most older adults. Smooth muscle changes mean decreased peristaltic action and reduced gastric acid secretion, which may affect gastric comfort and appetite. A concern of many older adults is *constipation*, which is usually defined as the lack of a bowel movement for 3 or more days. A lack of dietary fiber, low levels of physical activity, and lack of fluid are associated with constipation among healthy older adults (Annells & Koch, 2003). Constipation is also associated with Parkinson's disease and irritable bowel syndrome or as a side effect of medications, so it should always be investigated (Woodward, 2012). Although the problem of constipation does not always receive serious attention, a review reported that chronic constipation was associated with serious consequences including fecal impaction, incontinence, and delirium, leading to severe curtailment in ADLs and, in some cases, necessitating hospitalization (Tariq, 2007).

Assessment of gastrointestinal function begins with asking about the older adults' usual diet; appetite and changes in appetite; occurrence of nausea, vomiting, indigestion, or other stomach discomforts; and problems with bowel function, including constipation and diarrhea. In relation to constipation, the nurse should ask about exercise, diet, and fluid intake, and whether the older adult is using prescribed, over-the-counter, or herbal remedies to deal with constipation. A 3- to 7-day meal diary can illustrate eating habits that might have an impact on constipation. Older adults with limited incomes may be less likely to purchase fresh fruit and vegetables because of cost; this can lower the ingestion of fresh fruits and vegetables and fluids, which contributes to constipation, as does limited exercise and mobility. Older adults have a diminished sense of thirst, and fluid intake may be inadequate to maintain normal bowel function. Diagnostic testing can include barium enemas and X-rays, stool analysis, and examination of the colon. Older adults residing in nursing homes are especially at risk for dehydration and associated consequences for bowel function (Mentes & Wang, 2011).

Special attention should be directed to changes in appetite and specifically to loss of appetite. Poor appetite with related declines in body weight and energy is often seen as a warning sign that signals future health problems (Morley, 2003). Decreased body weight is associated with negative changes to the skin, making it prone to injury, and reduced caloric intake affects energy levels needed for mobility and other ADLs. Poor appetite is not solely embedded in gastrointestinal function and instead includes aspects of social and psychological function. Mealtime is also a social experience and often involves interaction with others. One study of community-dwelling older adults reported that impaired appetite was associated with depression, poor self-rated health, smoking, chewing problems, visual impairment, and weight loss (Lee et al., 2006).

Oral health assessment is an area often overlooked with older adults, and nurses should routinely ask about oral health practices including brushing, flossing, and regular contact with a dentist. Poor oral care leads to dental caries, dry mouth, and mouth infections as well as systematic infections that can affect cardiac and respiratory function. Examination of the mouth should include observing the condition of the tongue, teeth, and gums for dehydration, infection, and poor oral hygiene. Check dentures to be sure they are well-fitting, particularly if a weight change has occurred. Especially at risk for oral health problems are older adults with limited incomes who cannot manage regular contact with a dentist and older adults in long-term care facilities who lack the physical or cognitive ability to maintain self-care in oral health (Bawden, 2006).

Genitourinary Function

Age-related changes in the genitourinary system along with age-related diseases such as diabetes and hypertension can have a major impact on everyday life. Bladder muscles weaken and bladder capacity is lessened. Difficulties in sensing that the bladder has not emptied may mean that residual urine stays within the bladder, creating a medium for potential infection. Older women are more likely to experience incontinence, which is often related to a history of childbirth or gynecologic surgeries. Gynecologic assessment of older women is an area of assessment that is sometimes neglected. Older women and their caregivers may mistakenly believe that because the childbearing years have passed or because of sexual inactivity, a gynecologic exam is no longer needed (Richman & Drickamer, 2007). The nurse should be asking questions about abnormal bleeding, vaginal discharge, and any urinary symptoms. Pelvic examinations and Pap smears are usually carried out by physicians, but nurses have an important role in identifying the need for this further assessment.

Older men may develop problems with an enlarged prostate that impedes the flow of urine through the urethra. Incontinence is not a normal part of aging; when incidents of incontinence occur regularly, this can lead to embarrassment, restricted social activity, and skin problems. Urinary incontinence can be managed and improved by nursing interventions that involve behavioral *treatment options* (McGuire, 2006). More detailed content on urinary incontinence, assessment, and nursing interventions are presented in Chapter 15. Unmanaged incontinence can have significant consequences to daily life, and unmanaged incontinence in the home environment is a major factor in the decision for nursing home placement.

A serious medical problem, chronic renal failure can arise as a complication of age-related diseases such as diabetes and hypertension. This is a potentially life-threatening illness that requires specialized care and may ultimately mean support through kidney dialysis.

Health history questions should attend to any previous or current difficulties related to the frequency and voluntary flow of urine during either the day or night. If incontinence is a problem, then questions should focus on the type of incontinence: *stress*, *urge*, *functional*, or *overflow* (see Chapter 15). Older adults who have problems with continence may restrict their fluid intake, which will have implications for other body systems, including skin condition and the gastrointestinal system. The nurse should ask about fluid intake, especially caffeine and alcohol (because these substances affect bladder tone) and observe the skin for dehydration. The nurse also should ask about medication use (prescribed, over-the-counter, and herbal remedies). Diagnostic tests include urine analysis tests for blood, bacteria, and other components such as *ketones*. Other diagnostic tests may be ordered by the physician to assess bladder muscle tone and function and prostate size and potential obstructions.

Sexual Function

Two of the prevailing myths in our society are that older adults are neither sexually active nor interested in sexual relationships. This is not the case; however, several factors associated with aging do have an impact on sexual activity, including lack of partner (often through widowhood), chronic illnesses, and medication use that may negatively affect performance and sexual satisfaction. In conducting a comprehensive assessment with an older adult, asking about sexual function is appropriate. However, it is important to be knowledgeable about age-related and disease-associated changes in relation to sexual function and to be sensitive and respectful of privacy because this is clearly a very personal area of human function.

Age-related changes for men include a decrease in the speed and duration of erection; in women there is a decrease in vaginal lubrication. Health and social factors may have a great impact on sexual activity among older adults; chronic illness such as osteoarthritis and diminished positive self-image because of a societal emphasis on youthful beauty are two such factors. Lack of privacy inhibits the expression of sexuality; this in particular can be a deterrent in residential long-term care facilities (Richman & Drickamer, 2007).

Assessment questions should focus on sexual function and whether there have been any changes or concerns. Do not assume that older adults are sexually inactive. Instead, ask about sexual activity and whether there have been changes or concerns in relation to sexuality and sexual activity. Asking these questions can open the door to further dialogue. In the past few years, there has been a great deal of advertising by pharmaceutical companies for erectile dysfunction drugs. The advertising is aimed at middle-aged and older adults, and there may be some natural curiosity about these new drugs. An older adult's questions about enhancement medications might be best answered in consultation with a pharmacist because of potential side effects and interactions with other medications.

Neurological Function

The neurological system affects all other body systems. Age-related changes involve declines in reaction time, kinetic and body balance problems, and sleep disturbances. Age-related diseases such as Alzheimer's disease and Parkinson's disease and other health problems such as stroke can lead to cognitive changes including memory loss, lack of spatial orientation, *agnosia*, *apraxia*, *dysphagia*, *aphasia*, and delirium. Dementia is a collection of diseases where the changes in brain cells and activity lead to progressive loss of mental capacity. Alzheimer's disease is the most common disease of dementia. Cognitive assessment for dementia will be discussed in a later section of this chapter.

> **CLINICAL TIP**
>
> Alzheimer's disease is the most common type of dementia.

Neurological assessment of older adults includes several components. The nurse should ask about medications (prescribed, over-the-counter, and herbal remedies) and any medical diagnosis related to the neurological system, such as history or family history of stroke. The nurse should observe and ask about previous and current impairments in speech, expression, swallowing, memory, orientation, energy level, balance, sensation, and motor function. Other areas of assessment relate to the occurrence of sleep disturbance, tremors, and seizures.

Musculoskeletal Function

Several age-related changes occur in the musculoskeletal system and lead to decreased muscle tone, strength, and endurance. The stiffening of connective tissue (ligaments and tendons) and erosion of articular surfaces of joints create restrictions in joint mobility. Declines in hormone production contribute to bone loss, and the ability to heal is reduced. Common musculoskeletal health problems include *osteoarthritis* and *osteoporosis*. Of particular concern are the risk of falls and the potential for fractures with their associated morbidity and mortality. One commonly used assessment tool for the risk of falls is the Morse Fall Scale; a description of this scale is provided in Chapter 12. In assessing older adults who have a history of falls, the use of fall diaries is recommended, along with training to complete the diaries (Perry et al., 2012).

The most commonly reported illness among older adults is osteoarthritis, and it is more likely to occur in the weight-bearing joints, especially the hips and knees. Because sore and stiff joints are universally associated with aging, older adults and healthcare professionals often take an accepting attitude about these complaints. The nurse should be asking about the history of sore joints: Which joints are affected? How long has there been pain? What kind of pain is it? Does it interfere with everyday activities? Is the pain managed? If so, how is it managed? Is there a history of bone and muscle injuries? Has there been surgery? Have alternative and complementary therapies such as acupuncture or herbal remedies been explored? What are the pertinent lifestyle factors for this older adult, including participating in exercise and physical activity?

Observation of posture, balance, and walking can assist in asking the appropriate questions: Does the older adult favor one side of the body while walking? Are assistive devices such as canes and walkers being used? Canes and walkers should be at the appropriate height in relation to body height. Ask whether an assessment was done by a therapist in selecting the height, weight, and type of cane or walker. In observing walking and rising from a chair, attend to body language and facial expressions that indicate discomfort. Observe and examine the kind of footwear being worn. Does the footwear offer adequate support while promoting good circulation?

The Up and Go Test provides a quick assessment of an older persons mobility and overall function. The nurse should measure a distance of 10 feet from the persons chair and ask the patient to rise, walk to the line, turn, walk back, and sit down. An average time to do this is 10 seconds; greater than 10 seconds may indicate functional problems with ambulation (Reuben et al., 2008).

> **CLINICAL TIP**
>
> The Timed Up and Go Test (TUG) is a reliable measure of overall physical function and mobility for older adults.

Osteoporosis is a major health problem and has an increasingly large impact on disability and the need for supportive and rehabilitative health services (Stone & Lyles, 2006). Osteoporosis causes a gradual loss of bone mass, and bones become porous and vulnerable to fracture. It is associated with aging, heredity, poor calcium and vitamin D intake, hormonal changes, and a sedentary lifestyle. Older adults with osteoporosis experience symptoms of chronic back pain, muscle weakness, joint pain, loss of height, and decrease in mobility. Bone density tests can compare bone mass with individuals of comparable or younger ages as a marker. If needed, calcium and vitamin D intake can be increased through diet or supplements. The nurse should ask about symptoms and whether a bone density test has been carried out; if so, what were the subsequent recommendations? Often the plan of care for osteoporosis is pain control and treatment, so it is important to assess current pain management strategies.

Sensory Function

Age-related and disease-related changes in sensory function can have profound effects on older adults and their day-to-day functioning. Of the five senses—hearing, vision, smell, taste, and touch—it is the occurrence of diminished vision and hearing that seems to have the greatest impact on older adults. Problems with vision or hearing can have negative effects on social interaction and hence on social and psychological health. A study sited in complex continuing care facilities demonstrated that hearing impairment and mood were associated, and that improved hearing was directly related to improved mood and quality of life (Brink & Stones, 2007).

Presbyopia refers to an age-related change in vision. The lens of the eye becomes less elastic and this creates less efficient accommodation of near and distant vision. *Presbycusis* refers to age-related progressive hearing loss. Decrements in vision and hearing can affect communication ability, with potential consequences to older adults' health, safety, everyday activities, socialization, and quality of life. Screening tools for vision and hearing are of two types: self-report and performance-based.

Specifically for vision, difficulty in reading has implications for *health literacy* and safety in relation to reading instructions on prescription bottles and following other written directions for health care. Age-related *macular degeneration*, the deterioration of central vision, is the leading cause of severe vision loss in older adults in the United States. Older adults should undergo regular eye examinations for changes in vision (including the formation *of cataracts*) and screening for ocular pressure (for *glaucoma*). The American Academy of Ophthalmology recommends periodic eye examinations at 1- to 2-year intervals for older adults who do not experience symptoms or high risk factors (Jung, Coleman, & Weintraub, 2007). These performance-based tests are conducted by other health professionals—optometrists and ophthalmologists—but nurses are often in a key position to screen for vision problems and to encourage older adults to initiate and maintain regular visits with other health professionals to assess vision changes.

The following two screening procedures are simple tests for functional vision:

1. Ask the older adult to read a newspaper headline and story and observe for difficulty and accuracy.
2. Ask the older adult to read the prescription bottle and, again, observe for difficulty and accuracy.

It is important to follow up with specific questions that explore the vision problem from the perspective of the individual: Is vision a problem? Does it interfere with everyday activities or with hobbies and social life? Are magnification aids or enlarged printed material useful strategies? Is home lighting contributing to the problem? Is it more difficult to see in the evening compared with other times of the day?

Hearing loss is a major concern for many older adults. Furthermore, the perceived stigma of hearing loss and attendant shame may lead some older adults to deny this loss and reject hearing assessment and the use of hearing aids (Wallhagen, 2009). According to the U.S. Census Bureau (Bureau of the Census, 1997), about 30% of older adults between 65 and 74 years of age and 50% of those between 75 and 79 years of age experience some hearing loss. Most hearing loss in older adults is both symmetric and bilateral, and hearing problems are exacerbated in a noisy environment. Non-aging-related hearing loss can be attributed to *cerumen* impaction, infection, occurrence of a foreign body, or *otosclerosis*. Assessment questions should ask about any hearing problems and how these problems affect the older adults' everyday life. The following question is useful in assessing ear and hearing problems: Are you experiencing a hearing problem or any ear pain, ringing in the ears, or ear discharge? One study reported that asking, "Do you have a hearing problem now?" was effective in screening for hearing loss among older adults (Gates, Murphy, Rees, & Fraher, 2003). An initial assessment question might be, "When is your hearing loss the biggest problem for you?" The nurse who assesses hearing function is in a good position to recommend further diagnostic testing with an audiologist.

CLINICAL TIP

Never overlook the obvious and most simple explanation for confusion—it could be impacted wax in the ears.

For older adults who wear hearing aids, the condition and working order of these aids is often overestimated and should be regularly assessed and monitored. One study conducted in a retirement community reported that for most of those wearing hearing aids, a visual check indicated problems with either broken or missing components, inappropriate volume setting, or weak or dead batteries, and this was especially true for those older adults who were relatively dependent on nursing care (Culbertson, Griggs, & Hudson, 2004).

The other senses are taste, smell, and touch. Taste and smell are interrelated; the sense of smell influences the sense of taste for food as well as appetite. Although there are some age-related changes (e.g., fewer taste receptors), older adults who are experiencing a noticeable loss of taste and smell generally have other medical conditions (Ferrini & Ferrini, 2012). Medical conditions, especially those affecting the nose; medication side effects; nutritional deficiencies; poor oral hygiene; alcohol use; and smoking can all detrimentally affect the senses of smell and taste. Assessments should ask generally about satisfaction with taste and smell, the duration and extent of the problem, and the impact of the problem on everyday life.

Integumentary Function

Age-related changes to the skin include loss of elasticity, slower regeneration of cells, diminished gland secretion, reduced blood supply, and structural changes, including loss of fat. This means that the skin of older adults is more susceptible to injury and infection and less resilient in terms of repair. Older adults with decreased mobility and extended bed rest are at high risk for skin damage and breakdown. For many older adults, skin dryness and itching are two common complaints. Emollients and powders can bring relief for most minor skin conditions.

Asking questions about skin problems and concerns and inspecting the skin are basic elements of assessment and should be done on a regular basis. If skin injury has already occurred, close monitoring and treatment are essential. The nurse should ask about rashes, itching, dryness, frequent bruising, and any open sores. Skin conditions can be linked with nutritional status and body weight, and the nurse can work with a nutritionist to promote a healthy diet and appropriate weight. Any loss of sensation, particularly in extremities, is a cause of concern. Impeded circulation with lack of sensation can lead to untreated skin breakdown, and prevention is preferable to the more serious consequences of infection and disability. In the event of wounds, there are assessment tools to gauge the extent and level, The NPUAP-EPUAP Pressure Ulcer Classification System, which is described in more detail in Chapter 18. Nurses with expertise in wound care, a specialized area of nursing practice, are usually available in acute and long-term care for consultation and advice.

The older adults' skin should be observed for color, hydration, circulation, and intactness. Fluid intake may be less than optimal and result in severe dryness. The nurse should be asking questions about skin changes, signs and symptoms of infection, usual skin care, and problems with healing. The nurse should also observe the fingernails and toenails for splitting and tears.

Endocrine and Metabolic Function

Age-related changes in endocrine function include decreased hormone secretion and breakdown of metabolites. Of special concern for older adults is the onset of diabetes mellitus or thyroid disease because these diseases can be insidious and silent: Much damage to the body can occur even before these conditions are diagnosed. Diabetes mellitus becomes more prevalent with age, but the symptoms *of polydipsia, polyphagia,* and *polyuria* may go unnoticed for several years. Because the thirst sensation diminishes with age, older adults may not be aware of their polydipsia. By the time the disease is diagnosed, more serious complications such as impaired circulation, foot ulcers, and vision disturbances may have ensued.

The more common form of diabetes mellitus among older adults is type 2 or non-insulin-dependent diabetes mellitus. With age, there is an increased resistance to the action of insulin within the body, and this change, in combination with lifestyle choices, places some older adults at inordinate risk for developing this disease. Age-related changes, heredity, obesity, poor nutrition, inadequate physical activity, and other illnesses increase the likelihood of type 2 diabetes among older adults. Given that the disease may be silent for many years, it is critical that nurses be attuned to assessing for the risk for developing diabetes among older adults and monitor changes and symptoms at every opportunity. As part of the health history, the following areas should be addressed:

> Family history of diabetes
> Changes in weight and appetite
> Fatigue
> Increased thirst and fluid intake
> Vision problems
> Slow wound healing
> Headache
> Gastrointestinal problems

More specific symptoms should be further assessed, including occurrence of polyphagia, polydipsia, and polyuria. Diagnostic tests such as fasting blood sugar can provide a definitive diagnosis. The oral glucose tolerance test is of little value by itself because the older adult may have impaired glucose tolerance but not diabetes (Armetta & Molony, 1999).

In terms of thyroid disease, the formation of nodules that interfere with normal thyroid functioning becomes more common with age. Unfortunately, hypothyroidism and associated symptoms of fatigue, forgetfulness, and cold sensitivity may be seen as normal "slowing down" with age and go undetected. Hyperthyroidism is much more likely in the older years, but among older adults, the typical symptoms of restlessness and hyperactivity may be lacking.

For older adults, hyperthyroidism, or an overproduction of thyroid hormone, does not usually mean major changes to everyday life. Nursing observation and assessment questions should address the occurrence of nervousness, heat intolerance, weight loss, tremor, and palpitations. Hypothyroidism, or below normal levels of thyroid hormone, causes several changes that can be uncomfortable and distressing. In the health history, the nurse should be assessing for skin changes (dry, flaky), fluid retention (edema and weight gain), fatigue, forgetfulness, constipation, and unusual sensitivity to the cold. Diagnostic tests (TSH test, TRH test, and radioimmunoassay) provide definitive diagnosis.

Hematologic and Immune Function

Several factors affect older adults' hematologic and immune systems. In relation to hematologic function, anemia is a common disorder among older adults, especially among those in nursing homes: About 40% of adults age 60 or older have iron-deficiency anemia. Although a slight decrease in hemoglobin occurs with aging, more often the anemia is attributable to an iron deficiency or another illness. Assessment should focus on observation of the color and quality of the skin and nail beds, and address food choices and food habits. Of a more serious nature, iron deficiency can occur because of blood loss, and the nurse should ask questions about occurrence of blood in stools. Diagnostic tests include hemoglobin, hematocrit, complete blood count (CBC), and red blood cell (RBC) count.

The immune system functions to protect the body from bacteria, viruses, and other microorganisms. Age-related changes to the immune system include diminished lymphocyte function and antibody immune responses. These changes put older adults at risk for infections. Vaccines for influenza and pneumonia are given in the fall and are available in physicians' offices, public health agencies, and other sites. As part of the assessment, the nurse should ask about recent and current infections and access to and use of vaccines to prevent infections. In terms of the symptoms of infection, it is important to remember that when evaluating vital signs, older adults tend to have a diminished febrile response to infection.

Some nurses are uncomfortable talking with older adults about sexual activity, prophylaxis, and sexually transmitted diseases (STDs), but these questions are an essential part of the health assessment process. Sexually active older adults, particularly those with more than one partner, are at risk for STDs. Of particular concern is the lack of STD education ("safe sex") programs focused on older adults, specifically HIV education. Human immunodeficiency virus (HIV) is a human retrovirus that causes acquired immune deficiency syndrome (AIDS). The disease is spread through parenteral and body fluids. It can be sexually transmitted through anal, oral, and vaginal intercourse.

AIDS is an epidemic in the United States, and the Centers for Disease Control and Prevention (CDC) reports that 11% of those infected are 50 years of age or older. Older adults may not be tested for HIV because they do not believe that they are at high risk or they may be unwilling to discuss their risky sexual behaviors. In terms of assessment, it is important to address the topic of sexual activity and ask the same questions that would be asked of a younger person. Open-ended questions are preferable, and it will be more productive to say, "Tell me about your sex life" rather than simply asking, "Do you have sex?" (Anderson, 2003). Depending on the status of sexual activity, other questions related to sexual preference and number of partners should be pursued. Signs and symptoms associated with HIV, such as weight loss, dehydration, ataxic gait, or fatigue, may go unnoticed or be attributed to age-related changes. However, once risk factors are identified, diagnostic testing will confirm a diagnosis.

Cognitive Assessment

Changes in cognitive function with age vary among older adults and are difficult to separate from other comorbidities (physical and psychological conditions), other age-related changes (e.g., hearing and vision) (see **Box 6-4**), the side effects of medications, and changes in intellectual activity. Generally speaking, older adults manifest a gradual and modest decline in short-term memory and experience a reduction in the speed with which new information is processed.

Cognitive function is usually understood in relation to the qualities of attention, memory, language, visuospatial skills, and executive capacity. The most extensively used cognitive assessment tool is the Mini Mental State Examination (MMSE) (Folstein, Folstein, & McHugh, 1975). The MMSE was originally developed to differentiate organic from functional disorders and to measure change in cognitive impairment, but it was not intended to be used as a diagnostic tool. It measures orientation, registration, attention and calculation, short-term recall, language, and visuospatial function. It does not measure executive function, and the results of the MMSE can vary by age and education, with older individuals and those with fewer years of formal education having lower scores (Crum, Anthony, Bassett, & Folstein, 1993). In addition, some of the MMSE items may be less relevant for older adults who are hospital inpatients or who are living in long-term care facilities (Stewart, O'Riley Edelstein, & Gould, 2012). For example, orientation-based questions regarding dates and day or time may be less relevant for long-term care residents compared with questions that ask about location of their room in the facility. A sample of items from the MoCA is given in **Box 6-5**.

BOX 6-4 Research Highlight

Methods: A sample of 15 community-dwelling women (aged 44–70 years) were interviewed and asked about how they had taken care of themselves since the onset of their visual problems. The qualitative content analysis was guided by the definition of health literacy from the Institute of Medicine (2004) as the ability to "obtain, process, and understand basic health-related information and services needed to make appropriate health decisions."

Findings: The women reported that healthcare workers made the following assumptions: that they could not provide their own self-care, that they were being cared for by personal caregivers,

and they were dependent on government assistance. In addition, women reported that healthcare workers focused on their disability and not on them as persons.

Application to practice: In assessing the health literacy of older adults with visual impairment, nurses should ensure that the assessment is based on identifying ability, respecting personhood, and not making assumptions related to independence and pathology.

Harrison, T. C., Mackert, M., & Watkins, C. (2010). Health literacy issues among women with visual impairments. *Research in Gerontological Nursing*, *3*(1), 49–60.

BOX 6-5 Montreal Cognitive Assessment (MoCA)

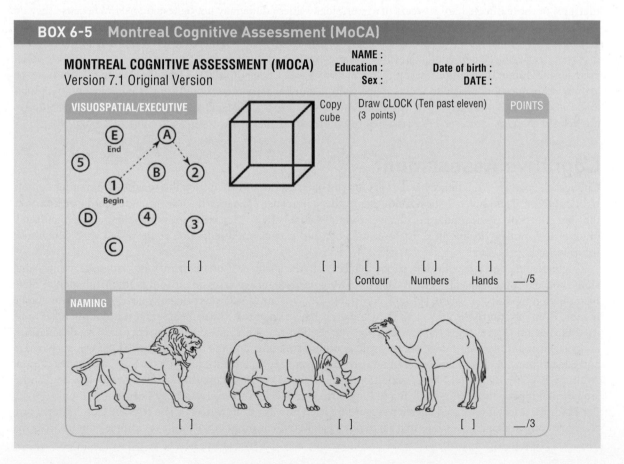

MEMORY	Read list of words, subject must repeat them. Do 2 trials, even if 1st trial is successful. Do a recall after 5 minutes.		FACE	VELVET	CHURCH	DAISY	RED	No points
		1st trial						
		2nd trial						

ATTENTION	Read list of digits (1 digit/sec.).	
	Subject has to repeat them in the forward order [ ] 2 1 8 5 4	
	Subject has to repeat them in the backward order [ ] 7 4 2	___/2

Read list of letters. The subject must tap with his hand at each letter A. No points if ≥ 2 errors.	
[ ] F B A C M N A A J K L B A F A K D E A A A J A M O F A A B	___/1

Serial 7 subtraction starting at 100 [ ] 93 [ ] 86 [ ] 79 [ ] 72 [ ] 65	
4 or 5 correct subtractions: **3 pts**, 2 or 3 correct: **2 pts**, 1 correct: **1 pt**, 0 correct: **0 pt**	___/3

LANGUAGE	Repeat: I only know that John is the one to help today. [ ]	
	The cat always hid under the couch when dogs were in the room. [ ]	___/2

Fluency/Name maximum number of words in one minute that begin with the letter F [ ] (N ≥ 11 words)	___/1

ABSTRACTION	Similarity between e.g. banana - orange = fruit [ ] train - bicycle [ ] watch - ruler	___/2

DELAYED RECALL	Has to recall words **WITH NO CUE**	FACE [ ]	VELVET [ ]	CHURCH [ ]	DAISY [ ]	RED [ ]	Points for UNCUED recall only	___/5
Optional	Category cue							
	Multiple choice cue							

ORIENTATION	[ ] Date [ ] Month [ ] Year [ ] Day [ ] Place [ ] City	___/6

© **Z.Nasreddine MD**   **www.mocatest.org**   Normal ≥ 26/30

Administered by: _____

TOTAL	___/30
Add 1 point if ≤ 12 yr edu	

The Mini-Cog is another screening tool that can be administered in 5 minutes or less and requires minimal training (Doerflinger, 2007). The screening consists of a three-item recall and a clock-drawing test (CDT). This reliable tool can assist nurses with early assessment of cognitive problems. Through the clock test component, the Mini-Cog is used to assess language comprehension, visual—motor skills and executive function while the three-item component assess recall. Because it is a short test, it is seen as less stressful for older adults compared with other tools. A full-text article about the Mini-Cog can be accessed through http://www .consultgerirn.org

Dementia is a permanent progressive decline in cognitive function, and Alzheimer's disease is the most common form of dementia. The *Diagnostic and Statistical Manual of Mental Disorders (DSM-V),* 5th edition (American Psychiatric Association, 2013), used by both the psychiatric and psychological communities, states

BOX 6-6   Recommended Readings

American Geriatrics Society, AGS Panel. (Updated annually). *Geriatrics at your fingertips.* New York, NY: Blackwell.

Baldwin, S., & Capstick, A. (2007). *Tom Kitwood on dementia: A reader and critical commentary.* Buckingham, UK: McGraw-Hill Open University Press.

Kane, R. L., Ouslander, J. G., Abrass, I. B., & Resnick, B. (2013). *Essentials of clinical geriatrics* (7th ed.). New York, NY: McGraw-Hill.

Mast, B. T. (2011). *Whole person dementia assessment.* Baltimore, MD: Health Professionals Press.

that dementia of the Alzheimer's type typically is manifested by both impaired memory (long-or short-term) and inability to learn or recall new information, and is distinguished by one (or more) of the following cognitive disturbances: aphasia, apraxia, agnosia, or disturbance in executive functioning (i.e., planning, organizing, sequencing, abstracting). These cognitive limitations have broad and major implications for occupational and social interaction, as well as safety. The declines associated with Alzheimer's disease are progressive and irreversible. Definitive diagnosis is possible only on autopsy, but diagnosis is made in the absence of alternatives (e.g., brain tumor and other neurological conditions or diseases). Several tools are available to assess cognitive function, and the common element of most is the assessment of memory function (see **Box 6-6**).

For nurses, assessing cognitive function is a challenging task because of the combination of factors that may be interacting: physical and psychological comorbidities, age-related changes, the side effects of medications, and changes in environment, as some examples. Added to this is the concern that for older adults and their families, even the suspicion of Alzheimer's disease can be a frightening and discouraging experience. The behaviors associated with dementia are stigmatizing and concerns arise related not only to the loss of memory, but even more so to the potential loss of the "person" as the disease progresses (Dupuis, Wiersma, & Loiselle, 2012). An influential individual in our understanding of the course and nature of cognitive decline in dementia was Tom Kitwood, who defined *personhood* and pioneered the theory and practice of "person-centered care." Personhood is "a standing or status that is bestowed upon one human being by others, in the context of relationship and social being . . . it implies recognition, respect and trust" (Kitwood, 1997). Kitwood and Bredin (1992) argued that older persons with dementia should be recognized for their uniqueness, their experiential being, and their relatedness with others. Taking this perspective, nursing assessment emphasizes individualization, asking about and taking into account previous preferences for care directly expressed by the older adult with dementia or from family members as proxies, when necessary.

An area of assessment of older adults with dementia that has not been well attended to is that of "social ability." Social abilities include giving and receiving attention, participating in conversation, recognizing social stimuli, appreciating humor, and being helpful to others (Baum, Edwards, & Morrow-Howell, 1993; Dawson, Wells, & Kline, 1993; Sabat & Collins, 1999). Dawson and her colleagues have developed and validated a social abilities assessment subscale that can be used as a basis for supporting and maintaining ability in social life as much as possible. This area of assessment is much neglected and there is an opportunity for nurses to expand thinking in this area and develop ways of assessing the social abilities of older adults with dementia.

Psychological Assessment

Psychological assessment of older adults presents a wide continuum from positive mental health to mental health problems, and the tendency seems to be weighted toward assessment of mental health disorders. In this section we will be looking at two areas of psychological assessment: quality of life, which may include several positive mental health constructs, and depression, a common mental health problem.

Quality of Life

Quality of life and successful aging are two central concepts in assessment and care of older adults. Broadly speaking, quality of life encompasses all areas of everyday life: environmental and material components as well as physical, mental, and social well-being (Fletcher, Dickinson, & Philp, 1992). Quality of life among older adults is highly individualistic, subjective, and multidimensional in scope. With respect to what constitutes quality of life, what is important to one person may be quite unimportant to another. Related to quality of life is the concept of successful aging. Long associated with community living, successful aging has traditionally been linked with physical health, independence, functional ability, and *longevity*. However, other elements such as engagement in social life, self-mastery, optimism,

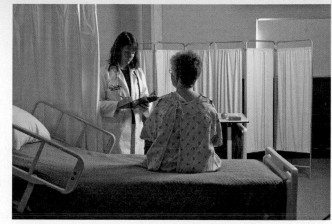

Figure 6-1 Quality care begins with comprehensive assessment.
Photo courtesy of Don Battershall (Hartford Foundation).

personal meaning in life, and attainment of goals have been suggested as vital to the idea of successful aging (Reker, Peacock, & Wong, 1987; Rowe & Kahn, 1997). Elements of successful aging can include self-acceptance, positive relationships with others, and personal growth. A broad conceptualization of successful aging means broad applicability to older adults with varying abilities and disabilities. If we can go beyond the idea of physical health as the primary criterion for successful aging, then we can remove the labeling of frail older adults as being "unsuccessful" in their aging (Guse & Masesar, 1999).

Assessment of quality of life and successful aging can assist in better understanding the psychological health of older adults. Simply put, the following assessment questions will open dialogue on attitude, beliefs, and feelings about aging and mental health (see **Figure 6-1**). For example, the nurse can ask, "How would you describe your quality of life?" and "What would add to your quality of life?" Questions on successful aging are also informative. For example, "Would you describe yourself as someone who is aging successfully?" and "What would help you to age successfully?"

Depression

Clinical depression is the most common mental health problem among older adults, and it often goes undetected because clinicians attribute depressive symptoms to age-associated changes, chronic physical illness, medication side effects, or pain. The consequences of clinical depression can be serious and include suicidal ideation and suicide attempts. The prevalence of clinical depression in older Americans is estimated to be 14%–20% among community-dwelling individuals, 30%–40% among recently hospitalized individuals, and 15%–30% among older persons residing in long-term care facilities (Anstey, von Sanden, & Sargent-Cox, 2007; Lebowitz et al., 1997; Wilson, Mottram, & Sexsmith, 2007). Minor depression can precede clinical or major depression and can be a response to stressors such as widowhood, loss of independence, or other losses. Older Americans may experience minor depression on a chronic basis but not meet the established criteria for clinical or major depression as outlined in the DSM-V. To meet the DSM-V criteria, an older adult must experience five or more of the following symptoms during a 2-week period (American Psychiatric Association, 2013):

> Sadness
> Lack of enjoyment of previously enjoyed activities

> Significant weight loss
> Sleep disturbance
> Restlessness
> Fatigue
> Feelings of worthlessness
> Impaired ability to think clearly or concentrate
> Suicide ideation or attempt

Depressed older adults may experience difficulty with sleeping, loss of appetite, physical discomfort, anxiety, hopelessness, bouts of crying, and thoughts of suicide. They may feel uncomfortable in social situations and curtail their usual social contacts and events, creating a downward spiral of depression and isolation. A study conducted among rural older adults in public housing facilities reported an association among symptoms of depression, poverty, and social isolation (Fisher & Copenhaver, 2006).

Depression is associated with cognitive limitations, and depressed older adults can experience disorientation, shortened attention span, emotional outbursts, and difficulty in intellectual functioning. Differentiating between dementia and depression when several of the same symptoms are present is a challenge for nurses. An excellent source is the document "Delirium, Dementia and Depression in Older Adults: Assessment and Care" (Registered Nurses' Association of Ontario, 2016), found at the Website http://www.rnao.org. Chapter 11 provides more information on the relationship among dementia, depression, and delirium.

The Geriatric Depression Scale (GDS) is widely used by nurses to assess symptoms of depression. The interviewer asks the older person a set of 30 questions with possible answers of yes or no. A "negative" response, which depending on the question may be a yes or no answer, is scored as one point; a higher score indicates more symptoms of depression. A score of 0–30 is possible, with 0–9 being normal, 10–19 indicating mild depression, and 20–30 indicating severe depressive symptoms. The 30-item GDS is provided in **Box 6-7**, and the capitalized responses are to be used in the scoring of responses.

Clinical depression may be chronic or have a shorter duration, and it is not the same as experiencing temporary feelings of unhappiness, confused thinking, and somatic complaints. Nurses are in a good position, whether it be in community, acute care, or long-term care practice, to screen for potential depression (Bruno & Ahrens, 2003). One study found that questions asking about functional ability decline, visual impairment, memory impairment, and using three or more medications provided a reasonably good screen for depressive symptoms and consequential health service utilization (Dendukuri, McCusker, & Belzile, 2004). Even asking the question, "Do you often feel sad or depressed?" is likely to open discussion and lead to further assessment of feelings of depression (Mahoney et al., 1994). Treatment of depression requires the input and knowledge base of several disciplines (Wang, 2011).

Social Assessment

Social functioning affects health and disease outcomes, and health status affects the ability to socialize and interact with others (Tomaka, Thompson, & Palacios, 2006). As people age, they may find that their social networks become smaller, and this may place them at risk in several ways. Decades of research have told us that individuals with low quantity and quality of social relationships have a higher morbidity and mortality risk compared with those who have a good quantity and quality of social contacts. A supportive social network and in particular the presence of a spouse can act to maintain an older adult in the community; the lack of a partner is a predictor of nursing home placement.

Social assessment of older adults includes collecting information on the presence of a social network and on the interaction between the older adult and family, friends, neighbors, and community. Kane, Ouslander, and

BOX 6-7   Geriatric Depression Scale (1983)

1. Are you basically satisfied with your life? Yes/No
2. Have you dropped many of your activities or interests? Yes/No
3. Do you feel that your life is empty? Yes/No
4. Do you often get bored? Yes/No
5. Are you hopeful about the future? Yes/No
6. Are you bothered by thoughts you can't get out of your head? Yes/No
7. Are you in good spirits most of the time? Yes/No
8. Are you afraid that something bad is going to happen to you? Yes/No
9. Do you feel happy most of the time? Yes/No
10. Do you often feel helpless? Yes/No
11. Do you often get restless and fidgety? Yes/No
12. Do you prefer to stay at home, rather than going out and doing new things? Yes/No
13. Do you frequently worry about the future? Yes/No
14. Do you feel that you have more problems with memory than most? Yes/No
15. Do you think that it is wonderful to be alive now? Yes/No
16. Do you often feel downhearted and blue? Yes/No
17. Do you feel pretty worthless the way you are now? Yes/No
18. Do you worry a lot about the past? Yes/No
19. Do you find life very exciting? Yes/No
20. Is it hard to you to get started on new projects? Yes/No
21. Do you feel full of energy? Yes/No
22. Do you feel that your situation is hopeless? Yes/No
23. Do you think that most people are better off than you are? Yes/No
24. Do you frequently get upset over little things? Yes/No
25. Do you frequently feel like crying? Yes/No
26. Do you have trouble concentrating? Yes/No
27. Do you enjoy getting up in the morning? Yes/No
28. Do you prefer to avoid social gatherings? Yes/No
29. Is it easy for you to make decisions? Yes/No
30. Is your mind as clear as it used to be? Yes/No

Reproduced from Yesavage, J. A., Brink, T. L., Rose, T. L., Lum, O., Huang, V., Adey, M. M., Leirer, V. O. (1983). Development and validation of a geriatric depression scale: A preliminary report. *Journal of Psychiatric Research, 17,* 37–49. Reprinted with permission.

Abrass (2013) developed a broad-based social assessment that includes asking questions about recent life events (such as death of a spouse), living arrangements, everyday activities requiring help (and who usually provides help), potential isolation (frequency of leaving the house and having visitors), adequacy of income, and sources of healthcare coverage (see **Box 6-8** for additional resources). Posed by the nurse, these general questions can identify areas of limitation in social contact and social support.

Having a social network of friends and family does not necessarily mean that there are social supports. However, the Lubben Social Network Scale contains 10 items, 3 of which have been found to differentiate those who are isolated from those who are not (Kane, 1995). These questions are:

> Is there any one special person you could call or contact if you needed help?
> In general, other than your children, how many relatives do you feel close to and have contact with at least once a month?
> In general, how many friends do you feel close to and have contact with at least once a month?

BOX 6-8   Resource List

Hospital Elder Life Program (http://www .hospitalelderlifeprogram.org): The Hospital Elder Life Program (HELP) is a patient-care program, developed by doctors and nurses at the Yale School of Medicine, that is designed to prevent delirium among hospitalized older patients.

The John A. Hartford Foundation Institute for Geriatric Nursing (http://www.hartfordign.org and http://www.consultgerirn.org): These Websites offer links to several assessment tools, including SPICES (an overall assessment tool), Fall Risk Assessment, and the Geriatric Depression Scale.

National Institute for Health and Clinical Excellence (NICE) (http://www.nice.org.uk): This

agency is an excellence-in-practice organization responsible for providing national guidance on the promotion of good health and the prevention and treatment of ill health in the United Kingdom. The Website offers assessment and prevention tools in relation to falls and older adults.

Registered Nurses' Association of Ontario (http://www.rnao.org): This is the professional association of registered nurses in Ontario, Canada. It provides several best practices including assessment guidelines, for example, in the areas of pain; stage I to IV pressure ulcers; foot ulcers for people with diabetes; and screening for delirium, dementia, and depression in older adults.

The more important aspects of social support may be the number of supportive persons and the various types of support (emotional, instrumental, and informational) that are available. Seeman and Berkman (1988) have identified four questions that assess the adequacy of social support. These questions are:

> When you need help, can you count on anyone for house cleaning, groceries, or a ride?
> Could you use more help with daily tasks?
> Can you count on anyone for emotional support (talking over problems or helping you make a decision)?
> Could you use more emotional help (receiving sufficient support)?

Asking these kinds of questions will help assess the adequacy and range of support available to an older adult. Nurses should be asking questions about social support and social function as part of the comprehensive assessment. The questions developed by Lubben can be used with older adults generally across settings (community and acute and long-term care settings), whereas some of the questions posed by Seeman and Berkman (1988) clearly relate to older adults living in the community.

Spiritual Assessment

Spiritual assessment is an integral part of comprehensive assessment and provides a basis for an individualized plan of care (Forbes, 1994). Although there is a link between religiosity and spirituality, the two concepts are not synonymous. Religiosity refers to believing in God, organized rituals, and specific dogma; spirituality refers more broadly to ideas of belief that encompass personal philosophy and an understanding of meaning and purpose in life. Having religious beliefs may foster spirituality, but those without formal religious beliefs still can experience spirituality. Most health service intake forms have a place for collecting information on formal religious affiliation, but this does not necessary mean that the older adult is practicing his or her faith, or is active in a place of worship.

CLINICAL TIP

A spiritual assessment is equally important as assessing other body systems.

One of the earliest guidelines for spiritual assessment was developed by Stoll (1979), and it contains questions that address both religiosity and spirituality. The guidelines are divided into four areas:

1. The concept of God or deity (e.g., "Is religion or God significant to you?")
2. Personal source of strength and hope (e.g., "What is your source of strength and hope?")
3. Significance of religious practices and rituals (e.g., "Are there any religious practices that are important to you?")
4. Perceived relationship between spiritual belief and health (e.g., "Has being sick made any difference in your feelings about God or the practice of your faith?")

Nurses may not be comfortable conducting a spiritual assessment because it may seem inappropriately invasive or because it is an area that some nurses do not feel adequately prepared to address as an unmet need. If the intake record indicates a formal religious affiliation, then it is fairly straightforward to ask, "Do you have any religious needs?" or "Would you like to speak with a pastoral care worker?" Questions that address spirituality can begin by asking, "Are you having a spiritual need? Is there some way that I might help with your spiritual needs?" Another spiritual assessment question asks, "Have your health problems affected your feelings of meaning or purpose?" Spiritual assessment is an area that would benefit greatly from more research.

Other Assessment: Obesity

Obesity has become a major health problem among Americans, including older Americans, and it is associated with chronic disease and disability (Jensen, 2005). Given the obesity prevalence in middle-aged adults, the proportions and numbers of obese older adults are expected to increase substantially over the next decade (Arterburn, Crane, & Sullivan, 2004). Providing care to obese persons places caregivers, both family and staff members, at risk for injury. In 1998, the National Institutes of Health released the first federal overweight and obesity guidelines, which are based on the body mass index (BMI), a ratio of weight (in pounds) to height (in inches squared), as an assessment tool. The BMI is a number usually between 16 and 40; a BMI between 25 and 29 is considered "overweight" and more than 30 is considered "obese."

The adverse effects of obesity in relation to cardiovascular disease, diabetes, osteoarthritis, and gallbladder disease are well documented (Fields & Strano, 2005). Obese older adults are likely to experience balance and mobility problems that place them at risk for falls. One study reported obesity as being a risk factor for decline in functional ability (as assessed by needing assistance with ADLs and IADLs) (Jensen & Friedmann, 2002). Unfortunately, there has been little research conducted on obese older adults, and this remains an area for further research and tool refinement. It is not clear whether the markers for overweight and obesity are relevant to older adults who may experience illness-related weight gain or loss. It has been suggested that for many older adults, an emphasis on weight maintenance might be the best approach until more evidence is accumulated through research (Jensen & Friedmann, 2002).

Nurses can assess for overweight and obesity using the BMI and by asking about a history of weight change. If food intake is a concern, a common approach is to begin with a 3-to 7-day meal diary. This information can assist in determining a person's food habits. This is an area of assessment where nurses could benefit from working with the nutritionist and the dietician, who have a specialized knowledge base.

Developing an Individualized Plan of Care

At the beginning of this chapter, we indicated that the basis of an individualized plan of care for an older adult is a comprehensive assessment, and we have reviewed functional, physical, cognitive, psychological, social, and spiritual assessment. **Box 6-9** provides 10 guidelines for comprehensive assessment that form a basis with which to develop an individualized plan of care. Additionally, **Box 6-10** provides a summary of the quality assessment tools recommended as best practices by the John A. Hartford Foundation and the Nurse Competence in Aging initiative (see http://www.consultgerirn.org) (**Box 6-11**).

BOX 6-9   Ten Principles of Comprehensive Assessment

1. The cornerstone of an individualized plan of care for an older adult is a comprehensive assessment.
2. Comprehensive assessment takes into account age-related changes, age-associated and other diseases, heredity, and lifestyle.
3. Nurses are members of the healthcare team, contributing to and drawing from the team to enhance the assessment process.
4. Comprehensive assessment is not a neutral process.
5. Ideally, the older adult is the best source of information to assess his or her health. When this is not possible, family members or caregivers are acceptable as secondary sources of information. When the older adult cannot self-report, physical performance measures may provide additional information.
6. Comprehensive assessment should first emphasize ability and then address disability. Appropriate interventions to maintain and enhance ability and to improve or compensate for disability should follow from a comprehensive assessment.
7. Task performance and task capacity are two difference perspectives. Some assessment tools ask, "Do you dress without help?" (performance) whereas others ask, "Can you dress without help?" (capacity). Asking about capacity will result in answers that emphasize ability.
8. Assessment of older adults who have cognitive limitations may require task segmentation, or the breaking down of tasks into smaller steps.
9. Some assessment tools or parts of assessment tools may be more or less applicable depending on the setting, that is, community, acute care, or long-term care settings.
10. In comprehensive assessment, it is important to explore the meaning and implications of health status from the older adult's perspective. For example, the same changes in visual acuity for two older adults may have quite different meanings and implications for everyday life.

BOX 6-10   Assessment Tools Available through the Try This Series

The following are available via http://consultgerirn.org/resources:

- SPICES: An Overall Assessment Tool of Older Adults
- Katz Index of Independence in Activities of Daily Living (ADL)
- The Mini Mental State Examination (MMSE)
- The Geriatric Depression Scale (GDS)
- Predicting Pressure Ulcer Risk
- The Pittsburgh Sleep Quality Index (PSQI)
- The Epworth Sleepiness Scale
- Assessing Pain in Older Adults
- Fall Risk Assessment
- Assessing Nutrition in Older Adults
- Sexuality Assessment
- Urinary Incontinence Assessment
- Hearing Screening
- Confusion Assessment Method (CAM)
- Caregiver Strain Index (CSI)
- Elder Mistreatment Assessment
- Beers' Criteria for Potentially Inappropriate Medication Use in the Elderly
- Alcohol Use Screening and Assessment
- The Kayser Jones Brief Oral Health Status Examination (BOHSE)
- Horowitz's Impact of Event Scale: An Assessment of Post-Traumatic Stress in Older Adults
- Preventing Aspiration in Older Adults with Dysphagia

- Immunizations for the Older Adult
- Assessing Family Preferences for Participation in Care in Hospitalized Older Adults
- The Lawton Instrumental Activities of Daily Living (IADL) Scale
- The Hospital Admission Risk Profile (HARP)
- Confusion Assessment Method for the Intensive Care Unit (CAM-ICU)
- Avoiding Restraints in Patients with Dementia
- Brief Evaluation of Executive Dysfunction: An Essential Refinement in the Assessment of Cognitive Impairment
- Assessing Pain in Persons with Dementia
- Therapeutic Activity Kits

- Recognition of Dementia in Hospitalized Older Adults
- Wandering in the Hospitalized Older Adult
- Communication Difficulties: Assessment and Interventions
- Assessing and Managing Delirium in Persons with Dementia
- Decision Making and Dementia
- Working with Families of Hospitalized Older Adults with Dementia
- Eating and Feeding Issues in Older Adults with Dementia: Part I: Assessment
- Eating and Feeding Issues in Older Adults with Dementia: Part II: Interventions

---

BOX 6-11   **Web Exploration**

Visit the Hartford Institute's Website and browse the tools, videos, and articles available at http://consultgerirn.org/resources/

Advanced Assessment for Graduate Students

Graduate students who are conducting thesis research in clinical areas will endeavor to find the best tool or tools to measure the constructs of interest. The assessment tools described in this chapter in relation to clinical practice also have been used in clinical research in two ways.

First, a tool might be used to identify a specific target group as eligible participants in the study, for example, the Geriatric Depression Scale (GDS) might be used to screen a target group of participants to identify those who are experiencing mild depression (exhibiting score of 10–19 out of a possible score of 30). So, one of the inclusion criteria would be a score indicative of mild depression and the GDS would identify eligible participants. As another example, the inclusion criterion might be related to functional ability and the capacity of older adults living in nursing homes to perform independently none, some, or all basic ADL tasks. Because it is capacity and not performance that is the criterion, the graduate student will focus on what these older adults can do for themselves if given the opportunity. To screen potential participants for recruitment, an assessment is conducted to identify those who fit the inclusion criterion and exclude those who do not. The second way that graduate students doing clinical research may use the tools described in this chapter are as the "variables" of interest in order to explore, describe, or test the relationships between or among variables. In clinical practice as well as in research, it is important that we can rely on the chosen assessment tool to measure what we intend to measure. In clinical practice, we refer to the specificity and sensitivity of a tool whereas in clinical research, we refer to the reliability and validity of the tool.

Earlier, it was stated that quality of life and successful aging are individualistic and highly subjective. These constructs are difficult to measure because one tool will not fit for all older adults. Several years ago, we conducted a study that explored the factors that older adults living in nursing homes identified as important to their quality of life (Guse & Masesar, 1999). The prior literature search had suggested that there were several categories of factors that had been associated with quality of life among older adults but little information existed on quality of life among those living in nursing homes. We measured ADLs using a basic ADL tool but to measure quality of life, we used the categories of factors from the literature but we also asked open-ended questions similar to the ones raised earlier in the chapter, asking participants, "What are the three of four things that you feel are absolutely essential for your living a good quality of life here?"

In our study, factors identified as important to quality of life included: interaction with family and friends, personal qualities of self and others (e.g., humor and honesty), "room and board" items (e.g., private room and good food), and aspects of well-being (e.g., mobility and feeling independent). Two other factors, enjoying nature and being helpful to others, had not been widely reported in the literature but were identified in our study.

To summarize, graduate students conducting clinical research can use assessment tools as screening tools for inclusion and exclusion criteria and these tools can also be used to measure the variables of interest in the study. When established tools are not available or where there is a large range of possible values, then an open-ended (question) approach is required.

Summary

Comprehensive assessment of the older adult is an essential component of geriatric nursing care that involves both objective and subjective data collection. Nurses may obtain information about the older adult patient from a variety of sources including the patient, family, friends, caregivers, nursing staff, other team members, charts, and other written documentation. All aspects of the older adult person should be considered, including physical, psychological, socioeconomic, and spiritual. Particular challenges may be encountered when assessing older adults with cognitive impairments. This chapter presented many tools and Websites that can assist the nurse in assessing older adults as the initial step in individualizing a plan of care.

Clinical Reasoning Exercises

1. **In this chapter, we have said that** comprehensive assessment is not a neutral process. Reflect on what that really means and what kinds of things might constitute an unwanted bias to the assessment process.

2. **In this chapter, we have emphasized that** comprehensive assessment makes use of nursing knowledge and understanding of the combined factors of age-related changes, age-associated and other diseases, heredity, and lifestyle choices. Think of an older adult for whom you have provided care and describe that person. Try to outline the factors (age-related changes, age-associated and other diseases, heredity, and lifestyle choices) that are relevant for his or her health assessment.

Personal Reflections

1. In this chapter, we have underlined the importance of the healthcare team and consultation with team members. Reflect on your understanding of the contributions of team members in relation to the assessment of older adults. What are some of your personal qualities in terms of working as a member of the healthcare team?

2. How would you define "successful aging" in relation to your own aging? What are the implications of your definition in relation to decisions you might make during your lifetime? How might this definition affect the way you view the aging process of others?

References

Adnan, A., Chang, A., Arseven, O. K., & Emanuel, L. L. (2005). Assessment instruments. In L. L. Emanuel (Ed.), *Clinical geriatric medicine* (pp. 121–146). Philadelphia, PA: Saunders.

American Psychiatric Association. (2013). *Diagnostic and statistical manual of mental disorders* (5th ed., text rev.). Washington, DC: Author.

Anderson, M. A. (2003). *Caring for older adults holistically* (3rd ed.). Philadelphia, PA: F. A. Davis.

Annells, M., & Koch, T. (2003). Constipation and the breached trio: Diet, fluid intake, exercise. *International Journal of Nursing Studies, 40,* 843–852.

Anstey, K. J., von Sanden, C., & Sargent-Cox, C. (2007). Prevalence and risk factors for depression in a longitudinal, population-based study including individuals in the community and residential care. *American Journal of Geriatric Psychiatry, 15*(6), 497–505.

Armetta, M., & Molony, C. M. (1999). Topics in endocrine and hematologic care. In S. L. Molony, C. M. Waszynski, & C. H. Lyder (Eds.), *Gerontological nursing: An advanced practice approach* (pp. 359–387). Stamford, CT: Appleton & Lange.

Arterburn, D. E., Crane, P. K., & Sullivan, S. D. (2004). The coming epidemic of obesity in elderly Americans. *Journal of the American Geriatrics Society, 52,* 1007–1012.

Baum, C., Edwards, D. F., & Morrow-Howell, N. (1993). Identification and measurement of productive behaviours in senile dementia of the Alzheimer's type. *The Gerontologist, 33,* 403–408.

Bawden, M. E. (2006). Clean those teeth. *Perspectives, 30*(4), 15.

Beck, C. (1988). Measurement of dressing performance in persons with dementia. *American Journal of Alzheimer's Care and Related Disorders and Research, 3,* 21–25.

Brink, P., & Stones, M. (2007). Examination of the relationship among hearing impairment, linguistic communication, mood and social engagement of residents in complex continuing care facilities. *The Gerontologist, 47*(5), 633–641.

Bruno, L., & Ahrens, J. (2003). The importance of screening for depression in home care patients. *Caring,* 54–58.

Bureau of the Census. (1997). *Statistical abstract of the United States 1997* (117th ed.). Washington, DC: U.S. Department of Commerce.

Chan, C. C., & Lee, T. M. (1997). Validity of the Canadian Occupational Performance Measure. *Occupational Therapy International, 4*(3), 229–247.

Crum, R., Anthony, J., Bassett, S., & Folstein, M. (1993). Population-based norms for the Mini-Mental State Examination by age and educational level. *Journal of the American Medical Association, 269*(18), 2386–2391.

Culbertson, D. S., Griggs, M., & Hudson, S. (2004). Ear and hearing status in a multilevel retirement facility. *Geriatric Nursing, 25,* 93–98.

Dawson, P., Wells, D. L., & Kline, K. (1993). *Enhancing the abilities of persons with Alzheimer's disease and related dementias.* New York, NY: Springer.

Dendukuri, N., McCusker, J., & Belzile, E. (2004). The Identification of Seniors at Risk screening tool: Further evidence of concurrent and predictive validity. *Journal of the American Geriatrics Society, 52,* 290–296.

Doerflinger, D. M. C. (2007). The Mini-Cog. *American Journal of Nursing, 107*(12), 62–71.

Dupuis, S. L., Wiersma, E., & Loiselle, L. (2012). Pathologizing behavior: Meanings of behaviors in dementia care. *Journal of Aging Studies, 26,* 162–173.

Ferrini, A., & Ferrini, R. (2012). *Health in the later years.* New York, NY: McGraw-Hill Higher Education.

Fields, S. D., & Stano-Paul, L. (2005). Preface: Obesity. *Clinics in Geriatric Medicine, 21*(4), xi–xiii.

Fisher, K. M., & Copenhaver, V. (2006). Assessing the mental health of rural older adults in public housing facilities. *Journal of Gerontological Nursing, 22*(9), 26–33.

Fletcher, A. E., Dickinson, E. J., & Philp, I. (1992). Review: Quality of life instruments for everyday use with elderly patients. *Age and Aging, 21,* 142–150.

Folstein, M. F., Folstein, S. E., & McHugh, P. R. (1975). A practical method for grading the cognitive state of patients for the clinician. *Journal of Psychiatric Research, 12*(3), 189–198.

Forbes, E. J. (1994). Spirituality, aging, and the community-dwelling caregiver and care recipient. *Geriatric Nursing, 15*(6), 297–302.

Gates, G. A., Murphy, M., Rees, T. S., & Fraher, M. A. (2003). Screening for handicapping hearing loss in the elderly. *Journal of Family Practice, 52*(1), 56–62.

Gill, T. M., Williams, C. S., & Tinetti, M. E. (1995). Assessing risk for the onset of functional dependence among older adults: The role of physical performance. *Journal of the American Geriatrics Society, 43,* 604–609.

Guralnik, J. M., Branch, L. G., Cummings, S. R., & Curb, J. D. (1989). Physical performance measures in aging research. *Journal of Gerontology: Medical Sciences, 44*(5), M141–M146.

Guse, L. W., & Masesar, M. (1999). Quality of life and successful aging in long-term care: Perceptions of residents. *Mental Health Nursing, 20*(6), 527–539.

Harrison, T. C., Mackert, M., & Watkins, C. (2010). Health literacy issues among women with visual impairments. *Research in Gerontological Nursing, 3*(1), 49–60.

Institute of Medicine. (2004). *Health Literacy: A Prescription to End Confusion.* Washington, DC: National Academies Press.

Jensen, G. L. (2005). Obesity and functional decline: Epidemiology and geriatric consequence. *Clinics in Geriatric Medicine, 21*(4), 677–687.

Jensen, G. L., & Friedmann, J. M. (2002). Obesity is associated with functional decline in community-dwelling rural older adults. *Journal of the American Geriatrics Society, 50,* 918–923.

Jung, S., Coleman, A., & Weintraub, N. T. (2007). Vision screening in the elderly. *Journal of the American Medical Directors Association, 8*(6), 355–362.

Kahn, R. S. (1964). Comments. In M. P. Lawton & F. G. Lawton (Eds.), *Mental impairment in the aged* (pp. 109–114). Philadelphia, PA: Philadelphia Geriatric Center.

Kane, R., Ouslander, J., & Abrass, J. (2013). *Social assessment: Essentials of geriatrics* (7th ed). New York, NY: McGraw-Hill.

Kane, R. A. (1995). Comment. In L. Z. Rubenstein, D. Wieland, & R. Bernabei (Eds.), *Geriatric assessment technology: The state of the art* (pp. 99–100). New York, NY: Springer.

Kane, R. L. (1993). The implications of assessment. *Journals of Gerontology, 48*(special issue), 27–31.

Katz, S., Down, T. D., Cash, H. R., & Grotz, R. C. (1970). Progress in the development of the index of ADL. *The Gerontologist, 10,* 20–30.

Katz, S., Ford, A., Moskowitz, R., Jackson, B., & Jaffee, M. (1963). Studies of illness in the aged: The index of ADL, a standardized measure of biological and psychosocial functioning. *Journal of the American Medical Association, 185,* 94–101.

Kearney, P. M., & Pryor, J. (2004). The international classification of functioning, disability, and health (ICF) and nursing. *Journal of Advanced Nursing, 46*(2), 142–170.

Kitwood, T. (1997). *Dementia reconsidered.* Buckingham, UK: Open University Press.

Kitwood, T., & Bredin, K. (1992). Towards a theory of dementia care: *Personhood and well-being. Ageing and Society, 12*(3), 269–287.

Law, M., Polatajko, H., Pollock, N., McColl, M. A., Carswell, A., & Baptiste, S. (1994). Pilot testing of the Canadian Occupational Performance Measure: Clinical and measurement issues. *Canadian Journal of Occupational Therapy, 61*(4), 191–197.

Lawton, M. P. (1972). Assessing the competence of older people. In D. Kent & R. Kastenbaum (Eds.), *Research, planning and action for the elderly.* Sherwood, NY: Behavioral Publications.

Lawton, M. P., & Brody, E. M. (1969). Assessment of older people: Self-maintaining and instrumental activities of daily living. *The Gerontologist, 9*(3), 179–186.

Lebowitz, B. D., Pearson, J. L., Schneider, L. S., Reynolds, C. F., Aleropoulos, G. S., Bruce, M. F., . . . Parmelee, P. (1997). Diagnosis and treatment of depression in late life: Consensus statement update. *Journal of the American Medical Association, 278,* 1186–1190.

Lee, J. S., Kritchevsky, S. B., Tylavsky, F., Harrie, T. B., Ayonayon, H. N., & Newman, A. B. (2006). Factors associated with well-functioning community-dwelling older adults. *Journal of Nutrition for the Elderly, 26*(1), 27–43.

Luborsky, M. (1997). Attuning assessment to the client: Recent advances in theory and methodology. *Generations, 21*(1), 10–15.

Mahoney F. I., & Barthel, D. W. (1965). Functional evaluation: The Barthel index. *Maryland State Medical Journal, 14*(2), 61–65.

Mahoney, J., Drinka, T., Abler, R., Gunter-Hunt, G., Matthews, C., Gravenstein, S., & Carnes, M. (1994). Screening for depression: Single question versus GDS. *Journal of the American Geriatrics Society, 42,* 1006–1008.

McGuire, K. (2006). Promotion of urinary continence: Management of urinary incontinence in the geriatric setting. *Perspective, 30*(2), 22–23.

Mentes, J. C., & Wang, J. (2011). Measuring risk for dehydration in nursing home residents. *Research in Gerontological Nursing, 4*(2),148–156.

Mesman, G. R., Buchanan, J. A., Husfeldt, J. D., & Berg, T. M. (2011). Identifying preference in persons with dementia: Systematic preference testing vs. caregiver and family member report. *Clinical Gerontologist, 34,* 154–159.

Morley, J. E. (2003). Anorexia and weight loss among older persons. *Journal of Gerontology Biological Sciences, 58*(2), 131–137.

Morris, J. N., & Morris, S. A. (1997). ADL assessment measures for use with frail elders. In J. A. Teresi, M. P. Lawton, D. Holmes, & M. Ory (Eds.), *Measurement in elderly chronic care populations* (pp. 130–156). New York, NY: Springer.

Olenek, K., Skowronski, T., & Schmaltz, D. (2003). Geriatric nursing assessment. *Journal of Gerontological Nursing, 29*(8), 5–9.

Ostbye, T., Tyas, S., McDowell, I., & Koval, J. J. (1997). Reported activities of daily living: Agreement between elderly subjects with and without dementia and their caregivers. *Age and Ageing, 26,* 99–106.

Parker, M. G., & Thorslund, M. (2007). Health trends in the elderly population: Getting better and getting worse. *The Gerontologist, 47*(2), 150–158.

Perry, L., Kendrick, D., Morris, R., Dinan, S., Masud, T., Skelton, D., & for the ProAct65+ Study Team (2012). Completion and return of fall diaries varies with participants' level of education, first language and baseline fall risk. *Journal of Gerontology: Medical Sciences, 67A*(2), 210–214.

Registered Nurses' Association of Ontario. (2016). *Delirium, dementia and depression in older adults: Assessment and Care.* Toronto, Canada: Author.

Registered Nurses' Association of Ontario. (2004). *Caregiving strategies for older adults with delirium, dementia and depression.* Toronto, Canada: Author.

Reker, G. T., Peacock, E. J., & Wong, P. T. P. (1987). Meaning and purpose in life and well-being: A life span perspective. *Journal of Gerontology, 42,* 44–49.

Reuben, D. B., Herr, K. A., Pacala, J. T., Pollock, B. G., Potter, J. F., & Semla, T. P. (2008). *Geriatrics at your fingertips.* Malden, MA: American Geriatrics Society.

Reuben, D. B., & Sui, A. L. (1990). An objective measure of physical function of elderly outpatients: The physical performance test. *Journal of the American Geriatrics Society, 38,* 1190–1193.

Reuben, D. B., Valle, L. A., Hays, R. D., & Sui, A. L. (1995). Measuring physical function in community-dwelling older persons: A comparison of self-administered, interviewer-administered and performance-based measures. *Journal of the American Geriatrics Society, 43,* 17–23.

Richman, S. M., & Drickamer, M. A. (2007). Gynecologic care of elderly women. *Journal of the American Medical Directors Association, 8*(4), 219–223.

Rowe, J. W., & Kahn, R. L. (1997). Successful aging. *The Gerontologist, 37,* 433–440.

Sabat, S. R., & Collins, M. (1999). Intact social, cognitive ability and selfhood: A case study of Alzheimer's disease. *American Journal of Alzheimer's Disease,* 112–119.

Seeman, T. E., & Berkman, L. F. (1988). Structural characteristics of social networks and their relationship with social support in the elderly: Who provides support? *Social Science and Medicine, 26*(7), 737–749.

Stewart, S., O'Riley, A., Edelstein, B., & Gould, C. (2012). A preliminary comparison of three cognitive screening instruments in long-term care: The MMSE, SLUMS, and MoCA. *Clinical Gerontologist, 35,* 57–75.

Stolee, P., Patterson, M. L., Wiancko, D. C., Esbaugh, J., Arcese, Z. A., Vinke, A. M., . . . Crilly, R. G. (2003). An enhanced role in comprehensive geriatric assessment for community nurse case managers. *Canadian Journal on Aging, 22*(2), 177–184.

Stoll, R. L. (1979). Guidelines for spiritual assessment. *American Journal of Nursing,* 1574–1577.

Stone, L. M., & Lyles, K. W. (2006). Osteoporosis in later life. *Generations, 30*(3), 65–70.

Tappen, R. M. (1994). Development of the refined ADL assessment scale. *Journal of Gerontological Nursing, 20*(6), 36–41.

Tariq, S. H. (2007). Constipation in long-term care. *Journal of the American Medical Directors Association, 8*(4), 209–218.

Tinetti, M. E., Speechley, M., & Ginter, S. F. (1988). Risk factors for falls among elderly persons living in the community. *New England Journal of Medicine, 319,* 1701–1707.

Tomaka, J., Thompson, S., & Palacios, R. (2006). The relation of social isolation, loneliness and social support to disease outcomes among the elderly. *Journal of Aging and Health, 18*(3), 359–384.

Uniform Data System for Medical Rehabilitation. (1996). *Guide for the Uniform Data Set for Medical Rehabilitation (including the FIM instrument).* Buffalo, NY: Author.

Verbrugge, L. M., & Jette, A. M. (1994). The disablement process. *Social Science and Medicine, 38,* 1–14.

Wallhagen, M. I. (2009). The stigma of hearing loss. *The Gerontologist, 50*(1), 66–75.

Wang, D. S. (2011). Interdisciplinary methods of treatment of depression in older adults: A primer for practitioners. *Activities, Adaptation & Aging, 35,* 298–314.

Wilson, K., Mottram, P., & Sexsmith, A. (2007). Depressive symptoms in the very old living alone: Prevalence, incidence and risk factors. *International Journal of Geriatric Psychiatry, 22,* 361–366.

Woodward, S. (2012). Assessment and management of constipation in older people. *Nursing Older People, 24*(5), 21–26.

World Health Organization. (2001). *International classification of function, disability, and health (ICF).* Geneva, Switzerland: Author.

Yesavage, J. A., Brink, T. L., Rose, T. L., Lum, O., Huang, V., Aday, M., & Leirer, V. O. (1983). Development and validation of a geriatric depression screening scale. *Journal of Psychiatric Research, 17,* 37–49.

For a full suite of assignments and additional learning activities, see the access code at the front of your book.

Unit III
Health Promotion, Risk Reduction, and Disease Prevention

(COMPETENCIES 3–6, 9, 17, 18)

CHAPTER 7   PROMOTING HEALTHY AGING, INDEPENDENCE, AND QUALITY OF LIFE
(COMPETENCIES 4, 5, 9, 17, 18)

CHAPTER 8   IDENTIFYING AND PREVENTING COMMON RISK FACTORS IN THE ELDERLY
(COMPETENCIES 3, 4, 6, 9, 17)

©Creativamarea/Venta/Getty

Promoting Healthy Aging, Independence, and Quality of Life

David Haber

(Competencies 4, 5, 9, 17, 18)

LEARNING OBJECTIVES

At the end of this chapter, the reader will be able to:

> Apply the health contract technique and nutritional bull's-eye for behavior change.
> Describe several model health promotion programs.
> Explain the concept of re-engagement and provide examples of it.
> Identify the components of Medicare prevention.
> Explain the importance of life review.
> Recognize the importance of exercise and nutrition for healthy aging.
> Discuss the importance of the Green House project to the future of long-term care.

KEY TERMS

Bariatric surgery
Center for Science in the Public Interest
Complementary and alternative medicine
Dependence
Depression
Exercise
Green House
Health behavior change
Health contract/calendar
Life review

Medicare prevention
Mediterranean diet
Mental health
Model health promotion programs
Nutrition
Nutrition bull's-eye
Quality of life
Re-engagement
Vietnam War

Health promotion works, no matter what one's age, and even after decades of practicing unhealthy habits. But it does not work for everyone, all the time. So what needs to be done to increase the odds of promoting healthy aging successfully? Certainly the entire burden cannot be placed on the guilt-ridden backs of individuals. The federal and state governments play a significant role, as do religious institutions, businesses, community centers, hospitals, medical clinics, health professionals, educational institutions, families, neighborhoods, and even shopping malls. In this chapter, some of these influences on healthy aging will be explored.

Exercise and *nutrition* are probably the two most widely publicized components of health promotion, and they will be given their due in this chapter as well. We will use a broad definition of health promotion in this chapter, one that includes such diverse topics as self-management through health contracts, promoting mental health through life reviews, promoting *re-engagement* rather than retirement, and promoting the health of frail elders through unique homes rather than through institutions that are merely called (nursing) homes.

One aspect of health promotion lies with the federal government, and its Medicare prevention initiatives.

Medicare Prevention

The federal government reimburses Medicare recipients for prevention activities (see **Table 7-1**). Some of Medicare's reimbursement policies have emerged from the research evidence reviewed by the U.S. Preventive Services Task Force (USPSTF). USPSTF was launched by the U.S. Public Health Service to systematically review evidence of effectiveness of clinical preventive services. This task force periodically updates its research guidelines on a wide variety of screening and counseling recommendations, such as breast cancer screening, colorectal cancer screening, and counseling to promote physical activity.

These updates are no longer compiled in written form and distributed; instead, the guide can be accessed online: www.ahrq.gov/orifessuibaks/clinicians-providers/guidelines-recommendations/guide/cpsguide.pdf.

If you review the USPSTF recommendations (see Chapter 8), however, you will notice that they are often out of sync with Medicare reimbursement policies. Some reimbursement policies appear to have been influenced more by medical lobbyists advocating for specific segments of the medical industry (e.g., oncology, urology, orthopedics) than by policy derived from evidence-based medicine (Haber, 2001, 2005).

Although the movement into *Medicare prevention*—with substantially expanded coverage in 1998, 2005, and then in 2010 when the Affordable Care Act was enacted—undoubtedly benefits older Americans, there is room for considerable improvement in the way the Medicare program promotes health and prevents disease. Lobbyists have promoted medical screenings that are reimbursed too frequently or over too long a period of time. Some screenings may not be worth the expense (e.g., fecal occult blood test, barium enema, sigmoidoscopy, routine prostate cancer screening, baseline EKG). Conversely, over the decades Medicare policy has been stingy toward risk reduction counseling, which, not surprisingly, has had little if any lobbying effort behind it.

Fortunately, this has changed in the last decade. The highlights follow:

1. An initial physical examination that includes prevention counseling.
2. Annual wellness visits.
3. Smoking cessation—no longer limited to those who have an illness caused by or complicated by tobacco use.
4. Comprehensive health programs that include complementary and alternative practices, developed by Dean Ornish and Herbert Benson for cardiac rehabilitation.
5. Screening and intensive behavioral therapy for obesity.
6. Depression screening in a primary care setting that can provide follow-up and referral;
7. Alcohol misuse counseling sessions, up to 4 per year, in a primary care setting with a qualified provider.
8. Elimination of all deductibles and copayments for prevention services to enhance access.

TABLE 7-1 Medicare Prevention

One-time "Welcome to Medicare Physical"

Within 6 months of initial enrollment.

Physician takes history of modifiable risk factors (coverage makes special mention of depression, functional ability, home safety, falls risk, hearing, vision), height and weight, blood pressure, EKG.

Cardiovascular screening

Every 5 years.

Ratio between total cholesterol and HDL, triglycerides.

Cervical cancer

Covered every 2 years.

Pap smear and pelvic exam.

Colorectal cancer

Covered annually for fecal occult blood test.

Covered every 4 years for sigmoidoscopy or barium enema.

Covered every 10 years for colonoscopy.

Lung cancer

Long history of heavy smoking (defined as at least a pack a day for 30 years or the equivalent, for example, 2 packs a day for 15 years.

Covered up to age 77.

Densitometry

Covered every 2 years.

Diabetes screening

Annually (those with prediabetes, every 6 months).

Not covered routinely, but includes most people age 65+ (if overweight, family history, fasting glucose of 100–125 mg/dl [prediabetes], hypertension, dyslipidemia).

Mammogram

Covered annually.

Prostate cancer

Covered annually.

Digital rectal examination and PSA test.

Smoking cessation

Two quit attempts annually, each consisting of up to four counseling sessions.

Clinicians are encouraged to become credentialed in smoking cessation.

Immunization

Influenza vaccination covered annually; two different pneumococcal vaccinations covered one time, revaccination after 5 years dependent on risk.

(continues)

TABLE 7-1   Medicare Prevention (*continued*)

Other coverage

Diabetes outpatient self-management training (blood glucose monitors, test strips, lancets; nutrition and exercise education; self-management skills: 9 hours of group training, plus 1 hour of individual training).

Medical nutrition therapy for persons with diabetes or a renal disease: 3 hours of individual training first year, 2 hours subsequent years.

Glaucoma screening annually for those with diabetes, family history, or African American descent.

Persons with cardiovascular disease may be eligible for comprehensive prevention programs by Drs. Dean Ornish and Herbert Benson: coverage 36 sessions within 18 weeks, possible extension to 72 sessions within 36 weeks.

Abdominal aortic aneurysm, one-time screening by ultrasound for men aged 65–75 years who have ever smoked.

Obesity screening and intensive behavioral therapy; face-to-face counseling weekly for a month by a medical provider in a primary care setting, then five more monthly sessions, and then six additional monthly sessions if progress is being made.

Depression screening annually if in a primary setting that can provide follow-up treatment and referrals.

Alcohol misuse counseling annually if screened positive in a primary care setting by a qualified provider, up to four brief face-to-face counseling sessions annually.

Frequency and duration

These are estimates of what researchers recommend, relying most heavily on the U.S. Preventive Services Task Force recommendations, but not exclusively.

Blood pressure: Begin early adulthood, annually, ending around age 80.

Cholesterol: Begin early adulthood, every 2–3 years, ending around age 80.

Colorectal cancer: Begin age 50, every 10 years for colonoscopy, ending around age 80.

Mammogram: Begin age 50, every other year, consult with physician after age 75.

Osteoporosis: Begin early adulthood for women with no frequency recommended; no consensus after age 65 on frequency.

Pap test: Begin at age 21, two normal consecutive annual screenings, followed by every 3 years; two normal consecutive annual screenings around age 65, then discontinue.

Prostate cancer: Do not do routinely, except if there is a family history or African American heritage.

Definitions

Hypercholesterolemia: LDL above 160/130/100 (depending on risk factors); HDL below 40; ratio (total/HDL) 4.2 or above.

Diabetes: Fasting glucose 126 mg/dl and above; prediabetes, 100–125 mg/dl.

High blood pressure: Over 140/90; between 120/80 and 140/90 is prehypertensive.

Osteopenia: 1–2.5 standard deviations below young-adult peak bone density.

Osteoporosis: 2.5 standard deviations or more below young-adult peak bone density.

Medical screenings and immunizations are undeniably important tools for disease prevention, but the data collected by the USPSTF (1996) resulted in a surprising conclusion that is still being resisted on the screening side, but slowly adopted on the counseling side: "Among the most effective interventions available to clinicians for reducing the incidence and severity of the leading causes of disease and disability in the United States are those that address the personal health practices of patients" (p. xxii) . . . and "conventional clinical activities (e.g., diagnostic testing) may be of less value to clients than activities once considered outside the traditional role of the clinician," namely, counseling and patient education (USPSTF, 1996, p. xxii).

Health Behavior Change

Theories help us understand what influences health behaviors and how to plan effective interventions. A theory of *health behavior change* attempts to explain the processes underlying the learning of new health behaviors. The two most widely cited theories of behavior change are social cognitive theory (Bandura, 1977) and stages of change (Prochaska & DiClemente, 1992). Other theories that have marshaled support are health locus of control (Wallston & Wallston, 1982), health belief model (Becker, 1974), reasoned action (Fishbein & Ajzen, 1975), community empowerment (Wallerstein & Bernstein, 1988), and community-oriented primary care (Nutting, 1987).

The author of this chapter is not an advocate of any single theory. Theories are broad and ambitious, attempting to relate a set of concepts systematically to explain and predict events and activities. Concepts, however, are the primary elements of a theory, and each theory has a concept or two that is particularly well developed and helpful in guiding a risk reduction intervention. Borrowing concepts from different theories can help one plan an intervention (**Box 7-1**).

One behavior-changing tool that borrows concepts from a variety of theories is the *health contract/calendar* (see **Exhibits 7-1** and **7-2**). The health contract/calendar relies on the self-management capability of a client, after initial assistance is provided by a clinician or health educator. The client is helped to choose an appropriate behavior change goal and to create and implement a plan to accomplish that goal. The statement of the goal and the plan of action are then written into a contract format.

A health contract is alleged to have several advantages over verbal communication alone, especially when the communication tends to be limited in direction (i.e., mostly from health professional to client). The alleged advantages of a contract, which still need additional empirical testing, are that it is a formal commitment that not

---

BOX 7-1   Recommended Readings

Birren, J., & Cochran, K. (2001). *Telling the stories of life through guided autobiography groups.* Baltimore, MD: Johns Hopkins University Press.

Freedman, M. (1999). *Prime time: How baby boomers will revolutionize retirement and transform America.* New York, NY: Public Affairs.

Gawande, A. (2014). *Being Mortal: Medicine and What Matters in the End.* NY: Metropolitan books.

Haber, D. (2016). *Health promotion and aging: Practical applications for health professionals* (7th ed.). New York, NY: Springer.

Lorig, K., Ritter, P., Stewart, A., Sobel, D., Brown, B., Bandura, A., et al. (2001). Chronic disease self-management program: 2-year health status and health care utilization outcomes. *Medical Care, 39* (11), 1217–1223.

Rabig, J., Thomas, W., Kane, R., Cutler, L., & McAlilly, S. (2006). Radical redesign of nursing homes: Applying the Green House concept in Tupelo, Mississippi. *The Gerontologist, 46*(4), 533–539.

Thomas, W. (2004). *What are old people for?* Acton, MA: VanderWyk & Burnam.

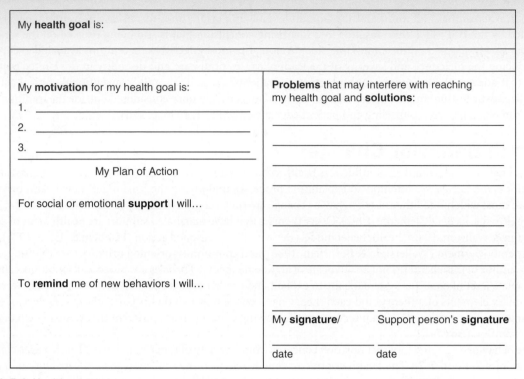

My **health goal** is: _____

My **motivation** for my health goal is:	Problems that may interfere with reaching my health goal and **solutions**:
1. _____	
2. _____	
3. _____	

My Plan of Action

For social or emotional **support** I will…

To **remind** me of new behaviors I will…

My **signature**/   Support person's **signature**

date   date

Exhibit 7-1 Health contract.
Reproduced from Haber, D. (2016). *Health promotion and aging: Practical applications for health professionals* (7th ed.). New York, NY: Springer Publishing Company.

only enhances the therapeutic relationship between provider and client, but also requires the active participation of the client. The contract also:

> Identifies and enhances motivation
> Clarifies measurable and modest goals
> Suggests tips to remember new behaviors
> Provides a planned way to involve support persons such as family and friends
> Provides a means to problem-solve around barriers that previously interfered with the achievement of a goal
> Suggests ways to design a supportive environment
> Provides incentives to reinforce behaviors
> Establishes a record-keeping system (i.e., a month-long calendar for the health contract/calendar technique)

The health contract/calendar technique includes a set of instructions (see Haber, 2007) that help older adults establish a goal, identify motivation, implement a plan of action, identify potential problems, and encourage solutions to overcome these barriers. The contract is signed and dated at the bottom by the older adult and a support person. Progress is typically assessed after one week, and the success of the contract is reviewed at the end of a month. There is also the potential for providing ongoing support.

Health contracts have been applied with varying degrees of success to a wide variety of behaviors, such as drug use, smoking, alcohol abuse, nutrition, and exercise (Berry, Danish, Rinke, & Smiciklas-Wright, 1989; Clark, Keukefeld, & Godlaski, 1999; Cupples & Steslow, 2001; Haber, 2007; Haber & Looney, 2000; Haber & Rhodes, 2004; Jette et al., 1999; Johnson, Nicklas, Arbeit, Webber, & Berenson, 1992; Leslie & Schuster, 1991; Lorig, Lubeck, Kraines, Seleznickm, Holman, 1996; Lorig et al., 2000; Moore, von Korff, Cherkin, Saunders, & Lorig, 2000; Neale, Singleton, Dupuis, & Hess, 1990; Schlenk & Boehm, 1998; Swinburn, Walter, Arroll, Tilyard, & Russell, 1998).

Fill in activities and make an X on each day you complete them.

Month: _____

Backup plan:

Sunday	Monday	Tuesday	Wednesday	Thursday	Friday	Saturday

Weekly Success #days completed/ #days contracted

Exhibit 7-2 Health calendar.

Permission from Haber, D. (2016). *Health promotion and aging: Practical applications for health professionals* (7th ed.). New York, NY: Springer Publishing Company.

There are many versions of health contracts ranging from the simple to the complex. Here is an example of a simple weight-loss contract developed by Dr. Joseph Chemplavil, a cardiac endocrinologist in Hampton, Virginia:

I, (patient's name), hereby promise to myself and to Dr. Chemplavil, that I will make every effort to lose my (agreed-upon) weight, and I will pay $1 to Dr. Chemplavil's Dollar for Pound Fund for every pound of weight that I gain, on each visit to the office, by cash. I also understand that I will receive $1 from the same fund for each pound of weight that I lose.

Dr. Chemplavil paid out $1,044 to 118 patients, received $166 from 30 patients, and 2 patients broke even (Kazel, 2004).

Research on health contracts has been limited and often marred by a lack of random assignment to treatment and control groups, small sample sizes, and lack of replication. In addition, there are several uncertainties about the effectiveness of health contracts in terms of one's ability to identify which components work better than others (e.g., health education, social support, the professional-client relationship, memory enhancement, motivation building, contingency rewards, etc.), whether contracts work better with one type of person than another, and how to determine the content and amount of training that is required for health educators or clinicians to help clients implement health contracts.

Even without a definitive body of research, health contracts are widely used. They are simple to administer, time-efficient, and even cost-effective when medical personnel assign the completion of health contracts to a health educator or trained office worker. The health contract can also be effectively taught to students in the classroom who are interested in health education, risk factor counseling, or program development (Haber, 2007).

Exercise

The 1996 *Surgeon General's Report on Physical Activity and Health* was an outstanding review of the research on the effects of physical activity on people's health, and it has yet to be improved upon. According to the Surgeon General's report, regular exercise, and physical activity improve health in a variety of ways, including a reduction in heart disease, diabetes, high blood pressure, colon cancer, depression, anxiety, excess weight, falling, bone thinning, muscle wasting, and joint pain.

However, 60% of adults did not achieve the recommended amount of physical activity, and 25% of adults were not physically active at all. Inactivity increased with age; by age 75, about one in three men and one in two women engaged in no physical activity. Inactivity was also more common among women and people with lower incomes and less education.

The most significant component of the Surgeon General's report was its advocacy for several tested exercise principles.

The report stresses the importance of motivation. To enhance it requires a large degree of modesty in setting goals and at least a small degree of enjoyment—hence, the emphasis on being more physically active rather than insisting on a narrow adherence to a rigid exercise regimen.

Americans should also get at least 30 minutes of physical activity or exercise most days of the week. This statement provided a major perspective shift from previous recommendations by government and exercise leaders. This new message recommended that Americans become more concerned about total calories expended through exercise or physical activity than about intensity level or duration of continuous exercise (Healthy People 2020, n.d.).

Regarding intensity level, the report stresses the importance of raising respiratory rate and body warmth—physiological changes that are apparent to the participant—but not to be too concerned about raising intensity level to a target heart rate—a practice many older adults find vexing. Regarding duration, it is no longer deemed essential to obtain 30 consecutive minutes of exercise. For Americans, the large majority of whom are not too active, accumulating shorter activity spurts throughout the day may be more effective. Taking a brisk walk in a shopping mall or climbing a few stairs in spare minutes can accumulate the benefits of exercise.

A review of the research literature concludes that accumulating several 5- or 10-minute bouts of physical activity over the course of the day provides beneficial health and fitness effects (DeBusk, Stenestrand, Sheehan, & Haskell, 1990; Jakicic, Donnelly, Pronk, Jawad, & Jacobson, 1995; Lee, Sesso, & Paffenbarger, 2000; Murphy, Nevill, Neville, Biddle, & Hardman, 2002; Pate et al., 1995). Bite-size portions of exercise may be more effective with controlling blood sugar throughout the day than a comparable longer session (Francois, Baldi, & Manning, 2014). One study also reported that if a person times these bouts of activity correctly they can gain the added benefit of replacing junk food snack breaks (Jakicic et al., 1995).

Regarding exercise itself, it is difficult for adults to go from inactivity to an exercise routine. Thinking about how to accumulate short bouts of activity is a useful way to get started on better health and fitness. For example, health educators can encourage older adults to vacuum the carpet more briskly than normally (even if it means doing it in segments throughout the day), or to put more energy into leaf raking or lawn mowing, gardening with enthusiasm, or dancing to music on the radio. In addition, health educators should not underestimate the ability of older adults to engage in adventurous or unusual sports (see **Figure 7-1**).

Finally, the Surgeon General's report urged Americans to be active most days of the week. We should aim for the habit of everyday physical activity or exercise, but should not allow the occasional lapse to discourage us.

Making physical activity or exercise a near-daily routine is more likely to become an enduring habit than the previously recommended three-times-per-week exercise routine.

For most older adults, a brisk walking program will provide sufficient intensity for a good aerobics program. An 8-year study of more than 13,000 people indicated that walking briskly for 30 to 60 minutes every day was almost as beneficial in reducing the death rate as jogging up to 40 miles a week (Blair et al., 1989). The authors of a study of 1,645 older adults reported that simply walking 4 hours per week decreased the risk of future hospitalization for cardiovascular disease (LaCroix, Veveille, Hecht, Grothous, & Wagner, 1996).

The National Center for Health Statistics (1985) reported that walking has much greater appeal for older adults than high-intensity exercise. A national survey indicated that a smaller percentage of persons age 65-plus (27%) engaged in vigorous activities, in comparison to 41% of the general adult population; however, people of all age groups (41%) were equally likely to walk for exercise.

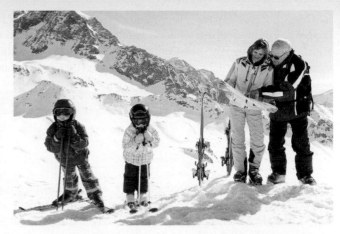

Figure 7-1 Grandparents can share active quality time with their grandchildren.
© Adie Bush/Cultura / Getty Images Plus/Getty.

Many older adults are concerned about unfavorable weather and may abandon their walking routine as a consequence. Prolonged hot or cold spells may sabotage a good walking program. Rather than discontinue this activity because of the weather, adults may choose to walk indoors at their local shopping malls. Many shopping malls—about 2,500 nationwide—open their doors early, usually between 5:30 and 10:00 a.m., for members of walking clubs.

There is also a relationship between one's neighborhood and one's health. Residents who depend on a car to get to most places and have few sidewalks for safe walking are likely to be more obese and have chronic medical conditions that impact health-related quality of life (Booth, Pinkston, & Boston, 2005; Sturm & Cohen, 2004). For every extra 30 minutes commuters drive each day, they have a 3% greater chance of being obese; in contrast, people who live within walking distance of shops are 7% less likely to be obese (Frank, Andresen, & Schmid, 2004). Older persons who believe their neighborhoods are favorable for walking are up to 100% more physically active (King, Brach, Killingsworth, Fenton, & Kriska, 2003; Li, Fisher, & Harmer, 2005). People at high risk for inactivity may increase their physical activity when they have access to walking trails (Brownson et al., 2000).

CLINICAL TIP

Remind older adults that they can accumulate the benefit of exercise throughout the day.

A sedentary person is estimated to walk about 3,500 steps a day, and the average American about 5,130 steps. Many advocates believe Americans should aim for 10,000 steps a day, or about 5 miles. Workplace physical activity, particularly among blue-collar occupations, helps many people reach the 10,000-step target, leaving older adults (and overweight office workers) most likely to be at risk (McCormack, Giles-Corti, & Milligan, 2006).

Pedometers are small devices that count steps, and are typically attached at the waist. They first appeared in Japan in 1965 under the name Manpo-meter—*manpo* in Japanese means 10,000 steps. Their introduction into America took another few decades, but they have been rapidly increasing in popularity—even McDonald's distributed them for a while as part of an adult Happy Meal called Go Active (salad, bottled water, and a pedometer for $4.99). Studies, though, have been equivocal about the benefits of using a pedometer to motivate individuals.

One study, for instance, reported that pedometers added no additional benefit to a coaching intervention (Engel & Lindner, 2006), whereas another publication noted that it increased the frequency of short walking trips (Stovitz, Van Wormer, Center, & Bremer, 2005). One study reported that cheap pedometers are likely to overestimate the actual number of steps taken (De Cocker, Cardon, & De Bourdeaudhuij, 2006).

CLINICAL TIP

Walking is one of the most beneficial exercises for older adults in preventing cardiovascular disease and decreasing mortality risk.

For the more tech-oriented boomers, and even some who are quite a bit older, there are fitness trackers. Rupert Murdoch, the 84-year-old international media mogul, told an Australian audience that he wore one. "I have a bracelet that keeps track of how I sleep, move, and eat—transmitting that information to the cloud." Fitness gadgets, like Fitbit Flex and the BodyMedia armband, measure total energy expenditure as well as intensity and duration of activity.

There are many ways in addition to the use of a pedometer or fitness tracker to add steps to a daily routine. For information and guidelines on this topic, contact America on the Move, at http://www.americaonthemove .org. Or join a noncompetitive walking, hiking or outdoor club. Two opportunities in this regard are the American Volkssport Association at 800-830-9255 or http://www.ava.org, and the local Sierra Club at http://www.sierraclub .org. If you want to add a mind-body dimension to walking, try ChiWalking, which combines walking with the principles of tai chi (http://www.chiwalking.com).

Traveling to another city can also be an excuse not to exercise, or it can be an opportunity to gather information from the local newspaper or chamber of commerce about a walking tour for an enjoyable way to get exercise and a unique way to learn about offbeat aspects of a city's history. Most if not all big cities have walking tours, and some sound particularly intriguing (such as Oak Park, Illinois's self-guided walking tours of Frank Lloyd Wright homes and the Big Onion walking tours of New York City's ethnic communities and restaurants [http://www.bigonion.com]).

Sarcopenia, or the gradual loss of muscle mass with age, is another exercise consideration. This loss is generally about. 5% to 1% a year after the age of 50, though it can begin as early as one's 30s. The primary intervention is strength-building, which can prevent much of this muscle deterioration. There are several interventions to choose from.

Weight machines can help with proper form but may be difficult to afford or access. Free weights add on the challenge of stabilizing muscles but are more associated with injury. Isometrics, the contraction of muscles without movement at the joint, can be implemented for free and at one's convenience, but can elicit the Valsalva maneuver, holding one's breath and raising one's blood pressure. Elastic bands are cheap and portable, though can challenge arthritic fingers and can snap (which can startle when it happens mid-exercise).

A joint effort by Tufts University and the CDC produced an online interactive program entitled *Growing Stronger: Strength Training for Older Adults*, and a booklet on strength training. Another resource on strength training is the website of Dr. Miriam Nelson, director of the John Hancock Center for Physical Activity and Nutrition, accessible at www.strongwomen.com.

There are also flexibility and balance considerations with age. Yoga and Tai Chi appear to be well-suited to the capabilities and interests of older adults. The most popular yoga activity is hatha yoga, a sequence of stretching, bending, and twisting movements that causes each joint to move slowly through its maximum range of motion, then is held for several seconds. Yoga improves body awareness, reduces stress, improves balance and coordination, and increases maximum range of motion by expanding joint mobility. The downside is that without proper instruction, injuries are not uncommon. Tai Chi consists of slow, graceful movements from a slight crouch position, and is effective with increasing body awareness and fall prevention (Wolfson et al., 1996).

> **CLINICAL TIP**
>
> Tai chi is considered one of the best activities to promote balance in older adults.

For a detailed description of a model exercise program that includes all the components previously examined, see Haber (2016).

Nutrition

Nutrition is only one component in the development and exacerbation of disease (heredity, environment, medical care, social circumstances, and other lifestyle risk factors also play a part), but eating and drinking habits have been implicated in 6 of the 10 leading causes of death—heart disease, cancer, stroke, diabetes, kidney disease, and liver disease—as well as in several debilitating disorders like osteoporosis and diverticulosis.

Older adults are in a particularly precarious position because they are more vulnerable to both obesity and malnutrition than other age groups. The highest percentage of obese adults is in the age group 50–69 years, with those ages 70–79 the next most obese (Squires, 2002). Also, older adults are at the highest risk of being malnourished (Beers & Berkow, 2000). Social isolation, dental problems, medical disease, and medication usage are among the risk factors for malnourishment in older adults.

Older adults are more conscientious about nutrition than other age groups, according to one national study (Harris, 1989). In this sample, a higher percentage of those over age 65 (approximately two-thirds) than of those in their 40s (one-half) reported trying "a lot" to limit sodium, fat, and sugar; eat enough fiber; lower cholesterol; and consume enough vitamins and minerals.

If older adults are paying more attention to their nutritional habits, one can only speculate that they may be motivated by more immediate feedback (heartburn, constipation, and so forth), or by feelings of greater vulnerability (higher risk of impairment from disease and of loss of independence). The next cohort of older adults—today's baby boomers—bring more than motivation to the table. They also bring a higher formal education level, including a strong interest in health education.

The federal government provides a modest amount of nutrition education for older adults and the rest of the American public. The 2005 Dietary Guidelines for Americans includes a 70-page blueprint for nutritional policy; a revised Food Guide Pyramid, dubbed MyPyramid; and a Website, http://www.mypyramid.gov The guidelines are supposed to be redrafted every 5 years by the U.S. Department of Agriculture (USDA) and the Department of Health and Human Services (DHHS). The Food Guide Pyramid, however, had not been updated for 13 years, and this website was a brand new initiative. The entire update was billed as an interactive food guidance system rather than a one-size-fits-all initiative.

The guidelines basically encourage Americans to eat fruits, vegetables, whole grains, and low-fat or fat-free dairy products, and there is much more detail on the consumption of these foods than was provided by previous guidelines. Fruits and vegetables are increased to 5 to 13 servings per day. Salt guidelines are specific for the first time, limiting it to one level teaspoon a day. Trans fat (to be banned nationally in 2018) is identified for the first time, and the advice is to keep intake as low as possible. Saturated fat limitations have become specific, keeping it to 10% of calories or less. Cholesterol level is to be less than 300 milligrams. Added sugars or sweeteners are discouraged for the first time, particularly in drinks. Whole grains are differentiated from the broad category of carbohydrates, and the recommendation is that one-half the grain servings should be whole grains.

In 2011 the MyPlate icon took over (see www.choosemyplate.gov). It is visually easy to grasp by using the image of a plate. On one side of the plate are vegetables (30%) and fruits (20%). On the other side of the plate are grains (30%) and protein (20%). The two easy dictums to remember from looking at the plate are: (1) half your plate should be vegetables and fruits, and (2) half your grains should be whole grains (with the nutritious and fibrous germ and bran coating intact).

This author prefers another educational tool that does not involve pyramids or plates, but a bull's-eye. The *nutrition bull's-eye* was developed by Covert Bailey (1996), and its goal is for people to consume the nutritious foods that are listed in the center of the bull's-eye. These foods are low in saturated fat, sugar, and sodium, and high in fiber. They include skim milk, nonfat yogurt, most fruits and vegetables, whole grains, beans and legumes, and water-packed tuna. As you move to the foods listed in the rings farther away from the bull's-eye, you eat more saturated fat, sugar, sodium, and low-fiber foods. In the outer ring of the bull's-eye, therefore, are most cheeses, ice cream, butter, whole milk, beef, cake, cookies, potato chips, and mayonnaise.

Unlike previous icons, Bailey's bulls-eye is focused on making distinctions within food categories. Whole-wheat products, for instance, are in the bull's-eye, whereas products made from refined white flour and those with added sugar are placed in the outer circles. Fresh fruits and vegetables are in the bull's-eye, but juiced vegetables and fruit that lose fiber and that concentrate sugars are placed in a ring just outside of the bull's-eye. Skim milk, low-fat and nonfat cottage cheese, and part-skim mozzarella are in the center ring, whereas whole milk and most cheeses are in the outer circles of the target.

The author has offered older clients a personalized version of the nutrition bull's-eye. In this version, you begin with a blank bull's-eye, and then add food and drink products that you usually consume to each of the rings. The foods and drinks in the personalized nutrition bull's-eye (see **Figure 7-2**) are clearly superior; the second ring is not as nutrient dense; the third ring is neutral, products that are not particularly harmful or helpful; and the outer ring includes the least nutritious foods and drinks that should be consumed sparingly.

In the center and innermost ring of the personalized bull's-eye, patients also add the foods and drinks that they are not currently consuming, but that they find sufficiently desirable and are considering adding to their diet (in italics in Figure 7-2). The assignment of food and drink products to each of the rings is likely best done with the aid of a dietitian who can assess their nutritional value. (Darson Rhodes and Mandy Puckett, former nutrition students at Ball State University identified products for the personalized nutrition bull's-eye in Figure 7-2.)

CLINICAL TIP

Encourage older adults not to waste their daily calories on sweetened drinks.

Mediterranean Diet

The *Mediterranean diet* became popular in America in 1997, as we discovered that the countries along the Mediterranean had among the lowest rates of coronary heart disease and many common cancers found in the Western world. This near-vegetarian diet was high on unrefined grains, potatoes, fruit, vegetables, fish, wine, and olive oil, and low on meat, cheese, refined sugar or flour, butter, and margarine.

Although the Mediterranean diet is more expensive than most Western diets, research reports that it reduces cardiovascular risk (Estruch, Ros, & Salas-Salvado, 2013), decreases stroke risk (Sherzai, Hei, & Boothby, 2012), lowers overall mortality rate (Levitan, Lewis, & Tinker, 2013), and slows cognitive decline (Feart et al., 2009). Moreover, these diets do not involve limits on calories, which has long been a barrier to success with low-fat approaches (Estruch et al., 2013).

Surprisingly, the diet is not low in fat, with about 37% to 40% of calories coming from it (versus the 30% or lower recommended by the American Heart Association)—primarily from olive oil, which consists mostly of monounsaturated fat. Thus, Americans began to extol the virtues of olive oil and other monounsaturated fats because they appear to slightly lower the unhealthy low-density lipoprotein (LDL) but leave the healthy, high-density

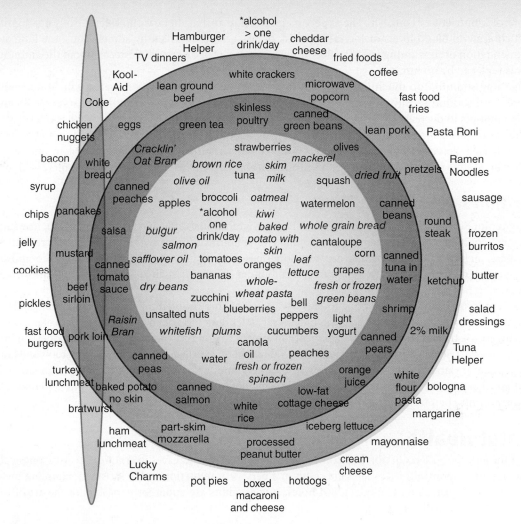

Italics indicate foods that client will consider adding to her typical diet.

Figure 7-2 Personalized nutrition bull's eye.

Permission from Haber, D. (2016). *Health promotion and aging: Practical applications for health professionals* (7th ed.). New York, NY: Springer Publishing Company.

lipoprotein (HDL) intact or may even raise it a little. The diet is also high in polyunsaturated Omega-3 fats, which are found in fish like salmon, and in nuts, green leafy vegetables, tofu, flaxseeds, and canola oil.

As stated by two respected experts in the nutrition field, limits on fat consumption are "an outdated concept, an obstacle to sensible change that promotes harmful low-fat foods [author's note: because they tend to substitute refined carbohydrates], undermines efforts to limit refined grains and added sugars, and discourages the food industry from developing products higher in healthy fats" (Mozaffarian & Ludwig, 2015, para. 11).

Dietary Implications for Older Adults

Many older adults in long-term care institutions are not only on low-fat diets, but low-cholesterol and low-sodium diets as well. Regarding cholesterol, in 2015 the Dietary Guidelines Advisory Committee no longer deemed dietary cholesterol a nutrient of concern. The expert panel concluded that dietary cholesterol does not significantly impact cholesterol blood levels or increase the risk of heart disease in healthy adults. Thus, the long-standing recommendation of consuming less than 300 milligrams per day of dietary cholesterol (about the amount in one egg) was replaced by no limits.

Regarding sodium, too much in the system causes the body to retain excess water, which increases blood pressure. And sodium sensitivity increases with age, as does blood pressure. Among persons age 85 and over, though, attempts to decrease hypertension can lead to *increased* mortality (Finestone, 2009; Rastas et al., 2006).

While not arguing for a high-fat, high-cholesterol, high-sodium diet for very old adults, it should be noted that highly restricted diets can lead to deficient dietary intake and malnutrition, a significant problem among those age 75 and over. Malnutrition is associated with impaired healing, prolonged hospital stays, and increased mortality.

Nutrition Advocacy and Education

The Center for Science in the Public Interest (CSPI) is an educational and advocacy organization. Its educational component consists of the *Nutrition Action Health Letter*, published monthly, which informs more than 800,000 subscribers, including this author. The organization is best known, however, for its advocacy accomplishments, under the leadership of its executive director and cofounder (in 1971), Michael Jacobson. More information can be obtained at https://cspinet.org/

The Center for Science in the Public Interest (www.cspinet.org) has led the fight for nutrition labels on food items in the supermarket; for exposing the hidden fat in Chinese, Mexican, Italian, and delicatessen food; for pressuring movie theaters to stop cooking popcorn in artery-clogging coconut oil; for warning labels on Procter & Gamble's fake fat, Olean, which may interfere with the absorption of nutrients and cause loose stools and cramping; for more accurate labeling of ground beef in supermarkets; and for the listing of trans fat on nutrition labels.

Perhaps their crowning achievement has been as a major player in spurring the government's Food and Drug Administration to ban trans fat in all food products in the United States by June, 2018.

Mental Health

Neither the average 50% reduction in income at retirement nor the increases in emotional losses, physical losses, and caregiving responsibilities in later life result in a persistent reduction in life satisfaction among most older adults. As sociologist Linda George (1986) notes, "Older adults are apparently masters of the art of lowering aspirations to meet realities" (p. 7).

Life Review

One tool for preserving or enhancing the *mental health* of older adults is the *life review*, which is an autobiographical effort that can be preserved in print, by tape recording, or on videotape. The review is guided by a series of questions in specific life domains, such as work and family, as well as memories further stimulated through a family photo album, other memorabilia, a genealogy, musical selections from an earlier time, or a trek back to an important place in one's past. It can be conducted by oneself, in a dyad, or as part of a group process. A life review is more likely to be conducted by or with an older adult who is relatively content with his or her life and not seeking therapy than it is to be used therapeutically with an older adult. Nonetheless, life reviews are believed to have therapeutic powers, and they are incorporated into a wide variety of counseling modalities (Haber, 2006).

The psychiatrist Robert Butler first extolled the benefits of the life review process to his colleagues and the public as early as 1961, as a way of incorporating reminiscence in the aged as part of a normal aging process. Dr. Butler described the life review as more comprehensive and systematic than spontaneous reminiscing, and perhaps more important in old age when there may be a need to put one's life in order and to come to an acceptance of present circumstances (Butler, 1995).

The review of positive and negative past life experiences by older adults has enabled them to overcome feelings of depression and despair (Butler, 1974; Butler, Lewis, & Sunderland, 1991; Watt & Cappeliez, 2000). Another study of the life review process reported positive outcomes in terms of stronger life satisfaction, psychological well-being, self-esteem, and reduced depression (Haight, Michel, & Hendrix, 1998).

Although life reviews are usually helpful for improving the mental health of most older adults who are seeking meaning, resolution, reconciliation, direction, and atonement, physicians, nurses, and other clinic personnel find it is too time-consuming to listen to the reminiscences of older clients in this era of medical care. Health professionals can, however, play a key role in referring older clients to appropriate forums or helping them obtain relevant life review materials.

One book, *Aging and Biography,* by the psychologist James Birren and colleagues (1996), helps guide and provide structure for the life review process by suggesting a focus on several themes, such as love, money, work, and family. Birren also suggests in another book, *Telling the Stories of Life Through Guided Autobiography Groups,* that incorporating life reviews into a small-group format can help in the retrieval as well as with the acceptance of memories (Birren & Cochran, 2001).

With careful monitoring, Birren noted that in his years of experience he has not had a group member report becoming depressed as a result of a life review (Birren & Deutchman, 1991). He warned, however, that persons who are already depressed or otherwise needing therapy should be under the supervision of a qualified professional.

Depression

Whether older adults participate in life reviews or not, they are vulnerable to *depression* due to losses that accompany aging such as widowhood, chronic medical conditions and pain, and functional *dependence* (Lantz, 2002). Not only can these emotional and physical losses lead to depression, but depression in turn can lead to more physical decline (Penninx et al., 1998b).

Although the mechanism is not understood, depression increases the likelihood of mortality from cancer (Penninx et al., 1998a) and heart disease (Frasure-Smith, Lesperance, & Talajic, 1995). The mortality rate for depressed patients with cardiovascular disease is twice that of those without depression (Lantz, 2002) and depression is an independent risk factor for cardiovascular disease (Coulter & Campos, 2012). Even mild depression can weaken the immune system in older persons if it goes on long enough (McGuire, Kiecolt-Glaser, & Glaser, 2002).

Depression also plays a significant role in suicidal behaviors, and older persons have the highest suicide rate of any age group. Older adults account for nearly 20% of all suicide deaths(American Foundation for Suicide Prevention, 2016). This elevated suicide rate, however, is largely accounted for by white men age 85 or older. The suicide rate of this age/gender category is four times higher than the overall national rate, with elderly males accounting for seven times the suicide rate of elderly females (Administration on Aging, 2015)

CLINICAL TIP

The suicide rate is highest among older white males, as depression is often undetected and underreported.

Depression in older adults often goes undetected until it is too late. Between 63% (Rabins, 1996) and 90% (Katon, von Korff, Lin, Bush, & Ormel, 1992) of depressed older patients go untreated or receive inadequate treatment. One retrospective study of older adults who had committed suicide revealed that 51 of the 97 patients studied had seen their primary care physician within 1 month of their suicide date. Of these 51, only 19 were even offered treatment, and only 2 of the 51 patients studied were provided adequate treatment (Caine, Lyness, & Conwell, 1996).

Barry Lebowitz (1995), formerly of the National Institute of Mental Health, estimated that 15% of Americans age 65 or over suffered from serious and persistent symptoms of depression, but only 3% were reported to be suffering from the clinical diagnosis of major depression. In other words, although depressive disorders that fulfill rigorous diagnostic criteria are relatively rare, subthreshold disorders are considerably more common, infrequently diagnosed, or treated with prescribed antidepressants, and because they usually go untreated, are likely to become chronic conditions (Beekman et al., 2002).

Detection of depression is hampered not only by the underreporting of symptoms by older patients, but also by biases on the part of physicians and family members. In one study, 75% of physicians thought that depression was understandable in older persons—that is, a normal facet of old age (Gallo, Ryan, & Ford, 1999). Family members may also view the signs and symptoms of depression as "normal aging," when in fact the persistence of depressive symptoms is not normal.

Dependency

The concepts that best capture the degree of dependency an individual must bear are Activities of Daily Living (ADLs) and Instrumental Activities of Daily Living (IADLs). ADLs measure the individual's ability to perform basic personal care tasks such as eating, bathing, dressing, using the toilet, getting in or out of a bed or chair, caring for a bowel-control device, and walking (the latter being the most common ADL limitation). The average nursing home resident needs help with five ADLs.

IADLs measure the individual's ability to perform more complex, multifaceted activities in one's environment, such as home management, managing money, meal preparation, making a phone call, or grocery shopping (the latter being the most common IADL limitation). These limitations typically precede the limitations associated with ADLs.

While ADLs and IADLs can reflect functional impairment on a temporary basis, such as during convalescence from surgery or a temporary disability, with age the limitations are typically chronic. This state of affairs presents not only a physical challenge to the older adults, but a mental health one as well. The primary mental health concern is focused on the quality of one's remaining life, rather than the quantity of years left to live (Haber, 2016). At age 65 we can expect about one-third of our remaining years to be dependent, but by age 85 that increases to two-thirds of our remaining years. With age, dependent living becomes increasingly problematic and is a big contributor to depression (Brenes et al., 2008).

Dependency is often described as frailty when there are three or more ADL deficiencies, combined with weakness and chronic exhaustion. To avoid or slow the descent into frailty, exercise is commonly recommended, even for the very old, but there are many other interventions as well. Smoking cessation, alcohol moderation, nutrition, fall and injury prevention, social support, medical screenings, immunizations, sleep hygiene, and medication management are just a few of the other factors to consider. There is plenty that we can control to lower the probability of a dependent life style or frailty, or at least to shorten this period of dependency as much as possible.

Quality of Life and Wellness

Life is more than the avoidance of dependency, however. We want to promote *quality of life*, which goes beyond mere autonomy in performing ADLs and IADLs. Quality of life may be defined as functional health combined with life satisfaction, a feeling of competency, and a perception of social support. About three-fourths of non-Hispanic Whites and almost two-thirds of African Americans and Hispanic Americans over the age of 65 report a good quality of life, according to the 2004–2006 National Health Interview Survey.

Older adult self-assessments are not always shared by others. Physicians, for instance, often rate the quality of life of older persons lower than do the elders themselves. Physicians are more influenced by objective health

BOX 7-2   Recommended Electronic Newsletter *Positive Aging*

Psychologists Ken and Mary Gergen edit this *electronic newsletter* devoted to positive approaches to aging. This newsletter not only offers a uniquely positive perspective, but summarizes a variety of research that is useful to practitioners. For a free subscription go to: taosinstitute.net/positive-aging-newsletter.

factors than are older adults, who tend to adapt to physical deficiencies over time. Even older persons in nursing homes tend to rate their health more positively than others do (Hooyman & Kiyak, 2011).

The broadest perspective on quality of life is reflected in the concept of wellness. Ironically, wellness as a term has not caught on in the medical world, but in both the corporate setting (Jacob, 2002) and the academic one (as evidenced by the name of this author's former employer: The Institute of *Wellness* and Gerontology at Ball State University), the concept finds fertile territory.

The most common conceptualization of wellness divides this term into seven components. These dimensions are:

Physical: Exercise, eat a well-balanced diet, get enough sleep, protect yourself
Emotional: Express a wide range of feelings, acknowledge stress, channel positive energy
Intellectual: Embrace lifelong learning, discover new skills and interests
Vocational: Do something you love, balance responsibilities with satisfying ways to occupy yourself
Social: Laugh often, spend time with family and friends, join a club, respect cultural differences
Environmental: Recycle daily, use energy-efficient products, walk or bike, grow a garden
Spiritual: Seek meaning and purpose, take time to reflect, connect with the universe.

The world of medicine fully embraces the legitimacy of the physical dimension of wellness, but gives much less emphasis to the other six domains. To access the full spectrum of wellness (see **Box 7-2**), you need to seek out the resources that are commonly available in community health. While exercise is the most ubiquitous health program in the community, the other domains of wellness are represented as well. This is the case with many of the model health promotion programs for older adults that are described in the next section.

Model Health Promotion Programs for Older Adults

Although there is no certain method for determining what constitutes a *model health promotion program*, there has been no shortage of attempts to identify them, develop a catalog that includes a summary of these exemplars, and distribute the catalog around the country in order to encourage their replication. Many of these model health promotion programs have been developed over the years with the aid of federal grants and other funding sources, have gone through multiple program evaluations, and can be helpful to health professionals who are interested in launching or improving their own program.

One of the more recent efforts in this regard has been organized by the Health Promotion Institute (HPI) of the National Council on Aging. The HPI started by summarizing 16 model programs or best practices and compiling them into a loose-leaf directory. The summaries included information on the planning process, implementation of the program, and program evaluations. Each year, new best practices have been added to this directory. If interested in obtaining a copy, contact the National Council on Aging, Health Promotion Institute, 300 D St., SW, #801, Washington, DC 20024; 202-479-1200 or contact online at www.ncoa.org.

Four model health promotion programs that have focused on older adults and have received national attention are summarized in the following sections. These programs have received federal funding and foundation support to evaluate their effectiveness and to encourage their replication.

Healthwise

The best-known older adult medical self-care program is Healthwise, located in Boise, Idaho. The Healthwise program relies mostly on the *Healthwise Handbook*, which provides information and prevention tips on 190 common health problems, with information periodically updated. The *Healthwise Handbook* (Healthwise, 2006) is now in its 17th edition. This handbook includes physician-approved guidelines on when to call a health professional for each of the health problems it covers. Some Healthwise community programs have supplemented the distribution of the handbook with group health education programs or nurse call-in programs. There is a Spanish language edition of the *Healthwise Handbook*, called *La Salud en Casa*, and a special self-care guide for older adults called *Healthwise for Life*.

With the assistance of a $2.1 million grant from the Robert Wood Johnson Foundation, Healthwise distributed its medical self-care guide to 125,000 Idaho households, along with toll-free nurse consultation phone service and self-care workshops. Thirty-nine percent of handbook recipients reported that the handbook helped them avoid a visit to the doctor (Mettler, 1997). Blue Cross of Idaho reported 18% fewer visits to the emergency room by owners of the guide.

Elements of the Healthwise program have been replicated in the United Kingdom, South Africa, New Zealand, Australia, and Canada. In British Columbia, the *Healthwise Handbook* was distributed to every household, and all 4.3 million residents had potential access to the Healthwise content through a website and a nurse call center. Additional information can be obtained from Donald Kemper or Molly Mettler, at www.healthwise.org.

Chronic Disease Self-Management Program

Kate Lorig, a nurse-researcher at the Stanford University School of Medicine, and her medical colleagues have been evaluating community-based, peer-led, chronic disease self-management programs for more than two decades, beginning with the Arthritis Self-Management Program (Lorig et al., 1996). This program has since evolved into a curriculum that is applicable to a wide array of chronic diseases and conditions.

Typically, each program involves about a dozen participants, led by peer leaders who have received 20 hours of training. The peer leaders, like the students, are typically older and have chronic diseases that they contend with. The program consists of six weekly sessions, each about 2.5 hours long, with a content focus on exercise, symptom management, nutrition, fatigue and sleep management, use of medications, managing emotions, community resources, communicating with health professionals, problem solving, and decision making. The program takes place in community settings such as senior centers, churches, and hospitals.

The theoretical basis of the program has been to promote a sense of personal efficacy among participants (Bandura, 1997) by using such techniques as guided mastery of skills, peer modeling, reinterpretation of symptoms, social persuasion through group support, and individual self-management guidance. In addition to improving self-efficacy, Lorig and colleagues (2001) reported reduced emergency room and outpatient visits, and decreased health distress, fatigue, and limitations in role function.

The Chronic Disease Self-Management Program is housed at Stanford University's Patient Education Research Center, 1000 Welch Road, #204, Palo Alto, CA 94304; 650-723-7935; http://patienteducation.stanford.edu/programs/cdsmp.html.

Project Enhance

Senior Services of Seattle/King County began the Senior Wellness Project (later renamed Project Enhance) in 1997 at the North Shore Senior Center in Bothell, Washington. It was a research-based health promotion program that included a component of chronic care self-management that was modeled after Kate Lorig's program

(Lorig, Sobel, & Stewart, 1999). The program also included health and functional assessments; individual and group counseling; exercise programs; a personal health action plan with the support of a nurse, social worker, and volunteer health mentor; and support groups. A randomized controlled study of chronically ill seniors reported a reduction in number of hospital stays and average length of stay, a reduction in psychotropic medications, and better functioning in ADLs (Leveille et al., 1998).

Project Enhance is a partnership among a university, an area Agency on Aging, local and national foundations, health departments, senior centers, primary care providers, older volunteers, and older participants. Versions of this model program are being replicated at senior wellness sites around the country (80+ sites in the United States) and two sites in Sweden to test its effectiveness in a variety of communities, in an assortment of sites, serving a diversity of clientele. Findings have demonstrated higher levels of physical activity and lower levels of depression among its participants (Dobkin, 2002).

Project Enhance is currently divided into two components: Enhance Fitness and Enhance Wellness. Enhance Fitness is an exercise program that focuses on stretching, flexibility, balance, low impact aerobics, and strength training. Certified instructors have undergone special training in fitness for older adults. Classes last an hour, involve 10 to 25 people, and participants can track their progress through a series of functional evaluations.

Participants who completed 6 months of Enhance Fitness improved significantly in a variety of physical and social functioning measures, as well as reported reduced levels of pain and depression. There was also a reduction in healthcare costs (Ackerman et al., 2003). The Enhance Fitness program has been replicated in 64 community sites across 6 states.

Enhance Wellness focuses on mental health, with an emphasis on lessening symptoms of depression and other mood problems, developing a sense of greater self-reliance, and lowering the need for drugs that affect thinking or emotions. Enhance Wellness typically consists of a nurse and social worker working with an individual. An analysis of the effectiveness of the program found that it reduced depression 1 year after the program and improved exercise readiness, physical activity levels, and self-reported health (Phelan et al., 2002).

To learn more about Project Enhance, contact Susan Snyder, Program Director at Senior Services of Seattle/King County, at susans@seniorservices.org.

Cardiac Wellness

There are two Medicare-reimbursable wellness programs for persons rehabilitating from heart disease or heart surgery, and both are unique in that they include several techniques that are considered to be *complementary and alternative medicine* that have not previously been covered by Medicare.

The first program is **Dean Ornish's Program for Reversing Heart Disease**. Dr. Dean Ornish, a physician at the University of California at San Francisco and founder of the Preventive Medicine Research Institute, has developed a program for reversing heart disease that has been replicated at several sites around the country. Dr. Ornish (1992) has recommended a vegetarian diet (see **Box 7-3**) with fat intake of 10% or less of total calories, moderate aerobic exercise at least three times a week, yoga and meditation an hour a day, group support sessions, and smoking cessation.

Dr. Ornish and his colleagues have reported that as a result of their program, blockages in arteries have decreased in size and blood flow has improved in as many as 82% of their heart patients (Gould et al., 1995). A 5-year follow-up of this program reported an 8% reduction in atherosclerotic plaques, while the control group had a 28% increase. Also during this time, cardiac events were more than doubled in the control group (Ornish et al., 1998).

The applicability of Ornish's program to the average patient is still of uncertain utility. It may take highly motivated individuals (e.g., patients with severe heart disease) and significant medical and health support

BOX 7-3   Research Highlight

The Mediterranean diet has been lauded as a key to living a longer, healthier life. Understanding this assumption, van den Brandt studied whether or not it could be supported by data. Sign into your database of nursing literature (CINAHL or PubMed, for example) and use the citation below to perform a search for this article. What were van den Brandt's findings? Is the Mediterranean diet a proven way to reduce the risk of mortality or premature death?

van den Brandt, P. A. (2011). The impact of a Mediterranean diet and healthy lifestyle on premature mortality in men and women. *American Journal of Clinical Nutrition, 94*, 913–920.

(requiring significant resources) for the model program to be useful to others. In addition, low-fat diets, and in this instance we are talking about very-low-fat diets, have fallen out of favor when they do not differentiate between the healthy and unhealthy fats. For additional information, contact Dean Ornish at http://www.pmri.org.

The second program originated at **Herbert Benson's Mind/Body Medical Institute**. Dr. Herbert Benson is a physician affiliated with Harvard Medical School and best known for his bestselling books on the relaxation response and for popularizing the term mind/body medicine. For individuals feeling the negative effects of stress, Benson's program teaches them to elicit the relaxation response, a western version of meditation. The Benson–Henry Institute for Mind/Body Medicine's clinical programs treat patients with a combination of relaxation response techniques, proper nutrition and exercise, and the reframing of negative thinking patterns.

Benson's nonprofit scientific and educational institute conducts research; provides outpatient medical services; and trains health professionals, postdoctoral fellows, and medical students. The Benson–Henry Institute for Mind/Body Medicine can be contacted at http://www.massgeneral.org/bhi/.

The research results from Benson's and Ornish's programs attracted the attention of Medicare, which funded a demonstration project to evaluate them. As a consequence of the demonstration project, in 2006 Medicare began to reimburse eligible patients for participation in these two cardiac wellness programs. These two programs have expanded the emphasis in Medicare from acute care medicine, rehabilitative medicine, and prevention to the inclusion of comprehensive wellness.

CLINICAL TIP

A healthy lifestyle, including a Mediterranean diet (for women particularly) lowers risk of premature death.

Re-Engagement Instead of Retirement

In 2011, baby boomers began turning age 65 and started becoming the gerontology boomers. Most of them will not retire, if "retirement" means a type of disengagement. Why will these gerontology boomers be different from the current crop of retirees?

First, the boomers will be the longest-lived cohort of older adults. They may have 25 or 30 years of life to negotiate after giving up their main line of work. How many of them will be comfortable with the idea of a quarter-century without additional earnings? How many will be comfortable letting go of education, exploration, and engagement?

The boomers will be the best-educated cohort of older adults. Between 1950 and 2000, the percentage of Americans age 65 or over with a high school diploma leaped from 18% to 66%; college graduates jumped from 4% to 15%. In 1991, 17% of Americans age 60–64 were involved in adult education; by 1999 that number had jumped to 32%. They say a mind—76 million minds, to be precise—is a terrible thing to waste, not only from the individual's standpoint, but from society's as well.

The boomers will be the healthiest cohort of older adults. Almost 90% of Americans ages 65–74 report that they have no disability, and the disability rate for older Americans continues to decline. An increasing number of older adults are exercising in late life, with brisk walking for exercise becoming commonplace among the old. Not only is a mind a terrible thing to waste, so is a healthy body.

Also, the boomers may become the most-engaged cohort of older adults. Fifty-four percent of boomers say helping others is important to them. A 2002 national survey by Hart Research Associates reported that about 60% of older Americans believe that retirement is a "time to be active and involved, to start new activities and to set new goals" (Hart, 2002). A 2005 survey by Civic Ventures and the MetLife Foundation (2005) reported that 58% of leading-edge baby boomers, those between ages 51 and 59, said they want to take jobs that serve their communities.

In addition, the boomers will be the largest cohort of retirees ever. The number of Americans age 65 or older will increase from 35 million in 2000 to more than 70 million in 2030. When these boomers came into the world they revolutionized hospitals and health care just through their sheer size. They did the same thing to public schools, the *Vietnam War*, and then the housing market, spurring a tremendous growth in building. A cohort this large is unlikely to pass into retirement and leave it unchanged, and boomers are unlikely to accept things as they are.

What might older adults do, if they decide to re-engage rather than retire? Here are two possibilities. The **Experience Corps** is one possibility. The Experience Corps is a foundation-supported program that has placed 2,000 older adults as tutors and mentors with 20,000 low-income children in urban public elementary schools and afterschool programs in 19 cities. These programs not only boost the academic performance of students, but enhance the well-being of the older volunteers in the process (Fried et al., 2004; Rebok et al., 2004; Tan, Xue, Li, Carlson, & Fried, 2006). Much work remains as two-thirds of the nation's fourth graders in major urban areas are reading below basic levels for their grade. For more information, contact Experience Corps at http://www .experiencecorps.org.

Green House

Nursing homes are not homes—they are institutions. No matter how well run they are, they are not places where most of us want to end up. We are at the beginning of revolutionizing the long-term care industry, and no one has been more innovative and successful at this early stage than William Thomas, MD, founder of the *Green House*. Dr. Thomas started out his career as a medical director in a nursing home and was saddened by how regimented and joyless the environment was.

In traditional nursing homes, residents are viewed as sick and dependent, which fosters learned helplessness and induced disability. Staff may encourage wheelchair dependency to serve the needs of staff members who are pressed for time. Dressing, feeding, bathing, and toileting need to be routinized and sped up for aides needing to stay on schedule. A staff member is more likely to rely on incontinence briefs than to take the time to develop individualized toileting routines.

Green Houses, in contrast, look like surrounding homes in a residential community. They are homes, not home-like, though they are bigger than the average home. The first ones were constructed in Tupelo, Mississippi, in 2003, and were 6,400 square feet. The rooms in these homes include extra expense, such as ceiling lifts, but these innovations can save costs over the long term by reducing back injuries, employee turnover, and workers' compensation.

Green House workers are paid more and are better trained than the typical nursing assistant, but the extra costs are offset by employee empowerment that reduces staff turnover and additional training expenses. The annual employee turnover rate in the average nursing home is 75%, whereas it was less than 10% in the first Green House in Tupelo. Moreover, not one staff person left during the house's first 3 years of existence.

About 10 people live in a Green House, each having a private room and bath, and access to a central hearth where cooking and socializing are done. There is a surrounding garden for contemplative walks and for growing vegetables and flowers. Doors can be opened to view the garden and hearth from an individual room or closed for privacy. With the circular nature of the individual rooms, both the garden and the central hearth are within 30 feet. There is strategically placed furniture to help with "cruising" to central areas and to help with gains in mobility (see **Case Study 7-1**).

Green Houses promote autonomy. Residents get up, eat, and go to bed when they want. They decide on which foods to eat, and that may even include pizza, wine, or ice cream. Medications are locked in individual rooms, rather than distributed by a cart that is wheeled from room to room. There are few features that are different from the typical home, and if there are unusual features, they are de-emphasized, like a ceiling lift that is recessed and used only when needed for transfer. Induction cooking in the kitchen prevents residents from burning themselves on a stove. Stoves have shut-off valves, with pot trappers to prevent hot pots from burning residents. A safety gate around the kitchen can be used when necessary.

Case Study 7–1

Dr. Brown is a retired superintendent of a large public school system in the Midwest. He has been widowed for 5 years and just recently retired at the age of 69 after experiencing a fall down a flight of stairs at his home that resulted in a fractured hip, skull fracture, and broken shoulder, for which he has been treated in the hospital and is being discharged soon. Dr. Brown's two adult children have encouraged him to sell his home and move somewhere where there is help available when he needs it. Dr. Brown hates the thought of a nursing home, especially since his wife spent about a year in one before her death. He is not certain whether an assisted living facility would work for him either. The family asks the hospital nurse for assistance in exploring living options for Dr. Brown.

Questions:

1. What questions should the nurse ask of Dr. Brown to help determine his preferences for living situations?
2. What other factors are essential to know about Dr. Brown in order to assist him with proper choices?
3. Are there any other team members who should be consulted within the hospital that could help with this decision? If so, who?
4. Would a Green House be a better option than assisted or independent living for Dr. Brown? Why or why not? What factors must be considered before answering this question?

People in the first 10 Green Houses were selected from nursing homes and represented a typical nursing home population. Of the first 40 selected, 12 had advanced dementia, and all Green House residents had the typical array of physical and cognitive limitations associated with the average nursing home resident.

Decision making is lodged in residents and workers, unless there are safety or budget issues that cannot be handled at that level. Aides are called shahbazim (derived from the mythical Persian royal falcon that protected the king), with the primary job responsibility to protect, nurture, and sustain.

Ideal staff ratio is 1 for every 5 residents; nurse ratio is 1 for every 2 houses (or 1 per 20 people), and administrator ratio (and one assistant) 1 for every 12 houses (or 1 per 120 people). Staff find replacements for themselves if sick, either through a substitute pool or through overtime (which is managed within the allowable budget).

Workers receive 120 hours of additional training in areas such as CPR, first aid, culinary skills, safe food handling, communication, and dementia care. They are better paid than the average long-term care worker ($11 per hour versus $7.50) and are given rotating responsibility (purchasing food and cooking, housekeeping, scheduling, budget, etc.). Unless the nonclinical work teams endanger safety or overspend budget, administrators cannot overrule their decisions.

Every Green House has been fully staffed so far, with never a day understaffed. Wheelchair use has declined, and the strength of residents has increased. Residents have the option to eat in a group or alone, with an individualized menu and pleasant surroundings—referred to as a convivium. A local cookbook is assembled to cater to the tastes of people born in a region. Shahbazim can eat with residents and participate in activities with them, along with family and friends.

Most of these ideas are summarized in William Thomas's book, *What Are Old People For?* and in a journal article titled, "Radical Redesign of Nursing Homes" (Rabig, Thomas, Kane, Cutler, & McAlilly, 2006). In a publication called CNS SeniorCare, Thomas (Rabig et al., 2006) sums up his philosophy:

Old age, like all the other phases of our lives, should be about life and living. Treating aging as a medical condition that must be managed with the professional distance prescribed by the medical model is wrong and leads to terrible suffering. For decades we have organized the life of the elder or disabled individual in a skilled nursing facility around the needs of the institution, rather than individuals who live there. (p. 14)

The Robert Wood Johnson Foundation provided a $10 million grant (from 2006 to 2010) to establish at least 30 Green Houses around the United States and to allow other long-term care owners and administrators to replicate them through training support and up to $125,000 in predevelopment loans.

Summary

Many exciting changes are taking place in the field of health promotion and aging (see **Box 7-4**). Perhaps it is time to establish a pro-aging movement—in contrast to the commercial and exploitive anti-aging movement. No longer needing to impress employers, in-laws, or peers, older adults are free to be themselves. Aging people have an opportunity to be freer, wiser, more engaged in helping others, and more willing to be an advocate not only for their own health, but for the well-being of society.

BOX 7-4   Web Exploration

Check out current nutrition recommendations at http://www.choosemyplate.gov/.

Clinical Reasoning Exercises

1. **What do you think is the most important health objective** that should be set for the future, and what should federal and state governments do to help?
2. **How familiar are you with the health-promoting resources** in your community? Find one that you are unfamiliar with but believe may be important for older persons. Summarize it sufficiently to answer most questions that older adults might have about it.
3. **What is your opinion** of the existing Medicare prevention coverage? What would you change, and why?
4. **Write a health contract/calendar** for yourself for 1 month. At the end of this time explain your success or lack of such with accomplishing your health goal.
5. **What has been your major barrier** when it comes to engaging in exercise on a regular basis, and have you attempted to overcome it? If so, how?
6. Check out the **nutrition guidelines at Choose My Plate http://www.choosemyplate.gov/**, and see what you can learn about nutrition that is interesting to you. Do you have any suggestions for improving this site?
7. **Research suggests that older adults are more conscious of their nutritional habits** than younger adults. Conduct your own survey of five older adults and five younger adults, asking them to rate how much attention they give to eating what is good for them, using a scale of 1 (not very often) to 10 (all the time). Does your convenience sample corroborate the positive relationship between age and good nutritional habits?

Personal Reflections

1. Create your own nutrition bull's-eye, filling in the foods and drinks that you consume or might consider consuming. Use it for a week to guide your eating choices. Take a list of the food products in the center of your bull's-eye to the supermarket with you. Did you find this technique to be helpful?
2. Have you ever conducted a life review with an older adult? If you have, how satisfying was it for you and for them? If not, why not? How do you feel about not having done one with an older family member?
3. Choose one of the model health promotion programs summarized in this chapter and find out something of interest to you about that program that is not mentioned in this chapter
4. The author believes that if we become more responsive to the healthcare needs of older adults, we will probably provide better health care for people of all ages in the United States. What do you think is the logic behind this belief?
5. What does this quotation by Henry Wadsworth Longfellow mean to you? "Age is opportunity no less than youth itself, though in another dress, and as the evening twilight fades away, the sky is filled with stars, invisible by day."
6. Describe a geriatric job, or an aspect of a job, that you would enjoy doing (related to nursing or not) and would be an important service for older adults, but is not currently being done.

References

Ackerman, R. T., Cheadle, A., Sandhu, N., Madsen, L., Wagner, E. H., & LoGerfo, J. P. (2003). Community exercise program use and changes in health care costs for older adults. *American Journal of Preventive Medicine, 25*(3), 232–237.

Administration on Aging. (2015). Older American's Behavioral Health Issue Brief 4: Preventing suicide in older adults. Retrieved from http://www.aoa.gov/AoA_Programs/HPW/Behavioral/docs2/Issue%20Brief%204%20 Preventing%20Suicide.pdf

American Foundation for Suicide Prevention (2016). Suicide statistics. Retrieved from http://afsp.org/about-suicide /suicide-statistics/

Bailey, C. (1996). *Smart eating.* Boston, MA: Houghton-Mifflin.

Bandura, A. (1977). *Social learning theory.* Englewood Cliffs, NJ: Prentice Hall.

Bandura, A. (1997). *Self-efficacy: The exercise of control.* New York, NY: W. H. Freeman.

Becker, M. (1974). The health belief model and personal health behavior. *Health Education Monographs, 2*(4), 236.

Beekman, A., Geerlings, S. W., Deeq, D. J., Smit, J. H., Schoevers, R. S., de Beurs, E., . . . van Tilburg W. (2002). The natural history of late-life depression: A 6-year prospective study in the community. *Archives of General Psychiatry, 59*(7), 605–611.

Beers, M., & Berkow, R. (2000). *The Merck manual of geriatrics* (3rd ed.). Whitehouse Station, NJ: Merck Research Laboratories.

Berry, M., Danish, S. J., Rinke, W. J., & Smiciklas-Wright, H. (1989). Work-site health promotion: The effects of a goal-setting program on nutrition-related behaviors. *Journal of the American Dietary Association, 89*(3), 914–920.

Birren, J., & Cochran, K. (2001). *Telling the stories of life through guided autobiography groups.* Baltimore, MD: Johns Hopkins University Press.

Birren, J., & Deutchman, D. (1991). *Guiding autobiography groups for older adults.* Baltimore, MD: Johns Hopkins University Press.

Birren, J., Kenyon, G. M., Ruth, J. R., Schroots, J. J. F., & Svensson, T. (Eds.). (1996). *Aging and biography: Explorations in adult development.* New York, NY: Springer.

Blair, S., Kohl, H. W. III, Paffenbarger, R. S. Jr., Clark, D. G., Cooper, K. H., & Gibbons, L. W. (1989). Physical fitness and all-cause mortality: A prospective study of healthy men and women. *Journal of the American Medical Association, 262*(17), 2395–2401.

Booth, K., Pinkston, M. M., & Poston, W. S. (2005). Obesity and the built environment. *Journal of the American Dietetic Association, 105* (5 Suppl. 1), S110–S117.

Brenes, G., Penninx, B. W., Judd, P. H., Rockwell, E., Sewell, D. D., & Wetherell, J. L. (2008). Anxiety, depression and disability across the life span. *Aging and Mental Health, 12,* 158–163.

Brownson, R., Housemann, R. A., Brown, D. R., Jackson-Thompson, J., King, A. C, Malone, B. R., Sallis J. F. (2000). Promoting physical activity in rural communities: Walking trail access, use, and effects. *American Journal of Preventive Medicine, 18*(3), 235–241.

Butler, R. (1974). Successful aging and the role of the life review. *Journal of the American Geriatrics Society, 22*(12), 529–535.

Butler, R. (1995). Foreword: The life review. In B. Haight & J. Webster (Eds.), *The art and science of reminiscing* (pp. xvii–xxi). Washington, DC: Taylor and Francis.

Butler, R., Lewis, M. I., & Sunderland, T. (1991). Aging and mental health: Positive psychosocial and biomedical approaches. Columbus, OH: Charles E. Merrill.

Caine, E., Lyness, J. M., & Conwell, Y. (1996). Diagnosis of late-life depression: Preliminary studies in primary care settings. *American Journal of Geriatric Psychiatry, 4*(1), S45–S50.

Civic Ventures and MetLife. (2005). *New faces of work survey.* Retrieved from http://civicventures.org/publications /surveys/new_face_of_work/new_face_of_work.pdf

Clark, J., Keukefeld, C., & Godlaski, T. (1999). Case management and behavioral contracting: Components of rural substance abuse treatment. *Journal of Substance Abuse Treatment, 17*(4), 293–304.

Coulter, S. A. & Campos, K. (2012). Identify and treat depression for reduced cardiac risk and improved outcomes. *Texas Heart Institute Journal, 39*(2), 231–234.

Cupples, S., & Steslow, B. (2001). Use of behavioral contingency contracting with heart transplant candidates. *Progress in Transplantation, 11*(2), 137–144.

DeBusk, R., Stenestrand, U., Sheehan, M., & Haskell, W. L. (1990). Training effects of long versus short bouts of exercise in healthy subjects. *American Journal of Cardiology, 65*(15), 1010–1013.

De Cocker, K., Cardon, G., & De Bourdeaudhuij, I. (2006). The validity of the inexpensive "stepping meter" in counting steps in free-living conditions. *British Journal of Sports Medicine, 40*(8), 714–716.

Dobkin, L. (2002). Senior wellness project secures health care dollars. *Innovations, 2,* 16–20.

Engel, L., & Lindner, H. (2006). Impact of using a pedometer on time spent walking in older adults with type 2 diabetes. *Diabetes Education, 32*(5), 98–107.

Estruch, R., Ros, E., Salas-Salvado, J. (2013). Primary prevention of cardiovascular disease with a Mediterranean diet. *New England Journal of Medicine, 368,* 1279–1290.

Feart, C., Samieri, C., Rondeau, V., Amieva, H., Portet, F., Dartigues, J. F., . . . Barberger-Gateau P. (2009). Adherence to a Mediterranean diet, cognitive decline, and risk of dementia. *Journal of the American Medical Association, 302,* 638–648.

Finestone, A. (2009). Definition of hypertension for the "old-old." *Journal of Gerontology: Medical Sciences, 64,* 1097.

Fishbein, M., & Ajzen, I. (1975). *Belief, attitude, intention and behavior: An introduction to theory and research.* Reading, MA: Addison-Wesley.

Francois, M., Baldi, J., & Manning, P. (2014). Exercise snack before meals: A novel strategy to improve glycemic control in individuals with insulin resistance. *Diabetologia, 57,* 1437–1445.

Frank, L., Andresen, M. A., & Schmid, T. L. (2004). Obesity relationships with community design, physical activity, and time spent in cars. *American Journal of Preventive Medicine, 27*(2), 87–96.

Frasure-Smith, N., Lesperance, F., & Talajic, M. (1995). Depression and 18-month prognosis after myocardial infarction. *Circulation, 91*(4), 999–1005.

Fried, L., Carlson, M. C., Freedman, M., Frick, K. D., Glass, T. A., Hill, J., et al. (2004). A social model for health promotion for an aging population: Initial evidence on the Experience Corps model. *Journal of Urban Health, 81*(1), 64–78.

Gallo, J., Ryan, S. D., & Ford, D. E. (1999). Attitudes, knowledge, and behavior of family physicians regarding depression in late life. *Archives of Family Medicine, 8*(3), 249–256.

George, L. (1986, Spring). Life satisfaction in later life. *Generations,* 5–8.

Gould, L., Ornish, D., Scherwitz, L., Brown, S., Edens, R. P., Hess, M. J., . . . Billings J. (1995). Changes in myocardial perfusion abnormalities by positron emission tomography after long-term, intense risk factor modification. *Journal of the American Medical Association, 274*(11), 894–901.

Haber, D. (2001). Medicare prevention: Movement toward research-based policy. *Journal of Aging and Social Policy, 13*(1), 1–14.

Haber, D. (2002). Health promotion and aging: Educational and clinical initiatives by the federal government. *Educational Gerontology, 28*(2), 1–11.

Haber, D. (2005). Medicare prevention update. *Journal of Aging and Social Policy, 17*(2), 1–6.

Haber, D. (2006). Life review: Implementation, theory, and future direction. *International Journal of Aging and Human Development, 63*(2), 153–171.

Haber, D. (2007). Health contract in the classroom. *Gerontology and Geriatrics Education, 27*(4), 41–54.

Haber, D. (2016). *Health promotion and aging: Practical applications for health professionals* (7th ed.), New York, NY: Springer.

Haber, D., & Looney, C. (2000). Health contract calendars: A tool for health professionals with older adults. *The Gerontologist, 40*(2), 235–239.

Haber, D., & Rhodes, D. (2004). Health contract with sedentary older adults. *The Gerontologist, 44*(6), 827–835.

Haight, B., Michel, Y., & Hendrix, S. (1998). Life review: Preventing despair in newly relocated nursing home residents' short-and long-term effects. *International Journal of Aging and Human Development, 47*(2), 119–142.

Harris, L. (1989). *The prevention index '89: Summary report.* Emmaus, PA: Rodale Press.

Hart, P. (2002). *The new face of retirement: An ongoing survey of American attitudes on aging.* Retrieved from http://www.experiencecorps.org/images/pdf/new_face_survey_results.pdf

Healthwise. (2006). *Healthwise handbook* (17th ed.). Boise, ID: Author.

Healthy People 2020. (n.d.) *iHealthy People 2020.* Retrieved from http://www.healthypeople.gov/2020/Connect/iHealthyPeople2020v25.pdf

Hooyman, N & Kiyak, H. (2011). *Social gerontology: A multidisciplinary perspective.* Boston, MA: Allyn & Bacon.

Jacob, J. (2002). Wellness programs help companies save on health costs. *American Medical News,* March, 32–33.

Jakicic, J., Donnelly, J. E., Pronk, N. P., Jawad, A. F., & Jacobsen, D. J. (1995). Prescription of exercise intensity for the obese patient: The relationship between heart rate, VO2 and perceived exertion. *International Journal of Obesity, 19*(6), 382–387.

Jette, A., Lachman, M., Giorgetti, M. M., Assmann, S. F., Harris, B. A., Levenson, C., . . . Krebs D. (1999). Exercise—It's never too late: The Strong for Life program. *American Journal of Public Health, 89*(1), 66–72.

Johnson, C. C., Nicklas, T. A., Arbeit, M. L., Webber, L. S., & Berenson, G. S. (1992). Behavioral counseling and contracting as methods for promoting cardiovascular health in families. *Journal of the American Dietetic Association, 92*(4), 479–481.

Katon, W., von Korff, M., Lin, E., Bush, T., & Ormel, J. (1992). Adequacy and duration of antidepressant treatment in primary care. *Medical Care, 30*(11), 67–76.

Kazel, R. (2004, June 28). Dieting for dollars. *American Medical News,* 17–18.

King, W., Brach, J. S., Killingsworth, R., Fenton, M., & Kriska, A. M. (2003). The relationship between convenience of destinations and walking levels in older women. *American Journal of Health Promotion, 18*(1), 74–82.

LaCroix, A., Leveille, S. G., Hecht, J. A., Grothaus, L. C., & Wagner, E. H. (1996). Does walking decrease the risk of cardiovascular disease hospitalization and death in older adults? *Journal of the American Geriatrics Society, 44*(2), 113–120.

Lantz, M. (2002). Depression in the elderly: Recognition and treatment. *Clinical Geriatrics, 10*(2), 18–24.

Lebowitz, B. (1995, Spring). Depression in older adults. *Aging and Vision News, 7,* 2.

Lee, I., Sesso, H. D., & Paffenbarger, R. S. (2000). Physical activity and coronary heart disease risk in men. *Circulation, 102*(4), 981–986.

Leslie, M., & Schuster, P. (1991). The effect of contingency contracting on adherence and knowledge of exercise regimen. *Patient Education and Counseling, 18*(3), 231–241.

Leveille, S., Wagner, E. H., Davis, C., Grothaus, L., Wallace, J., LoGerfo, M., Kent D. (1998). Preventing disability and managing chronic illness in frail older adults: A randomized trial of a community-based partnership with primary care. *Journal of the American Geriatrics Society, 46*(10), 1191–1198.

Levitan, E., Lewis, C., Tinker, L. (2013). Mediterranean and DASH diet scores and mortality in women with heart failure. *Circulation Heart, 6,* 1116–1123.

Li, F., Fisher, K. J., & Harmer, P. (2005). Improving physical function and blood pressure in older adults through cobblestone mat walking: A randomized trial. *Journal of the American Geriatrics Society, 53*(8), 1305–1312.

Lorig, K., Lubeck, D., Kraines, R. G., Seleznickm, M., & Holman, H. R. (1996). Outcomes of self-help education for patients with arthritis. *Arthritis and Rheumatism, 28*(2), 680–685.

Lorig, K., Ritter, P., Stewart, A., L., Sobel, D. S., Brown, B. W. J., Bandura, A., . . . Holman H. R. (2001). Chronic disease self-management program. *Medical Care, 39*(11), 1217–1223.

Lorig, K., Sobel, D., Holeman, M. D., Laurent, D., Gonzales, V., & Minor, M. (2000). *Living a healthy life with chronic conditions.* Palo Alto, CA: Bull.

Lorig, K., Sobel, D., & Stewart, A. (1999). Evidence suggesting that a chronic disease self-management program can improve health status while reducing hospitalization: A randomized trial. *Medical Care, 37*(1), 5–14.

Lorig, K., Stewart, A., Ritter, P., Gonzalez, V., Laurent, D., & Lynch, J. (1996). *Outcome measures for health education and other health care interventions.* Thousand Oaks, CA: Sage.

McCormack, G., Giles-Corti, B., & Milligan, R. (2006). Demographic and individual correlates of achieving 10,000 steps/day: Use of pedometers in a population-based study. *Health Promotion Journal of Australia, 17*(1), 43–47.

McGuire, L., Kiecolt-Glaser, J. K., & Glaser, R. (2002). Depressive symptoms and lymphocyte proliferation in older adults. *Journal of Abnormal Psychology, 111*(1), 192–197.

Mettler, M. (1997). *Unpublished update on the Healthwise Handbook program.* Healthwise, Inc., P.O. Box 1989, Boise, ID 83701.

Moore, J., von Korff, M., Cherkin, D., Saunders, K., & Lorig, K. (2000). A randomized trial of a cognitive-behavioral program for enhancing back pain self care in a primary care setting. *Pain, 88*(2), 145–153.

Mozaffarian, D. & Ludwig, D. S. (2015). The 2015 US dietary guidelines lifting the ban on total dietary fat. *Journal of the American Medical Association. 313*(24), 2421–2. doi:10.1001/jama.2015.5941.

Murphy, M., Nevill, A., Neville, C., Biddle, S., & Hardman, A. (2002). Accumulating brisk walking for fitness, cardiovascular risk, and psychological health. *Medical Science and Sports Exercise, 34*(9), 1468–1474.

National Center for Health Statistics. (1985). *National health interview survey.* Hyattsville, MD: U.S. Public Health Service, Advance Data, 13.

Neale, A., Singleton, S. P., Dupuis, M. H., & Hess, J. W. (1990). The use of behavioral contracting to increase exercise activity. *American Journal of Health Promotion, 4*(2), 441–447.

Nutting, P. (1987). Community-oriented primary care: From principle to practice. In P. Nutting (Ed.), *Community-oriented primary care* (pp. xv–xxv). Albuquerque: University of New Mexico Press.

Ornish, D. (1992). *Dr. Dean Ornish's program for reversing heart disease.* New York, NY: Ballantine.

Ornish, D., Scherwitz, L. W., Billings, J. H., Brown, S. E., Gould, K. L., Merritt, T. A., . . . Brand R. J. (1998). Intensive lifestyle changes for reversal of coronary heart disease. *Journal of the American Medical Association, 280*(23), 2001–2007.

Pate, R. R., Pratt, M., Blair, S. N., Haskell, W. L., Macera, C. A., Bouchard, C., . . . Wilmore J. H. (1995). Physical activity and public health. *Journal of the American Medical Association, 273*(5), 402–407.

Penninx, B., Guralnik, J. M., Pahor, M., Ferrucci, L., Cerhan, J. R., Wallace, R. B., Havlik R. J. (1998a). Chronically depressed mood and cancer risk in older persons. *Journal of the National Cancer Institute, 90*(24), 1888–1893.

Penninx, B., Guralnik, J. M., Ferucci, L., Simonsick, E. M., Deeq, D. J., & Wallace, R. B. (1998b). Depressive symptoms and physical decline in community-dwelling older persons. *Journal of the American Medical Association, 279*(21), 1720–1726.

Phelan, E., Williams, B., Leveille, S., Snyder, S., Wagner, E. H., & LoGerfo, J. P. (2002). Outcomes of a community-based dissemination of the health enhancement program. *Journal of the American Geriatrics Society, 50*(9), 1519–1524.

Prochaska, J., & DiClemente, C. (1992). Stages of change in the modification of problem behaviors. In M. Herson et al. (Eds.), *Progress in behavior modification* (pp. 184-218). CA: Sage.

Rabig, J., Thomas, W., Kane, R., Cutler, L., & McAlilly, S. (2006). Radical redesign of nursing homes: Applying the Green House concept in Tupelo, Mississippi. *The Gerontologist, 46*(4), 533–539.

Rabins, P. (1996). Barriers to diagnosis and treatment of depression in elderly patients. *American Journal of Geriatric Psychiatry, 4*(1), S79–S83.

Rastas, S., Pirttilä, T., Viramo, P., Verkkoniemi, A., Halonen, P., Juva, K., . . . Sulkava R. (2006). Association between blood pressure and survival over 9 years in a general population aged 85 and older. *Journal of the American Geriatrics Society, 54*, 912–918.

Rebok, G., Carlson, M. C., Glass, T. A., McGill, S., Hill, J., Wasik, B. A., . . . Rasmussen M. D. (2004). Short-term impact of Experience Corps participation on children and schools. *Journal of Urban Health, 81*(1), 79–83.

Schlenk, E., & Boehm, S. (1998). Behaviors in type II diabetes during contingency contracting. *Applied Nursing Research, 11*(2), 77–83.

Sherzai, A., Hei, L., Boothby, C. (2012). Stroke, food groups and dietary patterns. *Nutrition Reviews, 70,* 423–435.

Squires, S. (2002, October 14–20). We're fat and getting fatter. *Washington Post National Weekly Edition,* p. 34.

Stovitz, S., VanWormer, J. J., Center, B. A., & Bremer, K. L. (2005). Pedometers as a means to increase ambulatory activity for patients seen at a family medicine clinic. *Journal of the American Board of Family Practice, 18*(5), 335–343.

Sturm, R., & Cohen, D. (2004). Suburban sprawl and physical and mental health. Public Health, *118*(7), 488–496.

Swinburn, B., Walter, L. G., Arroll, B., Tilyard, M. W., & Russell, D. G. (1998). The green prescription study: A randomized controlled trial of written exercise advice provided by general practitioners. *American Journal of Public Health, 88*(2), 288–291.

Tan, E., Xue, Q. L., Li, T., Carlson, M. C., & Fried, L. P. (2006). Volunteering: A physical activity intervention for older adults—The Experience Corps program in Baltimore. *Journal of Urban Health, 83*(5), 954–969.

Thomas, W. (2004). *What are old people for?* Acton, MA: VanderWyk & Burnam.

U.S. Preventive Services Task Force. (1996). *Guide to clinical preventive services.* Baltimore, MD: Williams and Wilkins.

van den Brandt, P. A. (2011). The impact of a Mediterranean diet and healthy lifestyle on premature mortality in men and women. *American Journal of Clinical Nutrition, 94,* 913–920.

Wallerstein, N., & Bernstein, E. (1988). Empowerment education: Freier's ideas adapted to health education. *Health Education Quarterly, 15*(4), 379–394.

Wallston, K., & Wallston, B. (1982). Who is responsible for your health? The construct of health locus of control. In G. Saunders & J. Suls (Eds.), *Social psychology of health and illness.* Hillsdale, NJ: Erlbaum.

Watt, L., & Cappeliez, P. (2000). Integrative and instrumental reminiscence therapies for depression in older adults. *Aging & Mental Health, 4*(2), 166–183.

Wolfson, L., Whipple, R., Derby, C., Judge, J., King, M., Amerman, P., Schmidt, J., & Smyers, D. (1996). Balance and strength training in older adults: Intervention gains and Tai Chi maintenance. *Journal of the American Geriatrics Society, 44*(5), 498–506.

For a full suite of assignments and additional learning activities, see the access code at the front of your book.

CHAPTER 8

Identifying and Preventing Common Risk Factors in the Elderly

Joan M. Nelson

(Competencies 3, 4, 6, 9, 17)

LEARNING OBJECTIVES

At the end of this chapter, the reader will be able to:

> Discuss techniques for assessing and treating factors that lead to functional decline in the elderly.
> Describe recommended screening evaluations for the elderly population.
> Cite the expert recommendations for flu and pneumonia vaccines.
> Identify risk factors and signs of abuse in the elderly.
> Explain the protocol for reporting elder abuse.

KEY TERMS

Abuse	Functional decline
Activities of daily living	Guilt
Annoyance	Health promotion
Chronic Disease Self-Management Program	Health screening
	Healthy People 2020
Contracting	Instrumental activities of daily living
Cut down	Primary prevention
Dietary Approaches to Stop Hypertension diet	Secondary prevention
	Tertiary prevention
Eye opener	U.S. Preventive Services Task Force
Framingham Heart Study	

Health promotion activities can help prevent functional decline in older adults. Scientific evidence supports the fact that functional disability is not caused by aging, per se, but results from illnesses and diseases that are related to unhealthy lifestyle decisions. Unhealthy behaviors and lifestyles have been linked to physical decline in later life (Pluijm et al., 2007). This creates an exciting opportunity for nurses to improve the quality of life for the elderly client through evidence-based health promotion activities.

In this chapter, we will review the health promotion and disease prevention guidelines recommended by the following:

> *U.S. Preventive Services Task Force (USPSTF):* The USPSTF was convened by the U.S. Public Health Service to systematically review the evidence of effectiveness of clinical preventive services. The task force is an independent panel of private-sector experts in primary care and prevention whose mission is to evaluate the benefits of individual services and create age-, gender-, and risk-based recommendations about services that should routinely be incorporated into primary medical care. Its recommendations can be found at https://www.uspreventiveservicestaskforce.org/BrowseRec/Index/browse-recommendations

> *Healthy People 2020:* Healthy People 2020 is an initiative of a federal interagency workgroup with input from many governmental and private agencies. It is a set of healthcare objectives designed to improve the health of individuals and communities, eliminate health disparities, and improve access to care. Its recommendations can be found at http://www.healthypeople.gov/2020/about/objectiveDevelopment.aspx.

The recommendations presented in this chapter are guidelines for most patients, most of the time. Clinical judgment must be used in applying these guidelines to individual clients; for example, the risks and benefits of colonoscopy will be quite different for a healthy 75-year-old versus a frail 75-year-old with metastatic cancer. Individual variations in health status increase markedly with age, necessitating an individualized approach to health care.

Health Promotion and Disease Prevention Definitions

Health promotion activities are activities in which an individual is able to proactively engage in to advance or improve his or her health. *Primary prevention* activities are those designed to completely prevent a disease from occurring, such as immunization against pneumonia or influenza. *Secondary prevention* efforts are directed toward early detection and management of disease, such as the use of colonoscopy to detect small, cancerous polyps. *Tertiary prevention* efforts are used to manage clinical diseases to prevent them from progressing or to avoid complications of disease, as is done when beta-blockers are used to help remodel the heart in congestive heart failure.

Screening

Health screening is a form of secondary prevention and will be a focus of this chapter. In order to endorse screening for a specific disease, the USPSTF considers whether the disease occurs with enough frequency in a population to justify mass screening. The population is more likely to benefit from screening tests for a disease such as diabetes, which occurs frequently, than it is to benefit from screening for Addison's disease, which is uncommon. In order to justify the costs and inconvenience of screening, we must be able to detect the condition being screened at a relatively early stage and have effective treatments for the condition. Early detection of the disease has to result in improved clinical outcomes. The screening tests should be relatively noninvasive, acceptable to patients, cost effective, available, and highly sensitive and specific (see **Case Study 8-1**).

Case Study 8–1

You are working as a registered nurse (RN) for a community-based healthcare clinic. All adults over the age of 65 with Medicare insurance are encouraged to make a joint appointment with you and their provider for an annual Medicare Wellness Visit. You review the patient's individual risk factors and goals and develop a plan for all appropriate annual screening and health promotion activities as part of this visit.

You are visiting with Hilde M., an 82-year-old woman, who is accompanied by her daughter, Roxanne. Roxanne called you prior to the visit to inform you about her concerns about her mother's ability to live safely alone at home. She confides that her mother is forgetting many appointments and has fallen at least twice in the past 3 months. Although Mrs. M. had a

minor stroke 3 years ago, she has not been into the office for the past year because she lacks transportation since she gave up driving 2 years ago due to her poor vision. Roxanne has encouraged her mother to move into an assisted-living facility, but Mrs. M. does not want to sell her home of 50 years and give up her independence.

Questions:

1. What screening tests are appropriate for Mrs. M. at this time? Justify your choices.
2. What instruments will you use to perform the appropriate screening tests?
3. What counseling will you provide for Mrs. M. and her daughter, based on the limited information you have been provided?

Screening recommendations are graded by expert panels according to the strength of the supporting evidence and the net benefit. The USPSTF uses the following rating scale:

> *Level A:* The USPSTF recommends the service. There is high certainty that the net benefit is substantial based on rigorous experimental research with consistent results.
> *Level B:* The USPSTF recommends the service. There is high certainty that the net benefit is moderate or there is moderate certainty that the net benefit is moderate to substantial.
> *Level C:* Clinicians may provide this service to selected patients depending on individual circumstances. However, for most individuals without signs or symptoms there is likely to be only a small benefit from this service.
> *Level D:* The USPSTF recommends against the service. There is moderate or high certainty that the service has no net benefit or that the harms outweigh the benefits.
> *Level I:* The USPSTF concludes that the current evidence is insufficient to assess the balance of benefits and harms of the service. Evidence is lacking, of poor quality, or conflicting, and the balance of benefits and harms cannot be determined.

The Focus of Health Promotion Efforts

A major focus of health promotion efforts for the older adult is to minimize the loss of independence associated with illness and functional decline. Healthy People 2020 and the USPSTF suggest the following focus areas for nurses to promote health and prevent disability in the elderly client:

> Physical activity
> Nutrition

> Tobacco use
> Health screening
> Injury prevention
> Preventive medications and immunizations
> Caregiver support

Many of these foci show considerable overlap with recommendations for younger adults, but some, such as injury prevention and hearing and vision screening, are unique to older adults. It is important to consider the impact of health conditions on physical functioning and on quality of life in the older client. This is different from the focus in younger adults on treatment and cure of a single, acute condition. Multiple chronic illnesses are common in the elderly, and cure is often an unrealistic and inappropriate goal. These chronic illnesses can lead to disability and dependency. In fact, almost 38% of Americans over 65 years of age have some level of physical disability (Centers for Disease Control and Prevention [CDC], 2013). Symptoms that affect functional status should be the focus of interventions with this population. Maintaining independence in *activities of daily living* (ADLs) is an important goal for health-promoting activities.

By the time we are 85 years old, half of our remaining years of life are expected to be lived dependently, often in a nursing home. About 35 million American adults have some functional limitation, and over 60% of older adults have some difficulty in performing a basic action or complex activity (CDC, 2015a). Some of the preventive strategies that will be discussed in this chapter, such as smoking cessation, immunization, physical activity, weight control, blood pressure control, and arthritis and diabetes self-management programs, are known to be effective in lessening disability.

Assessment of functional status requires a multipronged approach. The ADLs scale and the *instrumental activities of daily living* (IADLs) scale are valid and reliable self-report tools to assess functional status (Lawton & Brody, 1969). Nurses can use these instruments to identify elderly individuals who are frail and may benefit from an increased level of care or additional in-home support. Fear of being advised to leave their home, however, can cause elderly individuals to deny difficulties. Because the ADL and IADL scales rely on self-reporting, they can fail to detect difficulties when clients are not forthcoming about their limitations.

Performance-based tools, such as the Get Up and Go test (Duxbury, 1997), can provide a more objective measurement of functional status and fall risk. This assessment requires clients to rise from a chair, walk 10 feet, turn around, return to the chair, and sit down. These actions are timed and compared with a historic sample of adults without balance problems who were able complete this test in less than 10 seconds. Older adults who are dependent in most ADLs and have poor balance and gait may take more than 30 seconds to complete the task. Clients are observed for sitting balance, transfers, gait, and ability to maintain balance while turning. If a gait abnormality is detected, weight-bearing exercise and physical rehabilitation may prevent further decline and lessen the risk of falls.

Frailty is a concept that is often discussed in the literature but is difficult to define and is the topic of much debate. Frailty involves visible changes such as weight loss, decreased physical activity, fatigue, weakness, and impaired mobility, as well as the accumulation of health conditions and deficits. There is agreement that frailty is associated with poor health outcomes, increased risk of hospitalization, and limited lifespan (U.S. Preventative Services Task Force [USPSTF], 2012a). Several frailty measures exist for use in practice, and tool selection should be guided by the skill of the person performing the assessment and the time allocated for the assessment (deVries et al., 2011).

Self-Management

What can nurses do to encourage clients to adopt health-promoting behaviors and manage their chronic illnesses? Kate Lorig, MD, has been instrumental in developing the concept of self-management and outlining the role of the healthcare provider in fostering the client's self-management of his or her chronic condition (Lorig &

Holman, 2000). Her research, which was sponsored by the Agency for Healthcare Research and Quality (AHRQ), supported the effectiveness of chronic disease self-management in preventing or delaying disability from chronic diseases. She has described how the self-management concept also may be applied to health promotion activities.

The *Chronic Disease Self-Management Program* (CDSMP) is a 17-hour course for patients with chronic diseases that is taught by trained laypeople (Stanford School of Medicine, 2016). The course goal is to teach patients to improve symptom management, maintain functional ability, and adhere to their medication regimens. The proven effectiveness of the intervention is, at least in part, attributable to the improved self-efficacy of clients who participate in the program. Clients come to believe that they can succeed in managing their illness and preventing disability.

Critical to the concept of self-management is an assessment of the client's goals and concerns, which may be different from the healthcare professional's goals and concerns. The nurse may think exercise will help lower a client's blood pressure, which may decrease stroke risk—certainly an important goal. The client's focus, however, may be that he does not want to go shopping for new clothes, needed as a result of his recent weight gain, and his goal is to continue to be able to use his current wardrobe. He will assess the value of his new exercise program in terms of his clothing budget, not in relation to his blood pressure readings.

Lorig & Holman (2000) identified five key elements of self-management programs: problem solving, decision making, resource utilization, forming a healthcare professional–client partnership, and taking action. In the problem-solving phase, a client may identify several barriers to initiating an exercise program and then list strategies for overcoming each barrier, to arrive at a workable strategy. Decision making helps to arm clients with the information needed to make the decisions they need to make on a daily basis. "How do I know when I am exercising too hard?" "Should I exercise when I don't feel well?" The provider plays an important role in providing accurate and sufficient information for clients to make informed decisions. Providers also teach clients to access and evaluate appropriate resources and create plans that are easily accomplished, limited in scope, and easily evaluated for success. A technique that has proven successful is to ask clients how confident they are on a scale of 1 to 10 (10 being maximally confident) that they will accomplish their objective. If the score is less than 7, encourage them to set a more realistic goal.

Contracting for health-promoting behaviors is another useful strategy. A successful contract for behavior change is very specific. The contract may begin with the overall behavioral goal ("I wish to lose 20 lb over the next year in order to improve my overall health, strength, and stamina"). The client determines his or her own short-term goal and means of achieving that goal for the next week ("I will exercise for 20 minutes, 3 times this week"). The nurse helps the client pinpoint exactly how and when that will occur. The client is encouraged to write the exact time the exercise will occur on a calendar, along with the exact form the exercise will take ("I will walk around my subdivision, which is 1.25 miles in length, at 10 a.m. on Tuesday, Thursday, and Saturday"). Ideally, the client and nurse will meet at the end of that period to evaluate and modify the plan for the next week or so. Barriers to implementing the plan are reviewed and taken into consideration to rewrite the following week's contract.

Self-management classes and contracting are strategies that can be incorporated through individual sessions or in group meetings, to help implement the health promotion and disease prevention ideas discussed in this chapter.

Physical Activity

Functional decline in the elderly is attributable, at least in part, to physical inactivity. Researchers have correlated physical activity through the lifespan with preservation of cognitive function. See **Box 8-1** for more information about this study. Physical activity can improve quality of life, decrease the risk of death from cardiovascular disease (CVD) and some cancers, and reduce the risk of bone fractures and falls (CDC, 2009, 2015b) (see **Box 8-2**).

BOX 8-1   Research Highlight

Middleton, Barnes, Lui, and Yaffe studied the impact of exercise throughout the life span to better understand the potential impacts on cognition in later stages of life. Sign into your database of nursing literature (CINAHL or PubMed, for example) and use the citation below to perform a search for this article. What were the results of this study? What kind of intervention can a caregiver offer on the basis of the information discovered?

Middleton, L. E., Barnes, D. E., Lui, L., & Yaffe, K. (2010). Physical activity over the life course and its association with cognitive performance and impairment in old age. *Journal of the American Geriatrics Society, 58*(7), 1322–1326.

BOX 8-2   Physical Activity Counseling

Level B recommendation: For adults with CVD risk factors, the USPSTF recommends intensive behavioral health counseling for adults who are overweight or obese and have additional CVD risk factors.

Level C recommendation: For adults without CVD risk factors, the USPSTF determined that although the correlation between physical activity and CVD is strong, existing evidence suggests only a small benefit for providing behavioral counseling in the primary care setting. Clinicians may choose to selectively counsel patients rather than incorporate counseling into the care of all adults in the general population.

Despite the well-documented benefits of exercise in reducing blood pressure and cholesterol, improving insulin resistance, reducing weight, strengthening bones, and reducing falls, one third of adults 65 years of age and older report that they do not engage in any leisure time physical activity (Partnership for Prevention, 2008). In order to receive health benefits from exercise, older adults should engage in 150 minutes of moderate intensity or 75 minutes of vigorous intensity exercise every week (CDC, 2009).

Physical inactivity causes increased healthcare costs to our nation. In fact, a CDC study has shown that the direct medical costs of inactive Americans are markedly higher than the costs for active Americans. The direct medical costs associated with physical inactivity were nearly $131 billion per year (Carlson, Fulton, Pratt, Yang, & Adams, 2015).

Scientific evidence supports the effectiveness of moderate physical activity in:

> Decreasing overall mortality
> Decreasing coronary heart disease (CHD), the leading cause of death in the United States
> Decreasing colon cancer
> Decreasing the incidence and improving the management of diabetes mellitus
> Decreasing the incidence and improving the management of hypertension
> Decreasing obesity
> Improving depression
> Improving quality of life
> Improving functional status
> Decreasing falls and injury

Moderate exercise is defined as 30 or more minutes of brisk walking on 5 or more days per week. Tai chi and yoga are helpful for improving balance and flexibility. Modified exercises, such as armchair exercises, can be helpful for the frail elderly or those with mobility restrictions. Sporadic, vigorous exercise should be discouraged.

Barriers to physical exercise that have been identified by the elderly include lack of access to safe areas to exercise, pain, fatigue, and impairment in sensory function and mobility. These barriers underscore the need to individualize your approach to helping clients develop an exercise regimen tailored to their needs and participate in community efforts to create environments that foster healthy lifestyles. The Partnership for Prevention (2008) developed an excellent community assessment guide with a list of strategies for communities to overcome barriers encountered by older adults to physical activities. This guide, called *Physical Activity Guidelines for Americans*, is accessible at http://www.health.gov/paguidelines/guidelines/chapter5.aspx.

What can be done to foster participation in physical exercise? Individuals can increase their chances of beginning and sticking with an exercise program if they identify activities that can be a regular part of their daily routine and identify individuals who can participate in the exercise with them. Nurses can help clients assess their current level of activity and barriers that prevent them from exercising. The nurse then can help the client with goal-setting, write a prescription for exercise, work with the client to develop an exercise program individually tailored to the client's needs, and follow by telephone at regular intervals to assess progress and barriers. Follow-up phone calls also can be used to assess how well the client has done with accessing community resources.

Nutrition

Of the 10 leading causes of death in the United States (cancer, diabetes, CHD, and cerebrovascular accidents [CVAs]), 4 are associated with unhealthy dietary patterns (CDC, 2015c). Most Americans do not eat enough fruits or vegetables and eat too much fat. Healthy People 2020 includes objectives to increase consumption of fruits, vegetables, and whole grains and decrease consumption of solid fats and sugars, as well as increasing the frequency with which healthcare providers counsel patients about nutrition and measure their body mass index (BMI).

Older adults may be at increased risk for poor nutrition due to the fact that they have multiple chronic illnesses, may have tooth or mouth problems that can interfere with their ability to eat, may be socially isolated, may have economic hardship, may be taking multiple medications that can cause changes in appetite or gastrointestinal (GI) symptoms, and may need assistance with self-care. Weight gain or loss may signal nutritional problems. A BMI less than 19 can signal undernutrition (Thomas, Ashmen, Morley, & Evans, 2000).

Measurement of body weight over time provides the simplest means of detecting nutritional risk. Unintended weight loss is highly correlated with mortality (Wannamethee, Shaper, & Lennon, 2005). The Mini Nutritional Assessment (MNA) is a tool that can be used by nurses to assess nutritional risk. It is available at http://www .mna-elderly.com/forms/mini/mna_mini_english.pdf. The MNA is a well-validated, six-item tool that can be administered quickly and used to predict poor health outcomes (Sieber, 2006).

Older adults residing in rehabilitation and long-term care facilities are at very high risk for inadequate nutrition. The Council for Nutritional Clinical Strategies in Long-Term Care developed an evidenced-based guideline for management of adults found to have nutritional compromise (Thomas et al., 2000). This guideline identifies adults with a BMI of less than 21 as potentially at risk and suggests that these adults be targeted for counseling and other interventions. The first step identified in this guideline is to clarify the patient and family's advanced directives. A comprehensive assessment is recommended to identify hydration status, medications, and medical conditions that could contribute to loss of appetite, swallowing difficulties, increased metabolic states, and decreased food intake. Nurses should notify the healthcare provider of the patient's dietary and fluid intake as well as any fevers; fecal impaction; constipation; mood disturbances; nausea, vomiting, or indigestion; signs of pain or infection; signs of swallowing problems; ill-fitting dentures; or dental problems. Nurses should check the chart for signs of nutritional inadequacy. These would include albumin less than 3.4 g/dL, cholesterol less than 160 mg/dL, hemoglobin less than 12 g/dL, and serum transferrin less than 180.

BOX 8-3   Nutrition Counseling

Level B recommendation: The USPSTF found good evidence to support counseling interventions among adults who are overweight or obese and have additional risk factors for the development of CVD.

Level C recommendation: For adults who are not overweight or obese without CVD risk factors.

Any adult with signs of undernutrition should be instructed to stop any special diets and encouraged to snack and use food supplements, such as protein shakes, between meals (not at meal times). Medications should not be administered with meals. Family can be encouraged to provide the older adult with favorite foods and provide socialization during mealtimes, when possible. A speech therapist can assist with adults who have dysphagia, and an occupational therapist is instrumental in identifying adaptive equipment to help older adults with the mechanics of eating. This guideline contains helpful algorithms for nurses and can be accessed at http://www.geroupr.com/nutri.pdf.

Being overweight or obese is also a health risk for older adults due to the associated risks for diabetes, heart disease, and some types of cancer. Adults with BMIs over 25 are considered to be overweight, and those with BMIs over 30 are considered obese. Overweight older adults should be counseled to avoid weight gain, whereas those who are in the obese category will benefit from weight loss strategies (see **Box 8-3**).

General dietary guidelines for older adults include (U.S. Department of Agriculture, 2010):

> Limit alcohol to one drink per day for women, two daily for men.
> Limit fat and cholesterol.
> Maintain a balanced caloric intake.
> Ensure adequate daily calcium, especially for women.
> Older adults should consume foods fortified with vitamins, such as fortified cereals or supplements.
> Older adults who have minimal exposure to sunlight or who have dark skin need supplemental vitamin D. Daily vitamin D intake should be 800 to 1000 IU and can be derived from fortified foods or supplements (Dawson-Hughes et al., 2010).
> Include adequate whole grains, fruits, and vegetables.
> Drink adequate water.

Tobacco Use

Cigarette smoking is the leading cause of preventable death in the United States. Approximately half of people who use tobacco can be expected to die from tobacco-related causes (CDC, 2008). Elderly Americans are just as likely as younger adults to benefit from quitting smoking. Quitting smoking can decrease the chance of having a myocardial infarction or dying from lung cancer or heart disease. Nonsmokers have improved wound healing, recovery from illness, and improved cerebral circulation.

A practice guideline for clinicians to help their patients quit smoking has been developed through the Public Health Service (Tobacco Use and Dependence Guideline Panel, 2008) and is available at http://www.ncbi.nlm.nih.gov/books/NBK63952/. The task force stresses that the most important step in helping a client quit smoking is to screen for tobacco use and assess the client's willingness to quit. It outlines the 5 As for clients who are ready to quit smoking and recommends that clinicians use motivational interviewing strategies to increase the likelihood of future quit attempts for those who are not ready to quit. Support to prevent relapse in those who have quit is also recommended (see **Box 8-4**).

BOX 8-4　Tobacco Cessation Counseling

Level A recommendation: The USPSTF found good evidence that screening, brief behavioral counseling, and pharmacotherapy are effective in helping clients quit smoking and remain smoke-free after 1 year. There are good data to support that smoking cessation lowers the risk for heart disease, stroke, and lung disease.

The 5 As:

Ask about smoking status at each healthcare visit.

Advise client to quit smoking.

Assess client's willingness to quit smoking at this time.

Assist client to quit using counseling and pharmacotherapy.

Arrange for follow-up within 1 week of scheduled quit date.

Practical tips for the nurse or provider to use in assisting patients who are ready to quit are provided in the guideline. One of the key strategies to use in any behavior change counseling is to encourage the patient to be very specific about what, when, and how he or she plans to make this change. In the case of smoking cessation, the older adult can be encouraged to mark a quit date on a calendar and to tell family and friends about plans to quit on that day. All tobacco products should be removed from the home in advance of this quit date. The "Quit Line" (1-800-QUIT-NOW) has additional counseling and support materials. Medications have been shown to increase success with long-term smoking cessation.

Safety

Many of the safety recommendations for older adults are similar to those for younger people: use lap and shoulder belts in motor vehicles, avoid driving while intoxicated, use smoke detectors in the home, maintain hot water heaters at or below 120°F. Falls, however, are a safety risk that are more common in the elderly.

Falls are the leading cause of unintentional injury death in older adults in this country. Approximately one in three adults over the age of 65 in the United States fall each year, and of these falls, one in five result in serious physical injury (CDC, 2015b). Twenty thousand Americans die as a result of a fall each year. Elderly adults are susceptible to falls as a result of postural instability, decreased muscle strength, gait disturbances and decreased proprioception, visual or cognitive impairment, and polypharmacy. Environmental conditions that contribute to falls are slippery surfaces, stairs, irregular surfaces, poor lighting, incorrect footwear, and obstacles in the pathway.

The American Geriatrics Society (AGS, 2010) and British Geriatrics Society have published a joint guideline on fall prevention for older adults (see **Box 8-5**). Nurses should ask all older adults three basic screening questions: "Have you fallen in the past year?"; "If so, what were the circumstances of the fall(s) and how often have you fallen?"; and "Do you have any difficulty with walking or balance?" Patients who have had more than one fall, have had an injury significant enough to require medical care, or have difficulty with walking or balance, require a full, multifactorial fall risk assessment. An algorithm useful in the assessment and treatment of fall risk can be accessed at http://www.medcats.com/FALLS/frameset.htm. Interventions aimed at reducing the risk of falls include a home safety evaluation with appropriate modifications, discontinuation of high-risk medications, management of postural hypotension, vitamin D supplementation, assessment and treatment of foot problems, and exercise. Strong data support the effectiveness of balance and strengthening exercises for fall reduction (Mitty & Flores, 2007), as well as research to support physiologic and environmental risk factor reduction.

BOX 8-5   Fall Prevention Counseling

Level C recommendation: The USPSTF does not recommend comprehensive risk assessment and management of these risks to prevent falls in all community-dwelling adults aged 65 years or older because the likelihood of benefit is small. This assessment and fall-risk plan should be provided for those with a history of falls, comorbid illnesses that place the patient at risk for falls, poor performance on the Get Up and Go test, and use of ambulatory devices.

Level B recommendation: The USPSTF recommends exercise or physical therapy and vitamin D supplementation to prevent falls in community-dwelling adults aged 65 years or older who are at increased risk for falls.

Polypharmacy and Medication Errors

Elderly adults are at increased risk of adverse drug effects compared to younger adults, as a result of the fact that they take more medications and the biologic effects of aging and chronic diseases. Medication underutilization and overutilization by this population has been shown to increase the number of hospitalizations and emergency room visits, worsen cognitive functioning, and contribute to falls.

The CDC (2015f) has developed a medication safety program with information for patients about high-risk medications and medication safety strategies. The U.S. Food and Drug Administration (2015) is spearheading a multiagency effort called the "Safe Use Initiative" that aims to coordinate efforts to improve the safe use of medications and to prevent harm by medication errors, *abuse*, and misuse. The American Pharmacists Association and the National Association of Chain Drugstores Foundation (2008) created a service model to help with medication management and included a sample format for a personal medication record; it can be accessed at http://www.pharmacist.com/sites/default/files/files/core_elements_of_an_mtm_practice.pdf.

Older adults comprise 12% of the population, but use about one third of all prescription and over-the-counter drugs sold in the United States. This number is markedly higher for hospitalized patients or those living in nursing homes or assisted-living facilities. Polypharmacy is not always inappropriate in this population of clients who have multiple chronic illnesses, but increased numbers of medications carry increasing risks. Budnitz, Lovegrove, Shehab, and Richards (2011) examined a large national database and discovered that almost 100,000 Americans over the age of 65 were admitted to the emergency department (ED) annually between 2007 and 2009 due to adverse drug events. Over half of these admissions were for patients over the age of 80, and four specific classes of medications accounted for over two thirds of these ED visits: warfarin, insulin, oral hypoglycemic medications, and oral antiplatelet medications.

The AGS has recently published an updated version of the Beer's Criteria for Potentially Inappropriate Medications in Older Adults (AGS, 2015). This update came from an extensive review of evidence relating to harm due to these agents and is available as an easy-to-use pocket card at http://www.americangeriatrics.org/files/documents/beers/PrintableBeersPocketCard.pdf. These medications include long-acting benzodiazepines, sedative or hypnotic agents, long-acting oral hypoglycemics, analgesics, antiemetics, and GI antispasmodics. Elderly clients who require home care services and are, therefore, among the more disabled, are prescribed these medications even more often than the healthier members of their cohort. See Chapter 11 for a thorough discussion on polypharmacy.

The Screening Tool of Older Persons' Prescriptions (STOPP) and the Screening Tool to Alert to Right Treatment (START) are new, validated tools for identification of inappropriate prescribing in the older adult; these are suggested to be used in conjunction with Beer's Criteria (O'Mahoney et al., 2015).

Immunizations

Annual vaccination against influenza is recommended for all adults 65 years of age or older, because more than 90% of the deaths from influenza occur in this population. Several studies suggest that flu vaccination is beneficial in preventing illness, hospitalization, and mortality in both community-dwelling and institutionalized elderly individuals (McElhaney, 2011). Due to the decreased immune function that accompanies older age, a new high-dose influenza vaccine is available for older adults. This vaccine contains four times the amount of antigen present in other forms of the influenza vaccine (CDC, 2015d) (see **Box 8-6**).

Older adults, especially those with chronic illnesses or who live in nursing homes, are susceptible to pneumococcal pneumonia, which results in death in over one third of clients over 65 years of age who acquire the disease. The emergence of drug-resistant strains of pneumococcal pneumonia underscores the importance of acquired immunization against the illness. The CDC recommends all adults 65 years and older receive a dose of PCV13 followed by a dose of PPSV23 at least 1 year later (see **Box 8-7**). Tetanus and diphtheria are uncommon diseases in the United States, but only 28% of adults age 70 or older are immune to tetanus. It is these adults who account for the majority of tetanus cases, a disease that results in death in more than one quarter of cases. The tetanus and diphtheria (Td) vaccine is highly efficacious against tetanus, but immunity may wane after 10 years. Periodic boosters of tetanus vaccine, traditionally given every 10 years in the United States, are recommended for older adults by the USPSTF. The Tdap vaccine, in addition to immunizing against tetanus and diphtheria, also contains pertussis vaccine and is recommended for any older adult who has close contact with infants younger than 12 months of age (CDC, 2015g).

Herpes zoster infection can occur at any age, but is far more common in older adults. Over 98% of American adults are believed to have serologic evidence of varicella zoster viral infection and could, at some time in their lives, experience an outbreak of shingles from this infection. An outbreak of herpes zoster causes a painful rash in one or two adjacent dermatomes in the body that lasts for 2 to 4 weeks. The most common complication of this condition is postherpetic neuralgia (PHN), severe pain that can last for months to years after resolution of the acute rash. It occurs in up to 50% of adults over the age of 60 who have a herpes zoster outbreak (CDC, 2014). For this reason, the CDC recommends one-time immunization against herpes zoster for adults 60 years of age and older regardless of whether they have had shingles (CDC, 2015g) (see **Box 8-8**).

BOX 8-6   Vaccination Recommendations from the CDC for Adults over Age 65 Years

Annual influenza vaccination—either standard dose trivalent vaccine or high dose (FluZone High Dose).

BOX 8-7   Vaccination Recommendations

All adults 65 years of age or older should receive a dose of PCV13 followed by a dose of PPSV23 at least 1 year later.

BOX 8-8   Vaccination Recommendations

Herpes zoster vaccine once after age 60, even if the older adult has had a prior episode of herpes zoster.

Tetanus vaccination—Td or Tdap—every 10 years Tdap recommended for older adults who have contact with infants younger than 12 months of age.

Mental Health Screening

Good mental health enables individuals to participate in productive activities and relationships and to adjust to change and loss. Mental disorders are characterized by alterations in mood, behaviors, or cognition and are associated with impaired functioning and/or distress. Mental disorders have been associated with complications resulting in disability or death, and they profoundly affect family members as well as patients. Mental disorders are as common in late life as they are during other stages of the lifespan, but some disorders are found relatively more frequently in elderly clients.

Depression

Although estimates of depression vary widely, up to 37% of community-dwelling older adults are depressed. Depression rates increase markedly among patients who have a chronic illness or disability and have been found to be 12% for hospitalized geriatric patients and over 50% for nursing home residents (Hoover et al., 2010). Elderly men have the highest rates of suicide in the nation.

The diagnostic criteria for depression, according to the *Diagnostic and Statistical Manual of Mental Disorders,* fifth edition (American Psychiatric Association, 2013) require that five or more of the following symptoms be present almost daily for a 2-week period and that they represent a change from baseline functioning and are not directly caused by a medical condition or drug: depressed mood, decreased pleasure or interest in activities, change in appetite or weight that is not a result of dieting, change in sleep pattern, psychomotor retardation or agitation, fatigue or loss of energy, feelings of worthlessness or guilt, recurrent thoughts of death or suicide, or diminished ability to think or concentrate.

There is good evidence to support screening for depression in adults, including older adults. Screening can improve identification of depressed elders and improve outcomes. Screening efforts must be coordinated with effective treatment and follow-up in order to have maximal benefit. Initial screening may be accomplished by asking two questions about mood and anhedonia: "Over the past 2 weeks, have you felt down, depressed, or hopeless?" and "Over the past 2 weeks, have you felt little interest or pleasure in doing things?" A positive response to this initial screen may be followed with the Geriatric Depression Scale, which has been found to have 92% sensitivity and 89% specificity for detecting depression in elderly adults (Kurlowicz & Greenberg, 2007). The PHQ-9 is another depression screen that has been validated for use with older adults (Kroenke, Spitzer, & Williams, 2001). The Cornell Scale for Depression in Dementia is a useful tool for cognitively impaired older adults (Alexopoulos, Abrams, Young, & Shamoian, 1988). A positive depression screen should be followed with an assessment of suicide risk and substance abuse.

> **CLINICAL TIP**
>
> Depression and anxiety often are seen together in older adults.

Dementia

Dementia affects almost 50% of Americans 85 years of age or older. Alzheimer's disease accounts for 60% to 70% of all cases of dementia and is associated with doubling of the death rate, compared to clients who are not affected, and markedly increased rates of nursing home admissions. Alzheimer's disease prevalence rates double every 5 years after the age of 65. Multiinfarct dementia accounts for 20% to 30% of dementias and is the second leading cause of dementia in the United States. Dementia is a chronic and progressive illness characterized by behavioral and cognitive changes that affect memory, problem solving, judgment, and speech and causes deficits in functional abilities.

Unfortunately, there is insufficient evidence at this time to suggest that population-wide screening of Americans 65 years and older for dementia is beneficial. It is difficult to recognize early Alzheimer's disease, and though it is difficult to quantify the deficit in dementia diagnosis by primary care providers, a study by Bradford, Kunik, Shultz, Williams, & Singh (2009) verified that missed diagnoses are common. Failure to diagnose early Alzheimer's disease may severely compromise client safety as a result of household and motor vehicle accidents. These clients are susceptible to financial losses through errors and scams that prey on the elderly. There is sufficient evidence to support the fact that medication delays the rate of cognitive impairment associated with Alzheimer's disease, which can lead to improved quality of life for individuals and families and decreased costs of care for our nation. Experts do recommend thorough screening for clients in whom cognitive impairment is suspected or when concerns are expressed by family members or friends.

Three screening tests are commonly used for all forms of dementia. The Mini-Mental State Examination (MMSE) is considered the gold standard diagnostic test to detect dementia. It has reasonable sensitivity and specificity and can be made more sensitive or specific depending on the cutpoint used to diagnose dementia (Folstein, Folstein, & McHugh, 1975). The clock-drawing test (CDT), in which the client is asked to draw a clock face and indicate a particular time, is a sensitive but nonspecific screening test (Sunderland et al., 1989). The use of informant reporting of an individual's cognitive status has been found to be a useful screening tool, as well.

It is important to distinguish between screening tools and tests used for the differential diagnosis of dementia (see **Box 8-9**). A thorough dementia evaluation involves systematic history and examination, laboratory testing, and brain imaging.

Alcohol Abuse

Forty percent of adults over the age of 65 drink alcohol and alcohol use can augment problems related to polypharmacy (National Institute on Alcohol Abuse and Alcoholism, 1998). It is very difficult to diagnose alcohol problems in the older adult for several reasons. Retired people do not have the lifestyle disruptions caused by heavy alcohol use that are commonly encountered in younger adults. They are less likely to be arrested for disorderly conduct or aggression related to their drinking. Alcoholics over the age of 65 are more likely to be living alone and drinking alone than younger adults. On the other hand, the older drinker is more likely to honestly report drinking to the healthcare provider and to comply with treatment strategies (see **Box 8-10**).

Older adults have alcohol-related complications that are not generally seen in younger adults, such as increased rates of hip fractures due to falls and medication reactions due to alcohol's effects on liver enzyme systems.

BOX 8-9   Depression and Dementia Screening

Level B recommendation: To support screening for depression, the USPSTF found good evidence that screening effectively identifies depressed patients and treatment of depression improves clinical outcomes as long as there is sufficient staff-assisted depression care to support diagnosis, treatment, and follow-up.

Level I recommendation: For dementia screening, the USPSTF found the clinical evidence to be insufficient to recommend screening for all elderly clients in a primary care setting. Most expert panels agree that clients who are suspected of having cognitive impairment or whose families express concern about their cognitive functioning should be screened.

BOX 8-10   Alcohol Screening

Level B recommendation: For screening, the USPSTF found good evidence that screening is beneficial in identifying patients whose alcohol consumption patterns place them at risk for increased morbidity and mortality and good evidence that counseling about alcohol reduction can produce sustained benefit over a 6- to 12-month period.

There is some evidence to suggest that light to moderate alcohol consumption in older adults may reduce the risk of CHD. The National Institute on Alcohol Abuse and Alcoholism (1998) recommends no more than 1 drink per day for this purpose. More than 7 drinks per week for women or 14 drinks per week for men has been defined as "risky" or "hazardous."

CLINICAL TIP

The CAGE questionnaire is a quick, reliable screening tool for alcohol abuse.

Several screening tools are commonly used to screen for alcohol abuse. The CAGE questionnaire is a self-report screening instrument that is easy and quick to administer (Ewing, 1984). It asks four yes/no questions and requires approximately 1 minute to complete. CAGE is a mnemonic for the following four key screening questions:

Cut down: Refers to attempts by the client to cut down on drinking

Annoyance: Related to suggestions by friends or family to cut down on drinking

Guilt: Relates to client guilt about drinking

Eye opener: Relates to the need for a drink in the morning to get going

The CAGE questionnaire has been found to have 75% sensitivity and 96% specificity. The 5 As and 5 Rs strategies, defined under the section on tobacco abuse in this chapter, are also suggested strategies for reducing alcohol consumption.

Another screening tool, the Alcohol Use Disorders Identification Test (AUDIT), is a 10-item screening test developed by the World Health Organization (WHO) and is sensitive for detecting alcohol dependence and abuse (Babor, Higgins-Biddle, Saunders, & Monteiro, 2001). You can learn more about this screening tool at http://whqlibdoc.who.int/hq/2001/WHO_MSD_MSB_01.6a.pdf

Elder Abuse and Neglect

Unfortunately, it is difficult to estimate the prevalence of elder abuse and neglect in this country, due, at least in part, to the lack of appropriate screening instruments and consequent underreporting of abuse and neglect by healthcare professionals. Reporting of elder abuse to the *adult protective services agency* is mandatory in almost all states, but it is estimated that only 1 in 14 cases of elder abuse and neglect is actually reported (National Center on Elder Abuse, n.d.). There is a paucity of studies to determine the effectiveness of interventions in decreasing abuse (see **Box 8-11**). Studies directed toward identification of both abuse victims and perpetrators are needed.

Elder abuse may include physical, sexual, psychological, and financial exploitation; neglect; and violation of rights. Physical abuse includes shaking, restraining, hitting, or threatening with objects. Sexual abuse includes

> **BOX 8-11   Elder Abuse Screening**
>
> **Level I evidence:** Insufficient evidence exists to support mass screening based on a lack of research to support the use of any particular screening too, and lack of evidence to support that identification of risk changes outcomes.

unwanted contact with the genitals, anus, or mouth. Clients who are psychologically abused experience threats, insults, or harassment or are recipients of harsh commands. Financial abuse occurs in the form of scams or can be perpetrated by family members who try to misuse a client's money or possessions. Neglect may be intentional or unintentional and occurs when required food, medication, or personal care is not provided. Abandonment is a form of neglect in which someone who has agreed to provide care for an elderly client deserts that client. Clients who are denied the right to make their own decisions, even though they are competent to do so, or are not provided privacy or the right to worship, are suffering from a violation of their inalienable rights.

> **CLINICAL TIP**
>
> Although many screenings, including elder abuse, have insufficient evidence to support routine mass screening, nurses should be knowledgeable about persons who are at high risk and perform appropriate screenings.

Self-neglect, wherein an older adult is unable to provide for his or her own care, is the most common provider-reported form of neglect (National Center on Elder Abuse, 1998). Most cases of elder abuse are perpetrated by a family member, and reasons for the abuse include caregiver burnout and stress, financial worries, transgenerational violence, and psychopathology in the abuser. Women and dependent elders tend to be the most vulnerable to abuse.

Assessment of abuse can be very difficult because the victim may be cognitively impaired and unable to describe the abuse. It is not unusual for elderly clients to have multiple bruises due to poor balance and loss of subcutaneous fat. Clues to abuse may include the following:

> The presence of several injuries in different stages of repair
> Delays in seeking treatment
> Injuries that cannot be explained or that are inconsistent with the client's history
> Contradictory explanations by the caregiver and the patient
> Bruises, burns, welts, lacerations, or restraint marks
> Dehydration, malnutrition, decubitus ulcers, or poor hygiene
> Depression, withdrawal, or agitation
> Signs of medication misuse
> A pattern of missed or canceled appointments
> Frequent changes in healthcare providers
> Discharge, bleeding, or pain in the rectum or vagina or a sexually transmitted infection (STI)
> Missing prosthetic device(s), such as dentures, glasses, or hearing aids

The USPSTF decided there is insufficient evidence to support mass screening of asymptomatic elderly clients for abuse or the potential for abuse. Suspected abuse should be evaluated through a thorough history with patients, caregivers, and other significant informants, taken separately. Home visits also can yield important clues to the situation. Physical examination, including mental status and evaluation of mood, is critical. Laboratory and imaging studies can support suspicions of dehydration, malnutrition, medication abuse, and fractures or other injuries.

Several assessment tools may help the nurse determine whether a client is being abused or is at risk for abuse, although none have been adequately tested for validity, reliability, and generalizability, according to the National Center on Elder Abuse (University of California at Berkeley, 2007). The Hwalek–Sengstock Elder Abuse Screening Test (H-S/EAST) (Neale, Hwalek, Scott, Sengstock, & Stahl, 1991) and the Vulnerability to Abuse Screening Scale (Schofield & Mishra, 2003) are commonly used screening instruments that are completed by the older adult.

If suspicions are strengthened through this assessment, a collaborative approach to management and prevention is required. Team members include the adult protective services agency, social workers, psychiatrists, lawyers, and law enforcement officials. It is important to ascertain whether the client is in immediate danger, in which case law enforcement will be helpful in removing the client from the dangerous situation. The approach to any abuse case should be coordinated with the adult protective services agency, as mandated by law. Abuse and neglect should be reported within 48 hours of the time you become aware of the situation. Elder abuse that occurs in nursing homes and assisted-living facilities must be reported to the Long-Term Care Ombudsman Program in most states.

In summary, guidelines for elder abuse treatment recommend that you (1) report abuse and neglect to adult protective services or other state-mandated agencies; (2) ensure that there is a safety plan and assess safety; (3) assess the client's cognitive, emotional, functional, and health status; and (4) assess the frequency, severity, and intent of abuse. It is important that the nurse's involvement does not end with the referral, but includes an ongoing plan of care because elderly persons referred to adult protective services are at increased risk of mortality in the decade following the referral. Chapter 24 provides additional information on the prevention and treatment of elder abuse.

Heart and Vascular Disease

CHD is the leading cause of death in the United States. Every year over 1 million Americans have a new or recurrent myocardial infarction (MI) or die from CHD. Almost 50% of patients who suffer MI or sudden death have no prior warning symptoms (Bolooki & Askari, 2010). Most of these unexpected cardiac events and cases of sudden death occur in patients over 65 years of age. For this reason, identification of clients at risk of MI, who may be able to benefit from primary prevention strategies, is desirable. National Health and Nutrition Examination Survey (NHANES) III data (National Center for Health Statistics, 2004) suggest that approximately 25% of U.S. adults may be at high risk for a coronary event and may be potential beneficiaries of primary prevention strategies. The *Framingham Heart Study* has elucidated many of the risk factors associated with CHD. This study began with over 5,000 male and female subjects about 50 years ago to study cardiovascular risk factors. As a result of decades of epidemiological work, the following risk factors have been identified:

> Age 50 or older for men and 60 or older for women
> Hypertension
> Smoking
> Obesity
> Family history of premature CHD
> Diabetes (considered to be a CHD risk-equivalent, i.e., carries the same risk of a coronary event as known CHD)
> Sedentary lifestyle
> Abnormal lipid levels

Other, nontraditional risk factors, including homocysteine, lipoprotein(a) and infectious agents also have been shown to contribute to the development of CHD (Boudi, 2015). A risk calculator to estimate an individual's 10-year risk for the development of CHD has been developed by the American Heart Association and the American College of Cardiology. It also incorporates USPSTF aspirin recommendations and Eighth Joint National Committee (JNC 8) guidelines for hypertension management. This calculator can be accessed at http://www.cvriskcalculator.com/.

Lipids

There is strong evidence to link elevations in total cholesterol (TC), low-density lipoprotein (LDL-C), and low levels of high-density lipoprotein (HDL-C) with coronary risk. Four large primary prevention trials documented a 30% reduction in cardiac events for clients whose cholesterol was reduced using statin therapy (USPSTF, 2008).

Unfortunately, there were very few subjects older than 65 years of age in primary prevention trials, but there have been studies of older adults with preexisting CVD who have shown a reduction in cardiovascular events with the use of statins (USPSTF, 2008). There is no age at which the Task Force recommends screening be stopped, but cholesterol levels are unlikely to increase after age 65 (see **Box 8-12**). For patients who have been tested and found to have normal levels of cholesterol before the age of 65, testing may not be necessary in later years.

The ratios of TC to HDL-C or LDL-C to HDL-C are better predictors of risk than TC alone. It is possible to accurately measure TC and HDL-C on nonfasting venous or capillary blood samples, but fasting blood samples are required for accurate LDL-C measurement. Two separate measurements are required for definitive diagnosis. The optimal interval for lipid testing has not been determined, but most expert guidelines support testing every 5 years, with shorter intervals for people who have elevated lipid levels and who may require therapy.

Hypertension

Fifty million Americans have high blood pressure. Older Americans have the highest prevalence of hypertension and are the least effectively treated. Framingham data suggest that clients who have normal blood pressure at age 55 have a 90% chance of developing hypertension at some time in their life. High systolic blood pressure, which is more strongly correlated with CVAs, renal failure, and heart failure than diastolic blood pressure, is the most common form of hypertension in the elderly and is less likely to be well controlled than diastolic blood pressure. The NHANES study found that among subjects 60 years of age or older, isolated systolic hypertension (systolic > 140 mmHg with diastolic > 90 mmHg) was present in 65% of cases of high blood pressure.

The 2014 Evidence-Based Guideline for the Management of High Blood Pressure in Adults report from the panel members appointed to the JNC 8 (James et al., 2014) is a national guideline for blood pressure screening and treatment. A summary algorithm describing this guideline can be accessed at http://jnc8.jamanetwork.com/. The systolic blood pressure goal for adults over the age of 60 was raised from 140 mmHg to 150 mmHg in the

BOX 8-12   Lipid Screening

Level A recommendation: For screening, there is strong evidence that correlates lipid abnormalities with cardiac risk. A simple blood test is a valid and reliable method of diagnosing lipid abnormalities, and diet and drug therapies are effective remedies. The USPSTF recommends screening all men over the age of 35 and women over age 45 who are at risk for CHD for lipid disorders.

JNC-8 guideline. This is the most controversial aspect of this new guideline and conflicts with another evidence-based guideline published by the American Society of Hypertension and the International Society of Hypertension who recommend a goal systolic blood pressure of 150 mmHg only for patients over the age of 80 (Weber et al., 2014).

It is important to diagnose and treat hypertension to reduce the incidence of cardiac disease (see **Box 8-13**). The correlation of cardiovascular risk and blood pressure is dramatic. Risk doubles with each increment of 20/10 mmHg after 115/75.

Blood pressure readings can be accurately determined by a properly calibrated sphygmomanometer using an appropriately sized cuff. (The cuff's bladder needs to encircle at least 80% of the client's arm.) Clients should have been seated in a chair for at least 5 minutes before blood pressure is measured. The client's feet should be uncrossed on the floor and the arm at heart level. Blood pressure measurements should be validated by measuring pressure in the contralateral arm. It is recommended that hypertension be diagnosed only after two or more elevated readings are obtained on at least two visits over a period of one to several weeks.

Lifestyle modifications are effective in preventing hypertension and lowering blood pressure in clients who have hypertension. These lifestyle changes include physical activity, weight loss, reducing dietary sodium, and following the *Dietary Approaches to Stop Hypertension (DASH) diet*, published by the National Institutes of Health (NIH) and downloadable at https://www.nhlbi.nih.gov/files/docs/public /heart/dash_brief.pdf. This is a comprehensive plan that can be given to patients and includes a summary of the DASH eating plan and its effectiveness in lowering hypertension, a diet and exercise journal, and meal plans using the DASH diet.

Aspirin Therapy

Aspirin therapy has long been known to be effective as a secondary prevention strategy for clients with heart disease, but the risks of GI bleeding and hemorrhagic stroke associated with aspirin therapy have delayed recommendations of aspirin as a means of primary prevention. A meta-analysis of five primary prevention trials (USPSTF, 2009a) that showed a 28% reduction of cardiac disease in subjects (most of whom were older than 50) has led experts to recommend aspirin chemoprophylaxis with men between the ages of 45 and 79 years and women between the ages of 55 to 79 at high risk for developing CHD and low risk for GI hemorrhage (see **Box 8-14**). GI bleeding occurred in approximately 0.3% of subjects given aspirin for 5 years, causing some

---

BOX 8-13   Blood Pressure Screening

Level A recommendation: Strong evidence exists that blood pressure measurement can identify adults at increased risk of cardiovascular disease due to high blood pressure. Treatment of hypertension substantially decreases the incidence of cardiovascular disease.

BOX 8-14   Aspirin Therapy

Level A recommendation: Good evidence exists that aspirin decreases the incidence of CHD in adults who are at increased risk of heart disease, but aspirin increases the incidence of GI bleeding and hemorrhagic strokes. The USPSTF concluded that evidence is strongest to support aspirin therapy in patients at high risk of CHD.

Level I recommendation: Insufficient evidence is unavailable to recommend for or against aspirin prophylaxis in men and women 80 years of age and older.

concerns about the risk versus benefit of aspirin for primary prevention of heart disease in patients who are at low risk for cardiac illness. The USPSTF states that there is insufficient evidence to recommend for or against aspirin prophylaxis in adults 80 years of age and older (USPSTF, 2009a).

Stroke

CVAs are the fifth leading cause of death in the United States, with more than two thirds of stroke occurring in persons age 65 years or older (CDC, 2015i). The physical, psychological, economic, and social costs of CVAs are enormously high, to clients as well as their families. Strokes are a significant cause of dependency among the elderly.

The primary risk factors for ischemic stroke are similar to those described in the previous section on heart disease: increased age, hypertension, smoking, and diabetes. Clients with coronary artery disease are at increased risk of stroke because atherosclerotic vessel disease is a common etiology for the two diseases. Lifestyle factors associated with CVA risk that have been identified by the National Stroke Association are heavy alcohol use, cigarette smoking, sedentary lifestyle, and a high-fat diet. In addition to these risk factors, atrial fibrillation and asymptomatic carotid stenosis place clients at high risk of CVD.

It is estimated that 36% of strokes suffered by clients 80 to 89 years of age are a result of nonvalvular atrial fibrillation (National Stroke Association, 1999). Adequate anticoagulation with warfarin therapy in patients with atrial fibrillation has been found to reduce stroke occurrence by 68%, whereas aspirin therapy was found to reduce CVAs by only 21%. It is based on these data that the American Heart Association guidelines recommend the use of oral anticoagulation for patients older than 75 years of age with nonvalvular atrial fibrillation. Patients 65 to 75 years old with atrial fibrillation, as well as other CVA risks, should be treated with warfarin or one of the newer factor Xa or direct thrombin inhibitors, and those without additional risk factors may be treated with anticoagulants or aspirin. The guideline underscores the importance of weighing the risk of hemorrhage against the benefit of therapy on an individual patient basis (Meschia et al., 2014).

Carotid stenosis is an important stroke risk factor. However, screening of asymptomatic persons for carotid artery stenosis, using either physical examination or carotid ultrasound, is not recommended by the USPSTF. Screening is justified if early treatment can change clinical outcomes and if there are effective, low-risk screening tests. The inability of experts to recommend screening is based on the fact that there is significant debate about the risks and benefits of carotid endarterectomy as a treatment for asymptomatic disease. The American Academy of Neurology (AAN) (2015) recommends carotid endarterectomy for asymptomatic stenosis when the artery is at least 70% occluded, but the USPSTF does not recommend carotid ultrasound for asymptomatic patients based on remaining questions about the risks and benefits of carotid endarterectomy as a result of varying surgical risks among studies. Physical findings that suggest stenosis auscultation of the carotid artery, are a poor predictor of subsequent stroke.

Experts agree that the risk of a stroke can be minimized through treatment of hypertension; using statin therapy after MI for normal and high cholesterol; using warfarin for patients with atrial fibrillation and specific risk factors, and for patients after MI who have atrial fibrillation, left ventricular thrombus, or decreased left ventricular ejection fraction; and modification of lifestyle-related risk factors such as smoking, alcohol use, physical activity, and diet.

Thyroid Disease

The USPSTF (2015) has found insufficient evidence to support screening for thyroid disease in adults. Older adults are far more susceptible to thyroid dysfunction than younger adults. Overt disease affects 5% of American adults, but the prevalence of subclinical hypothyroidism (elevated thyroid-stimulating hormone [TSH] with normal levels of thyroid hormone) is 17.4% among women older than age 75 and 6.2% among men over 65. Approximately 2% to 5% of these cases of subclinical hypothyroidism will progress to overt hypothyroidism each year (Cooper, 2001). The American Association of Clinical Endocrinologists (AACE) and the American Thyroid

Association (ATA) (Garber et al., 2012) published clinical guidelines for the diagnosis and management of thyroid disease that state that subclinical hypothyroidism may be associated with GI disorders, depression, dementia, lipid disorders, increased likelihood of goiter, and overt thyroid disease.

Subclinical hyperthyroidism is far less common in the population, affecting only a little more than 1% of adults over 60 years of age, but it is present in up to 20% of patients taking levothyroxine for hypothyroidism (Bahn et al., 2011).

Untreated hyperthyroidism can lead to atrial fibrillation, congestive heart failure, osteoporosis, and neuropsychiatric disorders. Hypothyroidism can cause constipation and ileus, lipid abnormalities, weight gain, decreased cognition, depression, and negative changes in functional status. The goal of screening would be to decrease the negative effects of overt thyroid disease.

The Task Force's inability to recommend for or against screening of asymptomatic persons for thyroid disease results (see **Box 8-15**) from the lack of clarity about the risks of subclinical disease. It is clear that both hypothyroidism and hyperthyroidism cause significant morbidity and need to be treated, but the negative consequences of these diseases appear to be present primarily in patients who present with symptoms of the disease. There are significant costs and risks associated with thyroid replacement that need to be considered before recommending mass screening. Many patients who receive thyroid hormone replacement develop subclinical hyperthyroidism, which may increase the risk of developing osteoporosis, hip fracture, and atrial fibrillation. The Task Force recommends that clinicians be cognizant of the signs and symptoms of thyroid disease and test symptomatic patients; evidence is lacking to justify screening of asymptomatic patients, however.

Osteoporosis

Half of all postmenopausal women will have a fracture related to osteoporosis at some point in their life. The risk for the development of osteoporosis markedly increases with age, and osteoporosis is responsible for 70% of the fractures that occur in older adults. Women ages 65 to 69 years have six times the risk of osteoporosis than younger postmenopausal women, and that rate increases to 14 times in women ages 75 to 79 (USPSTF, 2011). Age, low BMI, and failure to use estrogen replacement are the strongest risk factors for osteoporosis development (see **Box 8-16**). Other possible risks include white or Asian race, family history of compression or stress fracture, fall risk or history of fracture, low levels of weight-bearing exercise, smoking, excessive alcohol or caffeine use, and low intake of calcium or vitamin D. Certain medications, such as thyroid medication or prednisone, increase the chances of developing osteoporosis.

BOX 8-15   Thyroid Disease Screening

Level I recommendation: Insufficient evidence exists to recommend for or against screening based on limited evidence to establish health risks of subclinical disease and due to the risks of treatment.

BOX 8-16   Osteoporosis Screening

Level B recommendation: Osteoporosis is common in the elderly and is correlated with fracture risk. There are good screening tests to diagnose osteoporosis and effective treatments for the disease. Screening is recommended for all women 65 years and older and for women younger than 65 who are at high risk for fractures.

Level I recommendation: Related to screening for older men.

Some men are at increased risk of osteoporosis, and decisions about screening may be made on an individual basis. Men with chronic lung disease, have low testosterone levels, and require steroid medications for extended periods are at increased risk of bone loss (National Osteoporosis Foundation [NOF], 2010).

There is a strong association between bone mass and fracture risk, which continues into old age. Multiple studies demonstrate that therapies that slow bone loss are effective in reducing fracture risk, even if they are begun in old age. The USPSTF uses the Frax® tool, developed by the WHO, which determines an individual's risk for future fractures. Based on the risk factors, screening is recommended for all women over the age of 65 and for women between the ages of 50 and 64 if they meet the 9.3% probability of fracture in the next 10 years based on the Frax® tool (USPSTF, 2011). Bone density testing at the femoral, neck, and lumbar spine by dual-energy X-ray bone densitometry is the gold standard screening tool and the one most closely correlated with hip fracture risk, though heel measurements using ultrasonography are also predictive of short-term fracture risk. Men make up only 20% of the Americans with osteoporosis. Although they are at significantly less risk then women, one in four men over the age of 50 will incur a fracture due to osteoporosis (NOF, 2010). Despite these statistics, the USPSTF has deemed the available evidence insufficient to recommend osteoporosis screening for males (USPSTF, 2011).

Vision and Hearing

The prevalence of hearing and visual impairment increases with age and has been correlated with social and emotional isolation, clinical depression, and functional impairment. An objective hearing loss can be identified in 20% to 40% of adults over the age of 50 and in 80% of adults 80 years of age and older (USPSTF, 2012b). High-frequency loss is the most important contributor to this increase in hearing loss, though up to 30% of cases may be caused or compounded by cerumen impaction or otitis media, which are easily treated (Ivers, Cumming, Mitchell, Simpson, & Peduto, 2003).

Approximately 6.9% of adults over the age of 65 have severe visual impairment (American Federation for the Blind, 2015). Macular degeneration is the most common cause of visual loss in elderly whites, whereas African Americans are more likely to lose vision as a result of cataracts, glaucoma, and diabetes. Visual impairment has been correlated with falls and hip fractures in the elderly (Ivers et al., 2003).

The Snellen eye chart is a useful tool for detecting refraction errors but is, unfortunately, ineffective at detecting early macular degeneration. The USPSTF (2009b) has also found insufficient evidence to suggest that screening and treatment to improve visual acuity also improve functional outcomes in older adults. Ophthalmology referral may be useful for clients whose corrected vision is worse than 20/40 or who report visual problems that limit activities such as reading or driving. Many expert panels, including the American Academy of Ophthalmology, the American Optometric Association, and Prevent Blindness America, recommend regular ophthalmologic examinations for adults over 65 years of age (40 years of age for African Americans) based on the fact that effective glaucoma screening should be performed by eye specialists with specialized equipment to evaluate the optic disc and measure visual fields. The optimal frequency for glaucoma screening has not yet been determined.

The USPSTF (2012b) found insufficient evidence for screening for hearing impairment for older adults (see **Box 8-17**), based on a lack of demonstrated improvement in quality of life after improvement of hearing with hearing aids. Simple testing for hearing loss using a whisper voice test from a distance of 2 feet and

---

BOX 8-17   Hearing and Vision Screening

Level I recommendation: More research is needed to understand the benefits of hearing screening.

Level I recommendation: There is insufficient evidence to recommend for or against screening for visual acuity changes or for glaucoma in adults.

asking the older adult about his or her perceived hearing loss were effective at detecting hearing loss (see **Figure 8-1**).

Prostate Cancer

Prostate cancer is both the second most common form of cancer and the second most common cause of cancer death among U.S. men. The risk of developing prostate cancer increases with age and is the second leading cause of death overall in American men (American Cancer Society [ACS], 2015d). The disease is most prevalent in African Americans and least prevalent among Asian Americans.

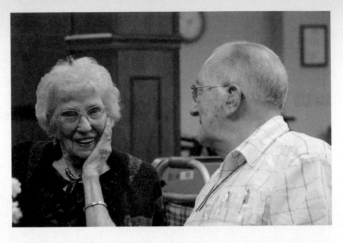

Figure 8-1 Nurses should be aware of the many sensory changes that come with advancing age.

Two tests are commonly used in prostate cancer screening: the digital rectal examination (DRE) and the prostate-specific antigen (PSA) blood test. "The pooled sensitivity, specificity, and positive predictive value for PSA were 72.1%, 93.2%, and 25.1%, respectively, and for DRE were 53.2%, 83.6%, and 17.8%, respectively" (Mistry & Cable, 2003, p. 95). Benign prostatic hypertrophy is common in older men, and the presence of this disease increases the likelihood of false-positive testing with the PSA. Most prostate cancers are slow-growing and unlikely to be a cause of significant morbidity and mortality in older men. The greatest controversy regarding screening for prostate cancer is the inability to accurately predict which cancers will be aggressive and require treatment and which are unlikely to metastasize.

CLINICAL TIP

Current medical treatment for prostate cancer in older males is often "watch and wait".

The ACS recommends that healthcare providers share decision making related to prostate cancer screening with male patients over 50 years of age who have at least a 10-year life expectancy (> 40 for select high-risk males). They suggest PSA-based screening with DRE for men who choose to be screened.

The USPSTF recommendation for prostate screenings differs from that of the ACS (2015d). The USPSTF recommends against screening for prostate cancer in all men, due to the high rates of false-positive tests with PSA screening and because many prostate cancers are slow growing. They cite the fact that PSA-based screening has failed to reduce prostate cancer mortality as additional rationale for their decision (ACS, 2015d). Discussion of this complex issue, including the pros and cons of screening, is recommended for men younger than age 75 (see **Box 8-18**). The CDC has a set of patient education materials designed to help guide this discussion, which can be found at http://www.cdc.gov/cancer/prostate/basic_info/infographic.htm

A large clinical trial sponsored by the National Cancer Institute, the Prostate, Lung, Colon and Ovarian (PLCO) Cancer Screening Trial, was designed to determine whether prostate screening and early detection of prostate cancer improved patient outcomes (National Cancer Institute, 2012). A report from this PLCO screening trial described a 7-year, controlled, multicenter trial of over 75,000 men who were randomized to receive either usual care or DRE and PSA testing. Men in the experimental group received more frequent prostate cancer screening than those in the control group but were not found to have any difference in prostate cancer-related death (Andriole et al., 2009).

BOX 8-18 Prostate Cancer Screening

Level D recommendation: The USPSTF recommends against PSA-based screening for men.

The ACS suggests discussing pros and cons of screening with men over age 50 with at least a 10-year life expectancy and providing PSA and DRE screening for those who choose to be tested.

BOX 8-19 Breast Cancer Screening

Level B evidence: For screening mammography, there is fair evidence to support benefit from breast cancer screening for women between the ages of 50 and 74 by mammogram every 2 years.

Level I recommendation: For screening of women 75 years and older.

Level D evidence: Clinical breast examination screening.

Level D evidence: Self-breast examination screening. The Task Force recommends against clinical breast examination or teaching women to do self-breast examination.

Level I evidence: A small group of women at high risk for breast cancer should be screened with MRI as well as mammography (ACS, 2015c).

Data from American Cancer Society (ACS). (2015) American Cancer Society recommendations for early breast cancer detection in women without breast symptoms. Retrieved from http://www.cancer.org/cancer/breastcancer /moreinformation/breastcancerearlydetection /breast-cancer-early-detection-acs-recs

---

Breast Cancer

Breast cancer is the most common cancer among U.S. women, and the prevalence of the disease increases with age. According to the CDC (2015e), 3% to 4% of women who are 60 years old today will get breast cancer by the age of 70. In 2015 there were over 230,000 new cases of breast cancer, with over 40,000 deaths (ACS, 2015c). In addition to age, risk factors for the disease include family history of breast cancer, atypical hyperplasia in breast tissue, obesity, use of postmenopausal hormones, and birth of a first child when a woman is over 30 years of age. The USPSTF recommends biennial breast cancer screening for women between the ages of 50 and 74 years; however, the Task Forces finds the evidence to be insufficient to rationalize screening by mammography for women over the age of 75 (USPSTF, 2015). This is despite the fact that women between the ages of 75 and 79 have the highest rate of breast cancer (CDC, 2015e). Although disease prevalence is high in this population, the Task Force wondered whether early detection of disease would improve health outcomes in a population that also has a higher incidence of other chronic illnesses. They wondered if there was an upper age limit at which breast cancer screening would no longer be beneficial (see **Box 8-19**).

Screening tests used to detect breast cancer include mammography and both mammography and magnetic resonance imaging (MRI) for women at very high risk of developing breast cancer (ACS, 2015c). The sensitivity of mammography to detect breast cancer varies widely, depending on a woman's age, whether she takes hormonal replacement, the technical quality of the testing equipment, and the skill of the radiologist. Overall, the test is more sensitive for older women than for younger women. Unfortunately, there are many false-positive tests, and up to one quarter of women who have annual mammograms may need to undergo unnecessary, invasive follow-up testing as a result of false-positive tests from mammography at some point in their lives. No studies have looked at the effectiveness of clinical breast examination without concurrent mammography to detect breast cancer. The USPSTF recommends against teaching the self-breast examination, concluding that the harms likely outweigh derived benefits and has found insufficient evidence for clinical breast examinations by healthcare providers or for diagnostic MRIs (USPSTF, 2009c).

Colorectal Cancer Screening

Colorectal cancer is both the third most common cancer in the United States and the third leading cause of cancer death in the United States (ACS, 2015a). The prevalence of the disease increases with age, and over 90% of colorectal cancer is diagnosed in clients over the age of 50 (ACS, 2015b). The American Cancer Society (ACS) released screening guidelines in 2008 that emphasize the importance of detecting precancerous growths as opposed to cancer itself. There are several good screening methods available to detect these precancerous lesions: annual fecal immunochemical test (FIT), stool DNA test (sDNA), annual fecal occult blood testing (FOBT), double-contrast barium enema, computed tomography colonography every 5 years, flexible sigmoidoscopy every 5 years, or colonoscopy every 10 years. Choice of screening test is determined based on client risk factors and preference. Patients who are at average risk for developing colorectal cancer should be screened regularly from the ages of 50 through 75 using one of these testing methods (USPSTF, 2015). The best method for FOBT is three consecutive stool samples collected at home by the patient on an annual basis. These tests should be examined without rehydration due to the decreased specificity of the test that is associated with rehydration of the samples. A single guaiac test, performed in the office with DRE, is not recommended as an adequate screening test (National Guideline Clearinghouse, 2009).

Patients who have a history of adenomatous polyps or inflammatory bowel disease or a family history of colorectal cancer or adenomatous polyps should receive colonoscopy. Screening for these high-risk clients is begun before age 50.

Colonoscopy is the most sensitive of the screening methodologies but is associated with the highest costs and risks. These risks include a small risk of perforation and bleeding and the risks associated with sedation, which is required for the procedure.

There is strong evidence to support colorectal screening for men and women age 50 or older, but insufficient evidence to determine which of the various screening options is preferred (see **Box 8-20**). As of 2011, only 50% of patients over the age of 50, for whom screening is recommended, report compliance with the ACS colorectal screening guidelines (ACS, 2011).

CLINICAL TIP

Colorectal cancer is treatable when caught early and screening by colonoscopy at age 50 (or earlier if family history is positive) is highly recommended.

BOX 8-20   Colorectal Screening

Level A recommendation: The task force strongly recommends colorectal screening by FOBT, sigmoidoscopy, or colonoscopy for adults between the ages of 50 and 75.

Level C recommendation: For adults between the ages of 76 and 85.

Level D recommendation: For adults over age 85.

Summary

In summary, there are many effective screenings for various diseases common to the elderly population. Nurses should utilize the appropriate resources to obtain and put into practice screening of aged patients according to the USPSTF guidelines. The USPSTF has created a mobile application to help you determine which screening services are appropriate for your patients. This web-based calculator can be accessed at http://epss.ahrq.gov/PDA/index.jsp. (**Table 8-1** contains a summary of guidelines.) Proper screening of older adults can save lives.

TABLE 8-1 Summary of USPSTF Screening Recommendations for Older Adults		
Screening Test	**Recommendation**	**Level of Evidence**
Physical activity	Physical activity has a positive impact on health, but the impact of counseling to improve physical activity is small. It is most effective for those with health problems directly related to lack of physical exercise.	Level B for adults who are overweight or obese or have CHD risk factors Level C for all other adults
Nutrition	Counseling clients with hyperlipidemia or CVD risk factors about nutrition is beneficial.	Level B
Tobacco use	Screening is helpful in identifying tobacco use, and counseling is effective in helping people quit smoking.	Level A
Depression	Screening is effective in identifying depression, and treatments are effective if adequate staff support is available.	Level B
Dementia	Insufficient evidence exists to support mass screening of elders for dementia, but there is good evidence to suggest screening to follow up on family or client's concerns about memory loss.	Level I
Alcohol abuse	Screening is beneficial and treatment is effective.	Level B
Elder abuse and neglect	No evidence exists that either screening or interventions are effective.	Level I
Lipids	Good evidence exists to support that treatment and screening are effective.	Level A
Hypertension	Good evidence to support that treatment and screening are effective.	Level A
Aspirin therapy for men over 45 years and women over 55 years of age	Good evidence exists to support aspirin therapy in clients at high risk for CVD.	Level A; Level I for adults over 80 years of age
Cerebrovascular disease	The USPSTF recommends against screening for asymptomatic carotid stenosis.	Level D
Thyroid disease	Insufficient evidence exists to support screening for thyroid disease.	Level I
Osteoporosis	Screening is recommended for all women over 65 years of age.	Level B

(continues)

TABLE 8-1 Summary of USPSTF Screening Recommendations for Older Adults *(continued)*		
Screening Test	**Recommendation**	**Level of Evidence**
Vision and hearing	Insufficient evidence exists that hearing screening and treatment actually improves function. Glaucoma testing by an ophthalmologist is recommended for adults at risk of developing glaucoma.	Level I
Prostate cancer	The USPSTF recommends against PSA screening to detect prostate cancer.	Level D
Breast cancer	Mammography is recommended every 2 years as a screening for breast cancer for older women.	Level B for women between the ages of 50 and 74 Level I for women age 75 and over
Colorectal cancer	Screening for colorectal cancer by FOBT, FIT, sigmoidoscopy, sDNA, double-contrast barium enema, or colonoscopy is recommended.	Level A for adults younger than 76 years of age Level C for those age 76 to 85 Level D for those over age 85

Clinical Reasoning Exercises

1. Iola R., a 72-year-old overweight woman, tells you she wishes she could exercise, but she can never bring herself to begin an exercise program. She knows that her hypertension, diabetes, and high cholesterol would benefit from regular exercise. She is caring for her grandchildren 3 days per week and cannot find the time to engage in regular exercise. She is not sure if it is safe to walk alone around her neighborhood, anyway. Explain how you could use the concepts of self-management of chronic illness and contracting to help Iola begin an exercise program. What benefits might she obtain through regular exercise? How frequently should she plan to exercise?

2. Mr. Gottlieb complains that he has been falling a lot recently. He can remember at least three falls in the past 6 months, but luckily none have resulted in injury yet. His friend is living in a nursing home as a result of complications and debility that followed a hip fracture, and Mr. Gottlieb does not want the same fate for himself. Describe how you will assess and manage Mr. Gottlieb's fall risk.

3. Mrs. Hall is a 94-year-old woman with Alzheimer's disease. Her daughter is her primary caregiver and calls to report that caring for her mother has become intolerable. "I can't make her eat, drink, or stop her incessant whining." You notice that Mrs. Hall has not been in to see her primary care doctor in over 3 years, but that she has been in to the emergency department four times in the past year for dehydration, urinary tract infections, and behavior management. You want to assess

the home situation for safety and provide caregiver support to the patient's daughter. What signs of abuse and neglect might you look for through a chart review? Through a clinic visit and evaluation of the client? Through laboratory testing? How could you get a better assessment of the actual home situation? If your suspicions are strengthened, how will you proceed to intervene with this case of suspected elder abuse and neglect?

Personal Reflections

1. In the case described in question 3 of the Critical Reasoning Exercises, which of the two clients described, Mrs. Hall or her daughter who initially called you, is your primary patient? Do you have loyalties to both? How could you address the care needs of Mrs. Hall's daughter?

2. Do you think you can counsel a client about health promotion if you do not adopt these behaviors yourself?

3. Mr. J., an 88-year-old gentleman, had a colonoscopy 6 years ago in which an adenomatous polyp was removed. His gastroenterologist has asked for your help in bringing Mr. J. back for follow-up testing. You call the patient, who tells you that although he recognizes the risk, he is not willing to undergo the procedure again. He believes his life expectancy is limited anyway and would prefer not to know if he has another polyp because he would not want to undergo surgery anyway. What do you do?

References

Alexopoulos, G. S., Abrams, R. C., Young, R. C., & Shamoian, C. A. (1988). Cornell Scale for depression in dementia. *Biological Psychiatry, 23*(3), 271–284.

American Academy of Neurology (AAN). (2015). Evidence-based guideline summary for clinicians: Carotid endarterectomy: An evidence-based review. Retrieved from http://tools.aan.com/professionals/practice/guideline/pdf/Clinician_guideline.pdf

American Cancer Society. (2011). *Colorectal cancer facts and figures 2014–2016.* Atlanta, GA: Author. Retrieved from http://www.cancer.org/acs/groups/content/documents/document/acspc-042280.pdf

American Cancer Society. (2015a). American Cancer Society recommendations for colorectal cancer early detection. Retrieved from http://www.cancer.org/cancer/colonandrectumcancer/moreinformation/colonandrectumcancerearlydetection/colorectal-cancer-early-detection-acs-recommendations

American Cancer Society. (2015b). *Breast cancer facts and figures 2015.* Atlanta, GA: Author. Retrieved from http://www.cancer.org/acs/groups/content/@editorial/documents/document/acspc-044552.pdf

American Cancer Society. (2015c). What are the key statistics about prostate cancer? Retrieved from http://www.cancer.org/cancer/prostatecancer/detailedguide/prostate-cancer-key-statistics

American Cancer Society. (2015d). American Cancer Society recommendations for prostate cancer early detection. Retrieved from http://www.cancer.org/cancer/prostatecancer/moreinformation/prostatecancerearlydetection/prostate-cancer-early-detection-acs-recommendations

American Federation for the Blind. (2015). Aging and vision loss fact sheet. Retrieved from http://www.afb.org/info/programs-and-services/professional-development/experts-guide/aging-and-vision-loss/1235

American Cancer Society. (2015e). American Cancer Society recommendations for early breast cancer detection in women without breast symptoms. Retrieved from http://www.cancer.org/cancer/breastcancer/moreinformation/breastcancerearlydetection/breast-cancer-early-detection-acs-recs

American Geriatrics Society. (2010). AGS/BGS clinical practice guideline: Prevention of falls in older persons. Retrieved from http://www.americangeriatrics.org/health_care_professionals/clinical_practice/clinical-guidelines-recommendations/prevention-of-falls-summary-of-recommendations

American Geriatrics Society 2015 Beers Criteria Update Expert Panel. (2015). American Geriatrics Society 2015 updated Beers Criteria for potentially inappropriate medication use in older adults. *Journal of the American Geriatrics Society, 63*(11), 2227–2246.

American Pharmacists Association, National Association of Chain Drug Stores Foundation. (2008). *Medication therapy management in pharmacy practice: Core elements of an MTM service model.* Retrieved from http://www.pharmacist.com/sites/default/files/files/core_elements_of_an_mtm_practice.pdf

American Psychiatric Association. (2013). *Diagnostic and statistical manual of mental disorders* (5th ed.). Arlington, VA: American Psychiatric Publishing.

Andriole, G. L., Crawford, E. D., Grubb, R. L. III, Buys, S. S., Chia, D., Church, T. R., . . . Berg, C. D. (2009). Mortality results from a randomized prostate cancer screening trial. *New England Journal of Medicine, 360,* 1310–1319.

Babor, T. F., Higgins-Biddle, J. C., Saunders, J. B., & Monteiro, M. G. (2001). *The alcohol use disorders identification test* (2nd ed.). Geneva, Switzerland: World Health Organization. Retrieved from http://www.talkingalcohol.com/files/pdfs/WHO_audit.pdf

Bahn, R. S., Burch, H. B., Cooper, D. S., Garber J. R., Greenlee M. C., Klein, I., . . . Stan, M. N. (2011). Hyperthyroidism and other causes of thyrotoxicosis: Management guidelines of the American Thyroid Association and American Association of Clinical Endocrinologists. *Endocrine Practice, 17*(3). Retrieved from https://www.aace.com/files/hyper-guidelines-2011.pdf

Bolooki, H. M., & Askari, A. (2010). *Acute myocardial infarction.* Lyndhurst, OH: Cleveland Clinic Publications, Disease Management Project. Retrieved from http://www.clevelandclinicmeded.com/medicalpubs/diseasemanagement/cardiology/acute-myocardial-infarction/#s0015

Boudi, B. (2015). *Risk factors for coronary artery disease.* Retrieved from http://emedicine.medscape.com/article/164163-overview

Bradford, A., Kunik, M. E., Schultz, P., Williams, S. P., & Singh, H. (2009). Missed and delayed diagnosis of dementia in primary care: Prevalence and contributing factors. *Alzheimer's Disease & Associated Disorders, 23*(4), 306–314.

Budnitz, D. S., Lovegrove, M. C., Shehab, N., & Richards, C. L. (2011). Emergency hospitalizations for adverse drug events in older adults. *New England Journal of Medicine, 365,* 2002–2012.

Carlson, S. A., Fulton, J. E., Pratt, M., Yang, Z., & Adams, E. K. (2015). Inadequate physical activity and health care expenditures in the United States. *Cardiovascular Diseases, 57,* 315–323.

Centers for Disease Control and Prevention. (2008). Smoking-attributable mortality, years of potential life lost and productivity losses—United States, 2000–2004. Retrieved from http://www.cdc.gov/mmwr/preview/mmwrhtml/mm5745a3.htm

Centers for Disease Control and Prevention. (2009). Fact sheet for health professionals on physical activity guidelines for older adults. Retrieved from http://www.cdc.gov/nccdphp/dnpa/physical/pdf/PA_Fact_Sheet_OlderAdults.pdf

Centers for Disease Control and Prevention. (2013). *The state of aging and health in America.* Atlanta, GA: Centers for Disease Control and Prevention, US Department of Health and Human Services.

Centers for Disease Control and Prevention. (2014). Shingles (Herpes Zoster). Retrieved from http://www.cdc.gov/shingles/hcp/clinical-overview.html

Centers for Disease Control and Prevention. (2015a). Disability and functioning (adults). Retrieved from http://www.cdc.gov/nchs/fastats/disability.htm

Centers for Disease Control and Prevention. (2015b). Falls among older adults: An overview. Retrieved from http://www.cdc.gov/homeandrecreationalsafety/falls/adultfalls.html

Centers for Disease Control and Prevention. (2015c). Fast stats: Leading causes of death. Retrieved from http://www.cdc.gov/nchs/fastats/leading-causes-of-death.htm

Centers for Disease Control and Prevention. (2015d). Fluzone high-dose seasonal influenza vaccine. Retrieved from http://www.cdc.gov/flu/protect/vaccine/qa_fluzone.htm

Centers for Disease Control and Prevention. (2015e). Breast cancer risk by age. Retrieved from https://www.cdc.gov/cancer/breast/statistics/age.htm

Centers for Disease Control and Prevention. (2015f). Medication safety program. Retrieved from http://www.cdc.gov/medicationsafety/

Centers for Disease Control and Prevention. (2015g). Recommended adult immunization schedule—United States. Retrieved from http://www.cdc.gov/vaccines/schedules/downloads/adult/adult-combined-schedule.pdf

Centers for Disease Control and Prevention. (2015i). Stroke facts. Retrieved from https://www.cdc.gov/stroke/facts.htm

Cooper, D. S. (2001). Subclinical hypothyroidism. *The New England Journal of Medicine, 345,* 260–265.

Dawson-Hughes, B., Mithal, A., Bonjour, J. P., Boonen, S., Burckhardt, P., Fuleihan, G. E. H., . . . Yoshimura, N. (2010). IOF position paper: Vitamin D recommendations for older adults. *Osteoporosis International, 21,* 1151–1154.

deVries, N. M., Staal, J. B., van Ravensberg, C. D., Hobbelen, J. S. M., Olde Rikkert, M. G. M., & Nijhuisvan der Sanden, M. W. G. (2011). Outcome instruments to measure frailty: A systematic review. *Ageing Research Reviews, 10,* 104–114.

Duxbury A. S. (1997). Gait disorders in the elderly: Commonly overlooked diagnostic clues. *Consultant, 37,* 2337–2351.

Ewing, J. A. (1984). Detecting alcoholism: The CAGE questionnaire. *Journal of the American Medical Association, 252,* 1905–1907.

Folstein, M. F., Folstein, S. E., & McHugh, P. R. (1975). "Mini-Mental State": A practical method for grading the cognitive state of patients for the clinician. *Journal of Psychiatric Research, 12,* 189–198.

Garber, J. R., Cobin, R. H., Gharib, H., Hennessey, J. V., Klein, I., Mechanick, J. I., . . . Woeber, K. A. (2012). Clinical practice guidelines for hypothyroidism in adults: Cosponsored by the American Association of Clinical Endocrinologists and the American Thyroid Association. *Endocrine Practice, 18*(6). Retrieved from https://www.aace.com/files/hypothyroidism_guidelines.pdf

Hoover, D. R., Siegel, M., Lucas, J., Kalay, E., Gaboda, D., Devanand, D. P., & Crystal, S. (2010). Depression in the first year of stay for elderly long-term nursing home residents in the USA. *International Psychogeriatrics, 22*(7), 1161–1171.

Ivers, R. Q., Cumming, R. G., Mitchell, P., Simpson, J. M., & Peduto, A. J. (2003). Visual risk factors for hip fracture in older people. *Journal of the American Geriatric Society, 51,* 356–363.

James, P. A., Oparil, S., Carter, B. L., Cushman, W. C., Dennison-Himmelfarb, C., Handler, J., . . . Ortiz, E. (2014). 2014 Evidence-based guideline for the management of high blood pressure in adults: Report from the panel members appointed to the Eighth Joint National Committee (JNC 8). *Journal of the American Medical Association, 311*(5), 507–520.

Kroenke, K., Spitzer, R. L., & Williams, J. B. (2001). The PHQ-9: Validity of a brief depression severity measure. *Journal of General Internal Medicine, 16*(9), 606–613.

Kurlowicz, L., & Greenberg, S. (2007). *The geriatric depression scale (GDS).* Hartford Institute for Geriatric Nursing, 4. Retrieved from https://consultgeri.org/try-this/general-assessment/issue-4.pdf

Lawton, M. P., & Brody, E. M. (1969). Assessment of older people: Self-maintaining and instrumental activities of daily living. *Gerontologist, 9,* 179–186.

Lorig, K., & Holman, H. (2000). Self management education: History, definition, outcomes, and mechanisms. *Annals of Behavioral Medicine, 26*(1), 1–7. Retrieved from https://www.ncbi.nlm.nih.gov/pubmed/12867348

McElhaney, J. (2011). Influenza vaccine responses in older adults. *Ageing Research Reviews, 10*(3), 379–388.

Meschia, J. F., Bushnell, C., Boden-Albala, B., Braun, L. T., Bravata, D. M., Chaturvedi, S., . . . Wilson, J. A. (2014). Guidelines for the primary prevention of stroke. *Stroke, 45*, 3754–3832.

Middleton, L. E., Barnes, D. E., Lui, L., & Yaffe, K. (2010). Physical activity over the life course and its association with cognitive performance and impairment in old age. *Journal of the American Geriatrics Society, 58*(7), 1322–1326.

Mistry K., & Cable, G. (2003). Meta-analysis of prostate-specific antigen and digital rectal examination as screening tests for prostrate carcinoma. *Journal of the American Board of Family Practice, 16,* 95–101.

Mitty E., & Flores, S. (2007). Fall prevention in assisted living: Assessment and strategies. *Geriatric Nursing, 28*(6), 349–357.

National Cancer Institute. (2012). Screening for prostate cancer in older patients (PLCO screening trial). Retrieved from http://clinicaltrials.gov/show/NCT00002540

National Center for Health Statistics. (2004). Third National Health and Nutrition Examination Survey (NHANES III) public-use data files. Retrieved from https://www.cdc.gov/nchs/nhanes/nhanes3/data_files.htm

National Center on Elder Abuse (with Westat, Inc.) (1998). The national elder abuse incidence study. The National Center on Elder Abuse. Retrieved from https://aoa.acl.gov/AoA_Programs/Elder_Rights/Elder_Abuse/docs/ABuseReport_Full.pdf

National Center on Elder Abuse. (n.d.). Elder abuse facts. Retrieved from https://www.ncoa.org/public-policy-action/elder-justice/elder-abuse-facts/

National Guideline Clearinghouse. (2009). Guideline synthesis: Screening for colorectal cancer. Retrieved from https://www.guideline.gov/syntheses/synthesis/50562

National Institute on Alcohol Abuse and Alcoholism. (1998). Alcohol and aging, alcohol alert #40. Retrieved from http://pubs.niaaa.nih.gov/publications/aa40.htm

National Osteoporosis Foundation. (2010). Clinician's guide to the prevention and treatment of osteoporosis. *Osteoporosis International, 25*(10), 2359–2381. Retrieved from https://www.ncbi.nlm.nih.gov/pmc/articles/PMC4176573/

National Stroke Association. (1999). Preventing a stroke. Retrieved from http://www.stroke.org/site/PageServer?pagename=prevent

Neale, A. V., Hwalek, M. A., Scott, R. O., Sengstock, M. C., & Stahl, C. (1991). Validation of the Hwalek-Sengstock elder abuse screening test. *Journal of Applied Gerontology, 10*(4), 406–418.

O'Mahoney D., O'Sullivan, D., Byrne, S., O'Connor, M. N., Ryan, C., & Gallagher, P. (2015). STOPP and START criteria for potentially inappropriate prescribing in older people, version 2. *Age and Aging, 44*(2), 213–218.

Partnership for Prevention. (2008). Physical activity guidelines for Americans, Chapter 5. Retrieved from http://www.health.gov/paguidelines/guidelines/chapter5.aspx

Pluijm, S. M., Vasser, M., Puts, M. T., Dik, M. G., Schalk, B. W., van Schoor, N. M., . . . Deeq, D. J. (2007). Unhealthy life styles during the life course: Association with physical decline in late life. *Aging Clinical and Experimental Research, 19*(1), 75–83.

Schofield, M. J., & Mishra, G. D. (2003). Validity of self-report screening scale for elder abuse: Women's Health Australia Study. *The Gerontologist, 43*(1), 110–120, Table 1.

Sieber, C. C. (2006). Nutritional screening tools: How does the MNA compare? Proceedings of the session held in Chicago, May 2–3, 2006 (15 years of mini nutritional assessment). *Journal of Nutrition Health and Aging, 10*(6), 488.

Stanford School of Medicine. (2016). Chronic disease self-management program. Retrieved from http://patienteducation.stanford.edu/programs/cdsmp.html

Sunderland, T., Hill, J. L., Mellow, A. M., Lawlor, B. A., Gundersheimer, J., Newhouse, P. A., & Grafman, J. H. (1989). Clock drawing in Alzheimer's disease: A novel measure of dementia severity. *Journal of the American Geriatric Society, 7*(8), 725–729.

Thomas, D. R., Ashmen, W., Morley, J. E., & Evans, W. J. (2000). Nutritional management in long-term care: Development of a clinical guideline. Council for Nutritional Strategies in Long Term Care. *The Journals of Gerontology Series A, Biological Sciences and Medical Sciences, 55A*(12), M725–M734.

Tobacco Use and Dependence Guideline Panel. (2008). *Treating tobacco use and dependence: 2008 update.* Rockville, MD: U.S. Department of Health and Human Services. Public Health Service.

University of California at Berkeley, School of Social Welfare. (2007). Instruments for assessing elder mistreatment: Implications for adult protective services. Retrieved from http://cssr.berkeley.edu/research_units/bassc/documents/C61602_9_web.pdf

U.S. Department of Agriculture. (2010). *Dietary guidelines for Americans, 2010. Washington, DC: U.S. Government Printing Office.* Retrieved from https://health.gov/dietaryguidelines/dga2010/dietaryguidelines2010.pdf

U.S. Food and Drug Administration. (2015). Safe use initiative. Retrieved from http://www.fda.gov/Drugs/DrugSafety/SafeUseInitiative/

U.S. Department of Health and Human Services, National Institutes of Health, & National Heart, Lung, and Blood Institute. (2006). DASH eating plan: Lower your blood pressure. Retrieved from http://www.nhlbi.nih.gov/health/public/heart/hbp/dash/new_dash.pdf

U.S. Preventive Services Task Force. (2008). Lipid disorders in adults (cholesterol, dyslipidemia): Screening. Retrieved from http://www.uspreventiveservicestaskforce.org/uspstf08/lipid/lipidrs.htm

U.S. Preventive Services Task Force. (2009a). Aspirin for the prevention of cardiovascular disease: Preventive medication. Retrieved from http://www.uspreventiveservicestaskforce.org/uspstf/uspsasmi.htm

U.S. Preventive Services Task Force. (2009b). Impaired visual acuity in older adults: Screening. Retrieved from https://www.uspreventiveservicestaskforce.org/Page/Document/UpdateSummaryFinal/impaired-visual-acuity-in-older-adults-screening1

U.S. Preventive Services Task Force. (2009c). Breast Cancer: Screening. Retrieved from http://www.uspreventiveservicestaskforce.org/uspstf/uspsbrca.htm

U.S. Preventive Services Task Force. (2011). Osteoporosis: Screening: Recommendations and rationale. Retrieved from http://www.uspreventiveservicestaskforce.org/3rduspstf/osteoporosis/osteorr.htm

U.S. Preventive Services Task Force. (2012a). Focus on older adults. Retrieved from https://www.uspreventiveservicestaskforce.org/Page/Name/focus-on-older-adults

U.S. Preventive Services Task Force. (2012b). Hearing Loss in Older Adults: Screening. Retrieved from http://www.uspreventiveservicestaskforce.org/uspstf11/adulthearing/adulthearart.htm

U.S. Preventive Services Task Force. (2015). Published recommendations. Retrieved from http://www.uspreventiveservicestaskforce.org/BrowseRec/Index/browse-recommendations

Wannamethee, S. G., Shaper, A. G., & Lennon, L. (2005). Reasons for intentional weight loss, unintentional weight loss and mortality in older men. *Archives of Internal Medicine, 165*(9), 1035–1040.

Weber, M. A., Schriffin, E. L., White, W. B., Mann, S., Lindholm, L. H., Kenerson, J. G., . . . & Harrap, S. B. (2014). Clinical practice guidelines for the management of hypertension in the community: A statement by the American Society of Hypertension and the International Society of Hypertension. *Journal of Hypertension, 32*(1), 3–15.

For a full suite of assignments and additional learning activities, see the access code at the front of your book.

Unit IV
Illness and Disease Management

(COMPETENCIES 9, 15–18)

© Creativaimage/iStock/Getty

CHAPTER 9

Management of Common Illnesses, Diseases, and Health Conditions

Kristen L. Mauk
Amy Silva-Smith

(Competencies 9, 15, 17, 18)

LEARNING OBJECTIVES

At the end of this chapter, the reader will be able to:

> Name the major risk factors associated with cardiovascular disease (CVD).
> Discuss the impact of the major CVDs seen in older adults on the health of the U.S. population.
> Recognize signs of myocardial infarction that may be unique to the older adult.
> Utilize resources and research to promote heart-healthy lifestyles in older adults.
> State the warning signs of stroke.
> Apply the Mauk model for poststroke recovery to the care of stroke survivors.
> Identify common treatments for pneumonia, tuberculosis (TB), and chronic obstructive pulmonary disease (COPD).
> Discuss how to minimize risk factors for common gastrointestinal problems in the elderly.
> Describe nursing interventions for patients dealing with gastroesophageal reflux disease (GERD).
> Discuss ways to prevent catheter-associated urinary tract infection (CAUTI).
> Identify signs, symptoms, and treatments for benign prostatic hyperplasia (BPH) and vaginitis.
> Recognize common treatments for several cancers in older adults: bladder, prostate, colorectal, cervical, and breast.
> List several medications that can contribute to male impotence.
> Recognize the clinical treatments for persons with Parkinson's disease (PD).
> Devise a nursing care plan for someone with Alzheimer's disease (AD).
> Discuss possible causes and solutions for dizziness in the elderly.
> List the modifiable risk factors for osteoporosis.
> Distinguish between osteoarthritis and rheumatoid arthritis in relation to typical presentation, treatment, and long-term implications.
> Contrast rehabilitative care for older adults with hip and knee replacement surgery.
> Describe the most effective way to condition a stump to promote use of a prosthesis.

> Distinguish the signs and symptoms of cataracts, glaucoma, macular degeneration, and diabetic retinopathy.
> Contrast management of the four most common eye disorders seen in the elderly.
> Distinguish among the three major types of skin cancer.
> Identify signs and symptoms of herpes zoster appearing in the elderly.
> Review prevention of the most common complications of diabetes in older adults.
> Devise a plan for good foot care for older adults with diabetes.
> Synthesize knowledge about hypothyroidism into general care of the older adult.

KEY TERMS

Activities of daily living

Age-related macular degeneration

Alzheimer's disease

Angina

Atherosclerosis

Benign paroxysmal positional vertigo

Benign prostatic hyperplasia

Biological therapies

Bone mineral density

Cardiovascular disease

Cataracts

Catheter-associated urinary tract infection

Cerebrovascular accident

Chemotherapy

Chronic bronchitis

Chronic obstructive pulmonary disease

Congestive heart failure

Continuous bladder irrigation

Corneal ulcer

Coronary artery disease

Coronary heart disease

Cystectomy

Demineralization

Diabetic retinopathy

Diverticulitis

Dysphagia

Emphysema

Erectile dysfunction

Gastroesophageal reflux disease

Glaucoma

Gonioscopy

Helicobacter pylori

Hemiparesis

Hemiplegia

Herpes zoster

Histamine 2 (H2) blockers

Hypertension

Immunocompromised

Incontinence

Instrumental activities of daily living

Intractable pain

Intraocular pressure

Mauk model for poststroke recovery

Meniere's syndrome

Metastasis

Myocardial infarction

Osteoporosis

Otoconia

Parkinson's disease

Peripheral artery disease

Peripheral vascular disease

Phantom limb pain

Proliferative retinopathy

Prostate-specific antigen

Proton pump inhibitors

Radiation therapy

Radical prostatectomy

Retinal detachment

Scatter laser treatment

Staging

Stroke

Survivor

Symptoms

Thrombocytopenia

Tinnitus

Tonometer

t-PA (tissue plasminogen activator)

Transient ischemic attack

Transurethral resection of the prostate

Tuberculosis

Urinary tract infection

Urostomy

Vitrectomy

The purpose of this chapter is to present basic information related to common diseases and disorders experienced by older adults. It is assumed that the reader of this text has fundamental nursing knowledge and will study disease processes more in depth in other courses. Extensive discussion of the nursing care and treatment of each disease is beyond the scope of this text, but nurses are encouraged to refer to traditional medical–surgical textbooks for further reading. The discussion in this chapter will use a systems approach to provide a "snapshot" of essential information regarding background, risk factors, signs and *symptoms*, diagnosis, and usual treatment, while emphasizing any important aspects unique to care of the elderly with each disorder. Unit 5 provides a thorough discussion of some additional common problems and geriatric syndromes.

Cardiovascular Problems

Several conditions and diseases related to the cardiovascular system are common in older adults. The specific conditions discussed in this section include *myocardial infarction* (MI), *hypertension*, *angina*, *heart failure* (HF), *coronary artery disease* (CAD), *stroke*, and *peripheral vascular disease*. Currently, 43.7 million Americans age 60 and older are affected by at least one cardiovascular health condition (Mozaffarian et al., 2015). In Canada, 28% of all male deaths and 29.76% of all female deaths in 2000 were due to heart disease and stroke (Heart and Stroke Foundation of Canada, 2009). The American Heart Association (AHA, 2012b) lists the following as the major cardiovascular diseases: hypertension (HTN), *coronary heart disease* (CHD; includes myocardial infarction and angina), heart failure (HF), and stroke. These will be discussed in the following sections.

Hypertension

Background/Significance

In 2011–2012, the prevalence of HTN among adults greater than 60 years of age was 65% though only 50% had adequate blood pressure (BP) control (Nwankwo, Yoon, Burt, & Gu, 2013). African Americans have a 1.6 times greater risk than Whites of having a fatal stroke, and a 4.2 times greater chance of developing end stage renal disease (Centers for Disease Control and Prevention [CDC], 2011). Over 95% of hypertension is called "essential" hypertension; that is, it has no known cause (Mayo Clinic, 2011).

Risk Factors/Warning Signs

Risk factors for hypertension are noted in **Table 9-1**. After age 50, isolated systolic HTN (i.e., a systolic BP > 140 and a diastolic BP <90) is the most common form and, by controlling systolic BP, overall mortality and events (e.g., stroke, MI, and HF) can be prevented (United States Department of Health and Human Services ([USDHHS], 2004). Complete information about the Joint National Committee's seventh report (James et al., 2014) for control of high blood pressure can be found at http://www.nhlbi.nih.gov/guidelines/hypertension/.

TABLE 9-1   Risk Factors for Hypertension
Heredity
Race (African American)
Increased age
Lack of physical activity
Male gender
High sodium intake
Diabetes or renal disease
Cushing's disease
Heavy alcohol consumption
Obesity
Some medications (steroids)
Sleep apnea

Data from American Heart Association (AHA). (2012e). High blood pressure. Retrieved from http://www.heart.org/idc/groups/heart-public/@wcm/@sop/@smd/documents/downloadable/ucm_319587 .pdf; National Institutes of Health [NIH]. (2008). The seventh report of the Joint National Committee on prevention, detection, evaluation, and treatment of high blood pressure (JNC 7). Retrieved from http://www.nhlbi.nih.gov/guidelines/hypertension/

TABLE 9-2   Strategies to Help Older Adults Control High Blood Pressure
Limit alcohol intake to one drink per day.
Limit sodium intake.
Stop smoking.
Maintain a low-fat diet that still contains adequate vitamins and minerals by adding leafy green vegetables and fruits.
Do some type of aerobic activity nearly every day of the week.
Lose weight. (Even 10 pounds may make a significant difference.)
Have blood pressure checked regularly. Report any significant rise in blood pressure to the physician.
Take medications as prescribed. Do not skip doses.

Assessment/Diagnosis

Accurate BP measurement is important both in the clinical and home setting and a diagnosis of HTN is made only after multiple readings taken at different times. Assessment for postural hypotension is needed prior to and after initiating treatment. Older adults with prehypertension, a systolic BP between 120 and 139 or a diastolic BP between 80 and 89 on multiple readings, should receive a recommendation to make lifestyle changes, because they often develop hypertension.

Interventions

Lifestyle modifications may help older adults to control blood pressure. **Table 9-2** lists recommended strategies for older adults. In addition, several medications may be used to treat hypertension in the elderly (see **Table 9-3**). According to JNC 8 guidelines, in the general population aged ≥60 years, pharmacological treatment should be initiated to lower systolic BP if ≥150 mm Hg or diastolic BP if ≥90 mm Hg and continue to treat to attain a systolic BP of <150 mm Hg and a diastolic BP of <90 mm Hg (James et al., 2014).

TABLE 9-3 Some Types of Medications Used to Treat Cardiovascular Disease		
Classification	**Action**	**Example**
*Diuretics	Decrease water and salt retention	Furosemide (Lasix)
*Beta-blockers	Lower cardiac output and heart rate	Atenolol (Tenormin)
*ACE inhibitors	Block hormone that causes artery constriction	Captopril (Capoten)
*Central alpha agonists	Block constriction of vessels	Clonidine (Catapres)
*Calcium channel blockers	Relax blood vessels to the heart	Amlodipine (Norvasc)
*Angiotensin II receptor blockers	Relax blood vessels by blocking angiotensin II	Irbesartan (Avapro)
*Vasodilators	Relax the walls of the arteries	Hydralazine (Apresoline)
+Digitalis	Strengthens and slows the heart	Digoxin (Lanoxin)
+Potassium	Helps control heart rhythm	K-Dur, K-Tab
+Blood thinners	Prevent clots	Warfarin (Coumadin); Heparin

*Medications used for both HF and HTN
+Medications used for HF

Thiazide diuretics and beta-blockers are drugs of choice for those elderly who do not have other coexisting medical conditions. Many older adults require several medications to achieve adequate control. In fact, combination therapy for older adults allows for smaller doses of each drug and may help avoid side effects. Some common combinations are a thiazide diuretic with either a potassium-sparing diuretic, a beta-blocker, a calcium channel blocker, angiotensin-converting enzyme inhibitors (ACEIs), or angiotensin receptor blockers (ARBs) (James et al., 2014), but nurses should refer to the most current JNC guidelines.

Older adults should work with their health professionals to achieve good control of their blood pressure, because it is a risk factor and contributor to many other serious health conditions including heart disease, stroke, and renal disease. Nurses may need to do extensive teaching about lifestyle modifications to assist older adults with smoking cessation and appropriate dietary choices. In addition to promoting nutrition, nurses should teach patients to read labels, avoid processed foods, prepare foods appropriately, and drink adequate amounts of fluids to stay hydrated.

Coronary Heart Disease

Coronary heart disease (CHD), also called coronary artery disease (CAD) or ischemic heart disease, affects millions of people each year in many countries. This condition is caused by hardening and narrowing of the blood vessels of the heart (*atherosclerosis*), resulting in an impaired blood supply to the myocardium. Nearly 16 million Americans are affected each year (Mozaffarian et al., 2015). The rates for older females after menopause are more than twice that of older females prior to menopause. Over 82% of people who die with CHD are age 65 years or over (AHA, 2012c). Angina and myocardial infarction (MI) are two consequences of CHD that will be discussed here.

Angina

Background/Significance

Angina pectoris is chest pain that results from lack of oxygen to the heart muscle. A small number of deaths are attributed to this cause each year, but mortality statistics related to angina are often included with CHD reports. Only about 18% of heart attacks are preceded by diagnosed angina (Harvard Men's Health Watch, 2009).

Risk Factors/Warning Signs

Among Americans ages 40–74, the prevalence of angina is slightly higher for females, significantly higher for Mexican American males and females, and slightly higher, though not significantly so, for African American females (AHA, 2012b). According to the AHA, the incidence of angina per 1,000 people aged 65–74 is highest for non-Black males (28.3), followed by Black males (22.4), Black females (15.5), and non-Black females (14.1) (AHA, 2012a, 2012b).

Angina is usually the first symptom of CAD in the older adult. Older adults with angina may first complain of dyspnea, dizziness, or confusion versus classic chest pain (O'Donnell, McKee, O'Brien, Mooney, & Moser, 2012).

Assessment/Diagnosis

Angina is classified as stable or unstable. Although the symptoms of angina may be similar to MI, there are several notable differences. Angina often occurs related to exercise or stress and is relieved by rest and/or nitroglycerin. The associated chest pain is generally shorter (less than 5 minutes) than MI, though the classic presentation is squeezing pain or pressure in the sternal area. A thorough history, assessment of vital signs, a 12-lead EKG to assess for ST segment changes and serum myocardial biomarkers (e.g., troponins) will help rule out or confirm an MI (Mozaffarian et al., 2015).

Intervention/Strategies for Care

Unstable angina may require hospitalization, whereas stable angina can be managed with medication and lifestyle modifications aimed at reducing the workload on the heart and the accompanying oxygen demand. Education for patients and families includes weight management, stress management, limiting caffeine, smoking cessation, an exercise regimen that considers the person's myocardial capacity, control of hypertension, and medical management of any coexisting endocrine disorder (such as hyperthyroidism). Beta-blockers and calcium channel blockers are often prescribed to decrease the oxygen demand on the heart. Patients should be alerted to side effects from these medications, such as fatigue, drowsiness, dizziness, and slow heart rate.

Myocardial Infarction

Background/Significance

Since 2000 there has been a decrease in the incidence of MI, from 224 per 1,000 to 208 per 1,000 (Yen et al., 2010) The risk of MI increases with age; men have the highest incidence of MI until approximately age 70, when the incidences of MI converge and the rate of MI for men and women equalizes (Zafari & Yang, 2012).

Risk Factors/Warning Signs

Risk factors for MI include HTN, race (especially African American males), high-fat diet, sedentary lifestyle, diabetes, obesity, high cholesterol, family history, cigarette smoking, excessive alcohol intake, and high levels of stress. Many risk factors are modifiable or controllable. Warning signs of MI are listed in **Table 9-4.** It is important to note that the warning signs are often very different for women than they are for men (see **Case Study 9-1**). Women often do not have substernal chest pain and instead may experience sharp pain, fatigue, weakness, and other nonspecific symptoms (Garas & Zafari, 2006). Symptoms may occur as much as 1 month prior to the occurrence of a myocardial infarction. These symptoms include chest pain, pain in the arm, neck, back or jaw, fatigue, stomach pain, shortness of breath, sweating, dizziness, or nausea (Fields, 2016).

Assessment/Diagnosis

Diagnosis may include electrocardiogram (ECG) and angiogram or cardiac catheterization to visualize areas of blockage. **Figure 9-1** shows the results of an angiogram with some degree of blockage in a major heart vessel. Following the angiogram, the nurse assists the cardiologist, in part, by keeping the leg straight with pressure on the femoral artery entry site per the facility's protocol. Patient and family education includes the importance of

TABLE 9-4   Warning Signs of Heart Attack
Chest pain appearing as tightness, fullness, or pressure
Pain radiating to arms
Unexplained numbness in arms, neck, or back
Shortness of breath with or without activity
Sweating
Nausea
Pallor
Dizziness
*Unexplained jaw pain
*Indigestion or epigastric discomfort, especially when not relieved with antacids

*Of particular significance in the elderly

Case Study 9-1

Mr. Jones is a 62-year-old man who lives next door to you. He comes over while you are out in your yard and says, "You're a nurse, so I have this question for you. I have had this annoying heartburn all day that just doesn't go away no matter what I do." He points to his epigastric area. "It just feels like this pressure right here and makes me a little sick to my stomach." Mr. Jones looks pale and a bit diaphoretic.

Questions:

1. What is your best response to this situation?
2. What could these signs and symptoms indicate?
3. What would you expect Mr. Jones to do at this point?
4. Are there any other questions you could ask that would provide additional information about the potential seriousness of his complaint?

monitoring the entry site for signs of hematoma, bleeding, or infection. Patients should be taught that bleeding at the site is considered an emergency and that firm, direct pressure must be applied to the site immediately. It is common for bruising to occur, and limits to lifting and driving should be strictly followed after the procedure to prevent complications.

Interventions

Thrombolytic therapy, if administered early in the course of MI, significantly reduces the morbidity and mortality associated with MI (Kulick, 2012). The following steps are recommended, if possible, while awaiting emergency treatment:

1. Have the patient rest.
2. Provide supplemental oxygen.
3. Give nitroglycerin sublingually every 5 minutes times three and monitor vital signs.
4. Give aspirin if not contraindicated.

Some nurses use the mnemonic MONA (morphine, oxygen, nitroglycerin, aspirin) to remember the steps in acute care treatment of MI. If neither oxygen nor nitroglycerin is available, proceed with giving aspirin.

CLINICAL TIP

Some nurses use the mnemonic MONA to remember the steps in acute care treatment of MI. If neither oxygen nor nitroglycerin is available, proceed with giving aspirin.

M = morphine

O = oxygen

N = nitroglycerin

A = aspirin

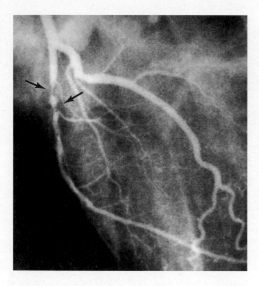

Figure 9-1 A coronary angiogram illustrating several areas of coronary artery narrowing (arrows). The individual demonstrated exertional chest pain (angina pectoris) on exercise.

Courtesy of Leonard V. Crowley, MD, Century College.

Usual medical treatment of MI includes several options, depending on the results of the diagnostic tests and extent of damage and blockage. Angioplasty is a common procedure that uses a balloon, stent, or other device to open the blocked vessel. Coronary artery bypass graft (CABG), commonly known as open-heart surgery, is often used for those with blockages in several major arteries in order to restore blood flow. Pharmacological treatment may include beta-blockers, angiotensin-converting enzyme (ACE) inhibitors, and antihypertensives. The recovery period includes careful monitoring in cardiac intensive care, then progression to outpatient cardiac rehabilitation, where patients will be closely monitored after discharge and assisted by specialized nurses to make lifestyle modifications to promote maximal recovery. It is important to encourage patients to follow-through with cardiac rehabilitation even though they may be feeling well.

Persons surviving a heart attack should be dedicated to reducing risk factors associated with heart disease. **Table 9-5** lists several strategies for older adults to prevent a first or subsequent heart attack. The American Heart Association Website has information about cardiac rehabilitation, its necessity in recovery from MI, and its ongoing importance for achieving optimal wellness. (AHA, 2012a). Support groups for *survivors* and families may also be helpful. Family members, particularly spouses, should be included in the rehabilitation process.

Heart Failure

Background/Significance

The incidence of heart failure (HF) varies among races and across age groups. For both males and females, non-Hispanic Blacks have the highest death rate from HF followed closely by non-Hispanic white males and non-Hispanic American Indians or Alaska Natives (James et al., 2015), The lifetime risk for someone to have HF is 1 in 5. The risk of CHF in older adults doubles for those with blood pressures over 160/90. Seventy-five percent of those with HF also have hypertension (James et al., 2015). The major risk factors for HF are diabetes and MI. Congestive heart failure often occurs within 6 years after a heart attack.

TABLE 9-5   Strategies for Older Adults to Reduce Risk of Heart Attack
Exercise regularly.
Do not smoke.
Eat a balanced diet with plenty of fruits and vegetables; avoid foods high in saturated fats.
Maintain a healthy weight.
Manage stress appropriately.
Control existing diabetes by maintaining healthy blood sugars and take medications as prescribed.
Limit alcohol intake to one drink per day for women and two drinks per day (or less) for men.
Visit the doctor regularly.
After a heart attack, participate fully in a cardiac rehabilitation program.
Involve the entire family in heart-healthy lifestyle modifications.
Report any signs of chest pain immediately.

TABLE 9-6   Signs and Symptoms of Chronic Heart Failure
Shortness of breath
Swelling of the legs, ankles, and feet
Coughing or wheezing
Fatigue
Lack of appetite or nausea
Confusion
Increased heart rate
Sudden weight gain
Decreased tolerance for physical activity

Data from Mayo Clinic (2012b). Heart failure symptoms. Retrieved from http://www.mayoclinic.com/health/heart-failure/DS00061/DSECTION=symptoms

Risk Factors/Warning Signs

Signs and symptoms of heart failure depend upon whether the left ventricular ejection fraction is preserved or reduced; see **Table 9-6** (Yancy et al., 2013). It is essential that older adults diagnosed with HF recognize signs of a worsening condition and report them promptly to their healthcare provider. Older adults may present with atypical symptoms such as decreased appetite, weight gain of a few pounds, or insomnia (Amella, 2004).

Assessment/Diagnosis

For in-home monitoring, daily weights at the same time of day with the same clothes on the same scale are essential. Based upon the severity of the HF and the relative stability/frailty of the patient, the primary care provider (PCP) will give guidelines for the patient to call if the weight exceeds his or her threshold for weight gain. This is usually between 1 and 3 pounds. Oxygen saturation levels can be monitored in any setting. An O_2 saturation of less than 90% is cause for concern and further investigation.

Intervention/Strategies for Care

Medications used to treat HF include ACE inhibitors, diuretics, vasodilators, beta-blockers, blood thinners, angiotensin II blockers, calcium channel blockers, and potassium. Digoxin, once a mainstay in the treatment of HF, is rarely used now although it may be seen on occasion. Heart failure is typically managed with lifestyle modifications and medications. Infrequently, surgery may be an option if valvular repair/replacement or heart transplant become necessary.

Treatment for HF involves lifestyle modifications discussed for promoting a healthy heart (see Table 9-7). In addition, nurses should teach older adults about lifestyle modifications that can decrease and/or help manage the workload on the heart (see **Box 9-1**). To minimize exacerbations, patient and family counseling should include teaching about the use of medications to control symptoms and the importance of regular monitoring with a healthcare provider (Agency for Healthcare Research and Quality [AHRQ], 2012; Hunt et al., 2009). These key points appear in **Table 9-7.** With the proper combination of treatments such as lifestyle changes and medications, many older persons can still live happy and productive lives with a diagnosis of heart failure and minimize their risk of complications related to this disease.

Stroke

Stroke, also known as *cerebrovascular accident* (CVA) or brain attack, is an interruption of the blood supply to the brain that may result in devastating neurological damage, disability, or death. Approximately 795,000 people in the United States have a new or recurrent stroke each year (Mozaffarian et al., 2015).

BOX 9-1   Resources about Cardiovascular Disease

American Heart Association
  1-800-AHA-USA1
  http://www.americanheart.org

American Society of Hypertension (ASH)
  http://www.ash-us.org

American Stroke Association
  1-888-4-STROKE
  http://www.strokeassociation.org

Heart and Stroke Foundation of Canada
  http://www.heartandstroke.ca

Heart and Stroke Foundation of Alberta, Canada
  http://www.heartandstroke.ab.ca

National Emergency Medicine Association
  http://www.nemahealth.org

National Institute of Neurological Disorders and Stroke
  http://www.ninds.nih.gov

National Stroke Association
  http://www.stroke.org

South African Heart Association
  http://www.saheart.org

TABLE 9-7   Lifestyle Modifications to Teach Older Adults with Heart Failure

Limit or eliminate alcohol use (no more than 1 oz. ethanol per day = one mixed drink, one 12-oz. beer, or one 5-oz. glass of wine).

Maintain a healthy weight. Extra pounds put added stress and workload on the heart. Weigh daily and report weight gains of 5 pounds or more to healthcare provider.

Stop smoking (no tobacco use in any form).

Limit sodium intake to 2–3 g per day—read the labels: avoid canned and processed foods. Take care with how foods are cooked or prepared at home (e.g., limit oils and butters).

Take medications as ordered—do not skip doses. Report any side effects to the physician.

Exercise to tolerance level—this will differ for each person. Remain active without overdoing it.

Alternate rest and activity. Learn energy conservation techniques.

Background/Significance

Stroke is the fifth leading cause of death in the United States (CDC/National Center for Health Statistics, 2015). A stroke occurs approximately every 40 seconds in the United States and death from stroke occurs more frequently among females. In Canada, stroke is the third leading cause of death (Statistics Canada, 2015).

There are two major types of stroke: ischemic and hemorrhagic. The vast majority of strokes are caused by ischemia (87%), usually from a thrombus or embolus (Mozaffarian et al., 2015). The symptoms and damage seen depend on which vessels in the brain are blocked. Carotid artery occlusion is also a common cause of stroke related to stenosis.

Risk Factors/Warning Signs

Some risk factors for stroke are controllable and others are not; risk factors appear in **Table 9-8.** The most significant risk factor for stroke is hypertension. Controlling high blood pressure is an important way to reduce stroke risk. Over three-fourths of persons with a first stroke had a BP > 140/90 (Mozaffarian et al., 2015). Smoking 40 or more cigarettes per day (heavy smoking) increases the stroke risk to twice that of light smokers. If a person quits smoking, their risk after 5 years mirrors that of a nonsmoker, so older adults should be particularly encouraged to stop smoking. Engaging in physical activity at least 4 times per week will reduce the risk of stroke by 20% compared to persons who reported exercising less than 4 times per week (McDonnell et al., 2013).

Several warning signs are common with stroke (see **Table 9-9**). Thromboembolic strokes are more likely to show classic signs than hemorrhagic strokes, which may appear as severe headaches but with few other prior warning signs. A quick initial evaluation for stroke can be performed by assessing for three easy signs: facial droop, motor weakness, and language difficulties.

TABLE 9-8   Risk Factors for Stroke

Controllable	Uncontrollable
Hypertension	Advanced age
High cholesterol	Gender (males more than females until menopause)
Heart disease	Race (African Americans more than Whites)
Smoking	Heredity
Obesity	
Stress	
Diabetes	
Depression	
Atrial fibrillation	

TABLE 9-9   Warning Signs of Stroke

- Sudden numbness or weakness of face, arm, or leg, especially on one side of the body
- Sudden confusion; trouble speaking or understanding
- Sudden trouble seeing in one or both eyes
- Sudden trouble walking, dizziness, or loss of balance or coordination
- Sudden severe headache with no known cause

Case Study 9–2

Your grandfather is 85 years old and tells you at a family gathering that yesterday he had some blurred vision and numbness down his right arm. He didn't tell his wife or anyone else because the symptoms went away within 10 minutes, but he wanted to tell you just in case he should have it checked out.

Questions:

1. What should you tell your grandfather? What do his symptoms possibly indicate?

2. What risk factor does he have for stroke?
3. What other questions should you ask to gain more information?
4. What is the next step of action that your grandfather should take?
5. Should anything be discussed with his wife? If so, what?
6. At this point, are there specific topics that should be taught to your grandfather?

Other warning signs of stroke include a temporary loss of consciousness or the appearance of the classic warning signs that go away quickly (see **Case Study 9-2**). *Transient ischemic attacks* (TIAs) are defined as those symptoms similar to stroke that go away within 24 hours (and usually within minutes) and leave no residual effects. Most TIAs are from atherothrombotic disease, with another 20% from cardiac emboli and 25% from occlusion of smaller vessels (Warlow, Sudlow, Martin, Wardlaw, & Sandercock, 2003). Having a TIA increases the risk of stroke tenfold compared to those who have not had a TIA (ASA, 2016b, 2016c).

Assessment and Diagnosis

There are several tools for assessing for signs and symptoms of stroke; one easy acronym is FAST:

F stands for facial droop. Ask the person to smile and see if drooping is present.

A stands for arm. Have the person lift both arms straight out in front of him. If one is arm is drifting lower than the other, it is a sign that weakness is present.

S stands for speech. Ask the person to say a short phrase such as "light, tight, dynamite" and check for slurring or other abnormal speech.

T stands for time. If the first F-A-S checks are not normal, then one is to remember F-A-S-T that time is important and the emergency medical system should be activated (National Stroke Association, 2015).

CLINICAL TIP

Use the acronym FAST as a quick check for stroke.

 F = facial droop

 A = arm

 S = speech

 T = time

Older adults experiencing the warning signs of stroke should note the time on the clock and seek immediate treatment by calling 911 (ASA, 2016b). Transport to an emergency medical facility for evaluation is essential for the best array of treatment options. A history and neurological exam, vital signs, as well as diagnostic tests including ECG, chest X-ray, platelets, prothrombin time (PT), partial thromboplastin time (PTT), electrolytes, and glucose are routinely ordered. Diagnostic imaging may include computed tomography (CT) without contrast, magnetic resonance imaging (MRI), arteriography, or ultrasonography to determine the type and location of the stroke. The CT or MRI should ideally be done within 90 minutes so that appropriate emergency measures may be initiated to prevent further brain damage.

Interventions

The first step in treatment is to determine the cause or type of stroke. A CT scan or MRI must first be done to rule out hemorrhagic stroke. Hemorrhagic stroke treatment often requires surgery to evacuate blood and stop the bleeding.

Acute Management

The American Heart/American Stroke Association has published numerous guidelines for the treatment of various types of stroke. These can be accessed through the ASA's Website at http://my.americanheart.org/professional /StatementsGuidelines/Statements-Guidelines_UCM_316885_SubHomePage.jsp. On this homepage for professionals, nurses can find stroke statements and guidelines based upon current evidence. Those hospitals that have been certified as Primary or Comprehensive Stroke Centers by the Joint Commission have met strict criteria for the treatment of stroke and may be preferred places for care.

The gold standard at present for treatment of ischemic stroke is *t-PA (tissue plasminogen activator)*. At this time, t-PA must be given within 3 hours after the onset of stroke symptoms. This is why it is essential that older adults seek treatment immediately when symptoms begin. Only about 3–5% of people reach the hospital in time to be considered for this treatment (ASA, 2012d). t-PA may be effective for a select group of patients after the 3-hour window (up to 4.5 hours), and this treatment window has been approved in Canada (Heart and Stroke Foundation of Canada, 2009). New treatments are being explored to extend the treatment window, including the use of a synthetic compound derived from bat saliva that contains an anticoagulant-type property. The major side effect of t-PA is bleeding. Other, much less common procedures such as angioplasty, laser emulsification, and mechanical clot retrieval may be options for treatment of acute ischemic stroke.

Additionally, the use of cooling helmets to decrease the metabolism of the brain is thought to preserve function and reduce ischemic damage (Hemmen & Lyden, 2007). The roles of hyperthermia, hyperglycemia, and hypertension are being explored, as these are associated with higher morbidity and mortality.

To prevent recurrence of thromboembolic stroke, medications such as aspirin, ticlopidine (Ticlid), clopidogrel (Plavix), dipyridamole (Persantine), heparin, warfarin (Coumadin), and enoxaparin (Lovenox) may be used to prevent clot formation. Once the stroke survivor has stabilized, the long process of rehabilitation begins. Each stroke is different depending on location and severity, so persons may recover with little or no residual deficits or an entire array of devastating consequences.

The effects of stroke vary, but may include *hemiplegia*, *hemiparesis*, visual and perceptual deficits, language deficits, emotional changes, swallowing dysfunction, and bowel and bladder problems. Ninety percent of all *dysphagia* results from stroke (White, O'Rourke, Ong, Cordato, & Chan, 2008). Although the deficits that present themselves depend on the area of brain damage, it is sometimes helpful to picture most strokes as involving one side of the body or the other. A person with left-brain injury presents with right-sided weakness or paralysis, and a person with right-sided stroke presents with left-sided weakness or paralysis. **Table 9-10** lists common deficits caused by stroke, seen in varying degrees, and some common problems associated with strokes on one side of the brain versus the other.

Poststroke Rehabilitation

Rehabilitation after a stroke focuses on several key principles. These include maximizing functional ability, preventing complications, promoting quality of life, encouraging adaptation, and enhancing independence.

TABLE 9-10 Common Deficits Caused by Stroke		
Common Characteristics Associated with Stroke of Either Side	**Right Hemisphere Stroke**	**Left Hemisphere Stroke**
Weakness/paralysis	Left hemiparesis or hemiplegia	Right hemiparesis or hemiplegia
Fatigue	Left homonymous hemianopsia	Right homonymous hemianopsia
Depression	Difficulty with cognitive tasks such as spatial-perceptual tasks, sequencing, following multistep instructions, and writing	Aphasia (especially expressive type)
Emotional lability		Reading/writing problems
Some memory impairment	Memory deficits related to performance	Dysarthria
Sensory changes	May not recognize or accept limitations or deficits	Dysphagia
Social isolation	Overestimating abilities	Anxiety when trying new tasks
Altered sleep patterns	Impulsive	Tendency to worry and be easily frustrated
	Quick movements	Slow, cautious
	Anosognosia or other forms of left-sided neglect	Memory deficits related to language
	Impaired judgment	
	Inappropriately low anxiety	
	Higher risk for falls due to lack of safety awareness	
	Deficits less easily recognized by others	

Rehabilitation emphasizes the survivor's abilities, not disabilities, and helps him or her to work with what he or she has while acknowledging what was lost.

If significant functional impairments are present, evaluation for transfer to an intensive acute in-patient rehabilitation program is recommended. In-patient rehabilitation units offer the survivor the best opportunity to maximize recovery, including functional return. An interdisciplinary team of experienced experts, including nurses, therapists, physicians, social workers, and psychologists, will help the survivor and the family to adapt to the changes resulting from the stroke. Although the goal of rehabilitation will usually be discharge back to the previous home environment, this is not always possible. Advanced age and functional capacity, particularly ambulatory ability, may be predictors of discharge to a nursing home (Pereira et al., 2014).

The *Mauk model for poststroke recovery* (Easton, 2001; Mauk, 2006) (see **Box 9-2**) can help guide nursing practice by suggesting focused interventions for each of the six phases of stroke recovery. **Tables 9-11** and **9-12** list the major concepts and subconcepts of the model (see **Figure 9-2**) and the major tasks for survivors and nurses. Complications common after stroke appear in **Table 9-13.**

Patient and Family Education

A large amount of teaching is often done by stroke rehabilitation nurses who work with older survivors. Many topics may need to be covered, depending on the extent of brain damage that has occurred. Some topics should be addressed with all survivors and their families (**Box 9-3**). These include knowing the warning signs of stroke and how to activate the emergency response system in their neighborhood, managing high blood pressure, understanding

BOX 9-2 Research Highlight

Aim: To test the accuracy of nursing students in assessing the phases of a stroke model.

Methods: A sample of 30 nursing student volunteers was provided a 15-minute overview and diagram of the Mauk model for poststroke recovery. Then they were asked to read five case studies and use the Mauk model to assess the phase of stroke being described.

Findings: The six phases of poststroke recovery emerging from the data were labeled in a model: agonizing, fantasizing, realizing, blending, framing, and owning. The majority of respondents (57%) were able to rate the correct phase of stroke recovery with 100% accuracy. Areas of the model that needed clarification were identified as the blending and owning phases.

Application to practice: Nursing students were able to quickly learn and correctly identify the phases of the Mauk model. Parts of the model can benefit with more clarification and increased testing. By using the Mauk model for poststroke recovery, nurses can more efficiently target their care by focusing nursing interventions unique to the phase of recovery in which survivors are. Nurses should assess the phase of recovery and focus on care interventions related to the essential tasks for each phase.

Mauk, K. L., Lemley, C., Pierce, J., & Schmidt, N. A. (2011). The Mauk model for poststroke recovery: Assessing the phases. *Rehabilitation Nursing, 36*(6), 241–247.

TABLE 9-11 The Six Phases (Concepts) of the Poststroke Journey with Characteristics

Phase/Concept	Characteristics/Subconcepts
Agonizing	Fear, shock/surprise, loss, questioning, denial
Fantasizing	Mirage of recovery, unreality
Realizing	Reality, depression, anger, fatigue
Blending	Hope, learning, frustration, dealing with changes
Framing	Answering why, reflection
Owning	Control, acceptance, determination, self-help

Reproduced from Easton, K. L. (2001). *The poststroke journey: From agonizing to owning* (Doctoral dissertation). Wayne State University, Detroit, MI: Author.

TABLE 9-12 Summary of Major Survivor and Nursing Tasks for Each Phase of the Poststroke Journey

Phase	Survivor Task	Nursing Task
Agonizing	Survival	Protection and physical care
Fantasizing	Ego protection	Reality orientation and emotional support
Realizing	Facing reality	Emotional and psychosocial support
Blending	Adaptation	Teaching
Framing	Reflection	Listening; providing reason for the stroke
Owning	Moving on	Enhancing inner and community resources

Reproduced from Easton, K. L. (2001). *The poststroke journey: From agonizing to owning* (Doctoral dissertation). Wayne State University, Detroit, MI: Author.

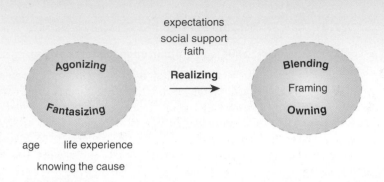

Figure 9-2 The Mauk model of poststroke recovery.

TABLE 9-13   Common Complications Related to Stroke
Common Medical Complications after Stroke
Depression
Deep vein thrombosis
Dysphagia (sometimes resulting in aspiration)
Pressure ulcers
Neurogenic bowel (especially constipation)
Neurogenic bladder (especially urinary incontinence)
Shoulder subluxation
Spasticity

BOX 9-3   Evidence-Based Practice Highlight

The author implemented a research utilization project with 35 female stroke survivors in a freestanding rehabilitation facility. A control group of 35 patients discharged from the same facility and not receiving the educational intervention were used as a control group. The interdisciplinary team at the rehabilitation facility agreed to implement the following four interventions that were shown in the literature to provide best evidence for practice: (1) enhanced bladder history, (2) timed and prompted voiding, (3) bathroom training programs, and (4) pelvic floor exercises. The outcomes of the project showed the women who received the interventions showed a significantly higher mean FIM change in bladder FIM score than the control group. Consistent implementation of evidence-based practice in the area of bladder management with female stroke survivors resulted in better bladder management for patients.

Data from Cournan, M. (2012). Bladder management in female stroke survivors: Translating research into practice. *Rehabilitation Nursing, 37*(5), 220–230.

---

what medications are ordered as well as how often to take them and why, the importance of regular doctor visits, preventing falls and making the home environment safe, available community education and support groups, and the necessity of maintaining a therapeutic regimen and lifestyle to decrease the risk of complications and recurrent stroke. All survivors will need assistance in re-integrating into the community. This is generally begun in the rehabilitation setting.

Family caregivers of stroke survivors must also deal with many issues. Studies have supported the need for family caregivers to have extensive support as the stroke victim and his or her family members transition from the acute care setting to home (Cameron & Gignac, 2008; Lefebure, Levert, Pelchat, & Lepage, 2008; Steiner et al., 2008). Lutz and Young (2010) suggested that a systematic, comprehensive assessment be done of the family, patient, and caregiver, including examining resources and implementing case management across the continuum of care that also considers the needs and preferences of the caregiver in addition to the stroke survivor.

Intensive rehabilitation programs enhance outcomes for geriatric stroke survivors, whether offered in rehabilitation units or in skilled nursing facilities (Duraski, Denby, Danzy, & Sullivan, 2012; Jett, Warren, & Wirtalla, 2005). **Table 9-14** presents general approaches to care for stroke survivors. Generally, advanced age is considered to be a negative factor in recovery from stroke, but factors such as motivation and hope must also be considered in the rehabilitation process. In addition, much of the research literature regarding functional level of recovery after stroke suggests that return of function peaked and did not significantly progress much after the 3- to 6-month mark poststroke. However, emerging research suggests that survivors can and do continue to make improvements in daily function even years after a stroke (Duraski et al., 2012). Much of this improvement may be in the area *of instrumental activities of daily living* (IADLs), or home activities that the survivor wished to resume after the stroke.

Peripheral Artery Disease (PAD)

Background/Significance

Peripheral artery disease (PAD), the most common type of peripheral vascular disease (PVD), affects 8–12 million Americans, 12–20% of those over the age of 65, and could reach as many as 9.6 million Americans by the year 2050 (Chin et al., 2013).

Risk Factors/Warning Signs

The risk factors for PAD are the same as those for CHD, with diabetes and smoking being the greatest risk factors (AHA, 2011). According to the American Heart Association, only 25% of those older adults with PAD get treatment.

Assessment/Diagnosis

The most common symptoms of PAD are leg cramps that worsen when climbing stairs or walking, but dissipate with rest, commonly called intermittent claudication (IC). The majority of persons with PAD have no symptoms (Hirsch et al., 2006). PAD is a predictor of CHD and makes a person more at risk for heart attack and stroke. Left untreated, PAD may eventually lead to impaired function and decreased quality of life, even when no leg symptoms are present. In the most serious cases, PAD can lead to gangrene and amputation of a lower extremity.

Interventions

Most cases of PAD can be managed with lifestyle modifications such as those discussed previously for heart-healthy living. Nurses should also encourage patients with PAD to discuss their symptoms with both their healthcare provider and a physical therapist, because some patients find symptom relief through a combination of medical and therapy treatments (Chin et al., 2013; Peach, Griffin, Jones, Thompson, & Hinchliffe, 2012).

Respiratory Problems

Respiratory problems are common among older adults and a leading contributor to mortality and morbidity. This section will present information on pneumonia, chronic obstructive pulmonary diseases (COPDs), and tuberculosis. There are many nursing interventions to enhance quality of life for older adults with breathing problems. These will also be reviewed.

TABLE 9-14 General Approaches to Traditional Nursing of the Stroke Survivor

Common Characteristics Associated with Stroke of Either Side	Right Hemisphere Stroke	Left Hemisphere Stroke
When working with the patient, encourage use of the affected side to reduce neglect.	Foster a calm and unhurried care environment.	Speak slowly and distinctly. Use simple sentences for those with aphasia.
When the person is alone, place items (such as the call light, tissues, and other personal items) on the unaffected side to promote self-care and safety and to avoid isolation.	Break tasks into simple steps.	Encourage all forms of communication.
Use a variety of teaching modalities during educational sessions to promote learning.	Be especially attentive to safety issues that may arise from poor judgment and lack of safety awareness. Protect the patient from injury.	Use a variety of communication techniques: gesturing, cues, pointing, writing, communication boards, yes/no questions (if appropriate). Find what is most effective for each person.
Minimize distractions during educational sessions. Keep these teaching items short and relevant.	Be alert for possible deficits that may not be overt. Avoid overstimulation.	Allow time for the person to respond to questions.
Use terms such as affected/unaffected side or weak/strong side instead of good/bad.		Provide teaching in a quiet, structured environment. Monitor the patient for swallowing difficulties.
Use critical pathways or care plans to promote consistency of care, but remember that each survivor is unique and be sure to adapt nursing care accordingly.		Promote a positive self-image by attention to good grooming, personal hygiene, and positive reinforcement.
Alternate rest and activity.		
Build endurance slowly. Remember that a stroke is exhausting to the entire body.		
Include the person and family in the plan of care.		
Assist the patient and family in setting reasonable goals.		
Make early referrals to stroke services or the specialized stroke team.		
Connect the family with a stroke support group or club.		
Use a discharge follow-up plan.		

Pneumonia
Background
According to the CDC (2015), over 53,000 deaths in 2013 were due to pneumonia. Adults 65 years and older were disproportionately affected by these disorders as compared to younger adults; the risk of mortality increases with age. The majority of serious pneumonia cases occurred in those age 65 and older, with this population having 5–10 times the risk of death from pneumonia as younger adults (Kennedy-Malone, Fletcher, & Plank, 2014).

Pneumonia is infection of the lung parenchyma that can be caused by a variety of organisms including bacteria, viruses, and mycoplasmas. There are about 30 causes of pneumonia (ALA, n.d.). The two most common pathways through which microorganisms invade the lung are inhalation of droplet particles carrying infectious pathogens and aspiration of oropharyngeal secretions (Weinberger, 2004). Older adults are considered at particularly high risk for pneumonia with a significantly increased risk for serious infection when they have comorbidities such as chronic obstructive lung disease, heart failure, immunosuppression, cerebrovascular disease, and poor mobility (ALA, n.d.). The incidence of community-acquired pneumonia (CAP) among older adults (≥65 years) is about 221.3 per 10,000 (ALA, 2008). When bacteria are the cause, the most common pathogen is *Streptococcus* with about 50% of people with CAP requiring hospitalization (ALA, n.d.). When hospitalized this population is at risk for poor health outcomes including respiratory failure requiring ventilator support; sepsis; and longer length of hospitalization, duration of antibiotic therapy, and other supportive treatment (ALA, n.d.).

Risk Factors/Warning Signs
The onset of bacterial pneumonia can be sudden or gradual; however, older adults may not present with typical symptoms of chills, fever, chest pain, sweating, productive cough, or dyspnea and instead they may have acute alerted mental status (confusion/delirium). Cases of viral pneumonia account for about half of all types of pneumonia and tend to be less severe than bacterial pneumonia. Symptoms of viral pneumonia include fever, nonproductive hacking cough, muscle pain, weakness, and shortness of breath.

Assessment and Diagnosis
Diagnosis is made through chest X-ray, complete blood count (CBC), and/or sputum culture to determine the type and causal agents (if bacterial). A thorough history and physical that includes assessment of dentition, swallowing ability, and eating (watch for coughing while eating) to evaluate for aspiration risk should be done. Crackles may be heard in the lungs through auscultation, and chest pain with shortness of breath may be present.

Interventions
Bacterial pneumonia can often be treated successfully when detected early, and viral pneumonia generally heals on its own (antibiotics are not effective if pneumonia is caused by a virus), though older adults may experience a greater risk of complications than younger adults. Oral antibiotics will significantly help most patients with bacterial pneumonia, and even though many older persons may require hospitalization, intravenous (IV) antibiotics have not been shown to be necessarily more effective than oral types, with IV treatment resulting in longer hospital stays and more hospital-acquired problems (ALA, n.d.(a)).

Aspiration pneumonia is caused by inhalation of a foreign material, such as fluids or food, into the lungs. This occurs more often in persons with impaired swallowing (see Chapter 17 for a discussion on dysphagia), those who have esophageal reflux disease, or who are unconscious. One particular danger to which nurses should be alert is those older adults receiving tube feedings. Care must be taken to avoid having the person in a laying position during and immediately after tube feeding because aspiration can occur; it is important to note that tube feedings do not reduce the risk of aspiration. Having the head of the bed elevated or, even better, the person in a sitting position when eating or receiving enteral nutrition helps to avoid the potential complication of pneumonia related to aspiration.

When recovering from pneumonia, the older adult should be encouraged to get plenty of rest and take adequate fluids to help loosen secretions (with accommodations made to support the added need to urinate due to the increased fluid intake, a common reason why older adults may not drink adequate fluids). Tylenol or aspirin (if not contraindicated by other conditions) can be taken to manage fever as well as aches and pains. Exposure to others with contagious respiratory conditions should be avoided. Respiratory complications are often what lead to death in the older adults, so they should be cautioned to report any changes in respiratory status such as increased shortness of breath, high fever, or any other symptoms that do not improve. Symptoms typically resolve before radiographic resolution of the infiltrate (what would be seen on the chest X-ray), so it is important to follow up with a chest X-ray to assure resolution of the pneumonia.

Prevention of pneumonia is always best. Adults over the age of 65 are advised to get a pneumonia vaccine (pneumococcal polysaccharide vaccine, or PPV), although its effectiveness may be somewhat diminished in higher risk groups than in healthy adults (ALA, 2008). This vaccine is generally given one time, though sometimes a revaccination is recommended after about 6 years for older adults with higher risk, yet the majority of older adults do not get a pneumonia vaccine (ALA, n.d.). A yearly flu vaccine is also recommended for older adults, because pneumonia is a common complication of influenza in this age group. Medicare will cover these vaccines for older persons, so cost should not be a prohibiting factor in prevention.

Chronic Obstructive Pulmonary Disease

Background

Chronic obstructive pulmonary disease (COPD) refers to a group of diseases resulting in airflow obstruction due to smoking, environmental exposures, and genetics. However, smoking is clearly the most common cause of COPD. The two disorders most commonly included under the umbrella of COPD are *emphysema* and *chronic bronchitis*. Although the pathophysiological mechanisms contributing to airflow obstruction is different in these two disorders, most patients demonstrate features of both emphysema and chronic bronchitis.

In 2008, the CDC released a report naming COPD as the third leading cause of death in the United States (ALA, 2016; Miniño, Xu, & Kochanek, 2008). There are more than 11 million people in the United States diagnosed with COPD (ALA, 2016). However, due to the underdiagnosis of the disease, only estimations of the prevalence of COPD are available, which suggest that approximately 24 million people are living with COPD (ALA, 2016). Slightly more females than males are affected, with female smokers having a greater chance of death from COPD than nonsmoking females (ALA, 2016).

Chronic Bronchitis

Chronic bronchitis is a common COPD among older adults. It results from recurrent inflammation and mucus production in the bronchial tubes. Repeated infections produce blockage from mucus and eventual scarring that restricts airflow. The American Lung Association (2012a) stated that about 8.5 million Americans had been diagnosed with chronic bronchitis as of 2005. Females are twice as likely as males to have this problem.

Emphysema

Emphysema results when the alveoli in the lungs are irreversibly destroyed. As the lungs lose elasticity, air becomes trapped in the alveolar sacs, resulting in carbon dioxide retention and impaired gas exchange. More males than females are affected with emphysema, and most (91%) of the 3.8 million Americans with this disease are over the age of 45 (ALA, 2004).

Risk Factors/Warning Signs

The major risk factor for COPD is smoking, which causes 80–90% of COPD deaths. Other risk factors appear in **Table 9-15**. Alpha-1-antitrypsin deficiency is a rare cause of COPD, but can be ruled out through blood tests.

TABLE 9-15   Risk Factors for COPD
Smoking
Air pollution
Second-hand smoke
Heredity
History of respiratory infections
Industrial pollutants
Environmental pollutants
Excessive alcohol consumption
Genetic component (alpha-1-antitrypsin deficiency)

Although COPD is almost 100% preventable by avoidance of smoking (Kennedy-Malone et al., 2014), environmental factors play a strong role in the incidence of COPD. Approximately 19.2% of people with COPD can link the cause to work exposure, and 31.7% have never smoked (ALA, 2008).

The signs and symptoms of chronic bronchitis include increased mucus production, shortness of breath, wheezing, decreased breath sounds, and chronic productive cough. Chronic bronchitis can lead to emphysema. Signs and symptoms of emphysema include shortness of breath, decreased exercise tolerance, and cough.

Assessment and Diagnosis

Persons with COPD often experience a decrease in quality of life as the disease progresses. The shortness of breath so characteristic of these diseases impairs the ability to work and do usual activities. According to a survey by the American Lung Association (2004), "half of all COPD patients (51%) say their condition limits their ability to work [and] limits them in normal physical exertion (70%), household chores (56%), social activities (53%), sleeping (50%), and family activities (46%)" (p. 3). Diagnosis is made through pulmonary function and other tests, a thorough history, and a physical.

Interventions

Although there are no easy cures for COPD, older adults can take several measures to improve their quality of life by controlling symptoms and minimizing complications. These include lifestyle modifications such as smoking cessation, medications (see below), oxygen therapy, and pulmonary rehabilitation (see **Table 9-16**). Older adults should have influenza and pneumonia vaccinations. Pneumococcal conjugate vaccine (PCV13) and Pneumococcal polysaccharide vaccine (PPSV23) are recommended for all adults 65 years or older (CDC, 2016c). Oxygen therapy is required in those individuals demonstrating hypoxemia based on resting, nocturnal, and ambulatory oximetry readings.

Medications are used to help control symptoms, but they do not change the downward trajectory of COPD that occurs over time as lung function worsens. Typical medications given regularly include bronchodilators through oral or inhaled routes. Antibiotics may be given to fight infections and systemic steroids for acute exacerbations.

In extreme cases, lung transplantation or lung volume reduction surgery may be indicated. Older persons with severely impaired lung function related to emphysema may be at higher risk of death from these procedures and have poorer outcomes.

Nurses working with older adults with COPD will find it challenging to assist them with a home maintenance program that addresses their unique needs with this chronic disease. Teaching should involve the patient and family and should plan for the long term. Reducing factors that contribute to symptoms, medication usage,

TABLE 9-16   Strategies for Symptom Management for Older Adults with COPD
Do not smoke.
Avoid second-hand smoke.
Avoid air pollutants and other lung irritants.
Exercise regularly as tolerated or prescribed.
Maintain proper nutrition.
Maintain adequate hydration—especially water intake.
Take medications as ordered: bronchodilators (antibiotics and steroids for exacerbations).
Use energy conservation techniques.
Alternate activities and rest.
Learn and regularly use breathing exercises.
Learn stress management and relaxation techniques.
Recognize the role of supplemental oxygen.
Receive yearly pneumonia and influenza vaccines to avoid serious infections.
Investigate pulmonary rehabilitation programs.
Join a support group for those with breathing problems and their families.
Explore any possible surgical options with the physician.

alternating rest and activity, energy conservation, stress management, relaxation, and the role of supplemental oxygen should all be addressed. Many older adults with COPD find it helpful to join a support group for those who are living with similar problems.

Tuberculosis

Background

Tuberculosis (TB), caused by *Mycobacterium tuberculosis,* is a contagious infection that involves the lungs but can attack any part of the body. Primary TB is caused by inhalation of air droplets from an infected person through coughing, sneezing, laughing, or other activities in which particles become airborne (NCBI, 2011). Older adults and *immunocompromised* persons are at the greatest risks. According to the CDC's Morbidity and Mortality Weekly Report [MMWR] (CDC, 2012b), the incidence of TB in 2011 has declined by 6.4% since 2010. There are a reported 3.4 cases per 100,000 populations in the United States, which translates to about 10,521 new TB cases in 2011. However, data continue to point to a trend of foreign-born or racial/ethnic minorities being disproportionately affected by TB compared to U.S.-born persons. This gap is continuing to widen despite an overall decreased number of cases in both groups (CDC, 2012b). The AIDS epidemic has contributed to the spread of TB, particularly in less developed countries; this may be due to the suppression of the immune system that is associated with AIDS.

Risk Factors/Warning Signs

Nursing home residents are considered an at-risk group due to the typically higher rates found in this population. General guidelines from the Advisory Committee for Elimination of Tuberculosis (Centers for Disease Control and Prevention [CDC], 1990) set a concrete strategy for prevention and management of TB in nursing homes to decrease the spread among this institutionalized and vulnerable population. Thus, older adults who may be discharged from acute care facilities to a nursing home will generally undergo TB skin testing prior to discharge.

Screening for TB is simple and can be done at the local health department, clinic, or doctor's office. A Mantoux test is an intradermal injection that is read for results 48–72 hours after administration. A result of 11 mm or greater of induration (not redness, but swelling) is considered a positive result. It is recommended that older adults undergo a two-step screening wherein the test is given again, because there are many false results in the older adults. A positive TB skin test should be followed up with a chest X-ray to rule out active disease.

It must be noted that persons who received a vaccine for TB may have a positive reaction. A TB vaccine is commonly given in many countries outside the United States.

A person can be infected with TB and have no symptoms; this means they may have a positive skin test, but cannot spread the disease. Such a person can develop TB later if left untreated. Those with active TB can spread the disease to others and should be treated by a physician or other healthcare provider. The signs and symptoms of TB appear in **Table 9-17**.

Assessment and Diagnosis

For older adults born in the United States, a positive skin test may prompt the healthcare provider to initiate preventative treatment. The medication isoniazid (INH) is generally given to kill the TB bacteria. Treatment with INH often lasts at least 6 months. Few adults have side effects from the medication, but those that are possible include nausea, vomiting, jaundice, fever, abdominal pain, and decreased appetite. Patients taking INH should be cautioned not to drink alcohol while on the medication.

Interventions

Patients with active TB can be cured, but the medication regimen is complex, with several different drugs taken in combination. Caution should be taken to avoid spread of the disease. This generally means isolation for patients in the hospital with active TB. There are 10 medications approved to treat TB (CDC, 2016f). Medications should be strictly taken for the entire period of time (usually 6–9 months) to kill all of the bacteria. Older adults may need assistance with keeping track of these medications; evaluation of medication management should be included in the assessment. The use of a medication box set up by another competent and informed family member to ensure compliance with the medication regimen may be helpful, because it can be overwhelming for some persons. Adequate rest, nutrition, and hydration, as well as breathing exercises, may help with combating

TABLE 9-17 Signs and Symptoms of Tuberculosis
A severe cough that lasts more than 3 weeks
Chest pain
Bloody sputum
Weakness
Fatigue
Weight loss
Poor appetite
*Chills
*Fever
*Night sweats

*May not be present in the elderly.
Modified from Centers for Disease Control and Prevention. (2016a). Tuberculosis (TB) disease: Symptoms & risk factors. Retrieved from http://www.cdc.gov/features/tbsymptoms/

the effects of TB. Since over half of all patients with actively diagnosed TB have come to the United States from other countries, language may be a barrier. Education requires understanding and may necessitate an interpreter to ensure understanding of the complex regimens required to eradicate the bacteria.

Gastrointestinal Disorders

Gastrointestinal problems are among the most frequent complaints of older adults. Several common disorders will be discussed here, including gastroesophageal reflux, peptic ulcer, *diverticulitis*, constipation, and several types of cancers.

Gastroesophageal Reflux Disease

Background/Significance

Although *gastroesophageal reflux disease* (GERD) is common among older adults, the true prevalence is not known, as many patients with GERD-related symptoms never discuss their problems with their PCP. GERD is thought to occur in 5–7% of the world's population, with 21 million Americans affected (International Foundations for Functional Gastrointestinal Disorders, 2008), and is found in both men and women.

Risk Factors/Warning Signs

Pathophysiological changes that occur in the esophagus (reduced lower esophageal pressure and length, impaired motility of the esophagus, and reduced salivary secretion), hiatus hernia, and certain medications and foods increase the risk for GERD. Obesity and activities that increase intra-abdominal pressure such as wearing tight clothes, bending over, or heavy lifting have also been linked to GERD (WebMD, 2011). The cardinal symptom of GERD is heartburn; however, older adults may not present with this, but rather complain of atypical symptoms such as pulmonary conditions (bronchial asthma, chronic cough, or chronic bronchitis), otorhinolaryngeal problems (hoarseness, pain when swallowing foods, or chronic laryngitis), or noncardiac chest pain (Pilotto & Franceschi, 2009). GERD can result in chronic mucosal inflammation with erosive esophagitis and ulceration, which can be further complicated by strictures and bleeding (Pilotto & Franceschi, 2009). The chronic back-flow of acid into the esophagus can lead to abnormal cell development (Barrett esophagus) that increases the risk for esophageal adenocarcinoma. Therefore, it is essential that nurses consider atypical presentations of GERD when caring for older adults.

CLINICAL TIP

Persons with GERD should avoid chocolate, peppermint, and caffeine, as these can loosen the LES and allow more acid into the esophagus.

Assessment and Diagnosis

Older adults often present with atypical symptoms, making the diagnosis of GERD very challenging. As people age the severity of heartburn can diminish, while the complications, such as erosive esophagitis, become more frequent. Therefore, endoscopy should be considered as one of the initial diagnostic tests in older adults who are suspected of having GERD (Pilotto & Franceschi, 2009). Examination of the esophagus, stomach, and duodenum through a fiber-optic scope (endoscopy) while the person receives conscious sedation allows the gastroenterologist to visualize the entire area, identify suspicious areas, and obtain biopsies as needed. *Helicobacter pylori*, a chronic bacterial infection in humans, is a common cause of GERD, affecting about

BOX 9-4   Resources for Those with GERD

American College of Gastroenterology (ACG)	American Gastroenterological Association (AGA)
4900-B South 31st Street	4930 Del Ray Avenue
Arlington, VA 22206-1656	Bethesda, MD 20814
703-820-7400	301-654-2055
http://www.acg.gi.org	http://www.gastro.org

30–40% of the U.S. population. Testing for *H. pylori* can be done during the endoscopy or by urea breath testing or stool antigen testing (Ferri, 2011).

Interventions

The objectives of treatment include: (1) relief of symptoms, (2) healing of esophagitis, (3) prevention of further occurrences, and (4) prevention of complications (Pilotto & Francheschi, 2009). Lifestyle and dietary modifications are important aspects of care. The nurse should recommend smoking cessation; limiting or avoiding alcohol; and limiting chocolate, coffee, and fatty or citrus foods. Medications should be reviewed and offending medications modified, as certain medications decrease the lower esophageal sphincter (LES), allowing acid to backflow into the esophagus. These include anticholinergic drugs, some hormones, calcium channel blockers, and theophylline. Avoidance of food or beverages 3–4 hours prior to bedtime, weight loss, and elevation of the head of the bed on 6- to 8-inch blocks are some other interventions that may help alleviate symptoms. Pharmacological treatments with antacids in conjunction with *histamine 2 (H2) blockers* (Tagmet, Zantac, Axid, and Pepcid) are used for mild GERD. If these are ineffective in controlling symptoms, then the *proton pump inhibitors* (PPIs) are the next drugs of choice, which include omeprazole, lansoprazole, rabeprazole, pantoprazole, and esomeprazole. The H2 blockers are often prescribed twice a day and the PPIs once a day; however, sometimes these may be ordered twice daily. These medications should be taken on an empty stomach. Laparoscopic fundoplication surgery, although controversial, may be indicated in adults who fail treatments and have severe complications (**Box 9-4**).

Peptic Ulcer Disease

Background/Significance

Each year, about 5 million people in the United States are affected by peptic ulcer disease (PUD), with about 12% occurrence in those over age 75 years and 9.6% in people ages 65–74. The overall trend for incidence of PUD has been declining in young men; however, the opposite is true for older women (Anand, 2013). Early identification and treatment is important, because about 25% of people with PUD have serious complications such hemorrhage, perforation, or gastric outlet obstruction (Mayo Clinic, 2016b). Ulcers are a common cause for hospitalizations for upper gastrointestinal (GI) bleeding in the United States (Laine & Jensen, 2012). Upper GI bleeds occur in about 15–20% of adults, with about 20% of episodes in older adults occurring with no symptoms of the disease. Although a small percentage of people experience perforation the risk of death is high in older adults when it does occur (Mayo Clinic, 2016b).

Risks/Warning Signs

The most common causes of PUD are *H. pylori* infection and use of nonsteriodal anti-inflammatory drugs (NSAIDS). Other risk factors include smoking, drinking alcohol, caffeine, and stress. In hospitalized adults, critical illness, surgery, or hypovolemia contribute to development of an ulcer (Mayo Clinic, 2016b). The most common symptom is dyspepsia (indigestion), which can classified as ulcer-like or food-provoked. Ulcer-like is the most common and is manifested by burning pain and epigastric, hunger-like pain that is relieved with food, antacids, and/or medications classified as antisecretory agents. Patients with food-provoked dyspepsia may present with epigastric discomfort and fullness after eating a meal, belching, early satiety, nausea, and occasional vomiting. These symptoms can overlap (Soll, 2011). Older adults may experience "silent" PUD, which makes it difficult to identify before complications occur (Barkun & Leontiadis, 2010).

Assessment and Diagnosis

The diagnosis is made through the history and physical. The typical symptoms are episodic gnawing or burning epigastric pain, often occurring 2 to 5 hours after meals. The older adult should be evaluated for anemia, hematemesis, melena, or heme-positive stool suggesting a GI bleed. Vomiting is suggestive of an obstruction, weight loss and anorexia of cancer, and persistent upper abdominal pain radiating to the back may indicate perforation. Adults 55 years and older presenting with any of these symptoms should promptly be referred to a gastroenterologist for further evaluation. Patients should be tested for *H. pylori* with a urea breath test, stool antigen test, or endoscopic biopsy. When there are acute problems, such as a GI bleed, older adults may have an atypical presentation of acute confusion, restlessness, abdominal distention, and falls (Mayo Clinic, 2016b)

Interventions

The treatment depends on the cause. If *H. pylori* is present, then eradication with antibiotics and antisecretory therapy for about 10 to 14 days is indicated. Administration of proton pump inhibitors (PPIs), bismuth, many antibiotics, and an upper GI bleed can lead to false-negatives. It is essential to address risk factors, as stated above (Ramakrishnam & Salinas, 2007). If the person is taking NSAIDs for pain, discuss alternatives such as acetaminophen and nonpharmacological treatments. Lifestyle modifications such as avoidance of late meals, elevation of head of bed, weight loss in overweight or obese people, smoking cessation, and avoidance of recumbency for 2 to 3 hours after meals (American Gastroenterology Association [AGA], 2008) should be taught. Medications, such as PPIs or histamine H2-receptor blockers, are used to heal an ulcer. If for some reason aspirin or NSAID cannot be discontinued, use of a PPI is more effective. Prevention should always be reinforced; it is important to identify those at risk (previous ulcer, use of NSAIDS, anticoagulant therapy, over 70 years of age, *H. pylori* infection, and use of oral corticosteroids) and then use PPIs and educate the person about prevention measures (Lockrey & Lim, 2011).

Diverticulitis

Background/Significance

Diverticulitis is an inflammation or infection of the pouches of the intestinal mucosa (see **Figure 9-3**). Diverticular disease is more common among older adults than younger people (Tursi, 2012). Sixty-five percent of older adults will develop diverticulosis, (which are protrusions of the intestinal mucosa in the weakened muscle wall of the large bowel) by 85, with some going on to develop diverticulitis (Kennedy-Malone et al., 2014), an infection or inflammation of the diverticuli. The exact cause of diverticulosis is not known, but it is speculated that a diet low in fiber and high in refined foods causes the stool bulk to decrease, leading to increased colon transit time. Retention of undigested foods and bacteria results in a hard mass that can disrupt blood flow and lead to abscess formation. The earlier the diagnosis and treatment, the better the outcomes will be; however, complications such as bleeding increase the risk of less-than-optimal outcomes.

Risks/Warning Signs

Risk factors for diverticulosis include obesity, chronic constipation, straining, irregular and uncoordinated bowel contractions, and weakness of bowel muscle due to aging. Other risk factors are directly related to the suspected cause of the condition; these include older than 40 years of age, low-fiber diet, and the number of diverticula in the colon (Thomas, 2011). Diverticulosis can present with pain in the left lower quadrant (LLQ), can get worse after eating, and may improve after a bowel movement. Warning signs of diverticulitis include fever, increased white blood cell count, bleeding that is not associated with pain, tachycardia, nausea, and vomiting.

Assessment and Diagnosis

Evaluation of the abdomen may reveal tenderness in the LLQ and there may be rebound tenderness with involuntary guarding and rigidity. Bowel sounds may be initially hypo-active and can be hyperactive if the obstruction has passed. Stool may be heme-positive. The initial evaluation is abdominal X-ray films, followed by a barium enema, though a CT scan with oral contrast is more accurate in diagnosing (Thomas, 2011). A CBC should be obtained to assess for infection and anemia.

Interventions

Diverticulosis is managed with a high-fiber diet or daily fiber supplementation with psyllium. Diverticulitis is treated with antibiotics, but in acute illness the person may require hospitalization for IV hydration, analgesics, bowel rest, and possible NG tube placement. Morphine sulfate should be avoided because it increases the intraluminal pressures within the colon, causing the symptoms to get worse (Thomas, 2011). In some cases, either where the person has complications that do not resolve with medical management or has several repeated episodes, a colon resection may be needed. Patient education should include information about diet, avoidance of constipation and straining during bowel movements, and when to seek medical care. The diet should include fresh fruits, vegetables, whole grains, and increased fluid intake, unless contraindicated.

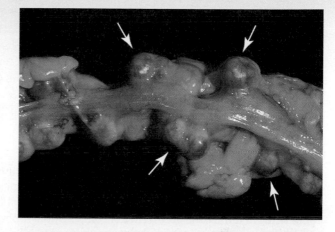

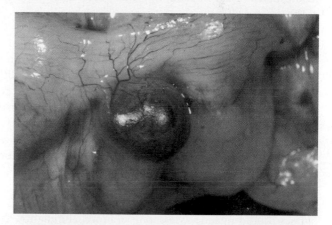

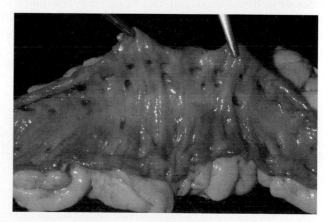

Figure 9-3 Diverticula of colon demonstrated by injection of barium contrast material into colon [barium enema]. Diverticula filled with contrast material appear as projections from the mucosa [arrows].
Courtesy of Leonard V. Crowley, MD, Century College.

> **CLINICAL TIP**
>
> About half of patients with diverticulitis will eventually have a bowel obstruction, and about 25% of patients with diverticulitis require surgery (Kennedy-Malone, Fletcher, & Martin-Plank, 2014).

Constipation

Background/Significance

Constipation is the most common bowel problem in older adults. The definition varies by patients and healthcare providers, but the ROME III criteria for chronic constipation provide a definition based on symptoms. Constipation is a preventable and treatable problem that requires identification of the risk factors (see **Table 9-18**) to reduce the occurrence of complications. Some of the complications that can occur include fecal incontinence, fecal impaction, urinary retention, rectal prolapse, diverticular disease, and impaired quality of life (Harari, 2009).

Risks/Warning Signs

Constipation is often multifactorial, with causes that can include a combination of systemic or local conditions. Some of the risk factors include impaired mobility, medications (anticholinergics, analgesics, iron supplements, and calcium supplements), depression, neurological conditions (dementia, Parkinson's disease, stroke, diabetes mellitus, and spinal cord injury), dehydration, low dietary fiber, metabolic disturbances (hypothyroidism, hypercalcemia, hypokalemia, and uremia), undergoing dialysis, mechanical obstruction, and decreased access to toilet (Harari, 2009). Warning signs include constipation with a family history of colon cancer, rectal bleeding, unexplained anemia, weight loss, or narrowed caliber of stool (Ham, Sloane, Warshaw, Bernard, & Flaherty, 2007).

Assessment and Diagnosis

Nurses should include assessment of bowel elimination that focuses on predisposing causes. History should include all over-the-counter medications, diet and fluid intake, and physical activity. Other assessments include psychosocial, mental health (mood), cognitive, and laboratory studies (CBC, electrolytes, glucose, and thyroid profile). The diagnosis is based on clinical presentation and physical examination. It is important to determine the onset and duration of the constipation, along with functional and nutritional status. Abdominal assessment and rectal exam should include checking stool for occult blood.

TABLE 9-18   Factors to Consider in Bowel Management

Uncontrollable Factors	Controllable Factors
Family history	Diet
Presence of neurogenic bowel	Fiber
Fluids	Fluids
Existence of prior bowel disease	Timing
	Activity
	Positioning
	Medications

Interventions

Initial interventions should focus on lifestyle and dietary modifications (see **Table 9-19**). Bulk agents (e.g., psyllium, methylcellulose) should be considered for those who do not respond to lifestyle changes, and for those who do not respond to bulking agents, osmotic laxatives (e.g., lactulose, sorbitol) should be considered. Residents of nursing homes appear to respond to stimulant laxatives (e.g., senna, bisacodyl). Enemas should not be used on a regular basis and should be reserved for those who do not respond to treatments or who have evidence of fecal impaction. Nonpharmacological interventions include regular exercise, establishment of a regular routine for toileting (assure privacy), and encouragement of a high-fiber diet with adequate fluid intake (unless contraindicated) (Mauk & Rye, 2012).

Cancers

Aging is a major risk factor for cancer. Cancer is the second-leading cause of death after heart disease. Esophageal, stomach, colorectal, and pancreatic cancers will be discussed here briefly, but readers are referred to the resources listed and traditional medical surgical textbooks for a more thorough discussion.

Colorectal

Background/Significance

Colorectal (CRC) cancer is the second most commonly diagnosed cancer and the second leading cause of mortality in the United States (Richardson, Tai, & Rim, 2011) yet the most curable form of cancer if the disease is localized to the bowel (National Cancer Institute [NCI], 2008). The vast majority of this type of cancer is adenocarcinoma arising from colonic polyps. Although most polyps do not become malignant, the risk of cancer increases as the polyp size increases (Edwards, 2002). Strong evidence supports that screening for CRC can reduce the incidence and the risk of mortality (Richardson et al., 2011).

Risks/Warning Signs

Risk factors include a first-degree relative with colorectal cancer, age 50 or older, hereditary disease such familial polyposis, and a history of ulcerative colitis or Crohn's disease. Other risk factors are high-fat diet, alcohol consumption, cigarette smoking, sedentary lifestyle, and exposure to environmental toxins. Warning signs such as

TABLE 9-19   Principles of Bowel Programs to Prevent Constipation

- Start with a clean bowel. (Administer needed medications or enemas to cleanse the bowel prior to initiating a program or protocol.)
- Try all-natural means first: fiber, fluids, activity, timing, positioning.
- Be sure the person is taking adequate fiber and fluids before adding medications.
- Change only one item at a time in the program. Allow several days to pass before evaluating the effectiveness of the change. If needed, add another intervention.
- Stool softeners are given for hardened stool, and the person must drink at least a liter of fluid per day for them to be effective.
- Peristaltic stimulators are useful when the person is unable to move the stool down into the rectum.
- Use the least caustic type of suppository that is effective for the older person.
- Avoid the use of bedpans—have the person sit upright on the toilet or commode.
- Avoid the regular use of enemas.

abdominal pain, palpable mass in lower right quadrant, anemia, and dark red or mahogany-colored blood mixed in the stools are indicative of tumors of right colon. Manifestations of tumors on the left include progressive abdominal distention, pain, vomiting, constipation, and bright red blood on the surface of the stool (McCance, Huether, Brashers, & Rote, 2010).

Assessment and Diagnosis

The nurse should evaluate bowel elimination patterns when obtaining the history to determine if there has been a change. According to the American Cancer Society, screening recommendations are based on the level of risk. Those with an average risk should begin screening at age 50 years with an annual fecal occult blood test and flexible sigmoidoscopy every 5 years or colonoscopy every 10 years. People at a high risk should have a colonoscopy every 3–5 years starting at age 40, or at least 10 years prior to when it appeared in any close relatives.

Interventions

Educate older adults about the risks of colorectal cancer and recommend screening as appropriate. Teach them how to lower their risks by maintaining a diet that is high in grains, fruits, and vegetables, and low in processed red meats; replacing vitamin D when deficient; adding calcium and folic acid supplements; avoiding excessive alcohol; and increasing their physical activity.

Gastric (Stomach)

Background/Significance

Despite a decline in the incidence of stomach cancer, this condition comprises about 2% (21,230) of all new cancers and causes about 10,960 deaths each year (American Cancer Society [ACS], 2017). The average age of diagnosis is t69 years; approximately two-thirds of people with stomach cancer are age 65 or older. There is a greater incidence among men than in women, as well as in Hispanics, African Americans, and Asian/Pacific Islanders as compared to Caucasians (ACS, 2017). If detected early, there is a good prognosis, but once a tumor has advanced, patients may quickly deteriorate.

Risks/Warning Signs

There are several risk factors for stomach cancer. *H. pylori* appears to be the major cause, especially in the distal aspect of the stomach. People who have been treated for mucosa-associated lymphoid tissue (MALT) lymphoma have an increased risk, which may be related to *H. pylori* bacteria. Consumption of large amounts of smoked foods, salted fish and meat, and pickled vegetables; smoking cigarettes (particularly of the upper portion of the stomach); obesity (not strong link); previous gastric surgeries; pernicious anemia; blood type A; and family history of gastric adenocarcinoma are other risk factors (ACS, 2017). Patients may not have signs of the cancer until later in the disease, when the prognosis is poor.

Assessment and Diagnosis

Early in the disease patients may be asymptomatic or experience vague symptoms such as loss of appetite (especially for meat), malaise, and "indigestion." As the disease progresses, they may have unintentional weight loss, upper abdominal pain, vomiting, change in bowel habits, and anemia due to occult bleeding (McCance et al., 2010). Diagnostic tests will depend on the symptoms the person is experiencing. The best way to diagnose is by performing an EGD so there is direct visualization and the ability to obtain a biopsy.

Interventions

Surgery is the standard treatment for gastric cancers. Nurses can help with primary prevention of stomach cancer by educating older adults about how to reduce risks and identify early symptoms. Dietary changes are a significant way to reduce risks; a diet lower in red meats and higher in antioxidants has a protective effect (ACS, 2017). In addition, weight loss and smoking cessation may also be beneficial. Encourage regular physical exams and reporting of suspicious symptoms, as early testing can help decrease the risk of mortality.

Esophagus

Background/Significance

The risk of cancer of the esophagus increases as a person ages; in 2005–2009, the median age at diagnosis was 68 years of age, while 69 years was the average age of death (Howlader et al., 2011). The two most common types of cancers of the esophagus are adenocarcinoma, followed by squamous cell carcinoma. Early detection is key because the prognosis for either type is relatively poor.

Risks/Warning Signs

Squamous cell carcinoma is associated with malnutrition. This can be related to lower socioeconomic status, poor dietary habits, alcoholism, tobacco use, obesity, radiation exposures, and chronic GERD (American Gastroenterology Association, 2008). Adenocarcinoma is related to reflux esophagitis and hiatal hernia; these both can cause erosive esophagitis and ulcerations, which can lead to Barrett esophagus and cancer (McCance et al., 2010). The most common warning sign is heartburn initiated by spicy or highly seasoned foods.

Assessment and Diagnosis

The nurse should assess for heartburn after eating spicy foods and when lying down. Dysphagia that can present as pressure-like and may radiate to the back between the scapulae is another common symptom. In older adults, symptoms may not appear until the cancer advanced, when the cancer has most likely metastasized. Older adults with dysphagia should undergo an EGD.

Interventions

Nurses can initiate primary prevention by encouraging smoking cessation and limitation of alcohol intake (a maximum of one drink per day for females and two for males). Older adults should be educated about risk factors and when to notify healthcare professionals of symptoms that may warrant further evaluation.

Pancreas

Background/Significance

The incidence of pancreatic cancer has increased over the past few years to the point where the lifetime risk of developing it is 1.47% (ACS, 2013a). Pancreatic cancer is found more often in older adults and is a leading cause of death in this age group. It is estimated that about 44,000 people will be diagnosed with and about 37,390 will die of pancreatic cancer in 2012 (Howlader et al., 2011). The prognosis is poor because there are often suboptimal responses to treatment.

Risks/Warning Signs

Risk factors include tobacco smoking and smokeless tobacco use (about twice as high for cigarette smokers as compared to nonsmokers), family history, diabetes mellitus, obesity, and possibly high levels of alcohol consumption. Unfortunately, early warning signs often are absent. Symptoms that require further evaluation are weight loss, pain in upper abdomen that radiates to the back, and high blood glucose levels. Sometimes tumors develop near the common bile duct, causing an obstruction that leads to jaundice; this may allow for earlier diagnosis.

Assessment and Diagnosis

Patients may present with vague, diffuse pain that is located in the epigastric area of the left upper quadrant. Diarrhea can be an early symptom, and weight loss can be a late finding. At the present time there are no early

---

BOX 9-5   Resources for Those with Common Cancers

American Cancer Society (all forms of cancer)

    I Can Cope (community support groups)

    1599 Clifton Road, N.E.

    Atlanta, GA 30329

    1-800-ACS-2345

    http://www.cancer.org

American Urological Association

    Online patient information resource http://
    www.urologyhealth.org

Bladder Health Council

    c/o American Foundation for Urologic

    Disease

    1000 Corporate Boulevard, Suite 410

    Linthicum, MD 21090

    800-828-7866

National Breast Cancer Foundation

    http://www.nationalbreastcancer.org

---

diagnostic methods. A CT scan can be done to identify pancreatic cancer; however, endoscopic ultrasonography is more sensitive in detecting the cancer (McPhee, Papadakis, & Rabow, 2012).

Interventions

Surgery, *radiation therapy*, and *chemotherapy* are all treatment options, but these are done with the hopes of extending survival or as part of palliative care. Less than 20% of people diagnosed with pancreatic cancer are candidates for surgery because the cancer often has metastasized by the time of diagnosis. For those people for whom the disease is localized and who have small cancers (<2 cm) with no lymph node metastases and no extension outside the capsule of the pancreas, the 5-year survival rate for surgical treatment is about 18–24%. Hospice should be considered as early as possible when the prognosis is terminal (see **Box 9-5**).

Genitourinary Problems

The elderly may experience several major problems related to the reproductive and urinary systems. This section will discuss some common problems, including urinary tract infection, bladder cancer, atrophic vaginitis, breast cancer, *benign prostatic hyperplasia* (BPH), prostate cancer, and erectile dysfunction. Urinary incontinence, which is common in older adults, is addressed in its own chapter (Chapter 15) under a section on geriatric syndromes.

Urinary Tract Infection

Background/Significance

Urinary tract infections (UTIs), also called cystitis (inflammation of the bladder), are common among older adults and are more frequent in women. They are a primary cause of urinary incontinence and delirium. *Catheter-associated urinary tract infections* (CAUTIs) are more common among older adults (Fakih et al., 2012) and are mainly attributed to the use of indwelling urinary catheters. Many indwelling catheters are thought to be unnecessary and one study noted that physicians were often not aware of the purpose for which their patients had a catheter inserted (Saint, Meddings, Calfee, Kowlaski, & Krein, 2009). UTIs have been show to increase morbidity and mortality, length of hospital stay, and cost of hospitalization (Kleinpell, Munro, & Giuliano, 2008). CAUTI is considered preventable and is not reimbursed by Medicare, so hospitals will largely assume the financial costs for preventable infections of this type. Since nurses play a key role in inserting, maintaining, and decision making regarding catheter use, it is essential that those working with older adults be alert to current guidelines for catheter use.

Risk Factors/Warning Signs

Several risk factors are associated with UTIs. These include being female, having an indwelling urinary catheter, the presence of urological diseases, and hormonal changes associated with menopause in women. Signs and symptoms of UTIs include urinary frequency and burning or stinging felt during voiding. Pain may be felt above the pubic bone, and a strong urge to void but with small amounts of urine expelled are also symptoms. The most significant risk factor for CAUTI is prolonged use of an indwelling catheter. In hospital-acquired UTIs, 75% are associated with the use of an indwelling catheter (CDC, 2012). In women, signs and symptoms of CAUTI may be more severe than those reported by patients in the community who do not have an indwelling catheter. Lethargy, malaise, onset or worsened fever, flank pain, and altered mental status have been associated with CAUTI (Hooton et al., 2010).

Assessment/Diagnosis

Nurses should thoroughly assess and document patients' urinary output, including amounts, color, odor, appearance, frequency of voiding, urgency, and episodes of incontinence. A urine specimen should be obtained if UTI is suspected. Laboratory results will show the type of organism causing the infection, and the sensitivity will tell what medication the organism is susceptible to. These results should be reported promptly to the physician or nurse practitioner caring for the patient so that a diagnosis and treatment plan can be made.

Interventions

Prevention of UTIs is considered a primary nursing strategy. Elderly female patients can be instructed to make lifestyle modifications such as increasing their fluid intake; emptying the bladder after sexual intercourse; practicing good perineal hygiene, including wiping front to back after toileting; getting enough sleep; and avoiding stress (PubMed Health, 2011). Although many of these common-sense strategies are recommended by PCPs, there is a lack of scientific evidence to support many of them. Many UTIs will clear up on their own, particularly if the person increases oral fluid intake during early symptoms. However, with many older adults, antibiotic treatment may be needed. In general, a course of 3 days for healthy adults is thought to be sufficient, but for more resistant bacteria, a longer course more than 5 days may be needed (PubMed Health, 2011). For those with repeated or chronic UTIs, a low dose of antibiotics taken for 6–12 months may be indicated (Hooton et al., 2010). Monitor the patient's temperature at least every 24 hours (Carpenito, 2013). Encourage fluids. If an indwelling catheter is in place, evaluate if continued use is necessary.

If the underlying cause is CAUTI, treatment will be more aggressive. To prevent CAUTI, nurses should thoroughly assess and document a patient's urinary output as with a suspected standard UTI. Appropriate uses of indwelling catheters may include those with acute urinary retention, the acutely ill who need more accurate monitoring of urinary output, perioperative patients having certain surgeries, those with sacral or coccygeal wounds and incontinence, those with prolonged immobility such as spinal injury, and persons at end of life (Health Care Infection Control Practices Advisory Committee [HICPAC], 2009). Alternatives to indwelling catheters should be considered for appropriate patients. Intermittent catheterization, if appropriate, is preferred over indwelling catheter use, especially for long-term maintenance of bladder management (Hooton et al., 2010). Condom catheters may be an appropriate choice for some males. If an indwelling urinary catheter is necessary, sterile technique on insertion should be strictly observed and asepsis maintained afterwards. The catheter should be removed as soon as possible to reduce the risk of CAUTI. Clear removal guidelines for catheters should be established and in place for all patients (American Nurses Association [ANA], 2016). Some suggested strategies to include in hospital protocols are electronic medical record reminders to the nurse or physician and automatic stop dates (Hooton et al., 2010). There are many resources for nurses and patients that can help prevent CAUTI: A simple FAQ page for patients and families can be found at http://www.cdc.gov/hai/pdfs/uti/CA-UTI_tagged.pdf and the HICPAC clinical practice guideline for professionals can be found at http://www.cdc.gov/hicpac/pdf/CAUTI/CAUTIguideline2009final.pdf. The ANA provides a CAUTI prevention tool. This can be found at http://nursingworld.org/ANA-CAUTI-Prevention-Tool

CLINICAL TIP

Staging of Bladder Cancer (Mayo Clinic, 2016a, para 7):

Stage I. Cancer at this stage occurs in the bladder's inner lining but hasn't invaded the muscular bladder wall.

Stage II. At this stage, cancer has invaded the bladder wall but is still confined to the bladder.

Stage III. The cancer cells have spread through the bladder wall to surrounding tissue.

Stage IV. By this stage, cancer cells may have spread to the lymph nodes and other organs, such as your bones, liver, or lungs.

Reproduced from Mayo Clinic. (2016a). Bladder cancer. Retrieved from http://www.mayoclinic.org /diseases-conditions/bladder-cancer/basics/tests-diagnosis/con-20027606

Bladder Cancer

Background/Significance

Bladder cancer occurs mainly in older adults, with an average age at diagnosis of 73 years, with 9 out of 10 cases of bladder cancer diagnosed in persons over age 55. The ACS (2016b) reported estimates that in 2016 there will be about 76,960 new cases of bladder cancer and about 16,390 deaths from bladder cancer (about 11,820 in men and 4,570 in women). Men are three times as likely to get cancer of the bladder as women (American Foundation for Urologic Disease, 2008) and the incidence increases with age. The incidence of new bladder cancers is about 5% of all cancers and the 4th leading cancer in men (ACS, 2016a).

Risk Factors/Warning Signs

Risk factors include chronic bladder irritation and cigarette smoking, the latter contributing to over half of cases (see **Case Study 9-3**). Male gender and age are also risk factors. The classic symptom of bladder cancer is painless hematuria, which may be a reason that older adults sometimes do not seek treatment right away.

Case Study 9-3

Dr. Johnson is a 62-year-old dentist who runs a busy practice in a large suburb of Chicago. He had been a smoker for over 30 years but recently quit. For some time he has noted little spots of blood in his urine, but he did not have pain, so he attributed it to some prostate problems he has had in the past. Dr. Johnson hears a couple of his patients discussing a mutual friend with bladder cancer who has similar symptoms, and this prompts him to visit his family physician for a checkup. After several tests and a cystoscopy, Dr. Johnson is diagnosed with early stage bladder cancer.

Questions:

1. What risk factors did Dr. Johnson have for bladder cancer?
2. What primary sign did he exhibit?
3. Since his cancer was detected early, what treatments might be options in his case?
4. If Dr. Johnson's cancer becomes invasive, what other options are available for treatment?
5. Describe the nursing implications and care required if Dr. Johnson needed to have a cystectomy.
6. How would you explain a cystectomy to his family?

Assessment/Diagnosis

Assessment begins with a thorough history and physical. Be sure to ask the patient if he/she has experienced any bleeding or observed blood with voiding; older adults may attribute the bleeding to hemorrhoids or other causes and feel that because there is no pain, it could not be serious. Diagnosis may involve several tests including an intravenous pyelogram (IVP), urinalysis, and cystoscopy (in which the physician visualizes the bladder structures through a flexible fiber-optic scope). This is a highly treatable type of cancer when caught early. In fact, the ACS (2012c) estimates that there were more than 500,000 survivors of this cancer in 2012.

Interventions

Once diagnosed, treatment depends on the invasiveness of the cancer. Treatments for bladder cancer include surgery, radiation therapy, immunotherapy, and chemotherapy (Mayo Clinic, 2016a). Specifically, a transurethral resection (TUR) may involve burning superficial lesions through a scope. Bladder cancer may be slow to spread, and less invasive treatments may continue for years before the cancer becomes metastatic, if ever.

Immune/*biological therapy* includes Bacillus Calmette-Guérin (BCG) wash, an immune stimulant that triggers the body to inhibit tumor growth. BCG treatment can also be done after TUR to inhibit cancer cells from re-growing. Treatments are administered by a physician directly into the bladder through a catheter for 2 hours once per week for 6 or more weeks (Mayo Clinic, 2017). The patient may be asked to lie on his/her stomach, back, or side throughout the procedure. The nurse should instruct the patient to drink plenty of fluids after the procedure and to be sure to empty the bladder frequently. In addition, because the BCG contains live bacteria, the patient should be taught that any urine passed in the first 6 hours after treatment needs to be treated with bleach: One cup of undiluted bleach should be placed into the toilet with the urine and allowed to sit for 15 minutes before flushing (Mayo Clinic, 2017).

If the cancer begins to invade the bladder muscle, then removal of the bladder (*cystectomy*) is indicated to prevent *metastasis*. Additional diagnostic tests will be performed if this is suspected, including CT scan or MRI. Chemotherapy and/or radiation may be used in combination with surgery. When the cancerous bladder is removed, the person will have a *urostomy*, a stoma from which urine drains into a collection bag on the outside of the body, much like a colostomy. Bleeding and infection are two major complications after surgery, regardless of type. Nursing care includes assessment and care of the stoma, emptying and changing collection bags as needed, monitoring output, and assessing for bleeding and infection. Significant education of the patient related to intake/output, ostomy care, appliances, and the like is also indicated.

CLINICAL TIP

Painless hematuria, as a primary sign of bladder cancer, may be ignored by the older adult or blamed on another possible condition. Any unexplained bleeding should be investigated.

Female Reproductive System

Two major problems common among older females will be discussed here. These include atrophic vaginitis and breast cancer.

Atrophic Vaginitis

Background/Significance

Normal aging changes in the female reproductive system (see Chapter 4) make elderly women more at risk for infection: Less vaginal lubrication and more alkaline pH due to lower estrogen levels put elderly women at increased risk of vaginitis, and the vaginal canal also becomes more fragile with age due to atrophy. Vaginitis, or inflammation of the vaginal canal and the external genitalia (vulva), may have several causes, including bacteria, yeast, viruses, organisms passed between sexual partners, chemical irritants (such a douches), or even clothing. Atrophic vaginitis (AV) is one of the most common problems, affecting 10–50% of postmenopausal women (Reimer & Johnson, 2010). Often, the symptoms are mistaken for a normal part of aging and women may not report them to their PCP.

Risk Factors/Warning Signs

Atrophic vaginitis is caused by low estrogen levels. It may be progressive in relationship to the time after the onset of menopause because of sustained low levels of estrogen. Signs and symptoms of AV include abnormal vaginal discharge, burning, itching, tenderness, dryness, soreness, sparse labial hair, and pain with sexual intercourse (WebMD, 2012).

Assessment/Diagnosis

Because there are many major causes of vaginitis, and more than one can be present at the same time, the underlying cause of vaginitis can be difficult to diagnose. Older women with the above symptoms should be referred to their PCP or gynecologist for appropriate treatment. However, since AV is relatively common among postmenopausal women, the nurse practitioner or physician examining the patient will largely rely on the patient's description of symptoms and a thorough history and physical examination for diagnosis. This includes inspection of the vaginal and cervical areas (with speculum use). No laboratory tests are generally needed to diagnose AV in the postmenopausal woman.

Interventions

Treatment for AV is prescribed on an individual basis. The Society of Obstetricians and Gynecologists of Canada (SOGC) and the North American Menopause Society (NAMS) "recommend the use of nonhormonal lubricants or moisturizers and maintenance of sexual activity as first-line treatment" (Reimer & Johnson, 2010, p. 26). If the patient does not respond to this, then hormone-based therapy is considered.

There are several different types of hormonal therapy to treat AV. Vaginal estrogen therapy comes in the form of creams, vaginal rings, or tablets. Treatments with creams may be messier than the rings or tablets, and may be prescribed daily or twice weekly depending on the medication used (Reimer & Johnson, 2010). The use of local estrogen therapy can significantly improve symptoms of vaginal dryness, and it promotes sexual and urogenital health (North American Menopause Society, 2012).

For general vaginal health, women should be instructed to avoid douching and the use of feminine deodorant sprays or perfumes. Wearing cotton undergarments may also help. A water-soluble lubricant, such as K-Y gel, should be used during intercourse if vaginal dryness is a problem; the use of other lubricants such as Vaseline contributes to cases of vaginitis other than atrophic. In addition, cigarette smoking can increase the potential for AV, so smoking cessation is encouraged.

Breast Cancer

Background/Significance

Breast cancer is the second leading cancer diagnosis for women after skin cancer. The ACS (2015) estimated 2231,840 new cases of invasive breast cancer in 2015, as well as over 60,000 cases of new in situ cancer in women and about 2,350 cases of breast cancer in men (2015). It was also estimated that over 40,000 women would die from breast cancer in 2015 (ACS, 2015). The incidence of breast cancer in women over 50 has declined since the year 2000, and this is attributed largely to the decrease in use of menopausal hormone therapy (MHT), previously known as hormone replacement therapy (HRT) (ACS, 2015; BreastCancer.org, 2012; McEneaney, 2012). Most breast cancers are diagnosed in women over the age of 65 (National Breast Cancer Foundation, 2012). White women have a higher incidence of breast cancer after age 45, while African American women have a higher

Case Study 9-4

Mrs. Valdez is a 65-year-old woman who comes to the physician's office after experiencing enlargement of her right breast upon self-exam. The nurse observes during the physician's physical examination that Mrs. Valdez's right breast is twice as large as the left one and has a puckered appearance. The physician tells Mrs. Valdez that she will need to have some tests and a biopsy and then he leaves the room. Mrs. Valdez looks at the nurse and asks, "What does he mean? What is wrong with me?"

Questions:

1. What should the nurse explain to Mrs. Valdez at this point? What educational materials might she need?
2. What tests would the nurse expect the physician to order?
3. Are there possible risk factors for breast cancer that Mrs. Valdez might have? If so, what are they?
4. Given the physical observations, what would the nurse expect to see done for this patient?

incidence rate prior to age 45 years and a higher likelihood of dying from breast cancer at any age (ACS, 2015; BreastCancer.org, 2012). Men may also develop breast cancer, though this is much less frequent, and they should not be excluded from education about the disease.

Risk Factors/Warning Signs

There are several risk factors for breast cancer, some controllable, some not. These include family history, late menopause, having the first child after age 30, obesity, high fat intake, and alcohol consumption. Of course, primary nursing care focuses on those factors that can be modified. Geriatric nurses should be particularly aware of the importance of early detection among those older women who are at higher risk.

Signs and symptoms of breast cancer include a breast mass or lump, breast asymmetry, dimpling of the skin or "orange peel" appearance, discharge, and nipple changes (ACS, 2012d; Kennedy-Malone et al., 2014). Early detection by screening is important since there may not be any pain or other symptoms associated with early stages of breast cancer.

Assessment and Diagnosis

An abnormality, such as a lump felt upon examination of the breasts either by the patient or PCP, may be the first indication of a problem. In general, however, most breast lumps are benign and could be due to factors other than cancer, such as fibrocystic disease.

A breast exam performed by a clinician, mammography, and biopsy, in addition to lab tests, chest X-ray, and bone scans, are indicated for diagnosis (see **Case Study 9-4**). Stage I breast cancer has a 98% survival rate at 5 years (National Breast Cancer Foundation, 2012), so early diagnosis and treatment is essential.

Interventions

Screening is an important intervention for prevention and early detection. Screening guidelines for older women have changed significantly in recent years, based on current evidence. The CDC guidelines (2016b) state that women who are not at high risk aged 50–74 years should have a screening mammography every 2 years. Current evidence is insufficient to support screening for breast cancer in women over 75 (U.S. Preventive Services Task Force, 2009).

CLINICAL TIP

Although clinical and self breast exams may not have sufficient evidence to suggest this type of screening for all women, anecdotal clinical evidence suggests that many women who perform self breast exam and discover an unusual finding report that this is what sent them to the physician for further assessment.

Nursing care is important at all levels of prevention. Nurses working with older adults should encourage appropriate screening according to recommended guidelines, and the elderly should be encouraged to have regular checkups with their physician. Although controversy exists over the use of mammography, it remains an effective means to detect many cancerous tumors at an earlier stage with minimal risk to the person, but screening should begin in middle adulthood.

Treatment for breast cancer depends on stage, but includes any combination of radiation, chemotherapy, or surgery. Depending on the type of tumor, hormone therapy may also be effective. Older women undergoing mastectomy as treatment for breast cancer may require more time for recovery. Promotion of the return of full range of motion to the arm on the operative side is essential. This may require physical therapy in addition to the psychosocial and emotional support involved in rehabilitation.

Male Reproductive System

The most common disorders related to the reproductive system among older men include benign prostatic hyperplasia (BPH), cancer of the prostate, and *erectile dysfunction* (ED).

Benign Prostatic Hyperplasia

Background

BPH, also known as prostatism, results from noncancerous enlargement of the prostate gland that is associated with advanced age. This condition affects nearly 50% of men ages 51–60 and up to 90% of men over 80 years (American Urological Association, 2017). Although the enlargement is benign, it is sometimes associated with prostate cancer, so men with this condition should be carefully monitored.

Risk Factors/Warning Signs

Reasons for why the prostate tends to enlarge as a man ages are unclear. Known risk factors for BPH are few, but include advanced age and family history; in fact, BPH is so common with advanced age that nearly all men would have some prostate enlargement if they lived long enough. BPH occurs when the enlarged prostate squeezes and compresses the urethra, causing symptoms such as a decreased urinary stream, increased frequency, increased urgency, nocturia, incomplete emptying, dribbling, a weak urine stream, and urinary *incontinence* (see **Table 9-20**). The urge to void may be so frequent in men with BPH (as often as every 2 hours) that it can interfere with sleep and *activities of daily living* (ADLs).

Assessment and Diagnosis

Diagnosis is made using any number or combination of tests and studies including digital rectal exam (DRE), urinalysis, postvoiding residual, *prostate-specific antigen* (PSA), urodynamic studies, ultrasound, and cystoscopy. The DRE and PSA are used to help rule out prostate cancer as a cause of the symptoms.

TABLE 9-20   Signs and Symptoms of BPH
Decreased urinary stream
Urinary frequency
Urinary urgency
Nocturia
Urinary incontinence
Incomplete bladder emptying
Urinary dribbling
Feelings of urge to void but difficulty starting urine stream
Decreased quality of life related to symptoms
Altered sleep patterns related to nocturia

Interventions

Watchful waiting is one of the recommended medical treatments for BPH that is not causing severe lower urinary tract symptoms (American Urological Association, 2017). Other medical treatment generally includes medications and surgery. The two most frequently used types of medications are alpha-blockers and 5-alpha-reductase inhibitors. Alpha-blockers, such as alfuzosin, doxazosin (Cardura), terazosin (Hytrin BPH), and tamsulosin (Flomax MR), work to relieve symptoms of BPH by relaxing the smooth muscle of the prostate and bladder neck to allow urine to flow more easily. None of the four medications listed has been convincingly shown to be more effective than the other (American Urological Association, 2017). A 5-alpha-reductase inhibitor such as finasteride (Proscar) works differently, by shrinking the prostate to promote urine flow, but has sexual side effects such as impotence (American Urological Association, 2017; Mead, 2005; U.S. Department of Health and Human Services, National Kidney and Urological Diseases Information Clearing House [NKUDIC], 2012).

There are several surgical procedures that can be used to treat BPH. One of the most common surgical interventions for BPH is a *transurethral resection of the prostate* (TURP). During this procedure, the urologist resects the enlarged prostate gland through a cystoscope (see **Figure 9-4**). Older men sometimes call this the "Rotor Rooter" surgery. Nursing care after this procedure is essential to avoid complications related to the heavy bleeding that may occur. The patient will have an indwelling urinary catheter with three ports. Postoperatively, *continuous bladder irrigation* (CBI) must be maintained to prevent dangerous clotting of the blood. The nurse is responsible for assessing the color of the urine draining from the catheter. The urine in the tube should be charted with specific terms such as bright red, brick red, tea colored, amber, yellow, or clear. The number and size of clots draining from the catheter should be described. The goal of the CBI is to flush the bladder, so the nurse must regulate the rate of the fluid to keep the urine yellow or as clear as possible. CBI will continue postoperatively until the bleeding stops. Bleeding complications may result if the CBI is allowed to go dry or the catheter is removed too soon after surgery. In the event that the patient is unable to void after removal of the catheter post-TURP, the catheter may need to be reinserted. If the nurse is unable to reinsert the catheter, the physician may need to be called in to do this. Nurses should be particularly alert to the potential for complications in older men after this procedure.

A newer procedure that has shown promising results is holmium laser enucleation of the prostate (HoLEP). Although the HoLEP procedure generally takes longer than the TURP, it has some added benefits, such as a low incidence of needing further surgery and the ability to take a larger and better tissue sample for examination than with TURP. However, most residents are still being taught TURP as the gold standard of treatment for treatment of BPH (Bhojani & Lingeman, 2011).

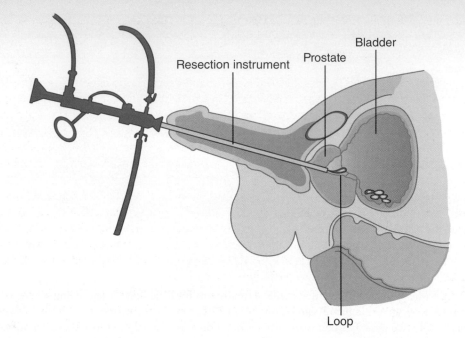

Figure 9-4 TURP.

Prostate Cancer

Background

Prostate cancer is the second leading cause of cancer death in U.S. males, with an estimated 241, 740 new cases and 28,170 deaths in 2012 (NCI, 2013). One in 6 men will have prostate cancer in his lifetime, but mortality (1 in 36) has declined (ACS, 2012b; NCI, 2013). When found in the local and regional stages, the 5-year survival rate is nearly 100% (ACS, 2012b). The incidence of prostate cancer increases with age. Over half of men 70 years and older show some histological evidence of prostate cancer, though only a small percentage die from this disease.

Risk Factors/Warning Signs

Older men with prostate cancer may be asymptomatic, so screening is still recommended but PSA screening is only recommended if symptoms of prostate cancer are present (National Center for Health Research, 2016). If present, symptoms of prostate cancer may include urinary urgency, nocturia, painful ejaculation, blood in the urine or semen, and pain or stiffness in the back or thighs (American Urological Association Foundation [AUAF], 2008; NCI, 2013). Risk factors for prostate cancer include advanced age, a diet high in saturated fats, family history, and race/ethnicity (African Americans slightly higher than Whites, and low incidence among Asian males) (ACS, 2013b; AUAF, 2008).

Assessment and Diagnosis

Screening for prostate cancer begins with a digital rectal exam and PSA test. The rectal exam may detect malignancy in the form of a hard, nodular prostate. A PSA of less than 4 ng/mL is considered normal for ages 60–69 years, whereas 7 ng/mL may be normal in the 70–79 age group because PSA rises with age. Sixty percent of men with a PSA above 10 ng/mL have prostate cancer, but most men with a PSA of over 4 ng/mL do not have prostate cancer (Mead, 2005; National Center for Health Research, 2016). There are many false negative and positives with the PSA test. Diagnosis can only be confirmed through biopsy.

Interventions

If a biopsy of the prostate is needed, the nurse can educate the patient on what to expect. The biopsy is often done in the urologist's office. Usually, local anesthetic is used. The physician will use a special needle to take samples of the prostate, which is accessed through the rectal wall. Several samples will be taken. The procedure generally takes around 10 minutes, and the patient may be ordered some antibiotics to take afterwards to prevent possible infection after the procedure (ACS, 2012b). The biopsy samples will be sent to a lab where the pathologist will examine them. If found to be cancerous, the tumor will be graded and discussion of treatment will be done with the physician and patient.

Treatment depends on the stage of cancer growth, but for more localized cancers it generally includes three major options: *radical prostatectomy*, radiation therapy, and active surveillance. The "decision to proceed to prostate biopsy should be based primarily on PSA and Digital Rectal Examination (DRE) results, but should take into account multiple factors including free and total PSA, patient age, PSA velocity, PSA density, family history, ethnicity, prior biopsy history, and comorbidities" (AUAF, 2009, pp. 5–6). The patient's age, health condition, and life expectancy should be considered when planning treatment.

Because a radical prostatectomy is major surgery and carries some inherent risks, all options should be considered with the older patient. The major problems after surgery to remove the prostate include urinary *incontinence* (which is often temporary) and impotence. The skill and experience of the surgeon can decrease the risk of urinary incontinence after surgery.

A holistic approach to care may include dietary changes such as a low-fat diet and the addition of vitamin E, selenium, and soy protein (Bradway & Yetman, 2002). It is important that a patient not adopt complementary medicine treatments without talking with his doctor.

Nursing care surrounding treatment for prostate cancer will involve helping families to explore their options, linking them to community resources, and providing education related to managing postoperative complications if surgery is indicated. Geriatric nurses should be informed as to the various options available for treatment of impotence that accompanies this type of surgery. Couples should be provided with support group information as well as information on penile implants and other devices that patients may wish to consider after recovery.

Erectile Dysfunction

Background

Erectile dysfunction (ED), also known as impotence, is defined as the inability to achieve and sustain a sufficient erection for intercourse. Erectile dysfunction is more common in men over age 75 (WebMD, 2017). About 30 million American men are affected by ED (NKUDIC, 2012). The incidence of ED increases with age, but it is not inevitable and is highly treatable in many cases.

Risk Factors/Warning Signs

The causes of ED may be many, including diabetes, hypertension, multiple sclerosis, spinal cord injury, thyroid disorders, alcoholism, renal failure, hypogonadism, other diseases, some medications (see **Table 9-21**), and psychological factors (such as fear, guilt, or depression). Smoking, alcoholism, and obesity may also contribute to ED. In men over age 75, ED has a positive correlation with prostate and urinary problems as well as advanced age (WebMD, 2017).

Assessment and Diagnosis

Assessment of ED should include a thorough patient history, physical and psychological exam, and lab tests. Interviewing the man's sexual partner may also provide clues as to the cause of ED. Determining whether the

TABLE 9-21 Medications That May Affect Sexual Function
Anticholinergics
Antidepressants
Antihypertensives
Digoxin
Hypnotics
Sedatives
Sleeping medications
Tranquilizers

cause is physical, psychological, or a combination of both is a good place to start. It is important for nurses to note that ED can also be an important predictor of overall health in older men (WebMD, 2015).

Interventions

Treatment for ED usually begins with the least invasive strategies. This could include lifestyle modifications such as smoking cessation, monitoring alcohol intake, dietary changes for weight control, and increasing exercise. If the problem seems more psychological than physical (after testing), referral to a qualified counselor or psychiatrist may be ordered. Medications should be examined for those contributing to ED, and adjustments or alternatives to those medications should be explored with the PCP.

CLINICAL TIP

Any male who is wanting to begin Viagra medication should have an eye exam.

Other treatment options for ED fall into several categories, including oral medications, vacuum pump devices, penile implants, and drugs injected into the penis. Sildenafil (Viagra) is an oral medication that is taken 1 hour prior to sexual activity. It is contraindicated in those with heart disease and may result in some cardiovascular-related side effects including headache, flushing, and nasal congestion. Other oral products on the market (Cialis, Levitra) are based on similar principles. A complaint about Viagra is the possibility of irreversible visual impairment in some men, but screenings for those at increased risk for this complication (those with certain characteristics in the inner eye being at higher risk) can be done by most primary care physicians or ophthalmologists.

Vacuum devices have a good acceptance in the elderly population, with a 70–90% success rate (Reuben et al., 2015). These devices work in various ways to pump or draw blood into the penis and use another mechanism, such as a ring around the base of the penis, to help sustain the erection for intercourse. Risks from use of this device would include bruising or bleeding (in extreme cases). Nursing instruction to couples on the use of such a device is essential to prevent harm. Other treatments for ED include medications that may be injected directly into the penis to cause temporary erection, and some persons may opt for having surgery to insert a penile implant. There are two types of penile implants: one that results in permanent erection and one that may be pumped to cause erection and then released. All options should be explored with persons wishing information on treatment of ED.

Neurological Disorders

Two of the most frequently occurring neurological diseases in the elderly are *Parkinson's disease* (PD) and *Alzheimer's disease* (AD). Chapter 10 is devoted entirely to nursing management of dementia, so the reader is referred there for a more thorough discussion.

Stroke also considered a neurological disorder, was discussed previously in the section on circulation problems. Complications that affect the neurological system as a result of a variety of causes may include seizures, tremor (see discussion on PD), peripheral neuropathy (see discussion on diabetes), and dizziness. These are also briefly presented in this section.

Parkinson's Disease

Background

Parkinson's disease is one of the most common neurological diseases, affecting at least 4 million people in the United States (National Parkinson Foundation, 2013). Parkinson's disease usually affects people over the age of 50, and the likelihood of developing PD increases with age (National Institute of Neurological Disorders and Stroke, 2008); the average age of onset is about 59 years of age (APDA, 2013). It affects both men and women, particularly those over the age of 60 years (National Parkinson Foundation, 2013). Parkinson's disease was first described by Dr. James Parkinson as the "shaking palsy," so named to describe the motor tremors witnessed in those experiencing this condition.

Parkinson's disease is a degenerative, chronic disorder of the central nervous system in which nerve cells in the basal ganglia degenerate. A loss of neurons in the substantia nigra of the brainstem causes a reduction in the production of the neurotransmitter dopamine, which is responsible for fine motor movement. Dopamine is needed for smooth movement and also plays a role in feelings and emotions. One specific pathological marker is called the Lewy body, which under a microscope appears as a round, dying neuron.

Risk Factors/Warning Signs

Parkinson's disease has no known etiology, though several causes are suspected. There is a family history in 15–25% of cases (National Institute of Neurological Diseases and Stroke [NINDS], 2015). Environmental toxins and neuroinflammation related to exposure to pesticides, solvents, and traumatic brain injury are being investigated (NINDS, 2015).

There are four cardinal signs of PD: bradykinesia (slowness of movement), rigidity, tremor, and gait changes such as imbalance or uncoordination. A typical patient with PD symptoms will have some distinctive movement characteristics with the components of stiffness, shuffling gait, arms at the side when walking, incoordination, and a tendency to fall backward. Not all patients exhibit resting tremor, but most have problems with movement; such as difficulty starting movement, increased stiffness with passive resistance, and rigidity, and freezing during motion (NINDS, 2012). Signs, symptoms, and associated characteristics of PD appear in **Table 9-22**. Advanced PD may result in Parkinson's dementia.

Assessment and Diagnosis

Diagnosis of PD is made primarily on the clinician's physical examination and thorough history taken from the patient and/or family. Nurses should note that several other conditions may cause symptoms similar to PD, such as the neurological effects of tremor and movement disorders. These may be attributed to the effects of drugs or toxins, Alzheimer's disease, vascular diseases, or normal pressure hydrocephalus, and not be true PD. There is no one specific test to diagnose PD, and labs or X-rays rarely help with diagnosis.

Interventions

Management of PD is generally done through medications. Levodopa, a synthetic dopamine, is an amino acid that converts to dopamine when it crosses the blood–brain barrier. Levodopa helps lessen most of the serious signs and symptoms of PD; however most who use levodopa will develop levodopa-induced dyskinesias such as tics and tremors (NINDS, 2015). Another side effect to note is hallucinations. A more common treatment, and generally the drug of choice, involves a medication that combines levodopa and carbidopa (Sinemet), resulting

TABLE 9-22   Signs, Symptoms, and Associated Problems Seen in Persons with Parkinson's Disease

Bradykinesia
Rigidity
Tremor
Pill rolling
Incoordination
Shuffling gait, arms at side
Freezing of movements
Balance problems (tendency to fall backward)
Vocal changes; stuttering
Swallowing problems
Drooling
Visual disturbances
Bowel and bladder dysfunction
Sexual dysfunction
Dizziness
Sweating
Dyskinesias
Sleep pattern disturbances
Dementia
Memory loss
Emotional changes
Confusion
Nightmares
Twitching
Handwriting changes
Depression
Anxiety
Panic attacks
Hallucinations
Psychosis

in a decrease in the side effect of nausea seen with Levodopa therapy alone, but with the same positive control of symptoms, particularly with relation to movement. Patients should not be taken off of Sinemet precipitously, so it is important to check all of a patient's medications if they are admitted to either acute or long-term care. Dopamine agonists trick the brain into thinking it is getting dopamine. This class of medications is less effective than Sinemet, but may be beneficial for certain patients. The most commonly prescribed dopamine agonists are pramipexole (Mirapex) and ropinirole (Requip) (Parkinson's Disease Foundation, 2012). Medications such as Sinemet show a wearing-off effect, generally over a 2-year period. During this time, the person must take larger doses of the medication to achieve the same relief of symptoms that a smaller dose used to bring. For an unknown reason, if the medication is stopped for about a week to 10 days, the body will reset itself and the person will be able to restart the medication at the lower dose again until tolerance is again reached. This time off from the medication is called a "drug holiday" and is a time when the person and family need extra support, because the person's symptoms will be greatly exacerbated without the medication. The earliest drugs used for PD symptom management were anticholinergics such as Artane and Cogentin, and these medications are still used for tremors and dystonias associated with wearing-off and peak dose effects (Parkinson's Disease Foundation, 2012).

For those affected by levodopa side-effects, deep brain stimulation (DBS), with electrode-like implants that act much like a pacemaker to control PD tremors and other movement problems, has become a widely used alternative. The person using this therapy will still have the disease and generally uses medications in combination with this treatment, but may require lower doses of medication (NINDS, 2012). Thalamotomy, or surgical removal of a group of cells in the thalamus, is used in severe cases of tremor. This will manage the tremors for a period of time, but is a symptomatic treatment, not a cure. Similarly, pallidotomy involves destruction of a group of cells in the internal globus pallidus, an area where information leaves the basal ganglia. In this procedure, nerve cells in the brain are permanently destroyed. Scientists are working on strategies to utilize both adult and fetal tissue stem cell transplants to regenerate brain tissue in persons with PD (Politis & Lindvall, 2012).

Other research includes areas in which nurses may advocate for evidence-based practice in their facilities or organization. For example, Tai Chi has been shown to be effective in improving balance and reducing falls for PD patients (NINDS, 2012). Rehabilitation units have been using Tai Chi for similar benefits in other patients with neurological deficits. Simple interventions such as using Wii games to promote activity and exercise may be explored. The role of caffeine in PD is also being examined. In a small randomized control study of 61 patients with PD, caffeine equivalent to 2–3 cups of coffee per day was given to subjects and compared with a control group of those taking a placebo. Those patients receiving the caffeine intervention showed little improvement in daytime sleepiness, but modest improvement in PD severity scores related to speed of movement and stiffness (Postuma et al., 2012). Further study with larger groups was recommended by the researchers.

Much of the nursing care in PD is related to education. Because PD is a generally chronic and slowly progressing disorder, patients and family members will need much instruction regarding the course of the disease and what to anticipate. Instruction in the areas of medications, safety promotion, prevention of falls, disease progression, mobility, bowel and bladder, potential swallowing problems, sleep promotion, and communication is important. Most of the problems seen as complications of PD are handled via the physician as an outpatient, but certainly complications such as swallowing disorders as the disease progresses may require periods of hospitalization. When persons suffer related dementia in the final phases of the disease, they are often cared for in long-term care facilities that are equipped to handle the challenges and safety issues related to PD dementia. Areas for teaching appear in **Table 9-23**. In addition, access to resources and support groups is essential. A list of helpful resources and agencies is provided in **Box 9-6**.

Dizziness

Background

Dizziness is quite common in older adults, affecting about 30% of those over age 65. It represents about 2% of the consultations in primary health care (Hansson, Mansson, & Hakanson, 2005) and is the most common complaint in those over 75 who are seen by office physicians (Hill-O'Neill & Shaughnessy, 2002). There are four major types of dizziness according to Hill-O'Neill and Shaughnessy: vertigo, presyncope (light-headedness), disequilibrium (related to balance), and ill-defined (i.e., it does not fit in any other categories). These are further explained under assessment and diagnosis.

TABLE 9-23 Patient/Family Teaching Regarding Parkinson's Disease Key Areas
Medication therapy (side effects, wearing off, drug holidays, role of diet in absorption)
Safety promotion/fall prevention
Disease progression
Effects of disease on bowel and bladder, sleep, nutrition, attention, self-care, communication, sexuality, and mobility
Swallowing problems
Promoting sleep and relaxation
Communication
Role changes
Caregiver stress/burden—need for respite
Community resources

BOX 9-6 Resources for Those with Parkinson's Disease

American Parkinson Disease Association
800-223-2732
http://www.apdaparkinson.org

Michael J. Fox Foundation for Parkinson's Research
212-509-0995
http://www.michaeljfox.org

National Institute of Neurological Disorders and Stroke (NINDS)
800-352-9424
http://www.ninds.nih.gov

National Parkinson Foundation
800-327-4545
http://www.parkinson.org

Parkinson's Disease Foundation
800-457-6676
http://www.pdf.org

Risk Factors/Warning Signs

Risk factors for dizziness include advanced age, sudden change in position, inner ear problems, orthostatic hypotension, cerebrovascular disease, cardiovascular disease, cervical spondylosis, vestibular diseases, Meniere's disease, and TIAs. The signs and symptoms of dizziness can vary from lightheadedness lasting seconds to dizziness lasting for days as in *benign paroxysmal positional vertigo* (BPPV). Certain medications can also cause dizziness.

Signs and symptoms of BPPV include dizziness, presyncope, feelings of imbalance, and nausea. The symptoms begin when the person changes head position, even something as usual as tipping the head back or turning the head in bed.

Assessment and Diagnosis

Vertigo—a false sense of motion or spinning—may be caused by BPPV, which is brought on by normal calcium carbonate crystals breaking loose and falling into the wrong part of the inner ear. It can also be caused by inflammation in the inner ear; *Meniere's syndrome;* vestibular migraine; acoustic neuroma; rapid changes in motion; or more serious problems such as stroke, brain hemorrhage, or multiple sclerosis.

Presyncope is when the older person complains of feeling faint or light-headed. It is associated with a drop in blood pressure such as occurs when the person sits up or suddenly changes to a standing position, or with an inadequate output of blood from the heart. It can also be caused by medications that induce orthostatic hypotension, hypovolemia, low blood sugar, or some other cause of lack of blood flow to the brain.

Disequilibrium is a loss of balance or the feeling of being unsteady when walking. Causes of disequilibrium include vestibular problems, sensory disorders, joint or muscle problems, or medications.

The fourth category is really a "catch all" for possible causes of dizziness not included in the first three categories. Problems in this category include such things as other inner ear disorders, anxiety disorders, hyperventilation, cerebral ischemia, side effects of medications, Parkinsonian symptoms, hypotension, low blood sugar, and benign positional vertigo.

Dizziness is generally treatable by addressing the cause. However, in some cases, such as dizziness associated with poststroke, it can be a permanent impairment.

Otological dizziness (a major classification in the elderly, according to Hain and Ramaswamy [2005]) refers to vertigo caused by changes in the vestibular system. The most common types in the elderly are Meniere's syndrome and BPPV. Meniere's syndrome is common in those over age 50. The cause is unknown, though it is often attributed to a virus or bacterial infection. Signs and symptoms include a rapid decrease in hearing; a sense of pressure or fullness in one ear, accompanied by loud *tinnitus* (ringing in the ears); and then vertigo (Hain, 2012; Hain & Ramaswamy, 2005; Hill-O'Neill & Shaughnessy, 2002). It may involve the excessive buildup of fluid in the inner ear, which is the cause of the feeling of fullness in the ear. A feeling of being unsteady or dizzy may last for as little as 30 minutes or for days after the episode (Mayo Clinic, 2012).

As mentioned previously, BPPV is the most common cause of dizziness in the older age group, accounting for as much as 50% of all dizziness, with an increasing incidence with age (Hain, 2003, 2012). BPPV occurs when debris called *otoconia* ("rocks in the ears") become dislodged from their usual place in the ear and get stuck elsewhere in the vestibular system. Although in most cases the underlying cause of BPPV is not known, the degeneration of the vestibular system in the inner ear that occurs with normal aging is thought to play a major role. In cases of vertigo that do not respond to traditional medication for dizziness (such as Antivert), BPPV should be suspected. A key to diagnosis of BPPV is Hallpike's maneuver, in which the patient is laid down quickly from a sitting position, with the head turned to the side and hung over the back of the exam table. This will produce a characteristic nystagmus if the cause is BPPV.

Interventions

Treatment for dizziness depends on the underlying cause. For dizziness caused by body position, behavioral modification is indicated. Depending on the cause of dizziness, medication may be helpful. For dizziness of acute onset, methylprednisolone may be used over a 3-week period to improve vestibular function. In Meniere's disease, meclizine may help with acute symptom relief. If the cause is TIAs, then aspirin therapy might be initiated to decrease vascular risk factors (Reuben et al., 2015).

BPPV can be treated in the office by the physician, advanced practice nurse, or even a physical therapist with knowledge of the proper maneuvers. The Epley maneuver is a technique by which the patient is put into a series of specific positions and head turns to promote return of the otoconia to their proper place in the ear. After this treatment, the patient must stay in the office for 10 minutes and then sleep in a recliner chair at 45 degrees for the following 2 nights. They should also be instructed to avoid head positions that cause BPPV for at least another week (Hain, 2003). Other maneuvers and even surgical treatment may be necessary in rare variations of BPPV; these would be recommended by the physician on a case-by-case basis.

Dizziness, whatever the cause, can be particularly distressing to the older adult. It can interfere with ADLs, the ability to drive, and the maintenance of independence. Elders may decrease activities and spend more time at home due to the fear of dizzy spells or of falling. It is a leading cause of elderly persons discontinuing driving, which may be depressing to them and limit their social activity. In other cases the fear of having to stop driving will keep a person from seeking medical attention. Early diagnosis of the cause of dizziness can result in better outcomes by starting treatment sooner and avoiding complications that can result from bouts of syncope or vertigo.

Nurses should encourage older adults with complaints of dizziness to seek medical help. Treatment may be with medication, simple maneuvers, or lifestyle changes. Emotional support during diagnosis and testing, and reassurance that most causes of dizziness are treatable, can be a comfort to the older adult with this problem.

Seizures

Background

One in 26 people will develop a seizure disorder (England, Liverman, Schultz, & Strawbridge, 2012). Epilepsy affects about 2.2 million Americans of all ages (England et al., 2012). Key differences between seizure occurrence in older versus younger adults include: the elderly have a higher incidence of seizures, stroke is the leading cause of seizures in older adults, and the symptoms are more vague in the elderly than in younger adults (Davidson & Davidson, 2012). In older adults, it can be more challenging to find appropriate treatment as a result of adverse drug reactions, drug interactions, altered absorption rates, and comorbidities (Davidson & Davidson, 2012).

Seizures can be caused by a variety of conditions in older persons, however the most common cause is stroke (Gilad, 2012). A list of potential causes of seizures in older adults appears in **Table 9-24**.

There are three major classifications of epilepsies, although there are many additional types. Generalized types are more common in young people and associated with grand mal or tonic-clonic seizures. A number of cases have an undetermined origin and may be associated with certain situations such as high fever, exposure to toxins, or rare metabolic events. In older adults, localized (partial or focal) epilepsies are more common, particularly complex partial seizures (Luggen, 2009). In contrast to young adults, Rowan and Tuchman (2003) cite other differences in seizures in the elderly: low frequency of seizure activity, easier to control, high potential for injury, a prolonged postictal period, and better tolerance with newer antiepileptic drugs (AEDs). Additionally, older adults may have coexisting medical problems and take many medications to treat these problems.

Risk Factors/Warning Signs

Risk factors for seizures in older adults include cerebrovascular disease (especially stroke), age, and head trauma. The most obvious signs and symptoms of epilepsy are seizures, although changes in behavior, cognition, and level of consciousness may be other signs. Also, note that exposure to toxins can cause seizures that are not epilepsy. Complex partial seizures in older adults may include symptoms such as "confusion, memory loss, dizziness, and shortness of breath" (Davidson & Davidson, 2012, p. 16). Automatism (repetitive movements), facial twitching with following confusion, and coughing are also signs of the more-common complex partial seizure (Luggen, 2009).

TABLE 9-24   Possible Causes of Seizures in the Elderly
Stroke or other cerebrovascular disease
Arteriosclerosis
Alzheimer's disease
Brain tumor
Head trauma
Intracranial infection
Drug abuse or withdrawal
Withdrawal from antiepileptic drug

Assessment and Diagnosis

Diagnosis is made by careful description of the seizure event, a thorough history, and physical. Eyewitness accounts of the seizure incident can be quite helpful, although many community-dwelling older adults go undiagnosed because their seizures are never witnessed. In addition, complete blood work, neuroimaging, chest X-ray, ECG, and electroencephalogram (EEG) help determine the cause and type of seizure (National Institute for Health and Clinical Excellence [NICE], 2012).

Interventions

Treatment for epilepsy is aimed at the causal factor. The standard treatment for recurrent seizures is antiepilepsy drugs (AEDs). The rule of thumb, "start low and go slow," for medication dosing in older adults particularly applies to AEDs. The elderly tend to have more side effects, adverse drug interactions, and problems with toxicity levels than younger people.

Research has suggested that older adults may have better results with fewer side effects with the newer AEDs than the traditional ones, though about 10% of nursing home residents are still medicated with the first-generation AEDs (Mauk, 2004). The most common older medications used to treat seizures include barbiturates (such as phenobarbital), benzodiazepines (such as diazepam/Valium), hydantoins (such as phenytoin/Dilantin), and valproates (such as valproic acid/Depakene) (Deglin & Vallerand, 2005; Resnick, 2008).

Several newer drugs are also used, depending on the type of seizure. Second-generation AEDs, including gabapentin (Neurontin), lamotrigine (Lamictal), oxcarbazepine (Trileptal), levetiracetam (Keppra), pregabalin (Lyrica), tiagabine (Gabitril), and topiramate (Topamax), are generally recommended over the older AEDs; however, older AEDS such as phenytoin (Dilantin), valproate (Depakote), and carbamazepine (Tegretol) are the most commonly prescribed treatment options (Resnick, 2008). Each of these medications has specific precautions for use in patients with certain types of medical problems or for those taking certain other medications. When assessing for side effects in older patients, be sure to be alert to potential GI, renal, neurological (ataxia), and hepatic side effects. Additionally, some newer extended-release AEDs are thought to be better tolerated and have a lower incidence of systemic side effects (such as tremors) (Uthman, 2004).

Musculoskeletal Disorders

Among older adults, there are several significant musculoskeletal problems that can significantly impact quality of life. Osteoporosis can lead to fractures. Arthritis is a major source of pain among older adults, and those who experience related decreased range of motion may have joint replacement surgery. Some of these common disorders will be discussed in this section.

Osteoporosis

Background/Significance

Osteoporosis is a bone disorder characterized by low bone density or porous bones. Over 44 million Americans, including 55% of adults age 50 or over, have this disease. Although often thought of as a woman's disease, by age 90 17% of men have osteoporosis as do 32% of women (Cawthon, 2011; Khosla, 2010). Older persons of all ethnic backgrounds may experience osteoporosis, though it is more common among Whites and Asians. The risk factors for this disorder are many and appear in **Table 9-25**.

Risk Factors/Warning Signs

A major complication of osteoporosis is fractures. These are especially common in the vertebral spine, hips, and wrists. The cumulative cost for treatment of osteoporosis and associated fractures and pain is expected to rise to $204 billion during the period of 2006–2015 and to exceed $228 billion during 2016–2025 (USPSTF, 2011).

TABLE 9-25   Risk Factors for Osteoporosis
Personal history of fracture after age 50
Current low bone mass
History of fracture in a first-degree relative
Being female
Being thin and/or having a small frame
Advanced age
A family history of osteoporosis
Estrogen deficiency as a result of menopause, especially early or surgically induced
Abnormal absence of menstrual periods (amenorrhea)
Anorexia nervosa
Low lifetime calcium intake
Vitamin D deficiency
Use of certain medications, such as corticosteroids and anticonvulsants
Presence of certain chronic medical conditions
Low testosterone levels in men
An inactive lifestyle
Current cigarette smoking
Excessive use of alcohol
Being White or Asian, although African Americans and Hispanic Americans are at significant risk as well

Data from National Institute of Arthritis and Musculoskeletal and Skin Diseases. (2014). What is osteoporosis? Fast facts: An easy-to-read series of publications for the public. Retrieved from http://www.niams.nih.gov/health_info/bone/osteoporosis/osteoporosis_ff.asp

Because there are sometimes no signs or symptoms during the early course of bone deterioration, osteoporosis is often undiagnosed and untreated until fracture occurs.

Assessment/Diagnosis

Osteoporosis-related fractures may lead to pain, immobility, and other complications. If signs and symptoms are present besides fractures, they may take the form of pain and kyphosis Diagnostic testing would reveal decreased bone density and any pathological fractures present via X-ray. On occasion, hairline fractures do not manifest themselves with the initial X-ray, but appear 5–10 days after the initial assault.

Interventions

Because this is a highly treatable and often preventable disease when detected early, all women over the age of 65 years should have *bone mineral density* (BMD) or bone mass measurement done, while women with risk factors for osteoporosis should have BMD at age 60 (AHRQ, 2013). Steps can be taken to prevent osteoporosis by habits that help build strong bones before the age of 20, when bones are fully developed. Preventing osteoporosis in adolescent years would include eating a well-balanced diet with plenty of calcium and vitamin D, no smoking or excessive alcohol intake, plenty of weight-bearing exercise, and discussing any needed treatments with the physician to minimize the risk of the disease. It should be noted that most of the calcium in the diet of American children comes from milk, though yogurt, broccoli, and certain enriched cereals may provide additional sources. Nurses can be active in primary prevention of osteoporosis through educating children in schools about the effects of this disease in later life and how to prevent it.

Treatment of existing osteoporosis takes many forms. Postmenopausal women are often prescribed biphosphonates (such as Fosamax), calcitonin (Miacalcin), or estrogen/hormone replacement medications (such as Estratab or Premarin). Some of these medications are aimed at promoting adequate amounts of calcium in the bones, whereas the hormone replacement therapies replace the estrogen not being produced after menopause, which helps create more of a balance between the delicate hormones that guide bone reabsorption and *demineralization*. The use of estrogen replacement therapy was once used to decrease the incidence of serious fractures in postmenopausal women, but now only selective estrogen receptor modulators are approved for this use (Gallagher & Levine, 2011) due to the associated side effects. Weight-bearing exercises and getting enough calcium in the diet or through supplementation are other treatments to consider. If vitamin supplementation is used, it is essential that the patient take not only calcium but also vitamin D to promote the absorption of the calcium. Nurses should encourage patients to discuss all treatment options with their physicians. Nutritional counseling and the role of sunlight (a source of vitamin D) and exercise should also be addressed. One potential exercise that is being explored for its benefit for both balance and promoting bone health is Tai Chi, a form of Eastern martial arts—one randomized controlled trial demonstrated that the Tai Chi group should increase balance (Shan et al., 2008).

Arthritis

Arthritis, or inflammation of the joint, is the number one chronic complaint and cause of disability in the United States (Arthritis Foundation, 2016), affecting over 50 million Americans (Arthritis Foundation, 2016; CDC, 2016a). There are over 100 types of arthritis, with the two most common being osteoarthritis (OA) and rheumatoid arthritis (RA). These will be discussed here in relationship to their impact on the lives of older adults. Rheumatic diseases affect approximately 21% of the US population, 1.3 million with RA (Helmick et al., 2008). Nearly 10% of Americans report having arthritis, with many experiencing functional limitations as a result (CDC, 2016a).

Osteoarthritis

Background/Significance

Osteoarthritis (OA) is also called degenerative joint disease, osteoarthrosis, hypertrophic arthritis, and degenerative arthritis (Arthritis Foundation, 2016). It affects about 13.9% of the U.S. population age 25 or older and 33.6% of those 65 or older, which equals an estimated 26 million adults (CDC, 2011). Bitton (2009) estimated that the cost of osteoarthritis to be approximately $89.1 billion, including both direct and indirect costs as well as lost wages due to time off from work.

Risk Factors/Warning Signs

The cause of OA is unknown, but it affects females more often than males, and risk increases with certain factors. Modifiable risks include obesity, joint injury, occupation, structural alignment, and muscle weakness. Nonmodifiable risks include gender (women are more at risk), age, race (White and Asian people are at higher risk), and genetic predisposition (CDC, 2011). At this point, it is unknown whether smoking increases risk.

Assessment and Diagnosis

This disease is characterized by chronic deterioration of the cartilage at the ends of the bones; eventually, the bones at the joint become inflamed due to cartilage breakdown, which released cytokines (inflammation proteins) and enzymes that further damage the cartilage. This results in a change in the shape and make-up of the joint so that it will not function smoothly. Bone fragments and cartilage may float in what joint fluid there is, causing irritation and pain, and often resulting in bone spurs (osteophytes) forming near the end of the bone (Arthritis Foundation, 2016).

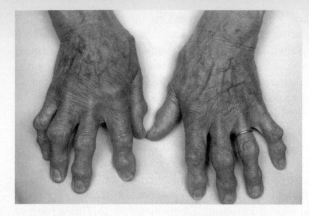

Figure 9-5 Bouchard's and Herberden's nodes.
© Mediscan/Visuals Unlimited, Inc.

Signs and symptoms of OA include pain, stiffness (especially in the morning), aching, some joint swelling, and inflammation. Osteoarthritis targets joints such as the fingers, feet, knees, hips, and spine. Heberden's nodes (bony enlargements at the end joints of the fingers) and Bouchard's nodes (bony enlargements at the middle joints of the fingers) are common (see **Figure 9-5).** Radiographs would show increased heat at the site of inflammation as well as bone deterioration. As OA progresses, the individual may experience crepitus, limping, limited range of motion, increased pain, and even fractures. Diagnosis is made through various lab tests, X-rays, MRIs, or CT scans to visualize areas of damage.

Interventions

The most common associated complication of OA is pain. Although there is no cure for OA, treatment is generally aimed at symptom reduction through lifestyle modifications, nonpharmacological therapies, and medication. For example, risk factors that can be modified, such as excessive stress to the joint (perhaps caused by sports or obesity), should be addressed with exercise programs for strengthening muscles and weight loss (see **Case Study 9-5).** Exercise programs that are holistic and interdisciplinary, particularly those offered in rehabilitation units, may help individuals cope with pain and increase functional levels. In addition, many persons use alternative methods of pain control in combination with medications. **Table 9-26** provides a summary of common treatments for pain for those with OA.

Medications used for treatment of OA include acetaminophen (Tylenol), aspirin, nonsteroidal anti-inflammatory drugs (NSAIDs) such as ibuprofen and naproxen, COX-2 inhibitors (such as celecoxib/Celebrex), tramadol (Ultram), and antidepressants. Other therapies include injection of steroids into the joint to decrease inflammation or injection of synthetic material (such as Synvisc) that acts as a lubricant in the absence of synovial fluid to provide comfort. Other therapies to preserve motion and decrease pain include heat or cold, splints, adaptive equipment, aquatic therapy, and nutrition. In cases of severe dysfunction and pain, surgery with joint replacement may be an option.

Case Study 9-5

Mrs. Chiu is a small, 100-pound, 90-year-old Chinese woman with fractures of the vertebral spine. Because of kyphosis and pain associated with osteoporosis, Mrs. Chiu has been bedbound in a nursing home for several months. Her family visits regularly and has many questions about her condition, especially if it is something that her teenage granddaughters might develop.

Questions:

1. What are Mrs. Chiu's known risk factors for osteoporosis and resulting fractures?
2. How should you answer the family's questions?
3. Are the granddaughters at risk because Mrs. Chiu has osteoporosis? If so, what can they do to prevent it?
4. What teaching should be done with this family?

TABLE 9-26 Treatments for Pain Associated with Osteoarthritis	
Pharmacological	**Nonpharmacological**
Acetaminophen	Moist heat
Aspirin	Warm paraffin wraps
NSAIDs	Stretch gloves or stockings
Capsaicin (topically, with other therapies)	Range of motion exercises
Nabumetone	Upper extremity activities (such as piano playing, typing, card-playing)
	Swimming
	Adaptive equipment
	Heat/cold applications
	Warm bath (limit to 20 minutes)
	Good posture
	Supportive shoes
	Well-balanced diet
	Maintenance of appropriate weight

Important for any nurse caring for older persons taking NSAIDs is the awareness of common side effects. The most common adverse effects of NSAIDs include gastrointestinal symptoms such as stomach upset, nausea, vomiting, and more seriously, gastric ulcers. COX-2 drugs were thought to minimize these effects. Currently all COX-2 medications except Celebrex have been pulled from the market due to associated cardiac risk (Frisco, 2013).

Rheumatoid Arthritis

Background/Significance

Rheumatoid arthritis is characterized by remissions and exacerbations of inflammation within the joint. It affects the fingers, wrists, knees, and spine. In contrast to OA, RA is caused by chronic inflammation that can cause severe joint deformities and loss of function over time (see **Figure 9-6**).

Rheumatoid arthritis affects over 2 million Americans and is more common in women than men. It is generally diagnosed between the ages of 40 and 50 and can cause significant disability for adults who live into old age with this disorder (Mayo Clinic, 2012c). Although the cause is unknown, researchers believe RA may be due to a virus or hormonal factors. In 1987, Peter Gregersen identified the relationship between five specific amino acids and RA, hypothesizing that the area of the genome known as the major histocompatibility complex was critical to RA susceptibility. Twenty years later the ability to fine-map the MHC was discovered. With this technique it is expected that scientists will be able to identify the specific area of the MHC and the triggering mechanism in the HLA proteins responsible for RA. Knowing the cause of the antigens that initiate RA will be the first step towards better treatment for the disease (Von Radowitz, 2012).

Risk Factors/Warning Signs

Risk factors for RA include being female, having a certain predisposing gene, and exposure to an infection. Advanced age is a risk factor until age 70, after which incidence decreases. Cigarette smoking over a period of years is another risk factor.

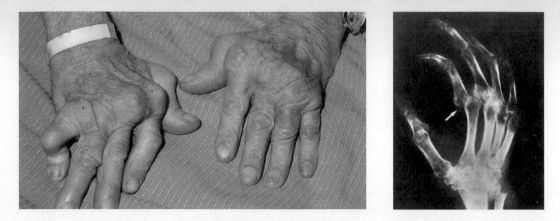

Figure 9-6 A, Advanced joint deformities caused by rheumatoid arthritis. B, Radiograph illustrating destruction of articular surfaces and anterior dislocation of base of index finger (arrow) as a result of joint instability.
Courtesy of Leonard V. Crowley, MD, Century College.

There are numerous potential complications with RA, including lung disease (Antin-Ozerkis, Evans, Rubinowitz, Homer, & Matthay, 2010), increased risk of diabetes (Solomon et al., 2010), and cardiac arrhythmias, specifically atrial fibrillation (Gabriel & Crowson, 2012). Patients with RA need to be educated and cautioned to pay attention to any signs and symptoms of these potential diseases and to seek medical attention, and not "write them off" to an RA exacerbation.

Assessment and Diagnosis

Signs and symptoms of RA are systemic and include malaise, fatigue, symmetrical patterns of joint inflammation, pain, stiffness, swelling, gelling (joints stiff after rest), elevated sedimentation rate, presence of serum rheumatoid factor, and elevated white blood cell count (WBC) in the synovial fluid of the inflamed joint. Radiographs will show erosion of the bone. Pain is more prevalent in RA, and joint deformities can cause more debilitation than is generally seen with OA. In addition, RA often strikes in young to middle adulthood, with more degeneration seen over time than with OA.

Interventions

The treatment for RA is similar to OA with the exception that anti-inflammatory and immune-suppressing drugs may play a more important role. DMARDs (disease-modifying antirheumatic drugs) are also used in RA. Historically these drugs were not used until all other medications had been tried; now, however, the DMARDs are often used within 3 months of diagnosis, the intention being to modify the disease process and prevent the deformities and pain associated with the disease (Reuben et al., 2015). These medications may not show results for several months, and nurses should teach patients to recognize signs of infections such as chills, pain, and fever.

Nurses should expect to see many complications associated with arthritis. Some potential nursing diagnoses are pain, impaired physical mobility, fatigue, decreased endurance, powerlessness, self-care deficits, sleep pattern disturbance, depression, impaired coping, social isolation, fear, anxiety, and body-image disturbance. Goals for care include promoting independence within limitations, pain management, and education.

Educational programs for persons with arthritis should include exercise and mobility, education, counseling, individual physical and occupational therapy, and a focus of independence in ADLs with self-care. These types of programs help decrease disability, pain, and the need for assistance, as well as reduce joint tenderness. Pain coping and exercise training may also enhance pain control.

Joint Replacement

Joint replacement is used for several different diagnoses, including fracture, immobility, and *intractable pain*. The two most commonly performed joint replacement surgeries are total hip arthroplasty and total knee arthroplasty. Knee replacements are mainly related to advanced arthritis that causes severe pain and decreased function. Hip replacements may also be done related to arthritis or due to fracture, usually from falling.

Steel, Clark, Lang, Wallace, and Melzer (2008) and Constantinescu, Goucher, Weinstein, and Fraenkel (2009) reported significantly fewer joint replacements done on Hispanics and Blacks than Whites, due to reasons beyond access and financial resources. The researchers suggested that cultural differences, values, and attitudes might also play a role in seeking joint replacement.

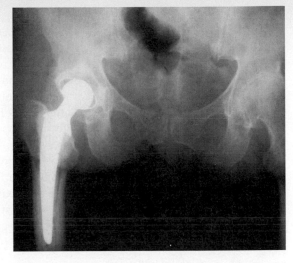

Figure 9-7 Total hip prosthesis.
Courtesy of Leonard V. Crowley, MD, Century College.

Total Hip Arthroplasty/Replacement

Background/Significance

Hip replacement surgery may be indicated when an older person demonstrates lack of function, trouble with ADLs, and continued pain that is not sufficiently addressed with traditional medical therapy. Certainly, those with certain types of hip fractures will be candidates for this surgery also. In women, body weight and older age have been found to be risk factors for needing hip replacement due to OA (National Institute of Arthritis and Musculoskeletal and Skin Diseases, 2003).

Interventions

During hip replacement, a prosthetic device made of metal, plastic, ceramic, or various other substances is substituted for the worn-out, damaged, or fractured portions of the hip. The implant is made of a ball-type device on a stem that fits into the femur. The socket of the pelvis helps hold the ball that is articulated onto the joint (see **Figure 9-7**). During surgery, physicians may choose to cement the prosthesis into the femur or not. Staples are generally used to close the wound, with a nonstick dressing applied. Staples are usually removed 7–10 days after surgery, depending on healing of the wound. Sometimes physicians will order half of the staples removed initially and the other half later. Steri-Strips may be applied to assist with wound edge approximation.

CLINICAL TIP

Although many newer prostheses do not set off metal detectors, patients who travel by airplane after joint replacement should inform TSA officials of their implant before going through metal detectors.

Postoperatively, the person will remain in acute care for several days to a week, and then many older adults may need rehabilitation services as in-patients or outpatients, depending on comorbidities, physical condition, and family support. Weight bearing is progressive and depends upon the physician's orders based on the condition of the bones observed during surgery. It is essential that the nurse and other team members strictly observe weight-bearing instructions (such as toe-touch, partial, or full) to avoid injury to the healing hip. Dislocation of the traditional prosthesis can also result from not following routine hip precautions after surgery. Routine hip precautions include not crossing the legs at the knees or ankles, not bending in a chair more than 90 degrees, keeping a pillow between the knees (to maintain abduction) until determined by the physician, and avoiding lying on the operative side until the physician gives permission to do so. Surgical procedures for total hip arthroplasty continue to advance. Minimally invasive surgery may require the same precautions as traditional surgery depending upon the approach of the surgeon. Single incision using a frontal approach is being done in select hospitals across the United States and has the advantage of not requiring mobility limitations immediately after surgery (Alcelik et al., 2012; Neville, Dvorkin, Chittenden, & Fromm, 2008; Wong et al., 2011).

Nursing instruction to patients and family members should include watching for signs and symptoms of wound infection. Patients should report any redness, swelling, drainage, or odor from the operative site. A small amount of brownish drainage from the site a few days postoperatively is normal. Fever or malaise could also be signs of infection and should be promptly reported to the physician. These nursing implications apply to all surgical procedures.

Additionally, reminders about routine hip precautions (as indicated by the procedure performed), exercises, and ambulation as indicated by the physical therapist, as well as traveling implications, should be given. Some prostheses will cause the alarm at airport security to go off. Teach patients to inform security personnel of their hip prosthesis prior to entering the security gate.

Total Knee Arthroplasty/Replacement

Background/Significance

Similar to hip replacement, knee replacement is done when a person is experiencing decreased range of motion, trouble walking or climbing stairs, and increased degeneration of the joint so as to impair quality of life. This most often occurs as a result of arthritis (either osteo-or rheumatoid arthritis).

Interventions

Total knee replacement (TKR) surgery involves resurfacing or removing the distal portion of the femur that articulates with the end of the shin bone. The prosthesis consists of metal and plastic or similar materials that are cemented onto the newly resurfaced areas of the articulating bones. Although often done under general anesthetic, this surgery can also be performed under spinal anesthesia. Sometimes blood loss is significant, so patients may be asked to donate their own blood ahead of time to be given back to them in the event it is needed. In addition, a growing trend is toward bilateral knee replacement in those persons requiring both knees to be surgically repaired. The benefits of this are the one-time operative anesthetic and room costs, and many physicians feel recovery from bilateral replacement is similar to single replacement. However, the pain and lack of mobility, as well as the significant increase in the assistance needed after surgery when a bilateral replacement is done, may make this less than ideal for most older patients. Surgical procedures for TKR have not evolved quite as rapidly as total hip arthroplasy; however, additional procedures include partial knee replacement, which might be performed in lieu of TKR. Despite the procedure, nursing care remains constant.

Discomfort after knee surgery is generally severe in the first few days. Nurses should encourage patients to use cold packs on the operative area for the first day and take pain and sleeping medications as ordered. In addition, alternative therapies such as guided imagery have been shown to help with pain management (Posadzi & Ernst, 2011). Many joint replacement patients feel a loss of control and independence. Nurses can help the recovery process by maintaining a professional therapeutic relationship with patients. This has been shown to assist older persons in regaining their sense of independence (Heikkinen, Helena, Taina, Anne, & Sanna, 2008).

CLINICAL TIP

When caring a patient with joint replacement, ask the therapist what the ideal extension and flexion for that particular patient should be.

Therapy will begin immediately in the acute care hospital. Although weight bearing does not usually occur until 24 hours after surgery, sitting in a chair and using a continuous passive motion machine (CPM), if ordered, will ease recovery. The use of a CPM is generally based on the surgeon's preference. There is research to support it, as well as studies indicating that walking soon after surgery has an equal effect and makes the CPM unnecessary. However, in cases of an older person who may not have the mobility skills initially after surgery that a younger person would, a CPM may be beneficial to keep the joint flexible and decrease pain.

Nursing implications include teaching the patient about signs and symptoms of infection, care of the surgical site (if staples are still present), pain management, and expectations for recovery. A range of motion from 0–90 degrees is the minimum needed for normal functioning. Most prostheses will allow up to about 120 degrees of flexion, though 110 degrees is considered satisfactory range of motion after knee replacement. After discharge, a walker is usually used in the first few weeks, followed by light activities 6 weeks after surgery. In addition, the patient's spouse may experience feelings of being overwhelmed due to role transitions that occur after surgery and during the recovery period. Nurses can help facilitate this transition by providing education and discussing realistic expectations (Walker, 2012).

Amputation

Background/Significance

Amputation is an acquired condition that results in the loss of a limb, typically from disease, injury, and/or associated surgery. Approximately 185,000 amputations occur each year in the U.S. There are almost 2 million people living with limb loss in the United States. The main causes of amputation are vascular disease (54%) and trauma (45%) (Amputee Coalition, 2016).

Risk Factors/Warning Signs

Most amputations involve the lower extremities, above or below the knee. The greatest risk factor for amputation is diabetes with accompanying peripheral vascular disease, with African Americans having a 4 times greater rate of amputation than Whites with diabetes (Amputee Coalition, 2016). Advanced age and the incidence of diabetes in the elderly make this a potential problem in the older age group. HgbA1c level may be a significant predictor of foot amputation.

Assessment/Diagnosis

In the acute phase of recovery after surgery, it is important to prevent contractures of the knee joint (if present) and attempt to maintain normal muscle power and range of motion in remaining joints. The limb should not be hung over the bedside or placed in a dependent position. Both in acute care and rehabilitation, the stump should be conditioned to prepare for the wearing of a prosthesis. In certain circumstances, an older person may choose, in consultation with the physician, not to wear a prosthesis. This generally occurs when there are other health issues, such as poor balance from another disease or disorder that would make falling and injury more likely with prosthetic use.

Interventions

Initially, there may be drainage from the surgical site, and a sterile dressing will be kept in place and changed at least daily. Eventually, the staples or sutures will be removed and a thick, black eschar will form at the amputation site and gradually come off. An Ace wrap or stump shrinker sock (elastic) is used to help prepare the stump for wearing the prosthesis. Several factors should be considered when preparing the stump to wear a prosthesis. These include a movable scar, lack of tenderness/sensitivity, a conical shape, firm skin, and lack of edema. All of these can be achieved by proper wrapping of the stump to maximize shrinkage and minimize swelling. The prone position, if tolerable, is an excellent way to promote full extension of the residual limb.

It is also important for the person to begin therapy right away. The higher/more proximal the amputation, the higher the energy expenditure to walk (Lusardi, Jorge, & Nielson, 2013). The elderly generally have a 40% decrease in speed and 80% more energy expenditure. When using the prosthesis at first, an older adult may tire easily. Be sure to take into account any coexisting problems, such as cardiopulmonary disease, when considering energy expenditure. The newest technologies allow prosthetics to be light, durable, and more comfortable.

Nurses will need to teach patients and families about stump care, mobility, adaptation, coping, and self-care. Home maintenance, dealing with complications and/or additional health problems, wear and tear on non-weight-bearing joints, adapting to the environment, accessibility, stigma, depression, role changes, decreased energy, and chronic pain are all issues to be aware of related to amputation. It is likely that the person with lower extremity amputation will experience some shoulder problems over time due to the additional stress on this non-weight-bearing joint. Remember that alteration in body image is a significant hurdle to overcome for some individuals. *Phantom limb pain,* or pain sensations in the nonexistent limb, is more common after traumatic amputations and may last for weeks after amputation. Massage and medications may help with this type of pain control (Reuben et al., 2015). Additionally, proper wrapping of the stump (in a figure-eight wrap) may help decrease the chance of phantom limb pain later (Kalapatapu, 2012).

In general, older persons with amputation may return to a normal quality of life with some adaptations. The care provided by nurses and physicians in rehabilitation after amputation may make the difference in the person's ability to cope with the changes that result after surgery. Geriatric nurses can facilitate the transition back into the community after amputation by educating patients and families about resources to assist with adaptation.

Sensory Impairments

Although many normal aging changes occur in the sensory system, most of the common abnormalities seen in the elderly are related to vision. The CDC (2016e) estimates that 3.4 million people in the U.S. are legally blind with 21 million having visual impairments. About 90% of the world's visually impaired persons are of low income (WHO, 2014). Some of the most common age-related vision problems for older adults are cataracts, glaucoma, macular degeneration, and diabetic neuropathy. This section will discuss these impairments and others. As diseases related to the senses of touch, hearing, and taste are rare, these will not be discussed here. The other most common sensory problem in older adults is chronic sinusitis, which will also be discussed.

Cataracts

Background

Cataracts are responsible for 51% of world blindness, representing about 20 million people (World Health Organization [WHO], 2010). More than 90% of cataracts are age-related. Cataracts are so common in older adults that some almost consider them an inevitable consequence of old age and often fail to report during the history and physical. According to the University of Washington, Department of Ophthalmology (2008), 400,000 new cases of cataract development are diagnosed each year, 1,350,000 cataract extractions are currently performed each year, 3,700,000 visits to a doctor related to cataracts occur each year, and 5,500,000 people have visual obstruction due to cataracts.

Risk Factors/Warning Signs

Advancing age is the biggest risk factor for the development of cataracts. Other risk factors include diabetes, uveitis, intraocular tumor, long-term use of medications such as corticosteroids, excessive exposure to sunlight, blunt or penetrating trauma, and excessive exposure to heat or radiation. Tobacco use, family history of cataracts, high alcohol intake, and lack of dietary antioxidants also puts the person at risk for cataract development (Gerzevitz, Porter, & Dunphy, 2011). The etiology is thought to be from oxidative damage to lens protein that occurs with aging. Although about half of people between 65 and 75 years of age have cataracts, they are most common in those over age 75 (70%).

Assessment and Diagnosis

Cataracts cause no pain or discomfort and may be manifested by gradual opacity of the lens, which affects the ability to see clearly. This causes decreased visual acuity, sensitivity to glare, and altered color perception. Older adults may not be aware of the problem until visual changes occur. They may report blurred or distorted vision or complain of glare when driving at night. The person may present with a fall due to visual changes. Some older adults will disclose that their reading vision has improved and they no longer need reading glasses, something called "second sight." Eventually the pupil changes color to a cloudy white. Generally, the most common objective finding is decreased visual acuity, such as that measured with a Snellen eye chart. The patient should be referred to an ophthalmologist for further evaluation and consideration of surgery.

Interventions

Although changes in eyeglasses are the first option, when quality of life becomes affected, the most effective treatment for cataracts is surgery. Surgery is relatively safe and usually is done as an outpatient procedure. The opaque lens is removed and replaced with an artificial intraocular lens. This is the most common operation among older adults, and more than 95% of them have better vision after surgery (WHO, 2014). The benefits of surgery include improved visual acuity, depth perception, and peripheral vision, leading to better outcomes related to ADLs, quality of life, and reduced risk of falls. Complications associated with surgery are rare but include retinal detachment, infection, and macular edema. The lens is removed through an incision in the eye and an intraocular lens is inserted. The surgical incision is either closed with sutures or can heal itself. After surgery, patients will need to avoid bright sunlight; wear wrap-around sunglasses for a short time; and avoid straining, lifting, or bending. Cataract surgery today offers a safe and effective treatment to maintain independence and improve quality of life for older adults.

Glaucoma

Background

Glaucoma is a group of degenerative eye diseases with various causes that leads to progressive optic neuropathy, in which the optic nerve is damaged by high *intraocular pressure* (IOP), resulting in blindness. Glaucoma is a leading cause of visual impairment and the second leading cause of blindness in the United States, and occurs more often in those over 40, with an increased incidence with age (3–4% in those over age 70) (Fingeret, 2009; Kennedy-Malone et al., 2001). It is the cause of 12% of the world's blindness (WHO, 2016).

Risk Factors/Warning Signs

Unlike cataracts, there are some ethnic distinctions with the development of glaucoma. African Americans tend to develop it earlier than Caucasians, and females more often than males. Glaucoma is more common in African Americans, Asian Americans, and Alaska Natives. Other contributing factors include eye trauma, small cornea, small anterior chamber, family history, cataracts, and some medications (Kennedy-Malone et al., 2014).

Assessment and Diagnosis

Although the cause is unknown, glaucoma results from pupillary blockage that limits flow of aqueous humor, causing a rise in intraocular pressure. Two major types are noted here: acute and chronic. Acute glaucoma is also called closed angle or narrow angle. Signs and symptoms include severe eye pain in one eye, blurred vision, seeing colored halos around lights, red eye, headache, nausea, and vomiting. Symptoms may be associated with emotional stress. Acute glaucoma is a medical emergency and the patient should seek emergency help immediately. Blindness can occur from prolonged narrow angle glaucoma.

Chronic glaucoma, also called open angle or primary open angle, is more common than acute (90% of cases are this type), affecting over 2 million people in the United States. One million people probably have glaucoma and don not know it, and 10 million people have above normal intraocular pressure that may lead to glaucoma if not treated (University of Washington, Department of Ophthalmology, 2008). This type of glaucoma occurs gradually. Peripheral vision is slowly impaired. Signs and symptoms include tired eyes, headaches, misty vision, seeing halos around lights, and worse symptoms in the morning. Glaucoma often involves only one eye, but may occur in both.

Interventions

Since there is no scientific evidence of preventative strategies, early detection in those at risk is important. Treatment is essential to prevent loss of vision, because once vision has been lost to glaucoma, it cannot be restored. Diagnosis is made using a *tonometer* to measure IOP; normal IOP is 10–21 mm Hg. Ophthalmological examination will reveal changes in the color and contour of the optic nerve when glaucoma is present. *Gonioscopy* (direct exam), which is performed by an optometrist or ophthalmologist, provides another means of evaluation.

Treatment is aimed at reducing IOP. Medications to decrease pressure may be given, and surgical iridectomy to lower the IOP may prevent future episodes of acute glaucoma. In chronic glaucoma, there is no cure, so treatment is aimed at managing IOP through medication and eyedrops. Nurses should regularly evaluate if the person is consistently using the eyedrops as prescribed and, if not, determine why and develop strategies to improve medication adherence. In some cases it may be appropriate to have patients demonstrate how they administer the eyedrops. In addition, older adults should be assessed for safety related to visual changes and also reminded to schedule and attend regular visits with their ophthalmologist.

Macular Degeneration

Background

Age-related macular degeneration (ARMD) is the most common cause of reading, close-up vision, and visual impairment for those over age 65, affecting about 1.8 million Americans over the age of 40 (CDC, 2016e). Macular degeneration occurs in approximately 10% of long-term care residents age 66–74 years and increases to 30% for those residents age 75–85 (Stefanacci, 2007).

Risk Factors/Warning Signs

Age is a major risk factor; 3.8% of Americans between the ages of 50 and 59 years have some form of ARMD, with about 14.4% of older adults ages 70–79 having the disease (American Health Assistance Foundation, 2012). Other risk factors include smoking, hypertension, diabetes mellitus, family history of macular degeneration, female gender, obesity, Caucasian, prolonged exposure to ultraviolet light, and diet high in fat and/or low in nutrients and antioxidants. Inactivity has also been linked to ARMD, which is most likely related to the increased risk for cardiovascular disease.

Assessment and Diagnosis

Macular degeneration results from damage or breakdown of the macula and subsequent loss of central vision. Generally associated with the aging process, it can also result from injury or infection. Two types are noted: dry (nonexudative) and wet (exudative). Dry macular degeneration affects 90% of those with the disease (CDC, 2016e) and has a better prognosis. The dry type progresses slowly, with more subtle changes in vision than the wet type, which comes on suddenly and may cause more severe loss in vision. The signs and symptoms of ARMD are decreased central vision, seeing images as distorted, decreased color vision, and sometimes a central scotoma (a large, dark spot in the center of vision).

Case Study 9-6

Mrs. Booker has recently been diagnosed with ARMD. She is distressed to feel she is going blind and there is nothing she can do about it. She expresses these frustrations to the nurse and asks for help.

Questions:

1. What should the nurse's response be?
2. What initial adaptations need to be made early in the disease process?
3. Are there any things that Mrs. Booker can do now to help modify her environment for this progressive vision loss? What would those things be?
4. To which resources should the nurse refer Mrs. Booker for further information and support?

Interventions

Although there is no cure for macular degeneration, some new therapies show promise (see **Case Study 9-6**). Photodynamic therapy uses a special laser to seal leaking blood vessels in the eye. Antioxidant vitamins (C, D, E, and beta-carotene) and zinc also seem to slow the progress of the disease (Age-Related Eye Disease Study Authors, 2001). Retinal cell transplantation or regeneration works by harvesting cells from the body and injecting them into diseased macular sites in the hope that new and healthy cells will grow, thus reversing the damage caused by ARMD.

New medications have been approved for the treatment of macular degeneration. Ranibizumab (Lucentis) was approved in 2006, and not only has it shown promise in stopping the progression of macular degeneration, but approximately 50% of the patients taking the medication have shown an improvement in their vision to 20/40. It is given by injection into the eye by an ophthalmologist every 4 weeks for 2 years. Bevacizumab (Avastin) has been used in the treatment of wet macular degeneration and was widely used prior to the advent of ranibizumab. In 2011 Eylea (aflibercept) injection was approved by the FDA to treat the wet form of ARMD. Pegaptanib (Macugen) was approved in 2004 for the treatment of neovascular macular degeneration. It is also injected directly into the eye and targets endothelial growth factor (Stefanacci, 2007).

Chances are that most gerontological nurses will care for older adults with ARMD. Initially, small changes in the environment should be encouraged, such as better lighting in hallways, minimizing glare from lamps or shiny floors, and decorating living spaces in contrasting colors (Kennedy-Malone, Fletcher, Martin-Plank, 2014). Visual adaptive devices such as magnifying glasses and reading lamps may provide temporary help as vision worsens. Auditory devices such as books on tape and adaptation of the environment to the visual impairment may help maintain independence. Nurses should be aware of the treatments being researched (see **Box 9-7**) and can assure patients that although there is no cure at present, there is hope for the future (see **Box 9-8**). Encourage patients to exercise; avoid overexposure to the sun; wear sunglasses and a hat; maintain a healthy weight; eat a nutritious diet that includes leafy green vegetables, fruit, fish, and foods containing vitamins D, E, and C, beta-carotene, and omega 3-fatty acids. It is also important that blood pressure and blood sugar are controlled.

It is crucial to remind patients not to just assume that visual changes are "due to aging," but that they may be treatable. Many people avoid seeking treatment for fear that nothing can be done and that they could lose their driver's license.

BOX 9-7   Resources for Those with Visual Impairments

American Academy of Ophthalmology

    P.O. Box 7424

    San Francisco, CA 94120-7424

    415-561-8500

    http://www.aao.org

American Council of the Blind

    1155 15th Street, NW, Suite 720

    Washington, DC 20005

    http://www.acb.org

American Printing House for the Blind

    P.O. Box 6985

    1839 Franklin Avenue

    Louisville, KY 40206

    http://www.aph.org

EyeCare America

    A Public Service Foundation of the American

    Academy of Ophthalmology

    1-877-887-6327

    1-800-222-3937

    http://www.eyecareamerica.org

Lighthouse International

    111 East 59th Street

    New York, NY 10022-1202

    1-800-334-5497

    1-800-829-0500

    http://www.lighthouse.org

Macular Degeneration Foundation

    http://www.eyesight.org

National Eye Institute

    31 Center Drive MSC 2510

    Bethesda, MD 20892-2510

    301-496-5248

    http://www.nei.nih.gov

BOX 9-8   Web Exploration

Visit Lighthouse International at http://www.lighthouse.org and read about new software that may assist persons with visual problems.

Diabetic Retinopathy

Background

Diabetes has become an epidemic in the United States. *Diabetic retinopathy,* a complication of diabetes mellitus, is a leading cause of blindness among adults age 25 to 74. Approximately 700,000 have proliferative diabetic retinopathy with an annual incidence of about 65,000 (Klein, Knudtson, Lee, Gangnan, & Klein, 2009). Blindness results from the breakage of tiny vessels in the retina as a complication of diabetes and generally affects both eyes. The exact mechanism is not known, but the longer a person has diabetes, the more likely he or she is to suffer visual impairment (WHO, 2016a). Currently approximately 7 million diabetics suffer from diabetic retinopathy, 700,000 are at risk for blindness, and 16 million are prime targets for blinding disorders (University of Washington, Department of Ophthalmology, 2008).

Risk Factors/Warning Signs

There are no early warning signs of diabetic retinopathy, so it is essential that older adults with diabetes have a dilated eye exam each year. Early diagnosis and treatment can prevent much of the blindness that occurs from this disorder. Risk factors include "duration of diabetes, level of glycemia, presence of high blood pressure, dependence on insulin, pregnancy, levels of selected serum lipids, nutritional and genetic factors" (WHO, 2016a, para 3).

Assessment and Diagnosis

During the eye exam the eye care professional will do a visual acuity test, a dilated eye exam, and tonometry. If a person complains of seeing spots floating in the visual field, bleeding may be occurring and the person should see an eye doctor as soon as possible.

There are four stages of diabetic retinopathy. These appear in **Table 9-27**. Of the four stages, *proliferative retinopathy* is the most severe. As new, fragile, and abnormal blood vessels grow to compensate for the blocked vessels in the retina, these vessels may leak blood into the eye, causing swelling of the macula and blurred vision. This is what causes much of the blindness seen with diabetic retinopathy (Kennedy-Malone, Fletcher, Martin-Plank, 2014).

Interventions

The first three stages of diabetic retinopathy are not treated. The first priority in treating proliferative retinopathy is to treat the cause of the vitreous hemorrhage itself. For patients with diabetes, glycemic control is essential. Those with hypertension should have a goals of a BP less than 130/80 for those with diabetes and 140/90 for those without diabetes (Kennedy-Malone, Fletcher, & Martin-Plank, 2014). For more severe cases of bleeding in the eye, a *vitrectomy* may be needed. When blood collects in the center of the eye, a vitrectomy allows removal of the vitreous gel that has blood in it through a small incision in the eye. The blood-contaminated vitreous gel is replaced with a saline-type solution. This is often done as an outpatient procedure. The patient will need to wear an eye patch for days to weeks and use medicated eyedrops to prevent infection. After a vitrectomy, the person's eye may be red and sensitive for some time.

The most important nursing consideration in caring for older persons who may be at risk for diabetic retinopathy is to emphasize prevention of this complication. Treatment becomes necessary with more severe cases, so the best treatment is prevention through regular eye exams, good control of blood sugars, monitoring hypertension, and controlling cholesterol levels. The nurse should encourage the older adult with diabetes to develop a good working relationship with a trusted eye care professional.

TABLE 9-27	Four Stages of Diabetic Retinopathy	
Stage	**Description**	**Pathophysiology**
Stage 1	Mild nonproliferative retinopathy	Microaneurysms in retina
Stage 2	Moderate nonproliferative retinopathy	Blockage of some blood vessels supplying retina
Stage 3	Severe nonproliferative retinopathy	Blockage of many blood vessels supplying retina; retina is deprived of needed circulation
Stage 4	Proliferative retinopathy	Advanced stage; new blood vessels that are abnormal and easily breakable form to compensate for blockage of circulation to retina; these vessels may break and leak to cause macular edema and blurred vision

Data from National Eye Institute. (2015). Facts about diabetic eye disease. Retrieved from https://nei.nih.gov/health/diabetic/retinopathy.

Retinal Detachment

Although not as common as the other visual problems discussed, *retinal detachment* may occur in the older adult. It can be the result of trauma to the eye. Symptoms may be gradual or sudden and may look like spots moving across the eye, blurred vision, light flashes, or a curtain drawing. If an older person presents with such symptoms, he or she should seek immediate medical help. Keep the person quiet to minimize further detachment. Surgery may be required to save vision.

Corneal Ulcer

Corneal ulcers are more common in the elderly than in younger age groups due to decreased tearing that occurs with normal aging. Also, many elderly patients have worn contact lenses, either for a very long time or as a result of cataract surgery; improper cleaning or accidents can occur when placing the lenses, which can cause corneal abrasions. The ulcers may also result from inflammation of the cornea related to stroke, fever, irritation, dehydration, or a poor diet. Corneal ulcers are difficult to treat and may leave scars that affect vision. Signs of corneal ulcer may include bloodshot eye, photophobia, and complaint of irritation. The nurse should encourage the older person to seek prompt assistance from an eye care professional.

Chronic Sinusitis

Background

One of the common health complaints of the elderly is chronic sinusitis. About 14.1% of Americans 65 and older report suffering from chronic sinusitis; for those 75 years and older, the rate is slightly lower at 13.5% (American Academy of Otolaryngology, 2012). Age-related physiological and functional changes that occur can cause restrictions to the airflow. This results from irritants blocking drainage of the sinus cavities, leading to infection.

Risk Factors/Warning Signs

Symptoms include a severe cold, sneezing, cough (that is often worse at night), hoarseness, diminished sense of smell, discolored nasal discharge, postnasal drip, headache, facial pain, fatigue, malaise, and fever (Rudmik & Soler, 2015).

Assessment and Diagnosis

Upon physical examination, the person may complain of pain on palpation of the sinus areas, and edema and redness of the nasal mucosa may be evident. Allergies, common cold, and dental problems should be ruled out for differential diagnosis. When symptoms continue over a period of weeks and up to 3 months and are often recurring, chronic sinusitis should be suspected. A CT scan of the sinuses will show areas of inflammation.

Interventions

Treatment for chronic sinusitis is with antibiotics, decongestants, and analgesics for pain. Inhaled corticosteroids may be needed to reduce swelling and ease breathing (Rudmik & Soler, 2015). Irrigation with over-the-counter normal saline nose spray is often helpful and may be done two to three times per day. The person with chronic sinusitis should drink plenty of fluids to maintain adequate hydration and avoid any environmental pollutants such as cigarette smoke or other toxins. Chronic sinusitis is a condition that many older adults wrestle with their entire life. Avoidance of precipitating factors for each individual should be encouraged.

Integumentary Problems

Many changes occur in the integumentary system with normal aging. These are discussed in Chapter 4. One of the most common problems in the elderly is a skin breakdown due to pressure ulcers. The treatment of pressure ulcers is discussed at length in Chapter 18. Skin cancer and herpes zoster infection (shingles) are also common ailments. These two disorders will be briefly addressed here.

Skin Cancers

Background

There are three major types of skin cancer: basal cell, squamous cell, and malignant melanoma (MM).

Basal cell carcinoma (see **Figure 9-8**) is the most common skin cancer, accounting for 65–85% of cases (Kennedy-Malone et al., 2014). According to the American Cancer Society (2016a), about 5,4 million cases of basal cell and squamous cell carcinoma are diagnosed each year. Squamous cell carcinoma is more common in African Americans and is also less serious than

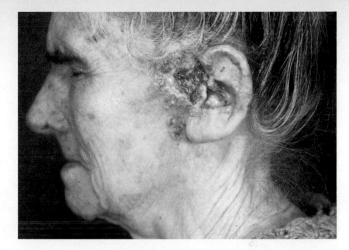

Figure 9-8 Basal cell carcinoma.
Courtesy of Leonard V. Crowley, MD, Century College.

malignant melanoma. It accounts for approximately 200,000–300,000 new cases yearly. Malignant melanoma accounts for only 3% of all skin cancers, but it is responsible for the majority of deaths from skin cancer. Older adults are 10 times more likely to get MM than adults under age 40 (Johnson & Taylor, 2012). About 8,420 people were estimated to die from malignant melanoma in 2008.

Risk Factors/Warning Signs

Older adults are more susceptible to skin cancers because of a variety of factors. These include exposure to carcinogens over time (such as UV radiation) and immunosenescence, or a decline in immune function. The major risk factor for all types of skin cancer is sun exposure.

Assessment and Diagnosis

Annual physical examinations should include inspection of the skin for lesions. Older adults should be taught to report any suspicious areas on their skin to the physician. Persons should particularly look for changes in shape, color, and whether a lesion is raised or bleeds.

Basal Cell Carcinoma

Basal cell carcinoma (BCC) is the most common kind of skin cancer. It is often found on the head or face, or other areas exposed to the sun. Although there are different forms of BCC, the nodular type is most common, and appears as a raised, firm, papule that is pearly or shiny with a rolled edge (Johnson & Taylor, 2012). Patients often complain that these lesions bleed and scab easily. When treated early, it is easily removed through surgery and is not life threatening, though it is often recurring.

Squamous Cell Carcinoma

Squamous cell carcinoma (SCC) also appears as lesion on areas of the body exposed to the sun, or from other trauma such as radiation. HPV is a risk factor of SCC, and metastasis is more common than with BCC. The lesions of SCC appear scaly, pink, and thicker than BCC. Their borders may be more irregular and the lesions may look more like an ulceration.

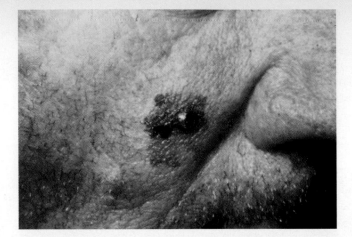

Figure 9-9 Malignant melanoma.
Courtesy of Leonard V. Crowley, MD, Century College.

Malignant Melanoma

Malignant melanoma has a more distinctive appearance than other types of skin cancer. The areas appear asymmetric with irregular borders, a variety of colors (including black, purplish, and pink), and size greater than 6 mm. Malignant melanoma is often identified with the ABCDE method (see **Figure 9-9**) and accounts for the vast majority of deaths from skin cancer.

Interventions

The best treatment for skin cancer in the elderly is prevention. All older persons, especially those with fair skin who are prone to sunburn, should wear sunblock and protective clothing. Most skin cancers, when treated early, have a good prognosis.

All skin lesions larger than 6 mm, or those with any of the ABCDE signs, should be referred for biopsy. There are many nonsurgical interventions. These include cryotherapy, radiotherapy (for superficial BCC or SCC) electrodessication and curettage, and topical treatments. Topical treatments are generally not as effective as more aggressive interventions, but research is ongoing in this area.

The prognosis for MM depends on the extent and staging of the tumor, but when caught very early, the cure rate is nearly 100%. Malignant melanoma presenting in older adults is often more advanced and aggressive. Malignant melanoma metastases sites are typically the lymph nodes, liver, lung, and brain (Johnson & Taylor, 2012). Surgical treatment is required in malignant melanoma, with chemotherapy and radiation. Adjuvant treatments for MM are also often used.

Herpes Zoster (Shingles)

Background

Commonly known as shingles, *herpes zoster* is the reactivation of the virus that causes chicken pox. The CDC (2016d) states that 1 in 3 people in the U.S. will get shingles in their lifetime and the risk increases over the age of 50. Older persons may be infected with this latent varicella virus after initial exposure to it in the form of chicken pox. The virus then lays dormant in the neurons until it is reactivated, often due to immunosuppression, when it appears in the form of painful vesicles along the sensory nerves. Herpes zoster occurs in both men and women equally, with no specific ethnic variations, but is more common in the elderly and those who are immunosuppressed

Risk Factors/Warning Signs

Risk factors for developing shingles are age over 50 years, stress, and a suppressed immune system. For many older women particularly, emotional or psychological stress can trigger reactivations.

Signs and symptoms of herpes zoster include painful lesions that erupt on the sensory nerve path, usually beginning on the chest or face. These weepy vesicles get pustular and crusty over several days, with healing occurring in 2–4 weeks (Kennedy-Malone et al., 2014).

Assessment and Diagnosis

Diagnosis can be made by clinical appearance of the lesions and a history of onset. A scraping will confirm some type of herpes virus. The most common complaint of those with herpes zoster is severe pain that usually subsides in 3–5 weeks (NINDS, 2015). Postherpetic neuralgia, a complication of herpes zoster, may last 6–12 months after the lesions disappear and may involve the dermatome, thermal sensory deficits, allodynia (the perception of pain where pain should not be), and/or severe sensory loss, all of which can be very distressing for the patient.

Interventions

Antiviral medications such as acyclovir are used to treat shingles, but must be given within 48 hours of the eruption of the lesion. Topical ointments may help with pain and itching. Pain medications, particularly acetaminophen, are appropriate for pain management in older adults. Persons with pain that lasts past 6 weeks after the skin lesions are gone and that is described as sharp, burning, or constant require reevaluation by a physician. As of March 2011, a preventive vaccine was approved for persons over age 50 (NINDS, 2015) that cuts risk of acquiring shingles in half. About 28% of older adults took the vaccine in 2014 (CDC, 2016d).

Nursing interventions for the older adult with shingles are largely to recommend rest and comfort. The patient should be advised to seek medical attention as soon as he or she suspects shingles, in order to receive the best results from acyclovir. The virus will run its course, but the person is contagious while vesicles are weepy. Persons should not have direct contact (even clothing) with pregnant women, people who have not had chicken pox, other elderly persons, or those with suppressed immune systems. The older person with shingles may experience concerns with pain management and feel a sense of isolation, particularly if they live alone. Arranging for a family member or friend who does not have a high risk of infection to check on the older person at home is advisable. Zostavax, a vaccine for shingles, has become available, and it is recommended for all persons age 60 or older. At this time it is covered by Medicare (see **Case Study 9-7**).

Case Study 9-7

Eloise Mitchell is a 90-year-old female who lives alone in a senior living apartment. She has three children, none of whom live nearby. Although she has been in good health, Ms. Mitchell has recently experienced weight loss and frequent "colds." She was recently diagnosed with shingles and comes to you, the nurse for the senior living complex, for some help. How would you respond to the following questions from Ms. Mitchell?

Questions:

1. What caused the shingles?
2. The doctor says it's like chicken pox, but I wasn't exposed to that, so how did I get it?
3. Why is there so much pain with this problem? Is there anything I can do to get relief? The medication doesn't help that much.
4. Can I really have sores on the bottom of my feet and in my mouth?
5. How long am I contagious?
6. When will I start to feel better? I had a friend who was under the weather for months! Is that usual?
7. Can I ever get this again? If so, how can I prevent it? It's awful!

Endocrine/Metabolic Disorders

Two of the most common disorders in this category among older adults are diabetes and hypothyroidism. These will be discussed in this section.

Diabetes Mellitus

Background

Diabetes mellitus is a common metabolic disorder that affects carbohydrate, lipid, and protein metabolism. It is estimated that about 8.3% (25.8 million) of persons in the United States have diabetes mellitus (American Diabetes Association, 2013). There are two major types of diabetes, type 1 (T1DM) and type 2 (T2DM). T1DM is characterized by autoimmune destruction of the insulin-producing beta cells of the pancreas, leading to a deficiency of insulin. New-onset of adult T1DM in older adults rarely happens; however, due to better treatment of T1DM, older adults who have been diagnosed at an earlier age are living longer. About 90% of older adults with diabetes have T2DM, which is often related to obesity. T2DM is characterized by hyperglycemia and insulin resistance; however, impaired insulin secretion may also be present. Diabetes mellitus is a major cause of disability and death in the United States, and is the seventh leading cause of death among older adults.

Risk Factors/Warning Signs

The risk of diabetes increases with age (45 years and older). Other risk factors include family history, obesity, race (African Americans, Hispanics, Native Americans, Asian Americans, Pacific Islanders), hypertension (blood pressure greater than or equal to 140/90 mm Hg), less "good" cholesterol (less than 35 mg/dl), lack of exercise, polycystic ovary syndrome, having a history of delivering large babies (≥9 pounds), personal history of gestational diabetes, and prediabetes (Laberge, Edgren, & Frey, 2011). Type 2 is the most common type. About 86 million Americans have prediabetes, which if not addressed, may result in Type 2 diabetes within 5 years (CDC, 2014). The risk of death from DM is significantly higher among older Mexican American, African American, and Native American women when compared to Whites. The CDC (2014) names obesity, weight gain, and physical inactivity as the major risk factors for DM among women.

Assessment and Diagnosis

The most common presentation for older adults with T1DM is hyperglycemia. Older adults may not have the classical symptoms such as polydipsia, polyuria, polyphagia, and weight loss; instead, they may have an atypical presentation (Chang & Halter, 2009). They may first present with falls, urinary incontinence, fatigue, or confusion. Because older adults may have T2DM for years before it is diagnosed, they often have macrovascular and microvascular complications at the time of diagnosis, so evaluation of these should be considered at this time.

Interventions

Prevention is the best approach to care, which involves identifying those at risk and encouraging lifestyle change. Older adults with diabetes mellitus have a high risk for complications related to macrovascular disease, microvascular disease, and neuropathy. Macrovascular diseases include coronary heart disease, stroke, and peripheral vascular disease, which can lead to amputation. Microvascular diseases are chronic kidney disease, which is the most common cause of end-stage renal disease, and diabetic retinopathy, which can lead to blindness. Peripheral neuropathy presents as uncomfortable, painful sensations in the legs and feet that are difficult to treat. A lack of sensation may also be present and contribute to the risk of falls. There is no cure for peripheral neuropathy, and it tends to be a complication for which patients experience daily challenges trying to manage the symptoms. A combination of medication to address pain and interventions by a physical therapist seems to be the best current treatment. Most of the complications of DM seen in the elderly have been discussed elsewhere in this chapter.

Treatment is aimed at helping patients to achieve and maintain glycemic control to decrease risk of complications. The initial treatment approach is to work with the older adult to establish treatment goals aimed at reducing long-term complications. This often requires working within an interprofessional team. Aggressive treatment may be appropriate for most older adults; however, the risk of hypoglycemia is higher in older adults. Older adults with hypoglycemia may have an atypical presentation with acute onset of confusion, dizziness, and weakness instead of tremors or sweating. The best measure of good blood glucose management and controlled blood sugars is HgbA1c levels (glycosylated hemoglobin). This measure of hemoglobin provides insight into the previous 3 months of blood sugar control. If HgbA1c is elevated, it indicates that the blood sugar has been high over time. For most people with diabetes, HgbA1c ≤7% indicates optimal glycemic control; however, due to poor health outcomes, for frail older adults or those with a life expectancy ≤5 years this may not be the best, and HgbA1c of 8% might be more appropriate.

Management is successful when a balance is achieved among exercise, diet, and medications. Medications may be oral hypoglycemics or insulin injection. Insulin injection is used in T1DM and may be prescribed for T2DM because as the person ages, beta-cell function declines. If insulin is needed, it is important to consider if there are visual problems or hand arthritis that limits the dexterity necessary to prepare and inject the medication. For some, a simple regimen such as premeasured doses and easier injection systems (e.g., insulin pens with easy-to-set dosages) is the best. Nurses will need to do a significant amount of teaching (see **Tables 9-28** and **9-29**) regarding the signs and symptoms of hyper-and hypoglycemia and the role of medications in managing blood sugar.

TABLE 9-28   The National Diabetes Education Program's Seven Principles for Management

Principle 1: Find out what type of diabetes you have.
Principle 2: Get regular care for your diabetes.
Principle 3: Learn how to control your diabetes.
Principle 4: Treat high blood sugar.
Principle 5: Monitor your blood sugar level.
Principle 6: Prevent and diagnose long-term diabetes problems.
Principle 7: Get checked for long-term problems and treat them.

Data from National Diabetes Education Program. (n.d.). National Diabetes Education Program (NDEP) guiding principles for diabetes care: For people with diabetes. Retrieved from https://web.stanford.edu/group/usvh/stanford/misc/Diabetes%202.pdf.

TABLE 9-29   Key Areas for Nursing Teaching of Older Persons with Diabetes

Proper nutrition
Exercise
Medications
Signs and symptoms of hyper- and hypoglycemia
Meaning of lab tests: FBS, blood glucose, HgbA1c
Use of a glucometer
Foot care
Importance of adherence to therapeutic regimen
Possible long-term complications
Prevention of complications
Develop a plan of action for when illness occurs

Although much of the teaching done with older adults is usually in the acute care hospital or rehabilitation setting, telephone follow-up calls have been shown to improve patient adherence to diet. Additionally, a significant finding of Kim and Oh's (2003) research was that patients receiving phone calls from the nurse about adherence to the prescribed regimen for diabetes management showed improved HgbA1c over those who did not have follow-up phone calls.

Thorough evaluation of readiness to learn and of the ability of an older person to manage his or her medications must be done. Older adults who need to give themselves insulin injections may experience anxiety about learning this task. Demonstration, repetition, and practice are good techniques for the older age group. Adaptive devices such as magnifiers may help if the syringes are hard to read. A family member should also be taught to give the insulin to provide support and encouragement, although the older adult should be encouraged to remain independent in this skill if possible. A plan for times of sickness and the use of a glucometer to monitor blood sugars will also need to be addressed. Additionally, the dietician may be consulted to provide education for the patient and family on meal planning, calorie counting, carbohydrate counting, and nutrition. Many patients benefit from weight loss, so the nutritionist can assist with dietary planning in this regard also.

CLINICAL TIP

Teach patients with diabetes the importance of checking their feet twice daily and to never go barefoot.

Due to the increased risk of infection and slow healing that result from diabetes, foot care is an essential component in teaching older adults to manage DM. Some experts believe that good preventive foot care would significantly reduce the incidence of amputation in the elderly. Older persons with DM should never go barefoot outside. Extremes in temperature should be avoided. Shoes should be well fitting and not rub. Socks should be changed regularly. Elders should be taught to inspect their feet daily, with a mirror if needed. Corns and ingrown toenails should be inspected and treated by a podiatrist, not by the patient. Older persons should see their podiatrist for a foot inspection at least yearly. Patients should be cautioned that even the smallest foot injury, such as a thorn or blister, can go unnoticed and unfelt—and often results in partial amputations that lead to a cascade of lower extremity problems.

Hypothyroidism

Background

Hypothyroidism results from lack of sufficient thyroid hormone being produced by the thyroid gland. Older adults may have subclinical hypothyroidism, in which the TSH (thyroid-stimulating hormone) is elevated and the T4 (thyroxine or thyroid hormone) is normal. In this condition, the body is trying to stimulate production of more thyroid hormone. Some older adults with this condition will progress to have primary or overt hypothyroidism, which is when the TSH is elevated and T4 is decreased. Hashimoto's disease is the most common cause and represents 90% of all patients with hypothyroidism (American Association of Clinical Endocrinologists, 2005; Woolever & Beutler, 2007), though certain pituitary disorders, medications, and other hormonal imbalances may be causal factors.

Risk Factors/Warning Signs

Older adults may present an atypical picture, but the most common presenting complaints are fatigue and weakness. **Table 9-30** provides additional classic signs and symptoms.

Assessment and Diagnosis

Best practice recommendations say that screening for hypothyroidism in asymptomatic older adults is controversial (Reuben et al., 2015). Diagnosis should include a thorough history and physical; bradycardia and heart

TABLE 9-30   Signs and Symptoms of Hypothyroidism
*Weakness
*Fatigue
Dry skin
Brittle hair
Hair loss
Weight gain (7–20 pounds)
Cold sensitivity
Puffy face
Headache
Difficulty sleeping
Goiter
Trouble breathing or swallowing
Constipation
Ataxia
Depression
Bradycardia
Anorexia

*Primary signs in the elderly; others may or may not be present.
Data from Kennedy-Malone, L. D., Fletcher, K. R., & Martin-Plank, L. (2014). *Advanced practice nursing in the care of older adults.* Philadelphia, PA: F. A. Davis; Reuben, D. B., Herr, K. A., Pacala, J. T., Pollock, B. G., Potter, J. F., & Semla, T. P. (2015). *Geriatrics at your fingertips* (10th ed.). Malden, MA: American Geriatrics Society.

failure are often associated factors. Lab tests should include thyroid and thyroid antibody levels (common to Hashimoto's), and lipids, because hyperlipidemia is also associated with this disorder.

Interventions

Treatment centers on returning the thyroid hormone level to normal. This is done through oral thyroid replacement medication, usually L-thyroxine. In older adults with coexisting cardiovascular disease, starting with the usual doses may exacerbate angina and worsen the underlying heart disease, so it is important to start low and go slow. Titration should be done cautiously, with close monitoring of the older adults response to the medication. The does should be adjusted on 6-week intervals until euthyroid (normal levels of thyroid hormone) is achieved. Once the TSH is within normal limits, checking the TSH should be done every 6 to 12 months to monitor effectiveness and blood levels, because hyperthyroidism is a side effect of this therapy and can have serious implications on the older person's health.

Nurses should teach patients about the importance of taking thyroid medication at the same time each day without missing doses. Sometimes older adults have other problems associated with hypothyroidism, such as bowel dysfunction and depression. Any signs of complicating factors should be reported to the physician, and doctors' appointments for monitoring should be religiously kept. Strategies for managing fatigue and weakness should also be addressed, because some lifestyle modifications may need to be made as treatment is initiated.

Summary

This chapter provided brief and concise snapshots of illnesses, diseases, and health conditions common to older adults. Students and health professionals may learn additional information about these problems in greater detail from other courses or sources. This chapter focused on a review of basic knowledge but added specific information related to older adults who may require interventions related to certain common conditions.

There are several notable conditions commonly seen in older adults that may be the result of a variety of factors, not just one physical problem or disease. These include depression, anxiety, delirium, dementia, and insomnia. Common geriatric syndromes are discussed in separate chapters in this text and readers are encouraged to refer to these for more specific information on these conditions.

Clinical Reasoning Exercises

1. This chapter discusses a great deal of content. Choose one health condition or disease that interests you most and search the Internet site of the organization dedicated to that cause. What resources are available for persons with this problem?

2. Volunteer through your local hospital to help with stroke and/or blood pressure screenings of older adults. Note any common risk factors you observe among the persons that are being screened.

3. Visit a support group related to one of the long-term conditions discussed in this chapter. It might be a stroke survivor's meeting, the breather's club, or a Parkinson's disease group. Listen to the participants and their family members. Write down anything new you learned about how people live with and manage this condition. Talk personally with a family who is living with the condition that you are further investigating. Talk to participants and their family members. Write down anything new you learned about how people live with and manage this condition.

4. Go to your local mall, church, shopping center, restaurant, or other place where seniors living in the community might gather. Listen to casual conversations between older adults. What types of health problems and concerns do they express?

5. Talk to a nurse who works in the emergency room, or to a local cardiologist. Ask what symptoms they have seen in older adult patients who were diagnosed with myocardial infarction. How are these symptoms different from or similar to a classic presentation?

Personal Reflections

1. Of the disorders presented in this chapter, which are the most familiar to you? Which do you feel you need to do more reading about? Have you ever cared for an older patient with any of these problems? Did the information in the text present what you saw as signs and symptoms in this patient?

2. Which of the diseases in this chapter do you feel are most common in the people you take care of? Have you noticed any ethnic or cultural differences in the geographic area where you work?

3. If an older person came to you and wanted to know about one of the diseases in this chapter, what would you tell the person? How is your comfort level with what needs to be taught for each of the disorders in this chapter?

4. Make a list of three diseases that you are least knowledgeable about and re-read that section of this chapter. Memorize the signs and symptoms, and think about the nursing interventions you should use.

References

Agency for Healthcare Research and Quality. (2012). Management of chronic heart failure. A national guideline. Retrieved from http://guideline.gov/content.aspx?id=10587

Agency for Healthcare Research and Quality. (2013). Routine osteoporosis screening recommended for all women over age 65. Retrieved from http://www.ahrq.gov/news/press/pr2011/tfosteopr.htm

Age-Related Eye Disease Study Authors. (2001). A randomized, placebo-controlled, clinical trial of high-dose supplementation with vitamins C and E, beta carotene, and zinc for age-related macular degeneration and vision loss. *Archives of Ophthalmology, 119,* 1417–1436.

Alcelik, I., Sukeik, M., Pollock, R., Misra, A., Naguib, A., & Haddad, F. S. (2012). Comparing the mid-vastus and medial parapatellar approaches in total knee arthroplasty: A meta-analysis of short term outcomes. *Knee, 19*(4), 229–236.

Amella, G. J. (2004). Presentation of illness in older adults. *American Journal of Nursing, 104*(10), 40–51.

American Academy of Otolaryngology. (2012). Head and neck. Retrieved from http://www.entnet.org/

American Association of Clinical Endocrinologists. (2005). Hypothyroidism. Retrieved from http://www.aace.com/publications/guidelines

American Cancer Society. (2017). About stomach cancer. Retrieved from https://www.cancer.org/cancer/stomach-cancer/about/key-statistics.html

American Cancer Society. (2012a). Cancer facts and figures. Retrieved from http://www.cancer.org/acs/groups/content/@epidemiologysurveilance/documents/document/acspc-031941.pdf

American Cancer Society. (2012b). Prostate cancer. Retrieved from http://www.cancer.org/Cancer/ProstateCancer/DetailedGuide/prostate-cancer-diagnosis

American Cancer Society. (2012c). Bladder cancer. Retrieved from http://www.cancer.org/Cancer/BladderCancer/DetailedGuide/bladder-cancer-key-statistics

American Cancer Society. (2012d). American Cancer Society recommendations for early breast cancer detection in women without breast symptoms. Retrieved from http://www.cancer.org/cancer/breastcancer/moreinformation/breastcancerearlydetection/breast-cancer-early-detection-acs-recs

American Cancer Society. (2013a). Pancreatic cancer. Retrieved from http://www.cancer.org/acs/groups/cid/documents/webcontent/003131-pdf.pdf

American Cancer Society. (2013b). Prostate cancer. Retrieved from http://www.cancer.org/cancer/prostatecancer/detailedguide/prostate-cancer-risk-factors

American Cancer Society. (2015). Breast cancer: Facts and figures 2105–2016. Retrieved from http://www.cancer.org/acs/groups/content/@research/documents/document/acspc-046381.pdf

American Cancer Society. (2016a). Key statistics on basal and squamous cell skin cancers. Retrieved from http://www.cancer.org/cancer/skincancer-basalandsquamouscell/detailedguide/skin-cancer-basal-and-squamous-cell-key-statistics

American Cancer Society. (2016b). Key statistics on bladder cancer. Retrieved from http://www.cancer.org/cancer/bladdercancer/detailedguide/bladder-cancer-key-statistics

American Diabetes Association. (2013). Diabetes statistics. Retrieved from http://www.diabetes.org/diabetes-basics/diabetes-statistics/

American Foundation for Urologic Disease. (2008). Bladder cancer. Retrieved from http://www.urologyhealth.org/urology/index.cfm?article=100

American Gastroenterology Association. (2008). Gastroesophageal reflux disease. Retrieved from http://www.gastro.org/wmspage.cfm?parm1=848#GERD?

American Health Assistance Foundation. (2012). About glaucoma. Retrieved from http://www.ahaf.org/glaucoma/

American Heart Association (2011). About peripheral artery disease. Retrieved from http://www.heart.org/HEARTORG/Conditions/More/PeripheralArteryDisease/About-Peripheral-Artery-Disease-PAD_UCM_301301_Article.jsp

American Heart Association. (2012a). Cardiac rehabilitation. Retrieved from http://www.heart.org/HEARTORG/Conditions/More/CardiacRehab/Cardiac-Rehab_UCM_002079_SubHomePage.jsp

American Heart Association. (2012b). *Heart disease and stroke statistics. 2012 update.* Retrieved from http://my.americanheart.org/professional/General/Heart-Stroke-2012-Statistical-Update_UCM_434526_Article.jsp

American Heart Association. (2012c). *Statistical fact sheet 2012 update: African Americans and cardiovascular diseases.* Retrieved from http://www.heart.org/idc/groups/heart-public/@wcm/@sop/@smd/documents/downloadable/ucm_319568.pdf

American Heart Association. (2012e). High blood pressure. Retrieved from http://www.heart.org/idc/groups/heart-public/@wcm/@sop/@smd/documents/downloadable/ucm_319587.pdf

American Lung Association. (2004). Chronic obstructive pulmonary disease (COPD) fact sheet. Retrieved from http://www.lung.org/lung-disease/copd/resources/facts-figures/COPD-Fact-Sheet.html

American Lung Association. (2008). *Pneumonia fact sheet.* Retrieved from http://www.lung.org/lung-disease/influenza/in-depth-resources/pneumonia-fact-sheet.html

American Lung Association. (2016). Lung health and diseases. Retrieved from http://www.lung.org/lung-health-and-diseases/lung-disease-lookup/copd/learn-about-copd/how-serious-is-copd.html

American Lung Association. (n.d. (a)). Learn about pneumonia. Retrieved from http://www.lung.org/lung-health-and-diseases/lung-disease-lookup/pneumonia/learn-about-pneumonia.html

American Lung Association. (n.d. (b)). Pneumonia. Retrieved from http://www.lung.org/lung-health-and-diseases/lung-disease-lookup/pneumonia/

American Lung Association. (n.d. (c)). Understanding COPD. Retrieved from http://www.lung.org/lung-disease/copd/about-copd/understanding-copd.html

American Nurse's Association. (2016). ANA CAUTI prevention tool. Retrieved from http://nursingworld.org/ANA-CAUTI-Prevention-Tool

American Parkinson Disease Foundation. (2013). Basic information about PD. Retrieved from http://www.apdaparkinson.org/publications-information/basic-info-about-pd/

American Stroke Association. (2012b). *Stroke risk factors.* Retrieved from http://www.strokeassociation.org/STROKEORG/AboutStroke/UnderstandingRisk/Understanding-Stroke-Risk_UCM_308539_SubHomePage.jsp

American Stroke Association. (2012c). *Stroke treatments.* Retrieved from http://www.strokeassociation.org/STROKEORG/AboutStroke/Treatment/Treatment_UCM_310892_Article.jsp

American Stroke Association. (2016). *Warning signs.* Retrieved from http://www.strokeassociation.org/STROKEORG/WarningSigns/Stroke-Warning-Signs-and-Symptoms_UCM_308528_SubHomePage.jsp

American Urological Association. (2017). Benign prostatic hyperplasia. Retrieved from https://www.auanet.org/education/guidelines/benign-prostatic-hyperplasia.cfm

American Urological Association Foundation. (2008). The management of localized prostate cancer. Retrieved from http://www.auanet.org/content/media/pc08.pdf

American Urological Association Foundation. (2009). Prostate specific antigen best practice statement: 2009 update. Retrieved from http://www.auanet.org/content/guidelines-and-quality-care/clinical-guidelines/main-reports/psa09.pdf

Amputee Coalition. (2016). Limb loss statistics. Retrieved from http://www.amputee-coalition.org/limb-loss-resource-center/resources-by-topic/limb-loss-statistics/limb-loss-statistics/

Anand, B. S. (2013). Peptic ulcer disease. Retrieved from http://emedicine.medscape.com/article/181753-medication

Antin-Ozerkis, D., Evans, J., Rubinowitz, A., Homer, R. J., & Matthay, R. A. (2010). Pulmonary manifestations of rheumatoid arthritis. *Clinics in Chest Medicine, 3*(3): 451–478.

Arthritis Foundation. (2016). About arthritis. Retrieved from http://www.arthritis.org/about-arthritis/

Bhojani, N., & Lingeman, J. E. (2011). Surgery for BPH/LUTS: Is TURP still the gold standard? *Urology Times, 39*(13), 38–39.

Bitton, R. (2009). The economic burden of osteoarthritis. *American Journal of Managed Care, 15*(8 Suppl), S230–S235.

BreastCancer.org. (2012). *U.S. breast cancer statistics.* Retrieved from http://www.breastcancer.org/symptoms /understand_bc/statistics.jsp

Cameron, J., & Gignac, M. A. M. (2008). "Timing it right": A conceptual framework for addressing the support needs of family caregivers to stroke survivors from the hospital to home. *Patient Education and Counseling, 70*(3), 305–314.

Carpenito, L. J. (2013). *Nursing diagnosis: Application to clinical practice.* Philadelphia, PA: Wolters Kluwer/ Lippincott Williams & Wilkins.

Cawthon, P. (2011). Gender differences in osteoporosis and fractures. *Clinical Orthopaedics & Related Research, 469*(7), 1900–1905. doi:10/1007s11999-011-1780-7

Centers for Disease Control and Prevention. (1990). *Prevention and control of tuberculosis in facilities providing long-term care to the elderly: Recommendations of the Advisory Committee for Elimination of Tuberculosis.* Retrieved from http://www.cdc.gov/niosh/topics/tb/

Centers for Disease Control and Prevention. (2011a). National diabetes fact sheet: National Estimates and general information on diabetes and prediabetes in the United States.

Centers for Disease Control and Prevention. (2011b). *Summary health statistics for US Adults, 2010, Table 2.* Retrieved from http://www.cdc.gov.nchs/data/series/rs_10/sr10_252.pdf

Centers for Disease Control and Prevention. (2012b). Trends in Tuberculosis—United States, 2011. *Morbidity and mortality Weekly Report, 61*(11), 181–185.

Centers for Disease Control and Prevention. (2014). National diabetes statistics report. Retrieved from http:// www.cdc.gov/diabetes/data/statistics/2014statisticsreport.html

Centers for Disease Control and Prevention/National Center for Health Statistics (2015). Deaths and mortality. Retrieved from http://www.cdc.gov/nchs/fastats/deaths.htm

Centers for Disease Control and Prevention. (2016a). Arthritis. Retrieved from https://www.cdc.gov/arthritis /data_statistics/

Centers for Disease Control and Prevention. (2016b). Breast cancer screening. Retrieved from http://www.cdc .gov/cancer/breast/basic_info/screening.htm

Centers for Disease Control and Prevention. (2016c). Pneumococcal vaccination. Retrieved from https://www .cdc.gov/vaccines/vpd-vac/pneumo/

Centers for Disease Control and Prevention. (2016d). Shingles surveillance. Retrieved from http://www.cdc.gov /shingles/surveillance.html

Centers for Disease Control and Prevention. (2016e).TB disease: Symptoms and risk factors. Retrieved from http://www.cdc.gov/tb/topic/treatment/tbdisease.htm/

Centers for Disease Control and Prevention. (2016f). Treatment for TB disease. Retrieved from http://www.cdc .gov/features/tbsymptoms

Centers for Disease Control and Prevention. (2016g). Vision health initiative. Retrieved from http://www.cdc .gov/visionhealth/basic_information/vision_loss.htm

Chang, A. M., & Halter, J. B. (2009). Diabetes mellitus. In Halter, J. B., Ouslander, J. G., Tinetti, M. E., Studenski, S., High, K. P., & Asthana, S, *Hazzard's geriatric medicine and gerontology* (6th ed., pp. 1308–1332). New York, NY: McGraw-Hill.

Chin, T., Sawamura, S., Shiba, R., Oyabu, H., Nagakura, Y., Takase, I., . . . Nakagawa, A. (2013). Peripheral artery disease. Retrieved from http://my.clevelandclinic.org/health/articles/peripheral-arterial-disease

Constantinescu, F., Goucher, S., Weinstein, A., & Fraenkel, L. (2009). Racial disparities in treatment preferences for rheumatoid arthritis. *Medical Care, 47*(3), 350–355. doi:10.1002/rnj.054

Cournan, M. (2012). Bladder management in female stroke survivors: Translating research into practice. *Rehabilitation Nursing, 37*(5), 220–230.

Davidson, P., & Davidson, K. (2012). Electroencephalography in the elderly. *Neurodiagnostic Journal, 52*(1), 3–19.

Duraski, S. A., Denby, F. A., Danzy, L. V., & Sullivan, S. (2012). Stroke. In K. L. Mauk (Ed.), *Rehabilitation nursing: A contemporary approach to practice* (pp. 215–254). Sudbury, MA: Jones & Bartlett Learning.

Easton, K. L. (2001). *The post-stroke journey: From agonizing to owning* (Doctoral dissertation). Wayne State University, Detroit, MI.

England, M. J., Liverman, C. T., Schultz, A. M., & Strawbridge, L. M. (2012). Epilepsy across the spectrum: Promoting health and understanding: A summary of the Institute of Medicine report. *Epilepsy & Behavior, 25*(2), 266–276.

Fakih, M. G., Greene, M. T., Kennedy, E. H., Meddings, J. A., Krein, S. L., Olmsted, R. N., & Saint, S. (2012). Introducing a population-based outcome measure to evaluate the effect of interventions to reduce catheter-associated urinary tract infection. *American Journal of Infection Control, 40*(4), 359–364.

Ferri, F. F. (Ed.). (2011). *Ferri's clinical advisor, 2011.* Philadelphia, PA: Elsevier Mosby.

Fields, L. (2016). 6 symptoms of women's heart attacks. Retrieved from http://www.webmd.com/heart-disease/features/womens-heart-attack-symptoms#1

Fingeret, M. (2009). The management of glaucoma. *Chilton's Review of Optometry, 113,* 7.

Frisco, D. J. (2013). About Celebrex (celecoxib) COX-2 inhibitor. Retrieved from http://wwwspine-health.com/treatment/pain-medication/about-celebrex-celecoxib-cox-2-inhibitor

Gabriel, S. E., & Crowson, C. S. (2012). Risk factors for cardiovascular disease in rheumatoid arthritis. *Current Opinion in Rheumatology, 24*(2), 171–176.

Gallagher, J. C., & Levine J. P. (2011). Preventing osteoporosis in symptomatic postmenopausal women. *Menopause, 18*(1), 109–118.

Garas, S., & Zafari, A. M. (2006). Myocardial infarction. eMedicine. Retrieved from http://www.emedicine.com/MED/topic1567.htm

Gerzevitz, D., Porter, B. O., & Dunphy L. M. (2011). Eyes, ears, nose and throat. In Dunphy, L. M., Winland-Brown, J. E., Portor, B. O., Thomas, D. J., *Primary care: The art and science of advanced practice nursing* (3rd ed., pp. 245–330). Philadelphia, PA: F. A. Davis.

Gilad, R. (2012). Management of seizure following a stroke: What are the options? *Drugs and Aging, 29*(7), 533–538.

Hain, T. C. (2003). Benign paroxysmal positional vertigo. Retrieved from http://www.tchain.com

Hain, T. (2012). Dizziness in older people. Retrieved from http://www.dizziness-and-balance.com/disorders/age/Dizziness%20in%20the%20Elderly.htm

Hain, T. C., & Ramaswamy, T. (2005). Dizziness in the elderly. Retrieved from http://www.galter.north-western.edu/geriatrics/chapters/dizziness.cfm

Ham, R. J., Sloane, P. D., Warshaw, G. A., Bernard, M. A., & Flaherty, E. (2007). *Primary care geriatrics: A case-based approach* (5th ed.). Philadelphia, PA: Elsevier Mosby.

Hansson, E. E., Mansson, N.-O., & Hakansson, A. (2005). Balance performance and self-perceived handicap among dizzy patients in primary healthcare. *Scandinavian Journal of Primary Health Care, 23,* 215–220.

Harari, D. (2009). Constipation. In J. B. Halter, J. G. Ouslander, & M. E. Tinetti (Eds.), *Hazzard's geriatric medicine and gerontology.* (6th ed., pp. 1103–1122). New York, NY: McGraw-Hill.

Harvard Men's Health Watch. (2009). Premature heart disease. Retrieved from http://www.health.harvard.edu/heart-health/premature-heart-disease

Health Care Infection Control Practices Advisory Committee. (2009). Guideline for prevention of catheter-associated urinary tract infection. Retrieved from http://www.cdc.gov/hicpac/pdf/CAUTI/CAUTIguideline2009final.pdf

Heart and Stroke Foundation of Canada. (2009). Stroke treatments. Retrieved http://www.heartandstroke.com/site/c.ikIQLcMWJtE/b.3483943/k.DA86/Stroke___Treatment.htm

Helmick, C. G., Felson, D. T., Lawrence, R. C., Gabriel, S., Hirsch, R., Kwoh, C. K., . . . National Arthritis Data Workgroup. (2008). Estimates of the prevalence of arthritis and other rheumatic conditions in the United States. *Arthritis & Rheumatism, 58*(1), 15–25.

Heikkinen, K., Helena, L., Taina, N., Anne, K., & Sanna, S. (2008). A comparison of two educational interventions for the cognitive empowerment of ambulatory orthopaedic surgery patients. *Patient Education and Counseling, 73*(2), 272–279.

Hemmen, T. M., & Lyden, P. D. (2007). Induced hypothermia for acute stroke. *Stroke, 38*(2), 794–799.

Hill-O'Neill, K. A., & Shaughnessy, M. (2002). Dizziness and stroke. In V. T. Cotter & N. E. Strumpf (Eds.), *Advanced practice nursing with older adults: Clinical guidelines* (pp. 163–182). New York, NY: McGraw-Hill.

Hirsch, A. T., Haskal, Z. J., Hertzer, N. R., Bakal, C. W., Creager, M. A., Halperin, J. L., . . . White, R. A. et al. (2006). ACC/AHA 2005 Practice guidelines for the management of patients with peripheral arterial disease (lower extremity, renal, mesenteric, and abdominal aortic): executive summary: a collaborative report from the American Association for Vascular Surgery/Society for Vascular Surgery, Society for Cardiovascular Angiography and Interventions, Society for Vascular Medicine and Biology, Society of Interventional Radiology, and the ACC/AHA Task Force on Practice Guidelines. *Circulation, 113,*1474–1547. doi:10.1161/CIRCULATIONAHA.106.173994

Hooton, T. M., Bradley, S. F., Cardenas, D. D., Colgan, R., Geerlings, S. E., . . . Nicolle, L. E. (2010). Diagnosis, prevention, and treatment of catheter-associated urinary tract infection in adults. *Clinical Infectious Diseases, 50*(5), 625–663.

Howlader, N., Noone, A. M., Krapcho, M., Neyman, N., Aminou, R., Waldron, W., & Edwards, B. K. (2011). *SEER cancer statistics review, 1975–2008* (p. 19). Bethesda, MD: National Cancer Institute.

Hunt, A. H., Abraham, W. T., Chin, M. H., Feldman, A. M., Francis, G. S., Ganiats, T. G. . . . Yancy C. W. (2009). 2009 focused update incorporated into the ACC/AHA 2005 Guidelines for the diagnosis and management of heart failure in adults. *Journal of the American College of Cardiology.* Retrieved from http://content.onlinejacc.org/article.aspx?articleid=1139601

International Foundations for Functional Gastrointestinal Disorders. (2008). About GERD. Retrieved from http://www.aboutgerd.org/

James. P. A., Oparil, S., Carter, B. L., Cushman, W. C., Dennison-Himmelfarb, C., Handler, J., . . . Ortiz, E. (2014). Evidence-based guideline for the management of high blood pressure in adults: Report from the panel members appointed to the Eighth Joint National Committee (JNC 8). *Journal of the American Medical Association, 311*(5),507–520. doi:10.1001/jama.2013.284427.

Jett, D. U., Warren, R. L., & Wirtalla, C. (2005). The relation between therapy intensity and outcomes of rehabilitation in skilled nursing facilities. *Archives of Physical Medicine and Rehabilitation, 86*(3), 373–379.

Johnson, S. R., & Taylor, M. A. (2012). Identification and management of malignant skin lesions among older adults. *The Journal for Nurse Practitioners, 8*(8), 610–161.

Kalapatapu, V. (2012). Lower extremity amputation. Retrieved from http://www.uptodate.com/contents/lower-extremity-amputation

Kennedy-Malone, L. D., Fletcher, K. R., & Martin-Plank, L. (2014). *Advanced practice nursing in the care of older adults.* Philadelphia, PA: F. A. Davis.

Kim, H., & Oh, J. (2003). Adherence to diabetes control recommendations: Impact of nurse telephone calls. *Journal of Advanced Nursing, 44(3),* 256–261.

Khosla, S. (2010). Update in male osteoporosis. *Journal of Clinical Endocrinology and Metabolism, 95*(1), 3–10.

Klein, R., Knudtson, M. D., Lee, K. E., Gangnon, R., & Klein, B. E. (2009). The Wisconsin Epidemiologic Study of Diabetic Retinopathy XXIII. The twenty-five-year incidence of macular edema in persons with type 1 diabetes. *Ophthalmology, 116*(3), 497.

Kleinpell, R. M., Munro, C., & Guiliano, K. K. (2008). Targeting health care-associated infection: Evidence-based strategies. In R. G. Hughes (Ed.), *Patient safety and quality: An evidence-based handbook for nurses* (AHRQ Publication No. 08-0043). Retrieved from www.ahrq.gov/qual/nurseshdbk/

Kulick, D. L. (2012). Heart attack treatment. Retrieved from http://www.medicineNet.com

Laberge, M., Edgren, A. R. & Frey, R. J. (2009). Diabetes mellitus, type 1. In Longe, J. L. (Ed.), *The Gale encyclopedia of medicine* (3rd ed.). Detroit, MI: Gale.

Laine, L., & Jensen, D. M. (2012). Management of patient with ulcer bleeding. *American Journal of Gastroenterology, 107:*345–360. doi:10.1038/ajg.2011.480

Lefebure, H., Levert, M., Pelchat, D., & Lepage, J. (2008). Nature, sources and impact of information or the adjustment of family caregivers: A pilot project. *Canadian Journal of Nursing Research, 40*(1), 143–160.

Lockrey, G., & Lim, L. (2011). Peptic ulcer disease in older people. *Journal of Pharmacy Practice and Research, 41*(1), 58.

Luggen, A. (2009). Epilepsy in the elderly. *The Clinical Advisor*. Retrieved from http://www.clinicaladvisor.com /epilepsy-in-the-elderly/article/129590/3/

Lusardi, M. M., Jorge, M. M., & Nielson, C. (2013). *Orthotics and prosthetics in rehabilitation*. St. Louis, MO: Elsevier.

Lutz, B., & Young, M. E. (2010). Rethinking intervention strategies in stroke family caregiving. *Rehabilitation Nursing, 35*(4), 152–160.

Mauk, K. L. (2004). Pharmacology update: Antiepileptic drugs. *ARN Network, 20*(5), 3, 11.

Mauk, K. L. (2006). Nursing interventions within the Mauk model for poststroke recovery. *Rehabilitation Nursing, 31*(6), 257–263.

Mauk, K. L., Lemley, C., Pierce, J., & Schmidt, N. A. (2011). The Mauk model for poststroke recovery: Assessing the phases. *Rehabilitation Nursing, 36*(6), 241–247.

Mauk, K. L., & Rye, J. (2012). Bowel and bladder management. In K. Mauk (Ed.), *Rehabilitation Nursing: A Contemporary Approach to Care* (pp. 121–135). Sudbury, MA: Jones & Bartlett Learning.

Mayo Clinic. (2011). Essential hypertension. Retrieved from http://www.Mayoclinic.com/health=high=blood=pressure /ds00100/DSECTION=causes

Mayo Clinic. (2012b). Heart failure symptoms. Retrieved from http://www.mayoclinic.com/health/heart-failure /DS00061/DSECTION=symptoms

Mayo Clinic. (2012c). Rheumatoid arthritis. Retrieved from http://www.mayoclinic.com/health/rheumatoid-arthritis /DS00020/tab=InDepth

Mayo Clinic. (2013). Benign paroxysmal positional vertigo (BPPV). Retrieved from http://www.mayoclinic.com /health/vertigo/DS00534

Mayo Clinic. (2016a). Bladder cancer. Retrieved from http://www.mayoclinic.org/diseases-conditions/bladder-cancer /basics/tests-diagnosis/con-20027606

Mayo Clinic. (2016b). Peptic ulcer. Retrieved from http://www.mayoclinic.org/diseases-conditions/peptic-ulcer /symptoms-causes/dxc-20231407

Mayo Clinic. (2017). Bacilllus of Calmette and Guerin vaccine live (intravesical route). Retrieved from http://www .mayoclinic.org/drugs-supplements/bacillus-of-calmette-and-guerin-vaccine-live-intravesical-route/description /drg-20062163

McCance, K. L., Huether, S. E., Brashers, V. L., & Rote, N. S. (2010). *Pathophysiology: The biologic basis for disease in adults and children* (6th ed.). Maryland Heights, MD: Mosby Elsevier.

McDonnell, M. N., Hillier, S. L., Hooker, S. P., Le, A., Judd, S. E., & Howard, V. J. (2013). Physical activity frequency and risk of incident stroke in a national US study of blacks and whites. *Stroke, 44,* 2519–2524. doi:10.1161 /STROKEAHA.113.001538.

McEneaney, M. J. (2012). Individualizing management for common concerns of postmenopausal women. *The Journal for Nurse Practitioners, 8*(6), 470–474.

McPhee, S. J., Papadakis, M. A., & Rabow, M. W. (2012). Current Medical Diagnosis & Treatment 2012. *LANGE McGraw-Hill Medical, 50.*

Mead, M. (2005). Assessing men with prostate problems: A practical guide. *Practice Nurse, 29*(6), 45–50.

Miniño, A.M., Xu, J., & Kochanek, K. D. (2010). Deaths: Preliminary Data for 2008. *National Vital Statistics Reports, 59* (2), 1–52. Retrieved from http://www.cdc.gov/nchs/data/nvsr/nvsr59/nvsr59_02.pdf

National Breast Cancer Foundation. (2012). Breast cancer. Retrieved from http://www.nationalbreast-cancer.org/edp/

National Cancer Institute. (2008). Cancer fact sheet. Colon and rectal cancer. Retrieved from http://www.cancer .gov/cancertopics/types/colon-and-rectal

National Cancer Institute. (2013). Prostate cancer. Retrieved from http://www.cancer.gov/cancertopics/types /prostate

National Center for Health Research. (2106). Are annual prostate cancer screenings necessary? Retrieved from http://center4research.org/child-teen-health/general-health-and-mental-health/are-annual-prostate-cancer-screenings-necessary-should-early-stage-prostate-cancer-be-treated/

National Diabetes Education Program. (2005). Guiding principles for diabetes care: For healthcare providers. Retrieved from http://www.ndep.nih.gov/diabetes/pubs/GuidPrin_HC_Eng.pdf

National Institute of Arthritis and Musculoskeletal and Skin Diseases. (2003). Scientists identify two key risk factors for hip replacement in women. Retrieved from http://www.niams.nih.gov

National Institute of Neurological Disorders and Stroke. (2005). NINDS shingles information page. Retrieved from http://www.ninds.nih.gov

National Institute of Health and Clinical Excellence. (2012). *The epilepsies: The diagnosis and management of the epilepsies in adults and children in primary and secondary care. Clinical guideline no. 137.* London: Author.

National Institute of Neurological Disorders and Stroke. (2008). Parkinson's disease. Retrieved from http://www.ninds.nih.gov

National Institute of Neurological Disorders and Stroke. (2012). Parkinson's disease information page. Retrieved from http://www.ninds.nih.gov/disorders/parkinsons_disease/parkinsons_disease.htm

National Institute of Neurological Disorders and Stroke. (2015, September). Parkinson's disease: Challenges, progress, and promise. Retrieved from http://www.ninds.nih.gov/disorders/parkinsons_disease/parkinsons_research.htm#about

National Osteoporosis Foundation. (2008). Fast facts on osteoporosis. Retrieved from http://www.nof.org/professionals/Fast_Facts_Osteoporosis.pdf

National Parkinson Foundation. (2013). Parkinson disease. Retrieved from http://www.parkinson.org/parkinson-s-disease.aspx

National Stroke Association. (2015). Act FAST. Retrieved from http://www.stroke.org/understand-stroke/recognizing-stroke/act-fast

Neville, D. A., Dvorkin, M., Chittenden, M. E., & Fromm, L. (2008). The new era of total hip replacement. *OR Nurse, 2*(10), 18–25.

National Institute of Neurological Disorders and Stroke. (2015). Shingles: Hope through research. Retrieved from https://www.ninds.nih.gov/Disorders/Patient-Caregiver-Education/Hope-Through-Research/Shingles-Hope-Through-Research#3223_10

North American Menopause Society. (2012). Menopause. *The Journal of the North American Menopause Society, 19*(3), 257–271. doi:10.1097/gme.0b013e31824b970a

Nwankwo, T., Yoon, S. S., Burt, V., & Gu, Q. (2013). Hypertension among adults in the United States: National Health and Nutrition Examination Survey, 2011–2012. *NCHS Data Brief, 133*, 1–8.

O'Donnell, S., McKee, G., O'Brien, F., Mooney, M., & Moser, D. K. (2012). Gendered symptom presentation in acute coronary syndrome: A cross sectional analysis. *International Journal of Nursing Studies, 49*(11), 1325–1332.

Parkinson's Disease Foundation. (2012). Prescription medications. Retrieved from http://www.pdf.org/parkinson_prescription_meds

Peach, G., Griffin, M., Jones, K. G., Thompson, M. M., & Hinchliffe, R. J. (2012). Diagnosis and management of peripheral arterial disease. *British Medical Journal, 345*, e5208.

Pereira, S., Foley, N., Salter, K., McClure, J. A., Meyer, M., Brown, J., . . . (2014). Discharge destination of individuals with severe stroke undergoing rehabilitation: A predictive model. *Disability and Rehabilitation, 36*(9), 727–731.

Pilotto, A., & Franceschi, M. (2009). Upper gastrointestinal disorders. In Halter, J. B., Ouslander, J. G., Tinetti, M. E., Studenski, S., High, K. P., & Asthana, S, *Hazzard's geriatric medicine and gerontology* (6th ed., pp. 1075–1090). New York, NY: McGraw-Hill.

Politis, M., & Lindvall, O. (2012). Clinical application of stem cell therapy in Parkinson's disease. *BMC Medicine, 10*(1), 1. Retrieved at http://bmcmedicine.biomedcentral.com/articles/10.1186/1741-7015-10-1

Posadzi, P., & Ernst, E. (2011). Guided imagery for musculoskeletal pain: A systematic review. *Clinical Journal of Pain, 27*(7), 645–653.

Postuma, R. B., Lang, A. E., Munhoz, R. P., Charland, K., Pelletier, A., Moscovich, M., . . . Shah, B. (2012). Caffeine for treatment of Parkinson disease. *Neurology.* Retrieved from http://www.neurology.org/content/early/2012/08/01/WNL.0b013e318263570d.short#cited-by

PubMed Health. (2011). Fact sheet: Cystitis in women. Retrieved from http://www.ncbi.nlm.nih.gov/pubmedhealth/PMH0005174/

Ramakrishnam, K., & Salinas, R. C. (2007). Peptic ulcer disease. *American Family Physician, 76,* 1005–1012.

Reimer, A., & Johnson, L. (2010). Atrophic vaginitis: Signs, symptoms, and better outcomes. *The Nurse Practitioner, 36*(1), 22–28.

Resnick, B. (2008). Treatment options for seizures in older adults. *Assisted Living Consult.* Retrieved from http://www.assistedlivingconsult.com/issues/04-01/alc12-Seizure-121.pdf

Reuben, D. B., Herr, K. A., Pacala, J. T., Pollock, B. G., Potter, J. F., & Semla, T. P. (2015). *Geriatrics at your fingertips* (10th ed.). Malden, MA: American Geriatrics Society.

Richardson, L. C., Tai, E., & Rim, M. P. H. (2011). Vital signs: Colorectal cancer screening, incidence, and mortality-United States, 2002–2010. *Morbidity and Mortality Weekly Report, 60*(26).

Rowan, J., & Tuchman, L. (2003). Management of seizures in the elderly. *Seizure Management, 2*(4), 10–16.

Rudmik, L., & Soler, Z. M. (2015). Adult chronic sinusitis. *Journal of the American Medical Association, 314*(9), 964. doi:10.1001/jama.2015.7892.

Saint, S., Meddings, J., Calfee, D., Kowlaski, C., & Krein, S. (2009). Catheter-associated urinary tract infection and the Medicare rule changes. *Annals of Internal Medicine, 150,* 877–884.

Shan, C. L., James, C. R., Chyu, M. C., Brismee, J. M., Zumualti, M. A., & Paklikuha, W. (2008). Effects of tai chi on gait kinetic, physical function and pain in elderly with knee. Retrieved from http://www.medicinenet.com/osteoporosis/article.htm

Soll, A. H. (2011). Overview of the natural history and treatment of peptic ulcer disease. Retrieved from http://www.uptodate.com/contents/overview-of-the-natural-history-and-treatment-of-peptic-ulcer-disease

Statistics Canada. (2015). Leading causes of death, by sex. Retrieved from http://www.statcan.gc.ca/tables-tableaux/sum-som/l01/cst01/hlth36a-eng.htm

Steel, N., Clark, A., Lang, W., Wallace, R. B., & Melzer, D. (2008). Racial disparities in the receipt of hip and knee joint replacements are not explained by need: The health & retirement study 1996–2004. *Journal of Gerontology Series A: Biological Sciences and Medical Sciences, 63*(6), 629–634.

Stefanacci, R. G. (2007, March/April). Let's not lose sight of residents' visual health. *Assisted Living Consult,* 23–26.

Steiner, V., Pierce, L., Drahuschak, S., Nofziger, E., Buchanan, D., & Szirony, T. (2008). Emotional support, physical help and health of caregivers of stroke survivors. *Journal of Neuroscience Nursing, 40*(1), 48–54.

Thomas, D. J. (2011). Abdominal problems. In Dunphy, L. M., Winland-Brown, J. E., Portor, B. O., Thomas, D. J, *Primary care: The art and science of advanced practice nursing* (3rd ed., pp. 492–581). Philadelphia, PA: F. A. Davis.

Tursi, A. (2012). Advances in the management of colonic diverticulitis. *Canadian Medical Association Journal, 184,* 14770–14776.

United States Preventive Services Task Force. (2009). Screening for breast cancer. Retrieved from http://www.uspreventiveservicestaskforce.org/uspstf/uspsbrca.htm

United States Preventive Services Task Force. (2011). Osteoporosis. Retrieved from http://uspreventiveservicestaskforce.org/3rduspstf/osteoporosis/osteoor.htm

University of Washington, Department of Ophthalmology. (2008). Cataract statistics. Retrieved from http://www.universityofwashington/ophthalmology.org

U.S. Department of Health and Human Services, National Kidney and Urological Diseases Information Clearing House. (2012). Prostate enlargement: Benign prostatic hyperplasia. Retrieved from http://kidney.niddk.nih.gov/kudiseases/pubs/prostateenlargement/#common

United States Department of Health and Human Services. (2004). The Seventh Report of the Joint National Committee on Prevention, Detection, Evaluation, and Treatment of High Blood Pressure. Retrieved from https://www.nhlbi.nih.gov/files/docs/guidelines/jnc7full.pdf

Uthman, B. M. (2004). *Successfully using antiepileptic drugs in the elderly.* Paper presented at the 6th annual U.S. Geriatric and Long Term Care Congress, Orlando, FL.

Von Radowitz, J. (2012). New research claims rheumatoid arthritis breakthrough. *The Independent.* Retrieved from http://www.independent.co.uk/life-style/health-and-families/health-news/new-research-claims-rheumatoid-arthritis-breakthrough-7537207.html

Walker, J. (2012). Care of patients undergoing joint replacement. *Nursing Older People, 24*(1), 14–20.

Warlow, C., Sudlow, C., Martin, D., Wardlaw, J., & Sandercock, P. (2003). Stroke. *Lancet, 362*(9391), 1.

WebMD. (2011). Heartburn/GERD health center. Retrieved from http://www.webmd.com/heartburn-gerd/news/20111222/study-acid-reflux-prevalence-increasing

WebMD. (2012). Women's health. Retrieved from http://women.webmd.com/guide/sexual-health-vaginal-infections

Weinberger, S. E. (2004). *Principles of pulmonary medicine* (4th ed.). Philadelphia, PA: Saunders.

White, N. G., O'Rourke, F., Ong, B. S., Cordato, D. J., & Chan, D. K. Y. (2008). Dysphagia: Causes, assessment, treatment and management. *Geriatrics, 63*(5), 15–18.

Wong, J. M., Khan, W. S., Chimutengwende-Gordon, M., & Dowd, G. S. E. (2011). Recent advances in designs, approaches and materials in total knee replacement: Literature review and evidence today. *Journal of Perioperative Practice, 21*(5), 165–171.

World Health Organization. (2014). Visual impairment and blindness. Retrieved from http://www.who.int/mediacentre/factsheets/fs282/en

World Health Organization. (2016a). Glaucoma. Retrieved from http://www.who.int/blindness/causes/priority/en/index6.html

World Health Organization. (2016b). Diabetes. Retrieved from http://www.who.int/mediacentre/factsheets/fs312/en/

Woolever, D. R., & Beutler, A. I. (2007). Hypothyroidism: A review of the evaluation and management. *Family Practice Recertification, 29*(4), 45–52.

Yancy, C. W., Jessup, M., Bozkurt, B., Butler, J., Casey, D. E., Drazner, M. H., . . . Wilkoff, B. F. (2013). 2013 ACCF/AHA guideline for the management of heart failure: executive summary: A report of the American College of Cardiology Foundation/American Heart Association Task Force on practice guidelines. *Journal of the American College of Cardiology, 62*(16), 1495–1539.

Yen, R. W., Sidney, M. S., Chanra, M., Sorel, M. M., Selby, J. V., & Go, A. S. (2010). Myocardial infarction. *American Journal of Medicine, 363*, 2155–2165.

Zafari, A. M., & Yang, R. H. (2012). Myocardial infarction. Retrieved from http://emedicine.medscape.com/article/155919-overview

For a full suite of assignments and additional learning activities, see the access code at the front of your book.

CHAPTER 10

Nursing Management of Dementia

Prudence Twigg
Christine E. Schwartzkopf

(Competencies 9, 15, 16)

LEARNING OBJECTIVES

At the end of this chapter, the reader will be able to:

> Differentiate among dementia, depression, and delirium.
> Identify the stages and clinical features of dementia.
> Describe procedures for diagnosing dementia.
> Recognize and address the common causes of delirium.
> Discuss the theoretical foundations of nursing care for persons with dementia.
> Contrast pharmacological and nonpharmacological interventions for dementia, delirium, and depression.
> Apply basic principles to provide safe and effective care for persons with dementia.
> List specific nursing interventions for behavioral and psychological symptoms of dementia.
> Recognize the role of adult day services in the care of persons with dementia.
> Identify the role that palliative care and hospice care play for individuals with dementia and their families.

KEY TERMS

Acetylcholine
Agnosia
Alzheimer's disease
Anticholinergic
Aphasia
Apolipoprotein E-e4
Apraxia

Beta-amyloid plaques
Cholinesterase
Cholinesterase inhibitor
Delirium
Dementia
Depression
Executive function

Hallucinations

Hospice

Major neurocognitive disorder

Neurofibrillary tangles

Neurotransmitter

Palliative Care

Paranoia

The purpose of this chapter is to present basic information about dementia, delirium, and depression. These conditions are sometimes referred to as the "3 Ds" of geriatrics because they are fairly common in older adults and their signs and symptoms often overlap. Additionally, this chapter includes information on pharmacological and nonpharmacological treatments and care approaches to improve care for older adults with dementia (see **Box 10-1**).

Dementia

Dementia is a general term that refers to progressive, degenerative brain dysfunction, including deterioration in memory, concentration, language skills, visuospatial skills, and reasoning, that interferes with a person's daily functioning. Although dementia is much more common in older adults than in younger persons, it is not considered a normal part of aging. The most common type of dementia (see **Box 10-2**) is *Alzheimer's disease* (AD), named after Dr. Alois Alzheimer, who first described the condition about 100 years ago. AD did not begin to be commonly diagnosed and systemically studied until the 1970s (Alzheimer's Association, 2016). The most recent edition of the *Diagnostic and Statistical Manual for Mental Disorders* (DSM-V) classified AD as one type of *major neurocognitive disorder*, and this term is often used by mental health care providers (American Psychiatric Association, 2013).

Currently, approximately 5.4 million people in the United States have AD. With the changing demographics of the U.S. population leading to a higher percentage of older adults, the number of Americans with AD is projected to nearly triple to about 13.8 million by the year 2050. Dramatic increases in the number of "oldest-old" (those whose age is > 85 years) across all racial and ethnic groups contributes to this increased prevalence. As will be discussed throughout this chapter, the needs of persons with dementia are complex and costly, both financially and psychologically, with families providing most of the care. There are no specific interventions for the prevention of AD, and the current treatments offer only modest benefits (Alzheimer's Association, 2016).

Although the aging brain undergoes many developmental changes, mild cognitive impairment (MCI), an intermediate state between normal aging and dementia, is characterized by acquired cognitive deficits; these changes *do not* significantly interfere with the daily functioning of most older adults. Studies conducted on MCI have introduced new concepts regarding the possible distinctions between normal and pathologic aging of the

---

BOX 10-1   Web Exploration

Review the following resources about dementia, delirium, and depression:

- Alzheimer's Association:
  http://www.alz.org
- American Association for Geriatric Psychiatry:
  http://www.aagpgpa.org

- National Institute of Mental Health:
  http://www.nimh.nih.gov
- National Institute of Neurological Disorders and Stroke:
  http://www.ninds.nih.gov
- National Institute on Aging:
  http://www.nia.nih.gov

> **BOX 10-2   Most Common Types of Dementia in Older Adults**
>
> Alzheimer's disease (AD) (most common)
>
> Vascular dementia (considered the second most common form of dementia, after AD)
>
> Mixed dementia (two or more types of coexisting dementias)
>
> Parkinson's dementia
>
> Lewy body dementia (LBD)
>
> Frontotemporal lobe dementia (FTLD)

brain. The hippocampus, a region of the brain important to learning and memory, gradually loses volume as part of the normal aging process. This loss is significantly accelerated in older people with AD, especially if they have vascular problems or diabetes. An international team of researchers has identified four genes that may play a role in the age-related decline of hippocampal volume, a finding that may provide insight to risk for cognitive decline and AD (Bis et al., 2012).

Persons with AD, however, have numerous pathological brain changes that contribute to their symptoms. The pathological hallmarks of AD are *beta-amyloid plaques* and *neurofibrillary tangles*. The plaques are dense deposits around neurons. The tangles build up inside nerve cells. Together, the plaques and tangles interfere with normal nerve cell function and lead to neuronal death (National Institute on Aging, 2007). Plaques made up of abnormal deposits of beta-amyloid protein are a hallmark of AD. The toxic buildup begins when the beta-secretase enzyme, working in concert with a partner enzyme, snips a small fragment of amyloid precursor protein and releases beta-amyloid from the cell membrane of neurons. The beta-amyloid can then gradually clump together to form the well-known plaques that may cause damage to brain cells (Obregon et al., 2012). See the section on the nervous system in Chapter 4 for more specific information about brain changes with aging and AD.

AD dementia is the most common type of dementia, accounting for an estimated 60% to 80% of cases, although several other types of dementia are also commonly seen in older adults. Vascular dementia (previously known as multiinfarct or poststroke dementia) is the second most common type of dementia, and combinations of Alzheimer's and vascular dementia are also quite common (called "mixed dementia"). Vascular dementia may occur rather acutely after a cerebrovascular accident (CVA, or stroke) or more insidiously due to chronic atherosclerosis of cerebral arteries. Much like the coronary arteries, cerebral arteries are negatively affected by factors such as hyperlipidemia, smoking, and hypertension, causing decreased blood flow to the brain and neuronal death (Alzheimer's Association, 2016). The clinical signs and symptoms of dementia due to Alzheimer's and vascular causes are similar, and generally the assessment of and interventions for these dementias are similar.

Parkinson's disease (PD) is a chronic neurodegenerative disease characterized by motor symptoms in the early stages, but cognitive symptoms and dementia may develop in the later stages of PD. Lewy body dementia (LBD) is a variant of dementia with a specific pathological finding in the brain (abnormal deposits of the protein alpha-synuclein). Clinically, LBD can be distinguished from AD by:

> Motor symptoms in the early stage of LBD (which occur in the late stage of AD)
> Visual hallucinations in early LBD (which occur in the middle stage of AD, if at all)
> Fluctuating mental status as a feature of LBD (which usually occurs only due to delirium in AD)

It is not uncommon for persons with LBD to initially be thought to have PD, due to their motor symptoms (e.g., decreased range of motion and gait instability), although their motor symptoms do not respond to dopaminergic agents given for PD.

Frontotemporal lobe dementia (FTLD) affects the frontal and temporal lobes of the brain and is often characterized by early deficiencies in *executive function* (e.g., planning and making decisions), whereas memory may initially remain fairly intact. There are three types of frontal lobe dementia (FLD):

> **Progressive behavior/personality decline:** Characterized by changes in personality, behavior, emotions, and judgment (e.g., behavioral variant frontotemporal dementia).
> **Progressive language decline:** Marked by early changes in language ability, including speaking, understanding, reading, and writing (e.g., primary progressive aphasia).
> **Progressive motor decline:** Characterized by various difficulties with physical movement, including shaking, difficulty walking, frequent falls, and poor coordination.

Persons with FTLD often experience personality changes and disinhibition (saying and doing inappropriate things) much earlier than persons with AD (Alzheimer's Association, 2016).

Normal pressure hydrocephalus (NPH) is a relatively rare type of dementia, but an important subtype, primarily because, if identified early, it may be partially reversible with surgical intervention. The symptoms of NPH are related to an abnormal accumulation of cerebrospinal fluid (CSF) and are clinically distinguishable from those of other dementias by a triad of symptoms: slowed cognitive processes, gait disturbances, and urinary incontinence with a relatively acute onset (Alzheimer's Association, 2016).

Other, less common dementias include Huntington's disease (hereditary), Wernicke-Korsakoff's syndrome (most commonly caused by chronic alcoholism), and Creutzfeldt–Jakob disease (a very rare, rapidly progressing fatal dementia related to "mad cow disease"). Down's syndrome is also associated with the eventual development of dementia. Approximately 75% of persons with Down's syndrome who are over 65 years old will have dementia. Although there are many types of dementia, the majority of cases are attributable to Alzheimer's, vascular dementia, or both (Alzheimer's Association, 2016).

CLINICAL TIP

There are many types of dementia, but Alzheimer's Disease is the most common.

Risk Factors for Dementia

The main risk factor for developing Alzheimer's-type dementia is age, but AD is not a normal part of aging. One in nine people age 65 and older have AD, and about one third of people age 85 and older have AD. Family history also plays a role in the risk of developing dementia. Having a first-degree relative (parent, sibling, or child) with AD increases the risk, and the risk increases even more if more than one first-degree relative has had the disease. Some of the increased risk is heredity (genetics), and some risk is related to shared environmental and lifestyle factors (see **Box 10-3**), though both may play a role in the increased risk within families (Alzheimer's Association, 2016). Neuroimaging and genetic testing have aided in the identification of individuals at increased risk for dementia.

BOX 10-3   Risk Factors for Dementia

- Age
- Family history
- Genetic factors
- History of head trauma
- Vascular disease
- Certain types of brain infections

One gene that increases the risk of AD in the general population is the presence of *apolipoprotein E-e4* (APOE-e4). The other common forms of the *APOE* gene (e2 and e3) are not associated with AD. Each person inherits two *APOE* genes, so some people will have no *APOE-e4,* some may have one *APOE-e4* (higher risk of AD), and a few may have two copies of *APOE-e4* (highest risk for AD). The *APOE-e4* gene has varying penetrance, however, so even persons at the highest risk may never develop the disease. The *APOE* gene codes for proteins associated with cholesterol transport in the body. There are rarer genes that are associated with the risk of AD, but these genes tend to be concentrated within a few hundred well-identified families (Alzheimer's Association, 2016). Although many people worry about having the *APOE-e4* gene, routine genetic screening is not recommended. The value of having such knowledge is questionable because of the varying predictive ability and lack of treatment for the presence of the gene.

CLINICAL TIP

The most significant risk factor for developing AD is advancing age.

On the other hand, several modifiable risk factors can lower risk of developing AD and vascular dementia. Persons with a history of head injury, head trauma, and traumatic brain injury are associated with increased risk of developing dementia later in life. Groups that routinely experience head injuries, such as boxers, football players, and combat veterans, may be at risk of dementia, late-life cognitive impairments, and evidence of tau tangles (a hallmark of AD) at autopsy. Protecting the head from injury by using seatbelts and bicycle and motorcycle helmets throughout the life span is one way to lower the risk of dementia. Vascular disease contributes to the risk of dementia, so taking care of one's brain, in much the same way that one can prevent heart disease, is another good way to lower the risk of dementia. Some data indicate that cardiovascular disease risk factors such as physical inactivity, high cholesterol, diabetes, smoking, and obesity are associated with a higher risk of developing dementia. Unlike genetic risks, cardiovascular risk factors are modifiable. Therefore, maintenance of ideal body weight, exercising, avoiding smoking, and controlling hyperlipidemia and hypertension may all help lower the risk of dementia. Finally, exercising the brain with lifelong cognitive activity, along with consuming a diet low in saturated fats and rich in vegetables, may support brain health (Alzheimer's Association, 2016).

Medical Diagnosis of Alzheimer's Disease and Dementia

When an older adult and/or the family members suspect memory problems and possibly dementia (see **Box 10-4**), the first step is a visit to the primary care provider (PCP). It is not uncommon for family members and friends to notice changes and request an evaluation even though the older adult may not think there are any problems. Conversely, some older adults without significant cognitive problems may be overly concerned about mild memory lapses and request evaluations. Whenever the cognitive function of an older adult is in question, the best course of action is to seek a medical evaluation. An increasing number of PCPs are routinely screening for

BOX 10-4   Possible Warning Signs of Dementia

- Frequent forgetfulness, especially of recent events
- Difficulty with common tasks (e.g., cooking)
- Forgetting common words
- Becoming lost in familiar areas
- Poor judgment, especially with finances
- Misplacing objects in unusual places (e.g., puts clothes in bathtub, puts purse in oven)
- Changes in mood, behavior, or personality
- Lack of interest or involvement in life activities

cognitive impairment in older adults using short questionnaires at office visits for other medical problems. The goal of this practice is to identify and treat dementia in the early stage, before the symptoms are more apparent and when interventions tend to be more successful. A new Medicare benefit, added under the Patient Protection and Affordable Care Act, is the Annual Wellness Visit (AWV). The AWV for older adults requires that a cognitive assessment be conducted, and the Alzheimer's Association has published recommendations for operationalizing the detection of cognitive impairment during the Medicare AWV in the primary care setting (Cordell et al., 2013).

AD has several clinical features, including, but not limited to, memory impairment (see **Box 10-5**). Memory impairment alone does not indicate AD; rather, the cognitive deficits and memory impairment must significantly interfere with functioning. Additionally, the diagnostic criteria require that one of the following features also be present: impaired executive function, aphasia, apraxia, or agnosia. Executive function refers to higher level functions such as the ability to think abstractly, plan, organize, complete sequences of action, and make decisions. Impaired executive function significantly affects a person's ability to complete day-to-day tasks. Even an activity as simple as getting dressed in the morning requires planning, decision making, and sequencing. *Aphasia* refers to language deficits, typically a lack of complex language (e.g., less vocabulary) and word finding difficulties (e.g., cannot think of the right word to speak) early in AD. *Apraxia* is the inability to carry out motor activities, even though there are no motor deficits (e.g., unable to comb one's hair even though the arms have full range of motion). *Agnosia* refers to the failure to recognize sensory stimuli (e.g., cannot look at a wristwatch and name what it is). In AD, the history of the cognitive deficits is that they have occurred gradually over a relatively long period (months to a few years).

BOX 10-5   Diagnostic Criteria for Alzheimer's Disease

Criteria for dementia: The patient has cognitive or behavioral (neuropsychiatric) symptoms that:

1. Interfere with the ability to function at work or at usual activities
2. Represent a decline from previous levels of functioning and performing
3. Are not explained by delirium or major psychiatric disorder

Cognitive impairment is detected through history taking and objective cognitive assessment.

The cognitive or behavioral impairment involves a minimum of two of the following domains:

- Impaired ability to acquire and remember new information (memory problems)
- Impaired reasoning and handling of complex tasks, poor judgment
- Impaired visuospatial abilities
- Impaired language functions
- Changes in personality, behavior, or comportment

Criteria for probable AD: The patient meets the above criteria for dementia and has the following:

- Insidious onset: Symptoms have developed over months to years
- Clear-cut history of worsening of cognition by report or observation
- The most prominent cognitive deficits are in one of the following categories:
  - Amnestic presentation: Impairment in learning and recall of recent information
  - Nonamnestic presentations:
    - Language presentations, such as word finding difficulties, aphasia
    - Visuospatial presentations, such as object agnosia, impaired facial recognition
    - Executive presentations, such as impaired reasoning, judgment, problem solving

The diagnosis should not be made (1) if there is substantial concomitant cerebrovascular disease, such as recent stroke; (2) if there are key features of other dementias, such as LBD or FTLD; (3) if there is evidence for another concurrent active neurological disease or nonneurological medical comorbidity; or (4) if there is a use medication that could be affecting cognition.

In addition to having the preceding deficits, to make a diagnosis of AD, the clinician must ensure that nothing else but AD accounts for the deficits observed. Therefore, a significant part of diagnosing AD is ruling out other possible causes of cognitive deficits such as delirium, depression, other central nervous system disorders, medication side effects, and numerous medical conditions that affect cognitive function.

The PCP evaluating cognitive problems in an older adult will conduct a history and physical examination. The medical history, particularly the onset, type, and duration of symptoms, may help distinguish chronic from acute cognitive changes. A thorough physical examination, including laboratory tests, may help identify possible reversible causes of the cognitive changes. Several medical disorders that can be identified with laboratory tests can contribute to cognitive problems in older adults, including severe liver disease, hypothyroidism, vitamin B_{12} deficiency, hypercalcemia, and latent syphilis. The patient's medication list should be carefully reviewed to determine any current medications that may be causing or worsening cognitive impairment. (A pharmacist may be enlisted to help with this review.) **Box 10-6** lists common medications that may cause or worsen cognitive impairment. Many of these medications appear on a list that is famous, or perhaps infamous, in the world of geriatrics: Beers Criteria for potentially inappropriate drugs in older adults (American Geriatrics Society, Beers Criteria Update Expert Panel, 2015). Medication issues will be discussed in more detail later in this chapter.

In 2011, the National Institute on Aging and the Alzheimer's Association revised the criteria for diagnosing AD, the first such revision since 1984 (McKhann et al., 2011). The new criteria distinguish among MCI, possible AD, and probable AD. Criteria for both dementia and more specifically for AD are included.

Usually, imaging of the head and brain will be conducted. Although AD cannot be directly diagnosed by computed tomography (CT) of the head or magnetic resonance imaging (MRI) of the brain, these studies may identify or rule out other possible causes of cognitive decline (e.g., the presence of a tumor or evidence of a stroke) and may confirm the presence of vascular disease. Use of positron emission tomography (PET) imaging and CSF assays of biomarkers are not recommended as part of the diagnostic workup, although these procedures are frequently a part of research studies.

Any possible medical problems contributing to cognitive changes will usually be treated before concluding that the older adult has dementia. Notably, delirium should be excluded and depression should be excluded or diagnosed and treated before a diagnosis of dementia can be firmly established.

BOX 10-6 Common Medications That Can Cause or Worsen Confusion

- Any anticholinergic agents or those with significant anticholinergic effects
- Analgesics
- Propoxyphene (found in Darvon and Darvocet)
- Meperidine (Demerol)
- Opiates in excessive doses
- Antiemetics
- Promethazine (Phenergan)—anticholinergic
- Antihistamines
- Diphenhydramine (Benadryl)—anticholinergic
- Antihypertensives—Clonidine (Catapres)
- Antipruritics
- Hydroxyzine (Atarax)—anticholinergic
- Antiseizure medications (most, to some degree)
- Phenobarbital
- Anxiolytics
- Meprobamate (Equanil)
- Benzodiazepines (Ativan, Xanax, Valium)
- Bladder relaxants
- Oxybutynin (Ditropan)—anticholinergic
- Gastrointestinal antispasmodics
- Dicyclomine (Bentyl)—anticholinergic
- Hyoscyamine (Levsin)—anticholinergic
- Histamine-2 antagonists
- Cimetidine (Tagamet)—anticholinergic
- Muscle relaxants
- Cyclobenzaprine (Flexeril)—anticholinergic
- Tricyclic antidepressants
- Amitriptyline (Elavil)—anticholinergic

(Alzheimer's Association, 2016).

The PCP may do simple "paper and pencil" screening tests to determine the presence and degree of cognitive impairment. If the screening tests are suspicious for cognitive impairment, the PCP may refer the older adult to a psychologist and/or psychiatrist for further testing, although many PCPs are comfortable making the diagnosis of dementia without referral to a specialist. There are several common neuropsychological screening tests that can be administered to older adults. Examples include the Mini-Cog (Borson, Scanlan, Brush, Vitallano, & Dokmak, 2000), the Montreal Cognitive Assessment (Nasreddine et al., 2005), and the Saint Louis University Mental Status (SLUMS) examination (Tariq, Tumosa, Chibnall, Perry, & Morley, 2006). (See **Box 10-7** to access these and other assessment tests referred to in this chapter.) Psychologists and/or psychiatrists administering neuropsychological tests for cognitive impairment may administer much more complicated and time-intensive tests to determine the exact nature of the cognitive deficits.

Many persons with a new diagnosis of (see **Box 10-8**) dementia and/or their families may think that the diagnosis is incorrect. Receiving a diagnosis of dementia is almost uniformly devastating to the client and/or family, and initially, denial is a common psychological coping mechanism. Clients and families who remain uncertain about the diagnosis should be counseled to seek a second opinion from a physician specializing in the diagnosis and treatment of dementia. From a medical, psychosocial, and financial planning perspective, acceptance of the diagnosis by the client and family and subsequent steps to act on the knowledge can positively influence care outcomes. Prolonged denial of the diagnosis tends to worsen the situation for both the client and family and delay necessary treatment. Older adults with dementia and their families should be referred to the Alzheimer's Association (http://www.alz.org), a national organization with local chapters, for support services.

BOX 10-7   Resources for Assessment Available on the Internet

Assessing and Managing Delirium in Older Adults with Dementia:
http://consultgeri.org/try-this/dementia/issue-d8

Assessing Pain in Persons with Dementia:
http://consultgeri.org/try-this/dementia/issue-d2

Avoiding Restraints in Patients with Dementia:
http://consultgeri.org/try-this/dementia/issue-d1

2015 Updated Beers Criteria for Potentially Inappropriate Medication Use in Older Adults
http://consultgeri.org/try-this/general-assessment/issue-16

Brief Evaluation of Executive Dysfunction:
http://consultgeri.org/try-this/dementia/issue-d3

Communication Difficulties: Assessment and Interventions in Hospitalized Older Adults with Dementia:
http://consultgeri.org/try-this/dementia/issue-d7

Confusion Assessment Method (CAM):
http://consultgeri.org/try-this/general-assessment/issue-13

Decision Making and Dementia:
http://consultgeri.org/try-this/dementia/issue-d9

Eating and Feeding Issues in Older Adults with Dementia: Parts I and II:
http://consultgeri.org/try-this/dementia/issue-d11.1
https://consultgeri.org/try-this/dementia/issue-d11.2.pdf

Geriatric Depression Scale (GDS):
http://consultgeri.org/try-this/general-assessment/issue-4

Mental Status Assessment of Older Adults: The Mini-Cog:
http://consultgeri.org/try-this/general-assessment/issue-3.1

Mental Status Assessment of Older Adults: Montreal Cognitive Assessment:
http://consultgeri.org/try-this/general-assessment/issue-3.2

The Palliative Performance Scale
http://consultgeri.org/try-this/general-assessment/issue-32

Functional Assessment Staging Tool (FAST)
http://geriatrics.uthscsa.edu/tools/FAST.pdf

BOX 10-8   Diagnosis of Dementia

- History and physical examination
- Review of medications
- Laboratory tests: Complete blood count (CBC), complete metabolic panel (CMP), thyroid-stimulating hormone (TSH), vitamin B_{12} level, syphilis serology
- Neuropsychological testing
- Imaging studies: CT scan and/or MRI, PET scan (not routinely)

BOX 10-9   Characteristics of Alzheimer's Disease by Stage

Mild Stage

- Memory loss
- Getting lost in familiar places
- Having more difficulty doing normal daily tasks
- Difficulty with managing finances
- Making bad decisions
- Not being as talkative or verbally fluent
- Being more moody or anxious

Moderate Stage

- Increased memory loss and confusion
- Short attention span
- Difficulty with language, numbers
- Difficulty with reasoning
- Inability to learn new things or to adapt to new situations
- Restlessness, agitation, anxiety, tearfulness, wandering—especially in the late afternoon or at night ("sundowner syndrome")

- Repetitive statements, questions, or movements
- Hallucinations, delusions, paranoia, irritability
- Impulsivity (saying or doing things he or she normally would not)
- Perceptual-motor problems (interfering with ADLs)

Severe Stage

- Weight loss
- Seizures in some patients
- Dysphagia (difficulty swallowing)
- Vocalizations, but speech usually unintelligible
- Increased time spent sleeping
- Bowel and bladder incontinence
- Loss of recognition of family
- Pressure ulcers
- Neuromuscular symptoms (contractures)

Stages of Alzheimer's Disease

AD is commonly divided into three stages for the purpose of clinical management: mild, moderate, and severe (National Institute on Aging, 2016) (see **Box 10-9**). During the mild stage of AD, symptoms are often subtle and may go unnoticed by the person and his or her family and friends or may be attributed to "just getting older," resulting in a delay in diagnosis and appropriate treatment. Behavioral and psychological symptoms of dementia (BPSD) are most commonly exhibited during the moderate stage (see **Figure 10-1**) and often lead to institution-alization due to the need for 24-hour supervision. BPSD will be discussed in more detail later in this chapter. The person with severe AD requires total care for all needs and will most often die of complications (aspiration pneumonia) related to dysphagia, unless another medical condition causes death sooner.

Reisberg et al. (2002) identified seven stages of AD using the FAST (Functional Assessment Staging Tool) (ranging from Stage 1: "no impairment" to Stage 7: "very severe cognitive decline"). The FAST is often used by

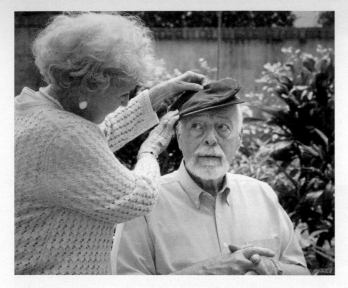

Figure 10-1 Family members may be the first to notice signs of cognitive decline.
© iStockphoto/Thinkstock.

palliative and hospice services to determine the stage of dementia to qualify for specialized end-of-life services. Regardless of the staging system employed, persons with AD may pass through the stages of the disease at varying rates, but generally die within 4 to 6 years of diagnosis, although most have had the disease for some time before diagnosis. However, the course of AD is quite variable and can range from 3 to 20 years (Alzheimer's Association, 2016).

Pharmacological Intervention for Dementia

The International Psychogeriatric Association (IPA) has published principles for care for persons with AD, including principles of pharmacological management (IPA, 2012). Ideally, pharmacological therapy for AD would prevent beta-amyloid plaques and/or ameliorate the neuronal damage caused by the plaques and *neurofibrillary tangles*.

Unfortunately, currently no medications are available that have this mechanism of action, although many new promising agents are being studied. Two classes of medications currently are approved for the treatment of Alzheimer's dementia: *cholinesterase inhibitors* (CEIs) and *N*-methyl-D-aspartate (NMDA) receptor antagonists. Both classes provide therapeutic effect by acting on neurotransmitters. Several neurotransmitters in the brain are affected by the pathological changes associated with AD.

Acetylcholine is a *neurotransmitter* in the brain, known to be important for memory. Medications or diseases that inhibit acetylcholine interfere with memory. Early in the course of AD, neuronal loss causes a decrease in the acetylcholine available for normal neurotransmission. Direct supplementation with acetylcholine is not currently feasible. Acetylcholine is naturally degraded in the brain by the enzyme acetylcholinesterase. CEIs exert therapeutic effect by blocking the enzyme, resulting in a net increase in acetylcholine.

Four drugs are currently approved for treatment of AD (see **Box 10-10**). The first CEI developed was tacrine (Cognex); however, this agent is no longer commonly used due to its dosing schedule (four times daily) and potential liver complications. The three remaining CEIs that are commonly prescribed for AD are donepezil (Aricept), rivastigmine (Exelon), and galantamine (Razadyne). The CEIs are generally started as early as possible in AD and continued throughout the disease course until no longer effective based on clinical judgment. The CEIs are generally well tolerated, although, when they are initiated, clients may complain of gastrointestinal (GI) side effects (nausea, diarrhea), due to the cholinergic effects of the medication on the GI tract. For this reason, the CEIs are usually started at low doses and then gradually titrated up (usually over a period of about 6 weeks) to the target dose to lessen side effects. Rivastigmine is also approved for use in mild to moderate Parkinson's dementia. All of the CEIs, however, are often prescribed off-label for dementias other than AD.

Glutamate is the main excitatory neurotransmitter in the brain. Glutamate excitotoxicity (due to excess glutamate) has been implicated in the pathogenesis of AD. When neurons die due to plaques and tangles, glutamate is released in large amounts into the extracellular fluid, increasing NMDA receptor activation and intracellular calcium influx into adjacent neurons. Excess intracellular calcium kills the remaining healthy neurons. Although excess glutamate is not the cause of AD per se, the cascading effect of neuronal death, excess glutamate, and further neuronal loss is believed to play a role in the progression of the disease.

BOX 10-10   Medication Treatment for Alzheimer's Disease

Medication	Target Dose
Cholinesterase inhibitors (CEIs)	
Donepezil (Aricept)	10 mg po q. daily
Galantamine (Razadyne ER) 2	4 mg po q. daily
Rivastigmine (Exelon)	6 mg po bid or 9.5-mg patch daily
***N*-methyl-ᴅ-aspartate (NMDA) receptor antagonists**	
Memantine (Namenda)	10 mg po bid
or Namenda XR	28 mg daily
Memantine/Donepezil (Namzaric)	28 mg/10 mg or 14 mg/10 mg daily

Refer to a pharmacology text for more specific information about medications for dementia.

BOX 10-11   Research Highlight

Aim: This review study evaluated the evidence for the effectiveness of the available pharmacologic treatments for dementia: cholinesterase inhibitors (CEIs) and memantine.

Methods: A systematic literature search for all English language randomized trials and observational studies on the treatment of dementia yielded 257 studies included in the review.

Findings: CEIs produce small, relatively short-lived (about 1 year) benefits in cognitive, functional, and global domains in mild to moderate dementia, but the clinical significance of these effects is unclear. Only marginal benefits are seen with severe disease, long-term treatment, and advanced age (>85 years old). Cholinergic side effects of weight loss, syncope, and debility are clinically significant and potentially detrimental for frail older adults, for whom the risks of treatment may outweigh the benefits. Memantine monotherapy may have some cognitive benefits in moderate to severe dementia, with minimal adverse effects.

Application to practice: CEIs and memantine for the treatment of AD show statistically significant results but only marginal clinical significance in cognition assessment measures. Nurses should use this knowledge when teaching patients and families about the risks and benefits of medication treatment for AD.

Buckley, J. S. & Salpeter, S. R. (2015). Risk-benefit assessment of dementia medications: A systematic review of the evidence. *Drugs & Aging, 32*(6), 453–467. Copyright 2015, with permission of Springer.

Memantine (Namenda) is an NMDA noncompetitive receptor antagonist, currently the only medication in this class, and helps to protect neurons from glutamate excitotoxicity without completely eliminating the glutamate necessary for normal neurological function (see **Box 10-11**). Memantine is generally well tolerated, it can be safely administered with donepezil or other *cholinesterase* inhibitors, and the combination has been found to be more effective than cholinesterase inhibitors alone. Memantine is currently approved for moderate to severe AD, although some clinicians may prescribe the medication for early-stage AD or other dementias (off-label use). Memantine, like the CEIs, is generally started at a low dose and gradually titrated up to the target dose (usually over a period of about 4 to 6 weeks) to lessen side effects. A drug combining both donepezil and memantine, Namzaric, is now also available.

The CEIs and memantine slow the progression of dementia, but do not stop the decline. After several months or years of treatment, however, the person receiving treatment may have significantly higher function than if he or she had not been treated at all. For this reason, once the medications are started, they are usually not discontinued unless significant side effects develop (rare after continuous use). Suddenly discontinuing the medications may result in a significant observable decline that may not be reversed by restarting the medications. If the medications are stopped for some reason for a period of days or weeks, and then restarted, the lowest dose is restarted and then titration proceeds back up to the target dose. Eventually, when the client is in the most advanced stage of AD and is clearly no longer benefiting from the medications (nonambulatory, mute, unable to recognize family members), the medications are usually weaned off.

Indirectly, good treatment for other medical conditions, particularly the management of vascular disease and associated conditions such as hypertension, hyperlipidemia, hyperglycemia, and elevated homocysteine levels, may help slow the progression of dementia. Vitamin E supplementation, as an antioxidant, is available over the counter and may be recommended for AD by some clinicians, although the daily dose should not exceed 400 IU due to concerns about toxicity and cardiovascular side effects. Medications not currently recommended for the treatment of AD include estrogen replacement, antiinflammatory agents (e.g., ibuprofen), and gingko biloba, although estrogen and ibuprofen may be appropriate for other uses (American Association for Geriatric Psychiatry [AAGP], 2006).

Numerous new medications for AD are being investigated in drug trials. The next generation of drugs is designed to prevent and/or destroy deposits of beta-amyloid plaque that kill the brain's nerve cells, which leads to the devastating loss of cognition and function that characterizes Alzheimer's. Some trials are exploring the strong correlation between heart disease and diabetes as Alzheimer's risk factors.

Medications That Can Cause or Worsen Confusion

With an understanding of some of the neurotransmitters affected by AD and the medications used to treat dementia, one can imagine that some medications could worsen confusion in persons with dementia. This is, indeed, the case. Particularly problematic are agents that block acetylcholine. Medications classified as *anticholinergic* or medications otherwise classified but with significant anticholinergic effects can be expected to worsen cognitive function in persons with dementia (see Box 10-6). Additionally, any medications that have central nervous system effects have the potential to negatively affect cognitive functioning.

Delirium

Delirium is a syndrome (group of symptoms) that occurs relatively acutely and is often called acute confusion—unlike dementia, which is characterized as chronic confusion. Delirium typically develops over a period of hours or days and is caused by some other underlying medical problem. Delirium can present with a hyperalert state (in which the person attends to all environmental stimuli simultaneously), hypoactive state (in which the patient seemingly retreats into inner thoughts and experiences that are abnormal), or mixed presentation (Fong, Davis, Growdon, & Inouye, 2015). A person of any age, when acutely ill, may experience delirium or acute confusion; however, older adults are at higher risk than younger adults, and older adults with preexisting dementia are at highest risk of developing delirium when acutely ill or injured. Not surprisingly, there is a high incidence of delirium among older adults in acute care hospitals (Jackson & Khan, 2015). Causes of delirium may include, but are not limited to, medication side effects, chronic alcoholism, tumors or infections in the brain, blood clots in the brain, vitamin B_{12} deficiency, and/or some thyroid, kidney, or liver disorders (see **Box 10-12**).

Inouye et al. (1990) developed an instrument, the Confusion Assessment Method (CAM), to assist nurses and others to identify delirium quickly and accurately using the four basic features of delirium: (1) acute onset or fluctuating course, (2) inattention, (3) disorganized thinking, and (4) altered level of consciousness. A diagnosis

BOX 10-12 Common Causes of Delirium in Older Adults

- Inadequate or inappropriate pain control
- Fecal impaction
- Medications (see also Box 10-7)
- Infections (urinary, respiratory, skin)
- Hypoglycemia or hyperglycemia
- Fluid or electrolyte imbalance
- Hypoxia
- Head trauma

of delirium is made if both features 1 and 2 are present, along with either of features 3 or 4. The CAM can be accessed online (see Box 10-7).

The nurse plays a critical role in identifying whether an older adult has experienced an acute change in mental status that could be delirium, assessing for delirium (using an instrument such as the CAM), reporting the change to the physician or nurse practitioner, implementing appropriate interventions, and continuing to evaluate the client for signs and symptoms of further decline or improvement.

CLINICAL TIP

Delirium has many causes and is associated with increased mortality.

The primary treatment for delirium is to discover and treat the etiology, or cause. The typical medical workup for the possible causes of delirium includes physical examination, laboratory tests (complete blood count, basic metabolic panel, and urinalysis), and imaging of the head and brain if trauma is suspected (e.g., delirium occurring after a recent fall). The medication list should be scrutinized for agents that are known to cause or worsen confusion (see Box 10-6). Particular attention should be paid to medications that have recently been started or increased. A pharmacist may be enlisted to assist with the review of medications.

Secondary interventions for delirium include keeping the patient comfortable, treating symptoms (e.g., with pain medication, oxygen, or intravenous fluids), and ensuring the safety of the client. Some persons with delirium may be quite lethargic (hypoactive delirium), whereas others may be very agitated (hyperactive delirium). Either situation presents a nursing challenge. For the lethargic client, oral intake may be compromised and the client is at risk of dehydration and aspiration pneumonia; impaired mobility increases the risk of pressure ulcers. The client with agitated delirium may be at risk of harming self or others and may require the judicious use of medications (e.g., benzodiazepines, antipsychotics). Physical restraints should be avoided if at all possible because they tend to cause more panic and agitation in older adults with delirium and can result in serious injury.

Other nursing interventions include moving the older adult to a room nearer the nursing station (for closer observation), implementing risk-of-falls protocols, providing one-to-one care and supervision, eliminating "tethers" when medically feasible (e.g., indwelling catheters, oxygen tubing), and eliminating confusing external stimuli (e.g., television). Generally, a calm, quiet environment is the most beneficial for a client with delirium. With appropriate medical care, delirium will eventually clear. One of the main goals of nursing care for delirium is to prevent further complications from developing during this acute syndrome. Delirium is further discussed in Chapter 13.

Depression

The risk of depression increases in older adults with chronic illnesses, including dementia. Content in Chapters 13 and 14 also discussed delirium and depression. *Depression* in the older adult is often not as obvious or as easily diagnosed as in young or middle-aged adults. Older adults may deny depression due to the stigma that this cohort

BOX 10-13   Diagnostic Criteria for Major Depression (DSM V Criteria)

At least five of the following symptoms for at least 2 weeks:

- Depressed mood*
- Diminished interest or pleasure*
- Significant involuntary weight loss or gain or appetite change
- Insomnia or hypersomnia
- Psychomotor agitation or retardation
- Fatigue or loss of energy
- Feelings of worthlessness or guilt

*Must have one of these symptoms

- Impaired concentration
- Recurrent thoughts of death or suicide

The symptoms must cause significant distress or impaired function and cannot be better accounted for by other medical conditions, substances, or bereavement.

Data from American Psychiatric Association. (2013). *Diagnostic and statistical manual of mental disorders* (5th ed.). Arlington, VA: Author.

often attaches to mental illness. Older adults, their families, or healthcare providers may incorrectly attribute depressive symptoms to normal aging. Many older adults do not meet the strict criteria for a diagnosis of major depression (see **Box 10-13**) and yet have significant depressive symptoms.

CLINICAL TIP

Nurses should recognize the difference between delirium, depression, and dementia to ensure appropriate treatment is being implemented.

The nurse can play an important role in recognizing possible symptoms of depression and reporting them to the PCP, screening for depression, and educating older adult clients and their families about depression. The most commonly used screening tool for depression in older adults is the Geriatric Depression Scale (GDS), a 30-item yes/no questionnaire developed by Yesavage et al. (1983) and subsequently shortened to a 15-item scale (Sheikh & Yesavage, 1986). See Box 10-7 to access the GDS online. The GDS and other screening tools, however, do not replace the need for a clinical examination to diagnose the condition. Many clinicians are qualified to diagnose and treat geriatric depression, including PCPs, psychiatrists, and psychiatric clinical nurse specialists.

Symptoms of depression may overlap with symptoms of dementia. For example, persons with depression frequently have poor concentration that may worsen performance on cognitive tests. Ordinarily, older adults with cognitive symptoms will be evaluated for both dementia and depression. If depressive symptoms are present, treatment with antidepressants and/or psychotherapy will be initiated. Mild cognitive symptoms in older adults often improve with the treatment of depression; however, some older adults will eventually be diagnosed with both dementia and depression.

Depression in older adults (**Box 10-14**) (with or without dementia) often includes symptoms of anxiety (see Chapter 14), agitation, and insomnia. Therefore, an important step in evaluating these symptoms in older adults is to screen for depression. Unfortunately, some older adults with depression are inappropriately treated for months or years with sedating medications to control these symptoms without ever being treated for the primary cause of their symptoms, depression. A complete discussion of geriatric depression is beyond the scope of this text; the reader is referred to mental health nursing texts for more information on the evaluation for and treatment of depression. The symptoms of dementia, delirium, and depression often overlap. See **Table 10-1** for a summary of some of the key similarities and differences.

BOX 10-14   Important Points about Depression in Older Adults

- Prevalent condition
- Often underrecognized
- Often undertreated
- May not meet strict diagnostic criteria
- May present with anxiety, agitation, or insomnia
- Symptoms may overlap with those of dementia
- Common cause of excess disability
- Potentially life threatening
- Treatable

TABLE 10-1   Comparison of Signs and Symptoms of Dementia, Depression, and Delirium

	Dementia	Depression	Delirium
Onset	Gradual over months to years.	Usually gradual.	Acute over hours to days.
Course	Slowly progressive, irreversible, minimally treatable.	Chronic, but sometimes abrupt with psychosocial stressors. Treatable.	Fluctuating. Reversible with identification and treatment of cause.
Level of Consciousness	Alert.	Alert.	Altered, cloudy, fluctuating.
Memory	Impaired. Initially short-term memory loss, eventually long-term memory loss.	Intact, but my exhibit poor effort on memory tests.	Short-term memory loss.
Orientation	Impaired to time, then place, and eventually person, including self.	Intact.	Impaired, fluctuating.
Psychomotor Speed	Normal. Slowed in advanced stages.	May be normal, hypoactive, or hyperactive.	Hypoactive, hyperactive, or mixed.
Language	Word-finding difficulties. Impairment increases with disease progression.	Normal. May not initiate much conversation.	Often incoherent.
Hallucinations	Usually visual if present. Most common in middle stage.	None less psychotic depression.	Common, tend to be tactile and visual.

Caring for the Person with Dementia
Theories of Dementia Care

Several theories of dementia care have been developed and tested. The Progressively Lowered Stress Threshold (PLST) model of Hall and Buckwalter (1987) focuses on the relationship between environmental stimuli and the lowered stress threshold of the person with dementia, identifying common stressors that may lead to behavioral and psychological symptoms—for example, misleading or inappropriate stimuli, excessive external demands, physical stressors, and changes in the environment, routine, or caregiver (Hall, 1994). Using this model, nurses focus on supporting the personal resources of the person with dementia (e.g., providing rest periods) and controlling that person's environment (e.g., assigning the same nursing assistant to care for the person when possible).

The Enablement Model of dementia care (Dawson, Wells, & Kline, 1993) focuses on supporting the remaining abilities of the person with dementia to avoid excess disability (i.e., functional impairment above and beyond what should be expected based on degree of dementia). Using this model, when abilities are still present (e.g., self-feeding), nurses focus on promoting the use of the retained abilities (e.g., setting up the meal tray for the client). When abilities have been lost due to progressive dementia (e.g., drinking from a glass without spilling), nurses focus on assisting the client and manipulating the environment to support the client (e.g., providing a "sippy" cup with a lid).

The Need-Driven Dementia-Compromised Behavior (NDB) model has conceptualized BPSD as resulting from background and proximal factors (Algase et al., 1996; Kolanowski, 1999). Background factors are person-related and more enduring; these include neurological factors, cognitive abilities, health status, and psychosocial history. Proximal factors are more amenable to change and include physiological and psychological need states, and the physical and social environment. The background and proximal factors interact to produce need-driven behaviors. The nurse considers the background factors in providing care and intervenes to change proximal factors that may be contributing to behavioral symptoms.

The antecedent-behavior-consequence (ABC) model can be used to analyze and understand the behavioral symptoms of persons with dementia (Smith, Buckwalter, & Mitchell, 1993). Using the ABC model, the nurse would first observe and describe the behavior. Next, the nurse would identify the antecedents or "triggers" that occurred before the behavior. Common triggers for behavioral symptoms in persons with dementia include, but are not limited to, personal care discomfort or embarrassment (e.g., bathing, toileting), the person with dementia misinterpreting environmental cues (e.g., a misplaced personal item must have been stolen), and caregiver approaches (e.g., rushing tasks). Finally, the nurse considers the consequences or reactions that may have worsened the behavior (e.g., yelling at the person with dementia who is resisting a bath). After analyzing the behavior using the ABC model, the nurse can plan changes to the antecedents and consequences to help prevent the behavioral symptom from recurring.

Retrogenesis theory, sometimes referred to as "reverse Piaget theory," describes the decline in cognition and function of persons with dementia in terms of reverse development (Reisberg et al., 2002). Retrogenesis theory posits that persons with dementia tend to lose cognition and function in the reverse order of acquisition. Using this theory, the nurse would understand why a person with severe dementia may put nonfood items in the mouth (analogous to Piaget's sensorimotor stage of infant development). The nurse would focus on providing an environment and activities consistent with the client's cognitive developmental stage. An important caveat to the use of this theory is that we do not want to fall into the habit of treating persons with dementia like children or referring to them as "babies." Persons with dementia should always be treated as adults, but knowledge of their cognitive stage of development can enhance understanding and promote more appropriate interventions.

Lawton's Person–Environment (P–E) Fit theory (1982) can be used as a theoretical basis for providing care to persons with dementia. (See the discussion of this theory in Chapter 3.) The environmental docility hypothesis, formulated by Lawton, posits that persons with a disability, including dementia, will be more dependent upon the physical and social environment. An appropriate environment will support higher functioning. "Environmental press" is the degree to which the environment challenges the individual. If the environment is too complex, a person with dementia may become frustrated and withdraw from activity; conversely, if the environment is too trivial, the person with dementia will not be challenged to maintain cognitive and functional abilities. Using the P–E Fit theory, the nurse can formulate plans of care that adjust the environmental conditions to challenge, without frustrating, the person with dementia.

Person-centered care, based on the work of Kitwood (1997), is not a true theory, but an approach to dementia care that incorporates several principles: (1) learning about the history and preferences of the person with dementia, (2) developing genuine relationships between persons with dementia and caregivers, (3) promoting physical and emotional comfort, and (4) respecting the choices of persons with dementia and their families (Talerico, O'Brien, & Swafford, 2003). In a review of person-centered care in long-term care, there were significant effects on decreasing behavioral symptoms and psychotropic medication use, though the authors note that there is a need for better definitions of the interventions and more rigorous study designs (Junxin & Porock, 2014).

Behavioral and Psychological Symptoms of Dementia

In the past, persons with AD and other dementias were often labeled as having "problem behaviors." You may still hear some clinicians using this term. A consensus group of the International Psychogeriatric Association (IPA, 2012), however, has recommended that the term *behavioral and psychological symptoms of dementia* (BPSD) (see **Box 10-15**) be used instead, emphasizing the understanding that such symptoms are disease-related. BPSD includes symptoms of disturbed perception, thought content, mood, or behavior. Behavioral symptoms typically can be assessed objectively by observing the person with dementia. Psychological symptoms are usually assessed by talking to the person with dementia and/or their families and caregivers.

The estimated frequency of BPSD varies considerably, with 5-year periods of prevalence reported as follow: delusions 60%, hallucinations 38%, agitation/aggression 45%, depression/dysphoria 77%, anxiety, 62%, and disinhibition 31%. If left untreated, BPSD contributes to premature institutionalization, increased financial costs, increased caregiver stress, excess disability for the person with dementia, and decreased quality of life for the person with dementia and the caregivers (IPA, 2012). The frequency of BPSD tends to peak in the middle stages of dementia and wane in the later stages.

Some types of BPSD are more common in certain types of dementia. For example, visual hallucinations and sexual disinhibition are more common in LBD and FTLD, respectively. Common delusions in dementia include the belief that others are stealing things, that one's spouse is having an affair, that one's spouse or other loved one is an imposter, or that one has been abandoned. One of the more difficult situations nurses employed in nursing homes often encounter is trying to find out if a particular item really was stolen from an older adult (a crime) or if the belief is falsely held by the older adult (a delusion). Visual *hallucinations* are more common than auditory hallucinations in persons with dementia and are more common in persons with visual deficits, who are presumably misinterpreting visual stimuli. Close attention to lighting, eliminating confusing visual stimuli, and providing visual aids may decrease visual hallucinations. When a person with dementia has ongoing disturbing hallucinations, delusions,

---

CLINICAL TIP

Agitated behaviors in the person with dementia are often a sign of unmet physical needs such as toileting or pain.

BOX 10-15 Behavioral and Psychological Symptoms of Dementia (BPSD)

Behavioral Symptoms

- Physical aggression (hitting, kicking, biting)
- Verbal agitation (screaming, meaningless vocalizations)
- Physical agitation (restlessness, purposeless movements)
- Wandering (continuous walking around aimlessly)
- Sexual disinhibition (exposing genitals, masturbating in public)
- Hoarding (keeping/hiding unusually large amounts of what are often useless items)

- Verbal aggression (swearing at, threatening others)
- Shadowing (following another person around closely for long periods of time)

Psychological Symptoms

- Anxiety
- Depressive symptoms (feeling sad, poor sleep and/or appetite, lack of interest in life)
- Hallucinations (seeing or hearing things that others do not)
- Delusions (holding false beliefs)
- Paranoia (having unreasonable fears)

BOX 10-16   Suggested Interventions for Delusions and Paranoia

- Assist the person to keep track of personal items.
- Avoid defensiveness if accused.
- Do not argue with the person.

- Maintain a simple, noncluttered environment.
- Avoid whispering in front of the person.

Note: Antipsychotic medications are often required.

BOX 10-17   Common Behavioral Triggers

- Hunger
- Thirst
- Toileting needs
- Feeling too hot or too cold
- Pain

- Boredom
- Overstimulation
- Certain people
- Certain activities (meals, baths)

---

and/or *paranoia* (see **Boxes 10-16** and **10-17**), a diagnosis of "psychosis of AD" may be made and the condition may be treated with antipsychotic medication.

Agitation is a nonspecific term often applied to the behavior of persons with dementia. Cohen-Mansfield (1996) studied agitation extensively and identified four subtypes of agitation: physically nonaggressive behaviors (e.g., restlessness, pacing), verbally nonaggressive behaviors (e.g., complaining, interrupting), verbally aggressive behaviors (e.g., screaming, swearing), and physically aggressive behaviors (e.g., hitting, kicking, biting). When a person with dementia becomes agitated, the possibility of delirium should be considered.

CLINICAL TIP

Suggested Interventions for Agitation and Aggression

- Avoid provoking situations.
- Intervene early, before the behavior escalates.
- Remain calm; speak in a soft voice.
- Approach slowly from the front.
- Avoid startling the person.
- Stay at the eye level of the person.
- Avoid touching initially; wait until the person is calmer.
- Distract the person.
- Avoid rational arguments.
- Avoid physical restraint if at all possible.
- Identify and address unmet needs (food, fluid, toileting).

Pharmacological Treatment for Behavioral and Psychological Symptoms of Dementia

Generally, nonpharmacological treatments for BPSD are initiated first and preferred due to potential medication side effects in older adults. When symptoms are uncomfortable for the person with dementia or the behaviors

BOX 10-18 Common Medications Prescribed for Behavioral and Psychological Symptoms of Dementia

Class/Medications	Common Uses
Selective Serotonin Reuptake Inhibitors Fluoxetine (Prozac) Sertraline (Zoloft) Paroxetine (Paxil) Citalopram (Celexa)	Depression, agitation, or anxiety attributed to depression
Serotonin norepinephrine reuptake inhibitors Venlafaxine (Effexor) Duloxetine (Cymbalta)	Depression, agitation, and/or anxiety attributable to depression
Other antidepressants Mirtazapine (Remeron) Trazadone (Desyrel)	Depression, used at lower doses for insomnia and appetite stimulation
Mood Stabilizers Divalproex (Depakote) Benzodiazepines	Low doses for insomnia, bipolar-type depression, agitation Anxiety, agitation
Antipsychotics Risperidone (Risperdal) Olanzapine (Zyprexa) Quetiapine (Seroquel) Aripiprazole (Abilify) Ziprasidone (Geodon)	Psychotic symptoms, mania, adjunct therapy for depression, violent behavior
Conventional/typical antipsychotic Haloperidol (Haldol)	Delirium, violent behavior

*Check the Beer Criteria list for cautions in older adults.

endanger self or others and have not responded to nonpharmacological treatments, then medications are prescribed. See **Box 10-18** for a list of medications commonly prescribed for BPSD.

Older antidepressants, such as amitriptyline (Elavil), are generally avoided in older adults with dementia due to their adverse side effect profiles (anticholinergic). Generally, the selective serotonin reuptake inhibitors (SSRIs) and serotonin norepinephrine reuptake inhibitors (SNRIs) are safe and effective with minimal side effects. The most common side effect of these classes is GI upset when the medications are started, so starting doses are usually low and gradually titrated upward. Paroxetine (Paxil) is often avoided because this agent has the most anticholinergic side effects in its class. Although gradual dose reductions, unless contraindicated, of all psychotropic medications are mandated in the nursing home setting, many clinicians continue antidepressants indefinitely due to the high rate of recurrence of geriatric depressive symptoms when medications are withdrawn (IPA, 2012).

Antipsychotics are generally reserved for psychotic or serious behaviors endangering self or others. Antipsychotics are not considered effective for dementia per se. The atypical antipsychotics carry a "black box warning" concerning the increased risk of adverse cardiovascular events. Generally, the atypical antipsychotics are preferred over the conventional antipsychotics due to the side effect profiles, although haloperidol (Haldol) is commonly used in acute care for delirium. Benzodiazepines are used cautiously in older adults due to their side effect profile, particularly increased risk of falls. Psychotropic drug use in the nursing home setting is highly regulated. Regular review of the

BOX 10-19   General Approaches to Managing Behavioral and Psychological Symptoms of Dementia

- Try nonpharmacological before pharmacological interventions.
- Maintain a calm, familiar environment and routine.

For specific BPSD:

- Identify and describe the behavior in as much detail as possible.

- Identify the antecedents (triggers) and consequences of the behavior (per the ABC model).
- Identify the desired behavioral outcome.
- Implement interventions.
- Evaluate the effectiveness of interventions.

risks and benefits along with trials of periodic gradual dose reductions are mandated unless clinically contraindicated. It is important to note that no medications have been approved by the U.S. Food and Drug Administration for the treatment of behavioral symptoms of dementia. The use of all such medications is considered "off label" prescribing.

A more complete discussion of pharmacological therapy (see **Box 10-19**) for persons with dementia is beyond the scope of this chapter. For more information, please consult psychiatric nursing and pharmacology texts.

Nonpharmacological Treatment for Dementia

Nurses, as an interdependent intervention, administer medications prescribed for persons with dementia. The largest role for nurses in dementia care, however, is applying the nursing process to promote comfort, function, and dignity for persons with dementia. The nurse uses theories about dementia care to guide assessment, nursing diagnosis, planning, intervention, and ongoing evaluation. The role of the nurse is particularly important in assessing and treating BPSD. When evaluating any acute changes in the cognition, behavior, and mood of persons with dementia, recall that delirium is a common cause of these changes. Systematic reviews of the literature have found that nonpharmacological treatments for dementia can improve outcomes (Livingston et al., 2014; Ortega, Qazi, Spector, & Orrell, 2015); however, more rigorous studies are needed and also more attention to the implementation of psychosocial interventions, particularly in the long-term care setting (Boersma, Weert, Lakerveld, & Droes, 2015).

General Interventions

Reality orientation is a technique that presents information to persons with dementia about themselves and their orientation in time and place. Nurses using reality orientation frequently remind the person with words and other cues (e.g., clocks, calendars). A systematic review of studies of reality orientation found that the technique could improve both cognitive and behavioral outcomes (Carmago, Justus, & Retzlaff, 2015). Reality orientation, however, may actually increase distress in some persons with dementia, who may be convinced of some other reality and resent being "corrected."

Validation therapy (VT), which was developed by Naomi Feil (1993), is a systematic method for communicating with and caring for persons with dementia in an empathic and individualized manner. VT recognizes that older adults with dementia are unique, valuable individuals who should be accepted nonjudgmentally. Within the VT framework, the behavior of persons with dementia is viewed as having meaning and is not just caused by physical and functional changes in the brain (the medical model of dementia). Furthermore, VT posits that older adults with impaired memory are often trying to resolve uncompleted developmental tasks from earlier in life, thus accounting for their tendency to dwell more on remote rather than recent memories. Feil developed her own classification of chronic confusion in older adults called the four stages of resolution: malorientation, time confusion, repetitive motion, and vegetation. Communication and care are based on the stage of resolution. The goals of VT are to reduce anxiety, restore a sense of self-worth, and improve function for the person with dementia. A systematic review of VT for persons with dementia concluded that there were too few good studies and relatively small numbers of subjects to draw any conclusions about the effectiveness of VT (Neal & Barton Wright, 2008).

VT and reminiscence therapy (RT) share several principles and approaches, though VT relies less on cognitive ability and thus can theoretically be used into much later stages of dementia. RT was developed for use with older adults by Norris (1986), based on Butler's (1963) work on life review. The purpose of RT is to promote adjustment and integrity for older adults through structured remembering and reflecting on the past. RT may be conducted individually, but is frequently a group activity for persons with dementia living in institutions, often incorporating refreshments. A systematic review of RT for persons with dementia concluded that there were too few good studies and too many variations in treatment protocols to evaluate the effectiveness of RT (Woods, Spector, Jones, Orrell, & Davies, 2008).

Environmental Interventions

Managing the environment of the person with dementia is a component of most theories of dementia care. The acute care environment, with its multiple and competing stimuli, can be very stressful for persons with dementia, who have decreased ability to adapt to change. Nurses should assess and modify the environment to control the information the patient is receiving (see **Box 10-20**).

The impact the environment has on patient behavior may fluctuate, depending on the degree of activity occurring at any given time. Behavioral symptoms are more likely to occur during periods of high activity: 7 to 10 a.m., 12 to 2 p.m., and 4 to 7 p.m. In an acute care environment, these times represent periods of high activity: shift changes, meal times, sending and receiving patients from operating rooms, doctor rounds, and visiting hours. Carefully planning activities to minimize additional procedures and demands during peak periods may prevent unnecessary stress and behavioral outbursts (Gitlin, Liebman, & Winter, 2003).

Physical Comfort Interventions

Interventions to promote elimination, comfort, sensory function, and adequate sleep and nutrition (discussed in other areas of this text) will contribute to overall well-being for persons with dementia and reduce the risk for BPSD.

Pain Management and Alzheimer's Disease

Many people with AD are unable to report their pain. In such cases, nurses must rely on observation to assess for pain behaviors. Each person might have a "pain signature," which means that one person's pain may cause him or her to become agitated and combative, whereas another may withdraw. Failure to recognize and treat pain can lead to sleep disturbances, malnutrition, depression, decreased mobility, needless suffering, and inappropriate psychotropic medication use (Corbett et al., 2014).

One of the most important steps in evaluating any patient, especially for those with AD, is to obtain a baseline pain assessment. Changes in baseline are then used to determine the need for adjustments in the treatment plan, such as the addition of an analgesic or dose adjustment. Because self-report is the single most reliable indicator

---

BOX 10-20   **Examples of Environmental Interventions**

Physical Environment
- Areas for safe wandering.
- Alarms on exits and/or the person to detect elopement.
- Adequate, but not harsh, lighting during the day.
- Low lighting at night.
- Soft background music.

- Appropriate, nonconfusing sensory stimuli.
- Comfortable room temperature.

Temporal Environment
- Establish a meaningful routine.
- Alternate activity and rest periods.

BOX 10-21   Possible Nonverbal Expressions of Pain

- Agitation
- Increased confusion
- Decreased mobility
- Combativeness
- Resistance to care
- Guarding
- Grimacing

- Restlessness
- Changes in eating and sleeping habits
- Withdrawal
- Aggression
- Rubbing or holding a particular area of the body
- Rapid breathing

BOX 10-22   Nonpharmacological Interventions for Pain

- Distraction
- Massage
- Heat or cold application

- Gentle movement and repositioning
- Participation in normal activities as able

of pain, those who are able to communicate verbally should be asked about their pain level. A pain assessment, such as a 0 to 10 scale or the Wong-Baker FACES pain rating scale, should be used to determine pain intensity. For more impaired clients, the nurse should assess for crying, moaning, groaning, and other verbalizations that may be indicative of pain, along with possible nonverbal expressions of pain (see **Box 10-21**). It is important to assess pain at rest and during activity. Pain behaviors are often more obvious during activities such as repositioning and bathing. See Box 10-7 for more information on how to assess for pain in persons with dementia.

The principles of good pain management for adults with Alzheimer's apply universally to those with the disease. Nonpharmacological interventions (see **Box 10-22**) should be tried first for mild pain and used along with pharmacological interventions in moderate to severe pain. Nonopioid analgesics should be considered for mild to moderate pain. Opioid analgesics are added to the treatment plan for more severe pain. If neuropathic pain is suspected, adjuvant analgesics such as local anesthetics, anticonvulsants, and antidepressants may be indicated. Opioid analgesics are generally started at very low doses and titrated upward based on continuing evaluation. When opioids are administered, it is particularly important to assess bowel function, because the person with dementia may not be able to report constipation.

Activity Interventions

Persons with dementia need a balance between stimulating and calming activities. Too much or too little activity may lead to behavioral and psychological symptoms. When evaluating behavioral symptoms, note the time of day and the level of activity at the time the symptoms occurred.

Interdisciplinary teamwork (see **Figure 10-2**) between nursing and the activities service is

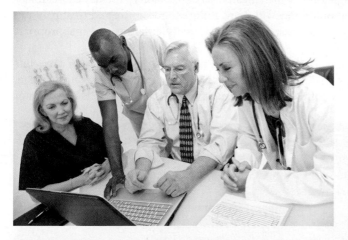

Figure 10-2 Interdisciplinary teamwork is important in providing quality care for older adults with dementia.
© iStockphoto.com/asiseeit

needed to assess the person's normal schedule of activities, looking for prolonged periods of activity or inactivity. Adjustments can be made to increase or decrease activity. In addition to the quantity of activity, the quality of activity is important. Generally, persons with dementia respond most positively to meaningful activities that are connected to their personal history and preferences. Lifelong personality characteristics also may be used to help choose appropriate activities (Kolanowski & Buettner, 2008). More extroverted individuals may prefer small group activities; more introverted individuals may prefer one-on-one or individual activities. Group physical activity can help meet both exercise and socialization needs (Netz, Axelrad, & Argov, 2007).

CLINICAL TIP

Try these techniques when caring for persons with dementia:

- Approach slowly from the front (so they can see you), then stand at their side (indicates support).
- Squat down at their level (less threatening) and call them by name (more personal and comforting).
- Use the hand-under-hand technique (tactile stimulation and warmth) to help them perform tasks or even when walking with you.

Data from Snow, T. (2016). A voice for dementia: Basics for success. Retrieved from http://teepasnow.com/subscriptions/16jan/BasicsForSuccess.htm; DementiaCareCentral. (2013). Basic tips for caregiving. Retrieved from http://www.dementiacarecentral.com/caregiverinfo/tips

Communication Interventions

Language and speech become progressively impaired in dementia, but maintaining communication is critical to effective care for persons with dementia. Keep in mind that behavior is a form of communication, and as dementia progresses it becomes increasingly more important for the nurse to analyze and interpret the behavior of a person with dementia in that context. For example, a person with dementia who is exhibiting a behavioral symptom may just need food, fluids, or to be toileted but unable to express that need. Nurses who routinely care for persons with dementia in long-term care become experts at interpreting the meaning of particular behaviors.

CLINICAL TIP

Suggested Communication Techniques
- Speak to the person distinctly and in simple phrases and sentences.
- Speak as one adult to another.
- Smile.
- Avoid "elderspeak" (sing-song baby talk).
- Keep the pace of the conversation slow.
- Listen.
- Allow sufficient time for responses.
- Be calm, remain patient, and speak softly.
- Maintain eye contact.
- Use nonverbal cues: Point or demonstrate what you want done.
- Repeat instructions as often as necessary.
- Lower voice to accommodate age-related hearing changes.
- For persons with limited speech, try using yes/no questions.
- Observe carefully for a person's nonverbal cues.

Interventions for Particular Behaviors

Nurses caring for persons with dementia are often challenged to address particular behaviors. Keeping in mind that these behaviors are most often symptoms of the disease process, the nurse can analyze the behaviors using the ABC model. An important step in this process is examining the possible antecedents, causes, or triggers for the behavior (see **Box 10-23**). When the antecedents of the behavior have been identified, the nurse can plan care to help prevent that behavior in the future. For example, if a person with dementia becomes agitated every time he or she has to void, scheduled toileting could be implemented to avoid this behavior. Nursing care for the behavioral symptoms of dementia is quite individualized because the cause of and approach to the behavior are very much dependent on the personal and contextual factors. There are, however, some general approaches to particular behaviors (see **Boxes 10-24** through **10-26**).

BOX 10-23   Key Points for Pain Control

- Persons with dementia may not be as able to report pain.
- Always consider pain as a possible cause of behavioral symptoms.
- Assess for possible objective indicators of pain.
- Administer analgesics routinely for painful conditions when the person cannot ask.

BOX 10-24   Suggested Interventions for Resistance to Bathing

- Remain calm.
- Use a soft voice.
- Choose a time when the person is most rested and least confused.
- Consider the person's lifelong preferences:
- Shower vs. bath
- Morning vs. evening
- Maintain a leisurely pace. Avoid rushing the person.
- Premedicate with analgesics if pain with movement is an issue.
- Allow the person to wear underwear or a patient gown, if desired.
- Avoid spraying water directly on the head or face.
- Pantomime the desired hygiene activities.
- Use distraction: Conversation, snacks, or music.
- When complete, give praise for clean appearance.

BOX 10-25   Suggested Interventions for Wandering

- Assess for unmet needs.
- Reassure the person that he or she is in the right place.
- Use identification bracelets (in case he or she gets lost).
- Place alarms on the person and/or doors to detect elopement.
- Provide a safe wandering "path."
- Provide alternative activities.
- Minimize medication use (to reduce risk for falls).
- Visually disguise exits.
- Provide daily exercise.
- Provide simple snack foods to be eaten "on the run."

BOX 10-26   Suggested Interventions for Inappropriate Sexual Behavior

- If disrobed, offer clothing.
- If masturbating:
  - Avoid laughing, scolding, or confrontation.
- Guide to a private place.
- Distract the person.

BOX 10-27   Suggested Interventions for Eating and Feeding Issues

- Thoroughly prepare meal trays (open cartons, cut food).
- Offer small, frequent meals and snacks.
- At meals, provide one food and one utensil at a time.
- Provide nutritious finger foods.
- Provide nutritional supplements, if indicated.
- Offer fluids in containers that can be self-managed ("sippy" cups, sports bottles).
- Request speech therapy (ST) and occupational therapy (OT) services, if needed.
- Provide adaptive utensils, if indicated. (OT will order.)
- Assist the client to feed self, rather than feeding, whenever possible.
- Use "hand-over-hand" feeding (your hand guides theirs).
- Gently cue the person to continue eating, chewing, and swallowing.
- Avoid making comments about manners or messiness.
- Provide the person with dignified protection for clothing.
- If agitation develops during feeding, stop and retry a little later.
- Avoid force feeding.
- Reassure the person that his or her food has been paid for (a common concern).
- Monitor body weight to detect gains or losses.

BOX 10-28   Suggested Interventions to Promote Continence and Toileting

- Ensure that toilets are visible.
- Keep bathroom doors open.
- Place signs/pictures as visual cues.
- Keep paths to the bathroom clear.
- Systematically assess voiding and bowel patterns.
- Offer toileting frequently.
- Use incontinence pads or briefs, as needed.
- For persons who can still toilet, use "pull-up"-type protective products.
- Provide adequate fluids during the day.
- Limit fluids at bedtime.
- Avoid beverages with caffeine.
- Ensure adequate fiber in diet.

Activities of Daily Living

As the disease progresses, persons with dementia become more dependent upon caregivers for assistance with activities of daily living (ADLs). See **Boxes 10-27** and **10-28** for suggested interventions in these areas.

Settings for Care: Focus on Adult Day Services

Adult day services are the cornerstone of community-based, long-term care alternatives. These services are designed to meet the needs of cognitively and functionally impaired adults through individualized plans of care (National Adult Day Services Association [NADSA], n.d.). Most frequently referred to as adult day care (ADC),

BOX 10-29   Typical Adult Day Services

- Recreational therapy and activities
- Meals
- Social services
- Transportation

- Personal care: Bathing, hair and nail care
- Nursing services
- Rehabilitation services (less commonly offered)
- Medical services (less commonly offered)

these services offer consumers the opportunity to continue living at home while receiving needed services in a safe, structured environment. They offer a comprehensive program that provides a variety of health, social, and related services in a protective setting during the daytime hours: midday meals, structured recreational activities, socialization opportunities, and appropriate cognitive stimulation (see **Box 10-29**). By 2014, the number of adult day services had increased to about 5,700 nationwide (NADSA, n.d.). Consumers of ADC increasingly have more healthcare and functional needs. Over 50% of ADC consumers have dementia.

As the older adult population increases, adult day services will undoubtedly become more appealing to consumers. Caregivers using ADC for older adults with dementia have more time to rest, run errands, and do other business. Adult day services assist persons with dementia to function at their highest level, strengthen caregivers' abilities and coping skills, and delay institutionalization.

Hospice/Palliative Care

End-of-life care is often fragmented among providers and provider settings, leading to a lack of continuity of care, which impedes the ability to provide high-quality, interdisciplinary care.

Dementia and cognitive impairment are on the rise. AD is the sixth leading cause of death in the United States overall and the fifth leading cause of death in Americans older than 65 years, although this may be an underestimation because AD may not have been listed as the cause of death on the death certificate, even though the patient may have been diagnosed with advanced dementia that significantly contributed to the death. AD is becoming a more common cause of death as the population of the United States and other countries age (Alzheimer's Association, 2016).

A blurred distinction exists between death *with* dementia and death *from* dementia. The different ways in which dementia eventually ends in death can create ambiguity about the underlying cause of death. Severe dementia frequently causes symptoms and complications of chronic disease and terminal illness, as immobility, bedsores, swallowing disorders, malnutrition, and delirium affect many people at the end of life. These can lead to the risk of pneumonia, which has been found as the most common cause of death among the elderly with dementia.

Realizing there is no "right" place to die, where we die is not usually something we get to decide. But, if given the choice, each person and/or his or her family should consider which type of care makes the most sense, where that kind of care can be provided, and whether family and friends are available to help. Enhanced communication among patients, families, and providers is crucial to high-quality end-of-life care.

Recently, the term *palliative care* has come to mean more than just treating symptoms. In the United States, palliative care refers to a comprehensive approach to improving the quality of life for people who are living with potentially fatal diseases. It provides support for family members, very similar to the more familiar concept of hospice care.

In a palliative care program, a multidisciplinary healthcare team works with both the patient and family to provide any support—medical, social, or emotional—needed to live with a chronic illness. Palliative care can be provided in hospitals, nursing homes, outpatient palliative care clinics, certain other specialized clinics, or

Case Study 10–1

Sam was retired from the U.S. Air Force. He was diagnosed with dementia at age 78. As the disease progressed and ADLs became more difficult, Sam's family wanted to explore more treatment options to slow the disease. Through palliative care provided by the Veterans Health Administration, Sam was able to receive the comfort care and emotional support he and his family needed to cope with his health problems. As Sam stabilized, he was discharged home. The program provided help around the house and other support for Sam's wife, making it easier for her to care for him at home.

at home. Medicare covers some of the treatments and medicine, and veterans may be eligible for palliative care through the Department of Veterans Affairs.

Who Can Benefit?

Palliative care is a resource for anyone with a long-term disease that will, in time, probably cause death, not just for people who might die soon. Those suffering from medical diseases, such as heart failure, chronic obstructive pulmonary disease, or chronic renal failure; individuals with disabilities such as PD; or patients with dementia can benefit with palliative care (see **Case Study 10-1**).

In time, if a doctor thinks the patient is not responding to treatment and is likely to die within 6 months, there are two possibilities:

> Palliative care could transition to hospice care.
> Palliative care could continue, with increasing emphasis on comfort care and less focus on medical treatment (See **Table 10-2**).

At this point, providing comprehensive comfort care to the dying person as well as support to his or her family makes more sense. *Hospice* is designed for this situation. The patient beginning hospice care understands that his or her illness is not responding to medical attempts to cure or to slow the disease's progress. Hospice care is beneficial, yet underutilized in advanced dementia. Patients dying with dementia who receive hospice care have better symptom management (Kiely, Givens, Shaffer, Teno, & Mitchell, 2010), fewer hospitalizations, and greater family satisfaction with care than those not receiving hospice care. Trends indicate that hospice enrollment is increasing. See Chapter 27 on end-of-life care for more specific information about hospice and palliative care.

Advance Directives

Although advance directives and advance care planning can be important tools to assist those facing the end of life, evidence suggests that end-of-life decision making in the United States is often poorly implemented. In a recent study, only 51.2% of adults older than 65 years had completed an advance directive (Rao, Anderson, Feng-Chang, & Laux, 2014).

Preparing an advance directive prior to the onset of cognitive impairment or conditions such as AD is very important. A person in the early stages of these conditions will likely still have the capacity to express their preferences and complete an advance directive if he or she had not already done so.

People with Alzheimer's have the legal right to limit or forgo medical or life-sustaining treatment, including the use of mechanical ventilators, cardiopulmonary resuscitation, antibiotics, and artificial nutrition and hydration. These wishes can be expressed through their advance directives.

TABLE 10-2 Some Differences Between Palliative Care and Hospice		
	Palliative Care	**Hospice**
Who can be treated?	Anyone with a serious illness	Anyone with a serious illness whom doctors think has only a short time to live, often less than 6 months
Will my symptoms be relieved?	Yes, as much as possible	Yes, as much as possible
Can I continue to receive treatments to cure my illness?	Yes, if you wish	No, only symptom relief will be provided
Will Medicare pay?	It depends on your benefits and treatment plan	Yes, it pays all hospice charges
Does private insurance pay?	It depends on the plan	It depends on the plan
How long will I be cared for?	This depends on what care you need and your insurance plan	As long as you meet the hospice's criteria of an illness with a life expectancy of months, not years
Where will I receive this care?	Home Assisted living facility Nursing home Hospital	Home Assisted living facility Nursing home Hospice facility Hospital

Nurses should:

> Urge preparation of advance directives early in adulthood
> Help families continue supporting the advance care wishes of their loved ones, especially when their cognitive health is declining
> Encourage review of prepared documents on an annual basis

Legislative Action

Reducing the burden of AD on patients and their families (see **Box 10-30**) is an urgent national priority. The National Alzheimer's Project Act was signed into law in January 2011, calling for the expansion and coordination of research and health service delivery across federal agencies for AD and related dementias.

The top priorities of the Act are to place significant focus on the millions of persons in the United States in the advanced stage of the disease, for whom there is a great need and opportunity to improve patient outcomes, contain healthcare expenditures, reduce disparities, and better coordinate care. It stresses the need for initiatives aimed at the prevention and early detection of dementia. These new efforts to fight AD included making an additional $50 million available for cutting-edge Alzheimer's research.

The additional NIH research funding will support both basic and clinical research. Investments will include research to identify genes that increase the risk of AD and testing therapies in individuals at the highest risk of the disease. On the clinical side, the funds may be used to expand efforts to move new therapeutic approaches into clinical trials and develop better databases to assess the nation's burden of cognitive impairment and dementia.

BOX 10-30   Research Highlight

Aim: To understand how spouses experience dementia in their loved one.

Method: Transcripts were analyzed of 19 90-minute support group meetings for spouses of those with dementia. Spouses were ages 67 to 82, caring for their partner with dementia within about the same age group. The 11 participants in the support group were all white, non-Hispanic and mostly female.

Results: Fourteen metaphors used by the participants were identified. These included the following: Journey, machine or circuit, basic orientation, harm or abuse, game metaphor, hand, child, container (caregiver feels trapped), image, struggle, weight, loss, story/performance, and honeymoon/dream.

Application to practice: Nurses can use these data to inform their conversations with spouses of those experiencing dementia. Listening for metaphoric conversation and understanding as a way of relating experiences and emotions can better inform the support health professionals provide for caregiving spouses.

Reproduced from Golden, M. A., Whaley, B. B., & Stone, A. M. (2012). "The system is beginning to shut down": Utilizing caregivers' metaphors for dementia, persons with dementia, and caregiving. *Applied Nursing Research, 25*(3), 146–151. Copyright 2012, with permission from Elsevier.

This announcement also includes an additional $26 million earmarked for support for caregivers in the community, improving healthcare provider training, and raising public awareness. The preliminary framework for the National AD Plan identifies key goals, including preventing and treating AD by 2025 (National Institute on Aging, 2012).

Summary

Many challenges face the gerontological nurse who is working with patients with dementia. As the population continues to age, the number of persons with dementia will also grow, so nurses need to be well informed about dementia care. Reliable assessment tools are available to assist nurses in recognizing dementia in earlier stages. The content of this chapter presented many suggestions of interventions for the common behaviors encountered among persons with dementia and for their caregivers.

Clinical Reasoning Exercises

1. Delirium may manifest as hypoactive or hyperactive. Which type of delirium do you think is more likely to be identified by nurses in the clinical setting and why?
2. Why do individuals with delirium tend to be unable to communicate appropriately? What are the characteristic features associated with delirium? What are the primary risk factors for the development of delirium? Is delirium a reversible disorder?
3. Evaluate the medication list of one of your clinical clients with dementia or delirium in relation to the Beers Criteria for potentially inappropriate medications for older adults.
4. Given the modest benefits of cholinesterase inhibitors and memantine in the treatment of dementia, debate the pros and cons of administering these medications for persons with dementia.
5. Choose a client in your clinical setting who has dementia. Practice communication strategies.

Personal Reflections

1. Have you ever cared for a patient or family member with dementia? How did you feel about this experience? What did you find most frustrating? How did you handle specific symptoms that caused changes in behavior?

2. What risk factors do you personally have for AD? Are there any activities that you can do to decrease your personal risk?

3. What do you consider the difference between chronic and acute illness?

4. This chapter focused on the nurse's role, but what challenges do you think family members face in caring for loved ones with AD?

References

Algase, D. L., Beck, C., Kolanowski, A., Whall, A., Berent, S., Richards, K., & Beattie, E. (1996). Need-driven dementia-compromised behavior: An alternative view of disruptive behavior. *American Journal of Alzheimer's Disease, 11*(6), 10–19.

Alzheimer's Association (2016). Alzheimer's disease facts and figures. *Alzheimer's and Dementia, 12*(4), 1–80.

American Association for Geriatric Psychiatry. (2006). Position statement: Principles of care for patients with dementia resulting from Alzheimer disease. Retrieved from http://www.aagponline.org/index.php?src=news&srctype=detail&category=Position%20Statement&refno=35

American Geriatrics Society Beers Criteria Update Expert Panel. (2015). American Geriatrics Society 2015 updated Beers Criteria for potentially inappropriate medication use in older adults. *Journal of the American Geriatrics Society, 63*(11), 2227–2246.

American Psychiatric Association. (2013). *Diagnostic and statistical manual of mental disorders* (5th ed.). Arlington, VA: American Psychiatric Publishing.

Bis, J. C., DeCarli, C., Smith, A. V., van der Lijn, F., Crivello, F., Fornage, M., . . . Cohorts for Heart and Aging Research in Genomic Epidemiology Consortium. (2012). Common variants at 12q14 and 12q24 are associated with hippocampal volume. *Nature Genetics, 44*(5), 545–551.

Boersma, P., vanWeert, J. C. M., Lakerveld, J., & Droes, R. M. (2015). The art of successful implementation of psychosocial interventions in residential dementia care: A systematic review of the literature based on the RE-AIM framework. *International Psychogeriatrics, 27*(1), 19–35.

Borson, S., Scanlan, J. M., Brush, M., Vitallano, P., & Dokmak, A. (2000). The Mini-Cog: A cognitive "vital signs" measure for dementia screening in multi-lingual elderly. *International Journal of Geriatric Psychiatry, 15*(11), 1021–1027.

Buckley, J. S. & Salpeter, S. R. (2015). Risk-benefit assessment of dementia medications: Systemic review of the evidence. *Drugs & Aging, 32*(6), 453–467.

Butler, R. N. (1963). The life review: An interpretation of reminiscence in the aged. *Psychiatry, 26,* 65–68.

Carmago, C. H., Justus, F. F., & Retzlaff, G. (2015). The effectiveness of reality orientation in the treatment of Alzheimer's disease. *American Journal of Alzheimer's Disease and Other Dementias, 30*(5), 527–532.

Cohen-Mansfield, J. (1996). Conceptualization of agitation results based on the Cohen-Mansfield Agitation Inventory and the Agitation Behavior Mapping Instrument. *International Psychogeriatrics, 8* (3 Suppl.), 309–315.

Corbett, A., Husebo, B. S., Achterberg, W. P., Erdal, A., & Flo, E. (2014). The importance of pain management in older people with dementia. *British Medical Bulletin, 111*(1), 139–148.

Cordell, C. B., Borson, S., Boustani, M., Chodosh, J., Reuben, D., Verghese, J., . . . & The Medicare Detection of Cognitive Impairment Workgroup (2013). Alzheimers' Association recommendations for operationalizing the detection of cognitive impairment during the Medicare Annual Wellness Visit in a primary care setting. *Alzheimer's & Dementia, 9*(2), 141–150.

Dawson, P., Wells, D. L., & Kline, K. (1993). *Enhancing the abilities of persons with Alzheimer's and related dementias: A nursing perspective.* New York, NY: Springer.

DementiaCareCentral. (2013). *Basic tips for caregiving.* Retrieved January 2, 2017 from http://www.dementiacarecentral .com/caregiverinfo/tips

Feil, N. (1993). *The validation breakthrough: Simple techniques for communicating with people with Alzheimer's-type dementia.* Baltimore, MD: Health Professions Press.

Fong, T. G., Davis, D., Growdon, M. E., & Inouye, S. K. (2015). The interface between delirium and dementia in elderly adults. *Lancet Neurology, 14*(8), 823–832.

Gitlin, L. N., Liebman, J., & Winter, L. (2003). Are environmental interventions effective in the management of Alzheimer's disease and related disorders? A synthesis of the evidence. *Alzheimer's Care Quarterly, 4*(2), 85–107.

Golden, M. A., Whaley, B. B., & Stone, A. M. (2012). "The system is beginning to shut down": Utilizing caregivers' metaphors for dementia, persons with dementia, and caregiving. *Applied Nursing Research, 25*(3), 146–151.

Hall, G. R. (1994). Caring for people with Alzheimer's disease using the conceptual model of Progressively Lowered Stress Threshold in the clinical setting. *Nursing Clinics of North America, 29*(1), 129–141.

Hall, G. R., & Buckwalter, K. C. (1987). Progressively lowered stress threshold: A conceptual model for the care of adults with Alzheimer's disease. *Archives of Psychiatric Nursing, 1*(6), 399–406.

Inouye, S., van Dyck, C., Alessi, C., Balkin, S., Siegal, A., & Horwitz, R. (1990). Clarifying confusion: The confusion assessment method. *Annals of Internal Medicine, 113*(12), 941–948.

International Psychogeriatric Association). (2012). Behavioral and psychological symptoms of dementia (BPSD). Retrieved http://www.bsa.ualberta.ca/sites/default/files/____IPA_BPSD_Specialists_Guide_Online.pdf

Jackson, P., & Khan, A. (2015). Delirium in critically ill patients. *Critical Care Clinics, 31*(3), 589–603.

Junxin, L., & Porock, D. (2014). Resident outcomes of person-centered care in long-term care: A narrative review of interventional research. *Int J Nurs Stud, 51*(10), 1395–1415.

Kiely, D. K., Givens, J. L., Shaffer, M. I., Teno, J. M., & Mitchell, S. L. (2010). Hospice use and outcomes in nursing home residents with advanced dementia. *Journal of the American Geriatric Society, 58*(12), 2284–2291.

Kitwood, T. (1997). *Dementia reconsidered: The person comes first.* Buckingham, UK: Open University Press.

Kolanowski, A. M. (1999). An overview of the need-driven, dementia-compromised behavior model. *Journal of Gerontological Nursing, 25*(9), 7–9.

Kolanowski, A., & Buettner, L. (2008). Prescribing activities that engage passive residents: An innovative method. *Journal of Gerontological Nursing, 34*(1), 13–18.

Lawton, M. P. (1982). Competence, environmental press, and the adaptation of older people. In M. P. Lawton, P. G. Windley, & T. O. Byerts (Eds.), *Aging and the environment: Theoretical approaches* (pp. 33–59). New York, NY: Springer.

Livingston, F., Kelly, L., Lewis-Holmes, E, Baio, G., Morris, S., Patel, N., . . . & Cooper, C. (2014). Non-pharmacological interventions for agitation in dementia: Systematic review of randomized controlled trials. *The British Journal of Psychiatry, 205*(6), 436–442.

McKhann, G. M., Knopman, D. S., Chertkow, H., Hyman, B. T., Clifford, R. J., Kawas, C. H., . . . & Phelps, C. H. (2011). The diagnosis of dementia due to Alzheimer's disease: Recommendations for the National Institute on Aging-Alzheimer's Association workgroups on diagnostic guidelines for Alzheimer's disease. *Alzheimer's & Dementia, 7*(3), 263–269.

Nasreddine, Z. S., Phillips, N. A., Bedirian, V., Charbonneau, S., Whitehead, V., Collin, I., ... & Chertkow, H. (2005). The Montreal Cognitive Assessment, MoCA: A brief screening tool for mild cognitive impairment. *Journal of the American Geriatrics Society, 53*, 695–699.

National Adult Day Services Association (NADSA). (n.d.). About adult day services. Retrieved from http://www .nadsa.org/learn-more/about-adult-day-services/

National Institute on Aging. (2007). Alzheimer's disease: Unraveling the mystery. Retrieved from https://www.nia
.nih.gov/alzheimers/publication/alzheimers-disease-unraveling-mystery/preface

National Institute on Aging. (2016). Alzheimer's disease fact sheet. NIH Publication No. 16-AG-6423. Retrieved
January 2, 2017 from http://www.nia.nih.gov/alzheimers/publication/alzheimers-disease-fact-sheet

Neal, M., & Barton Wright, P. (2008). Validation therapy for dementia. [Systematic review]. *Cochrane Dementia
and Cognitive Improvement Group Cochrane Database of Systematic Reviews, 2.*

Netz, Y., Axelrad, S., & Argov, E. (2007). Group physical activity for demented older adults: Feasibility and
effectiveness. *Clinical Rehabilitation, 21*(11), 977–986.

Norris, A. D. (1986). *Reminiscence with elderly people.* London, UK: Winslow.

Obregon, D., Hou, H., Deng, J., Giunta, B., Tian, J., Darlington, D., . . . & Tan, J. (2012). Soluble amyloid precursor protein-α modulates β-secretase activity and amyloid-β generation. *Nature Communications, 3,* 777.
doi:10.1038/ncomms1781

Ortega, V., Qazi, A., Spector, A., & Orrell, M. (2015). Psychological treatments for depression and anxiety in
dementia and mild cognitive impairment: Systematic review and meta-analysis. *British Journal of Psychiatry,
207*(4), 293–298.

Rao, J. K., Anderson, L. A., Feng-Chang, L., & Laux, J. P. (2014). Completion of advance directives among U.S.
consumers. *American Journal of Preventive Care, 46*(1), 65–70.

Reisberg, B., Franssen, E. H., Souren, L. E. M., Auer, S. R., Akram, I., & Kenowsky, S. (2002). Evidence and
mechanisms of retrogenesis in Alzheimer's and other dementias. *American Journal of Alzheimer's Disease and
Other Dementias, 17*(4), 202–212.

Sheikh, J. I., & Yesavage, J. A. (1986). Geriatric Depression Scale (GDS): Recent evidence and development of a
shorter version. In T. L. Brink (Ed.), *Clinical gerontology: A guide to assessment and intervention* (pp. 165–173).
New York, NY: Haworth Press.

Smith, M., Buckwalter, K., & Mitchell, S. (1993). Acting up and acting out: Assessment and management of
aggressive and acting out behaviors. In M. Smith, K. Buckwalter, & C. M. Mitchell (Eds.), *The geriatric mental
health training series.* New York, NY: Springer.

Snow, T. (2016). A voice for dementia: Basics for success. Retrieved from http://teepasnow.com/subscriptions/16jan
/BasicsForSuccess.htm

Talerico, K. A., O'Brien, J. A., & Swafford, K. L. (2003). Person-centered care: An important approach for 21st
century health care. *Journal of Psychosocial Nursing and Mental Health Services, 41*(11), 12–16.

Tariq, S. H., Tumosa, N., Chibnall, J. T., Perry, M. H., & Morley, J. E. (2006). Comparison of the Saint Louis University Mental Status Examination and the Mini-Mental State Examination for detecting dementia and mild
neurocognitive disorder: A pilot study. *American Journal of Geriatric Psychiatry, 14,* 900–910.

U.S. Department of Health and Human Services. (2008). *Advance directives and advance care planning: Report to
Congress.* Retrieved January 2, 2017 from http://aspe.hhs.gov/daltcp/reports/2008/adcongrpt.htm

Woods, B., Spector, A., Jones, C., Orrell, M., & Davies, S. (2008). Reminiscence therapy for dementia. [Systematic
Review]. *Cochrane Dementia and Cognitive Improvement Group Cochrane Database of Systematic Reviews, 2*
CD001120.

Yesavage, J. A., Brink, T. L., Rose, T. L., Lum, O., Huang, V., Adey, M. B., & Leirer, V. O. (1983). Development and validation of a geriatric depression screening scale: A preliminary report. *Journal of Psychiatric Research, 17*(1), 37–49.

For a full suite of assignments and additional learning activities, see the access code at the front of your
book.

Unit V
Management of Geriatric Syndromes

CHAPTER 16   SLEEP DISORDERS
(COMPETENCIES 7, 17, 18)

CHAPTER 17   DYSPHAGIA AND MALNUTRITION
(COMPETENCY 7)

CHAPTER 18   PRESSURE ULCERS
(COMPETENCIES 7, 17)

CHAPTER 11

Polypharmacy

Demetra Antimisiaris
Dennis J. Cheek

(Competencies 7, 17)

LEARNING OBJECTIVES

Evaluate the patient's medication list to formulate a plan to address medication-related problems before they occur.

> Recognize the symptoms of the syndrome of polypharmacy in elderly patients, acknowledging that the symptoms may be quite distant from the cause.
> Understand how goals of care influence appropriateness of medication choice.
> Identify drugs that are being used to treat side effects of other drugs.
> Explain how medications are tested for safety and efficacy with relationship to the elderly.
> Develop a personal system of addressing polypharmacy and medication-related problems in the clinical setting.
> Discuss how increasing medication burden can pose a hazard to the cognitively impaired elder.
> Describe why nurses have a unique perspective and role in the healthcare team when it comes to medication use and outcomes.

KEY TERMS

Accountability	Falls
Activities of daily living	Iatrogenic harm
Adverse drug reactions	Iatrogenesis
Beers Criteria	Instrumental activities of daily living
Brown bag assessment	Isolation
Delirium	Medication administration record
Dementia	Medication-related problem (MRP)
Depression	Morbidity
Geriatric syndrome	Mortality

National Transitions of Care Coalition
  (NTOCC)
Pharmacodynamics
Pharmacogenomics
Pharmacokinetics

Polypharmacy
Prescribing cascade
START criteria
STOPP criteria
Titration

Polypharmacy, or the concurrent use of multiple medications, fits the definition of a *geriatric syndrome* in that it is a common health condition in older adults that does not fit into the category of a discrete disease. Geriatric syndromes are highly prevalent within the older age group, multifactorial in etiology, and associated with substantial morbidity and mortality (Inouye, Stuenksi, Tinetti, & Kuchel, 2007). Four shared characteristics are associated with an increased risk of living with geriatric syndromes: older age, baseline cognitive impairment, baseline functional impairment, and impaired mobility. These are markers of frailty, and generally the more frail a person is, the higher the chance is that the person will experience multiple geriatric syndromes, including poor outcomes with medication use. An understanding of the relationship between frailty and medication misadventure will help clinicians identify and intervene to prevent potential polypharmacy-caused *morbidity* and *mortality*. Frailty alters *pharmacokinetics* (how drugs are absorbed, metabolized, and eliminated), *pharmacodynamics* (how drugs work in the body), and a person's ability to manage medications. Age is not necessarily a direct indication of frailty. Persons living with chronic disease who are under 65 years of age can be frail and face some of the same risks as an older frail person with respect to medication outcomes. Conversely, older people who are relatively healthy can tolerate and manage medications as well as a younger adult. A person's physiologic reserve is a strong determinant of one's ability to tolerate medications and resist medication harm. We will discuss polypharmacy as a geriatric syndrome; however, the principles presented are applicable to anyone using medications, especially the chronically ill and frail.

Statistics on the number of medications used per person in the United States are slow to appear in the literature. The Agency for Healthcare Research and Quality, a federally funded agency, in their May 2009 statistical brief noted that as of 2006, the average senior used approximately six prescriptions, which has increased from five noted in the past decade. This report also documents that the number of prescriptions per person increases with age (Stagnitti, 2009). The Kaiser Foundation Annual report on State Health Facts reveals that adults aged 19 to 64 filled an average of 12.6 prescriptions per person in 2014, whereas the elderly (65 years and older) filled an average of 27.9 prescriptions per person in 2014. Intuitively, this trend is likely to keep increasing over time. From the period of year 2000 to 2008, the number of people using one, two, and five prescription medications within the past month increased from 4% to 48%, 25% to 31%, and 6% to 11%, respectively (Gu, Dillon, & Burt, 2010). The total number of prescriptions per capita in the United States, including all age groups, is increasing over time; the number of scripts per capita as of 2014 was standing at 12.7, an increase from the 1997 level of 8.9 (Kaiser Foundation, 2014). There are many factors driving the trend toward increased medication use in the population at large. The most obvious is that there are just more medications available than ever before. The *Physicians' Desk Reference* (PDR, 1969) in 1969 consisted of 1,415 pages of monographs for every prescription and over-the-counter (OTC) product available in the United States. By 2012, the PDR consisted of 3,151 pages for just the prescription products alone, with a separate book approximately 800 pages in length to cover the OTC products (PDR, 2012). Additionally, an average of 27 products are approved by the U.S. Food and Drug Administration (FDA) annually, with very few taken off the market during the same period (Vandegrift & Datta, 2006).

The risks associated with multiple medication use are present at any age, but in the elderly who are frail and living with increasing multiple chronic diseases, that risk is more prevalent. Polypharmacy, like any other geriatric syndrome, can look on the surface like a specific disease state, while in actuality the symptoms observed are due to multiple and distant causes. A common example is when an elder is taking OTC nonsteroidal antiinflammatory drug (NSAID) pain medications and their blood pressure is mysteriously and suddenly elevated. Typically, the patient will be diagnosed as having worsening hypertension and a new hypertension medication will be prescribed, when the real cause is an OTC NSAID. This is usually not reported to the physician by the patient because the patient perceives OTC products as insignificant and is not aware of the connection between blood pressure and NSAID use.

How many medications used at the same time are enough to be labeled polypharmacy? As you can see in the previous example, it only takes one when viewing polypharmacy as a harmful syndrome. Although the word *polypharmacy* is derived from the Greek words "poly," meaning many, and "pharmakon," which means drug, polypharmacy as a syndrome can involve any one medication or multiple medications that in combination cause harm, are unnecessary, or are used inappropriately (Masoodi, 2008). Most medical literature commonly defines polypharmacy as the concomitant use of five medications; however, a particular number of drugs used at the same time do not always predict medication harm. Polypharmacy is seen among all age groups, but the combination of multiple chronic diseases, multiple doctors, multiple pharmacies, *isolation*, and advanced age increases the risk of medication harm. Consider polypharmacy in light of the following polypharmacy syndrome risk factors: 30% of elders live alone (which increases to 47% for women over 75), 41% of seniors reported taking five or more prescription medications, more than 50% have two or more physicians, and an estimated 64% of older individuals without *dementia* have some cognitive impairment (Caracciolo, Gatz, Xu, Perdersen, & Fratiglioni, 2012; Wilson, Schoen, & Neuman, 2007).

Polypharmacy poses a greater hazard for the elderly patient because of a diminished ability to eliminate medications as well as diminished physiological reserves. These issues, in combination with impairment in cognition, cause problems with an elder's ability to manage medications and report when adverse events occur.

Significance of the Problem
Morbidity, Mortality, and Costs

Inadvertent harm caused by the syndrome of polypharmacy accounts for numerous unnecessary costs to the healthcare system and patients (Budnitz, Lovegrove, & Shehab, 2011). It has been estimated that of hospitalized patients, 2,216,000 experience serious *adverse drug reactions* (ADRs), and of these patients 106,000 die annually from an ADR (Lazarou, Pomeranz, & Corey, 1998). To place this statistic in perspective, deaths from ADRs, if included in Centers for Disease Control and Prevention (CDC) rankings of causes of death, would place ADRs as the fifth leading cause of death annually, ahead of Alzheimer's disease (AD), diabetes, and kidney disease (CDC, 2012). However, statistics on ADRs are only as accurate as one's ability to recognize when an ADR is the cause. Most reported ADRs are incidents in which a medication was given and the person died shortly thereafter or a person was hospitalized for an ADR specifically and the result was death. The number of deaths attributed to organic causes such as kidney failure, which were actually caused by organ damage due to chronic or acute medication use, is still not well quantified. It is important to be aware that current statistics on the deaths or harm due to ADRs come mainly, if not all, from hospital records or institutional records such as nursing homes (where ADRs are often underreported due to lack of recognition of medication side effects). Therefore, the magnitude of ADR-related morbidity and mortality occurring in the ambulatory population at large is overlooked. The reported statistics on ADRs thus, are a potential underestimate of the true overall harm resulting from medication use.

In older patients (those over 65 years of age), up to 30% of the persons admitted to the hospital are admitted for *medication-related problems* (MRPs) (Marcum et al., 2012). In the nursing home setting, for every $1.00 spent on drugs, $1.33 in healthcare resources is consumed to treat drug-related problems (Bootman, Harrison, & Cox, 1997). A systemic review of observational studies found an overall 5.3% of hospital admissions associated with ADRs, with higher rates in the elderly (Kongkaew, Noyce, Ashcroft, 2008).

The risk of ADRs rises exponentially with the addition of each new medication to a person's drug regimen. Despite this, as a society, we are increasing our concomitant use of medication more each year (Denham, 1990).

An Important Historical Perspective

The stunning statistics on individual medication burden and medication-related harm associated with polypharmacy seems to have silently developed as our society rapidly increases the use of medications over a relatively short period of time. We are at an unprecedented time in history in which people are taking medications in a way as never before. Consider that our knowledge and ability to design drugs to fight disease is a relatively recent phenomenon. This means that an understanding of what happens when multiple medications are combined is in its infancy.

It was not until the mid-to-late 1800s that ether was determined to be a safer anesthetic than chloroform. Little discussion of specific dosing for specific patient types circulated in those days. It was one physician-scientist learning through trial and error and keeping notes in his corner of the world, in contrast to the way we derive and disseminate medical data and knowledge today. The first medication in the era of modern medicine use was in the early 1900s when aspirin was discovered to be a universal pain reliever. After that, in the 1930s and 1940s, penicillin and the first semisynthetic antibiotic, tetracycline, were developed. The field of pharmacokinetics was discovered in the 1960s and 1970s, and we started to understand that drugs are absorbed into the body, distributed, and eliminated primarily through the kidneys and liver.

In the late 1990s, with the mapping of the human genome for the first time, we then discovered that we all have a genetic, set-at-birth capacity to metabolize medications through numerous different pathways, each one working at a different rate in different people (*pharmacogenomics*). Yet for most medications we still have standard recommended doses for all adults regardless of individual pharmacogenomics. Today, knowledge of the physiology of aging is expanding, and even starting in our late 20s some people slowly move toward having less physiological reserve. As we lose muscle mass and our percentage of body fat increases, we become increasingly frail and our organs become more impaired. Medications can behave differently than they did in fairly healthy, carefully selected individuals the drugs were tested in for safety, efficacy, and FDA approval. In addition to new knowledge of the physiology of aging, the first clinical studies of polypharmacy and its relationship to morbidity, impaired function, and outcomes started to emerge just after the turn of this century.

Guidelines and Medical Literature on Polypharmacy

The guidance on recommended medication use to treat chronic disease and medical problems is designed to demonstrate efficacy and rarely designed to tell how drugs will perform in the frail elder. Drugs are brought to market through an FDA-guided safety and efficacy trial process, which often does not include the older patient or the patient who has multiple problems and takes multiple combinations of medications. For example, a medication being tested to treat Alzheimer's dementia (AD), which did not make it to market, had the following exclusion criteria: the patient would not qualify for the drug trial if they had "neurodegenerative disease and/or dementias other than AD, are a frequent smoker and/or frequent consumer of caffeine, have hypothyroidism, or folic acid deficiency or B12 deficiency, a history or presence of stroke or epilepsy, a history of an MI [myocardial infarction] within 5 years, severe hypotension or hypertension requiring therapy, uncontrolled atrial fibrillation or AV block higher than 1st degree" (Sunovion Pharmaceuticals, 2006). Most of the patients ineligible for this drug trial possessed many of the characteristics found in patients with dementia, who will ultimately use the medication, but the medication would be brought to market having been tried in a very different, and much healthier, group of patients. Additionally, how many patients are not going to smoke or consume coffee and soft drinks with caffeine? The take-home point is that most drugs studied in drug trials, including safety and efficacy trials for FDA approval and those aimed at proving drug efficacy in various disease states, do not include subjects who are likely to have poor or dangerous outcomes. Because the studies are designed mainly to look for efficacy, they are designed for success in proving efficacy, as opposed to looking for toxicity in the frailest patients. This means that most of the frail elders, the older old, or the people with multiple chronic disease and end organ damage will not be represented in our evidence-based guidance. It is easy to see why the elderly suffer poor outcomes caused by polypharmacy, given the way medications are tested for efficacy. Elders have multiple comorbidities, use more medication than younger patients and are not included in drug studies unless they are fairly healthy.

Another discrepancy between the literature on medication and the actual elderly medication user is that OTC drug and supplement use is not accounted for in the medical literature except on a case-by-case basis. It has been documented that 30% of elders take an analgesic medication and more than 60% of those individuals cannot identify the active ingredient in their brand of pain reliever. Overall, 40% of Americans believe that OTC medications are too weak to cause any real harm (Zagaria, 2009). These are alarming facts in light of the record number of medications going from prescription to OTC status.

The elder at large is not as carefully followed as the study subjects are by the study investigator physicians and team of clinical trial professionals. Older adult patients are faced with the challenges of aging and poor health such as multiple doctors, pharmacies, transitions of care, psychosocial isolation, and challenges performing their *activities of daily living* (ADLs) and *instrumental activities of daily living* (IADLs), all of which affect the ability to safely use medications but are not necessarily accounted for in the guidance. Thus, the assumption that what worked well in the medical literature, which produced guidelines or brought new drugs to market, will work well in the elderly patient is a false assumption under the current healthcare system.

We should assume that in elders, guidelines on disease state management are guidelines and not absolute benchmarks to reach to reap good outcomes. This is an important point because healthcare systems are increasingly moving toward rewards for meeting chronic disease management guidelines, and it is important to consider that those guidelines were not tested in the very old and very frail. An example would be the Centers for Medicaid and Medicare Services (CMS) PQRS program, which offers incentives to prescribers for meeting criteria for disease management; one example would be that a person with documented cardiovascular disease is prescribed a statin (PQRI, n.d). Additionally, there is the literature that makes sweeping health policy suggestions, such as a piece suggesting that statins should be served at fast food outlets in the condiments (Ferenczi, Asaria, Hughes, Chaturvedi, & Francis, 2010). Statins have not been tested in many older patients, and there are very few study subjects above the age of 72 in the studies from which the guidelines for statin use were derived. Even the JUPITER trial (Justification for the Use of Statins in Prevention: An Intervention Trial Evaluating Rosuvastatin), which was aimed at studying primary prevention in men over 50 and women over 60 years of age with elevated C-reactive protein, did not include any subjects over 71 years of age despite being conducted at 1,315 sites in 26 countries (Ridker et al., 2008).

An individualistic approach to each elder is necessary for safe medication use. This is not to suggest that guidance on adult disease management is not important, but rather to emphasize that guidance needs to be individualized for the frail elder until such time that more specific guidelines for elders becomes available. As we age, we become more physiologically diverse from one another through different environmental exposures, disease states, and genetic influences (see **Figure 11-1**).

Unfortunately, the individual approach takes time, for which the office visit typically does not allow. The average office visit consists of 15 minutes, of which 7 minutes is dedicated to greeting and social discussion, leaving a little over 7 minutes to address a patient's problems. According to one study, the result is an average of 3 minutes dedicated to discussion of medications per typical office visit (Tai-Seale, McGuire, & Zhang, 2007). If you are a frail elder on 20 medications, no one may be assessing the overall regimen for appropriateness, adherence, and side effects beyond the obvious, such as bleeds or abnormal laboratory values, which may be the only cue the prescriber has that something may be wrong with the medication regimen.

The healthcare community is beginning to study the impact of higher overall drug burden on elder function and well-being. From 1986 to 2011, there have been 19 studies using rigorous observational or interventional designs examining the relationship between medication use and functional status decline in the elderly. Of these,

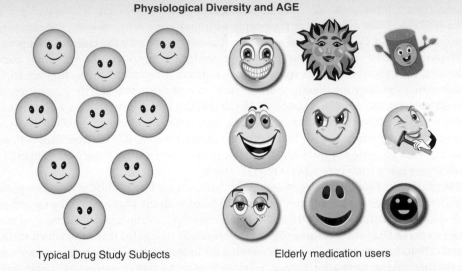

Physiological Diversity and AGE

Typical Drug Study Subjects   Elderly medication users

Figure 11-1 Cohort on the left represents the homogeneity of the typical study subject. Much of our study data and guidelines are built upon the study design seen on the left, but applied to the group on the right—the elderly, who are individually quite diverse.

three studies found an increased risk in functional decline among elders living with polypharmacy overall. Benzodiazepine use and functional decline were associated in four studies. As for antidepressants, one study found no relationship between antidepressant use and functional status, and another randomized trial found amitriptyline to impair some measures of gait. Anticholinergic burden was associated with worsening functional status in two studies. Several studies looked at multiple central nervous system drugs and found links to greater declines in self-reported mobility, with one study reporting hospitalized rehabilitation patients who used hypnotics/anxiolytics having a lower functional independence measure in motor gains than nonusers. Antihypertensive medications have been linked to impairment in functional status in two studies (Peron, Gray, & Hanlon, 2011). A review of 99,628 patients, over 65 hospitalized for ADRs, found that half were over 80 years of age, and four medications or medication classes were implicated alone or in combination. The high-risk medications were implicated in only 1.2% of cases, surprisingly. The four medication (classes) were warfarin, insulin, oral antiplatelets, and oral hypoglycemics (Budnitz et al., 2011). These are medications that we understand well and are commonly used, and, with appropriate monitoring, ADRs should be avoidable.

Risk Factors

Multiple Medications: The Prescribing Cascade—Is It the Medication or the Disease?

As mentioned earlier, the more medications a person takes concurrently, the higher is the risk of experiencing a MRP. Any one medication possesses multiple inherent risks (see **Figure 11-2**). There is the immediate risk of any medication causing anaphylaxis, and then there are the typical known side effects, the atypical side effects, the counterintuitive side effects, the dose limitations, the long-term use side effects, and the user error side effects. Take hydrochlorothiazide (HCTZ), a common "water" pill. Usually people think about monitoring for low potassium, but HCTZ requires ongoing monitoring not only of potassium, but also chloride, sodium, magnesium, lipids (can contribute to hyperlipidemia), uric acid (can lead to gout), complete blood counts (CBCs; can cause hemolytic anemia, *thrombocytopenia*), and glucose (can increase glucose resistance). HCTZ is a medication that patients sometimes take more than recommended because they diagnose themselves as needing to lose water, so adherence assessment is important in determining if side effects are relevant to regular use or hidden misuse of medication.

When medication side effects are treated with other medications, it is called the *prescribing cascade*. Usually, the practice of treating medication side effects with other medications is not intentional and is due to the mistaken identification of a medication side effect as organic in origin (caused by a disease or condition). Occasionally, in patients who necessitate extreme doses of a medication to control a condition for which there are no alternative treatments, side effects are anticipated and purposefully treated with other medications because the risk of discontinuation of the first medication outweighs the benefit. An example might

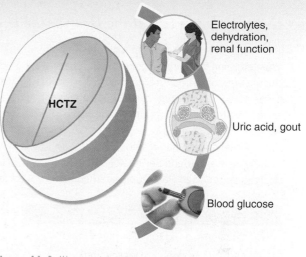

Figure 11-2 Illustration of the multiple monitoring issues that have to be addressed even in commonly utilized medications such as hydrochlorothiazide (HCTZ).
Blood glucose photo: © Dmitry Lobanov/Shutterstock

be a patient who demonstrates extreme agitation and aggression without high-dose antipsychotic therapy and would be unable to live successfully in the community or be part of an institutional setting appropriate for the patient's well-being without the risky antipsychotic use. Under such circumstances, the expected side effects of extrapyramidal syndrome (movement disorder) and metabolic syndrome might be treated with benztropine (a strong anticholinergic, used to address the drug-induced movement disorder) and glyburide. Benztropine can cause serious side effects itself, such as cardiac problems, impaired cognition, urinary retention, ocular issues, and temperature deregulation, as can glyburide, which can cause hypoglycemia and requires constant glucose monitoring. With the intentional use of medications to treat the side effects of another medication, the clinician should document the rationale for doing so, including the risks versus benefits, and the monitoring parameters along with the recommended intervals of monitoring. More times than not, the use of medications to treat the side effects of other medications is not intentional and, as a consequence, unnecessary and inappropriate use of medications occurs. The following prescribing cascade case illustrates a common polypharmacy scenario (see **Case Study 11-1**).

This was an actual case in which a patient had been diagnosed with and treated for Parkinson's disease (PD), despite the real cause of her movement disorder being the combination of drugs that are known (or not so well known) to induce movement disorders as a side effect (Alvarez & Evidente, 2008; Mellor, Ahme, & Thomson, 2009). The diagnosis of PD was made by her primary care doctor. She had moderate to severe dementia and lacked the verbal ability to describe the history of the onset of her movement disorder, which contributed to the inappropriate diagnosis that masked the true underlying cause of symptoms related to medication use.

Multiple Prescribers and Iatrogenic Harm

Today's healthcare system is very complex, and patients are handled by multiple physicians, facilities, healthcare agencies, and pharmacies. A well-known book entitled *To Err is Human* published statistics from a Harvard medical practice for the year 1984 and found that adverse events were responsible for 13.6% of all deaths and that 2.6% of errors resulted in permanent, disabling injury. It was determined by expert opinion that 56% of these adverse outcomes were preventable (Kohn, Corrigan, & Donaldson, 1999). This is known as *iatrogenic harm*

Case Study 11–1: Is It the Drug or the Disease

J. C. is an 84-year-old woman who presented to an assisted living home for assistance with her IADLs. Upon review of her admission medication orders, it was noted that she had some medications that are known to be inappropriate to use in the elderly, such as fluoxetine and metoclopramide (per the Beers Criteria). She had a significant amount of aphasia, tremor, and periods of agitation and aggression reportedly due to her dementia.

Past Medical History	
Hypertension	Vascular dementia
Parkinson's disease	Depression
Chronic atrial fibrillation	Osteoarthritis

Medications Upon Admission	
Warfarin 4 mg daily	Memantine 10 mg twice daily
Fluoxetine 20 mg daily	Tramadol 25 mg up to four times daily
Carbidopa-levodopa 25/100 mg three times daily	Metoprolol 25 mg XL daily
Metoclopramide 10 mg 30 minutes before meals	Hydrochlorothiazide 25 mg daily
Donepezil 10 mg daily	Quetiapine 25 mg twice daily
Acetaminophen 325 mg two tablets every 8 hours	

Medication Adjustments:

When the attending physician reviewed her case, she immediately recognized that the fluoxetine was too long acting for use in elders and discontinued it (American Geriatrics Society [AGS] Beers Criteria Update Expert Panel, 2015). The half-life of fluoxetine is about 48 to 70 hours, with an active metabolite that can remain in the body for another 15 days; in an elder, this can be longer. This long half-life elevates the risk that elders will build up too much fluoxetine due to impaired clearance. Most psychoactive medications cannot be abruptly stopped, but fluoxetine's half-life is so long that it self-tapers as it takes its time eliminating and is one of the only psychoactive medications that can be stopped immediately. The doctor's plan was to start citalopram in a few weeks instead of fluoxetine. She also immediately discontinued the metoclopramide, recognizing that its antidopaminergic effect is not safe to use in patients with movement disorders. She discontinued the tramadol due to its risk of not clearing efficiently in renally impaired patients, and J. C.'s estimated creatinine clearance was calculated at less than 30 mL/min. She instead prescribed routine acetaminophen for J. C.'s arthritis pain.

When the tramadol, fluoxetine, and metoclopramide were removed, her tremor went away and therefore, she did not need to take carbidopa-levodopa anymore. Her quality of life improved dramatically. J. C. was better able to walk and participate in activities and self-care. The elimination of the offending medications also revealed that her dementia-related behaviors of aggression and agitation were actually akathisia related to the use of fluoxetine, tramadol, and metoclopramide. Her orders for an antipsychotic agent twice daily were eliminated as a result. The patient lived the rest of her life pleasantly, with dementia as her primary problem, and was much more comfortable than when first presented.

or *iatrogenesis*, meaning doctor- or healthcare-created harm. Decades ago this complex dynamic in the healthcare system was less prevalent because there were fewer medications, interventions, and specialists. Elders are unfamiliar with how to safely negotiate their way through today's complicated healthcare system. When today's elders were younger, the medical system left the coordination of a person's health care to the physician's office. Generally, people would see one doctor for all their problems, and that doctor would spend a great deal of time with them, knew all of their history, came to the hospital when they were admitted, and knew their family and medications because that one doctor treated the whole family over their lifetime and was the sole prescriber. The average number of physicians that a patient over 65 years old today sees is 7. It would not be self-evident to an elder (or perhaps anyone) that bringing *all* of their medications to all 7 doctor visits and the hospital is a necessary precaution to foster safer medication assessment. For seniors living with five or more chronic conditions (approximately 20% of seniors), this number goes up to 14 different doctors at different addresses. This group also averages over 40 office visits in one year (Berenson, 2010).

Medication reconciliation by healthcare professionals is a serious challenge for numerous reasons. One of the most significant threats to sound medication reconciliation is the systemic problem of transitions of care. This leaves the patient as the healthcare provider's only witness to all of the medication changes. The patients themselves are perplexed by having to navigate a healthcare system that is very complex, difficult to understand, and hard to follow. Another threat to medication reconciliation is having to follow multiple providers' instructions and order changes, especially for elderly patients who are too ill to absorb so much constantly changing information. Serious MRPs can occur because of lack of coordination of care, lack of patient advocacy, and poor communication between providers. Today, the elder is faced with multiple physicians, multiple prescribers, and the obligation to coordinate their own care. The more an elder is exposed to the healthcare system, the higher the risk is for iatrogenic harm (Permpongkosol, 2011).

Despite multiple exposures to physicians' offices and hospitals and multiple missed opportunities to catch medication errors, most adverse drug events are rooted in the encounter with the prescriber, with a lesser part of the cause attributed to adherence. A study of the incidence and preventability of adverse drug events in community-dwelling elders found that 58.4% started at the prescribing stage, with 60.8% of these events having poor drug monitoring involved and only 21% attributed to problems with patient adherence. (The percentages do not add up to 100% because of overlap of causes per adverse drug event studied.) (Gurwitz et al., 1995). Healthcare providers such as nurses and clinical pharmacists can make a large impact by ensuring that the correct monitoring occurs as well as vigilant appraisal of dose and type of drug used. Monitoring for medication safety can include laboratory tests, drug interaction checks, physical assessment, and psychological assessment. Appropriate medication monitoring will be discussed in subsequent sections.

Multiple Pharmacies

With the advent of mail-order pharmacies and multiple chain stores at every corner, people are filling prescriptions at multiple pharmacies instead of filling all of their prescriptions at one pharmacy. The practice of using one pharmacy for all of a person's prescription, OTC, vitamin, and supplement purchases was an additional check of the overall medication regimen's safety. The virtual elimination of the single pharmacy model, in addition to studies demonstrating that patients are no longer receiving oral or written instructions from their physicians and pharmacists, leaves the prescription bottle label as the most important guide to medication use (Metlay et al., 2005; Morris, Tabak, & Gondek, 1997). Barriers to safe and effective medication use are both systemic and patient-centered. Health literacy is increasingly becoming recognized as a significant factor at any age. Ideally, the pharmacy would be an excellent point for patient education and counseling to help overcome literacy challenges. One study looked at nearly 400 English-speaking adults in three primary care clinics to study patient understanding of instructions on five prescription container labels. The investigators also assessed whether the subjects could actually demonstrate one of the label's dosing instructions using actual pills. The ability to correctly understand the five labels ranged from 67.1% to 91.1%, with people reading at or below sixth-grade level less likely to understand all five labels. Although 70.7% of the patients with low literacy correctly stated the instructions reading "take two tablets by mouth twice daily," only 34.7% could demonstrate the number of pills to be taken daily. In this study, as with many others, the greater the number of prescription medications, the greater is the likelihood of misunderstanding

(Davis et al., 2006). In elderly patients, literacy may be added to other challenges such as cognitive, sensory, and functional impairment.

Older Age: Frailty, Chronic Disease, Cognitive Impairment, and Altered Pharmacokinetics

There is irony in the fact that the population most likely to have a higher medication burden is the one facing increasing challenges to successful medication management—the elderly. Management of medications is not so different from other IADLs such as balancing a checkbook, planning to cook a meal, going to the grocery store, or doing the laundry. These activities require *intact* executive function, logical memory, verbal memory, attention, linguistic capacity, and other domains of cognitive function. To complete the ancillary tasks associated with medication management, such as shopping (procuring medication), finances (paying for medications), arranging transportation or driving (doctor's appointments), and using a telephone (calling pharmacies and physicians' offices), various domains of cognition in addition to intact executive function have to work well together (Hall, Hoa, Johnson, Barber, & O'Bryant, 2011).

Medications are additionally dangerous in the elderly because of frailty and the physiological changes that occur with age and have an impact on pharmacokinetics and pharmacodynamics. When we age, muscle turns to fat, altering the distribution of fat- and water-soluble drugs. The volume of distribution of fat-soluble drugs becomes larger and that of water-soluble drugs becomes smaller. This means, for example, that many medications that are psychoactive or target pain will take longer to work upon *initial* dosing because the volume of distribution is larger. However, once distribution is accomplished, the frail elderly patient will be more sensitive to the drug's effects. Conversely, water-soluble drugs will become active in the plasma faster due to smaller volumes of distribution in the elderly. Along with frailty comes protein wasting and typically lower albumen and protein levels. The medications that are highly protein- and albumin-bound in the plasma will be less bound in an older person, resulting in a high fraction of active drug or "free drug" floating around in the blood. What this means clinically is that when a subtherapeutic drug level result comes from the laboratory for a highly protein-bound drug, there may be no need to increase the dose, because the percentage of unbound or free (active) drug is still high.

Frailty is also accompanied by changes in the physiological function of the organs and tissues. Medications that are designed to work on various receptors may not find enough receptors to work on because they have diminished in number. One example of a common physiological change with age is altered baroreceptor activity. Orthostatic hypotension is common in elders, even without diuretic therapy or beta-blocker use, because baroreceptors become less sensitive to changes in posture, and the other compensatory systems that react to postural changes cannot respond because they are altered by frailty. Another example is the blood–brain barrier, an important structure that drugs are commonly designed around. Psychoactive medications are designed to be lipid- or fat-soluble because the brain is primarily made of lipids and the blood–brain barrier readily allows lipid-soluble compounds to enter the brain. Just as oil mixes with oil and not water, lipid-soluble drugs readily pass into the central nervous system and brain due to their fat-soluble properties, whereas water-soluble drugs do not. The blood–brain barrier works to let fat-soluble drugs into the brain and keep water-soluble (or polar) substances out. With age, this mechanism breaks down due to frailty, so, for example, some urinary incontinence (UI) medications (such as oxybutynin), which traditionally are well-known to cause confusion and memory impairment due to anticholinergic effects, have been redesigned to not cross into the brain by the addition of a polar entity, making them water soluble. Theoretically, this allows the newer UI medication to do its anticholinergic work in the periphery and not affect the brain. Unfortunately, these strongly anticholinergic drugs can cross into the frail brain through the compromised blood–brain barrier (Chancellor et al., 2012). Although newer UI medications are marketed to be safer and cause less confusion in the frail elder, the safety profile is not reliable because of age-related changes in the blood–brain barrier.

Transitions of Care

Earlier we discussed the increased risk of MRPs related to the increasing numbers of physicians and pharmacists that a patient utilizes. Transitions of care are another glaring source of medication misadventure. Increased transitions of care from one setting to another lead to a higher risk for MRPs. It has been estimated that up to 67% of medication histories taken in the healthcare setting have one or more errors in them, and that 46% of medication errors are made at admission or discharge with new prescriptions (National Audit Office [NAO], 2005; Sullivan, Gleason, & Rooney, 2005). It is easy to see how there can be a detrimental snowballing effect in elders transitioning frequently from one care setting to another, trying to rely upon the healthcare system to keep the medication list current and correct. **Case Study 11-2** illustrates the common scenario of a patient entering the hospital and being discharged on additional inappropriate and unnecessary medications.

Isolation

Isolation is a growing problem among the elderly, especially with the aging of the Baby Boomer generation. With the Boomers, there was a marked increase in the number of women not having children or families. Also, more than ever, families are geographically spread out as opposed to living and working in the same town in which they were born. The typical factors leading to isolation are gender (women more than men), health status, death of a spouse, disability, and loss of social network. These risk factors are additive (Holmen, Ericsson, & Winblad, 2000). When elders are isolated, it is difficult to assess their ability to self-care, their level of well-being, worsening health, and multiple other aspects of their lives. The absence of a social group makes medication side effects difficult to differentiate from new medical problems because no one is present to witness the onset of a problem, nor is anyone able to bear witness to the elder's ability to adhere to the prescribed regimen.

Warning Signs of Medication Misadventure

Nonspecific Complaints

The typical MRP manifests as a nonspecific complaint as opposed to an obvious reaction to a medication. In the case of anaphylaxis, it is easy to attribute the cause to the medication; however, many medication side effects reveal themselves insidiously, manifesting over time as problems such as an upset stomach, headache, dry mouth,

---

Case Study 11–2: Go to the Hospital and Come Back with Four More Medications

K. L. is an 84-year-old man who was sent to the hospital for treatment of possible urinary tract infection (UTI) and dizziness with fever. He has lived in assisted living at SHV assisted living facility for the past 4 years. K. L.'s hospital course was complicated by aggressive antibiotic treatment resulting in a *Clostridium difficile* infection and diarrhea. Geriatric Nurse Practitioner B. G. checked on K. L. the first day after he returned from the hospital. B. G. compared her chart records to the new posthospital discharge records and found several discrepancies and inappropriate medication changes:

Ht = 6 ft 1 in, Wt = 178 lb, BP = 125/65, RR = 18, HR = 72

PMH: DM2, HTN, OsteoArthritis, CAD, Afib, chronic UTI (colonization)

Labs: CMP within normal limits (WNL) except for creatinine 1.8, BUN = 32, glucose 72; K = 3.0

CBC WNL; Lipid panel TC = 70, LDL = 127, HDL = 65

Case Study 11-2: Go to the Hospital and Come Back with Four More Medications *(continued)*

From ALF to ED	Hospital DC summary	Current in ALF chart	Assessment and de-prescribing by GNP
Metoprolol XL 25 mg daily	Metoprolol XL 25 mg daily	Metoprolol XL 25 mg daily	
Digoxin 0.125 mg every other day	Amiodarone 200 mg twice daily	Amiodarone 200 mg twice daily	*Cardio consult placed him on amiodarone, purposefully avoided in the past, will switch back to digoxin every other day (Bahr, Lackner, & Pacala, 2008) DC amidarone.*
Warfarin 3 mg daily	Warfarin 3 mg daily	Warfarin 3 mg daily	
Lisinopril 20 mg daily	Lisinopril 20 mg daily	Lisinopril 20 mg daily	
Amlodipine 5 mg daily	Amlodipine 10 mg daily	Amlodipine 10 mg daily	Amlodipine dose increased by hospitalist targeting BP = 120/80; too low for K.L. due to orthostasis and age. Decrease to 5 mg.
Metformin 500 mg BID	Metformin 500 mg BID	Metformin 500 mg BID	
	Glyburide 5 mg daily	Glyburide 5 mg daily	Hypoglycemic and on glyburide. Glipizide a better choice in renal impairment (dose adjustment). Glyburide should be avoided in CrCl, 50ml/min. His est. CrCl = 33.3m/min. (American Geriatric Society Beers Criteria.) DC (discontinue, his BG likely went up due to acute infection)
	Simvastatin 40 mg daily	Simvastatin 40 mg daily	His lipid panel indicates that he does not need statin therapy, and amlodipine when given with simvastatin per FDA warning requires simvastatin dose of not more than 20 mg daily. DC
	Nitrofurantoin 100 mg daily	Nitrofurantoin 100 mg daily	Contraindicated in patients with CrCl < 60ml/min. (nitrofurantoin package insert) DC—patient known to have UT bacterial colonization.
Cranberry supplement	Vancomycin oral 250 mg every 8 hours for 10 days	Vancomycin oral 250 mg every 8 hours for 10 days	Not clear when vancomycin started, need to clarify how many days remain, then re-culture.
	Pantoprozole 20 mg daily prn	Pantoprozole 20 mg daily	This was a prn AST order (routine in hospital) carried forward to discharge which was mistranscribed to be routine. DC
	Diclofenac 75 mg twice daily prn	Diclofenac 75 mg twice daily	NSAIDS are contraindicated in patients on warfarin, and high risk for CV events in elders. (American Geriatrics Society Beers Criteria). DC.
Routine APAP	Same	Same	Same

decreased mental sharpness, agitation or edginess, a sudden change in appetite, insomnia, or hypersomnolence. This is one of the reasons polypharmacy occurs so easily. A patient goes into the 15-minute doctor's visit with a nonspecific complaint, and it typically is not recognized as a medication side effect, instead becoming another diagnosed condition and leading to another prescription (see **Figure 11-3**).

It is important to always remember that symptoms caused by medication side effects can seem quite unrelated to the actual medication. For example, the headache caused by a cardiac medication (due to vasodilation) is directly caused by the drug's intended action; another symptom, such as gout, is an indirect outcome of using diuretics, particularly thiazide diuretics. The separation between the actual presenting problem and the origin of the problem as a side effect of a drug leads to many misdiagnoses. More prescribing to "chase" the problem rather than fix it at the level of the cause occurs because of the lack of connection between drug use and new problems. Tracing a patient's problem back to the of-

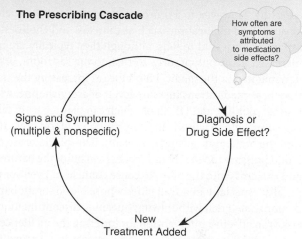

Figure 11-3 The Prescribing Cascade illustrated as a never-ending cycle of treating medication side effects that are inaccurately assessed as medical (or organic) problems rather than medication side effects, leading to more medications being prescribed, leading to more side effects.

fending drug is a challenge because it requires a high level of hands-on intervention, follow-up, and time. One way to ensure that a medication cause is not overlooked is to approach each problem a patient presents with as a possible MRP and do the research to see if any of the patient's medications have some connection, direct or indirect, to the presenting problem.

Timeline

Being aware of the emergence of a new problem (drug side effect) and the timing of the start of a new drug therapy is the most obvious method of detecting MRPs. The challenge comes with patients who are poor historians (and even cognitively intact elders can become confused about what they take and when if the number of medications they take is high). Another challenge that is often overlooked is the hidden use of OTC products, supplements, and herbal products. The presenting problem could be caused by unreported use of these products or sporadic use, which may cause a direct effect or compete with an existing stable regimen to destabilize the routine medications. An example of this could be warfarin users who occasionally use acetaminophen-containing products. It could be OTC cough and cold preparations, plain acetaminophen, or as-needed prescription opioid combination products that can raise the international normalized ratio (INR) unexpectedly. Usually a high dose of acetaminophen takes about 1 week to make an impact on INR. In this example, there is no direct toxicity from the acetaminophen, but the indirect change in INR can occur and be in effect even after the acetaminophen is discontinued. The clinician may not connect the two as the cause of the MRP because the OTC product is not in use anymore.

Falls

Falls are always of concern in the elderly in the community and in hospital settings. The drugs usually associated with falls are the benzodiazepines, muscle relaxants, first-generation antihistamines, and opioids. As with most aspects of MRP assessment, the importance of suspecting the unsuspected cannot be emphasized enough. In elders, especially with dementia, falls occur in the absence of benzodiazepines and other medications typically associated with falls. The reasons are numerous, including neurological changes affecting gait and balance, weakness due to frailty, and environmental factors. Some patients are fallers, regardless of what medications they are using. However, in a thorough assessment of medication-induced falls, all medications must be considered. Unsuspected medications such as diuretics and cholinesterase inhibitors (CEIs; donepezil, galantamine, or rivastigmine) can lead to falls, although they typically are not considered drugs that lead to falls. Diuretics cause increased urine output, urge to rush to the restroom, orthostatic problems, and dehydration. CEIs are actually documented in the medical literature as increasing the risk of falls, which would be predictable when you know that these medications increase levels of acetylcholine, which in turn can cause bradycardia, increased gastrointestinal motility, and UI, all of which can play a part in falls (Gill et al., 2009). Many cardiovascular medications can contribute to falls in elders by dropping blood pressure too low, causing orthostatic hypotension, or crossing into the brain and causing confusion. Beta-blockers are an example of this; if the blood pressure therapy drops blood pressure too low, beta-blockers can blunt the baroreceptor and cardiovascular response to postural changes and can cross into the brain to cause confusion. Even some lipophilic statins can cause confusion and contribute to falls, especially in a frail elder whose blood–brain barrier is no longer intact. One prospective cohort study demonstrated that withdrawing (meaning discontinuation of or decreasing in dose) medications that increase fall risk is an effective intervention for lowering the incidence of falls. Their list of target drugs included a majority of psychoactive medications and some cardiovascular medications, plus oral hypoglycemic agents. They found that this decrease in falls effect is more highly correlated with the withdrawal of cardiovascular drugs than in the other classes studied (van der Velde, Stricker, Pols, & van der Cammen, 2007). Awareness that other drugs in addition to the common list of fall-causing drugs, which mostly includes medications that cause drowsiness, better leads the clinician to connect the falls to unsuspecting medications causing falls (see **Box 11-1**).

Sudden Change in IADLs or ADLs

A global sign in the elderly that a problem or problems are developing is when their ability to carry out ADLs and IADLs changes, especially if there is an abrupt change. It was not until the mid-2000s that studies have shown a clear relationship among drug burden and functional impairment, increased hospitalization, and even death.

In particular, anticholinergic medications cause significant impairment in function and can accelerate progression of dementia, which results in increasingly less ability to participate in IADLs and ADLs (see **Exhibit 11-1**).

One study demonstrated that as anticholinergic medications are added, each additional unit of drug burden had a negative effect on physical function similar to that of three additional physical comorbidities, and a greater

---

BOX 11-1   Evidence-Based Practice Example

This meta-analysis aimed to examine the effectiveness of "cholinesterase inhibitors (CEIs) and memantine on the risk of falls, syncope, and related events, defined as fracture and accidental injury" (p. 1019). A meta-analysis of randomized controlled trials was conducted from numerous databases through 2009. The settings were the community and nursing homes. Participants yielded from the search included those from 54 placebo-controlled randomized trials that reported data on the factors of interest. CEI use was associated with greater risk of syncope than placebo, but not fractures, falls, or accidental injury. Memantine was not associated with falls, syncope, or accidental injury, but was correlated with fewer fractures. Gerontological nurses should realize that CEIs may increase the risk of syncope in older adults and memantine may have a favorable effect on fracture. The authors suggested that more research is needed to confirm and explain the observation of the reduction in number of fractures for those taking memantine.

Data from Kim, D. H., Brown, R. A., Ding, E. L., Kiel, D. P., & Berry, S. D. (2011). Dementia medications and risk of falls, syncope, and related adverse events: Meta-analysis of randomized controlled trials. *Journal of the American Geriatrics Society, 59,* 1019–1031.

effect than anxiety, *depression*, or cognitive impairment. In the same study, each additional unit of anticholinergic drug burden had a negative effect on cognitive task performance similar to that of four additional physical comorbidities and half the effect of anxiety, depression, or cognitive impairment (Hilmer et al., 2007). Another study demonstrated that chronic exposure to anticholinergic medications in patients who were taking CEIs to treat Alzheimer's disease experienced an acceleration of the worsening of the disease, which was double the rate of those who did not take anticholinergic medications (Lu & Tune, 2003). Lastly, a study looking at the most frail cohort of elders (nursing home patients) in which they "de-prescribed" or discontinued an average of 2.8 medications per patient in the intervention arm versus the usual care arm, found that the mortality rate in the intervention arm was 21% versus 45% in the usual care group. The intervention group's rate of referral to the emergency department was 11.8%, and the usual care group was sent to the emergency department at a rate of 30%. The 2.8 medications that the investigators chose to discontinue were conservative choices, with the aim of selecting just the most unnecessary medications (Garfinkel, Zur-Gil, & Ben-Israel, 2007). This and other studies have demonstrated that high medication burden, despite being used to improve health, can actually result in unnecessary functional impairment and even death, whereas decreasing drug burden can improve functionality significantly.

Dry Brain — confusion*
Dry Mouth — can't eat
Dry Eyes — blurry vision
Dries up urine — urinary retention
Dries up bowels — constipation

*Note that medications used for dementia, such as donepezil or Aricept, are procholinergic (opposite of anticholinergic) and anticholinergic medications can impair cognition.

(Campbell et al., 2009)

Exhibit 11-1 Anticholinergic side effects. Data from Campbell, N., Boustani, M., Limbil, T., Ott, C., Fox, C., Maidment, I., Schubert, C. C., Munger, S., Fick, D., Miller, D., & Gulati, R. (2009). The cognitive impact of anticholinergics: A clinical review. *Clinical Interventions in Aging, 4*, 225–233.

Assessment

Nurses have an exclusive place in the healthcare team when it comes to medications. They are the only member of the healthcare team that actually witnesses the patient's use and outcome of medications, at least in the institutional setting. One of the cornerstones of nursing education is patient assessment and the increased amount of time spent involved in face-to-face patient care, relative to other healthcare professionals. Nurses have extensive knowledge of the pharmacological aspects of the medication, including intended effect, side effects, administration, and monitoring parameters. Nurses have been administering, monitoring, educating, and documenting all components of medication use for decades. This is why nurses are in a position to make a significant contribution to combating the harms of medication misadventures. Many of the principles of medication and polypharmacy assessment are intuitive to nurses, and the following specific assessment skills can add to nursing's important role in minimizing polypharmacy harm.

Brown Bag Assessment

Many people have heard of the term "brown bag medication assessment," which means that patients bring in all of the medications they are currently taking, including OTCs, supplements, and herbals, to their clinic visits or hospitalizations for assessment. This method is far superior to relying on patient self-report, internal medical records, or transferred medical records from other providers. Even insurance claims data are not as accurate as face-to-face, brown bag medication assessment. The only consistent factor throughout the healthcare system is the patient, and having patients bring in what they are taking at that specific point in time is the most revealing way to assess and discuss medication use with the patient.

The benefit of the *brown bag assessment*, other than being superior to self-report, is that the clinician can see how many tablets or capsules are present versus the last time the medications were filled (date on label) to probe for adherence. If time permits, it is helpful to contact the patient's pharmacy (or pharmacies) and ask for a faxed drug list to compare to the medications brought in for the brown bag assessment. The patient also can be queried on how they take the medication and their knowledge of what the medications are for while viewing the medication, which is superior to asking about their medication use by name due to common memory and literacy challenges.

Gait and Frailty

Whenever possible, observation of the patient's functional ability is helpful in detecting potential MRPs. As discussed earlier, the physiological changes that occur with advanced age lead to changes in the way medications are metabolized, distributed, and take effect, and these changes can increase the risk of toxicity. Where an elder is on the spectrum of frailty is important to recognize when assessing for risk of poor medication outcomes. Observing ambulation is one of the most telling assessment tools in determination of frailty (Cesari et al., 2006). Geriatricians routinely use the Timed Up and Go (TUG) test, "which has an elder seated in a chair with arms get out of the chair, walk several paces, and return to the chair." The clinician observes for the patient's ability to support himself sitting, if he can stand without too much arm assistance, gait and balance, and ability to pivot and turn easily. Failure to perform any or all of these steps indicates possible sarcopenia and frailty.

Medication Adherence Rating Scales and Tests

Numerous clinical tests are available for assessment of medication adherence, which may be useful in identifying physical and cognitive barriers to successful medication management; however, each one has limits in terms of validation in the literature for universal applicability and clinical practicality. For example, there are instruments that utilize the patient's own medications and there are some that utilize simulated medications, but there are no studies comparing these different types head to head to determine which type is more universally valid. Some instruments take up to 30 minutes or longer to perform, and some take 15 minutes; whether these time requirements are clinically useful has not been studied. The instruments are measuring only cognitive and physical capacity to perform medication adherence; however, medication management and adherence is a very complex task that involves motivation and beliefs about each medication, perception of self-efficacy, ability to access medications, relationships with healthcare providers, and cultural and lifestyle factors. Thus, the assessment instruments found in the literature currently could be utilized as a screen for physical and cognitive barriers to medication adherence and management but not necessarily as predictive of poor medication outcomes. The brown bag assessment, in addition to assessment of cognitive status utilizing common standard clinical tests such as the Mini-Mental State Examination (MMSE) or CLOX (an executive clock-drawing task) (Folstein, Folstein, & McHugh, 1975; Royal, Cordes, & Polk, 1998), plus medication adherence rating scales, should be assessed periodically. The ultimate assessment is the in-home visit and assessment.

Take-Home Medical Administration Record

Occasionally, you will be faced with a patient for whom the brown bag assessment does not work. This patient may bring you all of the medications he or she ever had from 20 years ago to date and cannot tell you what he or she is currently taking; or a patient who, in the middle of the assessment, starts to describe the "pink" pill that he or she forgot to bring in; or you are unable to get a list of prescribed medications from other healthcare providers due to Health Insurance Portability and *Accountability* (HIPAA concerns), so you cannot complete the medication reconciliation. Is there an alternative method of medication reconciliation? There is: You can give the patient a homework assignment in the form of a take-home *medication administration record* (MAR). This exercise can provide you with a few important bits of data with respect to ability to complete the assignment. It will tell you that the patient has challenges with medication management (perhaps due to literacy, cognition, or just complexity of regimen) or, hopefully, clarify what the patient is actually taking. First, it forces the patient (or family) to list the medications taken daily and track days 1 to 31 regarding what was taken at what time of day. Instruct the patient or caregiver on how to fill it out, including how to document missed doses, and what efficacy and side effect items should be recorded, such as blood pressure, nocturia, sleeping patterns, or glucose levels. The patient and/or caregiver's ability to complete this record will give you some idea of their understanding of what the patient is taking, any problems with understanding the regimen, and how the medications are being used.

Literacy Screen

To successfully utilize today's healthcare system, the patient is required to understand, seek, and actively obtain health information, which can be rather complex at times. Add to that the described lack of one-on-one explanation and counseling about how to use medications, and the patient is left relying on one primary skill to follow instructions on how to safely use medications—reading. Reading labels and information provided from the pharmacy about medications (OTC or prescription) is the main source of guidance on medication use. Medication information presented on an OTC package or patient information handout accompanying a prescription is quite complex. Therefore, even if a patient is well educated, being able to digest the complex information provided in print about medications and act upon that information is quite a challenge; for the patient who has limited reading capacity, the challenge is even more formidable. Health literacy has multiple aspects, such as the ability to extract, understand, and use health-related information (Ishikawa, Takeuchi, & Yano, 2008). There are numerous health literacy assessments that are validated but not used in the practical clinical setting because they take too much time to administer. If time allows, the three-level HL Scale and the 3-brief SQs are the most comprehensive instruments to measure health literacy (Sayah, Williams, & Johnson, 2012). A brief screen that focuses on the reading component of health literacy is the Single Item Literacy Screener (SILS), which consists of one question: *"How often do you need to have someone help you when you read instructions, pamphlets, or other written material from your doctor or pharmacy?"* Possible responses are *1-Never, 2-Rarely 3-Sometimes, 4-Often, and 5-Always*. Scores greater than 2 are considered positive for some difficulty reading health-related material (Morris, MacLean, & Chew, 2006).

Swallowing Status

Swallowing status is a commonly overlooked aspect of assessment for MRPs. Screening for patients with swallowing difficulty should be a routine part of the assessment. The link between difficulty swallowing and medication crushing should be assessed. Patients often alter dosage forms at home by crushing and do not report it to their physicians. One study showed that one in every four doses administered in the nursing home setting contains an error (Haw, Stubbs, & Dickens, 2007), and the most common error was crushing medication inappropriately. When a patient is experiencing toxicity or inefficacy relative to their medications, it could be simply because they are altering their tablets and capsules to be able to swallow them or for other reasons. It is well-known to nurses that crushing a tablet, cutting a nonscored tablet in half, or breaking the seal of a capsule of long-acting products can result in a very high dose designed to be released over 12 to 24 hours being released all at once, resulting in toxicity. In general, long-acting products that are administered once daily or have an SR, XR, CR, or LA designation should not be crushed or split. Also, products that are toxic to the caregiver or patient upon contact should not be altered, such as chemotherapeutic agents (e.g., tamoxifen), hormonally active agents (e.g., finasteride), or an irritant (e.g., hydroxyurea). The following case illustrates two principles in assessment of MRPs: the importance of taking alterations of medication dosage form into account and how the signs of medication harm can seem very disconnected from the causative medication (see **Case Study 11-3**).

The challenge, even for healthcare professionals, is knowing which medications outside the obviously labeled SR, XR, SA, or CR are safe to crush. One place to look for information is the Institute for Safe Medication Practices (ISMP) at http://www.ismp.org. This Website is an excellent resource for safe medication use and includes information on medication administration timeliness, high-alert medications, and many other medication tools. Specifically, they have a frequently updated "Do Not Crush" medication list, which lists medications not to be crushed and the reasons why. Another place to seek information on which medications are crushable and which are not is to consult references pertaining to tube feedings, as you will find lists of liquid alternatives as well as reviews of which tablets and capsules are safe to alter. Lastly, you can put a request in to your pharmacists and have them find the information for you if it is not already clearly labeled on the medication itself.

Case Study 11-3: She Nearly Died from One Medication

M. C. was admitted to a skilled nursing facility for rehabilitation after a partial glossectomy for a recurrent carcinoma of the tongue. Her past medical history was significant for osteoarthritis, lupus, dizziness, syncope, falls, hypertension, osteoporosis, and hypothyroidism. Her medications were levothyroxine 75 mcg daily, Oyster-CalD 500 mg bid, Senna-S daily, alendronate 70 mg weekly, oxycodone/ acetaminophen prn, acetaminophen prn, and Milk of Magnesia. On 11/03/08, the nursing staff notified M. C.'s physicians of her complaints of a burning tongue and refusing food, resulting in weight loss and general decline. The team PharmD visited on 11/11/08 and when presented with the patient's complaint, noted the patient was refusing medication and food due to "bad taste" and "burning." Otherwise, she was cognitively intact with excellent postsurgical wound healing and absence of inflammation or exudates. Other common causes of glossitis had been excluded. Following a review of the nursing notes and medication record, a pattern of food refusal emerged. It appeared to be a weekly occurrence, coinciding with the scheduled dosing of alendronate, which can be caustic to the gastric and esophageal mucosa (Gonzalez-Moles & Bagan-Sebastian, 1999). The nursing staff confirmed adherence to appropriate alendronate administration, that is, before breakfast with 8 oz of water and remaining upright for 30 minutes. However, the staff then admitted that all tablets on two shifts were being crushed, despite lack of documentation of crushing in the MAR. The weekly dose of alendronate at 10 p.m. after dinner but right before going to bed was directly irritating the patient's buccal and esophageal mucosa. The nursing staff were unaware and lacked training about crushing sustained-release tablets, which was done routinely, and the dispensing pharmacy failed to provide any "Do Not Crush" labels. This is not surprising considering that one in every four doses administered in the nursing home setting contains an error, and the most common error was crushing medications inappropriately (Haw et al., 2007). Given the frequency with which patients in the long-term care setting have swallowing difficulties, coupled with the frequency of bisphosphonate use, this case is presented to alert others to this potentially life-threatening scenario.

Collateral History: Adult Child or Caregiver

When taking a medication history with an elderly patient, it is not always easy to determine the influence of possible cognitive impairment or psychosocial barriers. Whenever possible, try to get a caregiver or family member to corroborate the patient's report of medication use and side effects. Commonly, elders who are experiencing functional decline with or without cognitive impairment report they are having no problems out of fear that they may lose autonomy and independence. Falls are perceived as a sign that they are growing old and dependent, and therefore, elders hesitate to report falls to their family and physicians (Biderman, Cwikel, Fried, & Galinsky, 2002). Impaired ability to drive is another topic that can be medication-related that requires caregiver verification, as the elderly sometimes are unaware of their driving impairment or unwilling to report it. It may be necessary to ask the elderly patient's caregiver to keep an MAR or a log of symptoms, OTC use, and other medication-related data if they or the patient cannot accurately report this information.

Beers Criteria and START and STOPP Criteria

Some explicit criteria that provide information on potentially inappropriate medications (PIMs) for use in the elderly are available. The most popular of these are the *Beers Criteria*, the *START criteria* (Screening Tool to

Alert doctors to the Right Treatment), and the *STOPP criteria* (Screening Tool of Older People's potentially inappropriate Prescriptions). The Beers Criteria was updated in 2015, and since Mark Beers, the original author, is deceased, the American Geriatrics Society has carried on with expert panel authored updates roughly every 3 years. The Beers Criteria's purpose is to identify drugs to avoid in older adults independent of diagnosis and considering diagnosis, to reduce ADRs, and improve medication selection and use in older adults. It is designed for any clinical setting and to be used as an educational, quality, and research tool (American Geriatric Society, 2015). The 2015 release is quite robust and introduces a section on drug–drug interactions, renal dosing tables, how to use the Beers Criteria, and alternative agents section. The START and STOPP screening tools also address PIMs in the elderly and features a rather practical organizational structure that includes identification of excessive prescribing and prescribing oversight, categorized by physiological system, and recognizes high-risk groups such as patients with dementia or patients who fall. This criteria was produced as a European resource for identification of PIMs; although some medications are different from those of the U.S.-based Beers Criteria, it is nonetheless a well-written and useful list of 114 criteria. There are 80 STOPP criteria, which are medications that should be avoided or cautiously used in the elderly, and 34 START criteria, which are medications commonly underused in the elderly (O'Mahony et al., 2015). These are useful, educational references, and each brings a different perspective on various mechanisms of medication harm in elders. Although they do not list every single medication that can place an elder at risk, they cover the major categories, and by referring to them often, the clinician will eventually become familiar with the thought process behind identification of PIM use in the elderly.

Diagnosis

Polypharmacy-induced harm and MRPs are typically diagnosed through deductive means. When presented with a patient experiencing a problem and trying to ascertain whether that problem is caused by medications, there are several items that are important to rule out. These items should be a routine part of the medication differential diagnosis. First, patient adherence to the medication regimen should be documented and corrections to the patient medication list should be made. A common source of drug toxicity in the elderly—impaired renal drug clearance—should be assessed by calculating current estimated kidney function. Laboratory tests recommended in drug monographs should be performed routinely; however, due to time pressure in our healthcare system, the routine monitoring of laboratory tests is often overlooked. If obvious causes of MRPs cannot be detected and the problem persists, a trial drug discontinuation, if possible, may reveal the source of the problem.

Laboratory Results

The following are some of the common diagnostic laboratory parameters that are assessed in working up a case of MRPs.

Complete Metabolic Panel and Basic Metabolic Panel. The complete metabolic panel (CMP) and basic metabolic panel (BMP) are essential tests used to monitor therapy when taking just about any medication. The CMP monitors kidney and liver function, glucose, calcium, protein levels, and electrolyte and fluid balance, and the BMP monitors kidney function, glucose, calcium, and electrolyte and fluid balance. When medications known to cause electrolyte imbalances, such as diuretics, are being used, BMPs should be performed weekly for 2–3 weeks when starting therapy and periodically once stable on the new diuretic. Most recommendations on how often to monitor BMP while taking diuretics state "periodically" after the initial weeks of use (in which monitoring occurs frequently). This nonspecific time interval is confusing to clinicians and leaves the period in between electrolyte, fluid, and kidney function assessment open to individual clinician interpretation. In elderly and frail patients, the most conservative course of action is best because in the elderly, dangerous changes in electrolyte levels can occur abruptly, because elders have less homeostatic reserve, and because they are subjected to numerous new medications and sometimes have inconsistent food and fluid intake. Therefore, "periodically" in a relatively healthy younger adult taking a diuretic could safely be interpreted as

TABLE 11-1   Select Medications That Require Laboratory Monitoring

Medication	Tests	Reason
Amiodarone	Thyroid-stimulating hormone (TSH), liver function tests (LFTs), serum creatinine, and creatinine kinase (CPK)	Hypothyroid or hyperthyroid levels Hepatotoxicity (fatal at times) Rhabdomyolysis
Valproic acid	CMP, CBC, serum drug levels (albumin, serum protein)	Hyponatremia, syndrome of inappropriate secretion of antidiuretic hormone, pancytopenia, thrombocytopenia, and hepatotoxicity
Phenytoin	Serum creatinine (initiation of therapy), CBC, LFTs, serum drug levels (albumin, serum protein)	Hepatotoxicity, leukopenia, agranulocytosis, pancytopenia, megaloblastic anemia; no loading dose with renal impairment
ASA, naproxen, celecoxib	Serum creatinine, CBC, guaiac fecal occult blood test (FOBT)	Monitor international normalized ratio target, gastrointestinal bleeds
Statin therapy	CPK, lipid panel, baseline LFTs	Rhabdomyolysis, LFT at baseline, monitor need for statin and efficacy

See FDA drug monograph (package insert) under prescribing information for detailed explanation.

every 6 months to 1 year after stable on the diuretic therapy but in an elder could mean every 2–3 months depending on how many other comorbidities and medications are involved.

There are instances when an abnormality may show up on the BMP or CMP that seems very unrelated and distant from the medications the patient is taking. For example, you might expect that patients taking vitamin D do not need a CMP because the only laboratory monitoring necessary would be vitamin D levels, but a CMP still needs to be monitored because aggressive vitamin D supplementation can result in sudden changes in calcium.

Various laboratory tests are mandated per the FDA drug monograph for each particular medication. Some common medications requiring laboratory monitoring are listed in **Table 11-1**.

Lastly, one of the most common polypharmacy-related complaints is memory or cognitive impairment. If a patient presents with these complaints, in addition to assessment for the obvious medication-induced causes such as strongly anticholinergic medications, it is important to rule out common organic causes such as hypothyroidism and vitamin deficiencies. Elders should have their thyroid-stimulating hormone (TSH), vitamin B_{12}, and folate levels assessed when working up the complaint of cognitive impairment.

Cockroft and Gault Creatinine Clearance

Many medications have an FDA drug monograph recommendation for renal adjustment, even some that would not be expected, such as medications perceived to be of concern only for hepatic clearance, such as lovastatin, rosuvastatin, or simvastatin. On laboratory reports, the renal function is reported as glomerular filtration rate (GFR). It is important to recognize that the GFR reported on most laboratory reports is not the same as the renal function estimation that the FDA uses for drug dose adjustments. The FDA has adopted the Cockroft and

Gault method of creatinine clearance estimation as the standard upon which dose recommendations are based. Creatinine clearance can be calculated by several methods: the Modification of Diet in Renal Disease (MDRD) formula, which has been considered a very accurate estimate of GFR, although it underestimates GFR in obese patients and overestimates GFR in underweight patients. The important point when determining dose adjustments for medication is to use the Cockroft and Gault method because that is the basis for the FDA dose adjustment recommendations (U.S. Department of Health and Human Services [DHHS], 2012). It makes little sense to use other GFR estimations when they are irrelevant to the Cockroft and Gault–based dose adjustments values reported in the FDA recommendations (see **Exhibit 11-2**).

> **Cockroft and Gault Method**
> *A method of estimating renal function*
> **[creatinine clearance ml/min]**
>
> $$CrCl_{men} = \frac{(140 - Age)}{Scr \times 72} \times LBW^*$$
>
> $(CrCl_{women} = CrCl_{men} \times 0.85)$
>
> **Always use Cockroft and Gault equation because all FDA drug monographs are standardized to C&G.**
> *Use Lean Body Weight (Ideal Body Weight), especially in elders with poor muscle mass
> LBW: Lean Body Weight in Kg
> CrCl: Creatinine Clearance in mL/min
> SCr: Serum creatinine in mg/dL

Exhibit 11-2 Cockroft and Gault equation.

Diagnosing Problems with Medication-Taking Behavior

Medication adherence and behavior assessment is a key part of detecting MRPs and polypharmacy-related potential harm. Medication adherence is the degree to which the patient is actually taking the total prescribed medication regimen; medication-taking behavior involves the decisions a patient makes and acts upon related to the use of their medication regimen. Medication-taking behavior is influenced by patient beliefs, attitudes, preferences, experiences, and goals related to drug therapy.

The brown bag method is a time-consuming method of assessment, but should be performed at least annually, with results documented in the patient's chart, because it is the gold standard for office assessment of medication use. For brief patient encounters, a widely accepted medication-taking behavior screen that can be a means of assessing adherence is a four-item question sequence called the Abbreviated Morisky Scale (an eight-item scale exists as well) (Morisky, Green, & Levine, 1986).

CLINICAL TIP

The brown bag assessment is still a good tool to assess medication use. Although time-consuming, it provides more reliable information than a questionnaire alone.

Trial Discontinuations

A carefully considered trial discontinuation of a medication is one of the best ways to diagnose an MRP. For example, if a patient is experiencing generalized muscle pain or memory impairment while taking a statin, it would be of no harm to discontinue the medication for a few days and see if the muscle pain or cognition improves. A study showed that atorvastatin can be discontinued in patients who have stable cardiovascular status for up to 6 weeks, and it does not appear to increase the risk of cardiac events (McGowan, 2004). The type of medication considered is of most importance. For example, warfarin trial discontinuation would not be performed without very careful consideration of the risks versus benefits, and maintenance of psychoactive medication requires careful tapering to avoid precipitation of seizures. However, there are some instances in which a trial discontinuation would be easy to implement safely. If a patient were utilizing OTC products that seem to correlate with possible side effect symptoms, then trial discontinuation would be in order. The discontinuation of multiple medications at the same time is not a good practice and is ordinarily reserved for emergency situations such as life-threatening *delirium* in a frail elder, and then medications are typically cut down to a minimal number.

Interventions and Strategies for Care

Polypharmacy is one of the few reversible and preventable causes of iatrogenic harm. The challenge is that reversing and preventing MRPs requires careful monitoring, medication use, and prescribing. This ongoing process requires provider and patient awareness, education, and accountability; tracking and reconciliation of the processes of medication use; follow-up; information transfer; and patient and family engagement. There is a striking similarity to the challenge of coordinating transitions of care and the silent harm that lack of thoughtful transitions of care causes (**National Transitions of Care Coalition** [NTOCC], 2008). Strategies for intervention should include addressing psychological functioning, physiological functioning, cultural factors, health literacy and linguistic factors, financial factors, spiritual and religious functioning, physical and environmental safety, and family and community support. All of the above factors affect a person's relationship to medications and how utilization occurs.

The following strategies for intervention can help lower the risk of polypharmacy and medication misadventures.

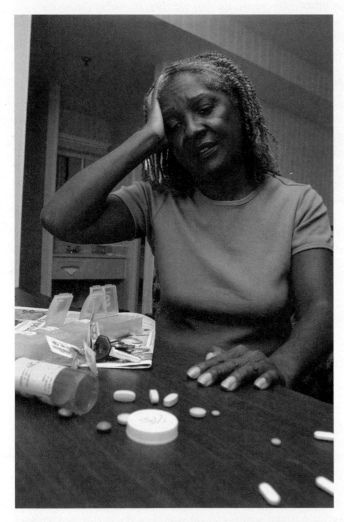

Figure 11-4 Failure to take medications or attend to other health needs can be a sign that an older adult lacks motivation to adhere to the medication regimen.
© Jones & Bartlett Learning. Courtesy of MIEMSS

Decrease the Number of Unnecessary or Harmful Medications

To decrease polypharmacy, start with matching each medication to one or more of the patient diagnoses and do your best to verify the right medication is being used for a valid purpose. There can be more than one medication for a particular diagnosis or more than one diagnosis for a particular medication; however, there should not be any medications being used without good reason (**Figure 11-4**). Any leftover or unmatched medication that the patient is taking should be considered for discontinuation after verification that it is not necessary. For example, patients often get started on stomach acid suppression therapy (AST) in the hospital as a precaution against stress ulcers; the AST often gets carried forward after hospitalization without a specific diagnosis such as peptic ulcer disease, gastroesophageal reflux, or esophagitis that necessitates AST use.

Occasionally, a diagnosis is attached to the discharge AST because clinic staff or a provider assumes it must be used for gastroesophageal reflux. The challenging facet of this exercise is to verify a diagnosis, which as described in Case Study 11-1 of this chapter, can be inaccurate.

Another common "diagnosis" which is often not accurate is a patient's allergy list. Sometimes people are listed as being allergic to a medication when they actually perceived a bad experience or had a transient upset stomach (or coincidental nausea) with a particular medication; they are not truly allergic in the sense of anaphylaxis, rashes, and hives. Just as medications have to be matched to a diagnosis, allergies should be verified. The reason this practice helps fight polypharmacy is that occasionally you will get a patient who has a list of 10 allergies, which means they have to take a dangerous alternative medication or multiple suboptimal medications when, in fact, one of the safer medications on the allergy list might actually be tolerable.

Another method for decreasing the number of medications is to question what is wanted versus needed. There are clearly medications that serve a necessary purpose and are needed for the well-being of the patient, such as a patient with atrial fibrillation who is taking warfarin to prevent a stroke. Sometimes, however, patients are taking medications that are not so necessary because their *family or friends* want them to take it and/or they harbor a false belief that the medication is necessary and/or safe. These drugs are more wanted than needed for patient well-being, and the clinician trying to lower MRP risk should evaluate the necessity. **Case Study 11-4** illustrates a situation in which, despite many compelling reasons to discontinue medications that the family wanted for the patient, ultimately the family would keep the questionable medications. This case also illustrates the limitations of managing medication use in the outpatient setting and the role of the clinician in attempting to implement ethical practices that are not always accepted by the patient or his or her caregiver. The clinician's role in this scenario is to take the effort to explain the risks and try to change the riskier medications to less risky medications. If that fails, it is important to document the attempt and outcome in the medical record. The use of consent forms for high-risk medications is a practice that is gaining in use, although it is not common. Consent forms are used more frequently in the nursing home setting, where lawsuits target use of antipsychotics or other high-risk medications.

The decision about which medications are necessary and which are not is a complex one. To help you understand more about appropriateness and risks of medications in the elderly, it is useful to make use of point-of-care applications on your smart phone or computer (e.g., Epocrates, Lexicomp, or Micromedex) or use online databases such as Drugs.com, or RxList. At first, it will be tedious to look up medications, but over time, you will become familiar with the common medications utilized by the elderly and how risks apply to their age group.

Appropriate Choices and Doses

How do clinicians know what are appropriate medications and doses for use in elders? Some medications are widely known as being high risk in the elderly. For example, medications new to market are notorious for bringing harm to the elderly and most geriatricians recommend waiting 5 to 7 years after marketing of a new drug before using in the elderly. This allows the FDA to gather postmarketing data, which include more elders than the safety and efficacy trials. Checking for appropriate dose in the elderly is a key way to catch medications at high-risk for poor outcomes in the elderly. Do not forget the saying "start low and go slow" when increasing doses in elders. The point-of-care applications and medication databases will often specifically state what doses are considered appropriate in the elderly, in addition to listing monitoring parameters of particular importance.

As described earlier, match the diagnosis list to the medications taken to help sort out unnecessary from necessary medication. The next thing to do is scan for medications that are known to cause problems in the elderly. Are there any Beers Criteria or START and STOPP criteria drugs present? Are there any medications that commonly cause electrolyte imbalances? Any that can cause confusion? Medication databases sometimes have the category "geriatric patients," and clinicians should look further at specific monitoring parameters and both common and uncommon side effects to extrapolate the reasons why cautions are issued with respect to the use in elders.

Case Study 11–4: When Drugs That Are a "Want" Are Used Over Drugs That Are a "Need"

K. L. is an 88-year-old woman living at home with her daughter, who is a single mother and works full time. K. L.'s daughter, L. C., is not ready to place her mother in a care home and says that she can handle her mother's rising need for hospitalization and increased care burden. K. L. was recently hospitalized for confusion and suffering a severe fall, which did not result in any broken bones. Her fall was due to multifactorial causes, including dehydration, overmedication for hypertension (inappropriate blood pressure goals), and the psychoactive medications she was taking. L. C. has come to take her mother home from the hospital. K. L.'s confusion has improved, and her fluid status has been addressed. L. C. did not accept the medication changes made by the medical team.

Medications upon admission	Medications upon discharge
Lisinopril 20 mg daily	Lisinopril 20 mg daily
Hydrochlorothiazide 25 mg daily	Metoprolol XL 25 mg daily
Atenolol 100 mg daily	Donepezil 5 mg (follow up in office next week)
Quetiapine 25 mg twice daily	Mirtazapine 7.5 mg at bedtime
Lorazepam 1 mg at bedtime	Trazodone 50 mg prn at bedtime
Amlodipine 10 mg daily	
Atorvastatin 40 mg daily	

L.C. stated that she would not take her mother home without the quetiapine and lorazepam because she cannot sleep at night due to her mother's behaviors, which included wandering. The medical team explained that quetiapine and lorazepam were discontinued due to their likely contribution to K. L.'s fall and the inappropriateness of indication. They explained that the use of antipsychotics, in particular in the elderly, for behaviors related to dementia is an off-label use and reserved for severe agitation, restlessness, and behaviors leading to potential harm of the patient. The increased mortality risk inherent with the use of antipsychotic agents in the elderly was explained, especially in light of her mother's compromised cardiac status due to age and lifelong history of cardiovascular disease. The team also explained that mirtazapine and trazodone would function to calm her mother in addition to starting donepezil, which may decrease her episodes of confusion.

Ultimately, L. C. stood by her desire to keep her mother on quetiapine and lorazepam because she felt that without those medications, she could not manage to keep her mother at home and still work herself. She also stated that K. L. had been taking them for 2 years already without incident, and that they left their new PCP because he tried to discontinue the same medications 2 months ago. The team had L. C. sign a consent form for the quetiapine discharge prescription (because it is an off-label use) and documented in the discharge summary that L. C. had been advised about the risks of using lorazepam despite K. L.'s fall risk and that L. C. stated she was going to get lorazepam anyway from her physician in the community if they did not provide it at discharge. The team then discontinued the trazodone and mirtazapine discharge orders.

CLINICAL TIP

Always ask about OTC medication use and what herbs or supplements the patient is taking.

Periodic assessment of the goals of care should be performed for the elderly. The goals of care in the elderly may be quite different from the goals of care in a middle-aged adult. Also, goals of care in an elderly patient can change from decade to decade or even year to year, so consideration of goals of care should be a part of all medication assessments. Commonly, elders are subjected to unnecessary medication risks because their prescribers have not taken into consideration that the goals of care for an elder may be quite different from those of a younger patient and that the risk-versus-benefit ratio may be unfavorable for an elder who is frail and taking a heavy medication burden. An example illustrating this point was the surprising outcome of the Action to Control Cardiovascular Risk in Diabetes (ACCORD) trial (Dluhy & McMahon, 2008). The ACCORD trial looked at blood pressure, lipids, and glucose control in patients with diabetes aged 40–79 who had been diagnosed with type 2 diabetes mellitus for an average of 10 years. One of the clinical questions they were trying to answer was: Would very tight control of blood glucose, HA_{1c} less than 6%, result in reduced cardiovascular events in patients with established cardiovascular disease or additional cardiovascular risk factors? The intensive glucose control group had a higher mortality rate than the standard care group, particularly the arm over 65 years of age. The higher mortality rate in the over–65 years' intensive therapy group resulted in a halting of the study in the over 65 years study arm. It is thought that the drug side effects and combinations were major contributors to the poor outcomes in this study arm. The ACCORD study outcome illustrates the risk of using any type of extreme, especially untested therapy, in older patients with varying degrees of disease and physiological compromise. Also, as a result of this and other studies, the American Diabetes Association and AGS have recommended that HA_{1c} targets be "individualized," whereas the AGS also recommends an HA_{1c} target of 8 for older, frailer patients with a life expectancy of less than 5 years, the reason being that the goals of preventing end organ damage due to diabetes mellitus (hyperglycemia) is not as important as protecting people in that group from hypoglycemia, which can lead to dementia, worsening of cognition, and other serious neurological impairments. In considering interventions for polypharmacy, for each medication, the questions of what is the long-term goal of the medication use versus the person's life expectancy, balanced with quality of life and potential risk of side effects, should be considered.

Foster Medication Literacy

During the assessment of your patient's understanding of medication purpose, dosing, and side effects, it may become evident that a medication literacy challenge exists. The traditional method of verbally reviewing the medication regimen before discharging the patient from care may or may not work. A few additional steps and repetition of information may provide improved medication understanding for success in home medication management. Patients who track their medication by color and pill size should be redirected toward the medication name and purpose, which should be repeatedly explained if necessary (and presented in written form) (see **Box 11-2**). The problem with identification of medications by size, shape, and color is that at any time a generic substitution could occur and the same medication may look totally different with the next refill. If size, shape, and color are the only means by which a patient can track medication, it would be advisable to set the patient up with routine medication checks in which they bring in all of their medications monthly and are coached on which one to take at the appropriate time and in the appropriate manner.

Creating a medication administration sheet that lists what should be taken when and any precautions, such as with or without food, is a useful tool to help patients increase their medication literacy. One place to find free downloadable medication record sheet templates is the Free Printable Medical Forms Website: http://www.freeprintablemedicalforms.com/category/medication

For patients who have very limited reading ability, it is advisable to use the simpler forms and draw symbols in wherever possible instead of words (i.e., instead of p.m., draw the moon, instead of a.m., draw the sun).

A patient's feelings of self-efficacy and beliefs about medication use have a profound impact on their success or failure in using medications. Medication prioritization is when patients adhere to the medications they perceive work or solve a prioritized problem, as opposed to those that seem to have no effect. Medications that are easily perceived

---

BOX 11-2   Research Highlight

Lam, Elliott, and George looked at self-administration medication programs (SAMP) and the ability of older adults to adhere to these programs while in the hospital. Working with a pharmacist and nurses, the older adults involved in the study were educated about SAMP and then allowed to participate in self-administration of medication under supervision. After proving success in the supervised program, they were permitted to begin independent use of a SAMP. Sign into your database of nursing literature (CINAHL or PubMed, for example) and use the citation below to perform a search for this article. What measurement tools were used to gauge an older adult's performance in adhering to his or her medication plan? What were researchers able to conclude from this study?

Lam, P., Elliott, R. E., & George, J. (2011). Impact of a self-administration of medications programme on elderly inpatients' competence to manage medications: A pilot study. *Journal of Clinical Pharmacy and Therapeutics, 36*, 80–86.

---

as effective by patients include pain medications or sleep aids, which, when taken, result in a noticeable effect of somnolence or relief from pain. A hypoglycemic agent used by a patient who measures blood glucose routinely can be seen as efficacious if the blood glucose measurements are on target when taking the medication and not when the medication dose is missed. Personal medication experience is very useful to elicit when assessing medication outcomes. Medications that do not provide a measurable obvious effect are more challenging when it comes to adherence (Rifkin et al., 2010).

Healthcare providers can promote health literacy regarding patient medications in terms of expected effects, monitoring for efficacy, and side effects of the medication, which in turn will foster adherence and more effective medication use.

Access to Medications

You might discover that patients skip medication doses because they cannot afford their medications. This occurs often during the Medicare D "doughnut hole" time of the year (typically July until the end of the year), when Medicare D beneficiaries hit a maximum prescription coverage spending limit that stops their coverage but then picks up above a much higher amount. The patient has to cover the costs of medications on their own for a few months and sometimes until the beginning of the new year, when the benefit cycle starts again. The "doughnut hole" coverage gap is supposed to be eliminated by the year 2020.

One cause of poor Medicare D coverage and a shorter time to reaching the "doughnut hole" is if an elder enrolled in Medicare D misses the opportunity every year from October 15 to December 7 for open enrollment. During open enrollment, it is prudent for community-dwelling seniors enrolled in Medicare D to go online with their current medication list at hand, at the following Website: https://www.medicare.gov/find-a-plan/questions/home.aspx.

This Website allows seniors or caregivers to compare plan coverage for their specific medications to find the plan that offers the best coverage. The coverage changes frequently (usually annually), which is why it is important to review coverage and make use of open enrollment to switch into a better plan if possible. Elders residing in long-term care facilities can switch plans on a monthly basis, as opposed to community dwellers who may only switch during open enrollment. (**Note:** Not all seniors have Medicare D, especially if their retirement benefits offer better coverage.)

There are other options to aid coverage of medications. The first is to make use of the pharmacies that offer a $4 or discount formulary. These formularies differ from pharmacy to pharmacy, but the lists for each pharmacy

---

CLINICAL TIP

Be sure to ask about the patient's ability to afford prescribed medications. Work with the interprofessional team to help patients find the most reasonable medication that will be both therapeutic and cost-effective.

---

should be online. Some offer a 30-day supply of some generics for $4, 90 days for $10, and there are even some pharmacies who offer a free 10-day supply of select antibiotics. Typically, mail order pharmacies offer a 90-day supply for a 1-month copay. For medications that are not on most formularies and are very expensive, there are patient assistance programs available through the pharmaceutical companies. There are also copay assistance programs and low-income subsidy programs that patients can apply for and are easily located by searching the Internet. Patients and providers can go to http://www.pacific.edu/Academics/Schools-and-Colleges/Thomas-J-Long-School-of-Pharmacy-and-Health-Sciences/Community-Health-Services/Medicare-Part-D.html (an outreach and education program led by California pharmacy schools) to learn more about Medicare Part D resources.

Summary

In elderly patients, the likelihood that a medication will cause some harm or impairment is heightened by impaired physiology, heavy medication burden, and increased inappropriate medication use by both the healthcare system and the patient. The complex considerations involved in fostering the appropriate use of each medication are often overlooked by all. Nurses are in a special place to make a positive impact by assessing for MRPs and intervening to improve medication outcomes. This chapter covers many aspects of medication misadventure, and it may seem overwhelming, but with application of even a few interventions to identify and fight MRPs, patient outcomes can be markedly improved. Individual clinicians can help fight MRPs by developing interventions that work in their practice setting and by teaching others about how to assess and affect MRPs using the techniques found in this chapter.

Clinical Reasoning Exercises

1. You are working in a nursing home and caring for two women with the same initials. They look alike and both have middle-stage dementia, so they are not reliable with giving their names. The nursing home does not allow name bands. How will you identify each resident when you go to deliver medications? What strategies could help prevent a medication error from occurring in this situation?

2. You observe the morning laboratories from one of your 89-year-old patients who is being assessed for renal failure. The serum creatinine is only slightly off normal. What is a better and more accurate way to estimate the patient's renal function prior to giving medications that are renally cleared and why?

3. What are the most likely times that an older person will experience side effects from a medication? Why are these times that the nurse should be extra vigilant?

Personal Reflections

1. Think about the American Nurses Association (ANA) Code of Ethics. According to the *Code of Ethics for Nurses,* what is your obligation if you know that a medication error has been made? What principles are upheld in the daily work of administering medications?

2. Have you ever made a medication error? What did you do about it? What effect did it have on

the patient or resident? On you as the care provider? Can you identify what you would have done differently to prevent the error?

3. How will you use the information in this chapter to provide better care related to medications and older adults? What helpful piece(s) of information can you immediately apply to your clinical practice?

References

Alvarez, M., & Evidente, V. (2008). Understanding drug-induced Parkinsonism: Separating pearls from oysters. *Neurology, 70*(8), e32–e34.

American Geriatrics Society. (2015). American Geriatrics Society 2015 updated Beers Criteria for potentially inappropriate medication use in older adults. *Journal of the American Geriatrics Society, 63*(11), 2227–2246.

Bateman, D. N. (2004). Digoxin-specific antibody fragments: how much and when? *Toxicology Review, 23*(3), 135–143.

Berenson, R. (2010). *The Medicare chronic care improvement program.* Retrieved from https://www.cms.gov/Medicare/Health-Plans/Medicare-Advantage-Quality-Improvement-Program/5CCIP.html

Biderman, A., Cwikel, J., Fried, A.V., & Galinsky, D. (2002). Depression and falls among community dwelling elderly people: A search for common risk factors. *Journal of Epidemiology Community Health, 56*(8), 631–636.

Bootman, J. L., Harrison, D. L., & Cox, E. (1997). The health care cost of drug-related morbidity and mortality in nursing facilities. *Archive of Internal Medicine, 157*(18), 2089–2096.

Budnitz, D. S., Lovegrove, M. C., & Shehab, N. (2011). Emergency hospitalizations for adverse drug events in older Americans. *New England Journal of Medicine, 365*(21), 2002–2012.

Campbell, N., Boustani, M., Limbil, T., Ott, C., Fox, C., Maidment, I., . . . Gulati, R. (2009). The cognitive impact of anticholinergics: A clinical review. *Clinical Interventions in Aging, 4,* 225–233.

Caracciolo, B., Gatz, M., Xu, W., Pedersen, N. L., & Fratiglioni, L. (2012). Differential distribution of subjective and objective cognitive impairment in the population: A nationwide twin-study. *Journal of Alzheimer's Disease, 29*(2), 393–403.

Centers for Disease Control and Prevention. (2012). *Centers for Disease Control leading cause of death 2010.* Retrieved from http://www.cdc.gov/nchs/fastats/lcod.htm

Cesari, M., Leeuwenburgh, C., Lauretani, F., Onder, G., Bandinelli, S., Maraldi, C., & Guralnik, J. M. (2006). Frailty syndrome and skeletal muscle: Results from the Invecchiare in Chianti study. *American Journal of Clinical Nutrition, 83*(5), 1142–1148.

Chancellor, M. B., Staskin, D. R., Kay, G. G., Sandage, B. W., Oefelein, M. G., & Tsao, J. W. (2012). Blood–brain barrier permeation and efflux exclusion of anticholinergics used in the treatment of overactive bladder. *Drugs & Aging, 29*(4), 259–273.

Davis, T. C., Wolf, M. S., Bass, P. F., 3rd, Thompson, J. A., Tilson, H. H., Neuberger, M., & Parker, R. M. (2006). Literacy and misunderstanding prescription drug labels. *Annals of Internal Medicine, 145*(12), 887–894.

Denham, M. J. (1990). Adverse drug reactions. *British Medical Bulletin, 46*(1), 53–62.

Dluhy, R. G., & McMahon, G. T. (2008). Intensive glycemic control in the ACCORD and ADVANCE trials. *New England Journal of Medicine, 358,* 2545–2559.

Ferenczi, E. A., Asaria, P., Hughes, A. D., Chaturvedi, N., & Francis, D. P. (2010). Can a statin neurtralize the cardiovascular risk of unhealthy dietary choices? *American Journal of Cardiology, 106*(4), 587–592.

Folstein, M. F., Folstein, S. E., & McHugh, P. R. (1975) "Mini-Mental State:" A practical method for grading the cognitive state of patients for the clinician. *Journal of Psychiatric Research, 12*(3), 189–198.

Garfinkel, D., Zur-Gil, S., & Ben-Israel, J. (2007). The war against polypharmacy: A new cost-effective geriatric-palliative approach for improving drug therapy in disabled elderly people. *Israel Medical Association Journal, 9*(6), 430–434.

Gill, S. S., Anderson, G. M., Fischer, H. D., Bell, C. M., Li, P., Normand, S. L., & Rochon, P. A. (2009). Syncope and its consequences in patients with dementia receiving cholinesterase inhibitors: A population-based cohort study. *Archive of Internal Medicine, 169*(9), 867–873.

Gonzalez-Moles, M. A., & Bagan-Sebastian, J. V. (1999). Alendronate-related oral mucosa ulcerations. *Journal of Oral Pathology and Medicine, 29*(10), 514–518.

Gu, Q., Dillon, C. F., & Burt, V. L. (2010). Prescription drug use continues to increase: U.S. prescription drug data for 2007–2008. *NCHS Data Brief, 42,* 1–8.

Gurwitz, J. H. (1995). Investigating polypharmacy presents numerous opportunities for problem solving. *Brown University Long-Term Care Quality Letter, 7*(9), 1.

Hall, J. R., Hoa, V. T., Johnson, L. A., Barber, R. C., & O'Bryant, S. E. O. (2011). The link between cognitive measures and ADLs and IADL functioning in mild Alzheimer's: What has gender got to do with it? *International Journal of Alzheimer Disease. 2011,* Article Id 276734, 6 pages. doi:10.4061/2011/276734

Haw, C., Stubbs, J., & Dickens, G. (2007). An observational study of medication administration errors in old-age psychiatric inpatients. *International Journal of Qualitative Health Care, 4*(19), 210–216.

Hilmer, S. N., Mager, D. E., Simonsick, E. M., Cao, Y., Ling, S. M., Windham, B. G., . . . Abernethy, D. R. (2007). A drug burden index to define the functional burden of medications in older people. *Archive of Internal Medicine, 167*(8), 781–787.

Holmen, K., Ericsson, K., & Winblad, B. (2000). Social and emotional loneliness among nondemented and demented elderly people. *Archives of Gerontology and Geriatrics, 31*(3), 177–192.

Inouye, S. K., Stuenski S., Tinetti, M. E., & Kuchel, G. A. (2007). Geriatric syndromes: Clinical, research and policy implications of a core geriatric concept. *Journal of the American Geriatric Society, 55*(5), 780–791.

Ishikawa, H., Takeuchi, T., & Yano, E. (2008). Measuring functional, communicative, and critical health literacy among diabetic patients. *Diabetes Care, 31*(5), 874–879.

Kaiser Foundation. (2014). Retail prescription drugs filled by pharmacies (annual capita per age). Retrieved from http://www.statehealthfacts.org/comparemapdetail.jsp?ind=268&cat=5&sub=66& yr=138&typ=1

Kim, D. H., Brown, R. A., Ding, E. L., Kiel, D. P., & Berry, S. D. (2011). Dementia medications and risk of falls, syncope, and related adverse events: Meta-analysis of randomized controlled trials. *Journal of the American Geriatrics Society, 59*(6), 1019–1031.

Kohn, L., Corrigan, J., & Donaldson, M. (1999). *To err is human: Building a safer health system.* Washington, DC: National Academies Press.

Kongkaew, C., Noyce, P. R., Ashcroft, D. M. (2008). Hospital admissions associated with adverse drug reactions: A systemic review of prospective observational studies. *Annals of Pharmacotherapy, 42*(7), 1017–1025.

Lam, P., Elliott, R. E., & George, J. (2011). Impact of a self-administration of medications programme on elderly inpatients' competence to manage medications: A pilot study. *Journal of Clinical Pharmacy and Therapeutics, 36*(1), 80–86.

Lazarou, J., Pomeranz, B. H., & Corey, P. N. (1998). Incidence of adverse drug reactions in hospitalized patients. *Journal of the American Medical Association, 279*(15), 1200–1205.

Lu, C. J., & Tune, L. (2003). Chronic exposure to anticholinergic medications adversely affects the course of Alzheimer's disease. *American Journal of Geriatric Psychiatry, 11*(4), 458–461.

Marcum, Z. A., Amuan, M. E., Hanlon, J. T., Aspinall, S. L., Handler, S. M., Ruby, C. M., & Pugh, M. J. (2012). Prevalence of unplanned hospitalizations caused by adverse drug reactions in older veterans. *Journal of the American Geriatric Society, 60*(1), 34–41.

Masoodi, N. A. (2008). Polypharmacy: To err is human, to correct divine. *British Journal of Medical Practitioners, 1*(1), 6–9.

McGowan, M. P. (2004). There is no evidence for an increase in acute coronary syndromes after short-term abrupt discontinuation of statins in stable cardiac patients. *Circulation, 110,* 2333–2335.

Mellor, K., Ahme, D., & Thomson, A. (2009). Tramadol hydrochloride use and acute deterioration in Parkinson's disease tremor. *Movement Disorders, 24*(4), 622–623.

Metlay J. P., Cohen, A., Polsky, D., Kimmel, S. E., Koppel, R., & Hennessy, S. (2005). Medication safety in older adults: Home-based practice patterns. *Journal of the American Geriatric Society, 53*(6), 976–982.

Morisky D. E., Green, L. W., & Levine, D. M. (1986). Concurrent and predictive validity of a self-reported measure of medication adherence. *Medical Care, 24*(1), 67–74.

Morris, L. A., Tabak, E. R., & Gondek, K. (1997). Counseling patients about prescribed medication: 12-year trends. *Medical Care, 35*(10), 996–1007.

Morris, N. S., MacLean, C. D., & Chew, L. D. (2006). The single item literacy screener: Evaluation of a brief instrument to identify limited reading ability. *British Medical Council Family Practice, 7,* 21. doi: 10.1186/1471-2296-7-21

National Audit Office. (2005). A safer place for patients: Learning to improve patient safety. Retrieved from http://www.nao.org.uk/publications/0506/a_safer_place_for_patients.aspx

National Transitions of Care Coalition. (2008). Transitions of care measures 2008. Retrieved from http://www.ntocc.org/Portals/0/PDF/Resources/TransitionsOfCare_Measures.pdf

O'Mahony, D., O'Sullivan, D., Byrne, S., O'Connor, M. N., Ryan, C., & Gallagher, P. (2015). STOPP/START criteria for potentially inappropriate prescribing in older people: Version 2. *Age and Ageing, 44*(2), 213–218.

Permpongkosol, S. (2011). Iatrogenic disease in the elderly: Risk factors, consequences and prevention. *Clinical Interventions in Aging, 6,* 77–82.

Peron, E. P., Gray, S. L., & Hanlon, J. T. (2011). Medication use and functional status decline in older adults: A narrative review. *The American Journal of Geriatric Pharmacotherapy, 9*(6), 378–391.

Physicians' Desk Reference (32nd ed.). (1969). Montvale, NJ: Thomson.

Physicians' Desk Reference (62nd ed.). (2012). Montvale, NJ: Thomson.

PQRI. (n.d.). Retrieved from http://www.qa.drfirst.com/pqrs.jsp

Ridker, P. M., Danielson, E., Fonseca, F. A., Genest, J., Gotto, A. M., Jr., Kastelein, J. J., . . . JUPITER Study Group. (2008). Rosuvastatin to prevent vascular events in men and women with elevated C-reactive protein. *New England Journal of Medicine, 359*(21), 2195–2207.

Rifkin, D. E., Laws, M. B., Rao, M., Balakrishnan, V. S., Sarnak, M. J., & Wilson, I. B. (2010). Medication adherence behavior and priorities among older adults with CKD: A semistructured interview study. *American Journal of Kidney Diseases, 56*(3), 439–446.

Royal, D. R., Cordes, J. A., & Polk, M. (1998). CLOX: An executive clock drawing task. *Journal of Neurology, Neurosurgery and Psychiatry, 64*(5), 588–594.

Sayah, F. A., Williams, B., & Johnson, J., A. (2012). Measuring health literacy in individuals with diabetes: A systematic review and evaluation of available measures. *Health Education & Behavior, 40*(1), 42–55.

Stagnitti, M. N. (2009). Average number of total (including refills) and unique prescriptions by select person characteristics, 2006. Retrieved from https://meps.ahrq.gov/data_files/publications/st245/stat245.pdf

Sullivan, C., Gleason, K., & Rooney, D. (2005). Medication reconciliation in the acute care setting: Opportunity and challenge for nursing. *Journal of Nursing Care Quality, 20*(2), 95–98.

Sunovion Pharmaceuticals. (2006). Safety and efficacy study of AC-3933 in adults with mild to moderate Alzheimer's disease. In ClinicalTrials.gov [Internet]. Bethesda, MD: National Library of Medicine. Retrieved from http://www.clinicaltrials.gov/ct2/show/NCT00359944

Tai-Seale, M., McGuire, T. G., & Zhang, W. (2007). Time allocation in primary care office visits. *Health Services Research, 42*(5), 1871–1894.

U.S. Department of Health and Human Services, Food and Drug Administration. (2012). Guidance for industry: Pharmacokinetics in patients with impaired renal function: Study design, data analysis, and impact on dosing and labeling. Retrieved from http://www.fda.gov/downloads/Drugs/GuidanceComplianceRegulatoryInformation/Guidances/ucm072127.pdf

van der Velde, N., Stricker, B., Pols, H., & van der Cammen T. J. (2007) Risk of falls after withdrawal of falls-risk-increasing drugs: A prospective cohort study. *British Journal of Clinical Pharmacology, 63*(2), 232–237.

Vandegrift, D., & Datta, A. (2006). Prescription drug expenditures in the U.S.: The effects of obesity, demographics and new pharmaceutical products. *Southern Economic Journal, 73*(2), 515–529.

Wilson, I. B., Schoen, C., & Neuman, P. (2007). Physician-patient communication about prescription medication nonadherence: A 50-state study of America's seniors. *Journal of General Internal Medicine, 22*(1), 6–12.

Zagaria, M. A. (2009). OTCs & seniors: Risks and safeguards. *US Pharmacopedia, 4*(34) (OTC Trends Suppl.), 12–15.

For a full suite of assignments and additional learning activities, see the access code at the front of your book.

CHAPTER 12

Falls in Older Adults

DeAnne Zwicker

(Competencies 3, 7, 12, 17)

LEARNING OBJECTIVES

At the end of this chapter, the reader will:

> Describe older adults with a predisposition for falls and falls with injury.
> Recognize intrinsic and extrinsic risk factors for falls in older adults.
> Incorporate a patient-specific fall risk assessment into an individualized plan of care.
> Describe screening tools to aid in assessment of fall risk.
> Identify nurse-led interventions within the interprofessional team to prevent falls specific to the patient's risk.

KEY TERMS

Environmental Hazards

Extrinsic risk factors

Fall prevention interventions

Fall risk assessment

Hendrich Fall Risk Model II

Hospital Elder Life Program

Intrinsic risk factors

Physical restraints

Safety promotion

STRATIFY scale

Timed Get Up and Go Test

Falls are one of the most common adverse events that threaten the quality of life of older adults. According to the Centers for Disease Control and Prevention (CDC), falls are the leading cause of death due to injury (CDC, 2012a) and result in 2.2 million emergency department visits, with almost 600,000 resulting in hospitalizations (CDC, 2012b). Falls can result in no injury, minor injury, or life-changing injuries. Almost 30% of those who fall experience moderate to severe injuries, including hip fracture, head trauma, and lacerations (CDC, 2012a). In 2013, the National Council on Aging reported falls at $34 billion, with the total cost expected to increase to over $67 billion by 2020.

Falls among older adults are *not* a normal consequence of aging and are most often due to multiple predisposing factors, including intrinsic (person specific) and extrinsic factors (environmental) (Panel on Prevention of Falls, 2011). The frequency of falls increases with age and frailty. A fall may represent an underlying acute illness or an impending new acute problem (urinary tract infection or arrhythmia), it may occur secondary to a chronic disease such as diabetic neuropathy), or it may represent worsening of progressing normal aging changes in vision, gait, and strength (Rubenstein & Josephson, 2006). Although there is no universal consensus on the definition of a fall (World Health Organization [WHO], 2010), a fall has been defined and accepted in the literature as "an event which results in a person unintentionally coming to rest on the ground or another lower level; not as a result of a major intrinsic event (such as a new stroke) or overwhelming hazard" (Tinetti, Speechley, & Ginter, 1988, p. 1703). A higher incidence of falls occurs in older, vulnerable, or frail adults (Anderson, Boshier, & Hannah, 2012; Cameron et al., 2012). Older adults are more likely to fall in all settings, but are at higher risk in hospital settings (Tinetti & Kumar, 2010). Also, those in the hospital often remain hospitalized up to 6 to 12 days longer after a fall (Oliver, Healey, & Haines, 2010).

Falls in the Hospital Setting

Falls are the most commonly reported incident in acute care hospitals (Anderson et al., 2012). Up to 50% of older hospitalized patients in the United States are at risk for falls, and almost half of those who fall suffer an injury (CDC, 2012b). Higher fall rates have been reported between 4 and 14 falls per 1,000 patient bed-days in older adults (Anderson et al., 2012), which roughly equals 1 million inpatient falls occurring in the United States each year (Oliver et al., 2010). The 2011 Institute of Medicine (IOM) report *The Future of Nursing: Leading Change, Advancing Health* reported that evidence links nursing to high-quality care for patients. When caring for hospitalized older adults, one of the primary responsibilities for nurses is to maintain patient safety and prevent iatrogenic events, including falls.

CLINICAL TIP

Falls are the most reported incident in acute care hospitals.

The complex hospital environment plays a role in older adult falls. Alarms, medical equipment, lack of personal assistance, assistive devices, furniture, and partial side rails have all proved to be *environmental hazards* associated with falls (Hendrich, 2006; Letts et al., 2010). Older adults in the hospital may have health conditions that place them at greater risk for falls; for example, an acute change in mental status (delirium) may develop secondary to an infection and cause the older adult to become confused or inattentive, which has been linked to hospital falls (Harrison, Ferrari, Campbell, Maddens, & Whall, 2010).

Falls occurring in the hospital represent a national measure of quality and safety in the National Database of Nursing Quality Indicators (NDNQI). According to the Center for Medicaid and Medicare Services (CMS), falls have been considered to be a hospital-acquired major complication or a consequence of being hospitalized. This makes falls potentially preventable (Radey & LaBresh, 2012). The American Nurses Association has included patient falls as one of the top 10 nurse-sensitive quality indicators (Montalvo, 2007) and the Joint Commission has designated patient falls as one of its National Patient Safety Goals (Joint Commission, 2016). The WHO has described falls and fall-related injuries as a "major public health challenge that calls for global attention. This problem will increase in magnitude as the number of older adults rises over the next decade and in many nations throughout the world" (WHO, 2010, p. 30).

Consequences of Falls

Older adults who experience a fall while hospitalized may experience physical and functional impairments, loss of independence, or even death and disability, often leading to placement in post-acute care or a nursing home after hospitalization (Helvic, Skancke, Selbaek, & Engedal, 2014; Oliver et al., 2010). In a study by Goodwin, Howrey, Zhang, and Kuo (2011), three of four older adults were admitted to the nursing home after being hospitalized for falls. In addition to physical injuries, there are psychological consequences after a fall, such as increased fear of falling, anxiety, helplessness, or depression (Boyd & Stevens, 2009; Painter et al., 2012). In a prospective study, older adults with continued concern about falling again had worse activities of daily functioning and participated less in social activities than those with less fall concerns; this was up to 14 months after the first fall (van der Muelen, Ziistra, Ambergen, & Kempen, 2014). These psychological consequences, particularly fear of falling again (fallophobia) can lead older adults to walk less, lose strength, and then curtail activities that aid in maintaining function and provide quality in their lives (Painter et al., 2012). Thus, fall prevention for hospitalized older adults is critically important to promote safety, quality care, and satisfaction for patients who must be hospitalized.

Fractures are the second most serious health consequence of falls after death due to serious injury from a fall. Of those who fall, 20% to 30% sustain moderate to severe injuries, 10% to 20% experience a fracture, and over 95% of fractures are due to a fall (CDC, 2015). The incidence of hip fracture is greater in older women, but death (mortality) from hip fracture is higher among older men (CDC, 2015). At least 50% of elderly persons who were ambulatory before fracturing a hip do not recover their pre-fracture level of mobility. Those with cognitive impairment have a much slower recovery than those without impairment (Beers & Berkow, 2005; Jones, Jhangri, Feeny, & Beaupre, 2015).

Aside from the impact falls have on patients, outcomes of falls also affect hospitals' cost per admission and length of stay. Older adults who sustain a fall while hospitalized utilize more healthcare resources than persons who do not fall. Policies set by the CMS, which provides payment coverage for older Medicare patients, have also established limits on hospital reimbursement for care due to a fall-related injury in the hospital (Inouye, Brown, & Tinetti, 2009). As of 2008, falls have not been reimbursed to the hospital for those occurring in the hospital (Inouye et al., 2009). Avoidance of the adverse outcomes associated with falls is especially important for judicious use of health-care resources. *Healthy People 2020* recommends implementation of interventions to decrease deaths and serious injury in hospitals (U.S. Department of Health and Human Services, 2014). The Agency for Healthcare Research and Quality (AHRQ, 2016) has developed toolkits for hospital-wide implementation of evidence-based programs to reduce falls, including training for hospital nurses (Zhao & Kim, 2015). Evidence-based fall prevention programs in hospital settings are paramount to reach these goals (see Resources for Hospital Fall Prevention Programs).

Fall Risk Factors

Falls rarely have one cause in older adults, but rather are multifactorial in origin or have more than one cause at a time. Falls are typically due to complex interactions of age-related decline, acute illness, chronic disease, postural control, and other factors such as intrinsic behaviors and mobility capacity (Flaherty & Resnick, 2011). Normal changes of aging commonly result in physiologic changes such as musculoskeletal weakness, change in cognition, or functional limitations.

CLINICAL TIP

Falls are usually multifactorial in origin, although certain medications (such as benzodiazepines) are an independent risk factor.

In order to accurately assess risk for falls, a comprehensive knowledge of factors that contribute to a fall is essential. Risk factors for falls can be categorized as intrinsic and extrinsic factors. *Intrinsic risk factors* are related to the patient's physiology and physical changes associated with aging, such as decreased vision and disorders affecting the physical function needed to maintain balance. These functions include vestibular (perception of body position/movement), proprioceptive (sense of body position), and cognitive and musculoskeletal function.

Many patients also experience multiple chronic diseases, gait and balance disturbances, and functional changes that may lead to falls, particularly when several of these factors exist together (Ambrose, Paul, & Hausdorff, 2013; Zhao & Kim, 2015).

Illnesses and disease states are also intrinsic risk factors for falls. For example, cognitive impairment—specifically impairment of executive function—is a risk factor for falls in older adults (Ambrose et al., 2013; Muir, Gopaul, & Odasso, 2012). Executive function is a mental skill that helps the person pay attention and manage daily activities such as shopping or driving. Lower extremity muscle weakness also has been shown to increase the risk of falls; and those with difficulty with knee extension strength, ankle dorsiflexion, and standing strength from a chair is also associated with fall risk (Ambrose et al., 2013). Balance deficits, cognitive impairment, age over 80 years, and visual impairment all have been shown to increase fall risk. Older adults with diabetes, low body mass index (BMI), depression, and foot problems are at higher risk for falls (WHO, 2010). Risk factors also can be categorized as modifiable and non-modifiable. Age over 80 is non-modifiable, age cannot be changed; however, balance, gait, and muscle weakness may be modified (Tinetti & Kumar, 2010).

Although many intrinsic risk factors usually contribute to the majority of falls in older adults, physical and/or cognitive impairments contribute most to falls and fall-related injuries (Muir et al., 2012). Research has shown a strong association between falls and cognitive changes, and fall risk is increased by 20% for every one-point decrease on the Mini-Mental State Exam. Tinetti and Kumar (2010) also report that the strongest risk factors for falling are use of specific medications, previous falls and strength, gait, and balance impairments. It is important to note, however, that most falls are multifactorial and thus include several different risk factors at once (Muir et al., 2012). (See **Table 12-1**.)

Older adults are vulnerable to drug-related falls for many reasons, including polypharmacy; aging changes, which may include change in ability to metabolize or excrete medications; anticholinergic burden; and comorbid illness (Huang, Mallet, Rochefort, Buckeridge, & Tamblyn, 2012). The most common medications increasing fall risk in older adults are benzodiazepines, atypical antipsychotics, antidepressants, antiparkinson medications,

TABLE 12-1   Intrinsic Risk Factors for Falls in the Hospital Setting

- Muscle weakness, decreased strength
- Cognitive impairment: Slow thinking, poor planning, memory loss; executive dysfunction issues
- Delirium: Acute cognitive impairment (reversible)
- Dementia: Chronic cognitive impairment (not reversible)
- Physical impairment or impaired mobility
- Use of assistive devices
- Gait and/or balance problems
- Age over 80 years
- Visual impairment
- Low body mass index
- Depression
- Foot problems
- Frailty
- Four or more medications
- Use of alcohol
- Use of pain or sleeping medications
- History of a fall in the past year
- Urinary or bowel problems (infection, incontinence, urgency)
- Sensory deficits, peripheral neuropathy, poor vision perception or peripheral vision

glucose-reducing medications, opioids, alcohol, and cardiovascular drugs, including antihypertensives. A multi-factorial risk assessment for falls needs to include a systematic review of all medications, over-the-counter drugs, and herbal remedies to identify those that may lead to a fall (Huang et al., 2012). Pharmacists are often a member of the interdisciplinary team (IDT) in hospitals and can review medications and make recommendations to the fall team regarding changing, reducing, or discontinuing high-risk medications (Cooper & Burfield, 2003). Astute nurses may recognize high-risk medications and report them to the primary provider or ask the pharmacist to review the medications. The American Geriatric Society (2012) has updated the Beer's Criteria, a list of medications that may be considered inappropriate in older adults due to the potential for falls or other adverse events. These include all benzodiazepines, sedatives and hypnotics (e.g., zolpidem), anticonvulsants (except in the presence of seizures), tricyclic antidepressants, and selective serotonin reuptake inhibitors (SSRIs) (see Resources).

Extrinsic risk factors are related to the physical environment, such as lack of grab bars, poor condition of floor surfaces, inadequate lighting, and inadequate or improper use of assistive devices. In the institutional care environments, extrinsic hazards include intravenous line poles, oxygen tubing, height of beds or stretchers, and side rails. In the home environment, extrinsic factors may include loose rugs, cords, or uneven walkways. Use of *physical restraints* and bed rails increase the risk of falls because patients attempt to free themselves from these constraints or climb over bed rails. For many years, physical restraints have been seen as potentially dangerous and may increase the risk of adverse events, such as entrapment between bed rail, bar, or bed frame, and often lead to serious injury. Raised side rails are at times avoided as they may increase the risk of serious injuries from falls. Low positioning also reduces the severity of injury (Healey, Oliver, Milne, & Connelly, 2008). There are also some benefits of bed rails if implemented appropriately, such as aiding in turning and prepositioning. Maintaining the bed in its lowest position will reduce the severity of injury if a fall occurs. Risks and benefits of side rails are outlined by the U.S. Federal Drug Administration (FDA) information on medical devices. Patients who are frail, confused, incontinent, experiencing pain, or unable to walk without assistance are at high risk for falls or adverse events due to bed rails (FDA, 2010). Assessing the individual patient's intrinsic and extrinsic risk factors will aid in developing the appropriate patient-specific interventions and plan of care to prevent falls (see Box 12-1).

CLINICAL TIP

Use a valid and reliable tool to assess fall risk.

Fall Risk Assessment

It is common for an older adult who was previously functioning independently to have a decline in physical or mental capacity during a new acute illness or during a long hospital stay. On admission, a baseline of cognitive and physical function should be ascertained by patient or family caregiver if the patient is cognitively impaired. Older adults admitted to acute care settings should have an initial *fall risk assessment* on admission, after any change in condition, and at regular intervals throughout their stay, such as at shift change. Older adults' risk factors may change at any time in the hospitalization; thus, reassessment of risk factors at regular intervals is important. A standardized risk assessment tool should be chosen to evaluate fall risk. Although there are several risk factors for falls, patients typically have different combinations of risk factors (AHRQ, 2013a).

Nurses often perform the initial and subsequent fall risk assessment using a tool that is evidence-based. There are many evidence-based tools available to evaluate falls risk. For patients who are able to rise from a seated position, the Timed Up and Go (TUG) (Mathias, Nayak, & Isaacs, 1986) may be used to evaluate strength, gait and balance, physical function, and fall risk. This instrument has a high sensitivity and specificity in identifying fallers from nonfallers (Shumway-Cook, Brauer, & Woolacott, 2000), and it takes about a minute to perform. (See **Box 12-1** for the *Timed Get Up and Go Test*.)

BOX 12-1　Timed Get Up and Go Test

Mark a line 3 meters (10 feet) away on the floor.

Instructions: Ask the patient to perform the following series of maneuvers:

1. Sit comfortably in a straight-backed chair.
2. Rise from the chair.
3. Stand still momentarily.
4. Walk a short distance (approximately 3 meters to the line).
5. Turn around.
6. Walk back to the chair.
7. Turn around.
8. Sit down in the chair.

Scoring: Observe the patient's movements for any deviation from a confident, normal performance. Use the following scale:

1 = Normal
2 = Very slightly abnormal
3 = Mildly abnormal
4 = Moderately abnormal
5 = Severely abnormal

Normal: Indicates that the patient gave no evidence of being at risk of falling during the test or at any other time.

Severely abnormal: Indicates that the patient appeared at risk of falling during the test.

Intermediate: Grades reflect the presence of any of the following as indicators of the possibility of falling: undue slowness, hesitancy, abnormal movements of the trunk or upper limbs, staggering, and stumbling.

A patient with a score of 3 or more on the Get Up and Go Test is at risk of falling. An older person who takes 12 seconds or more to complete the test is at high risk for falling.

This article was published in Mathias, S., Nayak, U. S. L., & Isaacs, B. (1986). Balance in elderly patients: The Get-up and Go test. *Archives of Physical Medicine & Rehabilitation, 67,* 387–389. Data from Centers for Disease Control and Prevention. (n.d.). *The Timed Up and Go (TUG) test.* Retrieved from https://www.cdc.gov/steadi/pdf/tug_test-a.pdf

There are many different fall risk assessment tools; however, the best tool should be selected for the population and setting and based on the reliability of the instrument, in particular as supported by evidence from randomized trials. A systematic review and meta-analysis of 14 studies revealed the *Hendrich Fall Risk Model II* showed high sensitivity, whereas the STRATIFY Risk instrument showed higher specificity. The STRATIFY tool was found to be the best tool for assessing the risk of falls by hospitalized acutely ill older adults (Aranda-Gallardo, Rodriguez, Canca-Sanchez, Moya-Suarez, & Morales-Asencio, 2013); therefore, this instrument would be the best choice for this population and hospital setting. Also, in a review of four fall risk assessment instruments the STRATIFY tool showed greater diagnostic ability than the others in the acute care setting (Aranda-Gallardo et al., 2013). Recent studies in hospitalized older adults show the need for more rigorous assessment of large population samples to determine the best tools to predict fall risk in older adults (Aranda-Gallardo, et al., 2013; Ivziku, Matrese, & Pedone. 2010). Other fall risk assessment tools can be found on the University of Iowa Website at https://www.healthcare.uiowa.edu.

In addition to the AGS medication guidelines for inappropriate medication in older adults, the Medication Fall Risk tool (Beasley & Patatanian, 2009) is an instrument designed to evaluate medication-related fall risk. The recommended use is in patients who are prescribed more than four different medications or over-the-counter products. The Medication Fall Risk Score can be calculated to determine risk of falls related to multiple medications. The evaluation is typically performed by a pharmacist but can be performed by other team members as well (see **Box 12-2** for a medication risk tool).

BOX 12-2   Evidence-based Practice Box: Medication Fall Risk Score

Background: This tool can be used to identify medication-related risk factors for falls in hospitalized patients. A pharmacist would perform this assessment.

Reference: Reproduced from Beasley, B., & Patatanian, E. (2009). Development and implementation of a pharmacy fall prevention program. *Hospital Pharmacy, 44*(12), 1095–1102. © 2009, Thomas Land Publishers, http://www.hosp-pharmacy.com.

How to use this tool: Evaluate medication-related fall risk on admission and at regular intervals thereafter. Add up the point value (risk level) for every medication the patient is taking. If the patient is taking more than one medication in a particular risk category, the score should be calculated by (risk level score) × (number of medications in that risk level category). For a patient at risk, a pharmacist should use the evaluation tools to determine if medications may be tapered, discontinued, or changed to a safer alternative.

Use this tool in conjunction with clinical assessment and a nursing risk scale (e.g., Tool 3H, Morse Fall Scale for Identifying Fall Risk Factors, or 3G **STRATIFY Scale** for Identifying Fall Risk Factors) to determine if a patient is at risk for falls and plan care accordingly. Note that this scale may not capture the medication risk factors that are most important on your hospital ward, so consider your local circumstances.* A hybrid approach is to have the nurse use a scale such as the one below and alert the pharmacist if the total score is 6 or greater.

If your hospital uses an electronic health record, consult the hospital's information systems staff about integrating this tool into the electronic health record.

Medication Fall Risk Score

Point Value (Risk Level)	American Hospital Formulary Service Class	Comments
3 (High)	Analgesics,* antipsychotics, anticonvulsants, benzodiazepines[†]	Sedation, dizziness, postural disturbances, altered gait and balance, impaired cognition
2 (Medium)	Antihypertensives, cardiac drugs, antiarrhythmics, antidepressants	Induced orthostasis, impaired cerebral perfusion, poor health status
1 (Low)	Diuretics	Increased ambulation, induced orthostasis
Score ≥6		**Higher risk for fall; evaluate patient**

*Includes opiates.
†Although not included in the original scoring system, the falls toolkit team recommends that you include non-benzodiazepine sedative-hypnotic drugs (e.g., zolpidem) in this category.

Orthostatic hypotension is common among older adults, specifically in the hospital setting. Orthostasis may worsen in the presence of aging changes in blood pressure regulation, particularly if the patient is taking cardiovascular medications or has cardiovascular disease (Milos, Bondesson, & Magnusson, 2014). An assessment for orthostatic hypotension should be performed in all older hospital patients (see **Table 12-2**). This is a very simple test to rule out fall risk related to orthostasis and should be performed in any patient who is potentially dehydrated, reporting dizziness on sitting up or standing, or taking cardiovascular medications, for example. There is often confusion in how to accurately perform orthostatic testing (see **Box 12-3** for directions).

TABLE 12-2   Nursing Assessments to Aid in Identifying Risk Factors for Falls

Assessment for Potential Clinical Problem Leading to Falls

- Pulse: Arrhythmias, bradycardia
- Orthostatic blood pressure: Postural hypotension (see Box 12-6)
- Oxygen saturation/pulse oxygen: Low oxygen saturation leads to confusion
- Vision screening deficits: Evaluate need to use glasses, visual acuity, depth perception, peripheral vision
- Muscle strength: Weakness in one or both sides
- Range of motion in neck, spine, and extremities: Limitations in range of motion
- Gait and balance: In postural control, balance, coordination, station, and gait (see Box 12-2)
- Pain level: Limits to obtain normal function (check pain level 1 to 10)
- Mental status deficits: Cognitive impairment, confusion, dementia, and delirium or LOC change
- Changes in thinking ability to maintain attention, planning ability
- Medical history: Stroke, hypertension, urinary incontinence, visual impairment
- Prolonged length of stay in hospital, care dependency
- Medications: Antipsychotic, antidepressants, benzodiazepines and other sedating drugs
- Memory: Ability to remember safety instructions
- Environmental: Wet floor, poor lighting in room, loose rugs, location in bathroom or patient room

*LOC = Level of consciousness: Alert, confused, drowsy, unresponsive.

BOX 12-3   Orthostatic Blood Pressure Measurement

Patient should be lying supine for 3 to 5 minutes prior to B/P measurement

Obtain blood pressure and pulse while supine

Assist patient to standing position

Obtain B/P and heart rate at 1 and 3 minutes

Document symptoms of dizziness and syncope in addition to vital signs; symptoms and vital signs together is a better indicator of volume loss

One or more of the following findings indicates volume loss:

- Decrease in systolic B/P >20 mm Hg or more
- Decrease in diastolic B/P of 10 mm Hg or more
- Increase in heart rate of 20 beats per minute or more

A position change from supine to standing is better diagnostic accuracy of volume depletion change from supine to sitting and then standing

Modified from AHRQ. (2013b). Tool 3F: Orthostatic Vital Sign Measurement. Retrieved from http://www.ahrq.gov/professionals/systems/hospital/fallpxtoolkit/fallpxtk-tool3f.html

B/P = Blood pressure

The IDT members may perform further evaluation of older adults, including a fall history, an examination of mental and mobility status, a checklist for the presence of sensory deficits such as hearing and vision screening, a comprehensive medication review, and a list of primary and secondary diagnoses. A review of the risk status may be performed at daily team rounds (Gillespie et al., 2012).

CLINICAL TIP

Many lawsuits for falls with injury could be prevented through proper assessment, evaluation, and documentation.

Post-Fall Assessment

Nurses and the IDT must assess older adults for risk of injury after a fall. Some patients may experience a serious adverse event after a fall. For example, if the patient is on warfarin (Coumadin) or another blood thinner, intracranial bleeding may occur if the patient sustains head trauma with the fall. After the patient is evaluated and deemed stable, the fall should be carefully reviewed for underlying contributing factors that led to the fall. The older adult should be asked to describe the sensations or events that preceded the fall, such as dizziness, and circumstances surrounding the fall, such as what activity the person was engaged in, the location of the fall, witnesses to the fall, and injuries sustained. A structured post-fall assessment is key to determining the underlying factors (Hempel et al., 2013). This typically requires an interdisciplinary team effort to identify modifiable risk factors (Ganz, Huang, & Saliba, 2013; Oliver et al., 2010). Identifying the causes of each fall is critical to preventing a future fall (Cameron et al., 2012). Modifiable risk factors such as bradycardia or orthostatic hypotension may be addressed immediately to modify the underlying causative factors and future falls. A fall IDT should provide a thorough evaluation of the patient to identify modifiable intrinsic risk factors in order to develop an accurate, patient-specific plan of care while an in-patient and after going home or to another level of care (Cameron et al., 2012).

Risk factors for serious injury after falling include a diagnosis of osteoporosis, previous joint replacement, and spinal abnormalities. Current use of anticoagulants such as warfarin or aspirin, a low platelet count, elevated international normalized ratio, or other clotting factors can result in acute bleeding. Most hospitals now have a post-fall protocol that includes assessment for signs or symptoms of fracture or potential for spinal injury before the patient is moved, and neurologic observations for all patients who may have sustained a head injury to improve outcomes. Some hospitals utilize a rapid response team to assess patients who have fallen, due to risk for serious injury and death. After a fall has occurred, it is important that a thorough medical assessment be done to identify any potential hidden injuries. An assessment of the patient who has fallen by a multidisciplinary team is another intervention that nurses can initiate to identify potential risk factors not previously identified to prevent further falls and injuries (Tinetti, Douchette, Claus, & Marottoli, 2015).

Case Study 12–1

Mr. Thompson is a 72-year-old African American man who lives alone, whose neighbors check in on him regularly as his daughter lives in California. His neighbor noticed he had not come out to get his mail or newspapers. She rang the doorbell and there was no answer, even though his car was in the driveway. She looked through the kitchen window and saw he was lying on the floor. She used the spare key he gave her to enter the house. The patient reported "I tripped over the dog, who was excited to get out, then could not get up." The neighbor called the ambulance, and Mr. Thompson was taken to the hospital. Later he was found to have a hip fracture sustained in the fall. Mr. Thompson admitted that his vision has been off and he has been "a little shaky walking lately." Mr. Thompson has a history of heart failure requiring diuretics, hypertension for many years, and prostate problems making him void frequently even at night.

Questions:

1. What are the potential fall risk factors for Mr. Thompson?
2. What assessment would you perform?
3. What are the likely findings?
4. What interventions might you discuss with Mr. Thompson?
5. What educational information would you provide?

Fall Prevention and Safety Promotion Strategies

The best approaches to fall risk prevention are patient-specific targeted interventions involving an IDT collaboration, specifically implementing targeted exercise, attention to coexisting medical conditions, environmental inspection, and hazard reduction (Rubenstein & Josephson, 2006; Wood et al., 2014). The 2003 IOM report *Keeping Patients Safe* defined surveillance as "observing changes in patient conditions that may signal a decline in condition along with taking an action to prevent complications" (p. 12). Surveillance is one of the primary proactive *safety promotion* interventions used by hospital nurses. Surveillance interventions include purposeful hourly rounding of mobile patients closer to the nurses' station, assignment of sitters, and observation devices. Surveillance is sometimes supported by technological devices such as alarms, pressure mats, video monitoring, and portable trigger alarms. However, alarm fatigue, or hearing alarms so often they get ignored, also can occur (Daniels, 2014). A recent study has shown some promise in monitoring patients electronically using a telemetry device, such as the Vital Signs Technologies transmitter, to monitor patients; however, more research is required (Dupree, Fritz-Campiz, & Musheno, 2014). The evidence for technological devices to reduce falls is limited in part because few studies have documented their effectiveness.

Patients who have a history of falls or a recent fall are often evaluated during nursing hourly rounds to ensure safety and may include the IDT (Halm, 2009). During rounds nurses evaluate pain, prompt patients to void, identify risks, and ensure precautions to avoid falls are in place. Ganz and colleagues (2013) found a 52% reduction in falls with hourly rounding, and thus when performed intentionally it can be very effective. Post-fall team huddles have shown to be helpful in identifying patient risks immediately after a fall (Ganz et al., 2013). Older adults often continue to fall in spite of interventions based on evidence. However, in an in-patient setting an immediate post-fall huddle of the IDT can quickly evaluate the potential underlying factors of the fall and ascertain modifiable risk factors to develop interventions right away to prevent further future falls (Cameron et al., 2012; Ganz et al, 2013).

Fall prevention strategies are likely to be more effective if they are supported by hospital senior leadership to implement a hospital falls prevention program. Likewise, the stakeholders need to know why it is important to employ an interdisciplinary approach. The most important factor in developing a fall prevention plan is to individualize the interventions that are specific to the patient's risk factors.

CLINICAL TIP

Universal fall precautions should be issued for all patients in the acute care setting.

Universal fall precautions should be implemented for all patients in the acute care setting regardless of risk. Universal precautions include orienting older adults to their environment, discussing rounding protocols, emphasizing safety measures (e.g., placing hospital bed in low position and locked), and educating the patient and family members of the risk of falling and the strategies needed to prevent falls. General strategies for all patients include use of nonskid slippers or shoes; removal of obstacles and clutter in the room; provision of easy access to toilet or bedside commode; and having the call light, bedside table, and other needs within easy reach (AHRQ, 2013a). Glasses and hearing aids should be worn prior to getting up, although caution is warranted with multifocal lenses during ambulation. The bed should be elevated to a comfortable height for transfers. The urgent priority in all settings, particularly acute care, is not only to reduce the number of falls, but also to eliminate falls with injury entirely. Individually tailored use of the fall prevention interventions based on risk factors discussed here will help reduce serious injuries.

Several medications are considered high risk in older adults due to their risk for falls. Psychotropic medication classes such as benzodiazepines, antipsychotics, pain medications, or other sedating medications may cause a patient to be drowsy or less alert and lead to a fall and possibly a hip fracture (Flaherty & Resnick, 2011). Benzodiazepines are an independent risk factor for older adult falls, meaning that the patient need have no other problems and is at significant risk taking benzodiazepines (Rochon, 2014). Although pain and other sedating medications may be required to treat a patient's condition, nurses need to evaluate the patient's response to these medications. Nurses can suggest dosage adjustments or medication changes to the primary provider when physical or cognitive impairment occurs after giving one of these medications. Surveillance for a change in a patient's condition may signal a significant decline in health status. An acute change should be reported to the primary provider immediately, as this change is often the first sign of an impending serious problem in older adults and may result in a fall. Changes in an older adult's status are very subtle, and even minor changes may indicate an acute impending event. Other surveillance interventions include making hourly rounds and checking on patients with altered cognition more frequently to reduce falls (AHRQ, 2013a). In general, scripted rounds usually include evaluation of pain, personal needs, placement of items in reach, and prevention of falls (e.g., use of call light to get up at night or prompted voiding as indicated). Proactive assessment of needs aids in improving safety and decreases call lights (AHRQ, 2013a; Halm & Quigley, 2011).

Fall prevention interventions include those that reduce the impact of known intrinsic risk factors. Ambulating persons with cognitive impairment helps maintain their mobility and strength, thus preventing functional decline and improving or maintaining functional capacity. Older adults with cognitive impairment are one of the highest risk groups for falls in the hospital setting (WHO, 2010). A program that aides in reducing falls in cognitively impaired older adults (particularly targeting prevention of delirium and functional decline) is the *Hospital Elder Life Program* (HELP; Inouye, 2000). This program employs volunteers to aid in walking patients to prevent delirium and maintain physical and cognitive function. The HELP program (Inouye, 2000) has been shown to reduce delirium by 23% and decrease length of stay by 7 days (Rubin, Neal, Fenlon, Hassan, & Inouye, 2011).

Calcium (1200 mg) and vitamin D (800 international units) supplementation has been recommended by the American Geriatrics Society (AGS) and the U.S. Preventive Task Force. Supplementation with vitamin D and calcium is recommended for reduction of osteoporosis and thus fractures if falls occur in older adults (Gillespie et al., 2009; Ross, Taylor, Yaktine, & Del Valle, 2011). A minimum of 12 months of treatment is recommended to maintain healthy bones and assist in prevention or slowing of osteoporosis, particularly in those shown to be deficient in vitamin D_3. Evidence suggests that vitamin D_3 supplementation also may decrease the risk of falling in older adults deficient in vitamin D_3. Nurses can recommend calcium and vitamin D be prescribed to older adults as there is evidence supporting its use to prevent falls (Gillespie et al., 2009, Kavyani et al., 2010).

The use of some medications is associated with falls. In 2012, the AGS released the updated Beer's Criteria, which identifies medications and doses of medication that may be harmful to adults age 65 and older. Judicious use of medications, avoiding inappropriate medications, and following the Beer's guidelines may reduce falls and/or fall injuries in older adults. Two key prescribing principles for older adults are "less is more" and "start low and go slow," which refers to starting doses at lowest levels to reduce potential overdose of medications. Cautious prescribing practices can lessen problems such as delirium, gastrointestinal bleeding, falls, and fractures in the older adult. The Beer's Criteria supports the CDC recommendations for medication reduction or withdrawal, especially for those taking four or more medications (AGS, 2012; CDC, 2012). Regular medication review and tapering off unnecessary therapy decreases the risk of adverse drug events (Rochon, 2006; Rochon, Schmader, & Sokol, 2015). The Beer's Criteria (2012) support the CDC recommendations for medication reduction or withdrawal, especially for those taking four or more medications (AGS, 2012; CDC, 2012). Regular medication review and tapering off unnecessary therapy decreases the risk of adverse drug events that may also result falls (Rochon, 2006; Rochon et al., 2015). Nurses give and monitor patient medications on a regular basis. Becoming familiar with high-risk medications and notifying the primary provider of these medications can help in reducing adverse drug events and falls (Zwicker & Fulmer, 2012). See **Table 12-3** for a list of nursing interventions to reduce falls.

TABLE 12-3   Nursing Interventions to Reduce Falls

- Implement Universal Precautions for all patients on admission
- Ensure adequate training is provided to assess for risk factors using an evidence-based instrument (nursing and IDT members)
- Inquire of patient/family information regarding past falls on admission
- Assess fall risk factors on admission, with significant change in condition, and with transfers
- Ensure risk and interventions are communicated between shifts, at transfers to radiology or other units, or on discharge to another facility or home
- Develop interdisciplinary, patient-individualized care plan interventions based on patients' specific fall risk assessment and include multiple factor evaluation related to falls:
  - High-risk medications: Collaborate with pharmacist and primary provider for those on four or more medications or those on inappropriate medications, such as benzodiazepines, psychoactive medications, or excess medications. Consider taper of high-risk or any unnecessary medications on consultation with primary provider and pharmacist
  - Gait and balance deficits: Recommend evaluation by physical therapist or occupational therapist
  - Cognition: Recommend evaluation of dementia, delirium, psychosis, or executive dysfunction by psychologist and primary provider
  - Prior falls: Significantly increases risk; recommend physical therapy and/or occupational therapy evaluation
  - Continence problems: Prompt voiding on rounds and nursing care
  - Orthostatic hypotension: Check orthostatic vital signs during nursing care
- Recommend a sitter or family member stay with the patient as needed for safety
- Inquire if family members have strategies that have been successful in reducing falls (patient preferences, etc.) or if they are able to stay with the patient if the patient is confused
- Evaluate environment for safety hazards in hospital and post-discharge setting, such as by a home evaluation
- Maintain baseline mobility while hospitalized
  - Recommend physical or occupational evaluation for exercise or strength and gait or balance interventions.
  - Implement recommended strategies on unit as well as in physical therapy department
  - Include patient and family education on mobility maintenance
  - Consider an algorithm for hospital ambulation program (e.g., http://www.AHRQ.gov/professionals/systems/hospital/fallpxtoolkit/fallpxtk7.html) or the HELP Program (Inouye, 2000).
- Ensure color-coded fall risk wrist bands and nonskid socks are applied, signage is in place, and patient/family understanding is verified
- Hourly rounds should ensure fall risk strategies are in place and Universal Precautions observed. Documentation may be logged on rounds when evaluation is performed
- Ensure appropriate assistive devices are in use for ambulating, transfers, and safe patient handling; consult with physical therapist or occupational therapist
- Ensure glasses and nonslip socks or low-heeled shoes are on for ambulation; multifocal glasses may increase risk
- Ensure environment is clear of clutter and light is adequate for ambulation. Monitor patients with intravenous poles
- Recommend interdisciplinary rounds on high-risk patients

Summary

Nurses hold a pivotal position in the acute care setting in assessing older adults for fall risk, developing and implementing patient-specific interventions in collaboration with the IDT, and providing education to the patient and family to reduce older adult falls, disability from fractures, head trauma, or even death (**Box 12-4**). There are several evidence-based guidelines that can be utilized by the nurse and IDT to provide preventive interventions for older adults; however, all nurses should be trained in the process so that assessments and interventions are based on evidence. By spending a few minutes to assess the older adult's risk for falls during routine care, the nurse can provide fall risk assessment and IDT-determined patient-specific interventions as well as patient and family education on prevention of falls. This will also help the older adult maintain functional status and quality of life. Interventions that reduce falls in older adults will also reduce the cost to the healthcare system by limiting the number of older adults who visit the emergency department or are hospitalized as the result of a fall that might have been prevented. Environmental and multifactorial patient assessments and interventions can make the difference between safety and falling. Nursing actions are key in helping prevent falls.

BOX 12-4   Resources for Fall Prevention

Degelau, J., Belz, M., Bungum, M., Flavin, P. L., Harper, C., Leys, K., . . . Webb, B.; for AHRQ (2013). Prevention of falls toolkit for providing quality of care in hospitals. Retrieved from http://www.ahrq .gov/professionals/systems/hospital/fallpxtoolkit/index.html

Institute for Clinical Systems Improvement (ICSI). (2012). Prevention of falls (acute care). Retrieved from https://www.icsi.org/guidelines__more/catalog_guidelines_and_more/catalog_guidelines /catalog_patient_safetyreliability_guidelines/falls/

Panel for Prevention of Falls in Older Persons, AGS/BGS. (2010). Geared for community setting. Retrieved from https://www.icsi.org/guidelines__more/catalog_guidelines_and_more/catalog_guidelines /catalog_patient_safetyreliability_guidelines/falls/

Center for Disease Control and Prevention. (2010). Compendium of effective fall interventions: What works for community-dwelling older adults (3rd ed.). Retrieved from http://www.cdc.gov /homeandrecreationalsafety/Falls/compendium/0.0_toc.html

---

Clinical Reasoning Exercises

1. Read the *Fall Prevention Center of Excellence* Website at http://www.stopfalls.org. Discuss your findings with another student nurse in one of your clinical groups.

2. Evaluate one fall-risk assessment tool and discuss its strengths and weaknesses. You can review fall-risk assessment tools at http://www.consultgerirn.org. Click on Topic Resources, Falls, then Assessment tools. Review the research of Zhao, Y. L., &

Kim, H. (2015). Older adult inpatient falls in acute care hospitals: Intrinsic, extrinsic, and environmental factors. *Journal of Gerontological Nursing, 41*(7), 29–43.

3. Read Boxes 12–1 to 12–5 on fall assessment. Describe how you would assess an 86-year-man with atrial fibrillation who has fallen at home. Describe how you would assess an 84-year-old woman with osteoporosis who has fallen getting out of bed in the hospital.

Personal Reflections

1. Have you ever cared for an older adult patient who fell in the hospital? How did it happen? How did the patient feel about that experience? What injuries occurred? Did the fall change how you think about the nursing role in surveillance or safety?

2. Have you ever cared for an older adult who fell at home? How did the patient feel about that experience? What injuries occurred? Did the patient experience a fear of falling after that? Did the fall change how you think about the nursing role in the home and community?

3. Have you ever had a family member who fell either at home or in the hospital setting? What resulted from the family member falling? Can you think of any ways that the fall could have been prevented?

4. What precautions are you aware of in the hospital or community setting in which you work that have been effective in reducing patient fall risks?

References

Agency for Healthcare Research & Quality. (2013a). Preventing Falls in Hospitals: A Toolkit for Improving Quality of Care. Retrieved from http://www.ahrq.gov/professionals/systems/hospital/fallpxtoolkit/index.html

Agency for Health Research & Quality. (2013b). Tool 3F: Orthostatic Vital Sign Measurement. Retrieved from http://www.ahrq.gov/professionals/systems/hospital/fallpxtoolkit/fallpxtk-tool3f.html

Agency for Healthcare Research & Quality. (2016). Toolkit for using the AHRQ quality indicators. Rockville, MD: Agency for Healthcare Research and Quality. http://www.ahrq.gov/professionals/systems/hospital/qitoolkit/index.html

Ambrose, A. F., Paul, G., & Hausdorff, J. M. (2013). Risk factors for falls among older adults: A review of the literature. *Maturitas, 75*(1), 51–61.

American Geriatrics Society & British Geriatrics Society. (2010). Clinical practice guideline: Prevention of falls in older persons. Retrieved from http://www.americangeriatrics.org/health_care_professionals/clinical_practice/clinical_guidelines_recommendations/prevention_of_falls_summary_of_recommendations

Anderson, O., Boshier, P. R., & Hannah, G. B. (2012). Interventions designed to prevent healthcare bed-related injuries in patients. *Cochrane Database of Systematic Reviews,* 1. doi:10.1002/14651858.CD008931.pub3

Aranda-Gallardo, M., Luna Rodriguez, E., Canca-Sanchez, J. C., Moya-Suarez, A. B., & Morales-Ascencio, J. M. (2015). Validation of the STRATIFY falls risk-assessment tool for acute-care hospital patients and nursing home residents: Study protocol. *Journal of Advanced Nursing, 71*(8), 1948–1957.

Beasley, B., & Patatanian, E. (2009). Development and implementation of a pharmacy fall prevention program. *Hospital Pharmacist, 44*(12), 1095–1102.

Beers, M., & Berkow, R. (2005). *The Merck manual of geriatrics* (5th ed.). Whitehouse Station, NJ: Merck.

American Geriatrics Society http://geriatricscareonline.org/ProductAbstract/american-geriatrics-society-updated-beers-criteria-for-potentially-inappropriate-medication-use-in-older-adults/CL001/?param2=search

Boyd, R., & Stevens, J. A. (2009). Falls and fear of falling: Burden, beliefs and behaviours. *Age and Ageing, 38*(4), 423–428.

Cameron, I. D., Gillespie, L. D., Robertson, M. C., Murray, G. R., Hill, K. D., Cumming, R. G., & Kerse, N. (2012). Interventions for preventing falls in older people in care facilities and hospitals. *Cochrane Database of Systematic Reviews,* 12.

Centers for Disease Control and Prevention. (n.d). The Timed Up and Go (TUG) test. Retrieved from https://www.cdc.gov/steadi/pdf/tug_test-a.pdf

Centers for Disease Control and Prevention, National Center for Injury Prevention and Control. (n.d.). Web-based Injury Statistics Query and Reporting System (WISQARS). Retrieved from https://www.cdc.gov/injury/wisqars/

Centers for Disease Control and Prevention. (2012a). Costs of falls among older adults. Retrieved from http://www.cdc.gov/HomeandRecreationalSafety/Falls/fallcost.html

Centers for Disease Control and Prevention. (2012b). Falls among older adults: An overview. Retrieved from from http://www.cdc.gov/HomeandRecreationalSafety/Falls/adultfalls.html

Centers for Disease Control. (2015). Injury prevention and control: Data & statistics (WISQARS™). Retrieved from http://www.cdc.gov/injury/wisqars/

Cooper, J. W., & Burfield, A. H. (2003). Medication interventions for fall prevention in the older adults. *Journal of the American Pharmacists Association, 49*(30), e70–e84.

DuPree, E., Fritz-Campiz, A., & Musheno, D. (2014). A new approach to preventing falls with injuries. *Journal of Nursing Care Quality, 29*(2), 99–102.

Flaherty, E., & Resnick, B. (Eds.). (2011). *Geriatric nursing review syllabus: A core curriculum in advanced practice geriatric nursing* (3rd ed.). New York, NY: American Geriatrics Society.

Ganz, D. A., Huang, D., Saliba, D. (2013). Preventing falls in hospitals: A toolkit for improving quality of care. Prepared by RAND Corporation, Boston University School of Public Health, and ECRI Institute under Contract No. HHSA290201000017I TO #1. AHRQ Publication No. 13-0015-EF. 2013. Rockville, MD: Agency for Healthcare Research and Quality.

Gillespie, L. D., Robertson, M. C., Gillespie, L. D., Lamb, S. E., Gates, S., Cumming, R. G., & Rowe, H. (2009). Interventions for preventing falls in older people living in the community. *Cochrane Database of Systematic Reviews*, (9):CD007146. doi:10.1002/14651858.CD007146.pub2

Goodwin, J. S., Howrey, B., Zhang, D. D., & Kuo, Y. F. (2011). Risk of continued institutionalization after hospitalization in older adults. *Journal of Gerontology Series A Biological Sciences and Medical Sciences, 66*(12), 1321–1327.

Halm, M., & Quigley, P. A. (2011). Reducing falls and fall-related injuries in acutely ill and critically ill patients. *American Journal of Critical Care, 20*(6), 480–484.

Harrison, B., Ferrari, M., Campbell, C., Maddens, M., & Whall, A. (2010). Evaluating the relationship between inattention and impulsivity-related falls in hospitalized older adults. *Geriatric Nursing, 31*(1), 8–16.

Healey, F., Oliver, D., Milne, A., & Connelly, J. B. (2008). The effect of bedrails on falls and injury: A systematic review of clinical studies. *Age and Ageing, 37*(4), 368–378.

Helvic., A. S., Skancke, R. G., Selbase, G., & Engedal, K. (2014). Nursing home admission during the first year after hospitalization: The contribution of cognitive impairment. *PLOS One, 9*(1) doi:10.1371/journal.pone.0086116

Hempel, S., Newberry, S., Wang, Z., Booth, M., Shanman, R., Johnsen, B., . . . Ganz, D. A. (2013). Hospital fall prevention: A systematic review of implementation, components, adherence, and effectiveness. *Journal of the American Geriatrics Society, 61*, 483–494

Hendrich, A. L. (2006). Inpatient falls: lessons from the field. Retrieved from http://www.psqh.com/mayjun06/falls.html

Hendrich, A. L., Bender, P. S., & Nyhuis, A. (2003). Validation of the Hendrich II fall risk model: A large concurrent case control study of hospitalized patients. *Applied Nursing Research, 16*(1), 9–21.

Huang, A. R., Mallet, L., Rochefort, C. M., Buckeridge, D. L., & Tamblyn, R. (2012). Medication-related falls in the elderly: Causative factors and prevention strategies. *Drugs & Aging, 1*(29) 359–376.

Inouye, S. (2000). *The hospital elder life program (HELP)*. Yale University School of Medicine. Retrieved from http://www.hospitalelderlifeprogram.org/public/public-main.php

Inouye, S., Brown, C., & Tinetti, M. (2009). Medicare nonpayment, hospital falls, and unintended consequences. *New England Journal of Medicine, 360*, 2390–2393.

Institute of Medicine. (2011). *The future of nursing: Leading change, advancing health*. Washington, DC: National Academies Press.

Institute of Medicine. (2003). *Keeping patients safe: Transforming the work environment of nurses.* Washington, DC: National Academies Press.

Ivziku, D., Matrese, M., & Pedone, C. (2010). Predictive validity of the Hendrich Fall Risk Model II in an acute geriatric unit. *International Journal of Nursing Studies, 48*(4), 468–474.

Joint Commission. (2016). *National patient safety goals.* Retrieved from https://www.jointcommission.org/assets/1/6/2016_NPSG_HAP_ER.pdf

Jones, C. A., Jhangri, G. S., Feeny, D. H., & Beaupre, L. A. (2015). Cognitive status at hospital admission: Postoperative trajectory of functional recovery for hip fracture. *Journal of Gerontology Series A Biological Sciences & Medical Science, 72*(1), 61–67.

Kavyani, R. R., Stein, B., Valiyil, R., Manno, R., Maynard, R. W., & Crews, D. C. (2010). Vitamin D treatment for the prevention of falls in older adults: Systematic review and analysis. *Journal of the American Geriatrics Society, 58*(7), 1299–1210.

Letts, L., Moreland, J., Richardson, J., Coman, L., Edwards, M., Ginis, K., . . . Wishart, L. (2010). The physical environment as a fall risk factor in older adults: Systematic review and meta-analysis of cross-sectional and cohort studies. *Australian Occupational Therapy Journal, 57*(1), 51–64.

Mathias, S., Nayak, U. S. L., Isaacs, B. (1986). Balance in elderly patients: The "get-up and go" test. *Archives of Physical Medicine & Rehabilitation, 67,* 387–389.

Meade, C. M., Bursell, A. L., Ketelesen, L. (2010). *Medsurg Nursing: Official Journal of the Academy of Medical-Surgical Nurses, 19*(1), 23–6, 36.

Milos, V., Bondesson, A., Magnusson, M. (2014). Fall risk-increasing drugs and falls: A cross sectional study among elderly patients in primary care. *BioMedCentral, 14,* 40.

Montalvo, I. (2007). The National Database of Nursing Quality Indicators™ (NDNQI®). *The Online Journal of Issues in Nursing, 12*(3), Manuscript 2.

Muir, S. W., Gopaul, K., & Montero Odasso, M. M. (2012). The role of cognitive impairment in fall risk among older adults: A systematic review and meta-analysis. *Age and Ageing, 41*(3), 299–308.

Murphy, T., Labonte, P., Klock, M., & Houser, L. (2008). Falls prevention for elders in acute care: An evidence-based nursing practice initiative. *Critical Care Nursing Quarterly, 31*(1), 33–39.

Oliver, D., Britton, M., Seed, P., Martin, F. C. and Hopper, A. H. (1997). Development and evaluation of evidence based risk assessment tool (STRATIFY) to predict which elderly inpatients will fall: Case-control and cohort studies. *BMJ, 315*(7115), 1049–1053.

Oliver, D., Healey, F., & Haines, T. P. (2010). Preventing falls and fall-related injuries in hospitals. *Clinics in Geriatric Medicine, 26,* 645–692.

Painter, J. A., Allison, L., Dhingra, P., Daughtery J., Cogdioo, K., & Trujillo, L. G. (2012). Fear of falling and its relationship with anxiety, depression, and activity engagement among community-dwelling older adults. *Journal of Occupational Therapy, 66*(2), 169–176.

Panel on Prevention of Falls in Older Persons, American Geriatrics Society/British Geriatrics Society (AGS/BGS). Summary of the updated American Geriatrics Society/British Geriatrics Society clinical practice guideline for prevention of falls in older persons. *Journal of the American Geriatrics Society, 59,* 148–157.

Radey, L. A., & LaBresh, K. A. (2012). *Evidence-based guidelines for selected and previously considered hospital-acquired conditions* (RTI Project Number 0209853.231.002.122). Baltimore, MD: Centers for Medicare and Medicaid Innovation.

Rubin, F. H., Neal, K., Fenlon, K., Hassan, S., Inouye, S. K. (2011). Sustainability and scalability of the Hospital Elder Life Program (HELP) at a community hospital. *Journal of the American Geriatric Society, 59*(2), 359–365. doi:10.1111/j.1532-5415.2010.03243.x

Rochon, P. (2014). Drug prescribing in older adults. Level V. Retrieved from http://www.uptodate.com/contents/drug-prescribing-for-older-adults

Rochon, P. A., Schmader, K. E., & Sokol, H. N. (2013). Drug prescribing for older adults. Retrieved from http://www.uptodate.com/contents/drug-prescribing-for-older-adults

Rochon, P. A. (2006). *Drug prescribing for older adults.* Retrieved from http://www.uptodate.com/contents/drug-prescribing-for-older-adults

Ross, A. C., Taylor, C. L., Yaktine, A. L., & Del Valle, H. B. (2011). *The Institute of Medicine (US) Committee to Review Dietary Reference Intakes for Vitamin D.* Washington, DC: National Academies Press.

Rubenstein, L. Z., & Josephson, K. R. (2006). Falls and their prevention in elderly people: What does the evidence show? *Medical Clinics of North America, 90*(5), 807–824.

Scott, V., Votova, K., Scanlan, A., & Close, J. (2007). Multifactorial and functional mobility assessment tools for fall risk among older adults in community, home-support, long-term, and acute care settings. *Age and Ageing, 36,* 130–139.

Shumway-Cook, A., Brauer, S., & Woollacott, M. (2000). Predicting the probability for falls in community-dwelling older adults using the Timed Up & Go Test. *Physical Therapy, 80*(9), 896–930.

Tinetti, M. E. (1986). Performance-oriented assessment of mobility problems in elderly patients. *Journal of the American Geriatric Society, 34*(2), 119–126.

Tinetti, M. E., & Kumar C. (2010). The patient who falls: It's always a trade-off. *Journal of the American Medical Association, 303*(3), 258–266.

Tinetti, M. E., Speechley, M., & Ginter, S. F. (1988). Risk factors for falls among elderly persons living in the community. *New England Journal of Medicine, 319*(26), 1701–1707.

U.S. Department of Health and Human Services. (2014). *Healthy people 2020.* Retrieved from https://www.healthypeople.gov/

U.S. Food and Drug Administration & Hospital Bed Safety Work Group (Revised 2010). *A guide to bed safety bed rails in hospitals, nursing homes and home health care: The facts.* Retrieved from http://www.fda.gov/MedicalDevices/ProductsandMedicalProcedures/GeneralHospitalDevicesandSupplies/HospitalBeds/ucm123676.htm

World Health Organization. (2010). *A global report on falls prevention: Epidemiology of falls.* Retrieved from http://www.who.int/ageing/publications/Falls_prevention7March.pdf

van der Muelen, E., Ziistra, G. A., Ambergen, T., & Kempen, G. I. (2014). Effect of fall-related concerns on physical, mental and social function in community-dwelling older adults: A prospective Cohort Study. *Journal of the American Geriatric Society, 62*(12), 2333–2338.

Wood, W., Tschannen. D., Trotsky, A., Grunawalt, J., Adams, D., Chang, D., . . . Diccion-MacDonald, S. (2014). A mobility program for an inpatient acute care medical unit. *American Journal of Nursing, 114*(10), 34–40.

Zhao, Y. L., & Kim, H. (2015). Older adult inpatient falls in acute care hospitals: Intrinsic, extrinsic, and environmental factors. *Journal of Gerontological Nursing, 41*(7), 29–43.

Zwicker, D., & Fulmer, T. (2017). Reducing adverse drug events. In M. Boltz, E. Capezuti, T. Fulmer, & D. Zwicker (Eds.), *Evidence-based geriatric nursing protocols for best practice* (5th ed.). New York, NY: Springer.

For a full suite of assignments and additional learning activities, see the access code at the front of your book.

CHAPTER 13

Delirium

Susan Saboe Rose

LEARNING OBJECTIVES

At the end of this chapter, the reader will be able to:

> Define delirium.
> Explain common causes of delirium in older adults.
> Describe signs and symptoms of delirium.
> Distinguish between delirium and dementia.
> Discuss appropriate treatment of delirium in a variety of settings.

KEY TERMS

Agitation	Mixed form
Attention	Orientation
Combativeness	Precipitating factors
Delirium	Predisposing factors
Hyperactive form	Reasoning
Hypoactive form	Thought process and content
Language	Wandering
Memory	

Delirium is one of the most common psychiatric conditions in frail older adults, and the most common complication of hospitalization among people ages 65 and older. Derived from the Latin term meaning "off the track," delirium refers to a transient global cognitive disorder or group of symptoms associated with complex medical comorbidities. Unlike dementia, which refers to a progressive trajectory of cognitive and functional decline, delirium is characterized by an acute onset of confusion, inattention, disordered thinking, and altered mentation that occurs in response to a medical condition. It is not uncommon for individuals to become delirious with a severe illness, and experience a dream-like state, complete with hallucinations and perceptual disturbances. In the research by Whitehorne, Gaudine, Meadus, and Solberg (2015), patients with delirium reported colorful delirium-related phenomena, such as seeing frozen turkeys, car lights on the wall, large black birds, monkeys, and fairies. This chapter will focus on delirium risk factors, prevention, assessment, and treatment.

Delirium comes in three forms: hyperactive, hypoactive, and mixed. The variation in presentation can create problems with recognition of delirium and lead to a missed diagnosis. The *hyperactive form* of delirium is the most recognized form of delirium and often manifests with psychomotor agitation, confusion, and perceptual disturbances such as hallucinations or delusions. Manifestations of the hyperactive form of delirium could include agitation, such as pulling at tubes or catheters, restlessness, attempts to climb out of bed or elope, physical aggression, or combativeness.

The *hypoactive form* of delirium may mimic a stupor or coma and occurs more commonly than the hyperactive form. Hypoactive delirium has a higher mortality rate than the hyperactive form, due to the complications of immobility. Referred to as a "quiet" delirium (Forrest et al., 2007), patients with this form of delirium are often not evaluated as thoroughly as those with agitation or combativeness, because their behavioral symptoms are not as problematic. Symptoms of hypoactive delirium may include lethargy, inattention, or severe somnolence. The prevalence of perceptual disturbances or delusions affects roughly half of patients with hypoactive delirium (Boettger & Breitbart, 2011).

The *mixed form* of delirium is the most frequent subtype of delirium and presents with both hyperactive and hypoactive features. It is not uncommon for delirious individuals to have daytime somnolence accompanied by nocturnal agitation and insomnia. Alternatively, individuals may fluctuate between the hyperactive and hypoactive forms during the course of a few hours.

Although delirium may mimic dementia, delirium is a separate syndrome and differs from dementia in key areas. One of the most important differences between delirium and dementia has to do with the onset of symptoms. In delirium, the onset of confusion and disordered thinking occurs fairly abruptly, within a short period of time, such as a few hours, days, or weeks. In contrast, dementia typically begins with minor symptoms that gradually progress over time, such as months to years. The ability to maintain attention or stay focused is also different. In delirium, attention is significantly impaired, while individuals with dementia are generally able to remain alert until latter stages of the disease. Finally, delirium is characterized by fluctuation in mentation and thinking throughout the day. Whereas individuals with dementia can have "good and bad periods" during the day, their memory and thinking skills tend to stay at a fairly constant level. Characteristics that differentiate delirium from dementia are described in **Table 13-1**.

CLINICAL TIP

Delirium is potentially reversible when detected early.

TABLE 13-1   Differentiating Delirium from Dementia

Delirium	Dementia
• Acute confusional state	• Chronic confusional state
• Abrupt onset (hours to days)	• Gradual decline (months to years)
• Impaired attention and focus	• Attention fairly preserved
• Fluctuating mentation and cognition	• Mentation is generally constant
• Potentially reversible	• Irreversible

The most important distinction between delirium and dementia is the potentially reversible attribute of delirium. Unlike dementia, which is a chronic, progressive, and ultimately fatal trajectory, delirium is an abrupt onset of confusion with an optimistic rate of reversibility. With aggressive treatment of underlying causes, it is possible to return the individual to his or her pre-delirium baseline. That said, the nature of delirium accelerates the pace of cognitive decline; therefore, the longer the delirium persists, the less robustly the individual will recover. Persistent delirium syndromes can last for months (Jans, Oudewortel, Brandt, & van Gool, 2015) and are associated with very poor outcomes. In fact, the duration of delirium is one of the strongest risk factors for length of stay in the hospital, cost of care, long-term cognitive impairment, and death. As Ely et al. (2004) pointed out, few developments in the course of critical illness portend a grimmer prognosis than development of delirium that does not readily resolve.

Background

The mechanism of delirium is not fully understood. Numerous etiologies are involved, and efforts to clarify the complexities often result in oversimplified explanations. One of the most predominant hypotheses describes delirium as a reversible impairment of cerebral oxidative metabolism plus multiple neurotransmitter abnormalities. Numerous neurotransmitters have been linked to delirium, such as acetylcholine, dopamine, serotonin, gamma-aminobutyric acid (GABA), and melatonin (Alagiakrishnan & Blanchette, 2012; Faught, 2014).

Acetylcholine plays a key role in delirium, explaining why anticholinergic medications, such as antihistamines, can cause delirium even in healthy individuals. Delirium is theorized to decrease acetylcholine synthesis in the central nervous system (CNS), and serum anticholinergic activity correlates with the severity of delirium (Campbell et al., 2009; Faught, 2014). The role of acetylcholine also explains the difficulty differentiating delirium from dementia: Alzheimer's disease is characterized by a loss of cholinergic neurons, illuminating why delirious individuals may exhibit symptoms similar to those of individuals with dementia. For this reason, many individuals with delirium can be inaccurately diagnosed as having dementia, which then decreases the likelihood of receiving a thorough medical evaluation to elicit reversible factors. When delirium is superimposed on underlying dementia, the pace of underlying cognitive decline is accelerated, often leading to death (Jans et al., 2015).

Significance of the Problem

Delirium is a medical emergency associated with increased morbidity and mortality. A wide variety of prevalence rates are available in the literature, underscoring the difficulty recognizing delirium due to the fluctuating nature of the condition. The prevalence of delirium has been reported to be from 10% to as high as 80% (Peritogiannis, Bolosi, Lixouriotis, & Rizos, 2015; Smulter, Lingehall, Gustafson, Olofsson, & Engstrom, 2015). Delirium occurs across all settings, but the highest prevalence occurs among critically ill individuals requiring mechanical ventilation (Rivosecchi, Smithburger, Svec, Campbell, & Kane-Gill, 2015). Delirium is commonly superimposed on underlying dementia, compounding both its symptoms and severity. Fick, Agostini, and Inouye (2002) found that the prevalence of delirium superimposed on dementia ranged from 22% to 89% and was associated with increased mortality.

Delirium is an independent predictor of death in older medical patients, and vigilant attention to identification and treatment is vital. Mortality rates for delirium are very high (Jans et al., 2015), and there is a high rate of death in the months following discharge (Bellelli et al., 2014; Melkas et al., 2012). Mortality rates aside, delirium in elders is a predictor of long-term cognitive and functional decline and is associated with falls, use of physical restraints, prolonged hospital stays, increased complications, increased cost, and long-term disability (Decrane, Culp, & Wakefield, 2012; Fick et al., 2002).

Risk Factors

Delirium is rarely caused by a single factor; rather, it represents an intrinsically multifactorial syndrome (Inouye, 2006). Individuals who are highly vulnerable to delirium at baseline may develop delirium with any precipitating factor,

TABLE 13-2   Predisposing and Precipitating Risk Factors in Delirium

Predisposing Factors (Baseline Vulnerability)	Precipitating Factors (Triggers)
• Advanced cancer	• Absence of a clock or watch
• Alcoholism	• Absence of reading glasses or hearing aids
• Cognitive impairment	• Acute cardiac or pulmonary events
• Certain medications or polypharmacy	• Bed rest, immobility
• Chronic pain	• Drug withdrawal
• Dehydration	• Fecal impaction
• Fluid and electrolyte imbalances	• Fluid or electrolyte disturbances
• Hypoxia	• Increased number of room changes
• Impaired cardiac or respiratory function	• Indwelling devices, such as urinary catheters
• Infection; usually urinary tract or pneumonia	• Medications
• Malnutrition	• Nosocomial or hospital-acquired infections
• Medical comorbidities	• Restraints
• Metabolic disturbances, electrolyte imbalance	• Severe anemia
• Sensory impairment, vision or hearing loss	• Sleep deprivation
• Unfamiliar surroundings	• Uncontrolled pain
	• Urinary retention

whereas patients with low vulnerability could be resistant to development of delirium, even with noxious insults. Risk factors of delirium are best understood as predisposing and precipitating factors, as illustrated in **Table 13-2**.

Predisposing factors are baseline vulnerabilities that are possessed by the patient prior to hospitalization. Predisposing factors include brain diseases or cognitive impairments such as dementia or stroke, sensory impairment such as vision or hearing loss, functional impairment, medical comorbidities, or history of alcohol abuse. Age is also a predisposing factor, as elderly patients are at the highest risk of delirium. Additional predisposing factors include infection, metabolic disturbances, dehydration, immobility, or malnutrition.

Precipitating factors are events or conditions that occur during hospitalization to trigger a delirium. Precipitating factors include acute cardiac or pulmonary events, bed rest, drug withdrawal, fecal impaction, fluid or electrolyte disturbances, and indwelling devices such as urinary catheters. Additional precipitating factors include infections, medications, restraints, severe anemia, uncontrolled pain, and urinary retention. An increased number of room changes, absence of a clock or watch, absence of reading glasses or hearing aids, and sleep deprivation also can precipitate delirium.

Certain medications can contribute to delirium in older adults, and are referred to as "deliriogenic." Anticholinergic medications (see **Table 13-3**), such as antihistamines, are particularly deliriogenic and well-known causes of acute and chronic confusional states. Anticholinergic effects on the peripheral nervous system include urinary retention and constipation, both of which are directly linked to delirium. Adding insult to injury, urinary retention and constipation are also linked to urinary tract infections (UTIs), which further increases risk of delirium, cumulating in a "vicious cycle" of treatment and side effects (Tune, 2001).

Updated frequently, the "Beers list" refers to a list of potentially inappropriate medications to avoid or use with caution in older adults, as they can exacerbate certain conditions and diseases. Originally developed and published by Beers and colleagues in 1991 (Beers et al., 1991), the list was subsequently revised in 1997, 2003, 2012, and 2015 (American Geriatrics Society, 2015). The Beers list is available from the American Geriatrics Society and can be downloaded at http://www.americangeriatrics.org.

TABLE 13-3   Common Anticholinergic Medications (with Examples) That Can Cause or Worsen Confusion

Analgesics: Propoxyphene, meperidine, excess doses of opiates
Antiemetics: Promethazine
Antihistamines: Diphenhydramine, chlorpheniramine, promethazine
Antihypertensives: Clonidine, beta-blockers
Antipruritics: Hydroxyzine
Anticonvulsants: Phenobarbital, carbamazepine
Antivertigo: Meclizine, scopolamine
Anxiolytics: Meprobamate or paroxetine
Benzodiazepines: Alprazolam, diazepam, lorazepam
Bladder relaxants: Oxybutynin propantheline, solifenacin, tolterodine
Gastrointestinal antispasmotics: Dicyclomine, hyoscyamine
Histamine-2 antagonists: Cimetidine, ranitidine
Muscle relaxants: Cyclobenzaprine, baclofen
Sedatives-hypnotics: Chloral hydrate
Tricyclic antidepressants: Amitriptyline, desipramine

Warning Signs

Agitation is a common delirium prodromal feature and a common warning sign of impending delirium. Prodromal symptoms often occur 1 to 3 days prior to the development of delirium and include restlessness, anxiety, irritability, distractibility, and disruption of sleep that may progress to daytime somnolence and nighttime wakefulness.

Behavior changes during the prodromal stage of delirium are common and can include anxiety, disorientation, and urgent calls for attention prior to the onset of delirium. De Jonghe et al. (2007) studied prodromal delirium symptoms in elderly patients and found that early symptoms of memory impairment, incoherence, disorientation, and underlying somatic illness predicted delirium.

Any sudden change in cognition or increase in agitation should be investigated. A person of any age, when acutely ill, may experience delirium; however, older adults with preexisting dementia are at highest risk of developing delirium when acutely ill or injured.

Assessment

Assessment of the frail elderly patient is complicated, particularly when advanced age is combined with comorbid conditions. In young and middle-aged adults, symptoms of fever or abnormal laboratory values are common indicators of illness. In older adults, however, geriatric syndromes such as confusion, weakness, lethargy, falls, and urinary incontinence are more common manifestations of illness. In fact, it is not uncommon for an older adult with a UTI to present with altered mental status as the sole symptom and with an absence of fever or any change in blood chemistry.

Arguably, the single most important factor in assessment is knowledge of the patient's baseline level of physical and cognitive functioning. The establishment of a baseline against which to compare assessment data is critical. If the patient is too confused to respond, data should be elicited from the patient's family or caregivers. All components of the patient's prior level of function, including basic activities of daily living (ADLs) such as bathing, dressing, toileting, and ambulation should be compared to those of current levels of functioning. The patient's baseline functional status for instrumental ADLs, such as food preparation, management of medications, house-keeping, bill-paying, and transportation, also should be queried.

Mental Status Examination

Nursing assessment is a key factor in recognition of delirium. The nature of delirium involves fluctuation of altered levels of consciousness throughout the day, so nurses are in the best position to observe this fluctuation over the course of a shift. The mental status examination is the most crucial portion of the nursing assessment, as a thorough evaluation of cognition is required to determine whether the patient meets the criteria for delirium. Assessment of mental status generally includes evaluation of basic domains of cognitive functioning: attention, orientation, language, memory, and reasoning, as well as *thought process and content*. A brief format for assessing domains of cognitive functioning in delirium is described in **Exhibit 13-1**.

Attention refers to the ability to disengage, reengage, and sustain focus and vigilance. This can be tested with exercises such as reverse weekdays, reverse month order, or subtraction. Attention is almost always impaired in delirium and provides a good benchmark for determination of improvement or decline.

Orientation is a function of memory and involves awareness of the dimensions of person, place, and time. This can be tested by asking the patient to state the name of the hospital, current age, or other indicators such as date, month, year, or approximate time of day. Orientation to person is rarely impaired, and even the most delirious individuals should be able to recall their name. Disorientation to place and time, however, are very common in delirium.

Language refers to the capacity for acquiring and using systems of communication. Comprehension can be assessed by asking questions to determine understanding. Comprehension is frequently impaired in delirium. In fact, the nature of delirium is characterized by fluctuating levels of cognition, so comprehension is likely to fluctuate accordingly. This is important to remember as the patient will have periods of lucidity that will alternate with periods of confusion and inattention. Patient teaching will need to be maximized during periods of lucidity.

Memory includes primary, secondary, and tertiary memory. Primary, or working, memory refers to the ability to register information. This can be tested by giving a patient several words or a phrase to remember. Secondary memory refers to the ability to recall that information and can be tested by asking the patient to recall the words or phrase after a few minutes. Tertiary or remote memory refers to recall of public events throughout history, or facts learned long ago. This can be tested by asking the patient about salient events that occurred during their lifetime, such as the death of President Kennedy. Primary, secondary, and tertiary memory are all likely to be impaired in delirium.

Reasoning refers to abstract concept formation and executive functioning. One of the most common ways to assess reasoning and executive functioning is with the clock drawing test (CDT). The following instructions are given: "Draw the face of a clock, place numbers on the clock, and put the hands at 10 minutes past 11 o'clock." The CDT assesses planning (circle size), organizing (placement of numbers), sequencing (inclusion of all numbers in the correct order), and abstraction (hand placement and length). Reasoning is frequently impaired and may fluctuate in accordance with the waxing and waning of mentation that is characteristic of a delirium.

The CDT is one of the most commonly used determinants of improvement or decline in delirium. As portrayed in **Figure 13-1**, the CDT provides a stark visual illustration of the disorganized cognition that accompanies delirium. This particular CDT also provides an example of the potential for cognitive improvement with aggressive treatment of delirium.

Confusion Assessment Method

Scales help us understand the level of symptomology of our patients, aid diagnosis, and help gauge treatment efficacy (Nash & Rose, 2012). The nurse plays a critical role in identifying whether an older adult has experienced an acute change in mental status that could be delirium.

Components	Characteristics	How to Assess	Changes in Delirium
Attention	Sustained focus Vigilance	"I'd like you to start at December, and say the months backwards."	Acute decline and impairment in attention
Orientation	Awareness of person, place, and time	"How old are you? What is the name of this building? What is today's date? What day of the week is this? About what time is it?"	Disorientation to time is a common finding. Disorientation to place may also occur.
Language	Object recognition and naming Verbal fluency Comprehension	Show the patient an object, such as a watch, and then less common parts of the watch. "What do you call this? And what do you call this part of the watch?" (Wristband, clasp or buckle, face or dial, stem or winder). "I'm going to give you one minute, and I'd like you to name as many of the United States as you can. Ck? Start."	Naming may be impaired. Verbal fluency may be diminished. Comprehension will fluctuate.
Memory	Registration and recall of recently presented information, remote memory for historical events	"I'm going to give you three words to remember. Say these words: Apple, penny, green. Say them again. Now I am going to distract you, and will ask you those words in a few minutes." "A few minutes ago, you memorized three words. What were they?" "Now I'm going to test your memory for things in the past. Do you remember when President Kennedy died? How did he die? Where did that happen? Who took his place as president?"	Registration and recall are likely to be grossly impaired in delirium. Recognition from a list may also be impaired. Remote memory is likely to be impaired in delirium.
Reasoning	Abstract concept formation, complex problem-solving	"Have you ever heard the phrase, 'People that live in glass houses shouldn't throw stones'? What does that mean?" "What would you do if you saw a small child in the middle of the road?" "I'd like you to draw the face of a clock, and place the hands at 10 minutes past 11:00."	Reasoning is likely to fluctuate, in accordance with waxing/waning of delirium.
Thought Process	Quality and coherence of thought	"Do you feel like your thoughts are jumbled, or moving at a different speed than normal?"	Thought process is disordered in delirium. Racing thoughts are common in hyperactive delirium, and cognitive slowing is common in hypoactive delirium.
Thought Content	Subject matter of thought	"Do you ever feel like your mind is playing tricks on you?" "Do you find that you've been having odd thoughts recently?" "Have you been having any unusual sensations or visions that just started in the past few days?"	Visual and tactile hallucinations are common in delirium. Auditory hallucinations are less common, and gustatory hallucinations are uncommon. Delusions are very common.

Exhibit 13-1 Brief Mental Status Examination for Delirium (Rose, 2010).

Reproduced from Rose. S. S. (2010). What's in your bag of tricks? Managing behavioral challenges in delirium and dementia. *Proceedings of the 11th Annual Oregon Geriatrics Society Conference*. Oregon Health & Sciences University: Portland, OR.

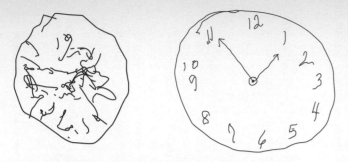

Figure 13-1 CDT during and after an episode of delirium.
Reproduced from Newton, P.A., Kuebrich, M. B., & Rose, S. S. (2012). Acute care of the elderly inpatient service. *Portland Area Geriatric Seminar Series: Excellence in Care, Research, and Education.* Portland, OR.

Inouye et al. (1990) developed the Confusion Assessment Method (CAM) to assist nurses and others to identify delirium quickly and accurately using the four basic features of delirium: (1) acute onset or fluctuating course, (2) inattention, (3) disorganized thinking, and (4) altered level of consciousness. A diagnosis of delirium is made if both features 1 and 2 are present, along with either features 3 or 4. The CAM is commonly used by both nursing and medical staff and considered by many to be the gold standard for recognition of delirium. CAM criteria is listed in **Table 13-4**.

Diagnosis

Any acute episode of confusion warrants a clinical evaluation. Once the determination of delirium has been obtained, the assessment shifts to a focus on investigating possible causes of delirium.

Nursing diagnostics include monitoring of vital signs. Oxygen saturation is important as hypoxia or carbon dioxide retention can contribute to delirium. Bladder scans are also important, as urinary retention is both a predictor and an outcome of delirium.

Nursing assessment skills are particularly needed to monitor for signs of infection. The two most common sources of infection in older adults are UTIs and pneumonia. Assess for symptoms of UTI, such as a new onset of urinary incontinence, urinary retention, foul or odorous urine, frequency, or dysuria. Monitor for symptoms of pneumonia by auscultating lung sounds and notifying the medical staff of aberrancies (Rosen et al, 2015).

Undertreated pain is a common contributor to delirium. Pain is particularly difficult to assess in older adults who also have cognitive impairment. Frequent vocalizations and repeated phrases such as "Help me, help me" are commonly associated with pain. Resistance to care, rubbing a particular body part, or combativeness when being bathed also can serve as indicators of pain.

Standard "delirium labs" include a complete blood count (CBC), comprehensive metabolic panel, and urinalysis. Additional laboratory tests generally include a vitamin B_{12} level; folate, magnesium, and phosphate levels; toxicology; and blood glucose levels to search for potential contributors to delirium. If indicated, a rapid plasma reagin (RPR) is included.

Delirium is a medical emergency, and neuroimaging is generally indicated. Computed Tomography (CT) of the head will help determine the presence of a stroke or if trauma related to a recent fall is suspected. Abdominal series are frequently performed to rule out medical culprits, such as constipation. Chest X-ray is indicated if there is a suspicion of pneumonia. An electrocardiogram (ECG) is important, especially if the patient requires treatment with neuroleptic medications, as they can contribute to cardiac arrhythmias.

TABLE 13-4   Confusion Assessment Method Criteria
1. Acute onset and fluctuating course
2. Inattention
3. Disorganized thinking
4. Altered level of consciousness
Diagnosis by CAM requires 1 and 2 and either 3 or 4.

Data from Inouye, S. K., van Dyck, C. H., Alessi, C. A., Balkin, S., Siegal, A. P., & Horwitz, R. I. (1990). Clarifying confusion: The confusion assessment method. *Annals of Internal Medicine, 113*(12), 941–948.

Other consultations include speech pathology for swallowing evaluations to assess risk of aspiration, as it relates to fluctuating mentation and levels of consciousness. Aspiration precautions are particularly important in the hypoactive or mixed forms of delirium. Medication review by a clinical pharmacist is commonly requested, as polypharmacy can contribute to delirium. Particular attention should be paid to medications that have recently been started or increased.

"I WATCH DEATH" is a commonly used mnemonic to evaluate for the presence of contributing factors for delirium (Wise, 1986). The reference to death in the mnemonic is a sobering reminder of the high mortality risks of delirium and the need for timely diagnosis and intervention.

Nursing assessment is a key factor and frontline concept, for both identification and reduction of delirium risk factors. Salient nursing diagnoses are included under the cognitive-Perceptual functional health pattern (Carpenito-Moyet, 2008) and may include confusion, disturbed sensory perception, impaired thought processes, and impaired comfort. Other common nursing diagnoses in the setting of delirium include constipation, urinary retention, anxiety, risk of aspiration, and risk for injury (Gordon, 1982).

Given the emergent nature of delirium, early identification of nursing diagnoses is important. It is necessary to be proactive and notify appropriate medical staff of any concerns about potential risks factors, immediately implement a plan of care, and continue close supervision.

Interventions

Just as delirium has a multifactorial etiology, the treatment of delirium is best accomplished with a multimodal approach. Attention to precipitating factors is vital, particularly in regard to avoiding the perils of immobility, promoting sleep and comfort, avoiding unnecessary tubes and catheters, and providing frequent cognitive stimulation and reorientation. Delirium treatment protocols that include mobilization, noise reduction, or sleep protocols are associated with reduction in delirium (Rivosecchi et al., 2015).

Treatment requires an almost obsessional attention to the patient. The nature of delirium is one of waxing and waning, and vigilance is required to recognize the overall pattern of delirium. Some fluctuations may be subtle, whereas others may have more of a circadian pattern, with nocturnal agitation. As a general rule, suspect that a delirium may be at play when your cognitive assessment differs from that performed by a nurse colleague at a different time of day.

One of the primary goals of treatment is management of delirium-related behaviors so that treatment of the underlying condition can be achieved. Behavioral and psychological symptoms occur in 90% of patients with cognitive impairment. Behavioral disorders in delirium tend to be more severe than those seen in dementia, but of shorter duration. The remainder of this chapter will focus on nursing interventions for specific behavioral challenges.

Pain

Management of pain is crucial, as undertreated pain is a precipitating factor for delirium (Schreier, 2010). Although postoperative pain may be a more recognizable condition, pain can occur from a variety of sources. Fundamentally, one of the most common sources of pain in hospitalized older adults is musculoskeletal pain related to immobility. Complicating things further, many clinicians incorrectly assume opioids are the cause of delirium in patients with pain, leading to a reduction in dosage or discontinuation of pain medications altogether. In fact, undertreated pain may be a stronger risk factor for delirium than pain medications (Robinson & Vollmer, 2012). Pain management regimens that involve scheduled analgesia are associated with lower incidence of delirium.

Agitation

One of the most common precipitants of delirium-related agitation is excess stimulation. The hospital environment is filled with extraneous noises, such as alarms, telephones, and pagers, that emit hundreds, if not thousands, of audible sounds each day. The cumulative effect of the overabundance of auditory and visual stimulation can be overwhelming to the individual with delirium. Delirium can be thought of as a "conceptual fog" in which every fragment of visual, auditory, tactile, and gustatory stimulation must be processed and interpreted by a fragile, delirious brain. Now think of the average hospital room, with all of the various sounds, shapes, colors, and smells. One of the best ways to reduce agitation is simply to remove excess stimulation. Eliminating extraneous noises, such as overhead paging; removing clutter from the patient's line of sight; removing excess equipment; turning off the television; and trying to limit as much stimulation as possible can go a long way toward reducing delirium-related agitation. Nicknamed "Feng Shui for the Frontal Lobe" (Rose, 2010), basic nursing interventions to reduce stimulation can significantly reduce agitation in individuals with cognitive impairment. Given that some forms of delirium may have a mortality rate of up to 76%, these basic nursing interventions can literally be lifesaving.

One of the best strategies for agitated and restless individuals is to help them out of bed and assist them with ambulation to burn off pent-up energy. Scheduled ambulation can go a long way toward reducing agitation, and the benefits of ambulation on sleep and well-being are well known. Mobilization can be as complex as full physical or occupational therapy treatments or as simple as passive range-of-motion exercises (Rivosecchi et al., 2015).

One common behavioral challenge is preventing delirious individuals from pulling out tubes and lines, which pose a safety issue. Camouflaging medical equipment can help discourage delirious patients from pulling out tubes. Consider double-gowning a patient with a telemetry box between layers to discourage removal. Abdominal binders are useful for discouraging self-removal of surgical tubes, and long pants are useful to help protect urinary catheters.

Combativeness

Whitehorne et al. (2015) underscore the fear that arises when the delirious individual is hallucinating and gives the example of a patient being a World War II veteran who thought the intensive care unit nurses were soldiers who were going to harm him.

One of the strongest predictors of *combativeness* in cognitively impaired elders is constipation (Leonard, Tinetti, Allore, & Drickamer, 2006). Delirious patients are particularly at risk of dehydration, as they may be confused and pull out intravenous tubes or may harbor delusions about food and drink. Patients with delirium are also prone to immobility, as they are less likely to ambulate independently. Prevention and treatment of constipation can go a long way toward reducing agitation and aggression.

CLINICAL TIP

When seeing combativeness in cognitively impaired older adults, check for constipation as a trigger.

It is important to monitor bowel status and aim for a daily bowel movement in the delirious patient. Provide stimulus to defecation, such as coffee or prune juice. Assist the patient to the bathroom to allow for suitable positioning instead of using a bedpan. Check for bowel impaction if no bowel movement is noted within 48 hours in the delirious patient.

Urinary retention is also a contributor to combativeness. Urinary retention is both a predictor and an outcome of delirium; it is also a precipitating factor that may trigger delirium due to a catecholamine surge from increased bladder-wall tension. At the same time, the role of acetylcholine in delirium increases the risk of urinary retention. This vicious cycle results in retention as both a risk factor for delirium and a common outcome of delirium. Although it may be tempting to try to avoid performing a bladder scan on a combative patient, vigorous monitoring for urinary retention is important—for both early detection of delirium and prevention of further delirium-related aggression. Additionally, a scheduled protocol of bladder scan and intermittent straight catheterization is preferable to the use of an indwelling urinary catheter.

Avoiding fatigue and sleep deprivation also can significantly reduce combativeness. Prevention is vital; it is important to avoid overstimulation, hunger, thirst, and frustration. Cluster activities at night to allow for maximum hours of sleep at night. Allow adequate rest periods during the day, and provide a calm and quiet environment when the delirious individual begins to show symptoms of aggression. A small snack can go a long way toward redirecting frustration and providing a calming distraction.

Inattentiveness

Inattentiveness is a key component of delirium and one of the defining characteristics; it may range from grossly disordered thinking to mildly disorganized thought processes. Inattentive behaviors may pose safety risks to delirious patients. For example, they may not remember to ask for help before getting out of bed or may not recognize that they are tethered to a cardiac monitor or oxygen regulator. They may have difficulty remembering patient instructions, such as how to use a call light. Frequent observation is necessary.

Nursing interventions to help with inattentiveness are geared toward increasing sustained focus. Giving a delirious patient some simple arithmetic problems to work on helps with sustained attention and focus and also provides cognitive stimulation. Sorting cards or folding laundry is a good activity for individuals with inattention, as it helps with sustaining focus over time. Family members can assist in this process; for example, ask the family of a delirious patient to bring in familiar photographs of family members and help the patient to organize the photos into family groups.

Wandering and Exit-Seeking

Wandering is a common symptom in individuals with cognitive impairment, including delirium. It is not uncommon for delirious patients to misjudge their level of wellness, think they are ready for discharge, and decide to try to leave the hospital setting while they are still fairly confused and disoriented.

There are numerous causes for wandering, including distorted memories of once-familiar surroundings or difficulty adapting to new surroundings. Delirium-related mental changes and disorientation can cause worsening of perceptual distortions that can prompt wandering and exit-seeking. Wandering that occurs at the same time every day may be linked to a lifelong routine, such as going to work. It is not uncommon for patients to become restless in the late afternoon, or try to elope at the change of shift as they see individuals leaving the unit.

Looking for a restroom is a common impetus for wandering in delirious individuals. Frequent toileting is a good way to prevent wandering, as is the use of signs and arrows to identify restrooms.

Sleep

Disruption of the sleep–wake cycle is common in delirium, as is nocturnal agitation. Even in the absence of delirium, sleep in older adults is problematic. In the seventh and eighth decades of life, the circadian rhythms tend to flatten and often lose the ability to maintain a functional sleep–wake cycle. In the presence of a delirium, sleep patterns become more fragmented and unpredictable. Sleep deprivation is common with the hyperactive form of delirium, and excessive somnolence is characteristic of the hypoactive form. The tenuous relationship

TABLE 13-5   When It's 3 AM . . . .

- Help the patient out of bed and assist with ambulation as needed to burn off excess energy
- Assist the patient to the bathroom
- Reduce as much stimulation as possible
- Turn off the television, turn off lights, provide a warm blanket, partially close door, and talk in a low monotone voice

between sleep and cognition affects the integrity of the circadian system, which results in degrading of sleep architecture and disrupted circadian rhythms.

Sleep hygiene is very important in delirium. Maximizing sunlight, especially during early morning, helps regulate sleep–wake cycles. Getting out of bed for all meals helps promote orientation and provides cognitive stimulation. Darkening the room and drawing the shades at night helps promote restfulness. Applying a warm blanket at bedtime helps promote comfort and sleep (see **Table 13-5**).

When a "Sitter" Is the Wrong Approach

One of the most common symptoms in delirium is psychosis, such as hallucinations or delusions. When delirium takes the form of paranoia and suspiciousness, direct supervision may become challenging. The nurse must balance the needs of patient observation with provision of stimulus for delusions. For the patient with severe paranoia, the presence of an unfamiliar observer can cause worsening of psychosis. Family members or familiar friends of the patient should be enlisted if the patient requires a constant companion.

Close supervision may be appropriate to prevent injury in the patient with acute agitation, alleviate fear, or provide comfort. Many hospitals and care facilities have trained individuals to provide one-to-one supervision, commonly referred to as "sitters." For the patient with delirium, it is imperative that use of a "sitter" supports the patient's plan of care, rather than be used solely to observe. In a syndrome with a mortality rate that may be as high as 80%, stringent vigilance to the plan of care is essential. Rather than "sitting," the one-to-one companion has an important role of assisting with hydration, monitoring for aspiration, providing cognitive stimulation during daytime hours and ensuring decreased stimulation at bedtime, providing frequent toileting, assisting with ambulation, and providing distraction and protection to avoid self-removal of tubes and devices.

CLINICAL TIP

Think about it: If you were suffering from paranoia, would you want a stranger staring at you for 24 hours a day?

Safety Concerns

Individuals with delirium are at higher risk of injury. Reduce the risk of burns secondary to patients with delirium handling hot liquids by opening containers of hot liquids and allowing them to cool before offering them to a delirious individual.

The nature of delirium is one of fluctuating levels of mentation. Individuals with the hypoactive form of delirium are at higher risk of aspiration because of decreased levels of consciousness. Maintain aspiration precautions and consider a mechanical soft diet until the delirium improves.

Delirious individuals are at high risk for falling. The human cost of a fall is immeasurable and life changing. Each year, at least 250,000 persons over age 65 have a hip fracture related to a fall and 2.5 million Americans are treated at the hospital for fall-related injuries, with a total healthcare cost of over $34 billion dollars for falls (Centers for Disease Control and Prevention [CDC], 2016).

Place the bed in the lowest position and employ a bed alarm for restless patients. The use of physical restraints as a fall-prevention device is inappropriate, as they are associated with increased agitation and panic in confused individuals and can result in serious injury or death.

Falls among delirious patients are commonly related to toileting. It is important to provide scheduled toileting to reduce the risk of agitation and urinary retention. It is also important to provide direct supervision of delirious individuals while they are in the restroom or on a bedside commode. Privacy during toileting must be modified sufficiently to ensure a quick response to avoid a potential fall or injury (see **Box 13-1**).

Home Management after Discharge

It is not unusual for delirium to take weeks to entirely resolve. Most patients are discharged from the acute care setting before the delirium has entirely resolved. During this period, the patient's mental status will continue to wax and wane. In general, rehabilitation in a skilled nursing facility is beneficial during the recovery period.

For patients discharged directly to the community, it is important that the patient and family know that the delirious individual needs 24-hour supervision until the delirium has completely resolved. Periods of inattention, disorganized thinking, and confusion may continue for several weeks. The patient recovering from delirium will need oversight of instrumental daily activities, including management of medications. They should refrain from driving until they have recovered. Family members may need to help the patient make complex or abstract decisions and help provide substituted judgment until the delirium fully clears.

Prognosis

The nature of delirium is one of potentially long-term waxing and waning of cognition. Eventually, the periods of lucidity will become longer, and the periods of confusion will become less frequent and less severe. A consistent baseline will emerge.

Delirium accelerates the pace of underlying cognitive decline. It is not unusual for an individual with mild cognitive impairment to manage fairly well in a familiar environment, but have more pronounced impairment after an episode of delirium. An underlying dementia may "declare itself" with persistent cognitive deficits that do not remit. Outpatient cognitive evaluation should be performed a few months after the delirium has resolved to evaluate for an underlying dementia.

Delirium distorts the person's sense of bodily and relational experiences. It is not uncommon to not remember an episode of delirium, and some individuals develop feelings of guilt and shame when told how they behaved during an episode of delirium. Further, patients reported feeling hurt when family members joked about the patient's behaviors while delirious (Whitehorne et al., 2015).

Although delirium is viewed as a temporary and reversible condition, many patients never return to their previous baseline. The longer the delirium persists, the poorer the outcomes, particularly when the delirium is superimposed on underlying dementia. Nursing assessment (see **Box 13-2**) and intervention are crucial (see **Case Study 13-1**).

BOX 13-2   Evidence-Based Practice Highlight

Go to https://consultgeri.org/geriatric-topics/delirium and review the resources available for assessing and treating delirium. A standard of practice guideline (Tullman, Fletcher, & Foreman, 2012), tools, and videos are available at this Website.

Case Study 13-1

Mr. Smith is a 79-year-old patient in the long-term acute care unit where you work. It is 3 o'clock in the morning, and Mr. Smith just pulled out his intravenous (IV) line. Investigating the reason for Mr. Smith's action is vital to determine the appropriate treatment.

Question: Why did he pull out the IV?	Strategy
Because he is restless?	Ambulate around the nursing station to burn off energy.
Because he is impulsive?	Try diversion, an activity vest, or meaningful activity.
Because he had to go to the bathroom?	Provide toileting every 2 hours, check for urinary retention.
Because he thought it was a worm or snake?	He may benefit from a low-dose antipsychotic for psychosis.

Summary

Delirium is a common problem among older adults, especially the frail and compromised elderly. Nursing care for the individual with delirium is aimed at discovering the underlying cause and treating it (see **Box 13-3**). Causes of delirium may be simple, such as a UTI, or complex and multifaceted. Although most delirium is considered an acute geriatric syndrome, untreated delirium can have harmful effects on the person's health and quality of life.

BOX 13-3   Research Highlight

With the understanding that delirium is often experienced by patients in intensive care, Whitehorne, Gaudine, Meadus, and Solberg sought to learn about delirium using interviews of ICU patients that reported living through the experience. Sign into your database of nursing literature (CINAHL or PubMed, for example) and use the citation below to perform a search for this article. On the basis of results of this study, what do we know about delirium and the impact it can have on a patient? What can a nurse do to recognize and assist patients experiencing delirium?

Whitehorne, K., Gaudine, A., Meadus, R., & Solberg, S. (2015). Lived experience of the intensive care unit for patients who experienced delirium. *American Journal of Critical Care, 24*(6), 474–479.

Clinical Reasoning Exercises

1. If an older adult in your care presents with sudden onset of confusion, how does this influence your assessment? What risk factors and warning signs for delirium will you look for?

2. Identify a patient that you are caring for, or have cared for in the past, who could be at risk for delirium. List the risk factors for this patient or resident and think about what interventions could be implemented to prevent delirium.

3. Go to http://www.consultgerirn.com and find the clinical guideline on delirium. Read through it, noting especially the statistics on delirium in older adults and the current standard of care.

Personal Reflections

1. Have you ever cared for a patient who had delirium? If so, did you recognize it at the time? Was it a hyperactive, hypoactive, or mixed form? How was it treated?

2. What behaviors associated with delirium do you see as most problematic? Which are the most difficult for you personally to handle in patients or residents?

3. How can you personally apply this information on delirium to your own clinical practice? Of what will you be more aware after studying the content of this chapter?

References

Alagiakrishnan, K., & Blanchette, P. (2012). Delirium. Medscape reference. Retrieved from http://www.emedicine.medscape.com

American Geriatrics Society, Beers Criteria Update Expert Panel. (2015). AGS updated Beers criteria for potentially inappropriate medication use in older adults. *Journal of the American Geriatric Society, 63*(4), 2227–2246.

Beers, M. H., Ouslander J. G., Rollingher I., Reuben, D. B., Brooks, J., & Beck, J. C. (1991). Explicit criteria for determining inappropriate medication use in nursing home residents. *Archives of Internal Medicine, 151,* 1825–1832.

Bellelli, G., Mazzola, P., Morandi, A., Bruni, A., Carnevali, L., Corsi, M., . . . Annoni, G. (2014). Duration of postoperative delirium is an independent predictor of 6-month mortality in older adults after hip fracture. *Journal of the American Geriatrics Society, 62*(7), 1335–1340.

Boettger, S., & Breitbart, W. (2011). Phenomenology of the subtypes of delirium: Phenomenological differences between hyperactive and hypoactive delirium. *Palliative and Supportive Care, 9*(2), 129–135.

Campbell, N., Boustani, M., Limbil, T., Ott, C., Fox, C., Maidment, I., . . . Gulati, R. (2009). The cognitive impact of anticholinergics: A clinical review. *Journal of Clinical Interventions in Aging, 4,* 225–233.

Carpenito-Moyet, L. J. (2008). *Nursing diagnosis: Application to clinical practice* (12th ed.). Philadelphia, PA: Lippincott Williams & Wilkins.

Centers for Disease Control and Prevention. (2016). Important facts about falls. Retrieved from http://www.cdc.gov/homeandrecreationalsafety/falls/adultfalls.html

Decrane, S. K., Culp, K. R., & Wakefield, B. (2012). Twelve-month fall outcomes among delirium subtypes. *Journal of Healthcare Quality, 34*(6), 13–20.

De Jonghe, J. F., Kalisvaart, K. J., Dijkstra, M., van Dis, H., Vreeswijk, R., Kat, M. G., . . . van Gool, W. A. (2007). Early symptoms in the prodromal phase of delirium: a prospective cohort study in elderly patients undergoing hip surgery. *American Journal of Geriatric Psychiatry, 15*(2), 112–121.

Ely, E. W., Shintani, A., Truman, B., Speroff, T., Gordon, S. M., Harrell F. E. Jr., . . . Dittus, R. S. (2004). Delirium as a predictor of mortality in mechanically ventilated patients in the intensive care unit. *Journal of the American Medical Association, 291*(14), 1753–1762.

Faught, D. D. (2014). Delirium: The nurse's role in prevention, diagnosis, and treatment. *MedSurg Nursing, 23*(5), 301–305

Fick, D. M., Agostini, J. V., & Inouye, S. K. (2002). Delirium superimposed on dementia: A systematic review. *Journal of the American Geriatrics Society, 50*(10), 1723–1732.

Forrest, J., Willis, L., Holm, K., Kwon, M., Anderson, M., & Foreman, M. (2007). Reducing risk: Recognizing quiet delirium—not all cases of delirium are of the familiar hyperalert-hyperactive subtype. *American Journal of Nursing, 107*(4), 35–39.

Gordon, M. (1982). *Nursing diagnosis: Process and application.* New York, NY: McGraw-Hill.

Inouye, S. K. (2006). Delirium in older persons. *New England Journal of Medicine, 354,* 1157–1165.

Inouye, S. K., van Dyck, C. H., Alessi, C. A., Balkin, S., Siegal, A. P., & Horwitz, R. I. (1990). Clarifying confusion: The confusion assessment method. *Annals of Internal Medicine, 113*(12), 941–948.

Jans, I. S., Oudewortel, L., Brandt, P. M., & van Gool, W. A. (2015). Severe, persistent and fatal delirium in psychogeriatric patients admitted to a psychiatric hospital. *Dementia and Cognitive Disorders Extra, 5,* 253–264.

Leonard, R., Tinetti, M. E., Allore, H. G., & Drickamer, M. A. (2006). Potentially modifiable resident characteristics that are associated with physical or verbal aggression among nursing home residents with dementia. *Archives of Internal Medicine, 166*(12), 1295–1300.

Melkas, S., Laurila, J. V., Vataja, R., Oksala, N., Jokinen, H., Pohjasvaara, T., . . . Erkinjuntti, T. (2012). Post-stroke delirium in relation to dementia and long-term mortality. *International Journal of Geriatric Psychiatry, 27,* 401–408.

Nash, M. C., & Rose, S. S. (2012). Using scales and measurement to improve quality in your geriatric practice. *Proceedings from the American Association for Geriatric Psychiatry 2012 Annual Meeting.*

Newton, P. A., Kuebrich, M. B., & Rose, S. S. (2012, January). Acute care of the elderly inpatient service. *Portland Area Geriatric Seminar Series: Excellence in Care, Research, and Education.* Portland, OR.

Peritogiannis, V., Bolosi, M., Lixouriotis, C., & Rizos, D. V. (2015). Recent insights on prevalence and correlations of hypoactive delirium. *Behavioural Neurology, 2015,* 416792. doi:10.1155/2015/416792

Rivosecchi, R. M., Smithburger, P. L., Svec, S., Campbell, S., & Kane-Gill, S. L. (2015). Nonpharmacological interventions to prevent delirium: An evidence-based systematic review. *Critical Care Nurse, 35*(1), 39–51.

Robinson, S., & Vollmer, C. (2012). Undermedication for pain and precipitation of delirium. *MEDSURG Nursing 19*(2), 70–83.

Rose, S. S. (2010). What's in your bag of tricks? Managing behavioral challenges in delirium and dementia. *Proceedings of the 11th Annual Oregon Geriatrics Society Conference.* Oregon Health & Sciences University: Portland, OR.

Rosen, T., Connors, S., Clark, S., Halpern, A., Stern, M. E., DeWald, J. L., . . . Flomenbaum, N. (2015). Assessment and management of delirium in older adults in the emergency department. *Advanced Emergency Nursing Journal, 37*(3), 183–196.

Schreier A. M. (2010). Nursing care, delirium, and pain management for the hospitalized older adult. *Pain Management Nursing, 11*(3), 177–185.

Smulter, N., Lingehall, H. C., Gustafson, Y., Olofsson, B., & Engstrom, K. G. (2015). Validation of the confusion assessment method in detecting postoperative delirium in cardiac surgery patients. *American Journal of Critical Care, 24*(6), 480–487.

Tullmann, D. F., Fletcher, K., & Foreman, M. D. (2012). Delirium. In M. Boltz, E. Capuezuti, T. Fulmer, & D. Zwicker (Eds.), *Evidence-based geriatric nursing protocols for best practice* (4th ed., pp. 186–199). New York: Springer Publishing Company, Inc.

Tune, L. E. (2001). Anticholinergic effects of medication in elderly patients. *Journal of Clinical Psychiatry, 62* (Suppl 21), 11–14.

Whitehorne, K., Gaudine, A., Meadus, R., & Solberg, S. (2015). Lived experience of the intensive care unit for patients who experienced delirium. *American Journal of Critical Care, 24*(6), 474–479.

Wise, M. G. (1986). Delirium. In R. E. Hales & S. C. Yudofsky (Eds.), *American Psychiatric Press textbook of neuropsychiatry* (pp. 89–103). Washington, DC: American Psychiatric Press.

For a full suite of assignments and additional learning activities, see the access code at the front of your book.

CHAPTER 14

Anxiety and Depression in the Older Adult

Lisa Byrd
Cynthia Luther

(Competencies 7, 17)

LEARNING OBJECTIVES

At the end of this chapter, the reader will be able to:

> Understand the behavioral changes associated with normal aging processes as related to mood.
> Recognize symptoms of anxiety and depression in older persons.
> Develop a plan of care for managing anxiety disorder in an older person.
> Distinguish between anxiety, sadness, and depression.
> Develop a plan of care for managing depression in an older person.
> Identify signs of suicidal risk in an older person.
> Explain an emergency plan for older persons who exhibit suicidal ideation.

KEY TERMS

Agoraphobia	Music therapy
Anhedonia	Obsessive-compulsive disorder
Antidepressant	Panic disorders
Anxiety	Phobic disorders
Anxiolytic	Posttraumatic stress disorder
Atypical antidepressants	Prayer
Cognitive behavioral therapy	Substance-induced anxiety disorder
Depression	Sadness
Dysthymia	Selective serotonin reuptake inhibitors
General anxiety disorder	Selective serotonin-norepinephrine
Late-onset depression	reuptake inhibitors
Major depression	Suicidal ideation
Minor depression	Suicide

Anxiety and depression commonly affect older individuals, at nearly 20% of the older population (Friedman et al., 2013; Touhy & Jett, 2014). Symptoms are often underreported by and undertreated in older individuals. Some older adults feel some degree of *sadness* or mild anxiety, which can be considered normal due to multiple issues related to the aging process, as well as life circumstances. Older adults often try to diminish the impact of symptoms or dismiss these feelings, fearing they are developing some form of dementia such as Alzheimer's disease (AD) (Martin-Plank, 2014). Anxiety and depressive disorders can have an impact on a person's health as well as reduce compliance with prescribed treatment plans. Only 3% of older persons report being actively treated for mental health issues, but it is estimated that 63% of those individuals who are diagnosed with some form of mental illness do not receive appropriate care (Touhy & Jett, 2014; Trevisan, 2015). Many healthcare providers do not actively pursue investigating late-life mental health changes and lack insight concerning the atypical presentations of anxiety and depression in aging adults. Additional factors to consider are the culturally and ethnically diverse older populations that present barriers to appropriate diagnosis and management. A key role of the nurse is to be observant of the psychological health and examine the impact on function and independence to develop the best plan of care and obtain the help needed to produce an optimal health outcome. Persons who are insured by Medicare are entitled to screening for mental health issues as part of the Initial Preventive Physical Examination (IPPE) encounter, also known as the "Welcome to Medicare" visit. Annually, providers screen for mental health issues as part of the "Annual Wellness Visit" (Center for Medicaid and Medicare Services [CMS], 2016).

> **CLINICAL TIP**
>
> Physical symptoms may be the first chief indication of psychosocial problems (Martin-Plank, 2014).

Behavioral Changes Associated with Aging

Psychological changes in aging vary based on circumstances, life experiences, and behavioral makeup of an individual. Often psychological health revolves around a person's role in life, with some individuals assuming new caregiver responsibilities for a spouse or grandchildren, experiencing a loss of meaningful work (retirement), undergoing physical changes in function due to declining health, experiencing loss of independence due to health deterioration or onset of illness, undergoing increased stress due to financial concerns and/or limited income, and losing friends and relatives due to death. Those who are experiencing the death of their significant partner/spouse may have problems related to role adaptation; this often can have overwhelming effects leading to self-doubt and negative self-perception (Vink et al., 2008; Sozeri-Varma, 2012). As a common response to the challenges of aging, older adults may present with symptoms *of anxiety*, *depression*, or both (Fiske, Loebach-Weatherell, & Gatz, 2009). In many older adults the symptoms are manageable and the individual remains independent. But in others, the anxiety and/or depressive symptoms have a significant impact on health and independence.

Anxiety

Low levels of anxiety experienced in normal daily living may be beneficial in heightening an individual's alert state and awareness of surroundings. However, when anxiety interferes with health or day-to-day functioning, it can be an issue that requires evaluation and possibly management.

Anxiety can be difficult to diagnose in the older patient due to atypical presentations. Anxiety is one of the most common psychiatric complaints throughout the lifespan. Anxiety disorders occur in 10% to 20% of elders and are twice as common as the dementias (8%) and four to eight times more prevalent than major depressive disorder (1% to 3%) (Cassidy & Rector, 2008). Anxiety has the potential to decrease quality of life, increase isolation, decrease independence, worsen medical conditions, and hasten the onset of death. It also can cause an individual to be less observant, possibly develop a type of tunnel vision, and diminish a person's ability to hear, understand, or retain instructions and information. Individuals with excessive anxiety tend to be self-absorbed, possibly related to an attempt to protect one's body image and maintain a sense of control. Symptoms of anxiety may be caused by certain medical conditions as well as side effects of medications. Treatment of anxiety can be a challenge because medications used to manage anxiety may cause older individuals to have other health-related problems or adverse effects, especially if the older adult is frail or has chronic medical conditions. The nurse plays an important role in recognizing possible symptoms of anxiety in older patients, identifying the impact of symptoms and behaviors and intervening as needed to maximize health outcomes. Nurses play a key role in obtaining an accurate diagnosis for anxiety by being observant for symptoms of anxiety, reporting concerning symptoms, screening for anxiety, ruling out treatable causes of anxiety, and educating older individuals and their families about anxiety symptom management. Review the basic algorithm for identifying and managing mental health issues in the older patient (**Table 14-1**).

Understanding Anxiety

The expression of anxiety is a normal human reaction and part of a fear response in the human body. Controlled anxiety is a safety mechanism that alerts an individual to be cautious. Sometimes anxiety is prolonged and exaggerated; often interfering with functioning as well as independence; it is described as an unpleasant

TABLE 14-1 Identify, Assess, and Treat Mental Health Issues Identify Symptom(s), Frequency, Duration, Severity, and Impact on ADLs

Needs			
Pain	**Unmet Psychological Needs**	**Environmental Concerns**	**Psychiatric Concerns**
• Pain	• Loneliness	• Environment: Under- or Over-stimulating	• Depression
• Infection	• Boredom	• Caregiver issues	• Anxiety
• Dehydration	• Apprehension, worry, fear	• Expectations	• Delirium
• Sleep disturbance	• Emotional discomfort		• Psychosis
• Medication side-effects	• Lack of stimulation		• Dementia
• Constipation	• Lack of socialization		• Other Mental Issues
• Incontinence/Retention			• Bipolar disorder
			• Schizophrenia

Management
Rule out reversible conditions
Manage environment
Depression
• SSRI (if no improvement consider a different SSRI)
Anxiety
• SSRI which also manages anxiety
• Short acting benzodiazepine PRN (if no improvement, consider long acting benzodiazepine)
Dementia
• Anticholinesterase inhibitors
• NMDA receptor agonist
Delirium/Psychosis
• Treat the cause
• Short acting benzodiazepine

TABLE 14-2   Risk Factors for Developing Anxiety

- Family history of anxiety disorders
- Female gender
- Perimenopause (due to hormonal changes)
- Increased frailty
- History of falls
- Acute or chronic illness
- Chronic pain
- Loss of family members, friends, independence, or home (including being moved to another residence such as a nursing home)
- Lack of social supports
- Recent traumatic event
- Poor self-rated health
- Concurrent diagnosis of depression, dementia, bipolar disorder, or schizoaffective disorder
- Certain medications

feeling of dread, apprehension, foreboding, or tension resulting from a threat to one's self-esteem or well-being (Martin-Plank, 2014). Cognitive aspects of an anxiety disorder include hypervigilance to threat; seeing oneself as vulnerable; and perceiving the demands of life as exceeding the available skills, abilities, or resources to cope (Cassidy & Rector, 2008). Anxiety is associated with decreased physical activity and diminished functional status and often leads to more healthcare visits and increased length of visits (Touhy & Jett, 2014). Anxiety may be a chronic issue in an older person that becomes more exaggerated as the individual grows older. Symptoms of anxiety may develop late in life or may be related to chronic diseases, cognitive decline, or depression (Auerhahn, Capezuti, Flaherty, & Resnick, 2007). Risk factors for developing an anxiety disorder include increasing frailty; medical illness (both acute illness and chronic disease); and losses of relatives, friends, or independence (Table 14-1). **Table 14-2** discusses risk factors that increase the incidence of an older individual developing anxiety.

Common Causes of Anxiety

There are many causes of anxiety in the geriatric population, including declining abilities to perform self-care and declining social interaction due to aging, illness, and pain. Many chronic medical conditions can cause anxiety symptoms and may be a signal of worsening of a condition, such as hypoxia related to chronic obstructive pulmonary disease (COPD) or respiratory infection. Other causes of anxiety include psychological stress such as financial concerns for older individuals with limited incomes, including the inability to pay for health care and/or medications. Sensory changes that can increase anxiety symptoms include visual impairment, causing an older person to not assess a situation properly or to misinterpret shadows as animals or people; hearing loss, which can lead to hearing fragmented conversations or interpreting sounds as a threat, which could then lead to paranoia; and proprioception decline, in which older persons cannot sense where their body parts are located and can lead to unsure footing, imbalance, and falls. **Table 14-3** lists medications that can increase anxiety in an older individual.

TABLE 14-3   Medications That May Cause Anxiety in Older Adults

Nonpsychotropic medications

- Sympathomimetic: Cold and allergy medications such as those containing ephdrine, pseudoephedrine, norepinephrine or dobutamine
- Xanthene derivatives such as drinks containing caffeine (coffee, colas) or OTC pain medications with caffeine; also, medications such as aminophylline and theophylline
- Antiinflammatory agents
- Thyroid medications
- Insulin (potential for hypoglycemic reaction)
- Corticosteroids such as prednisone
- Others: Nicotine, ginseng root

Psychotropic medications

- Antidepressants and medications for treatment of AD or ADHD in some patients, drugs for treatment of attention deficit disorders
- Tranquilizing drugs: Benzodiazepines (should be used with caution in the elderly), antipsychotics
- Anticholinergic medications can cause delirium that, may be confused with anxiety: OTC sleep medications with antihistamine properties antiparkinsonian agents, tricyclic antidepressants, antipsychotics

Other causes

- Caffeine: overuse or withdrawal from regular use
- Nicotine: overuse or withdrawal
- Stimulants such as illicit drugs (cocaine, methamphetamines and the like)
- Alcohol intoxication or withdrawal

Data from Shah, R. (2012). Major types of anxiety neuroses. Retrieved from http://www.anxietyneurosis.com/app/types.asp

Anxiety Assessment

Studies indicate that anxiety disorders are common in older individuals, although relatively few are diagnosed (Touhy & Jett, 2014). The key to management of anxiety in the older patient is proper assessment and identification of the problem. The nurse must be observant of the individual as well as the family unit to develop an optimal plan of care. The nurse should allow the individual to discuss concerns in an open, nonjudgmental atmosphere. The nurse may begin an assessment of the older patient by examining the overall mood, affect, and ability to maintain a conversation. Assess the person's ability to maintain a logical frame of thought in a conversation and stay focused and the ability to discuss concerns about health and illness. Assess the individual's current state of mind, appearance, attitude, behavior, speech, thought processes, thought content, perception, cognition, insight, and judgment. An individual's overall health must be included in the assessment: all medical and psychiatric conditions, medication use, substance use and/or abuse, history of depression and/or anxiety, and support systems, including family assistance and financial resources (ability to afford health care, medications, and costs of living such as food, housing, and transportation). A thorough mental health assessment includes evaluating an older

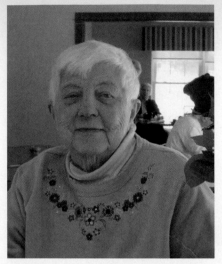

Figure 14-1 Many older adults live happy, fulfilled lives. Observing the person's demeanor and nonverbal behavior provides clues about mood.

individual's cognitive functioning, functional abilities, mood, and ability to appropriately answer questions. An anxiety assessment interview begins with a conversation to determine the following (Auerhahn et al., 2007):

> Patient's present mental status
> Patient's past mental status
> Patient's ability to manage daily activities and level of independence
> Impact of anxiety on an individual's life
> Course and nature of symptoms
> Individual's perception of his or her medical and psychiatric conditions on health
> Previous methods of managing symptoms

Instruments available to assess anxiety include the State-Trait Anxiety Inventory (STAI), the Hospital Anxiety Inventory, the Beck Anxiety Inventory, and the Hamilton Anxiety Scale. The nurse's assessment of the patient will assist in developing an appropriate diagnosis of anxiety. The following signs are common in many anxious individuals, and the person may exhibit one or more of the following symptoms:

> Rapid speech
> Restlessness or inability to sit still
> Uncooperative, hostile, guarded, or suspicious behaviors
> Avoidance of eye contact
> Repetitive, purposeless movements such as rocking, pill-rolling of the fingers, tapping of foot
> Staring and inability to answer questions or follow a commands
> Overexaggerated or blunted mood

Types of Anxiety and Symptoms of Anxiety

Anxiety disorders in older adults include *panic disorders, phobic disorders, obsessive-compulsive disorder* (OCD), *general anxiety disorder* (GAD), *posttraumatic stress disorder* (PTSD), and *substance-induced anxiety disorder* (see **Table 14-4**). Mixed anxiety and depression may occur simultaneously and is composed of at least four anxious or depressive symptoms:

> Irritability
> Anticipating the worst
> Concentration or memory difficulties
> Hopelessness
> Restlessness
> Sleep disturbance: Insomnia or hypersomnia
> Eating disturbances: Anorexia or overeating
> Fear of dying
> Fear of falling
> Fear of losing control or "going crazy"
> Physicals signs and symptoms: Muscle tension; headaches; dizziness or lightheadedness; sweating; dry mouth; feelings of choking; shortness of breath; chest pain; increased heart rate; trembling; frequent urination; abdominal distress, including nausea, vomiting, and/or diarrhea; and paresthesia (numbness or tingling sensations) (Byrd, 2011; Sozeri-Varma, 2012).

TABLE 14-4   Diagnostic Features: Anxiety Disorders

Generalized Anxiety Disorder (GAD)

- Excessive anxiety and worry (apprehensive expectation) about events or activities; intensity, duration, or frequency of anxiety or worry is out of proportion to likelihood or impact of the event
- Associated with restlessness, feeling keyed up or on edge, being easily fatigued, difficulty concentrating, irritability, muscle tension, or sleep disturbance

Agoraphobia

- Marked or intense fear or anxiety triggered by real or anticipated exposure to situations, such as public transportation, being in open spaces or enclosed spaces, being in a crowd, or being outside the home alone. The individual avoids situations related to fear of panic or other incapacitating or embarrassing symptoms.

Panic Disorder

- Abrupt surge of intense fear or discomfort with associated physical symptoms and cognitive symptoms
- Among the associated symptoms are palpitations, sweating, shortness of breath, chest discomfort, paresthesias, fear of loss of control or "going crazy," and fear of dying

Specific Phobia

- Marked fear or anxiety about a specific object or situation (flying, heights, animals, sight of blood, storms)

Posttraumatic Stress Disorder (PTSD)

- Development of characteristic symptoms following exposure to one or more traumatic events (war, physical abuse, violent crimes). Clinical symptoms may include flashbacks or fear-based reexperiencing; or emotional reactions such fear, helplessness, horror, or depressive symptoms. The individual has directly witnessed, experienced, learned of an actual or threatened violent or accidental event that occurred to a close family member or friend, or experienced repeated aversive details of traumatic events (such as first responders collecting human remains). Medical events such as waking during surgery, anaphylactic shock, and other events involving sudden, catastrophic medical events are considered traumatic events. Other behavioral characteristics include being quick-tempered and becoming aggressive.

Social phobia

- Marked fear or anxiety about social situations in which the individual is exposed to possible scrutiny by others. Examples of situations include having a conversation, meeting unfamiliar people, or performing in front of others. The individual fears that he or she will be humiliated, embarrassed, or negatively evaluated and that this will lead to rejection or offending others.

Substance- or Medication-Induced Anxiety Disorder

- Panic attacks or anxiety is predominant in the clinical presentation. Symptoms develop during or after substance intoxication or withdrawal or after exposure to a medication.
- Anxiety disorder due to another medical condition

Data from American Psychiatric Association. (2013). *Diagnostic and statistical manual of mental disorders* (5th ed.). Arlington, VA: American Psychiatric Publishing.

Differential Diagnoses for Anxiety

It is common for an older individual with a longstanding anxious personality to have an exacerbation of anxiety symptoms due to stress or illness. Anxiety also can exacerbate existing medical conditions, including cardiovascular disease leading to a cardiac event, pulmonary disorders leading to hypoxia, and skin disorders such as eczema leading to a flare-up. Anxiety may be a symptom of another problem in older adults, and other causes of anxiety must be ruled out to develop an appropriate plan of care.

Reversible causes of anxiety symptoms can include:

> Urinary tract infection (UTI)
> Upper respiratory tract infection (URI)
> Constipation
> Dehydration
> Hyperthyroidism
> Hypoglycemia
> Depression
> Endocrine or other neurological problem
> Caffeine or nicotine use
> Medication or substance use (both prescription and OTC)

Anxiety and Dementia

Older individuals with dementia commonly exhibit anxious symptoms. Occasionally, an individual with a diagnosis of dementia may present with an extreme episode of anxious or agitated behaviors and possibly aggression, often referred to as psychotic behaviors. Agitation may be displayed as an increase in wandering behaviors or as increased verbal or motor activity that is either appropriate but repeated frequently or inappropriate and exaggerated, suggesting lack of judgment. Anxious symptoms often manifest at some point in the progression of dementia in an older person.

CLINICAL TIP

Anxiety and depression often go together in older adults and should be treated together.

Managing Anxiety

There are a variety of ways the nurse can minimize the effects of anxiety, as well as multiple treatments available if an anxiety disorder is diagnosed and interfering with day-to-day functioning (**Table 14-5**):

> *Behavioral counseling.* A mental health professional can assist in obtaining a definitive diagnosis and provide a treatment plan. The nurse can assist with the initial diagnosis and help determine the cause of the anxious symptoms. The nurse also may help older individuals discuss their anxiety and develop strategies to identify the cause of their anxiety and manage the anxious symptoms.
> *Routine.* Encourage anxious older patients to establish a daily routine so the individual can develop a sense of security in his or her ability to accomplish tasks and safety in performing daily tasks. Engaging in routine activities will also assist the older person in developing familiarity in performance, which promotes independence. This is especially important in older patients with any degree of cognitive impairment, including AD and other dementias.
> *Cognitive-behavioral therapy.* The nurse may assist in *cognitive behavioral therapy* (CBT) to diminish anxiety in older patients—the cognitive part helps persons change their thinking patterns that support their fears, and the behavioral part helps change the way they react to anxiety-provoking situations. For example, if an individual has a fear of falling, exercise can improve balance and strength, while assistive devices may offer safety and security when walking. Physical and occupational therapists can help devise a plan to offer ways to ambulate and maneuver safely. If a person has a chronic medical condition or has had a traumatic medical event, the nurse may educate the person about the condition and ways to decrease problems, as well as provide strategies improve health. If an individual has chronic anxiety symptoms without an identifiable cause, the person may learn strategies to avert the anxious symptoms when they occur, including pursed breathing techniques and diversion maneuvers.

TABLE 14-5   Nursing Care for the Patient Experiencing Anxiety

- Decrease environmental stimuli
- Stay with the patient
- Make no demands and do not ask the patient to make major decisions
- Support current coping mechanisms (crying, talking, etc.)
- Do not confront or argue with the patient
- Speak slowly in a soft, calm voice (enunciate clearly)
- Avoid reciprocal anxiety (emotions can be contagious, and sensing anxiety in the nurse can worsen the patient's anxiety)
- Reassure the patient you will help develop a solution to managing the problem
- Reorient the patient to reality (unless this causes more anxiety)
- Respect the patient's personal space

> *Stress reduction.* Strategies to decrease stress as well as reduce the impact of illness or stress will assist in reducing anxiety. Stress reduction may be accomplished by distraction or diverting one's attention to a pleasant or non-anxiety-provoking topic. A monotonous sound may take someone's mind off what causes the individual anxiety—examples of monotonous sounds would be the whirl of a ceiling fan, the tick-tock of a clock, or a sound machine producing the sounds of ocean waves or rain. Stress management techniques include cognitive restructuring, imagery, meditation, *prayer*, relaxation exercises, and deep breathing exercises. Other methods include exercise, mindfulness meditation, yoga, and Tai Chi.

> *Getting adequate and efficient sleep.* Inadequate sleep, whether it is trouble getting to sleep, waking throughout the night, or early morning awakenings, can lead to impaired attention, slowed response time, impaired memory, impaired concentration, and decreased performance. The nurse can encourage an older individual with anxiety to develop a more efficient sleep pattern and establish a sleep routine: go to bed the same time each day and awaken at the same time, decrease daytime napping, and cease drinking fluids 2 to 3 hours prior to bedtime and urinate immediately before bedtime to prevent nighttime urination (nocturia).

> *Staying active.* Activity of any kind, whether physical or intellectual, can offer distraction and ease anxiety symptoms. The nurse can encourage the older patient to perform repetitive exercises or activities as well as to stay socially active. Relaxing activities and hobbies should be encouraged; common activities in older individuals include gardening, reading, fishing, art, and music.

> *Avoiding triggers.* The nurse should encourage an older person to avoid things that cause or aggravate the symptoms of anxiety. Also, individuals with anxiety issues should avoid substances that may increase anxious symptoms, such as caffeine, nicotine, OTC cold medications, and alcohol.

> *Support group therapy.* An older person and/or the family may benefit from support groups, which can offer not only psychological support but also be available for the person to discuss problems and concerns in a nonjudgmental atmosphere. Other advantages of support groups are that they allow individuals to vent their feelings and learn alternative methods to manage their issues from individuals who are experiencing similar problems.

> *Medication.* Medical management of anxiety disorders may be necessary if the anxious episodes are exaggerated, prolonged, and incapacitating or if they worsen an individual's ability to function or other medical conditions. The goals of medication management are aimed at controlling the symptoms of anxiety to diminish their impact on an individual's life. The main classes of medications used to treat anxiety disorders are antidepressants and antianxiety drugs, or *anxiolytics*.

Medication Management for Anxiety

Medications may be necessary if the anxious symptoms interfere with day-to-day functioning or independence, or are extremely distressing. Medication management of anxiety disorders in older individuals can be difficult because of the high incidence of side effects. Benzodiazepines have been the most commonly prescribed anxiolytic agent for managing anxious symptoms in the older population, but should be used very cautiously and only when absolutely necessary. Benzodiazepines do have the potential for abuse and dependence. Possible side effects of benzodiazepines in an elderly individual include motor incoordination, cognitive impairment, dizziness, amnesia, and falls. When symptoms are severe and a benzodiazepine is necessary, the ones preferred are those with a short duration, such as lorazepam or oxazepam. In certain individuals, longer-acting benzodiazepines may be required to manage chronic anxiety disorders.

Antidepressants are frequently used in older patients to assist in managing the symptoms of anxiety. They are recommended since some are efficacious in treatment of panic disorders, OCDs, GADs, and PTSD. The safest class of antidepressant agents, which is the most efficacious for use in older individuals with the least interactions with other medications and fewest side effects, is the *selective serotonin reuptake inhibitors* (SSRIs). Some are indicated for managing anxiety as well as depression (Auerhahn et al., 2007; Touhy & Jett, 2010). Commonly used antidepressants are discussed later in the section on managing depression (see **Case Study 14-1**).

CLINICAL TIP

SSRIs have a lower side effect profile than many other antidepressants and are often preferred over other classes of medications to treat depression.

All of these medications should be used with extreme caution in older individuals because they have anticholinergic properties, which can lead to cognitive decline, motor incoordination, dizziness, orthostatic hypotension, falls, urinary retention, and constipation (see **Table 14-6**).

Case Study 14-1

Ms. A is a 67-year-old woman who has experienced a fall that led to a fractured hip. After surgery to repair her fractured hip, she had a normal recovery period and was discharged to a rehabilitation center for improvement of balance and gait. However, her progression was extremely slow and she began crying hysterically during her physical therapy sessions. She stated she was extremely fearful of falling again. This fear of falling was justified, but would lead to incapacitation and further decline in her overall health if she became chair-bound or bed-bound. After the rehabilitation team discussed the problem of extreme anxiety with her healthcare provider, Ms. A. was placed on a low dose of escitalopram (Lexapro; an antidepressant that is also indicated for anxiety). Ms. A. also participated in CBT to assist in her understanding the cause of her anxiety attacks and helping her develop strategies to manage her fear of falling again. After 2 weeks, Ms. A. was still fearful but she did not become hysterical during her therapy sessions. She was able to participate in her walking and gait exercises and slowly become less anxious when trying to walk. Ms. A. was able to walk with the use of a walker and was discharged home again.

TABLE 14-6 Anxiolytics

Benzodiazepine: Short Acting	Action	Available Doses	Recommended to Use as Needed (prn)*
Lorazepam (Ativan)	Onset of action in 20 minutes Peak action at 1–1½ hours Frequency of dosing: Every 6 hours	0.5 mg, 1 mg, 2 mg	Recommended initial dose: 0.5 mg every 6 hours Forms available: Pills Also available in rapid onset formulations: Sublingual, cream, injectable (intramuscular)
Oxazepam (Serax)	Onset of action is slow Peak action at 2–3 hours Frequency of dosing: Every 8 hours	15 mg, 30 mg	Recommended initial dose: 15–30 mg at bedtime, may dose up to 3 times a day
Temazepam (Restoril)	Onset of action is slow Peak action at 45 minutes to 1½ hours Frequency of dosing: Every 24 hours (maximum dosing every 12 hours)	7.5 mg, 15 mg, 22.5 mg, 30 mg	Recommended to dose at bedtime lowest dose that achieves desired effect
Diazepam (Valium)	Onset of action in 20 minutes Peak action at 1–1½ hours Frequency of dosing: Every 6 hours	2.5 mg, 5 mg, 10 mg	Recommended initial dose: 2.5 mg twice a day
Benzodiazepine: Long acting			
Alprazolam (Xanax)	Onset of action in 45 minutes Peak action at 1 to 1½ hours Frequency of dosing: Every 8 hours	0.25 mg, 0.5 mg, 1 mg, 2 mg	Recommended initial dose: 0.25 mg twice a day
Chlordiazepoxide (Librium)	Onset of action in 1 hour Peak action at 45 minutes to 1½ hours Frequency of dosing: Every 12 hours	10 mg	Recommended initial dose: 25 mg twice a day
Clonazepam (Klonopin)	Onset of action in 30 minutes Peak action in 2–4 hours Frequency of dosing: Every 12 hours (maximum frequency 3 times a day)	0.125 mg, 0.25 mg, 0.5 mg, 1 mg	Recommended initial dose: 0.25–0.5 mg twice a day Maximum daily dose 20 mg
Clorazepate (Tranxene)	Onset of action in 1 hour Peak action in 2–4 hours Frequency of dosing: Every 12 hours	3.75 mg, 7.5 mg, 15 mg	Recommended initial dose: 3.75 mg twice a day
Flurazepam (Dalmane)	Onset of action in 30 minutes Peak action at 1–2 hours Frequency of dosing: Every 24 hours	15 mg, 30 mg	Recommended initial dose: 15 mg at bedtime

*Potential side effects: Ataxia, memory impairment, hypotension, falls, tremors, and hallucinations.

Behavioral Interventions for Managing Anxiety

Behavioral interventions to reduce stress and anxiety should be implemented to optimize treatment success in the older patient (see **Boxes 14-1** and **14-2**). Environmental structuring will assist in decreasing stress as well as diminishing triggers of anxiety. Techniques generally fall within three categories: relaxation, cognitive structuring, and exposure-response prevention.

Relaxation techniques make an older person focus on sounds, smells, or thoughts other than the ones that make the individual nervous or anxious.

BOX 14-1   Calming Maneuvers for Anxiety

Deep Breathing Exercises: Have the patient sit in a comfortable chair, with hands on the abdomen. Ask the patient to inhale slowly and deeply, feeling the abdomen rise. Hold the breath for a few seconds. Ask the patient to exhale slowly, allowing the abdomen to deflate. Repeat several times. Always speak in a soft, calm manner to assist the patient through the process.

Progressive Muscle Relaxation: The patient should lie down in a comfortable position. Ask the patient to tighten the muscles in his or her hand for a few seconds and then completely release the tension to relax the muscle. Focusing on a specific muscle by tightening and releasing tension provides greater relaxation response to the area. Progressively concentrate on the muscles of the arms, shoulders, face, chest, back, abdomen, legs, and feet. Again, use a soft, calm voice to assist the patient through the process.

BOX 14-2   Behavioral Strategies to Manage Anxiety

- Quiet environment, relaxed position.
- Have the individual focus on a monotonous sound or image to divert their attention and forget the anxious symptoms (clocks, fans, and sound machines offering ocean waves or rain).
- *Music Therapy*: Listen to music the individual enjoys to distract the person's thoughts.
- Art therapy: Participate in an activity that is nondemanding to distract the individual's thoughts.
- Exercise therapy: Engage in repetitive exercises that do not exacerbate the anxious symptoms to offer distraction.
- Other: Aromatherapy, guided imagery.
- Identify dysfunctional attitudes and beliefs that lead to anxiety symptoms.
- Explore the validity of the fear or causative agent leading to anxiety by verbalizing statements about the anxiety.
- Replace dysfunctional attitudes and beliefs about the problem with more positive statements that are based on reality or ways to manage the problem.
- Allow time to "worry"—set aside a worry-time—a designated time the individual is allowed to think about his or her fear. Do not allow the individual to worry about the problem outside of the designated worry time.
- Write down thoughts (brainstorm).
- Order priorities for attention.
- Develop problem-solving strategies.

Data from Ebersole, P., Hess, P., Touhy, T., Jett, K., & Schmidt-Luggen, A. (2008). *Toward healthy aging: Human needs & nursing response* (7th ed.). St. Louis, MO: Mosby; Touhy, T., & Jett, K. (2014). Mental health. In *Ebersole and Hess' gerontological nursing & healthy aging* (4th ed., pp. 336–353). St. Louis, MO: Mosby; Merck Manual of Geriatrics Online. (2012). Overview of anxiety disorders. Retrieved from http://www.merckmanuals.com/professional/psychiatric_disorders/anxiety_disorders/overview_of_anxiety_disorders.html; Merck Manual Professional Version. (2015). Online resource. Retrieved from http://www.merckmanuals.com/professional

Cognitive restructuring helps the person identify the trigger or stimulus that causes or maintains anxiety within the individual, making the person aware of the trigger so he or she may slowly gain control over the effect of the stimuli to develop a range of coping strategies and tools.

Exposure-response prevention may be used with individuals with both panic disorders and OCD. The individual is exposed to thoughts of the trigger that causes his or her anxiety, is given strategies to cope with the problem, and eventually becomes desensitized to the trigger.

Depression

A significant number of older individuals experience depression, which can affect individual health and overall quality of life as well as decrease an individual's lifespan. Many older adults experience chronic medical conditions along with chronic pain and fatigue, all of which can lead to depression. Common causes of depression include the following:

> Decline in health or new onset of illness
> Exposure to multiple medications and their associated side effects, as well as drug–drug interactions, can cause elders to feel physically and mentally "down"
> Having outlived spouses, loved ones, and friends
> Having to move from private homes to assisted living or long-term care because of decreasing ability to live independently

Isolating oneself, becoming more sedentary, and experiencing pervasive feelings of sadness are not normal when growing older. When these symptoms are present, seem severe, or last longer than expected, a diagnosis of depression must be considered.

Prevalence of Depression in the Aging Population

Approximately 10% of men and 18% of women over the age of 65 in the United States report current symptoms associated with clinically significant depression. These findings have been relatively unchanged since 1998. Between men and women, men in the over-85 age group are at highest risk for depression (18%), and white males in this category are at the highest risk for suicide (National Institute of Mental Health [NIMH], 2012). Among women over the age of 65, those between the ages of 75 and 79 are noted to be at the highest risk (20%) for depression (Centers for Disease Control and Prevention [CDC], 2015; Older Americans, 2010). In long-term care facilities the prevalence of depression has been reported as high as 29% (Seitz, Purandare, & Conn, 2010).

Types of Depression and Presentation

Major Depression, Minor Depression, and Dysthymia

The American Psychiatric Association's (APA's) *Diagnostic and Statistical Manual of Mental Disorders* (5th ed.) (2013), also known as the *DSM-V,* defines *major depression* as a depressive episode in which an individual experiences pervasive feelings of anxiety and sadness that coincide with *anhedonia*, or loss of pleasure and interest in daily activities. Concurrently, at least five or more of the following symptoms must be present most of the day, nearly every day for a minimum of 2 consecutive weeks: increased fatigue with loss of energy, irritability and/or restlessness, oversleeping or trouble sleeping, poor concentration or difficulty with mental processing and decision making, inappropriate guilt or perception of worthlessness, changes in appetite that lead to weight gain or weight loss not related to dieting, and thoughts of suicide or death and/or attempts at suicide. Symptoms consistent with depression that occur for the first time later in life are referred to as *late-onset depression*, whereas older adults who report a history of depression at an earlier stage in life are often diagnosed with "recurrent" depression. An older adult who presents with severe symptoms of sadness or other symptoms consistent with major depression will often report a history of one or more major depressive events at some point in their lifetime.

Major depression can change or distort the way older adults view themselves, their lives, and those around them. In addition, older adults with major depression often display functional activity impairments such as changes in regular activities of daily living (ADL), decreased socialization, and poor compliance with medication therapy and healthcare recommendations (Substance Abuse and Mental Health Services Administration, 2011).

Symptoms that are indicative of depression include the following (APA, 2013):

> No interest or pleasure in enjoyable activities
> No interest in sexual activities
> Feeling sad or numb
> Crying easily or for no reason
> Feeling slowed down
> Feeling worthless or guilty
> Change in appetite; unintended change in weight
> Trouble recalling things, concentrating, or making decisions
> Problems sleeping, or wanting to sleep all of the time
> Feeling tired all of the time
> Thoughts about death or suicide

Minor depression is a subset of major depression and is defined as an episode of depressive thoughts that is less severe than major depression, but has a similar 2-week time frame for presentation. Individuals show evidence of only one to four of the eight cardinal symptoms of major depressive disorders. Minor depression may be a precursor to a major depressive illness (APA, 2013; Soriano, 2007).

Dysthymia is a chronic form of depression that is often diagnosed in older adults with prolonged illness or those who experience long-term challenges in their daily living. Older adults who present with dysthymia experience mild to moderate depressive symptoms that are present throughout most days over a 2-year period. In order to receive a diagnosis of dysthymia, individuals must also report two of the following symptoms: poor concentration or difficulty making decisions, poor appetite or overeating, fatigue, low energy, excessive sleep, or insomnia (APA, 2013).

Manifestations of Depression

Depression is manifested in both affective and somatic responses in varying patterns based on gender. Men often blame others for their current depressed mood, display increased irritability and anger, and intentionally create conflicts. Males may act suspicious and guarded, display restlessness and agitation, display an extreme desire to be in control, and perceive that admitting self-doubt and despair are inherent weaknesses. In contrast, depressed women often blame themselves for their depressed state, feeling anxious, scared, apathetic, slowed down, and worthless. They often have trouble setting boundaries and avoid all conflicts, but do not have trouble talking with others about their self-doubt and despair (Helpguide.org, 2012).

Because the onset of depression in older adults can often coincide with onset of an illness, it is frequently misattributed to a somatic cause and not properly diagnosed (Fiske et al., 2009). Somatic symptoms such as persistent muscle aches, chronic headaches, palpitations, or insidious changes in stomach, bowel, or bladder function should be considered as possible symptoms of depressive disorders unless clearly attributable to a medical condition (Grohol, 2012).

CLINICAL TIP

Depression often coincides with illness, so it may not be recognized or properly diagnosed. Somatic symptoms, unless attributable to a medical condition, should prompt investigation into possible depression.

Different Presentations of Depression

Symptoms of depression also can manifest in varying patterns of thought and behavior.

> *Catatonic depression:* Individual is very withdrawn; thinking, speech, and general activity may slow down, as well as the cessation of all voluntary activities; may not take care of himself or herself, household, or pets; and may also mimic others' speech (echolalia) or movements (echopraxia).
> *Melancholic depression:* Individual does not receive pleasure from usual activities; may appear sluggish, sad, and withdrawn; may speak little, stop eating, and lose weight; often shows no emotions or may feel excessively or inappropriately guilty.
> *Psychotic depression:* Individual has false beliefs (delusions) about having committed unpardonable sins or crimes, having incurable or shameful disorders, or being watched or persecuted; may have hallucinations, usually of voices accusing them of various misdeeds or condemning them to death; and some individuals may imagine that they see coffins or deceased relatives.
> *Atypical depression:* Individual may appear anxious and fearful (especially in the evening); may have an increased appetite, resulting in weight gain, and although initially unable to sleep, transitions to sleeping for increasingly longer periods of time; depressed mood may be lessened in response to positive events, but individual is excessively sensitive to perceived criticism or rejection; may become agitated or very restless while exhibiting behaviors such as frequent wringing of the hands, rocking back and forth, or talking continuously.

Relationship of Depression to Chronic Disease

Chronic diseases remain pervasive in older adult populations and the incidence of morbidity and mortality from chronic disease increases with each decade of life. Currently, 80% of individuals over the age of 65 have one or more chronic conditions such as heart disease, vascular disease, hypertension, diabetes, cancer, arthritis, or lung disease (CDC, 2011). Depressed individuals who present with heart disease, cancer, COPD, or stroke have the highest incidence of mortality associated with their disease (Murphy, Jiaquan, & Kochanek, 2012). Concurrent depression in the presence of these four chronic diseases is strongly related to increased burden of illness and worsening overall outcomes.

CLINICAL TIP

Approximately 80% of older adults have at least one chronic health condition.

Diagnosing Depression

Nurses providing care for older adults are currently being called to strongly consider screening for depression and assisting in the initiation of treatment as part of comprehensive holistic care for their patients. Primary screening of all at-risk older adults is the first step in diagnosing depression. A diagnosis of major depression in older adults is made with documentation of positive findings on a reliable depression screening tool (Low & Hubley, 2007). These findings revolve around eight cardinal symptoms: expression of guilt, loss of sexual interest, changes in nutritional intake, alterations in sleep patterns, decreased energy, poor concentration, agitation or apathy, and suicidality (Soriano, 2007). Symptoms must have been consistently present over the previous 2-week period prior to the screening (Grohol, 2012).

The use of appropriate screening tools such as the 15-item Geriatric Depression Scale (GDS) (Camus, Kraehenbuhl, Preisig, Bula, & Waeber, 2004; Sheikh & Yesavage, 1986) or the Patient Health Questionnaire nine-item screening tool (PHQ-9) (Spitzer, Kroenke, & Williams, 1999) demonstrate adequate sensitivity and specificity for older adults and provide avenues for intervention or referral depending on severity scores and suicidal risks.

Interpreting the Patient Health Questionnaire 9-Item Test

The PHQ-9 questions are designed to reflect the onset, in the previous 2 weeks at time of screening, of specific depression-related symptoms reported by individuals. Scoring is completed using a simple point system of 0 to 3, where 0 correlates with having no prior symptoms and 3 indicates having experienced the symptom almost every day (see **Exhibit 14-1**). The total score for the PHQ-9 is 27.

The scoring guide for the PHQ-9 is summarized below (The MacArthur Initiative on Depression and Primary Care, 2009):

The total point score helps determine the severity of the depression, which can help guide the treatment plan and also suggest possible suicide risk. Scoring is as follows:

5–9 = minimal depressive symptoms; supportive education and observation is recommended

10–14 = minor depression, dysthmia, or mild major depression; treatment may include psychotherapy, antidepressants, or watchful waiting

15–19 = moderately severe major depression; requires psychotherapy or antidepressants

20 and above = need psychotherapy and antidepressants in combination

After completing the screening, assess the time period that the patient has reported having symptoms. If symptoms have lasted over a 2 year period, this may indicate chronic depression, which may require ongoing CBT for the best treatment outcomes.

Older adults who score 2 or higher on one or both PHQ-2 questions often require some form of treatment for their depressed symptoms (MacArthur Initiative on Depression and Primary Care, 2009). A positive two-item screening warrants further testing using expanded screening tools and can be completed and reviewed by a nurse practitioner or other clinician for treatment planning. Data collected in the screening tool also can be used to ensure that appropriate referral for specialized interventional care is completed.

CLINICAL TIP

Older adults who score 2 or higher on one or both PHQ-2 questions often require some form of treatment for their depressed symptoms.

Differential Diagnoses for Depression

A thorough medical and cognitive assessment is necessary to determine whether the symptoms of depression are due to underlying neurologic diagnoses such as AD or dementia. Depressive disorders also must be distinguished from other disorders such as anxiety disorders and late-life schizophrenia. Depression rating scales, cognitive screening instruments, and structural and functional neuroimaging studies may be implemented as determined by the individual patient.

Physical disorders, such as anemia, hypothyroidism, Parkinson's disease (PD), and other neurologic disorders must also be ruled out because they may present with symptoms similar to depression (*Merck Manual—Home Health Handbook*, 2008a).

There are no definitive laboratory tests or neurologic imaging tests to diagnose depressive disorders; however, laboratory and radiographic testing should be performed to rule out other occult disorders that can be associated

PATIENT HEALTH QUESTIONNAIRE-9 (PHQ-9)

Over the last 2 weeks, how often have you been bothered by any of the following problems? *(Use "✓" to indicate your answer)*	Not at all	Several days	More than half the days	Nearly every day
1. Little interest or pleasure in doing things	0	1	2	3
2. Feeling down, depressed, or hopeless	0	1	2	3
3. Trouble falling or staying asleep, or sleeping too much	0	1	2	3
4. Feeling tired or having little energy	0	1	2	3
5. Poor appetite or overeating	0	1	2	3
6. Feeling bad about yourself — or that you are a failure or have let yourself or your family down	0	1	2	3
7. Trouble concentrating on things, such as reading the newspaper or watching television	0	1	2	3
8. Moving or speaking so slowly that other people could have noticed. Or the opposite — being so fidgety or restless that you have been moving around a lot more than usual	0	1	2	3
9. Thoughts that you would be better off dead or of hurting yourself in some way	0	1	2	3

FOR OFFICE CODING_____ + _____ + _____ + _____

=Total Score: _____

If you checked off _any_ problems, how _difficult_ have these problems made it for you to do your work, take care of things at home, or get along with other people?

Not difficult at all	Somewhat difficult	Very difficult	Extremely difficult
☐	☐	☐	☐

Exhibit 14-1 Patient Health Questionnaire-9 (PHQ-9).

Reproduced from Pfizer. (n.d). Patient Health Questionnaire (PHQ) Screeners. Retrieved from http://www.phqscreeners.com/select-screener/36. Developed by Drs. Robert L. Spitzer, Janet B.W. Williams, Kurt Kroenke and colleagues, with an educational grant from Pfizer Inc. No permission required to reproduce, translate, display or distribute.

with depressive symptoms. Completion of a full laboratory screening includes a complete blood count (CBC), thyroid-stimulating hormone (TSH), complete metabolic panel (CMP), vitamin B_{12}, serum folate, and urinalysis. Also magnetic resonance imaging (MRI) of the brain to detect changes consistent with a mass or vascular lesion that may be causing depressive symptoms is also helpful in the diagnosis of depression (Lyness, 2012).

Depression and Dementia

Current estimates of mild cognitive impairment (MCI) manifesting in older adults between the ages of 70 and 89 range from 15% to 20% (Petersen et al., 2008; Su et al., 2014). Of those individuals with MCI, 25% will be diagnosed with progressive Alzheimer's-type dementia each year (Kaduszkiewicz et al., 2014). Symptoms consistent with depression have been shown to precede dementia in both men and women (Goveas, Espeland, Woods, Wassertheil-Smoller, & Kotchen, 2011). Furthermore, as the number of recurrent depressive episodes increases throughout older adulthood, the prevalence of permanent cognitive changes suggestive of dementia also appears to increase. These neurological changes are thought to be similarly related to metabolic-induced hippocampal brain injury that can occur with traumatic brain injury and cerebrovascular insults. Early onset of treatment for depression may have important implications in decreasing onset and progression of dementia in older adult populations in the future (Dotson, Beydoun, & Zonderman, 2010).

Managing Depression

Effective treatment of depression begins with evaluating the situation and the individual's social support system (Kiosses et al., 2015). The plan of care involves using an interdisciplinary team (IDT) approach, which includes the use of adaptive disease management to maximize quality of life, CBT, and pharmacologic therapy, as indicated, with antidepressants such as SSRIs, selective serotonin-norepinephrine reuptake inhibitors (SNRIs), and atypical antidepressants.

Counseling and Therapy

CBT is best performed by advanced- practice mental health clinicians who specialize in geriatric care. Specialized counselors who are trained in senior care are able to assist older adults and their caregivers in reframing internal and external constructs in order to stabilize concepts of self in the presence of depression. CBT, in combination with problem-solving therapy, is also effective in helping depressed older adults identify problems in their daily living that contribute to depression and formulate strategies for lifestyle and social modifications in the presence of chronic illness to improve overall quality of life (Arean et al., 2010).

Medication Management for Depression

Effective pharmacotherapy is necessary to manage major depression or depression that lasts for a prolonged period in older adults. Some individuals may be difficult to manage with medications due to resistance to certain antidepressants or side effects, but the key is to find the right medication with the greatest reduction in symptoms and with the least amount of side effects.

SSRI Therapy. There are multiple classes of antidepressant medications; however, the SSRIs are considered first-line therapy for managing depression in elders due to their limited side effect profile and overall performance in effectively treating depression. SSRIs inhibit cortical presynaptic serotonin (5HT) reuptake in the brain (**Table 14-7**). This pharmacologic response increases the amount of circulating serotonin in the neurosynapses, improves receptor binding to positively affect neurotransmission of serotonin (a potent mood-stimulating neurotransmitter), and ultimately decreases symptoms of depression (Lundbeck Institute CNS forum, 2012).

Selective Serotonin-Norepinephrine Reuptake Inhibitor Therapy. Selective serotonin-norepinephrine reuptake inhibitors (SNRIs) is another class of antidepressants commonly prescribed in older adults (Table 14-3). SNRIs affect both serotonin and norepinephrine in the brain, through neuroregulation that helps brain cells send and receive messages important for improving mood. Medications in this group of antidepressants are sometimes called dual reuptake inhibitors and may also assist with managing the symptoms of fibromyalgia and chronic fatigue syndrome, thought to be related to low levels of serotonin and norepinephrine (Lee & Chen, 2010).

TABLE 14-7   Antidepressants
Selective Serotonin Reuptake Inhibitors
Medication
Citalopram (Celexa)
Escitalopram (Lexapro)
Fluoxetine (Prozac)
Paroxetine (Paxil)
Sertraline (Zoloft)
Serotonin and norepinephrine reuptake inhibitors
Venlafaxine (Effexor XR)
Duloxetine (Cymbalta)
Others
Bupropion (Wellbutrin XR)
Mirtazapine (Remeron)

Data from Drugs.com. (2015). Retrieved from http://www.drugs.com/drug_information.html; Weise, B. (2011). Geriatric depression: The use of antidepressants in the elderly. *BC Medical Journal, 53*(7), 341–347.

Atypical Antidepressants. Another class of antidepressants commonly used in elders, often referred to as *atypical antidepressants*, includes dopamine-norepinephrine reuptake inhibitors (DNRIs), which work by primarily blocking the reuptake of dopamine and norepinephrine, with no direct action on the serotonin system. DNRIs may be utilized in the treatment of major depressive disorders (Byatt & Lundquist, 2012).

Nursing Interventions

As part of developing an optimal plan of care, nurses are responsible for completing assessments for evidence of depression in all older adults in their care, making sure that other somatic conditions have been ruled out, and developing strategies to optimize function, independence, and promote psychological health.

A comprehensive treatment plan may include the following (Halverson & Bienenfield, 2015; Kurlowicz & Havath, 2008):

> Providing a nonjudgmental atmosphere
> Instituting safety precautions for suicide risk for any patient who presents with severe symptoms or expresses suicidal ideation
> Monitoring and promoting nutrition, elimination, sleep/rest patterns, and physical comfort (especially pain control)
> Maintaining and/or enhancing physical function
  • Structuring regular exercise/activity
  • Considering referral to physical, occupational, and/or recreational therapies when necessary
  • Encouraging the older patient to develop a daily routine/activity schedule
> Encouraging utilization of social support systems
  • Identifying/mobilizing a support person(s) such as family, confidants, friends, hospital resources, support groups, or patient visitors

- Identifying if there is a need for spiritual support and contacting appropriate clergy, while being respectful of the patient's values and being cautious not to impart the one's personal and/or religious values upon a patient
> Maximizing independence and autonomy/personal control/self-efficacy by including the patient as an active participant in making daily schedules and short-term goals
> Identifying and reinforcing the patient's strengths and capabilities
> Providing structure to allow some familiarity in routine
> Encouraging daily participation in relaxation therapies or pleasant activities (art therapy, music therapy, etc.)
> Monitoring and documenting responses to medication and other therapies
  - Readministering the depression-screening tool used initially to determine efficacy of medication(s)
> Assisting the patient with problem-solving strategies
> Providing emotional support
  - Being empathic
  - Engaging in active and supportive listening
  - Encouraging expression of feelings and working toward fostering hope
  - Supporting adaptive coping
  - Encouraging pleasant reminiscence
> Providing information about any physical illnesses and treatment(s)
> Providing information about depression, reinforcing that depression is common, treatable, and not the person's fault
> Educating the patient and family about the importance of adherence to the prescribed treatment regimen for depression (especially medication) to prevent recurrence
> Teaching about specific antidepressant side effects
> Ensuring mental-health community support, including psychiatric, nursing-home-care intervention

Education is paramount to the success of all treatment programs for depression (Halverson & Bienenfield, 2015; Saver, Van-Nguyen, Keppel, & Doescher, 2007). Depressed patients in all phases of treatment need to understand the biological and psychological indicators for depression associated with chronic illness and aging. A comprehensive education program provided by the nurse should encompass the beliefs that older adults are self-aware, are dynamic, and use patterns of thought based on long-lived experiences to analyze, decide, and act on treatment recommendations. It is essential for nurses to understand and incorporate each patient's enduring patterns of living to enhance treatment outcomes, improve life satisfaction, and promote adaptation to changes associated with illness and aging. Using this knowledge will greatly assist nurses in helping patients assimilate depression care into their unique frameworks for optimal quality of life.

Suicide

Older adults who are experiencing major depression are at risk for suicide. *Suicide* is defined as taking one's own life. An older person may be at risk for harm to self, which can lead to immediate or hastened death. Thoughts of death and ways to hasten death or even commit suicide are among the most serious symptoms of depression. Many depressed individuals want to die or feel extreme worthlessness and feel they should die. Fifteen percent of untreated depressed older adults end their own life by suicide. Men over the age of 70 have the highest rate of completed suicides (Merck Manual—Home Health Handbook, 2008b; Merck Manual Professional Version, 2015).

A suicide threat is an emergency situation and requires immediate action. It is imperative that the nurse recognizes suicidal ideation and seeks prompt intervention. When an older person presents with severe symptoms of depression, expresses thoughts of being better off dead, or threatens to kill him/herself, the individual may require hospitalization. This will provide supervision of the person until treatment reduces depression and the risk of suicide. The risk of an older person committing suicide is especially high in the following situations:

> When depression is not treated or is inadequately treated
> After initially beginning treatment (when an individual is becoming more active mentally and physically but their mood is still extremely sad)
> When people continue to feel excessively sad even while returning to normal routine and activities
> When the person has a significant anniversary such as the death of a spouse or during a holiday season
> When an individual alternates between depression and mania (bipolar disorder)
> When the person feels very anxious
> When an individual is drinking alcohol or taking recreational or illicit drugs

Assessing Suicidal Risks

When assessing an older person's risk for suicide (**Box 14-3**), the nurse must determine if the patient has developed a plan. It is essential to directly ask the person if the individual has thought about what it would be like to be dead or if he/she has thoughts of killing him/herself, and, if so, have they thought about how they would accomplish this (see Case Study 14-2). If the person has developed a plan, this is an emergent situation and the nurse should assist in getting the person immediate help.

Suicidal behavior may include three main types of self-destructive acts: completed suicide, attempted suicide, and suicide gestures. Thoughts and plans related to suicide are called *suicidal ideation*. Suicidal behavior includes the following:

> Completed suicide: Intentional acts of self-harm that result in death
>   • Overmedicating self
>   • Omitting medications
>   • Lifestyle choices that lead to worsening of health, which could lead to death
>   • Overt suicidal maneuvers such as shooting self with a gun or cutting self with a sharp object
> Attempted suicide: Acts of self-harm that are intended to result in death but do not. Frequently, many older persons who attempt suicide may have some ambivalence about wishing to die and the behaviors may be a cry for help.
> Suicide gesture: Acts of self-harm that are unlikely to result in death. For example, people may scratch their wrists only superficially or take an overdose of vitamins.

BOX 14-3   Risk Factors for Suicide

- Over age 65 years of age
- Male
- Painful or disabling illness
- Living alone
- Perceived or real perception of inability to afford living expenses, medications, or other healthcare costs; debt or poverty
- Bereavement or loss
- Humiliation or disgrace
- Depression, especially when accompanied by psychosis or anxiety
- Persistent sadness even when other symptoms of depression are lessening

- A history of drug or alcohol abuse
- A history of prior suicide attempts
- A history of suicide in family members
- Traumatic childhood experiences, including physical or sexual abuse
- Preoccupation with and talk about suicide
- Well-defined plans for suicide

Modified from Merck Manual—Home Health Handbook (2008b). Suicidal behavior. Retrieved from http://www.merckmanuals.com/home /mental_health_disorders/suicidal_behavior /suicidal_behavior.html

For successful or completed suicides, guns are most frequently used by both men (74%) and women (31%). The next most common methods include hanging for men and drug overdose for women.

CLINICAL TIP

White males over the age of 85 still comprise the highest group for suicide. They may visit their primary care provided (PCP) within a month prior to the suicide, not reveal their suicidal ideations, not leave a note for family members, and use a more lethal means. Men in this age group warrant specific attention to mental health issues.

The nurse should report any suicidal-type behaviors to the patient's primary healthcare provider, who may hospitalize the individual. Sometimes an older adult will not agree to hospitalization; in most states, a physician is allowed to hospitalize certain individuals against their wishes if they are at believed to be at high risk of harming themselves or others (Merck Manual—Home Health Handbook, 2008b; Merck Manual Professional Version, 2015).

Suicide Prevention

Any older person who presents with threatening suicide or attempts at suicide should be taken very seriously, and these behaviors regarded as a plea for help. If a threat or attempt is ignored, there is risk that a life may be lost. Once an older person is determined to have a high potential for suicide, help should be sought immediately and care should be taken to engage the individual by speaking in a calm, supportive manner while waiting for emergency interventional care (see **Case Study 14-2**).

Case Study 14–2

Mr. B is a 72-year-old male whose wife died 6 months ago. He presents to his healthcare provider's clinic for routine examination having lost 15 pounds since his last visit 1 year ago (he denies trying to lose weight). He states he lives by himself since his children live out-of-town. He states he doesn't like to cook because "it is so hard to make a meal for just one person." He looks at his feet and does not make eye contact. Mr. B states it has become really hard to keep going since he lost "the love of his life." The nurse is extremely concerned, as Mr. B is exhibiting signs of thoughts of suicide. The next step was to ask Mr. B if he had thought about dying; he states "Everyone would be better off if I were not around." The nurse asks if Mr. B had thought about hurting himself or killing himself; he states that he has. The nurse next asks Mr. B if he has thought about how he would accomplish this. Mr. B states that he owns a gun and has been contemplating about shooting himself. The nurse initiates an emergency plan to have Mr. B admitted to the hospital for emergency treatment since he has a concrete plan to commit suicide and knows that elderly males who attempt suicide are often successful in accomplishing their goal of death. Mr. B is placed on paroxetine (Paxil) [an antidepressant] and is treated by a psychiatrist with individual as well as group therapy sessions. After 10 days of in-hospital management in a Geriatric-Psychiatric unit, he is discharged to live with his daughter and close supervision. Mr. B is still sad but his suicidal ideation has diminished and he is slowly improving. The nurse in this case saved Mr. B's life.

An attempt should be made to develop a rapport with the individual by discovering common interests and repeatedly using their name in conversation. Allow the suicidal person to discuss their feelings and worries and, if appropriate, offer constructive suggestions for solving the problem that brought on the crisis. Remind the individual of loved ones who care about him or her and reinforce his or her value and importance to others. Finally, the nurse must ensure that the at-risk individual receives face-to-face interventional help as quickly as possible (Merck Manual—Home Health Handbook, 2008b; Merck Manual Professional Version, 2015). **Box 14-4** provides additional resources for nurses assisting persons with depression and anxiety.

Summary

Depression and anxiety are common among older adults, particularly those with limited social support or resources. Geriatric nurses play a role in examining all aspects of an older patient, including his or her mental and emotional health, to make appropriate referrals for treatment (**Box 14-5**). Early recognition and intervention for anxiety and depression can improve quality of life and help prevent unnecessary complications.

BOX 14-4   Recommended Resources

ConsultGeriRN: Provides free resources, including assessment instruments and specialty nursing web links (http://www.consultgerirn.org)

Try This: Best practices in nursing care to the older adult. Offers assessment tools on a variety of topics relevant to the care of older adults. The *How to Try This* series comprises articles and videos presenting cases studies. (http://www.hartfordign.org)

Help Guide—Depression in Older Adults and the Elderly: Offers ways to recognize the signs and find treatment that works (http://www.helpguide.org/articles/depression/depression-in-older-adults-and-the-elderly.htm)

Anxiety Disorders Association of America (ADAA): Has as its mission to promote the prevention, treatment, and cure of anxiety, depression, and stress-related disorders through education, practice, and research. Excellent Website for resources about understanding anxiety disorders and treatment strategies. (http://www.adaa.org)

My Mental Health Medication Workbook by Fran Miller RN, MSN, BC: Offers patients an excellent interactive resource for understanding their mental illness and medication treatment. Provides information for a wide variety of mental illnesses. Published by PESI, LLC, Eau Claire, WI

Nursing Standard of Practice Protocol: Depression: A resource for evidence-based and authoritative information about nursing care of older adults. ConsultGeriRN.org is the geriatric clinical nursing Website of the Hartford Institute for Geriatric Nursing (HIGN), New York University College of Nursing. ConsultGeriRN.org is an evidence-based online resource for nurses in clinical and educational settings. ConsultGeriRN.org is funded in part by a grant from The Atlantic Philanthropies (USA) Inc. and The John A. Hartford Foundation. https://consultgeri.org/geriatric-topics/depression

Personal Health Questionnaire-9: Screening tool for depression and how to interpret the results. http://www.cqaimh.org/pdf/tool_phq9.pdf

Try This Series: GDS: Screening tool for depression. https://consultgeri.org/try-this/general-assessment/issue-4

BOX 14-5   Research Highlight

Fear of falling is a reality for many older adults. Painter, Allison, Dhingra, Daughtery, Cogdill, and Trujillo sought to acquire a deeper understanding of this fear and its relationship to anxiety, activity levels, and depression. Sign into your database of nursing literature (CINAHL or PubMed, for example) and use the citation below to perform a search for this article. What did this research team find? What was the conclusion of this study, and how does it impact care of the older adult?

Painter, J. A., Allison, L., Dhingra, P., Daughtery, J., Cogdill, K., & Trujillo, L. (2012). Fear of falling and its relationship with anxiety, depression, and activity engagement among community-dwelling older adults. *American Journal of Occupational Therapy, 66*(2), 169–176.

Clinical Reasoning Exercises

1. Mrs. Simmons, a 72-year-old widow living alone in her home, was recently admitted to the hospital after falling and fracturing her hip in her driveway. She underwent surgery to repair her hip fracture and was admitted to a nursing home for rehabilitation and gait training. She complains of not being able to sleep. She is not doing well in her rehabilitation—she states "I am afraid I am going to fall again." Should this be considered a problem? What additional information is needed to determine if changes should be made in her plan of care? What evidence can the nurse provide to Mrs. Simmons to support the need for further evaluation and treatment?

2. Mr. Brown is a 75-year-old man whose wife recently died of cancer. He presents to the emergency department with his daughter, who is concerned about his loss of 10 pounds since his wife's death. He does not make eye contact and appears to be in dirty clothes, the buttons on his shirt are not buttoned correctly, and he presents with poor hygiene. He states that his kids would be better off if he were no longer around. Is this an emergent situation? What is the most important information to attain from this patient? What other information is necessary to determine an appropriate plan of care? How can the nurse provide the support this patient requires?

Personal Reflections

1. You are involved in a motor vehicle accident. You awaken in the intensive care unit with both of your arms restrained. Discuss your emotions. What would you want the nursing staff to say or do?

2. Place the radio on a station, then set the dial where the station is not clear—there is a lot of background static and it is difficult to hear the announcer. Attempt to make a call or carry on a conversation with someone. Would you feel nervous? Would you be able to maintain the conversation? How does this experience affect your mood?

3. You present at an outpatient clinic where you are an established patient, to be seen for a routine follow-up visit. You are being assessed

by the nurse before being seen by your nurse practitioner. The nurse asks you how you are doing after the recent death of your spouse. You begin to cry. How would you want the nurse to respond? Would you feel comfortable being screened for depression at this time? Would you want to be educated about your risks for depression during this visit?

4. You are an older adult, living alone, and are aware that you are depressed. You have

had recent thoughts of suicide but have not made a plan to carry out the act yet. You are despondent and lacking energy to engage in any ADL. A home health nurse comes to your home for a visit. What interactions, assessments, and plan of care would be necessary for the nurse to engage in to keep you from carrying out a suicide plan?

References

American Psychiatric Association. (2013). *Diagnostic and statistical manual of mental disorders* (5th ed.). Washington, DC: American Psychiatric Association.

Arean, P. A., Rane, P., Mackin, R. S., Kanellopoulos, D., McCulloch, C., & Alexopoulos, G. S. (2010). Problem-solving therapy and supportive therapy in older adults with major depression and executive dysfunction. *American Journal of Psychiatry, 167*(11), 1391–1398.

Auerhahn, C., Capezuti, E., Flaherty, E., & Resnick, B. (2007). *The Geriatric nursing review syllabus.* New York, NY: American Geriatric Society.

Byatt, N., & Lundquist, R. (2012). Use of atypical antidepressants in elderly patients. Abhazia: Institute for Social and Economic Research. Retrieved from http://www.abkhazia.com/research-blogs/health/74-Therapeutic-Specialties/980-use-of-atypical-antidepressants-in-elderly-patients

Byrd, L. (2011). *Caregiver survival 101: Strategies to manage problematic behaviors in individuals with dementia.* Eau Claire, WI: PESI Publishing.

Camus, V., Kraehenbuhl, H., Preisig, M., Bula, C. J., & Waeber, G. (2004). Geriatric depression and vascular diseases: What are the links? *Journal of Affective Disorders, 81,* 1–16.

Cassidy, K., & Rector, N. (2008). The silent geriatric giant: Anxiety disorders in late life. *Geriatrics and Aging, 11*(3), 150–156.

Centers for Disease Control & Chronic Disease Prevention and Health Promotion. (2011). Healthy aging: Helping people to live long and productive lives and enjoy a good quality of life. Retrieved from http://www.aarp.org/content/dam/aarp/livable-communities/learn/health/Healthy-Aging-Helping-People-to-Live-Long-and-Productive-Lives-and-Enjoy-a-Good-Quality-of-Life-2011-AARP.pdf

Centers for Disease Control and Prevention. (2015). Healthy aging: Depression is not a normal part of growing older. Retrieved from http://www.cdc.gov/aging/mentalhealth/depression.htm

Centers for Medicaid and Medicare Services. (2016). Annual wellness visit benefits. Retrieved from https://www.cms.gov/Outreach-and-Education/Medicare-Learning-Network-MLN/MLNProducts/downloads/AWV_chart_ICN905706.pdf

Dotson, V. M., Beydoun, M. A., & Zonderman, A. B. (2010). Recurrent depressive symptoms and the incidence of dementia and mild cognitive impairment. *Neurology, 75*(1), 27–34.

Drugs.com. (2015). Retrieved from http://www.drugs.com/drug_information.html

Ebersole, P., Hess, P., Touhy, T., Jett, K., & Schmidt-Luggen, A. (2008). *Toward healthy aging: Human needs & nursing response* (7th ed.). St. Louis, MO: Mosby.

Fiske, A., Wetherell, J., & Gatz, M. (2009). Depression in older adults. *Annual Review of Clinical Psychology, 5,* 363–389.

Friedman, M., Furst, L., Gellis, Z., & Williams, K. (2013). Anxiety disorders in older adults. *Social Work Today, 13*(4), 10. Retrieved from http://www.socialworktoday.com/archive/070813p10.shtml

Goveas, J. S., Espeland, M. A., Woods, N. F., Wassertheil-Smoller, S., & Kotchen, J. M. (2011). Depressive symptoms and incidence of mild cognitive impairment and probable dementia in elderly women: The women's health initiative memory study. *Journal of the American Geriatrics Society, 59*(1), 57–66.

Grohol, J. M. (2012). Symptoms and treatments of mental disorders. *PsychCentral.* Retrieved from http://psychcentral.com/disorders/

Halverson, J., & Bienenfeld, D. (2015). Depression treatment and management. *Medscape.* Retrieved from http://emedicine.medscape.com/article/286759-treatment

Helpguide.org (2016). Depression in women: Causes, symptoms, and treatment. Retrieved from https://www.helpguide.org/articles/depression/depression-in-women.htm

Kaduszkiewicz, H., Eisele, M., Wiese, B., Prokein, J., Luppa, M., Luck, T., . . . Riedel-Heller, S. (2014). Prognosis of mild cognitive impairment in general practice: Results of the German AgeCoDe Study. *Annals of Family Medicine, 12*(2), 158–165.

Kiosses, D., Rosenburg, P., McGovern, A., Fonzetti, P., Zaydens, H., & Alexopoulos, G. (2015). Depression and suicide ideation during two psychosocial treatments in older adults with major depression and dementia. *Journal of Alzheimer's Disease, 48*(2), 453–462.

Kurlowicz, L., & Harvath, T. (2008). Nursing standard of practice protocol: Depression in older adults. *ConsultGeriRN.org: Hartford Institute for Geriatric Nursing.* Retrieved from https://www.guideline.gov/summaries/summary/43922/depression-in-older-adults-in-evidencebased-geriatric-nursing-protocols-for-best-practice

Lee, Y., & Chen, P. (2010). A review of SSRIs and SNRIs in neuropathic pain. *Expert Opinion in Pharmacotherapy. 17,* 2813–2825.

Low, G. D., & Hubley, A. M. (2007). Screening for depression after cardiac events using the Beck Depression Inventory II and Geriatric Depression scale. *Social Indicators Research, 82*(3), 527–543.

Lundbeck Institute CNS Forum. (2012). *The mechanism of action of specific 5-HT re-uptake inhibitors.* Retrieved from http://www.cnsforum.com/imagebank/item/Drug_SSRI_2/default.aspx

Lyness, J. M. (2012). Clinical manifestations and diagnosis of depression. *UpToDate.* Retrieved from http://www.uptodate.com/contents/clinical-manifestations-and-diagnosis-of-depression

MacArthur Initiative on Depression and Primary Care. (2009). Retrieved from http://www.depression-primarycare.org/clinicians/toolkits/

Martin-Plank, L. (2014). Psychological disorders. In L. Kennedy-Malone, K. R. Fletcher, & L. Martin-Plank (Eds.), *Advanced practice nursing in the care of older adults.* (pp. 545–600). Philadelphia, PA: F. A. Davis.

Merck Manual of Geriatrics Online. (2012). *Overview of anxiety disorders.* Retrieved from http://www.merckmanuals.com/professional/psychiatric_disorders/anxiety_disorders/overview_of_anxiety_disorders.html

Merck Manual—Home Health Handbook. (2008a). Depression. Retrieved from http://www.merckmanuals.com/home/mental_health_disorders/mood_disorders/depression.html

Merck Manual—Home Health Handbook (2008b). Suicidal behavior. Retrieved from http://www.merckmanuals.com/home/mental_health_disorders/suicidal_behavior/suicidal_behavior.html

Merck Manual Professional Version. (2015). Online resource. Retrieved from http://www.merckmanuals.com/professional

Murphy S. L., Jiaquan, X., & Kochanek, K. D. (2012). Deaths: Preliminary data for 2010. *National Vital Statistics Reports, 60*(4), 1–68.

National Institutes of Mental Health. (n.d.). Suicide. Retrieved from https://www.nimh.nih.gov/health/statistics/suicide/index.shtml

Older Americans. (2010). Key indicators of well-being. Federal Interagency Forum on Aging-Related Statistics. Retrieved from https://agingstats.gov/docs/PastReports/2010/OA2010.pdf

Painter, J. A., Allison, L., Dhingra, P., Daughtery, J., Cogdill, K., & Trujillo, L. (2012). Fear of falling and its relationship with anxiety, depression, and activity engagement among community-dwelling older adults. *American Journal of Occupational Therapy, 66*(2), 169–176.

Petersen, R. C., Roberts, R. O., Knopman, D. S., Geda, Y. E., Cha, R. H., Pankratz, V. S., . . . Rocca, W. A. (2008). Prevalence of mild cognitive impairment is higher in men: The Mayo Clinic Study of Aging. *Neurology, 75*(10), 889–897.

Saver, B. G., Van-Nguyen, V., Keppel, G., & Doescher, M. P. (2007). A qualitative study of depression in primary care: Missed opportunities for diagnosis and education. *Journal of the American Board of Family Medicine, 20*(1), 28–35.

Seitz, D., Purandare, N., & Conn, D. (2010). Prevalence of psychiatric disorders among older adults in long-term care homes: A systematic review. *International Psychogeriatrics, 22*(7), 1025–1039.

Shah, R. (2012). Major types of anxiety neuroses. Retrieved from http://www.anxietyneurosis.com/app/types.asp

Sheikh, J. I., & Yesavage, J. A. (1986). Geriatric Depression Scale (GDS): Recent evidence and development of a shorter version. In T. L. Brink (Ed.), *Clinical gerontology: A guide to assessment and intervention* (pp. 165–173). New York, NY: The Haworth Press.

Spitzer, R., Kroenke, K., & Williams, J. (1999). Validation and utility of a self-report version of PRIME-MD: The PHQ Primary Care Study. *Journal of the American Medical Association, 282*(18), 1737–1744.

Soriano, R. P. (2007). Depression, dementia, and delirium. In R. P. Soriano, H. M. Fernandez, C. K. Cassell, & R. M. Leipzig (Eds.), *Fundamentals of geriatric medicine: A case based approach.* New York, NY: Springer.

Sozeri-Varma, G. (2012). Depression in the Elderly: Clinical features and Risk Factors, *Aging and Disease, 3*(6), 465–471.

Su, X., Shang, L., Xu, Q., Li, N., Chen, J., Zhang, L., . . . Hua, Q. (2014). Prevalence and predictors of mild cognitive impairment in Xi'an: A community-based study among the elders. *PLOS One, 9*(1).

Substance Abuse and Mental Health Services Administration. (2011). *The treatment of depression in older adults: Depression and older adults: Key issues.* HHS Pub. No. SMA-11-4631, Rockville, MD: Center for Mental Health Services, Substance Abuse and Mental Health Services Administration, U.S. Department of Health and Human Services

Touhy, T., & Jett, K. (2014). Mental health. In *Ebersole and Hess' gerontological nursing & healthy aging* (4th ed., pp. 336–353). St. Louis, MO: Mosby.

Trevisan, L. (2015). Update on geriatric depression and anxiety. *Psychiatric Times.* Retrieved from http://www.psychiatrictimes.com/apa-2015-MDD/update-geriatric-depression-and-anxiety

Vink, D., Aartsen, M. J., & Schoevers, R. A. (2008). Risk factors for anxiety and depression in the elderly: A review. *Journal of Affective Disorders, 106*(1–2), 29–44.

Weise, B. (2011). Geriatric depression: The use of antidepressants in the elderly. *BC Medical Journal, 53*(7), 341–347.

For a full suite of assignments and additional learning activities, see the access code at the front of your book.

CHAPTER 15

Urinary Incontinence

B. Renee Dugger

(Competencies 7, 17)

LEARNING OBJECTIVES

At the end of this chapter, the reader will be able to:

> Describe the prevalence of urinary incontinence among older adults in community, acute care, and long-term care settings.
> Identify the negative social, psychological, physical, and economic implications of urinary incontinence.
> Understand that urinary incontinence is not a normal part of aging.
> Collect the appropriate data related to patients' urine control and plan evidence-based nursing care accordingly.
> Initiate evidence-based behavioral interventions to treat urinary incontinence and promote continence for those at risk for urinary incontinence.

KEY TERMS

Bladder diary
Bladder training
Established (chronic) incontinence
Functional urinary incontinence
Mixed urinary incontinence
Nocturia
Overflow urinary incontinence

Pelvic floor muscle exercises
Pelvic muscle rehabilitation
Prompted voiding
Stress urinary incontinence
Transient (acute) urinary incontinence
Urge suppression techniques
Urge urinary incontinence

Urinary incontinence (UI) is a common problem of the elderly and has tremendous impact on both the morbidity and quality of life of older adults (Godfrey, 2008; Ko, Lin, Salmon, & Bron, 2005; Teunissen, Van Den Bosch, Van Weel, & Lagro-Janssen, 2006). It is often associated with aging, being female, and particularly as a sequela to bearing children. Other contributory factors of UI include urinary retention, urinary tract infection (UTI), fecal impaction, diseases such as diabetes and Parkinson's disease, and certain classes of medications such as anticholinergics and narcotics (Newman, Gaines, & Snare, 2005; Qaseem et al., 2014; Wooldridge, 2000). Although UI may be a common problem, it is not a normal part of aging and requires evaluation.

UI, defined as the involuntary leakage of urine to a degree that it is troubling to the person, is a common health problem that affects more than 17 million Americans (Dowling-Castronovo & Bradway, 2008; Godfrey, 2008). This condition may exist in a variety of forms, including stress, urge, mixed, overflow, and functional UI (Dowling-Castronovo & Bradway, 2008; Godfrey, 2008). However, approximately 80% of adults with UI can experience significant improvement or resolution of their symptoms with evaluation and treatment (Lucas et al., 2012; Newman, Burgio, Markland, & Goode, 2014). The barrier to realization of UI improvement often is a failure of healthcare providers to (1) identify those with continence problems, (2) conduct a comprehensive assessment, and (3) initiate targeted interventions to address causes and contributing factors. Professional nursing has the knowledge, skills, opportunity, and responsibility to provide aspects of continence care such as screening patients, performing basic evaluation, and initiating treatment or referring patients to a specialist, if indicated (Dowling-Castronovo & Bradway, 2008; Newman et al., 2014).

Prevalence

UI affects men and women of all ages, at all levels of health, in all settings. Prevalence estimates vary widely, primarily due to differences in the definition of incontinence, the population studied, sampling approaches, and data collection methods (Godfrey, 2008). An estimated 10% to 15% of the total population will have UI (Milsom et al., 2014). Between 30% and 40% of community-dwelling middle-aged women experience UI, with prevalence increasing with age (Hunskaar et al., 2002). Among older women, prevalence is estimated at 13% to 46%, depending on the study (Faiena, Patel, Parihar, Calabrese, & Tunuguntla, 2015). Prevalence rates in community-dwelling men have a similar pattern, although the rates are lower, ranging from 1% to 5% in middle-aged men, and increasing to 9% to 28% in older men (Hunskaar et al., 2002).

The percentage of hospitalized elders expected to have UI is 35% (Dowling-Castronovo & Bradway, 2012), and more than 70% of residents in long-term care settings experience this condition (Lekan-Rutledge, 2004; McCliment, 2002; Newman et al., 2005; Palmer, 2008; Sparks, Boyer, Gambrel, & Lovett, 2004). A National Institutes of Health (NIH) consensus and state-of-the-science paper places the prevalence of UI in nursing homes at 60% to 78% for women and 45% to 72% for men (Landefeld et al., 2008).

Although UI is not a normal consequence of aging, certain physiological changes that accompany aging increase the risk for voiding problems, and certain conditions that predispose to continence problems are more likely to occur in older persons. The reader can find information about normal aging changes in the urinary system and their significance in the older adult in Chapter 4.

Implications of Urinary Incontinence
Physical, Psychological, and Social Implications

The vast majority of incontinent persons in the community do not seek help for their incontinence because they consider it a normal part of aging (McIntosh, Andersen, & Reekie, 2015; Newman et al., 2014). However, it is clear that as the degree of incontinence increases, the negative impact on lifestyle and social isolation also increases. It is likely that the total UI impact picture is unknown, because community-dwelling people with UI keep it to themselves and simply stay home.

Depression and anxiety are potential causes and consequences of incontinence (Coyne et al., 2012; Dugan et al., 2000; Hajjar, 2004; Heidrich & Wells, 2004). Relationships, activities of daily living (ADLs), socialization, and self-concept are affected by UI (Godfrey & Hogg, 2007). UI increases the risk of hospitalization and substantially increases the risk of admission to nursing homes in persons over 65 (Dowling-Castronovo & Bradway, 2012; Newman et al., 2005). Urge incontinence occurring at least weekly is associated with increased fall risk and nonspine, nontraumatic fractures in community-dwelling women age 65 years or older (Brown et al., 2000). Studies have repeatedly shown a negative impact on quality of life when elderly persons experience UI (Coyne et al., 2012; DuBeau, 2005; DuBeau et al., 2006; Ko et al., 2005; Teunissen et al., 2006). Sitoh et al. (2005) found from their research with elderly persons that the following conditions were most detrimental to health-related quality of life: "degree of frailty, . . . history of strokes, diagnosis of Parkinson's disease, previous falls or fractures and the presence of urinary incontinence" (p. 132). The International Continence Society recommended that any study involving UI should include assessing and measuring quality of life (Robinson & Shea, 2002).

Elderly persons who experience UI often suffer from physical and psychological distress. Some of the negative physical outcomes include dermatitis and possible skin ulceration, disruption of sleep patterns, UTIs and falls, which can lead to fractures (Doughty et al., 2012; Jacobson & Wright, 2015; Lekan-Rutledge, 2004; Newman et al., 2005; Wooldridge, 2000). Common psychological issues as a result of UI include feelings of loss of control, dependency, shame and guilt, social isolation, avoidance of activities, anxiety, impaired self-esteem, and depression (Bradway, 2003; DuBeau et al., 2006; Ko et al., 2005; MacDonald & Butler, 2007; Teunissen et al., 2006) (see **Box 15-1**).

BOX 15-1   Research Highlight

Aim: An aspect of this pre–post quasi-experimental prospective design study was examination of urinary incontinence (UI) impact on nursing home residents' health-related quality of life.

Method: A multidisciplinary team conducted a study in four Midwestern nursing homes with 33 nursing home residents. The team examined the residents' health-related quality of life utilizing the Incontinence Stress Questionnaire for Patients (ISQ-P) instrument before and after interventions. The interventions included staff education and bladder scanner placement in each nursing home.

Findings: Figure 15-1 depicts relationships found between the following ISQ-P instrument variables (*try to hide UI from others, am worried about urine leakage, urine smell causes me to avoid others, having bedsores because of it*, and *keep myself clean*) with two additional ISQ-P variables (*am a burden to others* and *blue or*

depressed). Calculation of Pearson correlation coefficient showed a strong positive correlation, suggesting a linear relationship between the first five variables culminating in feelings of being a burden and depression. These residents had an increased ISQ-P stress score leading to an assumption of decreased health-related quality of life (Coudret et al., 2009). During the interview process, residents made the statements shown in **Table 15-1** about their UI experience.

Application to practice: The relationships identified among the ISQ-P instrument variables show the residents with UI experience feelings of being a burden and depression. The resident comments captured in Box 15-2 also point to considerable stress and psychological pain. These findings give additional credence to the importance of caregiver sensitivity to these feelings and proper UI assessment and management to preserve or improve resident health-related quality of life.

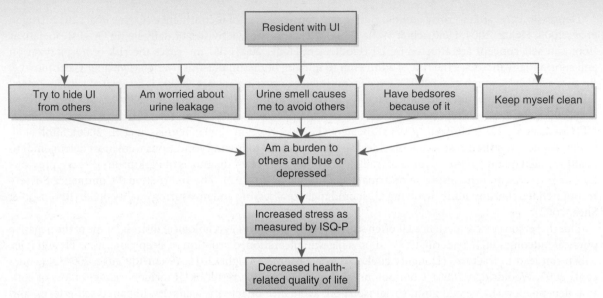

UI = Urinary incontinence   ISQ-P = Incontinence stress questionnaire for patients

Figure 15-1 Model of relationships of ISQ-P variables and resident health-related quality of life based on ISQ-P instrument.

Reproduced from Coudret, N., Ehlman, K., Dugger, R., Eggleston, B., Wilson, A., Harrison, E., & Mathis, S. (2009). *Assessing the benefits of bladder ultrasound scanners in nursing homes: Project funded by the Indiana State Department of Health-Final Report*. Unpublished manuscript, Evansville, IN: College of Nursing and Health Professions, University of Southern Indiana.

TABLE 15-1   Comments from Nursing Home Residents during Interviews

- I get used to it and it doesn't bother me most of the time.
- It's inconvenient.
- I can't help it.
- This condition is the reason I am in the nursing home.
- I just accept it.
- I don't talk about it much.
- I don't want to see it or anybody else to see it.
- I felt everything was taken away. It's sad.
- I feel like a pest if I have to keep calling.
- Not too many people like talking about that.
- I have irritation all the time but nobody does nothing.

Comments from Nursing Home Residents about the Variable I Cry When I Think or Talk about the Incontinence

- I want to, but I can't.
- I feel that is something a person can't help.
- I do it softly.
- Inside when I'm alone.
- I am past that.

Reproduced from Coudret, N., Ehlman, K., Dugger, R., Eggleston, B., Wilson, A., Harrison, E. & Mathis, S. (2009). *Assessing the benefits of bladder ultrasound scanners in nursing homes: Project funded by the Indiana State Department of Health—Final Report*. Unpublished manuscript, Evansville, IN: College of Nursing and Health Professions, University of Southern Indiana.

Economic Implications

UI carries a significant economic impact. The costs associated with UI management often are not covered by insurance and become an out-of-pocket expense (Coyne et al., 2014; Milsom et al., 2014; Wilson, Brown, Shin, Luc, & Subak, 2001). These expenses can interfere with the ability of persons on a fixed income to purchase medications and supplies to manage other health problems. In the United States, the direct costs associated with UI run as high $16 billion per year (Landefeld et al., 2008).

In addition to the adverse outcomes of UI for the nursing home resident, there are negative and costly effects for the nursing home facility as well. Estimated costs of UI care run as high as $5.2 billion annually for nursing homes in the United States (Frenchman, 2001; Landefeld et al., 2008). The cost of UI containment includes pads (both disposable and reusable), diapers, briefs, gloves, laundry products, and catheters, not to mention the time required by staff to provide care.

Frenchman (2001) estimated UI labor and materials costs as $17.21 per nursing home resident per day when examining two facilities in New Jersey. This resulted in over $6,200 of expense tied to UI per year per resident. Estimates are that 3% to 8% of nursing home costs and as much as 1 hour per day go toward each resident's incontinence care (Hu et al., 2004). The financial impact is even greater if residents experience falls, fractures, and pressure ulcers (Newman et al., 2005; Wooldridge, 2000). Wooldridge (2000) estimates institutions spend approximately $680 for each episode of UTI.

Assessment of Urinary Incontinence

An understanding of the types of incontinence and the factors associated with incontinence is necessary to guide evaluation and the development of appropriate targeted interventions. UI is categorized as *transient (acute)* or *established (chronic)* based on onset and etiology. Transient or acute incontinence is caused by the onset of an acute problem that once successfully treated should result in the resolution of incontinence. However, if transient UI is not appropriately assessed and managed in a timely manner, it can become established or chronic UI, which is much more difficult to treat.

Multiple causative and contributory factors have been associated with the development or exacerbation of voiding problems, in particular UI (Dowling-Castronovo, 2007). These causative factors include **d**elirium/**d**ementia, **i**nfection, **a**trophic vaginitis/urethritis, **p**sychological, **p**harmaceutical, **e**xcessive urine output, **r**estricted mobility, and **s**tool impaction and are identified by the mnemonic DIAPPERS (Resnick & Yalla, 1985). Delirium and dementia can interfere with the ability to recognize the need for toileting. A UTI can result in urinary frequency and urgency. Atrophic vaginitis and urethritis resulting from decreased estrogen causes thin, dry, friable vaginal and urethral mucosa. Psychological issues, especially depression, can interfere with the motivation to perform ADLs and attention to continence. Any pharmaceutical agent that affects bladder function or cognitive status change can contribute to UI. Pharmaceuticals such as narcotics can lead to constipation and stool impaction, which obstruct the bladder neck, leading to urine retention, overflow incontinence, and urgency. Narcotics also decrease bladder muscle contraction, resulting in urine retention and incomplete bladder emptying, which increases the risk of UTI. Excessive urine output resulting from hyperglycemia, hypercalcemia, hypoalbuminemia, and heart failure increase the risk of urge and stress UI. Restricted mobility interferes with the ability to reach the toilet in time to prevent leakage. The major types of UI include *stress*, *urge*, *mixed*, *overflow*, and *functional incontinence*. Information about these five major types of UI along with their characteristics are located in **Table 15-2** with a mnemonic as a memory aid.

Diagnosis of the type(s) of UI experienced is essential in the development of appropriate interventions. These interventions should be designed to address the varying levels of cognitive and physical functioning of the patient. The elements of a basic evaluation of UI are outlined in **Table 15-3** and discussed in greater detail below with respect to the older patient.

TABLE 15-2   Urinary Incontinence Types and Characteristics

The mnemonic SUMO-FUN is utilized to assist with remembering the major UI types (Mathis, Ehlman, Dugger, Harrawood, & Kraft, 2013).

Urinary Incontinence Type	Characteristics
Stress Incontinence	Involuntary loss of urine during activities that increase intraabdominal pressure (e.g., lifting, coughing, sneezing, and laughing). Bladder contractions and overdistention are absent. Hypermobility of the bladder neck and urethral sphincter defects are common causes. Weakness of the pelvic floor muscles leads to loss of support to the bladder neck, which disrupts the normal pressure gradient between the bladder and urethra and urine leakage.
Urge Incontinence	Strong, abrupt desire to void and the inability to inhibit leakage in time to reach a toilet. Uninhibited bladder contractions usually are a precipitating factor. Central nervous system disorders, such as stroke or multiple sclerosis, bladder infection, and caffeine ingestion are potential causes.
Mixed Incontinence	Presence of stress and urge incontinence
Overflow Incontinence	Overdistention of the bladder due to abnormal emptying. The leakage may be continuous or resemble that in stress or urge incontinence. Associated with diabetes, spinal cord injury below T10-11, and obstruction of the urethra, often due to an enlarged prostate gland.
FUNctional Incontinence	Results from problems external to the lower urinary tract, such as cognitive impairment, physical disability, and environmental barriers.

Reproduced from Mathis, S., Ehlman, K., Dugger, B. R., Harrawood, A., & Kraft, C. M. (2013). Bladder buzz: The effect of a 6-week evidence-based staff education program on knowledge and attitudes regarding urinary incontinence in a nursing home. *The Journal of Continuing Education in Nursing, 44*(11), 498–506. Reprinted with permission of SLACK Incorporated.

TABLE 15-3   Components of a Basic Evaluation for Urinary Incontinence

History
- Focused medical, neurologic, and genitourinary history
- Risk factor assessment
- Medication review
- Detailed exploration of incontinence symptoms

Physical examination
- General examination
- Abdominal examination
- Rectal examination
- Pelvic examination in women
- Genital examination in men

Postvoided residual volume

Urinalysis

Data from Dowling-Castronova, A., & Bradway, C. (2007). *Assessment and management of older adults with urinary incontinence.* [white paper]. Presented at The National Gerontological Nursing Association and American Association of Colleges of Nursing Conference in St. Louis, MO in October 2008.

Data Gathering

History and Other Pertinent Data

The first evaluation step is a discussion of voiding patterns and problems. Initiating questions focusing on usual number of voids during the day and night, as well as symptoms such as burning, hesitancy, pain, or low pelvic pressure, provides a less-threatening opening to this topic. It may be necessary to reword questions about the presence of incontinence to determine the occurrence of wetting accidents, their frequency, and volume of urine lost. Asking about the use of padding or protective garments may provide important clues to the presence of incontinence or the fear of an accident. Gather information about voiding problems onset and duration and activities that precipitate or are associated with their occurrence. Of particular relevance is determining bowel function status and usual bowel habits, because constipation and fecal impaction can precipitate UI.

A recall of daily food and fluid intake also provides important information about urological functioning and aids in treatment plan development. It is typical for patients with urgency and urge incontinence to report a fluid intake that consists primarily of bladder irritants (e.g., diet drinks, carbonated and/or caffeinated beverages) and minimal to no water.

The initial interview should help identify potentially reversible causative and contributing factors for UI. The history should provide clues to the type(s) of incontinence involved. It may be necessary for the patient to complete a detailed bladder diary (discussed in the next section, see **Figure 15-2**) over a period of 3 days to obtain a complete picture of UI-related factors.

Your Daily Bladder Diary

This diary will help you and your healthcare team. Bladder diaries show the causes of bladder control trouble. The "sample" line (below) will show you how to use the diary.

ACCIDENTS

Time	Drinks		Urine	Accidental Leaks	Did you feel a strong urge to go?	What were you doing at the time?
	How much?	What kind?	How much? Circle one	How many times? How much? Use measuring cups (ml's or oz's)	(check one)	Sneezing, exercising, having sex, lifting, etc.
Sample	2 cups	Coffee	sm (med) lg	2 oz or 2 ml	Yes No	Running
6-7 a.m.					Yes No	
7-8 a.m.					Yes No	
8-9 a.m.					Yes No	
9-10 a.m.					Yes No	
10-11 a.m.					Yes No	
11-12 noon					Yes No	
12-1 p.m.					Yes No	
1-2 p.m.					Yes No	
2-3 p.m.					Yes No	
3-4 p.m.					Yes No	
4-5 p.m.					Yes No	
5-6 p.m.					Yes No	
6-7 p.m.					Yes No	
7-8 p.m.					Yes No	
8-9 p.m.					Yes No	
9-10 p.m.					Yes No	
10-11 p.m.					Yes No	
11-12 mid					Yes No	
12-1 a.m.					Yes No	
1-2 a.m.					Yes No	
2-3 a.m.					Yes No	
3-4 a.m.					Yes No	
4-5 a.m.					Yes No	
5-6 a.m.					Yes No	

Your name:
Date:

Figure 15-2 A sample voiding diary.

BOX 15-2   Evidence-Based Practice Highlight

The UDI-6 and IIQ-7 assessment instruments and a sample bladder diary are available at: https://consultgeri.org/geriatric-topics /urinary-incontinence

These resources are part of the *Try This: Best Practices in Nursing Care to Older Adults* series

made available through the Hartford Institute for Geriatric Nursing at the http://www .ConsultgeriRN.org website. The website is an excellent source of evidence-based practice information and resources specific to multiple geriatric clinical nursing issues.

Awareness of the specific symptoms experienced and the degree of discomfort associated with each can be useful in determining the priority for intervening. Identifying those aspects of daily life that UI or the fear of UI disrupts can provide the outcomes to evaluate. For example, if UI interferes with exercise, participation in an exercise regimen three times a week might be the goal set with the patient. Once this goal is set, the nurse and patient would develop a specific plan to achieve the exercise goal.

Urinary Incontinence Interview Instruments

Interviews with persons experiencing incontinence reveal the difficulty persons experience when thinking about and discussing this very personal, private matter. The use of a tool that provides words and choices for responses frequently facilitates the exchange of information. Short form versions of the Urogenital Distress Inventory/Incontinence Impact Questionnaire (UDI/IIQ) provide objective measurement of the life impact and symptom distress, respectively, of UI and related conditions for women. With minor wording modifications of some items, the tool is appropriate for men and from hospitalization through reintegration into the community. If the patient has communication or cognitive deficits, obtain information from family members, when possible. At times, previous medical records or observation of current behaviors may be the only data source available. An instrument specific to the nursing home setting that measures stress associated with UI is the Incontinence Questionnaire for Patients (ISQ-P) (see **Box 15-2**) (Yu, 1987; Yu, Kaltreider, Hu, & Craighead, 1989).

Bladder Diary

The *bladder diary* is a critical component of a basic evaluation, regardless of the setting (Dowling-Castronovo, 2007; MayoClinic.com, 2008). By outlining the timing, amount, and type of fluid intake with the timing, amount, and continence status for each void, key UI data are collected, including severity, irritating or associated symptoms, precipitating events, and voiding problem patterns (Dowling-Castronovo, 2007). The patient should record bladder diary findings over 3 to 7 days; however, 72 hours typically provides sufficient data and is a more reasonable time frame for data collection (Doughty, 2000; Newman et al., 2014). See **Figure 15-3** for a sample bladder diary. Patients or caregivers can also collect the bladder diary data. Many times patients or informal caregivers completing these records identify patterns to the incontinence episodes and can begin to make positive changes. The bladder diary is a reliable method for assessing the frequency of voluntary voiding and UI and can be a particularly important data source to differentiate factors contributing to nocturia.

CLINICAL TIP

A bladder diary is one of the essentials tools of assessment of urinary incontinence.

Nocturia, the awakening from sleep to urinate, is a frustrating and common problem for many older persons. Nocturia may result from alterations in normal circadian rhythm of urine output, may be caused by lower urinary tract physiological changes that interfere with storage, or may indicate sleep apnea (Aristide, Weinstein, & Nair, 2013; Tyagi et al., 2014). Sleep apnea can be the root cause of nocturia in this population. Comorbidities of diabetes and hypertension greatly increase the risk of sleep apnea (Umlauf & Chasens, 2003). The serious nature of sleep apnea necessitates careful evaluation of the etiology (Aristide et al., 2013).

Cognitive Status

A client's insight into voiding status, recall of pertinent health information, and ability to participate in an interview are the first clues to cognitive status. Objective cognitive data can be obtained with the Mini-Mental State Examination (MMSE) (Folstein, Folstein, & McHugh, 1975), Mini-Cog (Borson, Scanlan, Brush, Vitallano, & Dokmak, 2000) and/or the Confusion Assessment Method (CAM) (Inouye et al., 1990; Inouye, 2006). See **Box 15-3** for additional information about the Mini-Cog and CAM assessments. The cognitive impairment severity level alerts the healthcare professional to the client's increased risk of persistent incontinence. It also guides selection of intervention options.

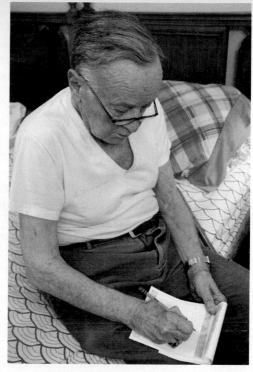

Figure 15-3 Keeping a bladder diary helps both the client and the nurse with assessment and management of UI.
© iStockphoto/Thinkstock

Physical Assessment

It is tempting to base the determination of incontinence type solely on the clinical signs and symptoms obtained during the history; however, clinical symptoms alone are not sufficient to determine the pathophysiology of voiding problems. Aspects of a general physical examination, with implications for voiding dysfunction, include focused physical examination of the genitourinary system, abdominal and rectal areas, and neurological system.

General Physical Assessment

An overall physical examination is appropriate to detect conditions that contribute to incontinence, such as peripheral edema, or neurologic abnormalities that suggest stroke, Parkinson's disease, or other neurologic disorders. Gross

---

BOX 15-3   Evidence-Based Practice Highlight

Proper cognitive status assessment of the patient experiencing UI is critical. Two evidence-based instruments to utilize for this assessment include the Confusion Assessment Method (CAM) and Mini-Cog assessments. A copy of the CAM instrument, along with information about and proper use of the instrument, is at https://consultgeri.org/try-this /general-assessment/issue-13

The availability of these instruments and accompanying assessment information, along with additional resources to support evidence-based practice, is part of the *Try This: Best Practices in Nursing Care of Older Adults* series of resources at the http://www .ConsultgeriRN.org website.

motor skills (e.g., locomotion, transfer skills, sitting, and balance), dexterity (e.g., managing buttons, zippers, and toilet paper), and the ability to communicate the need for assistance or reliably respond to verbal or written words must be assessed. Evaluate functional deficits and capabilities to determine barriers and/or assets in continence promotion. Calculating the average time it takes the patient to access a toilet while suppressing the urge to void will assist in identification of therapeutic interventions to facilitate continence, specific intervention goals, and the degree of continence possible.

Hydration Assessment

Initial and ongoing evaluation of hydration is essential to diagnose dehydration and minimize its complications. Dehydration complications range from urine becoming concentrated and triggering UI due to bladder contractions from bladder wall irritation to more systemic problems including confusion and lethargy (Dowling-Castronovo & Bradway, 2012). Physical parameters of hydration status include condition of oral mucous membranes, sublingual saliva pool, weight changes, confusion, and muscle weakness. Monitoring the balance between fluid intake and urine output, urine color, and urine specific gravity (SG) for the second void of the day are useful indicators of fluid status (Mentes & Iowa Veterans Affairs Nursing Research Consortium [Iowa Veterans Affairs], 2000, 2004). Urine SG of greater than 1.020 and dark yellow or brownish-green urine indicate the need for increased fluid intake (Armstrong, 2000). Blood tests such as blood urea nitrogen (BUN)/creatinine ratio, serum osmolality, and serum sodium are predictors of actual dehydration (Mentes & Iowa Veterans Affairs, 2000, 2004). Calculate body mass index (BMI) to identify persons at risk for hydration problems. Older adults with BMI of 21 or lower and 27 or higher are at risk for hydration issues (Mentes & Iowa Veterans Affairs, 2000 & 2004). In addition, the BMI will provide an indication of the extent of obesity, which also contributes to voiding problems.

Genitourinary Examination

In women, the pelvic examination should include assessment of the perineal skin integrity, specifically looking for lesions, irritation, or inflammation. Evidence of atrophic vaginal changes including pale, thin, dry, friable mucosa with complaints of vaginal itching, dryness, burning, and dyspareunia are notable. Vaginal pH levels 5 or above in women without evidence of a vaginal infection are also indicative of poorly estrogenized tissues (Qaseem et al., 2014; Shamliyan, Wyman & Kane, 2012). A urethral carbuncle, a cherry-red lesion at the urinary meatus, is another indicator of estrogen deficiency. Atrophic urethritis and vaginitis contribute to urge and stress UI and topical estrogen therapy is often the treatment of choice. The presence of perineum sensation indicates intact sacral nerve roots for the external urethral and anal sphincters. Check for pelvic organ prolapse. If the organ prolapse is beyond the vaginal introitus or symptomatic, refer the woman for further evaluation and treatment. Multiple types and sizes of pessaries are available for correction of prolapse. In men, examination of the external genitalia should include inspection of the skin, location of the urethral meatus, and retractability of the foreskin, if present.

An evaluation of pelvic floor muscle strength is an important component of the examination. This is a particularly important evaluation for diabetic patients due to possible neuropathy, which can interfere with normal sensory input resulting in bladder over-distention and urinary retention (Qaseem et al., 2014; Shamliyan et al., 2012). However, consider the appropriateness of performing an invasive, uncomfortable, and embarrassing vaginal digital examination, particularly in frail older women and cognitively impaired elders (Lekan-Ruteledge, 2004). This evaluation also provides key information about the patient's ability to isolate and identify the correct muscles. In men, and in women with vaginal stenosis, pelvic floor muscle strength can be evaluated rectally. If the individual is capable of using pelvic muscles to inhibit urge or suppress urine flow, a vaginal or rectal digital examination may not be needed to evaluate pelvic muscle control.

Rectal Examination

Assess both resting and active anal sphincter tone. The ability to contract the anal sphincter indicates a functional pelvic floor with intact innervation (Qaseem et al., 2014; Shamliyan et al., 2012). In men, palpate the prostate proximal to the internal anal sphincter through the anterior rectal wall, noting size, consistency, and tenderness. During the digital rectal examination, evaluate pelvic floor muscle strength and assess the rectal vault for large-caliber, hardened stool, suggesting constipation or impaction. If found, treat the impaction prior to initiating a bladder program.

Abdominal Examination

Palpate the abdomen for tenderness, fullness, or masses that may be indicative of fecal impaction. Auscultate bowel sounds to evaluate bowel motility. Palpate the suprapubic area to detect bladder tenderness or distention (Qaseem et al., 2014; Shamliyan et al., 2012).

Bladder Volume Evaluation

Evaluate for difficulties starting the urine stream, intermittent urine flow, strength of the urine stream, and the presence of post-void dribbling. Measure the patient's postvoid residual (PVR) urine volume by in-and-out catheterization or with a bladder ultrasound scanner post-void. A portable bladder ultrasound scanner can identify the patient's ability to empty the bladder and is the preferable method since it is noninvasive (McCliment, 2002). A PVR bladder volume of less than 150 milliliters in an elderly patient is considered normal. Consistent PVRs over 150 milliliters indicates incomplete bladder emptying and the need for further evaluation (Borrie et al., 2001).

Urine Examination

Urinalysis by dipstick or laboratory testing is a component of the initial evaluation of UI. Check urine for white blood cells, nitrites, glucose, and blood (Qaseem et al., 2014; Shamliyan et al., 2012). A UTI should be treated prior to initiation of other UI treatment because resolution of the UTI may eliminate the urine leakage, frequency, and/or urgency.

Environmental Assessment

Evaluate the environment as a potential factor in UI development and treatment. Structural characteristics such as the number, location, and accessibility of toileting facilities, the availability of physical assistance, and the availability of adaptive equipment and supplies for toileting are major considerations (Godfrey, 2008). Evaluate environmental characteristics of the hospital and potential discharge destinations and integrate the results into the treatment plan to achieve the optimal continence level.

Interventions and Care Strategies

Categories of Urinary Incontinence Treatment Strategies

Guidelines by national and international panels, based on extensive literature reviews, outline assessment and treatment of various UI types in specific populations (Dowling-Castronovo & Bradway, 2008, 2012). The three primary categories of UI treatment are behavioral management, pharmacological intervention (see **Box 15-4**), and surgical intervention (Godfrey, 2008).

Behavioral management refers to interventions that modify the patient's behavior or environment. Strategies included in a behavioral approach are voiding scheduling regimens, dietary management, urge suppression techniques, and *pelvic floor muscle exercises* (PFME) with and without the addition of biofeedback, vaginal cones, and electrical stimulation. Pharmacological intervention involves medications that alter detrusor muscle activity or bladder outlet resistance. Surgical interventions primarily address increasing bladder outlet resistance resulting from intrinsic sphincter deficiency, as well as removal of bladder outlet obstruction, relieving overflow incontinence (Bo & Hilde, 2013; Shamliyan, Wyman, Ramakrishnan, Sainfort, Kane, 2012; Shamliyan et al., 2012).

CLINICAL TIP

Pelvic floor muscle exercises (PFME) are a noninvasive strategy for urinary incontinence.

BOX 15-4   Clinical Practice Example

"No Pads, No Pills, No Hurry, and No Leaks" is the title of a 3-hour class taught by Audrey Cochran, MSN, GCNS-BC, CCCN. One of their assignments was to keep a diary of what they ate and drank and how it affected their bladder. In addition to learning how to do pelvic floor muscle exercises, the self-analysis helped all of them improve their bladder control.

Some findings from the group included that no one was bothered by coffee, but one person had to rush to the bathroom more often after drinking tea. Another had a "twitchy bladder" when she ate tomatoes in any form, whether in salad or pizza or spaghetti sauce. Another had problems with honeydew melon. In Cochran's clinical practice, some patients report that if they eat watermelon they "had just better plan on staying home the rest of the day." After keeping track of what she ate and drank, another patient discovered when she had her usual cereal with milk, coffee and orange juice for breakfast she had trouble controlling her bladder, but not when she substituted apple juice for the orange juice. A post-prostatectomy patient discovered when he drank a diet soft drink (containing aspartame) he leaked more than when he drank a regular soft drink. Increased problems with UI after ingesting sugar substitutes were also reported by several patients. These examples show the importance of patients keeping a diary of what goes in and when it comes out before and while making changes.

Patient-Centered Urinary Incontinence Treatment Goals

Clarify all UI treatment goals with the patient first. It is important to keep in mind that the patient's expectations for treatment outcomes should guide intervention choices. Patient goals are multidimensional and do not necessarily require total continence for patient satisfaction and improved health-related quality of life (Dowling-Castronovo & Bradway, 2007).

Behavioral Management

Behavioral approaches should be the first line of treatment for UI. Eliminating reversible factors is a first step in treatment to optimize urological functioning. Clinical practice guidelines identify dietary modifications (hydration and avoidance of bladder irritants), scheduled voiding, *prompted voiding*), *bladder training*, *pelvic muscle rehabilitation*, and *urge suppression techniques* as useful approaches in a comprehensive UI treatment regimen (Dowling-Castronovo & Bradway, 2008, 2012; Godfrey, 2008; Ostaszkiewicz et al., 2013).

Behavioral strategies differ in their mechanisms of action, the required patient participation level, and the technology involved. Interventions should be selected for patients based on the patient's UI type, mental and physical abilities, any other limitations, and environmental resources available. The versatility of behavioral therapy enables the care providers to adapt and individualize the treatment plan according to the patient's level of functioning. If successful, behavioral approaches eliminate the added expense and potential risk of an adverse drug reaction from pharmacological intervention and the complications associated with surgery (McIntosh et al., 2015).

Hydration Management

Managing hydration focuses on maintaining fluid balance. Ensuring an adequate, timely, appropriate fluid intake is essential to a successful continence program (see **Box 15-5** for hydration management resources). Older adults concerned about UI may intentionally reduce their fluid intake, which can lead to concentrated urine and irritability of the bladder wall, resulting in increased UI (Dowling-Castronovo & Bradway, 2007).

An individualized fluid goal must first be determined. To calculate fluid intake according to this standard, take 100 mL/kg for the first 10 kg of weight, 50 mL/kg for the next 10 kg, and 15 mL for the remaining kilograms

(Mentes & Iowa Veterans Affairs, 2000, 2004). Because this includes fluid from all sources, take 70% of the total to determine the goal for fluid volume intake alone (Mentes & Iowa Veterans Affairs, 2000, 2004).

Providing fluids throughout the day will help ensure meeting the fluid goal, yet minimize frequency and urgency resulting from rapid bladder filling from large fluid volume ingestion over a short period. The suggested percentage of fluid delivery is 75% to 80% of fluid at meals and 20% to 25% during nonmeal times, such as with medications and planned nourishment (Mentes & Iowa Veterans Affairs, 2000, 2004). For patients in a residential setting, this schedule offers the additional advantage of supervision for patients with swallowing problems. Fluid rounds midmorning and midafternoon, in conjunction with offers of assistance with toileting, have been effective in reducing incontinence and decreasing dehydration in nursing home residents. Fluids should be limited in the evening hours prior to bedtime, especially if nocturia is present (Mentes & Iowa Veterans Affairs, 2000, 2004).

A final consideration in fluid intake concerns the type of fluids consumed. The fluids should be limited to those without a diuretic or irritant effect. Many common foods and beverages may be irritating to the bladder, causing or contributing to UI. Carbonated and caffeinated beverages, citrus juices, acidic foods, alcoholic beverages, and aspartame are among the products commonly considered bladder irritants or having a diuretic effect (Dowling-Castronovo & Bradway, 2012). A review of the bladder diary (see Figure 15-2) is especially useful in detecting possible agents that precipitate urgency or incontinence. Reducing the intake of caffeinated beverages to no more than two servings a day is recommended for individuals experiencing urgency or urge incontinence (Arya, Myers, & Jackson, 2000). Postum is a potential alternative for coffee. However, water is the better choice of a liquid because it is not an irritant or diuretic and does not interfere with diabetes control.

For patients with swallowing problems, providing the appropriate consistency can prevent choking or aspiration. Nectars and thick liquids such as buttermilk and V8 juice are usually acceptable alternatives. Any liquid may be thickened with commercial products or by mixing it with natural thickeners such as baby food, mashed bananas, or wheat germ (M. Kain, personal communication, September 6, 2001).

Bowel Function Management

Maintaining bowel regularity prevents bladder emptying problems that may result from constipation and fecal impaction (see **Box 15-6**). Irregular bowel habits, immobility, dehydration, decreased fiber intake, medication side effects, and emotional factors contribute to the development of constipation. Maintaining hydration is critical in promoting bowel function, which in turn aids bladder function. Many hospitalized patients identify lack of privacy and change in daily routine as major factors contributing to constipation. Consider adding fiber with adequate fluids, if stools are hard. A mild stimulant such as prunes or prune juice 6 to 8 hours prior to planned defecation can assist removal of stool that is difficult to pass. A mixture of applesauce, prune juice, and bran has been effective in decreasing constipation and for laxative use in nursing home patients (Smith & Newman, 1989) (see **Table 15-4** for the recipe). Its thick texture may facilitate administration to patients with swallowing problems. The use of regular grocery store items to prepare the mixture should decrease the overall cost of the bowel program when compared to prescription or OTC products.

BOX 15-6   Evidence-Based Practice Highlight on Preventing Constipation

Best Practice Guideline: Prevention of
Constipation in the Older Adult Population

is available at http://rnao.ca/bpg/guidelines/
prevention-constipation-older-adult-population

TABLE 15-4   Bran Mixture Recipe for Treating or Preventing Constipation

1 cup applesauce
1 cup unprocessed coarse wheat bran
1/2 cup unsweetened prune juice
Mix together. Give 2 tablespoons a day with a glass of water or juice. May increase to 3 tablespoons twice a day gradually (weekly) until good bowel function is achieved. May be given in hot cereal or added to mashed bananas.
Refrigerate the bran mixture up to 5 days.

Prompted Voiding

Prompted voiding is an intervention for patients unable to recognize and act on the sensation of the need to void and exert neuromuscular control over voiding initiation. Prompted voiding has been successful in decreasing the frequency of UI in clinical trials with physically and cognitively impaired nursing home residents (Ostaszkiewicz et al., 2013; Skelly et al., 2011). The use of prompted voiding is also effective in home settings. Persons with urge, stress, and mixed UI have responded positively to this intervention (Ostaszkiewicz et al., 2013). Prompted voiding also has strong support for reducing UI in individuals with cognitive and physical deficits (Ostaszkiewicz et al., 2013; Skelly et al., 2011).

Prompted voiding is a scheduling regimen that initially focuses on the caregiver's behavior in order to change the incontinent person's voiding behavior. This methodology involves the consistent use of three caregiver behaviors: monitoring, prompting, and praising. The caregiver adheres to a schedule of regular monitoring, asking if the incontinent individual needs to use the toilet and checking to see if he or she is dry or wet. Prompting involves reminding the person to use the toilet and wait until the caregiver returns to void. Praise is the positive response or feedback given by the caregiver for appropriate toileting or dryness. The best predictor of an individual's likelihood to benefit is success during a therapeutic trial, usually lasting 3 days (Ostaszkiewicz et al., 2013; Skelly et al., 2011). A prompted voiding trial involves assessing the patient's ability to recognize the need to void and respond to the need appropriately, either by asking to toilet or by agreeing to toilet when the bladder is full. (See **Box 15-7** and **Table 15-5** for information and resources about prompted voiding.)

Bladder Training

Bladder training is an important component for continence and focuses on the ability to delay urination and suppress urgency. Bladder training is an educational program of scheduled voiding to provide patients with the skills to improve the ability to control urgency, decrease frequency of incontinent episodes, and prolong the interval between voiding (Dowling-Castronovo & Bradway, 2007)

The steps in a bladder-training program include setting a voiding schedule, teaching strategies for controlling urgency, monitoring voiding, and positive reinforcement. The initial voiding schedule is determined from baseline

---

BOX 15-7   Evidence-Based Practice Highlight

The Long-Term Care Best Practice Initiative— available at http://rnao.ca/bpg/guidelines
Promoting Continence Using Prompted Voiding is /promoting-continence-using-prompted-voiding.

TABLE 15-5   Steps in the Prompted Voiding Protocol

1. Greet the patient by name. Remember to always knock for resident privacy. Close the door and/or privacy curtain.

2. Ask the patient if she or he is wet or dry. Ask a second time if the patient does not respond.

3. Check clothes, bedding, or body to determine if he or she is wet or dry. Tell the patient if he or she is correct.

4. If the patient asks for help in toileting:

   a. Praise the resident. Be careful to not engage in "baby talk."

   b. Assist him or her to the toilet.

5. If the patient does not ask for help toileting, ask the patient if he or she wants to toilet.

   a. Ask a second time if he or she doesn't say yes the first time.

   b. Ask a third time if his or her response is other than yes or no.

6. Assist to toilet only if he or she says yes to your offer.

   a. Praise for appropriate toileting.

   b. Record outcome.

7. Ask if he or she wants something to drink and provide appropriate liquids.

8. Tell the resident when he or she can expect you to return.

Data from Lyons, S. S., Pringle Specht, J. K. (2000). Prompted voiding protocol for individuals with urinary incontinence. *The Journal of Gerontological Nursing, 26*(6), 5–13.

voiding data and prescribed according to the guidelines presented in **Table 15-6**. A 5- to 10-minute window on either side of the scheduled voiding time is allowed for flexibility. The training regimen is followed during waking hours, and the time between voiding is gradually increased by 15 to 30 minutes until the goal interval between voiding is reached (Dowling-Castronovo & Bradway, 2007). Although a 3- to 4-hour voiding interval is considered a maximal goal, most patients report they best tolerate an interval of 2 to 2.5 hours. Strategies to suppress urge include relaxation and distraction techniques such as slow deep breathing, concentrating on a task such as talking to someone, and pelvic muscle contractions.

Bladder training has been evaluated and implemented primarily with independent, community-dwelling elderly women. Persons with physical and cognitive impairment have been considered unlikely candidates for bladder training techniques. However, the potential benefit to voiding supports an effort to try this approach. In addition, an exercise program to improve walking in cognitively impaired nursing home residents can reduce daytime incontinence (Jivorec, 1991).

Pelvic Muscle Rehabilitation

Pelvic muscle rehabilitation involves the use of pelvic floor muscle exercise to increase strength, tone, and control of pelvic floor muscles to facilitate urine flow control and suppress urgency. The pelvic floor muscles support the

TABLE 15-6   Steps in Bladder Training

1. Complete a 72-hour bladder diary.

2. Review the bladder diary. Calculate the number of voids and bladder accidents in a 24-hour period. Determine fluid intake.

3. Examine data for patterns. Does UI occur only during certain times of day? Are accidents associated with certain events (activities, intake of specific type of fluids, medications)? What is the average time between voids and what is the longest interval?
   Are behaviors different for weekdays or weekends, or workdays vs. non-workdays, or time when you are at home or out of the home?

4. Establish an initial voiding interval and consider the optimal interval to be achieved. The typical interval for adults is every 4 hours during the day; however, data suggest for older persons every 2 to 2.5 hours may be optimum.
   The objective is to start the voiding routine when it is comfortable to separate urgency from voiding; then, utilize urge suppression skills, to increase the time between voiding until the goal is reached.

5. Urinate when you wake, after meals, before bedtime, and at the prescribed intervals.

6. If you get the urge to void and it is too soon to void, use the relaxation technique to make the urge go away. Remember, this involves taking very slow deep breaths until the urge goes away. Relax and concentrate when doing this. Contract the pelvic floor muscles quickly 3 to 5 times. Relax. Contract again.

7. Void at the prescribed time even if you do not feel the need.

8. If after a week it is very easy to wait the assigned time interval, lengthen the time by 15 to 30 minutes.

9. Begin by only practicing this technique at home, when you are relaxed and the bathroom is nearby.

10. Fluid intake should be kept at six 8-ounce glasses per day. If you awaken frequently during the night to void, drink the majority of your 8 ounces before 6 p.m.

Hints to remember
- Never rush or run to the bathroom—walk slowly.
- Use the relaxation technique in situations that cause you to have the urge to void before the assigned time interval. For example, if you get the urge to void whenever you start to unlock your front door, stop, relax, and take three slow deep breaths to let the urge pass. Then unlock the door and walk slowly to the bathroom.
- When you walk slowly to the bathroom, do some pelvic muscle exercises to prevent an accident.

pelvic organs. The proposed mechanism of action for pelvic muscle training is that strong and fast pelvic muscle contractions close the urethra, increases urethral pressure, and inhibits bladder contractions, which prevents leakage (Dowling-Castronovo & Bradway, 2007).

To teach the individual to identify and isolate the correct muscles, instruct him or her to "draw in" and "lift up" the rectal/anal sphincter muscles. Instruct patients to lift up the perivaginal muscles (from the pubic bone to the tailbone) and avoid contracting the abdominal, gluteal, and thigh muscles. Instruct the patient to either hold their hand over their lower abdomen or hum while contracting with no waver in the sound to determine if they are contracting their abdominal muscles. To help the patient avoid a bearing down motion, have him or her practice pushing down to feel what not to do. Start with contracting for 2 seconds, and then gradually increase the length of the contraction to a maximum 10-second hold. A repetition includes relaxing or resting the pelvic floor muscles between contractions for the same amount of time the muscle is contracted. A typical training regimen involves 10 repetitions 2 or 3 times a day.

Instruct the patient to use pelvic muscle contraction to prevent urine flow once the correct technique is mastered. If leakage occurs with activities that increase intraabdominal pressure, a muscle contraction should precede the activity. If urgency is the primary problem, the pelvic floor muscles can be used to suppress the urge. Contracting the muscles of the pelvic floor should occur repeatedly and rapidly if the patient is experiencing urgency. To aid in teaching the patient, ask him to tap his finger rapidly five times and let him know this is how often and rapid the muscle contractions should occur.

> ### CLINICAL TIP
>
> PFME need to be done frequently for maximal effectiveness. Reminding clients to do these exercises with each commercial while watching television is one strategy.

Biofeedback

Biofeedback is an adjunct to pelvic muscle rehabilitation and bladder contraction inhibition and has been effective with stress and urge UI (Herderschee, Hay-Smith, Herbison, Roovers & Heineman, 2011; Mendes, Rodolpho, & Hoga, 2016; Parker & Griebling, 2015). The use of biofeedback-assisted bladder training has particular advantages since it is very low risk and has no documented side effects; however, because it relies on learning new behaviors, it may have limited application for cognitively impaired patients (Herderschee et al., 2011).

Biofeedback, through either surface electrodes or vaginal or rectal probes, provides visual and/or auditory cues to facilitate incontinent patients' ability to isolate and identify pelvic floor muscles. It also helps decrease patients' tendency to use abdominal or gluteal muscles.

Pelvic Floor Electrical Stimulus

Pelvic floor electrical stimulation (PFES) is another adjunct to PFME. Pelvic floor electrical stimulation refers to the application of electric current to sacral and pudendal afferent fibers via a nonimplantable vaginal or anal probe (Parker & Griebling, 2015). Variable rates of current are used to improve urethral closure by activating pelvic floor muscles, thus exercising and strengthening the pelvic floor. Pelvic floor electrical stimulation also can facilitate an individual's ability to identify and isolate pelvic floor musculature. The Health Care Financing Administration (HCFA) review panel concluded that PFES is effective for patients with stress and/or urge incontinence and considers its use necessary and reasonable if PFMEs have been unsuccessful (Tunis, Whyte, & Bridger, 2000). In addition, the ability of PFES to passively exercise the pelvic floor is a potentially valuable treatment for individuals unable to perform the exercises.

Pharmacological Management

Medications are available to help treat stress and urge incontinence. Because many older persons have multiple chronic health problems, medications to treat incontinence should primarily serve as an adjunct to behavioral interventions. Medications prescribed for stress UI target the internal urinary sphincter or the urethral/vaginal tissues. The alpha agonist pseudoephedrine acts at the bladder neck, increasing urethral tone, which may decrease leakage and is often prescribed for mild cases of stress UI. However, pseudoephedrine potential side effects include insomnia, restlessness, nervousness, headache, and increased blood pressure and heart rate, which limit its usefulness in the older population. Duloxetine, a serotonin and norepinephrine reuptake inhibitor, increases external urethral sphincter tone and is used to treat stress UI. Estrogen is prescribed to treat urogenital atrophy, which increases stimulation of urogenital estrogen receptors and may increase urethral resistance. Evidence of its usefulness in stress UI is inconclusive; however, estrogen's effectiveness in treating atrophic tissues can help alleviate irritation and symptoms of urgency, which may decrease urge UI. The primary agents for uninhibited bladder contractions are anticholinergics or antispasmodics that decrease contraction of the detrusor muscle. **Table 15-7** presents an overview of the medications used for UI treatment.

TABLE 15-7   Medications Commonly Used to Treat Urinary Incontinence

Medication	Dosage	Comments
Hyoscyamine	0.375 mg twice daily orally	Has prominent anticholinergic side effects; available in alternative forms
Oxybutynin	2.5–5.0 mg three times daily orally (short-acting) 5–30 mg daily orally (long-acting) 3.9 mg over a 96-hour period (transdermal)	Long-acting and transdermal preparations have fewer side effects than short-acting preparations. Transdermal patch can cause local skin irritation in some patients
Propantheline	15–30 mg 4 times daily orally	Noted anticholinergic side effects
Tolterodine	1–2 mg twice daily orally (short-acting) 4 mg daily orally (long-acting)	Similar efficacy with long-acting and short-acting preparations.
Estrogen (for women)		
Vaginal estrogen preparations	Approximately 0.5 g cream applied topically nightly for 2 weeks, then twice per week Estradiol ring, replaced every 90 days Estradiol, 1 tablet daily for 2 weeks, then 1 tablet twice a week	Local vaginal preparations are probably more effective than oral estrogen.
Alpha-Adrenergic Antagonists (for men)		
Alfuzosin	2.5 mg three times daily orally	Useful in men with benign prostatic enlargement.
Doxazosin	1–16 mg daily orally	Postural hypotension can be a serious side-effect.
Prazosin	4–8 mg twice daily orally, begin with 0.5 mg once daily and titrate up	Check blood pressure regularly.
Tamsulosin	0.4–0.8 mg daily orally	Take 30 minutes after the same meal each day.
Terazosin	1–10 mg orally each day at bedtime	Doses must be increased gradually to facilitate tolerance.
Imipramine	10–25 mg three times daily orally	May be useful for mixed urge-stress incontinence; can cause postural hypotension and bundle-branch block.
Desmopressin	10–40 mcg of intranasal spray daily at bedtime 0.1–0.4 mg orally 2 hours before bedtime	Hyponatremia may occur in older adults; monitor serum sodium levels closely.

Data from Ouslander, J. G. (2004). Management of the overactive bladder. *The New England Journal of Medicine, 350,* 786–799.

Overflow incontinence in men that is the result of bladder neck obstruction from benign prostatic hypertrophy (BPH) may resolve with treatment of the prostate. Alpha antagonists (doxazosin, tamsulosin, and terazosin) relax the urinary sphincters, improving urine flow and decreasing urine retention and overflow incontinence. However, dizziness and orthostatic hypotension are potential side effects that must be addressed. Other options for BPH treatment are the 5-alpha reductase inhibitors finasteride and dutasteride. This class of medications blocks the conversion of testosterone to dihydrotestosterone, the form needed for prostate growth. The 5-alpha reductase inhibitors require about 3 to 6 months to take effect.

Devices and Products

A variety of absorbent products are available to contain urine. It is important that patients use products designed for urine; menstrual pads are a popular choice, but are not specifically designed to absorb and contain urine. The absorbent inner core of continence garments wicks the urine away from the skin and spreads it throughout the pad, increasing the volume of urine absorbed (Dingwall, 2008; Lekan-Rutledge, Doughty, Moore, Wooldridge, 2003; Mueller, 2004; Newman, 2002). The volume of urine that needs to be contained and the need for help toileting are important considerations in product selection. The use of briefs developed specifically for men and for women have several advantages to the traditional adult diaper. These garments are easier to manipulate to prepare for toileting and for repositioning clothing afterward. They also are more like usual underclothes, facilitating the expectation of a return to continence and promoting comfort. The introduction of products to accommodate moderate to heavy levels of incontinence has broadened the possibilities for successful containment. Many patients and family have been relieved (especially from an economic perspective) to learn of the availability of nondisposable garments that can be washed and reused.

Toileting equipment and collection devices are available for men and women to promote self-toileting, including female urinals, wheelchair urinals, and male reusable urinal/pant garments (Dingwall, 2008; Lekan-Rutledge et al., 2003; Mueller, 2004). The National Association for Continence (2015) is an excellent resource for patients and caregivers managing UI and can be accessed at http://www.nafc.org/.

Skin Care

Meticulous skin care is essential in the care of persons with incontinence. Moisture barriers and no-rinse incontinence cleansers are recommended over soap and water alone in preventing skin breakdown (Beeckman et al., 2015; Dowling-Castronovo & Bradway, 2007). It is important to gently dry the skin after cleansing and apply moisturizers. Petroleum-based products may be incompatible with some adult briefs, causing skin irritation (Newman, 2002).

Incontinence-associated dermatitis (IAD) describes skin irritation and impairment from exposure to urine and feces (Beeckman et al., 2015; Doughty et al., 2012). This condition is unique from pressure ulcer formation since it is caused by exposure to moisture and is not ischemic in nature. However, the presence of IAD increases the risk of pressure ulcer development (Doughty et al., 2012).

Environmental Intervention

Evaluation of the home may be helpful in modifying the environment to facilitate rapid access to the toilet. Consulting with an Occupational Therapist for the environmental evaluation can be very helpful.

Indwelling Urinary Catheters

Indwelling urinary catheters, once the primary means for managing UI, are no longer accepted as the first step in an incontinence treatment regimen. However, there are situations that may require catheter use. The Centers for Medicare and Medicaid Services (CMS) developed regulations for guidance of long-term indwelling catheter use (see **Table 15-8**). With long-term use, care must be taken to monitor for common complications of polymicrobial bacteriuria, fever, nephrolithiasis, bladder stones, epididymitis, and chronic renal inflammation

TABLE 15-8   Centers for Medicare and Medicaid Services Rules for Guidance of Indwelling Catheter Utilization

Urinary retention that cannot be treated or corrected medically or surgically, for which alternative therapy is not feasible, and which is characterized by:
• Documented PVR volumes in a range over 200 milliliters
• Inability to manage the retention/incontinence with intermittent catheterization
• Persistent overflow incontinence, symptomatic infections, and/or renal dysfunction
• Contamination of stage III or IV pressure ulcers with urine, which has impeded healing, despite appropriate personal care for the incontinence
• Terminal illness or severe impairment, which makes positioning or clothing changes uncomfortable, or which is associated with intractable pain

Reproduced from Centers for Medicare & Medicaid Services. (2005). *CMS Manual System. Publication 100-07.* Retrieved from http://www.cms.gov/Regulations-and-Guidance/Guidance/Transmittals/downloads//r8som.pdf

and pyelonephritis (Benvenuti et al., 2002). Maintaining hydration, urine flow, and cleanliness of the system are important components of care. Minimizing urethral trauma by using small-caliber catheters, a 5-cc retention balloon, and securing the catheter with a thigh strap will promote comfort and may help decrease complications. Emptying the catheter every 4–6 hours to avoid migration of bacteria up the lumen, cleaning the insertion site gently with soap and water daily, and avoiding irrigations may help decrease symptomatic UTI. Whenever the patient's status changes, such as healing of pressure ulcers, then a trial without the indwelling catheter should be attempted.

Intermittent urinary catheterization is another supportive measure to manage urinary retention (see Table 15-8). In and out catheterization allows regular bladder emptying, which reduces pressure within the bladder and improves circulation to the bladder wall, making the mucosa more resistant to infection (Newman, 2002). Sterile technique is used in institutions, and clean technique is used for catheterizations at home. Dexterity and mobility problems may interfere with self-catheterizations, as well as caregiver comfort with the procedure.

Summary

UI is a serious, potentially disabling condition with negative social, physical, psychological, and economic impacts. Incontinence is a common condition in the older population, but is not a part of the normal aging process. The majority of older adults who have UI can be successfully treated and experience improved health-related quality of life. The introduction of early, targeted behavioral interventions should improve urological functioning and limit the impact of uncontrolled incontinence. Therefore, older adults and their caregivers need education about evidence-based interventions to combat this all too prevalent health problem. Nurses are in a key position to assess, plan, intervene, and evaluate to ensure older adult patients prevent UI and maintain optimal urinary function. (**Figure 15-4**).

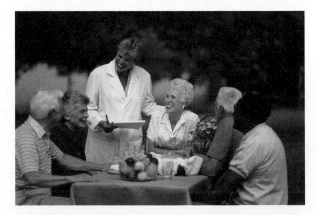

Figure 15-4 Nurses are in an ideal position to help educate older adults about current treatment for UI.
© Jupiterimages/Photos.com/Thinkstock

Clinical Reasoning Exercises

1. Mrs. O'Dell is having a problem with constipation since turning 70 years of age. She asks for advice about this. What would you suggest? What needs to be assessed before providing advice about this?
2. Choose one of the clinical practice guidelines provided in this chapter and review it. What can you take away from that guideline and apply to your clinical practice?
3. If you had to give a talk on urinary incontinence to a ladies' group from a church, what would you cover as the most important points on this topic? How could you make it interesting and engaging for the audience?

Personal Reflections

1. Have you ever cared for a person with urinary incontinence? If so, what was the setting and how did you feel about providing this care? What from this chapter might make you look at that situation differently?
2. Imagine that you have become an older adult and are beginning to experience problems with UI. What is the first action you would take after an incontinence episode? What, if anything, could you do earlier in your adult life to prevent UI?
3. Urinary incontinence is often thought of as more of a woman's problem than a man's. What would you recommend to a male who is experiencing UI as a result of prostate enlargement?

References

Aristide, G., Weinstein, M., & B Nair, G. (2013). Nocturia in obstructive sleep apnea-hypopnea syndrome: An unappreciated symptom. *Current Respiratory Medicine Reviews, 9*(3), 217–224.

Armstrong, L. E. (2000). *Performing in extreme environments.* Champaign, IL: Human Kinetics.

Arya, L. A., Myers, D. L., & Jackson, N. D. (2000). Dietary caffeine intake and the risk of detrusor instability: A case-control study. *Obstetrics and Gynecology, 96*(1), 85–89.

Beeckman, D., Van Damme, N., Schoonhoven, L., Van Lancker, A., Kottner, J., Beele, H., . . . & Van Hecke, A. (2015). Interventions for preventing and treating incontinence-associated dermatitis in adults. Retrieved from http://www.cochrane.org/CD011627/INCONT_interventions-for-preventing-and-treating-incontinence-associated-dermatitis-in-adults

Benvenuti, F., Cottenden, A., DuBeau, C., Kirshner-Hermanns, R., Miller, K., Palmer, M., & Resnick, N. (2002). Urinary incontinence and bladder dysfunction in older persons. In P. Abrams, L. Cardozo, S. Khoury, & A. Wein (Eds.), *Incontinence* (pp. 627–695). Plymouth, UK: Health Publication.

Bo, K., & Hilde, G. (2013). Does it work in the long term? A systematic review on pelvic floor muscle training for female stress urinary incontinence. *Neurourology and Urodynamics, 32*(3), 215–223.

Borrie, M. J., Campbell, K., Arcese, Z. A., Bray, J., Labate, T., & Hesch, P. (2001). Urinary retention in patients in a geriatric rehabilitation unit: Prevalence, risk factors, and validity of bladder scan evaluation. *Rehabilitation Nursing, 26*(5), 187–191.

Borson, S., Scanlan, J., Brush, M., Vitallano, P., & Dokmak, A. (2000). The Mini-Cog: A cognitive "vital signs" measure for dementia screening in multi-lingual elderly. *International Journal of Geriatric Psychiatry, 15*(11), 1021–1027.

Bradway, C. (2003). Urinary incontinence among older women: Measurement of the effect on health-related quality of life. *Journal of Gerontological Nursing, 29*(7), 13–19.

Brown, J. S., Vittinghoff, E., Wyman, J. F., Stone, K. L., Nevitt, M. C., Ensrud, K. E., & Grady, D. (2000). Urinary incontinence: Does it increase risk for falls and fractures? *Journal of the American Geriatrics Society, 48*(7), 721–725.

Centers for Medicare and Medicaid Services. (2005, December 15). *CMS Manual System-Pub. 100-07 State Operations Provider Certification.* Retrieved from http://www.cms.gov/Regulations-and-Guidance/Guidance /Transmittals/downloads//r8som.pdf

Coudret, N., Ehlman, K., Dugger, R., Eggleston, B., Wilson, A., Harrison, E., & Mathis, S. (2009, October 30). *Assessing the benefits of bladder ultrasound scanners in nursing homes: Project funded by the Indiana State Department of Health-Final Report.* Unpublished manuscript, Evansville, IN: College of Nursing and Health Professions, University of Southern Indiana.

Coyne, K. S., Kvasz, M., Ireland, A. M., Milsom, I, Kopp, Z. S., & Chapple, C. R. (2012). Urinary incontinence and its relationship to mental health and health-related quality of life in men and women in Sweden, the United Kingdom, and the United States. *European Urology, 61*(1), 88–95.

Coyne, K. S., Wein, A., Nicholson, S., Kvasz, M., Chen, C. I. & Milsom, I. (2014). Economic burden of urgency urinary incontinence in the United States: A systematic review. *Journal of Managed Care Pharmacy, 20*(2), 130–140.

Dingwall, L. (2008). Promoting social continence using incontinence management products. *British Journal of Nursing, 17*(9), 12–19.

Doughty, D. (2000). *Urinary and fecal incontinence: Nursing management.* St. Louis, MO: Mosby.

Doughty, D., Junkin, J., Kurz, P., Selekof, J, Gray, M., Fader, M., . . . Logan, S. (2012). Incontinence-associated dermatitis: Consensus statements, evidence-based guidelines for prevention and treatment, and current challenges. *Journal of Wound, Ostomy, Continence Nursing, 39*(3), 303–315.

Dowling-Castronovo, A. (2007). Urinary incontinence assessment in older adults part 1: Transient urinary incontinence. *Try This: Best Practices in Nursing Care to Older Adults,* Issue 11.1, Retrieved from http://www .casenex.com/casenet/pages/cases/aCure/Urinary_Incontinence.pdf.

Dowling-Castronovo, A., & Bradway, C. (2003). Urinary incontinence. In M. Mezey, I. Abraham, D. A. Zwicker, (Eds.), *Geriatric nursing protocols for best practice* (2nd ed., pp. 83–98). New York, NY: Springer.

Dowling-Castronovo, A., & Bradway, C. (2007). *Assessment and management of older adults with urinary incontinence* [white paper]. Presented at The National Gerontological Nursing Association and American Association of Colleges of Nursing Conference in St. Louis, MO in October 2008.

Dowling-Castronovo, A., & Bradway, C. (2008). Urinary incontinence in older adults admitted to acute care. In E. Capezuti, D. Zwicker, M. Mezey, & T. Fulmer. (Eds.). *Evidence-based geriatric nursing protocols for best practice* (3rd ed., pp. 309–336). New York, NY: Springer.

Dowling-Castronovo, A., & Bradway, C. (2012). Urinary incontinence in older adults admitted to acute care. In M. Bolz, E. Capezuti, T. Fulmer, & D. Zwicker. (Eds.), *Evidence-based geriatric nursing protocols for best practice* (4th ed., pp. 363–387). New York, NY: Springer.

DuBeau, C. E. (2005). Improving urinary incontinence in nursing home residents: Are we FIT to be tied? *Journal of the American Geriatrics Society, 53*(7), 1254–1256.

DuBeau, C. E., Simon, S. E., & Morris, J. N. (2006). The effect of urinary incontinence on quality of life in older nursing home residents. *Journal of the American Geriatrics Society, 54*(9), 1325–1333.

Dugan, E., Cohen, S. J., Bland, S. R., Priesser, J. S., Davis, C. C., Suggs, P. K., & McGann, P. (2000). The association of depressive symptoms and urinary incontinence among older adults. *Journal of the American Geriatrics Association, 48*(4), 413–416.

Faiena, I., Patel, N., Parihar, J. S., Calabrese, M., & Tunuguntla, H. (2015). Conservative management of urinary incontinence in women. *Reviews in Urology, 17*(3), 129–139.

Folstein, M. F., Folstein, S. E., & McHugh, P. R. (1975). "Mini-Mental State": A practical method for grading the cognitive state of patients for the clinician. *Journal of Psychiatric Research, 12*(3), 189–198.

Frenchman, I. B. (2001). Cost of urinary incontinence in two skilled nursing facilities: A prospective study. *Clinical Geriatrics, 9*(1), 49–52.

Godfrey, H. (2008). Older people, continence, and catheters: Dilemmas and resolutions. *British Journal of Nursing 1*(3), S4–S11.

Godfrey, H., & Hogg, A. (2007). Links between social isolation and incontinence. *British Journal of Nursing, 1*(3), S1–S8.

Heidrich, S., & Wells, T. J. (2004). Effects of urinary incontinence: Psychosocial well-being and distress in older community dwelling women. *Journal of Gerontological Nursing, 39*(5), 47–54.

Herderschee, R., Hay-Smith, E. J. C., Herbison, G. P., Roovers, J. P., & Heineman, M. J. (2011). Feedback or biofeedback to augment pelvic floor muscle training for urinary incontinence in women. *Cochrane Datebase of Systematic Reviews, 7.* doi:10.1002/14651858.CD009252.

Hu, T. W., Wagner, T. H., Bentkover, J. D., Leblanc, K., Zhou, S.Z., & Hunt, T. (2004). Costs of urinary incontinence and overactive bladder in the United States: A comparative study. *Urology, 63*(3), 461–465.

Hunskaar, S., Burgio, K., Diokno, A. C., Herzog, A. R., Hjalmas, K., & Lapitan, M. C. (2002). Epidemiology and natural history of urinary incontinence (UI). In P. Abrams, L. Cardozo, S. Khoury, & A. Wein (Eds.), *Incontinence* (pp. 167–201). Plymouth, UK: Health Publication.

Inouye, S.K. (2006). Delirium in older persons. *New England Journal of Medicine, 354*(11), 1157–65.

Inouye, S. K., van Dyck, C. H., Alessi, C. A., Balkin, S., Siegal, A. P., & Horwitz, R. I. (1990). Clarifying confusion: The confusion assessment method. *Annals of Internal Medicine, 113*(12), 941–948.

Jacobson, T. M., & Wright, T. (2015). Improving quality by taking aim at incontinence-associated dermatitis in hospitalized adults. *MedSurg Nursing, 24*(3), 151–158.

Ko, Y., Lin, S., Salmon, J. W., & Bron, M. (2005). The impact of urinary incontinence on quality of life of the elderly. *The American Journal of Managed Care, 11*(4), S103–S111.

Landefeld, C. S., Bowers, B. J., Feld, A. D., Hartmann, K. E., Hoffman, E., Ingber, M. U, . . . Trock, B. J. (2008). National Institutes of Health state-of-the-science conference statement: Prevention of fecal and urinary incontinence in adults. *Annals of Internal Medicine, 148*(6), 449–458.

Lekan-Rutledge, D. (2004). Urinary incontinence strategies for frail elderly women. *Urologic Nursing, 24*(4), 281–301.

Lekan-Rutledge, D., Doughty, D., Moore, K. N., Wooldridge, L. (2003). Promoting social continence: Products and devices in the management of urinary incontinence. *Urologic Nursing, 23*(6), 416–428.

Lucas, M. G., Bedretdinova, D., Bosch, J. L. H. R., Burkhard, F., Cruz, F., Nambiar, A. K., . . . Pickard, R. S. (2012). Guidelines on urinary incontinence. *European Association of Urology.* Retrieved from http://uroweb.org/wp-content/uploads/20-Urinary-Incontinence_LR1.pdf

MacDonald, C. D. & Butler, L. (2007). Silent no more; Elderly women's stories of living with urinary incontinence. *Journal of Gerontological Nursing, 33*(1), 14–20.

Mathis, S., Ehlman, K., Dugger, B. R., Harrawood, A., & Kraft, C. M. (2013). Bladder buzz: The effect of a 6-week evidence-based staff education program on knowledge and attitudes regarding urinary incontinence in a nursing home. *The Journal of Continuing Education in Nursing, 44*(11), 498–506.

MayoClinic.com. (2008). *Kegel exercises: A how-to guide for women.* Retrieved from http://www.mayoclinic.com/health/kegel-exercises/WO00119

McCliment, J. (2002). Non-invasive method overcomes incontinence: Programs retrains residents to recognize the urge to void. *Contemporary Longterm Care, 25*(5), 15.

McIntosh., L., Andersen, E., & Reekie, M. (2015). Conservative treatment of stress urinary incontinence in women: A 10-year (2004-2013) scoping review of the literature. *Urologic Nursing, 35*(4), 179–187.

Mendes, A., Rodolpho, J. R. C., & Hoga, L. A. K. (2016). Non-pharmacological and non-surgical treatments for female urinary incontinence: An integrative review. *Applied Nursing Research*, 31, 146–153.

Mentes, J. C., & Iowa Veterans Affairs Nursing Research Consortium. (2000). Hydration management protocol. *Journal of Gerontological Nursing, 26*(10), 6–15.

Mentes, J. C., & Iowa Veterans Affairs Nursing Research Consortium. (2004). *Evidence-based practice guideline: Hydration management.* Iowa City, IA: The University of Iowa Gerontological Nursing Interventions Research Center Research Translation and Dissemination Core.

Milsom, I., Coyne, K. S., Nicholson, S., Kvasz, M., Chen, C. I., & Wein, A. J. (2014). Global prevalence and economic burden of urgency urinary incontinence: A systematic review. *European Urology*, 65(1), 79–95.

Mueller, N. (2004). What the future holds for incontinence care. *Urologic Nurse, 24*(3), 181–186.

National Association for Continence. (2015). Retrieved from http://www.nafc.org/

Newman, D. K. (2002). *Managing and treating urinary incontinence.* Baltimore, MD: Health Professions Press.

Newman, D. K., Burgio, K. L., Markland, A. D., & Goode, P. S. (2014). Urinary incontinence: Nonsurgical treatments. In *Geriatric Urology* (pp. 141–168). New York: Springer.

Newman, D., Gaines, T., & Snare, E. (2005). Innovation in bladder assessment: Use of technology in extended care. *Journal of Gerontological Nursing, 51*(12), 33–41.

Norris, A. (2001). HCFA correspondence, January 1, 2001.

Ostaszkiewicz, J., Eustice, S., Roe, B., Thomas, L. H., French, B., Islam, T.,. . .& Cody, J. D. (2013). Toileting assistance programmes for the management of urinary incontinence in adults. *The Cochrane Library*. Retrieved from http://www.cochrane.org/CD010589/INCONT_toileting-assistance-programmes-for-the-management-of-urinary-incontinence-in-adults

Ouslander, J. G. (2004). Management of the overactive bladder. *The New England Journal of Medicine, 350*, 786–799.

Palmer, M. H. (2008). Urinary incontinence quality improvement in nursing homes: Where have we been? Where are we going? *Urologic Nursing, 28*(6), 439–444.

Parker, W. P., & Griebling, T. L. (2015). Nonsurgical treatment of urinary incontinence in elderly women. *Clinics in Geriatric Medicine, 31*(4), 471–485.

Qaseem, A., Dallas, P., Forciea, M. A., Starkey, M., Denberg, T. D., . . . & Shekelle P. (2014). Nonsurgical management of urinary incontinence in women: A clinical practice guideline from the American College of Physicians. *Annals of Internal Medicine, 161*(6), 429–440.

Resnick, N. M., & Yalla, S. V. (1985). Management of urinary incontinence in the elderly. *New England Journal of Medicine*, 313(800–804).

Rich, S. A., & Panill, F. C. (1999). Urinary incontinence. In E. R. Black, D. R. Bordley, T. G. Tape, & R. J. Panzer (Eds.), *Diagnostic strategies for common medical problems* (2nd ed., pp. 527–539). Philadelphia, PA: American College of Physicians.

Robinson, J. P., & Shea, J. A. (2002). Development and testing of a measure of health-related quality of life for men with urinary incontinence. *Journal of the American Geriatrics Society, 50*(5), 935–945.

Shamliyan, T., Wyman, J. & Kane, R. L., (2012). Nonsurgical treatments for urinary incontinence in adult women: Diagnosis and comparative effectiveness. *Comparative Effectiveness Review,* No. 36, AHRQ Publication No. 11 (12)-EHC074-EF. Retrieved from http://www.effectivehealthcare.ahrq.gov/ehc/products/169/834/urinary-incontinence-treatment-report-130909.pdf

Shamliyan, T., Wyman, J. F., Ramakrishnan, R., Sainfort, F. & Kane, R. L. (2012). Benefits and harms of pharmacologic treatment for urinary incontinence in women: A systematic review. *Annals of Internal Medicine, 156,* 861–874.

Sitoh, Y., Lau, T., Zochling, J., Schwarz, J., Chen, J., March, L. M., . . . & Cameron I. D. (2005). Determinants of health-related quality of life in institutionalised older persons in northern Sydney. *Internal Medicine Journal, 35*, 131–134.

Skelly, J., Cowie, B., Galarneau, L., Moncherie, E., Northwood, M., Ploeg, J., . . . Fok, E. (2011). Promoting continence using prompted voiding: Guideline supplement. *RNAO Best Practice Guideline*. Retrieved from http://rnao.ca/sites/rnao-ca/files/storage/related/7719_BPG_Continence-Supplement-Only-2011.pdf

Smith, D., & Newman, D. (1989). Beating the cycle of constipation, laxative abuse, and fecal incontinence. *Today's Nursing Home,* 12–13.

Sparks, A., Boyer, D., Gambrel, A., & Lovett, M. (2004). The clinical benefits of the bladder scanner: A research synthesis. *Journal of Nursing Care Quality, 19*(3), 188–192.

Teunissen, D., Van Den Bosch, W., Van Weel, C., & Lagro-Janssen, T. (2006). "It can always happen": The impact of urinary incontinence on elderly men and women. *Scandinavian Journal of Primary Health Care, 24*(3), 166–173.

Tunis, S. R., Norris, A., & Simon, K. (2000). *Medicare coverage policy decisions: Biofeedback for treatment of urinary incontinence. (#CAG-00020).* Washington, DC: Health Care Financing Administration.

Tunis, S. R., Whyte, J. J., & Bridger, P. (2000). *Medicare coverage policy decisions. Pelvic floor electrical stimulation for treatment of urinary incontinence. (#CAG-00021).* Washington, DC: Health Care Financing Administration.

Tyagi, S., Resnick, N. M., Perera, S., Monk, T. H., Hall, M. H. & Buysse, D. J. (2014). Behavioral treatment of chronic insomnia in older adults: Does nocturia matter? *Sleep, 37*(4), 681–687.

Uebersax, J. S., Wyaman, J. F., Schumaker, S. A., Fantl, J. A., & Continence Program for Woman Research Group. (1995). Short forms to assess life quality and symptom distress for urinary incontinence in women: The incontinence impact questionnaire and the urogenital distress inventory. *Neurourology and Urodynamics, 14*(2), 131–139.

Umlauf, M., & Chasens, E. (2003). Sleep disordered breathing and nocturnal polyuria: Nocturia and enuresis. *Sleep, 7*(5), 373–376.

Wagg, A., Gibson, W., Ostaszkiewicz, J., Johnson, T., Markland, A., Palmer, M.H., . . . & Kirchner-Hermanns, R. (2015). Urinary incontinence in frail elderly persons. Report from the 5th International Consultation on Incontinence. *Neurourology and Urodynamics, 34*(5), 398–406.

Wilson, L., Brown, J. S., Shin, G. P., Luc, K., & Subak, L. L. (2001). Annual direct cost of incontinence. *Obstetrics & Gynecology, 98*(3), 398–406.

Wooldridge, L. (2000, June). Ultrasound technology and bladder dysfunction. *American Journal of Nursing,* 3–14.

Yu, L. C. (1987). Incontinence stress index: Measuring psychological impact. *Journal of Gerontological Nursing, 13*(7), 18–25.

Yu, L., Kaltreider, D., Hu, T. I., & Craighead, W. (1989). The ISQ-P tool: Measuring stress associated with incontinence. *Journal of Gerontological Nursing, 15*(2), 9–15.

For a full suite of assignments and additional learning activities, see the access code at the front of your book.

CHAPTER 16

Sleep Disorders

Carol Enderlin
Melodee Harris
Karen M. Rose
Lisa Hutchison
Ellyn E. Matthews

(Competencies 7, 17, 18)

LEARNING OBJECTIVES

At the end of this chapter, the reader will be able to:

> Discuss the importance of sleep to successful aging.
> Describe the potential impact of sleep disturbance on quality of life in older adults.
> Explain common theories of sleep regulation.
> Identify the general effects of neurotransmitters associated with sleep and wakefulness.
> Describe basic sleep architecture, including stages of sleep.
> Discuss changes in sleep associated with the normal aging process.
> Obtain a basic sleep history, including identification of risk factors for sleep disturbance.
> Use basic and selected specific sleep screening instruments to assess sleep in older adults.
> Describe selected diagnostic tests used by sleep professionals to diagnose sleep disorders.
> Discuss common sleep disorders in older adults, including those associated with geropsychiatric disorders.
> Identify geriatric implications of pharmacologic interventions for sleep disorders.
> Discuss nonpharmacological interventions used in the management of sleep disorders in older adults, including cognitive, behavioral, and complementary alternative therapies.

KEY TERMS

Actigraphy

Apnea

Circadian rhythm

Circadian rhythm disorders

Cognitive behavioral therapy

Complementary and alternative medicine

Daytime sleepiness

Homeostatic sleep drive

Hypersomnias

Hypopnea

Insomnia	Restless legs syndrome
Neurotransmitters	Sleep architecture
Non-rapid eye movement (NREM) sleep	Sleep cycle
Obstructive sleep apnea	Sleep efficiency
Parasomnias	Sleep fragmentation
Periodic limb movements	Sleep quality
Polysomnography	Sleep-related breathing disorders
Rapid eye movement (REM) sleep	Suprachiasmatic nucleus
REM sleep behavior disorder	Total sleep time

Healthy sleep plays an important role in successful aging. Decreased morbidity (Foley, Ancoli-Israel, Britz, & Walsh, 2004) and mortality (Dew et al., 2003) are associated with adequate sleep. In a cross-sectional study of nearly 2,800 people 100 years of age, 65% reported good or very good sleep quality and had a weighted average of 7.5 hours of sleep (Gu, Sautter, Pipkin, & Zeng, 2010). Although age-related changes predispose older adults to sleep disorders, according to the 2003 Sleep in America Poll (National Sleep Foundation, 2010), healthy older adults were less likely to report sleep disturbances compared with older adults with multiple comorbid conditions (Foley et al., 2004). The health benefits of adequate sleep and potential detriments of sleep disturbance should always be carefully considered in the nursing care of older adults.

Although adequate sleep may promote health, approximately 50% of older adults have reported difficulty sleeping (Foley, Monjan, Simonsick, Wallace, & Blazer, 1999). Sleep disturbance may be related to poor sleep hygiene, including an irregular sleep schedule, environmental noise or light, and the use of stimulants (Ancoli-Israel, 2009). Nocturia, whether as a cause of awakening or in response to awakening for other reasons, is commonly associated with perceived poor sleep quality in older adults. Although nocturia may result in part from aging, it also may represent an overlooked pathologic disorder (Bliwise et al., 2009). Older adults with multiple chronic diseases such as depression, pain, cognitive or neurological disorders, and heart or lung disease may have difficulty falling or staying asleep or experience abnormal respiratory events during sleep (Foley et al., 2004). Last, older adults taking numerous medications (polypharmacy) may have disturbed sleep as a side effect of drug therapy (Neikrug & Ancoli-Israel, 2010). Increasing use of over-the-counter (OTC) sleep medications such as diphenhydramine (Basu, Dodge, Stoehr, & Ganguli 2003) also may have an impact on nighttime sleep indirectly through increased daytime sleepiness. Even the presence of mild insomnia symptoms is associated with poorer self-reported health status and quality of life than that enjoyed by good sleepers (Leger, Scheuermaier, Philip, Paillard, & Guilleminault, 2001).

Sleep and Quality of Life

Sleep is a quality-of-life issue (Silva et al., 2009; Vitiello, 2006). Sleep affects the physical, psychosocial, spiritual, economic, social, and spiritual well-being of older adults. Thus, impaired sleep can have serious consequences in multiple quality-of-life domains, which may jeopardize function and independence in this population.

CLINICAL TIP

Sleep disturbance in older adults may lead to the loss of independence (Stone et al., 2008).

Older adults with sleep disturbances tend to have more difficulty meeting family, work, and self-care responsibilities. Poor sleep quality may contribute to decreased energy and motivation for the performance of everyday activities (Ancoli-Israel, 2009). Inadequate cognitive function to perform complex mental and decision-making tasks (Haimov, Hanuka, & Horowitz, 2008; Nebes, Buysse, Halligan, Houck, & Monk, 2009), as well as the development of delirium (Misra & Malow, 2008) are associated with sleep disturbance and may result in institutionalization. There are also safety implications of sleep disturbance for older adults, such as drowsy driving, medication administration errors, or falls (Stone et al., 2008). Consequently, sleep has major implications for the nursing care of older adults (Vance, Heaton, Eaves, & Fazeli, 2011).

Sleep Regulation

Sleep is thought to be regulated by multiple interacting processes, including a *homeostatic sleep drive* and *circadian rhythm* pacing. According to the Two-Process Model of Sleep (Borbely, 1982), sleep and wakefulness are theorized to exist in a homeostatic balance and are synchronized into circadian patterns of approximately 24-hour cycles. Sleep drive (propensity) is the proposed response to periods of extended wakefulness (Borbely, 1982), in concert with circadian response to environmental light stimulation of the retina and sleep pacemaker or *suprachiasmatic nucleus* (Chou et al., 2003; Scheer & Shea, 2009). The sleep pacemaker provides innervation of the ventrolateral preoptic and lateral hypothalamic areas, in which sleep- and wake-promoting cells are respectively located (McGinty & Szymusiak, 2003). The Flip-Flop Switch Model of Homeostatic and Circadian Regulation of Sleep and Wake proposes that these "sleep- and wake-promoting systems" function similarly to a continuous feedback loop (Jun, Sherman, Devor, & Saper, 2006).

CLINICAL TIP

Proposed Models of Sleep Regulation:

The Two-Process Model of Sleep (Borbely, 1982) and The Flip-Flop Model of Homeostatic and Circadian Regulation of Sleep and Wake (Jun et al., 2006).

Neurotransmitters are released as a result of interaction between the specialized nerve cells of these systems, which either inhibit or stimulate wakefulness (arousal) (Fuller, Gooley, & Saper, 2006). Serotonin, norepinephrine, histamine, orexin, acetylcholine, dopamine, and glutamate are some of the main neurotransmitters, and pharmacological therapies often target their actions or accessibility (McGinty & Szymusiak, 2011). Sleep and wake are also influenced by the hormones melatonin and cortisol. Melatonin promotes the initiation and maintenance of sleep. Levels of melatonin are highest before the sleep onset and are produced in response to sunlight exposure. In contrast, cortisol promotes wakefulness or arousal. Cortisol levels are inhibited during sleep and rise during wakefulness (Scheer & Shea, 2009). Disturbance of sleep homeostasis and circadian rhythms, such as through excessive daytime napping, frequent nighttime awakening, or decreased sunlight exposure, may result in sleep impairment. Neurological damage or deterioration also may alter sleep through reduced function or inability to produce adequate amounts of neurotransmitters, such as through strokes or degenerative disorders like Alzheimer's or Parkinson's disease. The general effects of neurotransmitters associated with sleep and wakefulness are summarized in **Table 16-1**.

Sleep Architecture

Sleep architecture refers to the "relative amounts of the different sleep stages composing sleep and timing of sleep cycles" (Berry, 2012, p. 649). Stage W (wake) refers to the shift from full alertness to drowsiness.

TABLE 16-1 General Effects of Neurotransmitters Associated with Sleep and Wakefulness

Neurotransmitters	General Effects
Acetylcholine	Associated with electroencephalogram desynchronization during wake and REM sleep
Adenosine	Increased levels associated with sleep deprivation; action blocked by methylxanthines such as caffeine
Dopamine	Lesions of dopamine neurons are associated with decreased arousal; D2 and D3 receptor agonists are associated with sedation
Gamma-aminobutyric acid (GABA)	Promotes sleep (acts as a central nervous syndrome [CNS] depressant); primary inhibitory CNS neurotransmitter
Glutamate (glutamic acid)	Promotes wakefulness; primary excitatory CNS neurotransmitter
Glycine	Produces REM sleep-related paralysis
Histamine	Promotes wakefulness; N-1 receptor blockers (antihistamines) increase sleepiness
Hypocretin (orexin)	Promotes wakefulness; hypocretin system dysfunction is associated with narcolepsy and cataplexy
Melatonin (MT)	Promotes sleep onset; peaks before sleep; produced daily in response to sunlight stimulation of the suprachiasmatic nucleus; production decreases with aging
Norepinephrine	Promotes wakefulness
Serotonin or 5-hydroxytryptamine (5-HT)	Promotes wakefulness; highest during wake and lowest during sleep; serotonin inhibitors decrease REM sleep

Data from Lee-Chiong, T. (2008). *Sleep medicine: Essentials and review.* Oxford, UK: Oxford University Press.

Non-rapid eye movement (NREM) sleep, stages N1, N2, and N3, represent the transition from light to increasingly deep sleep. *Rapid eye movement (REM) sleep*, stage R, is commonly referred to as "dreaming" sleep. NREM sleep comprises approximately 75% of total sleep time (N1 = 5% to 10%, N2 = 50% to 60%, N3 = 15% to 20%), and REM makes up the remaining 25% in adults. NREM sleep stages N1, N2, and N3, plus sleep stage R, make up one *sleep cycle*, and one night of sleep is composed of three to five 90- to 120-minute sleep cycles. The total minutes spent asleep during both NREM and REM is referred to as the *total sleep time* (Iber, Ancoli-Israel, Chesson, Quan, & The American Academy of Sleep Medicine [AASM], 2007).

During NREM sleep, responsiveness to environmental stimuli decreases but muscle tone is retained. REM sleep is characterized by dreaming with variable responsiveness to environmental stimuli, voluntary muscle paralysis, and variable autonomic activity. During REM sleep, vital signs and cerebral blood flow are increased; however, temperature regulation is diminished (Carskadon & Dement, 2000).

CLINICAL TIP

One night of sleep is composed of three to five 90- to 120-minute sleep cycles (Iber et al., 2007).

Sleep and the Aging Process

The normal aging process is associated with some change in the sleep patterns and architecture of healthy older adults (Vitiello, 2006). In general, the bedtime and wake time of older adults are earlier than those of younger adults (Vitiello, 2006), and napping may increase (Driscoll et al., 2008; Foley, Ancoli-Israel, Britz, & Walsh, 2004). Sleep stages are characterized by decreased restorative NREM sleep (Carskadon & Dement, 2005) and REM or dreaming sleep (Bliwise, 2005). *Sleep efficiency* falls approximately 3% per decade, reflecting less time spent asleep while in bed attempting to sleep (Ohayon, Carskadon, Guilleminault, & Vitiello, 2004). This may be partly in response to changes in endogenous circadian temperature oscillation in older compared to younger adults, including a 60% lower mean amplitude and 2-hour-earlier minimum value (Czeisler & Dumont, 1992). Overall, sleep changes are similar in men and women after the age of 60 (Ohayon et al., 2004) and are associated less with actual aging than with existing disorders (Vitiello, Moe, & Prinz, 2002). Other normal developmental challenges that may have an impact on the sleep of older adults include adaptation to retirement (Redeker, 2011) and grief (AASM, 2005). Overall, the normal aging process is not associated with a decreased need for sleep, but it is associated with decreased ability to sleep (Bliwise, 1993). This decreased ability to sleep is often related to the sleep, medical, or psychiatric disorders commonly found in this population (Crowley, 2011).

Assessment of Sleep

History

Assessment of sleep is important to the overall nursing care of the older adult. The SPICES (**S**leep disorders, **P**roblems with eating or feeding, **I**ncontinence, **C**onfusion, **E**vidence of falls, **S**kin breakdown) assessment tool (Fulmer, 2007) can be used to identify older adults with sleep disturbances. The onset, duration, and severity of the symptoms, along with previous treatments, should be determined. Risks for sleep disturbances should also be identified, including a personal or family history of sleep disturbance, obesity, smoking, hypertension, depression, and other factors. A subjective account about sleep quality should be elicited, and older adults should be asked to describe their usual sleep patterns and nighttime routines. Patient-maintained sleep diaries are helpful sleep assessment tools. Daytime work, exercise, and recreational activities should be included, as well as the older adults' perception of daytime sleepiness. A caregiver or partner is an important resource for the older adult who snores or who is a poor historian, such as older adults with a diagnosis of dementia (Ward, 2011).

    Additionally, a thorough medication review is needed. OTC medications, as well as herbal medications, supplements, alcohol, caffeine, and nicotine, and substance abuse should be included. Special attention should be given to sedating medications such as antidepressants or anxiolytics. A schedule of medication administration such as diuretics is also important (Ward, 2011).

> **CLINICAL TIP**
>
> A caregiver or partner is an important resource for the older adult who snores or who is a poor historian.

General Survey

An appearance of either hyperalertness or flattened affect in the older adult should be noted as a possible sign of anxiety or depression, respectively, both of which may be associated with *insomnia*. Excessive *daytime sleepiness* in the older adult may be suggested by yawning, rubbing of the face, dark circles under the eyes, lack of attentiveness, or dozing off during the assessment (Vaughn & D'Cruz, 2011).

Physical Assessment

During the physical assessment, the height and weight should be obtained and the body mass index (BMI) calculated. The neck circumference also should be measured. *Obstructive sleep apnea* (OSA) is associated with a BMI greater than 30 kg/m^2 and/or a neck circumference exceeding 40 cm (Kushida & Efron, 1997). Simple visual inspection revealing a small or recessed mandible, dental malocclusion, a large tongue, or enlarged tonsils may suggest overcrowding of the oropharynx, which may contribute to OSA (Friedman et al., 1999; Mallampati et al., 1985). Mouth-breathing or asymmetry of the nose may suggest nasal obstruction, which may also contribute to OSA (Cao, Guilleminault, & Kushida, 2011).

Basic Sleep Assessment Instruments

There are several basic sleep assessment instruments that registered nurses may use as general screening tools to identify areas of concern. The presence and severity of daytime sleepiness can be assessed using the Epworth Sleepiness Scale (ESS). The ESS, composed of eight items using a Likert-type scale, takes 5 to 10 minutes to complete. Although not diagnostic, high ESS scores suggest the possible presence of OSA or narcolepsy (Johns, 1991, 1992, 1993, 1994).

Subjective *sleep quality* (the perception of sleep as restorative) can be assessed using the Pittsburgh Sleep Quality Index (PSQI). The PSQI, composed of 10 items that assess sleep disturbance and medication use, as well as daytime dysfunction, can be administered in approximately 10 minutes. A total or global sleep quality score can be computed, indicating adequate to poor sleep quality (Buysse, Reynolds III, Monk, Berman, & Kupfer, 1989).

Both of these instruments, along with background information, references, and online videos, can be accessed for free through the Hartford Institute for Geriatric Nursing General Assessment Series (Hartford Institute for Geriatric Nursing, 2015). If findings indicate severe daytime sleepiness or poor sleep quality, follow-up evaluation should be arranged with the primary healthcare provider for possible referral to a sleep specialist.

Specialized Sleep Assessment Instruments

A number of sleep assessment instruments may be used to screen for specific sleep disorders. The STOP BANG screening questionnaire surveys reported snoring, tiredness, and observed apnea (STOP) in addition to high blood pressure, BMI, age, neck circumference, and gender (BANG). The presence of several of these risk factors suggests possible OSA. The STOP BANG takes less than 10 minutes to administer, and is often included in preoperative assessments to identify patients at risk for postoperative OSA (Chung & Elsaid, 2009; Chung et al., 2008).

The Cambridge-Hopkins Restless Legs Syndrome Questionnaire (CH-RLS-Q13) is used to screen for the presence of symptoms that suggest probable restless legs syndrome. The CH-RLS-Q13 consists of 13 items that survey the presence of a recurrent uncomfortable urge to move legs, the position in which this urge is experienced, influence of activity on symptoms, severity of distress with symptoms, frequency of symptoms, and age of symptom onset. This instrument takes 10–20 minutes to administer (Allen, Burchell, MacDonald, Hening, & Earley, 2009).

The Insomnia Severity Index (ISI) assesses the presence and severity of insomnia symptoms, including difficulty falling or staying asleep, waking up too early, satisfaction with sleep, extent of sleep interference with function, how noticeable sleep impairment is to others, and amount of distress over sleep problems. The ISI can be completed in 5 minutes, and symptoms in the moderate to severe range suggest possible clinical insomnia (Bastian, Vallieres, & Morin, 2001).

It should be noted that the instruments described are intended for screening rather than diagnosis and that positive findings should be evaluated by the primary care provider and possibly referred to a sleep medicine specialist for additional diagnostic testing.

Diagnostic Sleep Tests

Polysomnography (PSG), also referred to as an "overnight sleep test," records electroencephalographic changes during sleep and allows identification of sleep patterns and events (Dement, 2011). Multiple physiologic variables are also simultaneously recorded during sleep, including muscle activity, nasal airflow, chest and abdominal effort, oxyhemoglobin saturation, and limb (leg) movement. Stages of sleep and sleep-related events can be detected with PSG, such as frequencies and durations of arousals, awakenings, apneas, and hypopneas (Collop, 2006). *Apnea* refers to absence of airflow at the nose or mouth for 10 seconds or longer, and is classifiable by type. OSA is associated with persistent pulmonary effort, whereas central apnea is characterized by an absence of respiratory effort. *Hypopnea* is broadly defined as partial reduction in airflow for 10 seconds or longer (Berry, 2012). Patient preparation for PSG is depicted in **Figure 16-1**.

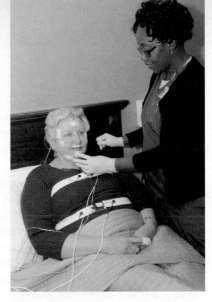

Figure 16-1 Dr. Carol Enderlin is prepared for overnight PSG by Valerie Wofford, registered PSG technologist (RPSGT).
Courtesy of the University of Arkansas for Medical Sciences (UAMS) Sleep Clinic.

Actigraphy (ACTG) detects motion as a proxy of wakefulness and the absence of motion as sleep (Tyron, 1991). An actigraph resembles a watch and is most commonly worn on the wrist during routine activity and sleep. Home monitoring of sleep for up to 60 days can be obtained with ACTG, depending upon the model used. More cost-effective and convenient than PSG, ACTG is a valid and reliable measure of sleep in normal healthy adults (Morgenthaler et al., 2007). The measurement of total sleep time is more accurate than of other sleep variables, and as sleep disturbance increases accuracy decreases (Ancoli-Israel et al., 2003). *Circadian rhythm disorders* (CGDs) and circadian rhythms, and sleep–wake patterns of adults with insomnia can be assessed using ACTG. It may be used to measure total sleep time in adults with OSA and as an alternative in populations such as elderly adults who may not tolerate PSG (Morgenthaler et al., 2007). Care should be taken to avoid use of wrist ACTG in older adults with an arteriovenous shunt or impaired lymphatic drainage. The frequency and pattern of periodic limb movements of sleep can be measured using ankle ACTG (Kazenwadel et al., 1995; Kemlink, Pretl, Sonka, & Nevsimalova, 2008); however, a history or risk of impaired peripheral perfusion or blood clots are contraindications to its use. Wrist ACTG is shown in **Figure 16-2**.

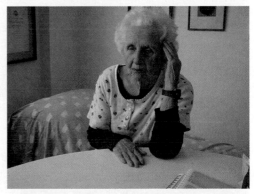

Figure 16-2 An actigraph resembles a watch and is most commonly worn on the wrist during routine activity and sleep. The actigraph detects motion as a proxy of wakefulness, and the absence of motion as sleep (Tyron, 1991).
Courtesy of Ambulatory Monitoring (Ardsley, NY).

Common Sources of Geriatric Sleep Disturbance

Common Sleep Disorders

In order to effectively screen for potential sleep disorders in older adults, geriatric nurses must have a basic knowledge of the most common sleep disorders found in this population. Broadly, sleep disorders may be subdivided into insomnia, sleep-related breathing disorders, hypersomnias, CRDs parasomnias, and sleep-related movement disorders.

Insomnia

Insomnia is defined as "persistent difficulty with sleep initiation, duration, consolidation, or quality that occurs despite adequate time & opportunity and circumstances for sleep, and results in some form of daytime impairment," (AASM, 2014, p.19). Insomnia is more common in women than in men, and its prevalence increases with age (Ohayon, 2002). It has been estimated that 50% of older adults have insomnia, often comorbid with other sleep, medical, or psychiatric disorders. Symptoms of insomnia may be present in other sleep disorders, including sleep-related breathing disorder, restless legs syndrome, and periodic limb movements (Morin, Mimeault, & Gagne, 1999).

PSG, or overnight sleep testing, records electroencephalographic changes during sleep (Dement, 2011). Muscle activity, nasal airflow, chest and abdominal effort, oxyhemoglobin saturation, and leg movements also can be recorded, and respiratory events (arousals, awakenings, apneas, hypopneas) detected (Collop, 2006).

Insomnia symptoms may also accompany psychiatric disorders such as depression (Benca, Ancoli-Israel, & Moldofsky, 2004) or chronic pain disorders (Taylor et al., 2007) and can lead to dependence on sedative-hypnotics or on alcohol as a form of self-medication (Bliwise, 1993). Although older adults may experience insomnia that is acute (transient), it is often chronic (lasting over 3 months) and persistent in up to 85% of cases (Morin, LeBlanc, Daley, Gregoire, & Merette, 2006).

Sleep-Related Breathing Disorders

Sleep-related breathing disorders are some of the most common sleep disorders found in the elderly population, and are characterized by "abnormalities of respiration during sleep," (AASM, 2014, p. 49). They include OSA (obstruction of the airway with continued respiratory effort but inadequate ventilation), central sleep apnea (CSA) syndromes (recurrent episodes of cessation of ventilation and ventilator effort), sleep-related hypoventilation and sleep-related hypoxemia disorders, and isolated symptoms and normal variants (AASM, 2014).

The prevalence of OSA increases with aging, is more common in men, and is associated with obesity, hypertension, and daytime sleepiness (AASM, 2014). A Swedish study of sleep apnea in community-dwelling elders reported that CSA was associated with cardiovascular disease and impaired systolic function in adults older than 75 years, whereas OSA was not (Johansson, Alehagen, Svanborg, Dahlstrom, & Brostrom, 2012). Diagnosis of OSA is based on patient/partner report and PSG (AASM, 2005), although daytime sleepiness scales and sleep apnea scales may be used as preliminary screening tools. Treatment of OSA depends upon its severity, but it most commonly includes continuous positive airway pressure (CPAP) (Neikrug & Ancoli-Israel, 2010). Although adherence to CPAP may present issues, older adults have demonstrated the ability to use it with multiple positive cardiovascular and cognitive benefits (Ancoli-Israel, 2007; Weaver & Chasens, 2007). Use of a CPAP device is shown in **Figure 16-3**.

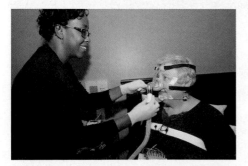

Figure 16-3 Multiple types of continuous positive airway pressure (CPAP) devices are available to maintain airway patency during sleep and are selected for patient comfort and maximum effectiveness.
Courtesy of the University of Arkansas for Medical Sciences (UAMS) Sleep Clinic.

CSA syndromes includes Cheyne-Stokes breathing pattern, which is associated with medical conditions such as congestive heart failure, stroke, or renal failure. This breathing pattern consists of a waxing and waning pattern of recurrent apneas (breathing cessation) and hypopneas (partial airflow reduction), which usually occur during

NREM sleep when assessed with PSG. CSA also may be associated with medications, among other causes (AASM, 2014).

Hypoventilation and hypoxemia disorders are nonobstructive and are characterized by decreased alveolar hypoventilation and decreased arterial oxygen desaturation, respectively during sleep. Hypoventilation and hypoxemia disorders may occur in the presence of normal pulmonary mechanical properties and may be precipitated by CNS depressants. These disorders often follow a slowly progressive course that can lead to pulmonary hypertension and cardiac failure. Hypoventilation and hypoxemia syndromes are diagnosed separately with PSG (AASM, 2014).

Sleep-related breathing disorders such as OSA are associated with frequent arousals from sleep, resulting in fragmented sleep and daytime sleepiness, which may be the presenting complaint (AASM, 2014). Patient education related to OSA is illustrated in **Figure 16-4**.

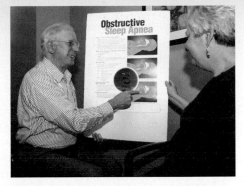

Figure 16-4 Dr. Greg Krulin discusses how the airway is closed in OSA, and how CPAP works to relieve the obstruction.
Courtesy of the University of Arkansas for Medical Sciences (UAMS) Sleep Clinic.

Central Disorders of Hypersomnia

Hypersomnias of central origin refer to sleep disorders with the main complaint of daytime sleepiness unrelated to other causes of sleep disturbance such as circadian rhythm or sleep-related breathing disorders. Hypersomnias include the sleep disorder narcolepsy, with or without cataplexy (sudden bilateral loss of muscle tone elicited by strong, usually positive emotions such as laughter). Narcolepsy is defined as "rapid transition from wakefulness to REM sleep" (AASM, 2005, p. 81), and its etiology includes both genetic and nongenetic factors. The pathology of narcolepsy is associated with loss of hypothalamic neurons, which contain hypocretin (an excitatory neuropeptide). The onset of narcolepsy is usually in late adolescence or early adulthood and is characterized by sleepiness and later by hypnagogic hallucinations (vivid perceptual experiences at sleep onset), sleep paralysis (a transient inability to move or speak during the sleep–wake transition), and disturbed nocturnal sleep. Diagnosis is based on patient-reported symptoms (AASM, 2005) and supported by a cerebrospinal fluid (CSF) hypocretin-1 level of less than 110 pg/mL. Other confirming sleep findings include a short sleep latency (under 8 minutes taken to fall asleep) on the Multiple Sleep Latency Test (Carskadon & Dement, 1982; Carskadon et al., 1986), and/or a sleep-onset REM period of 10 minutes or less after the onset of sleep, as measured by PSG. Narcolepsy can diminish quality of life by impairing school, work, and social functioning, and depression often develops (AASM, 2005). Treatment of narcolepsy includes pharmacologic agents; behavioral therapy, including sleep hygiene; and social support such as through groups (Guilleminault & Cao, 2011). Older adults who carry the human leukocyte antigen DQB1*0602 allele (associated with 95% of hypocretin-deficient narcolepsy) but who have no diagnosis of narcolepsy also have reported poorer perceptions of feeling rested than older adults without the allele with the same poor sleep efficiency. These findings suggest that there may be a "normal" phenotypic variation of REM sleep in DQB1*0602 allele carriers among older adults with insomnia (Zeitzer et al., 2011).

Other types of hypersomnias may be idiopathic (of unknown etiology). However, idiopathic hypersomnia must be distinguished from OSA, narcolepsy, and hypersomnia associated with medical and psychiatric disorders and medications (AASM, 2014). Prolonged sleep duration (9 hours or more per day) in adults 68 years or older has been associated with daytime sleepiness, in contrast to short sleep duration (6 hours or less), which was associated with night sleep disturbance and poor sleep quality. Older adults with hypersomnia should be referred to their primary care provider for further evaluation and determination of the need for consultation with a specialist.

CLINICAL TIP

OSA must always be considered in the presence of daytime sleepiness (Mesas et al., 2011).

Circadian Rhythm Disorders

A CRD is a disorder "caused by alternations of the circadian time-keeping system, its entrainment mechanisms, or a misalignment of the endogenous circadian rhythm and the external environment" (AASM, 2014, p.189). A CRD may be of the advanced or delayed phase type (ASPD or DSPD) based on the relative early or late onset patterns of sleep and wake time (Berry, 2012). Although a morningness type of sleep pattern is associated with increased aging and poorer objective sleep quality (less total sleep time and increased wake time during last 2 hours of sleep), the morningness type alone, rather than age, is associated with advanced sleep phase disorder (ASPD) (Carrier, Monk, Buysse, & Kupfer, 1997). Advanced phase–related complaints were twice those of delayed phase–related complaints in adults 40–64 years of age (Ando, Kripke, & Ancoli-Israel, 2002). Diagnosis is made based on sleep logs and ACTG, and treatment may include evening light therapy (Sack et al., 2007).

Delayed sleep phase syndrome (DSPD) is relatively rare among adults 40 to 64 years of age (Ando et al., 2002), although less is known of its frequency among older adults. DSPD is also diagnosed with sleep logs and ACTG and may be managed with prescribed sleep scheduling. Insomnia should be considered as a possible underlying problem, as persons with ASPD have symptoms of delayed sleep onset (Sack et al., 2007).

Parasomnias

Parasomnias are described as "undesirable physical events or experiences that occur during entry into sleep, within sleep, or during arousals from sleep" (AASM, 2014, p. 225). These may occur in NREM and REM sleep, or during transition to and from sleep. Parasomnias reflect activation of the CNS and may be characterized by abnormal movements, behaviors, emotions, perceptions, dreams, and autonomic nervous system activity. They also may be demonstrated through aggressive behavior, locomotion, sleep-related eating disorder, or sexual behaviors. Parasomnias disrupt sleep and may result in injuries, negative health, and social effects for the person with the disorder and their bed partner (AASM, 2014).

There are numerous REM-related parasomnias, including REM sleep behavior disorder. *REM sleep behavior disorder* (RSBD) is associated with the enactment of violent dreams, is most common in men older than 50 years with underlying neurological disorders (parkinsonism, dementia with Lewy bodies, narcolepsy, stroke), and is progressive in nature. Notably, 33% of persons newly diagnosed with Parkinson's disease have RSBD. Medications, including venlafaxine, selective serotonin reuptake inhibitors, mirtazapine, and other antidepressants may precipitate RSBD. This disorder is of particular concern in older adults due to the potential for self-injury or injury of the bed partner (AASM, 2014).

Sleep-Related Movement Disorders

Sleep-related movement disorders are usually characterized by stereotyped movements that interfere with sleep and sleep onset. These include various leg, limb, and jaw movements due to medical disorders, medications, or unknown causes (AASM, 2014).

Restless legs syndrome (RLS) is defined as "a sensorimotor disorder characterized by a complaint of a strong, nearly irresistible, urge to move the legs" (AASM, 2014, p. 283). Paresthesias (abnormal skin sensation without a noticeable cause) also may be reported. These worsen when sitting or lying down and are almost immediately relived by movement (AASM, 2014). Onset may be early (younger than 45 years of age) with slowly progressing symptoms or late in life (40 to 65 years of age) with rapidly progressing symptoms. The prevalence of RLS is higher in women and varies by race/ethnicity, with 5% to 10% of Northern Europeans reporting symptoms. The etiology of RLS includes familial inheritance, brain iron dysregulation, and dopamine abnormalities. Conditions or disorders associated with iron deficiency (renal failure, iron deficiency anemia) precipitate symptoms, as do antihistamines, dopamine receptor antagonists, and many antidepressants (AASM, 2014).

Periodic limb movements (PLMs), which are repetitive, involuntary jerks or twitches of the legs, are present in 80% to 90% of persons with RLS. Combined, RLS symptoms impair the ability to fall or return to sleep after awakening, and PLMs repeatedly provoke arousals and awakenings from sleep, resulting in sleep disturbance and daytime sleepiness.

The diagnosis of RLS is based on patient report and established criteria, and PLMs are measured using PSG (AASM, 2014). Both RLS and PLMs tend to increase with aging (Ancoli-Israel et al., 1991).

Geropsychiatric Disorders and Sleep

Sleep disturbance is a common problem in older adults with mental health conditions. Sleep disturbance in older adults is considered a geriatric syndrome, that often occurs with mental health disorders and substance abuse (Enderlin et al., 2013; Vaz Fragoso & Gill, 2007). It is estimated that 20% of older persons have a mental disorder (Karel, Gatz, & Smyer, 2012). Chronic illness and mental health disorders may overlap in older persons (Crystal, Sambamoorthi, Walkup, & Akincigil, 2003). Conditions such as depression, bipolar disorder, and schizophrenia often worsen with chronic conditions due to health disparities (De Hert et al., 2011). Therefore, it is critical that nurses are prepared to join the geropsychiatric workforce as leaders in the care of older persons with sleep disturbances and mental health disorders.

CLINICAL TIP

Sleep impairment in older adults is considered a geriatric syndrome that often occurs with mental health disorders and substance abuse (Enderlin et al., 2013; Vaz Fragoso & Gill, 2007).

According to the Centers for Disease Control and Prevention (CDC) (2015), the rate of depression ranges from 1% to 13.5% across healthcare settings. Sleep disturbance places the older adult at high risk for depression (Schutte-Rodin, Broch, Buysse, Dorsey, & Sateia, 2008), and deficiencies in neurotransmitters such as serotonin are associated with both sleep disturbance and depression (Peterson & Benca, 2011). Sleep characteristics of older adults with depression include taking longer to experience REM sleep and early morning wakefulness with difficulty falling back to sleep. In addition, depression is associated with insomnia, dreaming, and a loss of deep, restorative sleep (Enderlin et al., 2013; Peterson & Benca, 2011). Depression and anxiety often occur simultaneously in older adults. Findings of one study (n = 110) of older persons with generalized anxiety disorder alone or with depression resulted in greater severity of sleep disturbance than in older persons without a mental health disorder (Brenes et al., 2009). Although statistics vary, according to data from the National Comorbidity Survey-Replication (Gum, King-Kallimanis, & Kohn, 2009), there is a 7% prevalence of anxiety in older adults. Older adults with anxiety may experience nighttime panic attacks as well as the inability to fall asleep and stay asleep (Brenes et al., 2009; Ramsawh, Stein, & Mellman, 2011). It is estimated that 1.5–4.8% of older adults have severe and persistent mental health disorders (Institute of Medicine [IOM], 2012) such as bipolar or schizophrenia. Sleep disturbances are common in severe and persistent mental health disorders. For example, in the manic phase of bipolar disorder, older adults are likely to feel rested after only 3 hours of sleep (American Psychiatric Association, 2013). In schizophrenia there may be a reversal of the sleep–wake cycle or long episodes of complete sleeplessness and fragmented sleep (Benson & Feinberg, 2011; Enderlin et al., 2013).

Healthy, restorative sleep depends upon an intact CNS. In persons with dementia, neurodegeneration in the brain is responsible for homeostatic and circadian rhythm processes that regulate sleep (Bliwise, 2011). Abnormal patterns of decreased slow-wave sleep and less REM make it difficult to distinguish the stages of sleep on PSG studies. As a result of neurodegeneration, persons with dementia often present with nighttime wandering and daytime sleepiness (Petit, Montplaisir, & Boeve, 2011). In addition, there is subcortical damage to sleep-promoting neurons. The areas affected include the cholinergic basal forebrain nuclei, serotonergic raphe nuclei, dopaminergic nigrostriatial and pallidostriatal pathways, and noradrenergic locus coeruleus (Neubauer, 2003; Vitiello & Borson, 2001). Efferent pathways also may be damaged from the retina, hypothalamic nuclei, limbic forebrain, raphe nuclei, and reticular formation. Further, the hormonal response impairs sleep hormones such as melatonin (Vitiello & Borson, 2001). As neurons in the homeostatic mechanisms deteriorate, lesions are formed in the neuronal pathways causing the sleep–wake cycle response to weaken in the CNS (Cole & Richards, 2005).

Parkinson's disease caused by insufficient amounts of dopamine produced in the substantia nigra in the brain. Pathophysiology includes degeneration in the synucleinopathies that occur in Parkinson's disease and dementia with Lewy bodies (Petit et al., 2011; Postuma et al., 2009). REM sleep behavior disorder (RSBD) is an interesting sleep disturbance that is associated with syncleinopathies (Boeve, 2010). A diagnosis of RSBD includes both abnormal REM sleep electrophysiology and REM sleep behavior (Boeve, 2010; Enderlin et al., 2013). In RBD, there are sudden awakenings with vivid dreams, dream enactment behavior occurring during REM sleep, and physically aggressive behaviors that reflect the content of the dream (Boeve, 2010). The dreams may frighten and disrupt the sleep of caregivers making patient and caregiver safety a main nursing priority (Boeve, 2010; Enderlin et al., 2013). PSG studies are required in the diagnosis of RSBD (Boeve, 2010).

Sleep Management

Pharmacological management of sleep disorders in older adults is sometimes needed for relief of symptoms not amenable to nonpharmacological methods. However, older adults may be more sensitive to the potential side effects of sleep medications, especially those related to the CNS, which may predispose to cognitive impairment and falls.

As with other medications administered to this age group, the general rule is to start with a low dose and slowly increase it until the desired results are obtained. It should be noted that some medications have a risk profile that contraindicates their use in the elderly. Specialized references with geriatric doses and implications should always be consulted regarding the use of sleep medications in older adults. Medications often used to manage sleep disorders are summarized in **Table 16-2**, with current geriatric implications. Patient sleep medication counseling is critical to successful management of sleep disturbance or disorders (see **Figure 16-5**).

CLINICAL TIP

Older adults may be more sensitive to the potential side effects of sleep medications, especially those related to the CNS, which may predispose to cognitive impairment and falls.

TABLE 16-2 Geriatric Implications of Sleep Medications

Sleep Disorder	Drug Classification	Medications	Mechanism of Action	Geriatric Implications
Sleep-Promotion Enhancers (Walsh & Roth, 2011)				
Insomnia	Sedative-Hypnotics	Nonbenzodiazepines: Eszopiclone (Lunesta) Zaleplon (Sonata) Zolpidem (Ambien)	Theorized to enhance GABA	Avoid use in elderly; increased risk of delirium, falls, fractures (AGS, 2015; Semla Beizer, & Hibgee, 2015)
		Suvorexant (Belsomra)	Dual orexin-1 and orexin-2 receptor antagonist	At recommended dosages, no overall differences in safety/efficacy than in younger adults (Merck, 2014); side effects of somnolence, dizziness, possible additive CNS side effects; slightly increases levels of digoxin http://www.drugs.com/monograph/suvorexant.html Drowsiness and next-day sedation, dose-dependent and more common in women; lower doses recommended in older adults and women (Semla et al., 2015)
		Benzodiazepines Long-acting: Flurazepam (Dalmane) Quazepam (Doral)	Theorized to enhance GABA	Avoid use in elderly; extremely long half-life; prolonged sedation; increased risk of delirium, falls, and fractures (AGS, 2015; Semla et al., 2015)
		Benzodiazepines Short-acting: Temazepam (Restoril) Triazolam (Halcion)	Theorized to enhance GABA	Avoid use in elderly; increased sensitivity and risk of delirium, falls, fractures in elderly (AGS, 2015; Semla et al., 2015)
Other Sleep Promotion Enhancers (Krystal, 2011; 2015)				
	Antianxiety	Buspirone (BuSpar)	Unknown; high affinity for 5HT receptors; Moderate affinity for DA receptors	Recommended if anxiolytic is indicated (mild to moderate anxiety); less sedating than other anxiolytics (Semla et al., 2015)

(continues)

TABLE 16-2 Geriatric Implications of Sleep Medications (*continued*)

Sleep Disorder	Drug Classification	Medications	Mechanism of Action	Geriatric Implications
	Hormone	Melatonin *dietary supplement, OTC	MT1 and MT2 receptor agonist	No significant difference in safety for older as in younger adults (Semla et al., 2015)
		Ramelteon (Rozerem)		Total exposure of older adults to ramelteon is 86%–97% higher compared to in younger adults; does not exacerbate mild to moderate OSA http://www.drugs.com /pro/rozerem.html
Wake Promotion Blockers (Krystal, 2011)				
	Sedating antidepressants	Tricyclics: Amitriptyline (Elavil) Doxepin (Sinequan) doses > 6 mg/day (Silenor 6 mg) Trimipramine (Surmontil)	5HT and NE receptor blockers; antagonize 5HT and NE receptors	Avoid use in elderly; strong sedative, anticholinergic, and orthostatic hypotensive properties in elderly (AGS, 2015; Semla et al., 2015)
		Other: Trazodone (Desyrel) Mirtazapine (Remeron)	5HT reuptake inhibitor; H1 and alpha adrenergic receptor blockers	Very sedating; few anticholinergic effects; limited data published regarding use in elderly (Semla et al., 2015)
	Antihistamines	Diphenhydramine (Benadryl) *OTC Doxylamine succinate (Unisom) *OTC	H1 receptor antagonist Muscarinic cholinergic antagonist	Avoid use in elderly; highly anticholinergic; may cause confusion (AGS, 2015)
	Antipsychotics	Olanzapine (Zyprexa) Quetiapine (Seroquel)	Antagonize DA, H1, 5HT, muscarinic, cholinergic, and adrenergic receptors	Avoid use in elderly, not recommended for elderly except for actual diagnosis of psychosis; increased risk of stroke, death, tremors, and falls (AGS, 2015)

Wake-Promotion Enhancers (Guilleminault & Cao, 2011; Thorpy, 2015; Thorpy & Dauvilliers, 2015)

Narcolepsy	Stimulants	Amphetamines:	↑ MAO release (dopamine, norepinephrine, and 5-HT)	
		Methamphetamine	Similar to amphetamine, less peripheral side effects	Avoid use in elderly due to CNS stimulant effects (AGS, 2015); may cause cardiovascular effects, including palpitations, tachycardia, and hypertension; insufficient research in adults over 65 years of age http://www.drugs.com/sfx/methamphetamineside-effects.html
		Methylphenidate (Ritalin)	Blocks MAO uptake at lower dose than amphetamine	Avoid use in elderly due to CNS stimulant effects (AGS, 2015)
		Selegiline (Eldepryl)	MAO-B inhibitor; converts to amphetamine	Do not use capsule/tablet doses > 10 mg/day or orally disintegrating tablet (Zelapar) doses > 2.5 mg/day due to risk of nonselective inhibition of MAO; monitor for constipation and fluid/electrolyte imbalance in older adults (Semla et al., 2015)
		Modafinil (Provigil) Armodafinil (Nuvigil)	Unknown mode of action	Avoid use in older adults due to CNS stimulant effects (AGS, 2015); reduced excretion of modafinil and its metabolites in elderly; safety and effectiveness not established over 65 years of age (Semla et al., 2015)
	Anticataplectics	Venlafaxine (Effexor)	5HT and NE reuptake inhibitor	Avoid use in older adults (AGS, 2015); low anticholinergic and sedative properties; may be used in elderly when a stimulant is indicated; adjust dose for renal function (Semla et al., 2015)
		Sodium oxybate (Xyrem)	CNS depressant with anticataplectic activity	Side effects of dizziness, somnolence, disorientation, confusion, balance disorder, fecal/urinary incontinence, respiratory impairment; potential additive CNS effects; monitor for impaired motor and cognitive function in older adults http://www.drugs.com/ppa/sodium-oxybate.html

(continues)

TABLE 16-2 Geriatric Implications of Sleep Medications (*continued*)

Sleep Disorder	Drug Classification	Medications	Mechanism of Action	Geriatric Implications
		Fluoxetine (Prozac)	Selective 5HT reuptake inhibitor	Long half-life in elderly; associated with hyponatremia; (Semla et al., 2015); avoid in older adults with history of falls/fractures, syndrome of inappropriate secretion of antidiuretic hormone secretion (AGS, 2015)
		Protriptyline (Vivactil)	MAO uptake inhibitor	Avoid in older adults; highly anticholinergic, sedating, and orthostatic hypotension (AGS, 2015)
		Imipramine (Tofranil) Desipramine (Norpramin)	5HT and NE reuptake inhibitor; down-regulation of beta-adrenergic and 5HT receptors	Avoid in older adults; highly anticholinergic, sedating, and orthostatic hypotension (AGS, 2015)
		Clomipramine (Anafranil)	Affects 5HT and NE uptake	Avoid in older adults; highly anticholinergic, sedating, and orthostatic hypotension (AGS, 2015)

Dopamine Promoters or Enhancers and Opiate Receptor Binders (Allen et al., 2014; Hogl, 2015; Montplaisir, Allen, Arthur, & Ferini-Strambi, 2011; Trenkwalder et al., 2013)

Sleep Disorder	Drug Classification	Medications	Mechanism of Action	Geriatric Implications
Restless legs syndrome (RLS)	Dopamine agonists	Pramipexole (Miripex) Ropinirole (Requip)	Bind to DA receptors (D3) in place of DA; directly stimulate DA receptors	Half-life 1.5 times longer in elderly; renal clearance decreased in elderly; postural hypotension and confusion; dosage not adjusted for elderly; postural hypotension and daytime somnolence (Semla et al., 2015)
	Dopamine precursors:	Levodopa/carbidopa	↑ Available DA	Greater sensitivity to CNS side effects in elderly (confusion, somnolence, insomnia, nightmares) (Semla et al., 2015)

Benzodiazepines	Clonazepam (Klonopin) Temazepam (Restoril)	Depress nerve transmission in the motor cortex (decrease PLMs- and PLMs-associated arousals in RLS; given for insomnia symptoms secondary to dopaminergic agents)	Avoid in older adults (AGS, 2015) Potential decreased hepatic clearance and renal excretion in elderly; CNS (confusion, somnolence, insomnia, nightmares) and pulmonary (respiratory congestion and depression) toxicities; recommended (only) when indicated; use should be limited to 10–14 days (Semla et al., 2015)
Opiates	Oxycodone Codeine Oxycodone-naloxone	Possible opiate receptor binding and opioid levels to counterbalance endogenous opioid system dysfunction	Increased sensitivity to CNS and constipating effects in older as in younger adults (Semla et al., 2015) Side effects include falls, dizziness, sedation, urinary retention http://www.drugs.com/sfx/naloxone-oxycodone -side-effects.html
Anticonvulsants	Gabapentin (Neurontin)	↑ Brain DA levels directly (decrease peripheral neuropathy-related pain in RLS)	Decreased renal clearance with increasing age; CNS side effects of somnolence and fatigue in > 10% (not specific to elderly) (Semla et al., 2015)

5HT = serotonin, CNS = central nervous system, DA = dopamine, GABA = gamma-hydroxybutyrate, H = histamine, MAO = monoamine oxydase, MT1, MT2 = melatonin 1 and 2 receptors, NE = norepinephrine, OTC = over the counter, PLMs = periodic limb movements of sleep, RLS = restless legs syndrome.

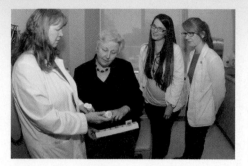

Figure 16-5 Dr. Lisa Hutchison, PharmD and pharmacy students provide sleep medication counseling.
Courtesy of Thomas and Lyon Longevity Clinic, Donald W. Reynolds Institute on Aging, UAMS.

Complementary and Alternative Medicine (CAM)

For all adults, national surveys indicate that as many as 38% use a *complementary* and/or *alternative medicine* (CAM) modality to improve some aspect of their health and well-being (Barnes, Bloom, & Nahin, 2008). CAM practices are used by older adults for reasons that may have implications related to improvement in sleep: to relive pain, to improve quality of life, and to maintain health and fitness (Williamson, Fletcher, & Dawson, 2003).

CAM practices are organized into several classifications according to the National Center of Complementary and Alternative Medicine (NCCAM), a component of the National Institutes of Health (NCCAM, 2015a). According to NCCAM, CAM practices and products are classified into these categories: whole medical systems (e.g., acupuncture); mind–body modalities (e.g., cognitive-behavior therapy); biological-based products (e.g., herbs and natural substances); manipulative and body-based modalities (e.g., massage, Tai Chi); and energy modalities (e.g., cranial electrical stimulation). Although not every CAM practice and product has been shown to be efficacious in improving sleep in older adults, there are promising results in some areas and these will be discussed.

Acupuncture

Acupuncture is practiced by providers who insert small needles into different points on the body, with or without the use of electrostimulation (NCCAM, 2014). Although acupuncture has shown promise in decreasing sleep disturbances in older adult females who are experiencing distressing symptoms related to menopause, including hot flashes that interrupt sleep; in insomnia in persons who have experienced a stroke; and in persons with fibromyalgia, there is insufficient evidence to support its widespread use to improve sleep in older adults (Borud, Grimsgaard, & White, 2010; Gooneratne, 2008). Further research in this area is ongoing and may provide more solid evidence for its use in older adults.

Mind–Body Modalities

Cognitive behavioral therapy (CBT) refers to a number of therapeutic approaches that focus on the effect of thinking on feelings and actions. Although approaches may differ, the common premise is that patients can learn to think differently, act on that learning, and change their behaviors. CBT is collaborative, time-limited in nature, and provides patients with the rationale and strategies necessary to develop self-management skills (National Association of Cognitive Behavioral Therapists, 2014). CBT approaches are often used to treat chronic sleep disturbances (Bootzin, 2005). Specifically, CBT for insomnia (CBTI), is a multicomponent approach aimed at modifying sleep schedules, habits, and maladaptive thoughts about sleep that can lead to the perpetuation of insomnia.

The most common, empirically supported, and standard components of CBTI are sleep restriction, stimulus control, cognitive therapy, and sleep hygiene education, with or without relaxation (Morgenthaler et al., 2006; Morin & Benca, 2012). Sleep restriction curtails the amount of time spent in bed each night to the patient's estimated average total sleep time. This reduction in sleep time increases the homeostatic sleep drive through mild sleep deprivation, which results in improved quality of sleep and decreased time to fall asleep. Stimulus control focuses on helping patients to reassociate the bed and bedroom with falling asleep, rather than bedtime being a stimulus for wakefulness (Bootzin & Perlis, 2011). Cognitive therapy assists patients to recognize maladaptive thoughts and beliefs about sleep and to reframe or "restructure" them more positively (Perlis & Gehrman, 2011). Sleep hygiene education promotes the following general practices: establish consistent bedtime and arise time, create a bedtime routine, and avoid stimulants close to bedtime; promote light snack before bed, regular exercise, and limited liquids in the evening; and initiate environmental modifications for a comfortable sleep environment (Posner & Gehrman, 2011). Although sleep hygiene is integrated into CBTI, evidence is insufficient to support its use as a stand-alone therapy (Schutte-Rodin et al., 2008; Wilson et al., 2010). Relaxation refers to a number of practices such as progressive relaxation and guided imagery. The aim of relaxation therapy is to reduce somatic and/or cognitive arousal and elicit a state of natural relaxation, characterized by slower breathing, lower blood pressure, and a feeling of calm and well-being (Berry, 2012).

CBTI is typically administered or supervised by a behavioral sleep specialist over 4 to 8 weeks. In addition to individual treatment, there is evidence that CBTI is effective via group settings (Jansson & Linton, 2005; Verbeek, Konings, Aldenkamp, Declerck, & Klip, 2006), telephone (Bastien, Morin, Ouellet, Blais, & Bouchard, 2004), Internet delivery (Vincent & Lewycky, 2009; Ritterband et al., 2012) and self-help education (Mimeault & Morin, 1999) methods. A shortened version, called Brief Behavioral Treatment of Insomnia (BBTI), has been administered in primary care settings (Espie et al., 2007; Germain & Buyssee, 2011).

CBT interventions for sleep disturbance offer some advantages for older adults who are at risk for polypharmacy and potential side effects of pharmacological interventions that may impair cognitive function or contribute to falls (Montgomery & Dennis, 2009b). CBTI has been successfully tested in older adults and is recommended as equivalent to pharmacological interventions, with sustained effectiveness over time for the treatment of insomnia (Epstein, Sidani, Bootzin, Belyea, 2012; Irwin et al., 2014; Morin et al., 2009; Riemann & Perlis, 2009). The majority of nonpharmacological interventions require specialized training in behavioral sleep medicine for safe and effective delivery, especially in older adults with medical or psychiatric comorbidities. However, standardized formats of CBTI have been recommended as appropriate for nurses to deliver under the supervision of a sleep specialist (Espie et al., 2007). Relaxation techniques and sleep hygiene education may be delivered by nurses familiar with the techniques and information. Nurses may also apply sleep hygiene to the care of hospitalized older adults by implementing relaxing bedtime routines (LaReau, Benson, Watcharotone, & Manguba, 2008), and minimizing adverse environmental noise and light (Missildine, 2008). Common methods of CBT and their purposes are summarized in **Table 16-3**.

A number of studies have described the effective use of various forms of CBTI for adults and older adults with insomnia (Brenes et al., 2012; Buysse et al., 2012; Irwin et al., 2014; McCrae, McGovern, Lukefahr, & Stripling, 2011). These approaches also have demonstrated some success in the treatment of older adults with insomnia and such comorbid disorders as chronic obstructive pulmonary disease (Kapella et al., 2011), coronary artery disease, osteoarthritis (Rybarczyk et al., 2005; Rybarczyk, Mack, Harris, & Stepanski, 2011; Vitiello, Rybarczyk, Von Korff, & Stepanski, 2009), and hot flushes and night sweats following breast cancer treatment (Mann et al., 2012). A case report recently described the favorable use of CBTI by an older woman, provided through a mobile application via a wearable device, which could tailor technology and enhance compliance for older adults (Chen, Hung, & Chen, 2016).

CLINICAL TIP

CBT is recommended as equivalent to pharmacologic interventions, with more sustained effectiveness over time, for the treatment of insomnia (Riemann & Perlis, 2009; Smith et al., 2002).

TABLE 16-3   Cognitive and Behavioral Therapies for Sleep Promotion

Therapy	Purpose
Sleep Restriction	Limits the time in bed to average total sleep time, then progressively increases time in bed through earlier bedtimes until it is equivalent to total sleep time (Spielman, Saskin, & Thorpy, 1987); contraindicated in persons requiring maximal vigilance for activities (e.g., driving), in conditions exacerbated by sleepiness (e.g., epilepsy, sleep-disordered breathing) (Epstein & Bootzin, 2002; Spielman, Yang, & Glovinsky, 2011), and lack of sleep (e.g., bipolar disorder) (Espie et al., 2007; Germain & Buysse, 2011).
Stimulus Control	Re-associates the bed and bedroom with falling asleep rather than with anxiety associated with prolonged sleep onset latency (Bootzin & Perlis, 2011).
Cognitive Therapy	Promotes identification and understanding of maladaptive cognitions or beliefs that stimulate worry (e.g., catastrophic thinking about the consequences of poor sleep) with more positive reframing (Buysse & Perlis, 1996; Perlis & Gehrman, 2011; Schutte-Rodin et al., 2008).
Sleep Hygiene Education	Increases knowledge of homeostatic and circadian processes, and sleep-promoting behaviors which influence sleep (Posner & Gehrman, 2011); most effective if individually tailored (Perlis, Jungquist, Smith, & Posner, 2005) and used in combination with other CBTI.
Relaxation	Decrease cognitive arousal and somatic tension (Berry, 2012; Lichstein, Taylor, McCrae, & Thomas, 2011). Includes multiple approaches (e.g., guided imagery, progressive muscle relaxation, mindfulness-based stress reduction, biofeedback).
Paradoxical Intention	Decreases or eliminates performance anxiety, through intentional avoidance of falling asleep (Espie, 2011).
Sleep Compression	An alternative to sleep restriction in older adults with serious medical co-morbidities; sleep is increasingly restricted in small increments over approximately 5 weeks through delayed bedtime or earlier wake time, until the time spent in bed is equivalent to the time asleep (Lichstein, Thomas, & McCurry, 2011).

BOX 16-1   Acupuncture, Valerian, Melatonin, Tai Chi, and Cranial Electrical Stimulation

Acupuncture, valerian, melatonin, Tai Chi, and cranial electrical stimulation need further research to support their use in older adults. A 3-minute slow-stroke back massage was associated with a 36-minute increase in minutes of nighttime sleep in persons with dementia residing in the nursing home (Harris, 2010).

Biological-Based Products

The two most widely studied biological-based products for sleep are melatonin and valerian (see **Box 16-1**). Melatonin is an endogenous neurohormone that is believed to play a role in the sleep–wake cycle. Lower levels of melatonin are found in older adults as compared to young adults (Sharma, Palacios-Bois, Schwartz, & Iskandar, 1989). A large meta-analysis on the efficacy of melatonin therapy concluded that melatonin did not have a significant benefit for insomnia in older adults, despite small improvements in sleep latency (Buscemi et al., 2004). Data on the efficacy of melatonin for sleep are mixed (Arendt, 2006). Valerian, an extract of the plant species *Valeriana officinalis,* has been studied to determine its effect on sleep–wake patterns. Although statistically significant results have been found in some clinical trials using valerian in older adults, additional study is warranted in this area as the authors of a meta-analysis of the use of the valerian compound concluded that it was safe but ineffective (Taibi, Landis, Petry, & Vitiello, 2007).

Manipulative Modalities

Back massage has been efficacious in a variety of older adult populations, including those in intensive care units (Richards, 1998), those with dementia in long-term care facilities (Harris & Richards, 2010), and in hospitalized patients following coronary artery bypass surgery (Nerbass, Feltrim, Souza, Ykeda, & Lorenzi-Filho, 2010). In a review of the evidence of massage for improvement of sleep in older adults, physiological and psychological indicators suggest the effectiveness of slow-stroke back massage and hand massage in promoting relaxation in older people across all settings (Harris & Richards, 2010). In a randomized controlled trial investigating the sleep effects of a 3-minute slow-stroke back massage in persons with dementia residing in the nursing home, Harris and colleagues (2010) found an increase of 36 minutes in the group receiving massage compared to controls. Slow-stroke back massage can be easily used by nurses and other patient care providers to promote sleep (see **Figure 16-6**).

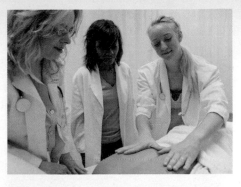

Figure 16-6 Dr. Melodee Harris instructs nursing students in the method of slow-stroke back massage.
Courtesy of Carr College of Nursing, Harding University.

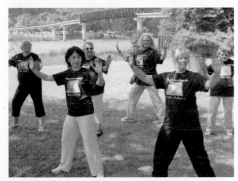

Figure 16-7 Dr. Pao-feng Tsai (front left), Alice An-Loh Sun Endowed Professor in Geriatric Nursing, provides instruction in Tai Chi.
Courtesy of UAMS College of Nursing.

Body-Based Modalities

Tai Chi is referred to as "moving meditation" as persons who use this modality move their bodies slowly, gently, and with awareness, while breathing deeply (NCCAM, 2015b). Tai Chi is a modality that is easily adaptable to a wide range of physical limitations, making it suitable for older adults. Tai Chi has been shown to be effective in improving self-reported sleep quality in older adults with sleep complaints (Irwin, Olmstead, & Motivala, 2008) and in older adults with heart failure (Yeh et al., 2008). A systematic review of the effects of Tai Chi, including those clinical trials that enrolled older adults, concluded that the strongest evidence for Tai Chi is in the prevention of falls and in improvement in psychological health, not in sleep parameters, per se (Lee, Ernst, & Choi, 2010). Tai chi can be adapted for use by older adults (see **Figure 16-7**).

Cranial Electrical Stimulation

Cranial electrical stimulation (CES) refers to the delivery of small, imperceptible amounts of microcurrent via clips to the ears. Although the precise mechanisms of action of CES are unknown, it is hypothesized that

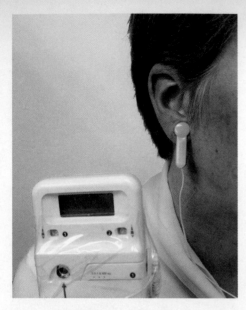

Figure 16-8 Dr. Karen Rose demonstrates the use of a cranial electrical stimulator device.
Courtesy of the University of Virginia, School of Nursing, and Alpha-Stim (Mineral Wells, TX).

CES may inhibit the reuptake of norepinephrine, serotonin, and dopamine (Shealy, Cady, Culver-Veehoff, Cox, & Liss, 1998). Studies of CES are mixed, with no conclusive evidence to suggest the widespread use of this modality to improve sleep in older adults. Rose, Taylor, and Bourguignon (2009) reported improvement of daily sleep disturbances trending toward statistical significance and clinical improvement in sleep onset latency in elders receiving CES, although overall findings were inconclusive. A CES device is shown in **Figure 16-8**.

Energy Fields

Light therapy is a form of CAM that involves the manipulation of energy or "biofields" (NCCAM, 2010). It is based on the circadian rhythm–related response to long-wavelength (green) light and short wavelength (blue) light levels (Gooley et al., 2010; NCCAM, 2010). Light therapy has been used for some time in the management of seasonal affective disorder (Terman, 2007), but there is limited high-quality evidence to support the use of light therapy for sleep disturbance in healthy older adults (Montgomery & Dennis, 2009a, 2009b). Early-morning awakening insomnia, subjective and objective sleep measures, and daytime functioning were improved for up to 1 month after two evenings of bright light therapy in a small sample of adults and older adults (Lack, Wright, Kemp, & Gibbon, 2005).

A number of small, randomized controlled trials have also explored light therapy in the management of sleep in older persons with dementia. Overall, their findings suggest no significant sleep improvements for this population (Forbes et al., 2009), although 1 hour of morning or evening bright light exposure did facilitate entrainment to the 24-hour day (Dowling, Mastick, Hubbard, Luxenberg, & Burr, 2005). A study using brief bright or dim morning light exposure in persons with dementia and their caregivers found improved sleep in the caregivers only, whether receiving bright or dim light therapy (Friedman et al., 2012).

Older adults may be intolerant of bright light therapy, and they should have ophthalmological eye examinations prior to its use. It should be used with caution in older adults with mania, retinal photosensitivity, or migraine headaches (Bloom et al., 2009).

Consequently, light therapy for sleep disturbance or circadian sleep disorders in either healthy older adults or those with dementia has not yet been clearly established as effective. Possible adverse consequences of light therapy also require further investigation.

Although other CAM modalities have been investigated to document their efficacy for improving sleep in older adults, because research is limited in these areas, no formal recommendations for use of these other modalities in older adults is warranted at this time.

Summary

Geriatric nurses should be aware of the positive implications of sleep for health promotion in older adults, as well as the potential negative implications of sleep disturbance for quality of life in this population. Disturbed sleep appears to have a bidirectional relationship with many common disease processes in older adults, such as depression, anxiety, heart disease, hypertension, and diabetes, as well as with many of the medications used to treat these disorders. Consequently, the care of older adults with sleep disturbance and multiple chronic diseases/disorders requires a holistic approach, in close collaboration with other healthcare providers. Sleep should be routinely included in nursing assessments of older adults and should be monitored periodically to detect changes that may indicate emerging alterations in health status or in response to therapy. **Boxes 16-2**, **16-3**, and **16-4** provide additional resources on sleep in older adults.

BOX 16-2   Research Highlight

This study investigated subjective sleep quality in women aged 50 years and older

Enderlin, Coleman, Cole, Richards, Kennedy, Goodwin, Hutchins, and Mack sought to better understand the quality of sleep obtained by women 50 years of age and older, factoring in their status with regard to illness and mood. They collected data by conducting interviews and various sleep and mood measurement and profiling tools. Sign into your database of nursing literature (CINAHL or PubMed, for example) and use the citation below to perform a search for this article. What did this research team find? How is sleep linked to mood? How can these findings help improve the care of older adults?

Enderlin, C.A., Coleman, E. A., Cole, C., Richards, K. C., Kennedy, R. L., Goodwin, J. A., Hutchins, L. F., and Mack, K. (2011). Subjective sleep quality, objective sleep characteristics, insomnia symptom severity, and daytime sleepiness in women aged 50 and older with nonmetastatic breast cancer. *Oncology Nursing Forum, 38*(4), E314–E325.

BOX 16-3   Recommended Resources

Resource Website

American Academy of Dental Sleep Medicine
http://www.dentalsleepmed.org

American Academy of Sleep Medicine
http://www.aasmnet.org/

American Sleep Apnea Association
http://www.sleepapnea.org/

American Sleep Association
http://www.sleepassociation.org/

Association for Behavioral and Cognitive Therapies
http://www.abct.org/Home/

Hartford Institute for Geriatric Nursing
https://consultgeri.org/geriatric-topics/sleepNarcolepsy Network
http://www.narcolepsynetwork.org/

National Sleep Foundation, Sleep in America Poll 2003
https://sleepfoundation.org/sleep-polls-data/sleep-in-america-poll/2003-sleep-and-aging

Oncology Nursing Society
http://www.ons.org/Research/PEP/Sleep

Restless Legs Syndrome Foundation
http://www.rls.org/

Society of Behavioral Sleep Medicine
https://www.behavioralsleep.org/index.php/society-of-behavioral-sleep-medicine-providers/member-providers

BOX 16-4   Evidence-Based Practice

The aim of this meta-analysis was to evaluate the effectiveness of current studies using dietary weight loss interventions to treat obstructive sleep apnea (OSA) in obese patients

This team of researchers from SUNY Buffalo examined the relationship between obesity and sleep apnea. These two conditions have long been associated with one another and Anandam, Akinnusi, Kufel, Porhomayon, and El-Solh combed the available literature to determine whether weight loss made an impact on the sleep apnea experienced by obese patients. Sign into

your database of nursing literature (CINAHL or PubMed, for example) and use the citation below to perform a search for this article. What did their investigation into the literature demonstrate? How do their findings help us understand the relationship between obesity, weight loss, and sleep apnea?

Anandam, A., Akinnusi, M., Kufel, T., Porhomayon, J., & El-Solh, A. A. (2012). Effects of dietary weight loss on obstructive sleep apnea: A meta-analysis. *Sleep and Breathing, 17*(1), 227–234.

Clinical Reasoning Exercises

1. Your patient is a 69-year-old widow who is having her routine blood pressure checked. In the conversation she mentions that she is exhausted and has been having trouble sleeping. You notice that she is very slow in her speech and movement and that her facial expression appears flat. How would you approach investigating her sleep disturbance further?

2. A 78-year-old gentleman has a follow-up visit for his congestive heart failure. While you are getting his vital signs you notice he appears sleepy. When questioned, he states that he has been very sleepy during the day, often dozes off when he gets still, and takes several naps a day. He reports no difficulty falling asleep, but does recall that he often awakens during the night for no specific reason in addition to getting up to urinate

several times. His wife adds that he snores loudly and sometimes stops breathing for a time. What screening assessments should you consider in assessing his daytime sleepiness and snoring?

3. A 62-year-old woman is being seen for difficulty falling asleep. She reports that although she feels tired and ready for sleep at night, her legs bother her and often keep her awake for hours. She describes "crawling" sensations in her legs that become most noticeable in the evening, and often require her to get up and walk around to obtain relief. Although walking relieves her discomfort, she states that the sensations in her legs return when she tries to lie down and sleep. What additional information do you need to ask regarding these problematic symptoms?

Personal Reflections

1. Maintain a sleep diary for your own sleep, by going to Sleep Diary NIH Office of Science Education, available at http://science. education.nih.gov/supplements/nih3/sleep/ guide/nih_sleep_masters.pdf

Scan through the materials provided at this site, and test your knowledge of sleep by taking the quiz: What Do You Know (or Think You Know) about Sleep?

References

Allen, R. P., Burchell, B. J., MacDonald, B., Hening, W. A., & Earley, C. J. (2009). Validation of the self-completed Cambridge-Hopkins questionnaire (CH-RLSq) for ascertainment of restless legs syndrome (RLS) in a population survey. *Sleep Medicine, 10*(10), 1097–1100.

Allen, R. P., Chen, C., Garcia-Borreguero, D., Polo, O., DuBrava, S., Micel, J., . . . Winkelman, J. W. (2014). Comparison of pregabalin with pramipexole for restless legs syndrome. *New England Journal of Medicine, 370*(7), 621–631.

American Academy of Sleep Medicine. (2005). *The international classification of sleep disorders: Diagnostic and coding manual* (2nd ed.). Westchester, IL: Author.

American Academy of Sleep Medicine. (2014). *The international classification of sleep disorders* (3rd ed.). Darien, IL: Author.

American Geriatrics Society & 2015 Beers Criteria Update Expert Panel. (2015). American Geriatrics Society updated Beers Criteria for potentially inappropriate medication use in older adults. *Journal of the American Geriatrics Society, 63*(11), 2227–2246.

American Psychiatric Association. (2013). *Diagnostic and statistical manual of mental disorders* (4th ed.). Washington, DC: Author.

Anandam, A., Akinnusi, M., Kufel, T., Porhomayon, J., & El-Solh, A. A. (2013). Effects of dietary weight loss on obstructive sleep apnea: A meta-analysis. *Sleep and Breathing, 17*(1), 227–234.

Ancoli-Israel, S. (2007). Sleep apnea in older adults: Is it real and should age be the determining factor in the treatment decision matrix? *Sleep Medicine Reviews, 11*(2), 83–85.

Ancoli-Israel, S. (2009). Sleep and its disorders in aging populations. *Sleep Medicine, 10*, S7–S11.

Ancoli-Israel, S., Cole, R., Alessi, C., Chambers, M., Moorcroft, W., & Pollak, C. P. (2003). The role of actigraphy in the study of sleep and circadian rhythms. *Sleep, 26*(3), 342–392.

Ancoli-Israel, S., Kripke, D. F., Klauber, M. R., Mason, W. J., Fell, R., & Kaplan, O. (1991). Periodic limb movements in sleep in community-dwelling elderly. *Sleep, 14*(6), 496–500.

Ando, K., Kripke, D. F., & Ancoli-Israel, S. (2002). Delayed and advanced sleep phase symptoms. *Israel Journal of Psychiatry and Related Sciences, 39*(1), 11–18.

Arendt, J. (2006). Does melatonin improve sleep? Efficacy of melatonin. *British Medical Journal (International Edition), 332*(7540), 550.1.

Barnes, P. M., Bloom, B., & Nahin, R. L. (2008). Complementary and alternative medicine use among adults and children: United States, 2007. *National Health Statistics Reports, 12*, 1–23.

Bastian, C. H., Vallieres, A., & Morin, C. M. (2001). Validation of the Insomnia Severity Index as an outcome measure for insomnia research. *Sleep Medicine, 2*(4), 297–307.

Bastien, C. H., Morin, C. M., Ouellet, M. C., Blais, F. C. & Bouchard, S. (2004). Cognitive-behavioral therapy for insomnia: Comparison of individual therapy, group therapy, and telephone consultations. *Journal of Consulting Clinical Psychology, 72*(4), 653–659.

Basu, R., Dodge, H., Stoehr, G. P. & Ganguli, M. (2003). Sedative-hypnotic use of diphenhydramine in a rural, older adult, community-based cohort: effects on cognition. *American Journal of Geriatric Psychiatry, 11*(2), 205–213.

Benca, R. M., Ancoli-Israel, S., & Moldofsky, H. (2004). Special considerations in insomnia diagnosis and management: Depressed, elderly, and chronic pain populations. *Journal of Clinical Psychiatry, 65*(Suppl 8), 26–35.

Benson, K. L., & Feinberg, I. (2011). Schizophrenia. In M. H. Kryger, T. Roth, & W. C. Dement (Eds.), *Principles and practice in sleep medicine* (pp. 1501–1511). St. Louis, MO: Saunders.

Berry, R. B. (2012). *Fundamentals of sleep medicine.* Philadelphia, PA: Elsevier.

Bliwise, D. L. (1993). Sleep in normal aging and dementia. *Sleep: Journal of Sleep Research & Sleep Medicine, 16*(1), 40–81.

Bliwise, D. L. (2005). Normal aging. In M. H. Kryger, T. Roth, & W. C. Dement (Eds.), *Principles and practice of sleep medicine* (pp. 24–38). Philadelphia, PA: Saunders.

Bliwise, D. L. (2011). Normal aging. In M. H. Kryger, T. Roth, & W. C. Dement (Eds.), *Principles and practice of sleep medicine* (pp. 27–41). St. Louis, MO: Saunders.

Bliwise, D. L., Foley, D. J., Vitiello, M. V., Farzaneh, P. A., Ancoli-Israel, S., & Walsh, J. K. (2009). Nocturia and disturbed sleep in the elderly. *Sleep Medicine, 10*(5), 540–548.

Bloom, H. G. Ahmed, I., Alessi, C. A., Ancoli-Israel, S., Buysse, D. J., Kryer, M. H., . . . & Zee, P. C. (2009). Evidence-based recommendations for the assessment and management of sleep disorders in older persons. *Journal of American Geriatric Society, 57*(5), 761–769.

Boeve, B. F. (2010). REM sleep behavior disorder: Updated review of the core features, the RBD-Neurodegenerative Disease Association, evolving concepts, controversies, and future directions. *Annals of the New York Academy of Sciences, 1184*, 15–54.

Bootzin, R. R. (2005). Preface. In M. L. Perlis, C. Jungquist, M. T. Smith, & D. Posner (Eds.), *Cognitive behavioral treatment of insomnia: A session-by-session guide.* New York, NY: Springer.

Bootzin, R. R., & Perlis, M. L. (2011). Stimulus control therapy. In L. Perlis, M. Aloia, & B. Kuhn (Eds.), *Behavioral treatments for sleep disorders: A comprehensive primer of behavioral sleep medicine interventions* (pp. 21–30). Boston, MA: Elsevier.

Borbely A. A. (1982). A two process model of sleep regulation. *Human Neurobiology, 1*(3), 195–204.

Borud, E., Grimsgaard, S., & White, A. (2010). Menopausal problems and acupuncture. *Autonomic Neuroscience: Basic & Clinical, 157*(1–2), 57–62.

Brenes, G. A., Miller, M. E., Stanley, M. A., Williamson, J. D., Knudson, M., & McCall, W. V. (2009). Insomnia in older adults with generalized anxiety disorder. *The American Journal of Geriatric Psychiatry, 17*(6), 465–472.

Brenes, G. A., Miller, M. E., Williamson, J. D., McCall, W. V., Knudson, M., & Stanley, M. A. (2012). A randomized controlled trial of telephone-delivered cognitive-behavioral therapy for late-life anxiety disorders. *American Journal of Geriatric Psychiatry, 20*(8), 707–716.

Buscemi, N., Vandermeer, B., Pandya, R., Hooton, N., Tjosvold, L., Hartling, L., . . . Klassen, T. (2004). Melatonin for treatment of sleep disorders. *Agency for Healthcare Research and Quality Evidence Report/Technology Assessments, 108*, 1–7.

Buysse, D. J., & Perlis, M. E. (1996). The evaluation and treatment of insomnia. *Journal of Practical Psychiatry and Behavioral Health, 2*(2), 80–93.

Buysse, D. J., Reynolds III, C. F., Monk, T. H., Berman, S. R., & Kupfer, D. J. (1989). The Pittsburgh sleep quality index: A new instrument for psychiatric practice and research. *Psychiatry Research, 28(2),* 193–213.

Buysse, D. J., Germain, A., Moul, D. E., Franzen, P. L., Brar, L. K., Fletcher, M. E., . . . Monk, T. H. (2012). Efficacy of brief behavioral treatment for chronic insomnia in older adults. *Archives of Internal Medicine, 171*(10), 887–895.

Cao, M. T., Guilleminault, C., & Kushida, C. A. (2011). Clinical features and evaluation of obstructive sleep apnea and upper airway resistance syndrome. In M. Kryger, T. Roth, & W. Dement (Eds.), *Principles and practice of sleep medicine* (5th ed., pp. 1206–1218). Philadelphia, PA: W.B. Saunders.

Carrier, J., Monk, T. H., Buysse, D. J., & Kupfer, D. J. (1997). Sleep and morningness-eveningness in the 'middle' years of life (20–59 y). *Journal of Sleep Research, 6*(4), 230–237.

Carskadon, M. A., & Dement, W. C. (2005). Normal human sleep: An overview. In M. H. Kryger, T. Roth, & W. C. Dement (Eds.), *Principles and practice of sleep medicine* (pp. 13–23). Philadelphia, PA: Elsevier/Saunders.

Carskadon, M. A., & Dement, W. C. (1982). The Multiple Sleep Latency Test: What does it measure? *Sleep: Journal of Sleep Research & Sleep Medicine, 5*(Suppl 2), 67–72.

Carskadon, M. A., Dement, W. C., Mitler, M. M., Roth, T., Westbrook, P. R., & Keenan, S. (1986). Guidelines for the multiple sleep latency test (MSLT): A standard measure of sleepiness. *Sleep, 9*(4), 518–524.

Centers for Disease Control and Prevention. (2015). Depression is not a normal part of growing older. *Healthy Aging.* Retrieved from http://www.cdc.gov/aging/mentalhealth/depression.htm

Chen, Y. X., Hung, Y. P. & Chen, H. C. (2016). Mobile application-assisted cognitive behavioral therapy for insomnia in an older adult. *Telemedicine and E Health, 22*(4), 332–334.

Chou, T. C., Scammell, T. E., Gooley, J. J., Gaus, S. E., Saper, C. B., & Lu, J. (2003). Critical role of dorsomedial hypothalamic nucleus in a wide range of behavioral circadian rhythms. *The Journal of Neuroscience, 23*(33), 10691–10702.

Chung, F., & Elsaid, H. (2009). Screening for obstructive sleep apnea before surgery: Why is it important? *Current Opinion in Anesthesiology, 22*(3), 405–411.

Chung, F., Yegneswaran, B., Liao, P., Chung, S. A., Vairavanathan, S., Islam, S., . . . Shapiro, C. M. (2008). STOP questionnaire: A tool to screen patients for obstructive sleep apnea. *Anesthesiology, 108*(5), 812–821.

Cole, C. S., & Richards, K. C. (2005). Sleep and cognition in people with Alzheimer's disease. *Issues in Mental Health Nursing, 26*(7), 687–698.

Collop, N. A. (2006). Polysomnography. In T. Lee-Chiong (Ed.), *Sleep: A comprehensive handbook* (pp. 973–976). Hoboken, NJ: Wiley-Liss.

Crowley, K. (2011). Sleep and sleep disorders in older adults. *Neuropsychology Review, 21*(1), 41–53.

Crystal, S., Sambamoorthi, U., Walkup, J. T., & Akincigil, A. (2003). Diagnosis and treatment of depression in the elderly Medicare population: Predictors, disparities, and trends. *Journal of the American Geriatrics Society, 51*(12), 1718–1728.

Czeisler, C. A., & Dumont, M. (1992). Association of sleep–wake habits in older people with changes in output of circadian pacemaker. *Lancet, 340*(8825), 933–936.

De Hert, M., Correll, C. U., Bobes, J., Cetkovich-Bakmas, M., Cohen, D., Asai, I., . . . Leucht, S. (2011). Physical illness in patients with severe mental disorders: Prevalence, impact of medications and disparities in health care. *World Psychiatry, 10*(1), 52–77.

Dement, W. C. (2011). History of sleep physiology and medicine. In M. Kryger, T. Roth, & W. Dement (Eds.), *Principles and practice of sleep medicine* (5th ed., pp. 3–15). Philadelphia, PA: W.B. Saunders.

Dew, M. A., Hoch, C. C., Buysse, D. J., Monk, T. H., Begley, A. E., Houck, P. R., . . . & Reynolds III, C. F. (2003). "Healthy older adults" sleep predicts all-cause mortality at 4 to 19 years of follow-up. *Psychosomatic Medicine, 65*(1), 63–73.

Dowling, G. A., Mastick, J., Hubbard, E. M., Luxenberg, J. S., & Burr, R. L. (2005). Effect of timed bright light treatment for rest-activity disruption in institutionalized patients with Alzheimer's disease. *International Journal of Geriatric Psychiatry, 20*(8), 738–743.

Driscoll, H. C., Serody, L., Patrick, S., Maurer, J., Bensasi, S., Houck, P. R., . . . Reynolds III, C. F. (2008). Sleeping well, aging well: A descriptive and cross-sectional study of sleep in "successful agers" 75 and older. *American Journal of Geriatric Psychiatry, 16*(1), 74–82.

Enderlin, C. A., Coleman, E. A., Cole, C., Richards, K. C., Kennedy, R. L., Goodwin, J. A., . . . & Mack, K. (2011). Subjective sleep quality, objective sleep characteristics, insomnia symptom severity, and daytime sleepiness in women aged 50 and older with nonmetastatic breast cancer. *Oncology Nursing Forum, 38*(4), E314–E325.

Enderlin, C. A., Kuhlmann, M. E., Harris, M., Hadley, M., Sullivan, A., Rose, K., & Mitchell, A. (2013). Sleep disturbance. In Tusaie, K. R. & Fitzpatrick, J. (Eds.), *Advanced practice psychiatric-mental health nursing: Integrating psychotherapy, pharmacotherapy and complementary/alternative approaches* (pp. 230–263). NY: Springer Publishing.

Epstein, D. R., Sidani, S., Bootzin, R. R., & Belyea, M. J. (2012). Dismantling multicomponent behavioral treatment for insomnia in older adults: A randomized controlled trial. *Sleep, 35*(6), 797–805.

Espie, C. A., MacMahon, K. M., Kelly, H. L., Broomfield, N. M., Douglas, N. J., Engleman, H. M., . . . Wilson, P. (2007). Randomized clinical effectiveness trial of nurse-administered small-group cognitive behavior therapy for persistent insomnia in general practice. *Sleep, 30*(5), 574–584.

Foley, D., Ancoli-Israel, S., Britz, P., & Walsh, J. (2004). Sleep disturbances and chronic disease in older adults: Results of the 2003 National Sleep Foundation Sleep in America Survey. *Journal of Psychosomatic Research, 56*(5), 497–502.

Foley, D. J., Monjan, A., Simonsick, E. M., Wallace, R. B., & Blazer, D. G. (1999). Incidence and remission of insomnia among elderly adults: an epidemiologic study of 6,800 persons over three years. *Sleep: Journal of Sleep Research & Sleep Medicine, 22*(Suppl 2), S366–S372.

Forbes, D., Culum, I., Lischka, A.R., Morgan, D. G., Peacock, S., Forbes, J., . . . & Forbes, S. (2009). Light therapy for managing cognitive, sleep, functional, behavioral, or psychiatric disturbances in dementia. *Cochrane Database of Systematic Reviews,* (4), CD003946.

Friedman, L., Spira, A. P., Hernandez, B., Mather, C., Sheikh, J., Ancoli-Israel, S., . . . & Zeitzer, J. M. (2012). Brief morning light treatment for sleep/wake disturbances in older memory-impaired individuals and their caregivers. *Sleep Medicine,* 13(5), 546–549.

Friedman, M., Tanyeri, H., La Rosa, M., Landsberg, R., Vaidyanathan, K., Pieri, S., Caldarelli, D. (1999). Clinical predictors of obstructive sleep apnea. *The Laryngoscope, 109*(12), 1901–1907.

Fuller, P. M., Gooley, J. J., & Saper, C. B. (2006). Neurobiology of the sleep-wake cycle: Sleep architecture, circadian regulation, and regulatory feedback. *Journal of Biological Rhythms, 21*(6), 482–493.

Fulmer, T. (2007). How to try this: Fulmer SPICES—A framework of six "marker conditions" can help focus assessment of hospitalized older patients. *American Journal of Nursing, 107*(10), 40–49.

Germain, A., & Buysse, D. J. (2011). Brief behavioral treatment of insomnia. In L. Perlis, M. Aloia, & B. Kuhn (Eds.), *Behavioral treatments for sleep disorders* (pp. 143–150). San Diego, CA: Academic Press.

Gooley, J. J., Rajaratnam, S. M., Brainard, G. C., Kronauer, R. E., Czeisler, C. A., & Lockley, S. W. (2010). Spectral responses of the human circadian system depend on the irradiance and duration of exposure to light. *Science Translational Medicine, 2*(31), 1–9.

Gooneratne, N. S. (2008). Complementary and alternative medicine for sleep disturbances in older adults. *Clinics in Geriatric Medicine, 24*(1), 121–138.

Gu, D., Sautter, J., Pipkin, R., & Zeng, Y. (2010). Sociodemographic and health correlates of sleep quality and duration among very old Chinese. *Sleep, 33*(5), 601–610.

Guilleminault, C., & Cao, M. T. (2011). Narcolepsy: Diagnosis and management. In M. Kryger, T. Roth, & W. Dement (Eds.), *Principles and practice of sleep medicine* (5th ed., pp. 957–968). Philadelphia, PA: W.B. Saunders.

Gum, A. M., King-Kalliimanis, B., & Kohn, R. (2009). Prevalence of mood, anxiety, and substance-abuse disorder for older Americans in the National Comorbidity Survey-replication. *American Journal of Geriatric Psychiatry, 17*(9), 769–781.

Haimov, I., Hanuka, E., & Horowitz, Y. (2008). Chronic insomnia and cognitive functioning among older adults. *Behavioral Sleep Medicine, 6*(1), 32–54.

Harris, M. (2012). The effects of slow-stroke back massage on minutes of nighttime sleep in persons with dementia in the nursing home: A pilot study. *Journal of Holistic Nursing, 30*(4), 255–263.

Harris, M., & Richards, K. C. (2010). The physiological and psychological effects of slow-stroke back massage and hand massage on relaxation in older people. *Journal of Clinical Nursing, 19*(7/8), 917–926.

Hartford Institute for Geriatric Nursing. (2015). *Assessment tools: Try this and how to try this resources.* Retrieved from http://consultgerirn.org/tools

Hogl, B. B. (2015). Therapeutic advances in restless legs syndrome (RLS). *Movement Disorders, 11*(11), 1574–1579.

Iber, C., Ancoli-Israel, S., Chesson, A., Quan, S. F., & The American Academy of Sleep Medicine. (2007). *The AASM manual for the scoring of sleep and associated events: Rules, terminology and technical specifications.* Westchester, NY: American Academy of Sleep Medicine.

Institute of Medicine. (2012). *The mental health and substance use workforce for older adults: In whose hands?* Washington, DC: The National Academies Press.

Irwin, M. R., Olmstead, R., & Motivala, S. J. (2008). Improving sleep quality in older adults with moderate sleep complaints: A randomized controlled trial of Tai Chi Chih. *Sleep, 31*(7), 1001–1008.

Irwin, M. R., Olmstead, R., Carrillo, C., Sadeghi, N., Breen, E. C., Witarama, T., . . . Nicassio, P. (2014). Cognitive behavioral therapy vs. tai chi for late life insomnia and inflammatory risk: A randomized controlled comparative efficacy trial. *Sleep, 37*(9), 1543–1552.

Jansson, M., & Linton, S. J. (2005). Cognitive-behavioral group therapy as an early intervention for insomnia: A randomized controlled trial. *Journal of Occupational Rehabilitation, 15*(2), 177–190.

Johansson, P., Alehagen, U., Svanborg, E., Dahlstrom, U., & Brostrom, A. (2012). Clinical characteristics and mortality risk in relation to obstructive and central sleep apnoea in community-dwelling elderly individuals: a 7-year follow-up. *Age and Ageing, 41*(4), 468–474.

Johns, M. W. (1991). A new method for measuring daytime sleepiness: The Epworth Sleepiness Scale. *Sleep, 14*(6), 540–545.

Johns, M. W. (1992). Reliability and factor analysis of the Epworth Sleepiness Scale. *Sleep: Journal of Sleep Research & Sleep Medicine, 15*(4), 376–381.

Johns, M. W. (1993). Daytime sleepiness, snoring, and obstructive sleep apnea: The Epworth Sleepiness Scale. *Chest, 103*(1), 30–36.

Johns, M. W. (1994). Sleepiness in different situations measured by the Epworth Sleepiness Scale. *Sleep: Journal of Sleep Research & Sleep Medicine, 17*(8), 703–710.

Jun, L., Sherman, D., Devor, M., & Saper, C. B. (2006). A putative flip-flop switch for control of REM sleep. *Nature, 441*(7093), 589–594.

Kapella, M. C., Herdegen, J. J., Perlis, M. L., Shaver, J. L., Larson, J. L., Law, J. A., & Carley, D. W. (2011). Cognitive behavioral therapy for insomnia comorbid with COPD is feasible with preliminary evidence of positive sleep and fatigue effects. *International Journal of Chronic Obstructive Pulmonary Disease, 6*, 625–635.

Karel, M. J., Gatz, M., & Smyer, M. A. (2012). Aging and mental health in the decade ahead: What psychologists need to know. *American Psychologist, 67*(3),184–198.

Kazenwadel, J., Pollmcher, T., Trenkwalder, C., Oertel, W. H., Kohnen, R., Kunzel, M., & Kruger, H. P. (1995). New actigraphic assessment method for periodic leg movements (PLM). *Sleep, 18*(8), 689–697.

Kemlink, D., Pretl, M., Sonka, K., & Nevsimalova, S. (2008). A comparison of polysomnographic and actigraphic evaluation of periodic limb movements in sleep. *Neurological Research, 30*(3), 234–238.

Krystal, A. D. (2011). Pharmacologic treatment: Other medications. In M. Kryger, T. Roth, & W. Dement (Eds.), *Principles and practice of sleep medicine* (5th ed., pp. 916–930). Philadelphia, PA: W.B. Saunders.

Krystal, A. D. (2015). Current, emerging, and newly available insomnia medications. *Journal of Clinical Psychiatry, 76*(8), 943–948.

Kushida, C. A., & Efron, B. (1997). A predictive morphometric model for the obstructive sleep apnea syndrome. *Annals of Internal Medicine, 127*(8), 581–587.

Lareau, R., Benson, L., Watcharotone, K., & Manguba, G. (2008). Examining the feasibility of implementing specific nursing interventions to promote sleep in hospitalized elderly patients. *Geriatric Nursing, 29*(3), 197–206.

Lack, L., Wright, H., Kemp, K., & Gibbon, S. (2005). The treatment of early-morning awakening insomnia with 2 evenings of bright light. *Sleep, 28*(5), 616–623.

Lee, M. S., Ernst, E., & Choi, T. Y. (2010). Tai Chi for breast cancer patients: A systematic review. *Breast Cancer Research and Treatment, 120*(2), 309–316.

Lee-Chiong, T. (2008). *Sleep medicine: Essentials and review.* Oxford, UK: Oxford University Press.

Leger, D., Scheuermaier, K., Philip, P., Paillard, M., & Guilleminault, C. (2001). SF-36: Evaluation of quality of life in severe and mild insomniacs compared with good sleepers. *Psychosomatic Medicine, 63*(1), 49–55.

Lichstein, K. L., Taylor, D. J., McCrae, C. S., & Thomas, S. J. (2011). Relaxation for insomnia. In L. Perlis, M. Aloia, & B. Kuhn (Eds.), *Behavioral treatments for sleep disorders: A comprehensive primer of behavioral sleep medicine interventions* (pp. 45–54). Boston, MA: Elsevier.

Mallampati, S. R., Gatt, S. P., Gugino, L. D., Desai, S. P., Waraksa, B., Freiberger, D., & Liu, P. L. (1985). A clinical sign to predict difficult tracheal intubation: a prospective study. *Canadian Anaesthetists' Society Journal, 32*(4), 429–434.

Mann, E., Smith, M. J., Hellier, J., Balabanovic, J. A., Amed, H., Grunfeld, E. A., & Hunter, M. S. (2012). Cognitive behavioural treatment for women who have menopausal symptoms after breast cancer treatment (MENOS 1): A randomised controlled trial. *Lancet Oncology, 13*(3), 309–318.

McCrae, C. S., McGovern, R., Lukefahr, R., & Stripling, A. M. (2011). Research Evaluating Brief Behavioral Sleep Treatments for Rural Elderly (RESTORE): A preliminary examination of effectiveness. *American Journal of Geriatric Psychiatry, 15*(11), 979–982.

McGinty, D., & Szymusiak, R. (2003). Hypothalamic regulation of sleep and arousal. *Frontiers in Bioscience, 1*(8s), 1074–1083.

McGinty, D., & Szymusiak, R. (2011). Neural control of sleep in mammals. In M. Kryger, T. Roth, & W. Dement (Eds.), *Principles and practice of sleep medicine* (5th ed., pp. 76–91). Philadelphia, PA: W.B. Saunders.

McNair, D. M., & Heuchert, J. W. P. (2005). *Profile of Mood States (POMS): Technical update.* North Tonawanda, NY: Multi-Health Systems.

Merck. (2014). *Belsomra (suvorexant) tablets prescribing information.* Whitehouse Station, NJ.

Mesas, A. E., Lopez-Garcia, E., Leon-Munoz, L. M., Graciani, A., Guallar-Castillon, P., & Rodriguez-Artalejo, F. (2011). The association between habitual sleep duration and sleep quality in older adults according to health status. *Age & Ageing, 40*(3), 318–323.

Mimeault, V., & Morin, C. M. (1999). Self-help treatment for insomnia: Bibliotherapy with and without professional guidance. *Journal of Consulting Clinical Psychology, 67*(4), 511–519.

Misra, S., & Malow, B. A. (2008). Evaluation of sleep disturbances in older adults. *Clinical Geriatric Medicine, 24*(1), 15–26.

Missildine, K. (2008). Sleep and the sleep environment of older adults in acute care settings. *Journal of Gerontological Nursing, 34*(6), 15–21.

Monk, T. H., Reynolds, C. F., Kupfer, D. J., Buysse, D. J. Coble, P. A., Hayes, A. J., Machen, M. A., . . . Ritenout, A. M. (1994). The Pittsburgh Sleep Diary. *Journal of Sleep Research, 3*, 111–120.

Montgomery, P., & Dennis, J. A. (2009a). Bright light therapy for sleep problems in adults aged 60+. *Cochrane Database of Systematic Reviews,* (1), CDC003403.

Montgomery, P., & Dennis, J. A. (2009b). Cognitive behavioral interventions for sleep problems in adults aged 60+. *Cochrane Database of Systematic Reviews,* (1), CD003161.

Montplaisir, J., Allen, R. P., Arthur, W., & Ferini-Strambi, L. (2011). Restless legs syndrome and periodic limb movements during sleep. In M. Kryger, T. Roth, & W. Dement (Eds.), *Principles and practice of sleep medicine* (5th ed., pp. 1026–1037). Philadelphia, PA: W.B. Saunders.

Morgenthaler, T., Alessi, C., Friedman, L., Owens, J., Kapur, V., Boehlecke, B., . . . American Academy of Sleep Medicine. (2007). Practice parameters for the use of actigraphy in the assessment of sleep and sleep disorders: An update for 2007. *Sleep, 30*(4), 519–529.

Morgenthaler, T., Kramer, M., Alessi, C., Friedman, L., Boehlecke, B., Brown, T., . . . Academy of Sleep Medicine. (2006). Practice parameters for the psychological and behavioral treatment of insomnia: An update. An American Academy of Sleep Medicine report. *Sleep, 29*(11), 1415–1419.

Morin, C. M. (1993). *Insomnia: Psychological assessment and management.* New York, NY: Guilford Press.

Morin C.M. & Benca, R. (2012). Chronic insomnia. *Lancet, 379*(9821),1129–1141.

Morin, C. M., Mimeault, V., & Gagne, A. (1999). Nonpharmacological treatment of late-life insomnia. *Journal of Psychosomatic Research, 46*(2), 103–116.

Morin, C. M., LeBlanc, M., Daley, M., Gregoire, J. P., & Merette, C. (2006). Epidemiology of insomnia: prevalence, self-help treatments, consultations, and determinants of help-seeking behaviors. *Sleep Medicine, 7*(2), 123–130.

Morin, C. M., Vallieres, A., Guay, B., Ivers, H., Savard, J., Mérette, C., . . . Baillargeon, L. (2009). Cognitive behavioral therapy, singly and combined with medication, for persistent insomnia: A randomized controlled trial. *JAMA 301*(19), 2005–2015.

National Association of Cognitive Behavioral Therapists. (2014). What is cognitive-behavioral therapy. Retrieved from http://www.nacbt.org/whatiscbt.htm

National Center for Complementary and Alternative Medicine. (2010). Light therapy: The intensity and duration of exposure to light can affect the circadian rhythm. Retrieved from http://nccam.nih.gov/research/results/spotlight/051710.htm

National Center for Complementary and Alternative Medicine. (2014). Acupuncture: In depth. Retrieved from http://nccam.nih.gov/health/acupuncture/introduction.htm

National Center for Complementary and Alternative Medicine. (2015a). Complementary, Alternative, or Integrative Health: What's In a Name? Retrieved from http://nccam.nih.gov/health/whatiscam

National Center for Complementary and Alternative Medicine. (2015b). Tai Chi and Qi Gong: In Depth. Retrieved from http://nccam.nih.gov/health/taichi/introduction.htm

National Sleep Foundation. (2010). *2003 sleep in America poll.* Washington, DC: Author.

Nebes, R. D., Buysse, D. J., Halligan, E. M., Houck, P. R., & Monk, T. H. (2009). Self-reported sleep quality predicts poor cognitive performance in healthy older adults. *Journal of Gerontology Psychological Sciences, 64B*(2), 180–187.

Neikrug, A. B., & Ancoli-Israel, S. (2010). Sleep disorders in the older adult: A mini-review. *Gerontology, 56*(2), 181–189.

Nerbass, F. B., Feltrim, M. I. Z., Souza, S. A. D., Ykeda, D. S., & Lorenzi-Filho, G. (2010). Effects of massage therapy on sleep quality after coronary artery bypass graft surgery. *Clinics (São Paulo, Brazil), 65*(11), 1105–1110.

Neubauer, D. (2003). *Understanding sleeplessness: Perspectives on insomnia.* Baltimore, MD: John Hopkins University Press.

Ohayon, M. M., Carskadon, M. A., Guilleminault, C., & Vitiello, M. V. (2004). Meta-analysis of quantitative sleep parameters from childhood to old age in healthy individuals: Developing normative sleep values across the human lifespan. *Sleep, 27*(7), 1255–1273.

Perlis, M. L., & Gehrman, P. R. (2011). Cognitive restructuring: Cognitive therapy for catastrophic sleep beliefs. In L. Perlis & B. Kuhn (Eds.), *Behavioral treatments for sleep disorders: A comprehensive primer on behavioral sleep medicine interventions* (pp. 119–126). Boston, MA: Elsevier.

Peterson, M. J., & Benca, R. M. (2011). Mood disorders. In M. H. Kryger, T. Roth, & W. C. Dement (Eds.), *Principles and practice of sleep medicine* (pp. 1488–1500). St. Louis, MO: Saunders.

Petit, D., Montplaisir, J., & Boeve, B. F. (2011). Alzheimer's disease and other dementia. In M. Kryger, T. Roth, & W. Dement (Eds.), *Principles and practice of sleep medicine* (pp. 1038–1047). St. Louis, MO: Saunders.

Posner, D., & Gehrman, P. R. (2011). Sleep hygiene. In L. Perlis, M. Aloia, & B. Kuhn (Eds.), *Behavioral treatments for sleep disorders: A comprehensive primer of behavioral sleep medicine interventions* (pp. 31–44). Boston, MA: Elsevier.

Postuma, R. B., Gagnon, J. F., Vendette, M., Fantini, M. L., Massicotte-Marquez, J., & Montplaisir, J. (2009). Quantifying the risk of neurodegenerative disease in idiopathic REM sleep behavior disorder. *Neurology, 72*(15), 1296–1300.

Ramsawh, H., Stein, M. B., & Mellman, T. A. (2011). Anxiety disorders. In M. Kryger, T. Roth, & W. Dement (Eds.), *Principles and practice of sleep medicine* (pp. 1473–1487). St. Louis, MO: Saunders.

Redeker, N. S. (2011). Developmental aspects of sleep. In N.S. Redeker & G. P. McEnany (Eds.), *Sleep disorders and sleep promotion in nursing practice* (pp. 19–32). New York, NY: Springer.

Richards, K. C. (1998). Effect of a back massage and relaxation intervention on sleep in critically ill patients. *American Journal of Critical Care: An Official Publication, American Association of Critical-Care Nurses, 7*(4), 288–299.

Riemann, D., & Perlis, M. L. (2009). The treatments of chronic insomnia: A review of benzodiazepine receptor agonists and psychological and behavioral therapies. *Sleep Medicine Reviews, 13*(3), 205–214.

Ritterband, L. M., Bailey, E. T., Thorndike, F. P., Lord, H. R., Farrell-Carnahan, L., & Baum, L.D. (2012). Initial evaluation of an Internet intervention to improve the sleep of cancer survivors with insomnia. *Psychooncology, 21*(7), 695–705.

Rose, K. M., Taylor, A. G., & Bourguignon, C. (2009). Effects of cranial electrical stimulation on sleep disturbances, depressive symptoms, and caregiving appraisal in spousal caregivers of persons with Alzheimer's disease. *Applied Nursing Research: ANR, 22*(2), 119–125.

Rybarczyk, B., Mack, L., Harris, J. H., & Stepanski, E. (2011). Testing two types of self-help CBT-I for insomnia in older adults with arthritis or coronary artery disease. *Rehabilitation Psychology, 56*(4), 257–266.

Rybarczyk, B., Stapanski, E., Fogg, L., Lopez, M., Barry, P., & Davis, A. (2005). A placebo-controlled test of cognitive-behavioral therapy for comorbid insomnia in older adults. *Journal of Consulting and Clinical Psychology, 73*(6), 1164–1174.

Sack, R. L., Auckley, D., Auger, R. R., Carskadon, M. A., Wright, K. P., Jr., Vitiello, M. V., & Zhdanova, I. V. (2007). Circadian rhythm sleep disorders: Part II, advanced sleep phase disorder, delayed sleep phase disorder, free-running disorder, and irregular sleep-wake rhythm: An American academy of sleep medicine review. *Sleep, 30*(11), 1484–1501.

Scheer, F. A., & Shea, S. A. (2009). Fundamentals of the circadian system. In C. J. Amlaner & P. M. Fuller (Eds.), *Basics of sleep guide* (2nd ed., pp. 199–221). Westchester, NY: Sleep Research Society.

Schutte-Rodin, S., Broch, L., Buysse, D., Dorsey, C., & Sateia, M. (2008). Clinical guideline for the evaluation and management of chronic insomnia in adults. *Journal of Clinical Sleep Medicine, 4*(5), 487–504.

Semla, T. P., Beizer, J. L., & Hibgee, M. D. (2015). *Geriatric dosage handbook* (20th ed.). Hudson, OH: Lexicomp.

Sharma, M., Palacios-Bois, J., Schwartz, G., & Iskandar, H. (1989). Circadian rhythms of melatonin and cortisol in aging. *Biological Psychiatry, 25*(3), 305–319.

Shealy, C. M., Cady, R. K., Culver-Veehoff, D., Cox, R., & Liss, S. (1998). Cerebrospinal fluid and plasma neuro-chemicals: Response to cranial electrical stimulation. *Journal of Neurological and Orthopaedic Medicine and Surgery, 18*(2), 94–97.

Silva, G. E., An, M. W., Goodwin, J. L., Shahar, E., Redline, S., Resnick, H., . . . Quan, S. F. (2009). Longitudinal evaluation of sleep-disordered breathing and sleep symptoms with change in quality of life: The Sleep Heart Health Study (SHHS). *Sleep, 32*(8), 1049–1057.

Smith, M. T., Perlis, M. L., Park, A., Smith, M. S., Pennington, J., Giles, D. E., & Buysse, D. J. (2002). Comparative meta-analysis of pharmacotherapy and behavior therapy for persistent insomnia. *The American Journal of Psychiatry, 159*(1), 5–10.

Stone, K. L., Ancoli-Israel, S., Blackwell, T., Ensrud, K. E., Cauley, J. A., Redline, S. S., . . . Cummings, S. R. (2008). Poor sleep is associated with increased risk of falls in older women. *Archives of Internal Medicine, 168*(16), 1768–1775.

Taibi, D. M., Landis, C. A., Petry, H., & Vitiello, M. V. (2007). A systematic review of valerian as a sleep aid: Safe but not effective. *Sleep Medicine Reviews, 11*(3), 209–230.

Taylor, D. J., Mallory, L. J., Lichstein, K. L., Durrence, H. H., Riedel, B. W., & Bush, A. J. (2007). Comorbidity of chronic insomnia with medical problems. *Sleep, 30*(2), 213–218.

Terman, M. (2007). Evolving applications of light therapy. *Sleep Medicine Reviews, 11*(6), 497–507.

Thorpy, M. J. (2015). Update on therapy for narcolepsy. *Current Treatment Options in Neurology, 17*(5), 347.

Thorpy, M. J., & Dauvilliers, Y. (2015). Clinical and practical considerations in the pharmacologic management of narcolepsy. *Sleep Medicine, 16*(1), 9–18.

Trenkwalder, C., Benes, H., Grote, L., Garcia-Borreguero, D., Hogl, B., Hopp, M., . . . RELOXYN Study Group (2013). Prolonged release oxycodone-naloxone for treatment of severe restless legs syndrome after failure of previous treatment: A double-blind, randomised, placebo-controlled trial with an open-label extension. *Lancet Neurology, 12*(12), 1141–1150.

Tyron, W. W. (1991). *Activity measurement in psychology and medicine.* New York, NY: Plenum Press.

Vance, D. E., Heaton, K., Eaves, Y. & Fazeli, P. L. (2011). Sleep and cognition on everyday functioning in older adults: Implications for nursing practice and research. *Journal of Neuroscience Nursing, 43*(5), 261–271.

Vaughn, B. V., & D'Cruz, O. F. (2011). Cardinal manifestations of sleep disorders. In M. Kryger, T. Roth, & W. Dement (Eds.), *Principles and practice of sleep medicine* (5th ed., pp. 647–657). Philadelphia, PA: W.B. Saunders.

Vaz Fragoso, C. A., & Gill, T. M. (2007). Sleep complaints in community-living older persons: A multifactorial geriatric syndrome. *Journal of the American Geriatrics Society, 55*(11), 1853–1866.

Verbeek, I. H., Konings, G. M., Aldenkamp, A. P., Declerck, A. C., & Klip, E. C. (2006). Cognitive behavioral treatment in clinically referred chronic insomniacs: group versus individual treatment. *Behavioral Sleep Medicine, 4*(3), 135–151.

Vincent, N., & Lewycky, S. (2009). Logging on for better sleep: RCT of the effectiveness of online treatment for insomnia. *Sleep, 32*(6), 807–815.

Vitiello, M. V. (2006). Sleep in normal aging. *Sleep Medicine Clinics, 1*(2), 171–176.

Vitiello, M. V., & Borson, S. (2001). Sleep disturbances in patients with Alzheimer's disease: Epidemiology, pathophysiology and treatment. *CNS Drugs, 15*(10), 777–796.

Vitiello, M. V., Moe, K. E., & Prinz, P. N. (2002). Sleep complaints cosegregate with illness in older adults: Clinical research informed by and informing epidemiological studies of sleep. *Journal of Psychosomatic Research, 53*(1), 555–559.

Vitiello, M. B., Rybarczyk, B. Von Korff, M. & Stepanski, E. J. (2009). Cognitive behavioral therapy for insomnia improves sleep and decreases pain in older adults with co-morbid insomnia and osteoarthritis. *Journal of Clinical Sleep Medicine, 5*(4), 355–362.

Walsh, J. K., & Roth, T. (2011). Pharmacologic treatment of insomnia: Benzodiazepine receptor agonists. In M. Kryger, T. Roth, & W. Dement (Eds.), *Principles and practice of sleep medicine* (5th ed., pp. 905–915). Philadelphia, PA: W.B. Saunders.

Ward, T. M. (2011). Conducting a sleep assessment. In N.S. Redeker & G. P. McEnany (Eds.), *Sleep disorders and sleep promotion in nursing practice* (pp. 53–70). New York, NY: Springer.

Weaver, T. E., & Chasens, E. R. (2007). Continuous positive airway pressure treatment for sleep apnea in older adults. *Sleep Medicine Reviews, 11*(2), 99–111.

Williamson, A. T., Fletcher, P. C., & Dawson, K. A. (2003). Complementary and alternative medicine: Use in an older population. *Journal of Gerontological Nursing, 29*(5), 20–28.

Wilson, S. J., Nutt, D. J., Alford, C., Argyropoulos, S. V., Baldwin, D. S., Bateson, A. N., . . . Wade, A. G. (2010). British Association for Psychopharmacology consensus statement on evidence-based treatment of insomnia, parasomnias and circadian rhythm disorders. *Journal of Psychopharmacology, 24*(11), 1577–1601.

Yeh, G. Y., Mietus, J. E., Peng, C. K., Phillips, R. S., Davis, R. B., Wayne, P. M., . . . Thomas, R. J. (2008). Enhancement of sleep stability with Tai Chi exercise in chronic heart failure: Preliminary findings using an ECG-based spectrogram method. *Sleep Medicine, 9*(5), 527–536.

Zeitzer, J. M., Fisicaro, R. A., Grove, M. E., Mignot, E., Yesavage, J. A., & Friedman, L. (2011). Faster REM sleep EEG and worse restedness in older insomniacs with HLA DQB1*0602. *Psychiatry Research, 187*(3), 397–400.

For a full suite of assignments and additional learning activities, see the access code at the front of your book.

CHAPTER 17

Dysphagia and Malnutrition

Neva L. Crogan

(Competency 7)

LEARNING OBJECTIVES

At the end of this chapter, the reader will be able to:

> Assess for dysphagia at the bedside.
> Develop a plan to meet the nutritional and hydration needs of a patient with dysphagia.
> Differentiate between anorexia of aging and malnutrition.
> Describe the steps necessary to adequately assess an older adult for malnutrition.
> Develop a plan to meet the nutritional needs of a homebound older adult suffering from weight loss and malnutrition.

KEY TERMS

Albumin	Fortified foods
Anorexia of aging	Leptin
Anthropometric measures	Malnutrition
Bioelectrical impedance analysis	Mid-upper arm circumference
Body mass index	Nasogastric tube
Cachexia	Oropharyngeal dysphagia
Deglutition	Percutaneous endoscopic gastrostomy
Diet history review	Prealbumin
Dysphagia	Sarcopenia
Dysphagia diet	Triceps skin fold
Esophageal dysphagia	Weight loss

Food is basic to life. For the older adult, food means family, togetherness, and quality of life. In response to a decrease in energy needs and expenditures, older age leads to a physiological change referred to as *anorexia of aging* (Morley, 2013). This physiological anorexia results from alterations in taste and smell, earlier satiation, and other changes related to normal aging (Morley, 2011b). The professional nurse needs to be able to successfully identify, evaluate, and treat problems affecting food intake. In this chapter, we will present the diagnoses and treatments of dysphagia and malnutrition. To start, we will pay special attention to the problem of dysphagia, a key causative and contributory factor of malnutrition for many older adults.

Dysphagia
Prevalence

We swallow approximately 600 times per day (Herskowitz, 2012). Swallowing is an automatic response to food or liquid in the mouth. *Dysphagia*, or problems with swallowing, is "an underrecognized, poorly diagnosed, and poorly managed health problem" that negatively affects the quality and potentially quantity of life (Ekberg, Hamby Woisard, Wuttge-Hanning, & Ortega, 2004, p. 143). Although dysphagia may occur at any age, it is more prevalent in the elderly. Prevalence data suggest that 68% of nursing home elders report dysphagia symptoms (Sura, Madhavan, Carnaby, & Crary, 2012). Approximately 30% of hospitalized patients and 13% to 38% of elderly who live independently experience dysphagia (Sura et al., 2012). Most importantly, the prevalence of dysphagia increases with age; thus, it is a major health problem in older adults.

Implications of Dysphagia

The physiological sequelae of dysphagia have traditionally received the greatest attention. Untreated dysphagia places a person at greater risk for nutritional deficiencies and respiratory problems. Dehydration and malnutrition from inadequate intake predispose persons to the development of many medical problems. Dehydration thickens secretions, increasing the risk for respiratory problems, and aspiration may lead to pneumonia and death. The ability and motivation to be active and involved in daily activities also may be adversely affected. The development of these complications is dependent on the nature and severity of the dysphagia and the overall health status of the individual.

   The social and psychological consequences of dysphagia also must be considered in the treatment and evaluation of care. The effects of dysphagia on quality of life were evaluated in 360 adults with subjective dysphagia complaints living in nursing homes or clinics in four European countries (Ekberg et al., 2004). The findings confirm the serious physiological impact of dysphagia. Fifty-five percent reported their eating habits were affected by their swallowing problems; over 50% ate less, 44% experienced *weight loss*, and over 30% were still hungry or thirsty after a meal. From a psychosocial perspective, 45% no longer found eating to be enjoyable, and more than half indicated dysphagia made life less enjoyable. Loss of self-esteem and an increasing sense of isolation also were reported. Over one third (36%) avoided eating with others, and 41% experienced anxiety or panic during meals. Of the individuals interviewed, 40% had a confirmed diagnosis, only 32% had received treatment, and just 39% believed dysphagia could be treated (Ekberg et al., 2004). An individual's ability to be nourished physically, emotionally, and socially is threatened by dysphagia. The findings from this study are supported by other literature (Bibi, Iqbal, Ayaz, Khan, & Matee, 2015).

Warning Signs and Risk Factors for Dysphagia

Deglutition is the act of swallowing in which a food or liquid bolus is transported from the mouth through the pharynx and esophagus into the stomach. Swallowing is a complex neuromuscular process that occurs in stages. Dysphagia is usually identified as being either oropharyngeal or esophageal, designating the phase in which dysfunction occurs. In the oropharyngeal phase, food is prepared for swallowing by mastication and mixing with saliva, and then is moved posteriorly, triggering the pharyngeal swallow reflex, which moves the bolus down the pharynx (Oropharyngeal dysphagia, 2009). During the pharyngeal swallow, the larynx closes and the epiglottis redirects the bolus around the airway, protecting the respiratory tract. The esophageal phase begins when the bolus enters the esophagus at the cricopharyngeal juncture or upper esophageal sphincter (UES). Peristaltic waves propel the bolus through the esophagus to the lower esophageal sphincter, which opens into the stomach (National Institute on Deafness and Other Communication Disorders (NIDCD), 2010). Because swallowing is a complex, coordinated event, causes of dysphagia are multiple and diverse. Each type of dysphagia is characterized by specific symptoms and associated with specific disorders.

Oropharyngeal dysphagia is usually related to neuromuscular impairments affecting the tongue, pharynx, and UES (Mayo Clinic, 2014). Stroke is the leading cause of oropharyngeal dysfunction (NIDCD, 2010). Persons experiencing oropharyngeal dysphagia often complain of difficulty initiating a swallow. A cough early in the swallow and nasal regurgitation are symptoms associated with oropharyngeal dysphagia (Udayakumar & Eubanks, 2015; Mayo Clinic, 2014). The oropharyngeal phase of dysphagia is voluntary and utilizes the motor and sensory pathways to move food posteriorly to the oropharynx, which then triggers the reflexive/involuntary phase in which the larynx and epiglottis are elevated and lowered, respectively, to prevent aspiration into the trachea. Dysphonia and dysarthria indicate motor dysfunction in the structures involved in the oral and pharyngeal phases and may be accompanied by dysphagia. Inadequate saliva production can also interfere with the formation and movement of the food bolus. Candidiasis, or thrush, a fungal infection identified by white plaques on the mucous membranes of the oral cavity, can cause pain and discomfort when swallowing.

Esophageal dysphagia results from motility problems, neuromuscular problems, or obstruction that interferes with the movement of the food bolus through the esophagus into the stomach (Udayakumar & Eubanks, 2015; Mayo Clinic, 2014). Common symptoms of esophageal dysphagia include complaints of food sticking after a swallow and coughing late in the swallow (Udayakumar & Eubanks, 2015). Muscular dystrophy, myasthenia gravis, scleroderma, achalasia, and esophageal spasms may cause motility problems. Inflammation of the esophagus, secondary to gastroesophageal reflux disease (GERD) or a retained pill, is another etiology for esophageal dysphagia. Medications associated with pill-induced irritation or injury include tetracycline, potassium chloride, quinidine, iron, nonsteroidal anti-inflammatory drugs, alendronate sodium, and vitamin C (Udayakumar & Eubanks, 2015). Common medical conditions associated with dysphagia are outlined in **Table 17-1**.

TABLE 17-1 Common Medical Conditions Associated with Dysphagia

Classification of Dysphagia	Neuromuscular Causes	Mechanical Causes
Oropharyngeal dysphagia	Cerebrovascular accident Parkinson's disease Multiple sclerosis Amyotrophic lateral sclerosis (ALS) Traumatic brain injury (TBI)	Tumors Inflammatory masses
Esophageal dysphagia	Zenker's diverticulum Achalasia Scleroderma	Tumors Strictures Tracheoesophageal fistula Foreign bodies Medication irritation Gastroesophageal reflux disease

Assessment

Clinical evaluation of swallowing skills in patients with conditions that predispose to dysphagia or who voice complaints that suggest a swallowing disorder should be a priority for nursing. Evaluation as it relates to dysphagia can refer to screening or diagnostic testing. Screening involves determining if the patient has signs or symptoms of dysphagia for the purpose of referring for diagnostic evaluation to identify physiological components of swallowing (Udayakumar & Eubanks, 2015; Mayo Clinic, 2014). Nursing plays a pivotal role in the early detection of swallowing problems and intervening to prevent complications from dysphagia. The findings from a screening evaluation allow prompt referral for diagnostic workup and implementation of interventions to promote safe eating and feeding practices.

Udayakumar and Eubanks (2015) suggest that 80% of dysphagia can be diagnosed through a history. A careful history of the dysphagia should be obtained during the nursing assessment. Open-ended questions that the nurse can ask of the patient or the caregiver might include: "How often do you cough after eating or drinking?" "How often do you feel that food is caught in your throat or chest?" "Show me where it sticks." "How long does it take for you to eat a meal?" "Is this a change for you?" The patient or caregiver should be asked about the presence of predisposing conditions or warning signs and symptoms. Additional questions might include: "What type of food causes the symptoms?" "Is the swallowing problem intermittent or progressive?" "Is heartburn present?" Specific signs and symptoms of both oropharyngeal and esophageal dysphagia are listed in **Table 17-2** (Paik, 2012).

The physical examination involves a cognitive, neuromuscular, and respiratory assessment. Important cognitive factors include interest in eating, ability to focus on and complete a meal, and the ability to remember and follow directions for safe eating. Neurological assessment involves testing sensory and motor components of the cranial nerves, in particular cranial nerves V, VII, IX, X, XI, and XII. Breath sounds, the strength of the person's cough, and his or her ability to clear the throat are clues to the integrity of the respiratory structures and the presence of protective mechanisms. Although commonly considered to be protective, the gag reflex is not an indication of the patient's ability to swallow (Gillen, 2016). However, detection of laryngeal elevation during a swallow maneuver grossly suggests airway closure (Gillen, 2016). Medications should be reviewed for those that can decrease saliva production (antihistamines, anticholinergics, antihypertensives, cold medications), decrease cognition (sedatives, hypnotics), and/or decrease the strength of the muscles involved in swallowing (antispasticity drugs).

TABLE 17-2   Signs and Symptoms of Dysphagia by Classification
Oropharyngeal
• Coughing or choking with swallowing
• Difficulty initiating swallowing
• Food sticking in the throat
• Sialorrhea
• Unexplained weight loss
• Change in dietary habits
• Recurrent pneumonia
• Change in voice or speech (wet voice)
• Nasal regurgitation
Esophageal
• Sensation of food sticking in the chest or throat
• Oral or pharyngeal regurgitation
• Change in dietary habits
• Recurrent pneumonia

CLINICAL TIP

Monitor abdominal distention by measuring the abdominal circumference from iliac crest to iliac crest. An increase in measurement of 8 to 10 cm beyond baseline is considered distention.

CLINICAL TIP

Older adults take more medications than any other age group. Medications can cause loss of appetite, reduced taste and smell, painful swallowing, and nausea and vomiting and can affect the absorption and use of nutrients.

Source: http://nutritionandaging.fiu.edu/aging_network/malfact2.asp

Bedside Poststroke Swallowing Tests

Oropharyngeal dysphagia following a cerebrovascular accident or stroke increases the likelihood of dehydration, malnutrition, aspiration pneumonia, persistent disablement, and even death (Poorjavad & Jalaie, 2014). In a multidatabase systematic review of journal articles targeting highly qualified screening tests for swallowing disorders following a stroke, Poorjavad and Jalaie identified and evaluated 264 journal articles to determine evidence level, presence of methodological bias, and reported sensitivity and specificity of each test. Screening test sensitivities ranged from 47% to 100%, and their specificities ranged from 63% to 100%. The researchers identified four simple, valid, reliable, sensitive and specific tests for screening swallowing at the bedside after a stroke (Poorjavad & Jalaie, 2014). The four identified tests were as follows:

> Oral pharyngeal and clinical swallowing examination
> Bedside aspiration test
> The Gugging Swallowing Screen
> The Toronto Bedside Swallowing Screening Test (TOR-BSST)

These bedside tests are highly sensitive and specific for the detection of dysphagia, and if conducted in a timely manner, can reduce the incidence of aspiration in at-risk older adults (Hassan & Aboloyoun, 2014).

The Nurses Role in Screening for Dysphagia

The effectiveness of trained nurses to screen for dysphagia after stroke was evaluated in the Collaborative Dysphagia Audit (CODA) Study. Nurses on a stroke unit received training in a simple water-screening test and screened acute stroke patients. The findings demonstrated a decrease in the number of patients who kept nothing by mouth (NPO), a decrease in the number of patients with inappropriate feeding orders, and improved referrals (Stroke Research Unit, 2001). The Gatehead Dysphagia Management Model (GDMM), developed from the results of the CODA, provides a decision tree to guide assessment and management of dysphagia (see **Case Study 17-1**).

CLINICAL TIP

Nearly half of the nation's low-income elders have lost all or most of their teeth, leading to problems with chewing and swallowing.

Source: http://nutritionandaging.fiu.edu/aging_network/malfact2.asp

Case Study 17-1

Mr. C., an 81-year-old widower, is admitted for stroke rehabilitation. He underwent a cystoscopy and transurethral resection of the prostate (TURP) for benign prostatic hypertrophy (BPH) 1 week ago. After the procedure he experienced a hypotensive episode and mental status changes. A workup revealed a large left middle-cerebral artery stroke. His stroke deficits include expressive aphasia, left neglect, dysphagia, and left hemiplegia. Concurrent health problems include coronary artery disease, hypertension, and hyperlipidemia under good control prior to surgery. Prior to transfer, Mr. C. had a low hematocrit level and Hemoccult-positive stool and received a blood transfusion. He was also suspected to have pneumonia and was started on an antibiotic.

On examination, Mr. C. is noted to be thin, pale, and lethargic. He has a weak cough, facial weakness, and a mild case of thrush. An indwelling urinary catheter is draining amber urine. Nonpitting edema is noted in his right hand; his arms have multiple bruises and dry, flaky skin. The transfer report indicates he requires minimal assistance with bed mobility and moderate assistance with transfers, including toilet transfers; his sitting balance is fair; and he can self-propel his wheelchair 150 ft. with standby assistance. His son and daughter live out of town and have had to return home. They were not able to accompany him at transfer and will not be able to visit until the weekend (4 days from now).

Orders on admission include a pureed texture diet with moderate thick liquids; Isosource 1.5 cans at 0800 and 1600 and 1 can at 1200 and 2000 with 325 cc free water flush every shift via PEG tube. One scoop of Benefiber is added to tube feeding three times a day. His medication orders

include Tenormin, 25 mg once a day; Lipitor, 20 mg at bedtime; Prevacid, 30 mg once a day; ASA, 81 mg once a day; Plavix, 75 mg once a day; amiodarone, 200 mg once a day; and clindamycin, 600 mg 3 times a day.

Questions:

1. Mr. C. presents multiple challenges. Which of the common health problems discussed in this chapter are relevant to his nursing care?
2. What are the priorities for Mr. C.'s care plan during his first week of rehabilitation?
3. What are key interventions to promote recovery and prevent complications?

After 3 days, the physician orders discontinuing his indwelling catheter. He experiences frequency, urgency, and incontinence. He has developed symptoms of an allergy—he is suffering from runny nose and dry cough. His tube feeding is being decreased as his dietary intake increases. When his family arrives, they ask about putting him on that medicine advertised on TV for overactive bladder and bring his over-the-counter (OTC) allergy medicine (Sudafed) for his cold. They also bring him his favorite soda.

Questions:

4. How would you respond to the family?
5. What actions would you take to address the problems and concerns raised?
6. How would your goals for care evolve over the next weeks of his stay?
7. What interventions would you institute to prevent the development of common health problems during his hospitalization and upon return to the community?

A careful assessment of the individual eating a meal also is an essential component of an evaluation, even if the initial screening does not suggest a swallowing problem (Udayakumar & Eubanks, 2015). Observations of a prolonged time required to complete a meal, "picking" at food, and active attempts to avoid eating (pushing the food away, turning away from offered food, refusing to open the mouth) may indicate a swallowing problem. Environmental factors that influence intake and eating behaviors, such as distractibility, fatigue, or even compatibility with dining companions or assistants, will not be apparent in a bedside evaluation. Gillen (2016) emphasizes the importance of contextual issues in an evaluation, pointing out that fatigue, pain, and anxiety may mask an older person's true abilities.

Assessment for aspiration is also important. Aspiration occurs when material passes into the larynx below the true vocal cords; silent aspiration refers to situations in which aspiration does not produce the typical cough or change in voice quality (Smith & Connolly, 2003). Pulse oximetry has been found to be an effective, efficient tool to detect aspiration while eating. In a review of trends in the evaluation and treatment of dysphagia after stroke, Smith and Connolly report that a 2% drop in oxygen saturation levels from baseline detects 86% of penetration/aspiration. When followed by a 10-mL water swallow test at the bedside, the ability to detect aspiration increases to 95%.

Persons at risk should be assessed upon admission to a facility or community caseload; if deterioration occurs after admission, the individual should be reassessed at that time. Persons with degenerative conditions should be reassessed on a regular basis and when the condition progresses. (Monitoring lung sounds, respiration rate and quality, and other vital signs remains an important component of ongoing assessment and evaluation of care.) If screening suggests dysphagia, a referral for diagnostic evaluation should be ordered. A speech–language therapist (SLT) will conduct a more focused examination, and occupational therapists (OTs) also may be requested to complete an extensive examination. Further testing to confirm the diagnosis and determine the presence of and conditions surrounding aspiration are conducted by radiology or gastroenterology subspecialists.

Interventions and Strategies for Care

Actual treatment of the dysphagia depends on the specific diagnosis and the level of dysfunction. Restoration of swallowing has been attempted using a variety of strategies ranging from electrical stimulation to thermal stimulation, muscle exercises, and even black pepper oil—all with varying success at restoring muscular function and normal swallowing. Another strategy was tested in a 2009 randomized clinical trial of 19 patients with oropharyngeal dysphagia. Patients were randomized into one of two groups, Shaker exercises or traditional therapy. Patients in the Shaker exercises group were found to have significantly less posttherapy aspiration than those in the traditional therapy group (Logemann, Rademaker, Pauloski, Kelly, & Stangl-McBreen, 2009). The Shaker technique is described here (Swigert, 2016, para 2):

> The patient lies flat and, keeping the shoulders on the bed/mat, raises the head to look at the toes. The patient maintains this position (the goal is 60 seconds) and then repeats this 2 more times. The second part of the exercise is a repetitive movement. In the same starting position, the patient raises the head to look at the chin, lowers the head back to the bed and then repeats this 30 times. Three sets of 30 are the goal.

Nursing interventions to manage dysphagia in order to minimize the risk of aspiration and promote nutrition and hydration involve compensatory eating techniques, diet modification, and oral care and may require adaptive equipment.

Compensatory Eating Techniques

Specific interventions are developed for persons with dysphagia based on the swallowing problems identified. The results of a diagnostic workup or referral to an SLT or OT should provide specific recommendations for eating techniques. However, appropriate positioning is critical for safe eating and swallowing for all individuals. An upright position with the arms and feet supported, the head midline in a neutral position, and the chin slightly tucked is recommended to minimize the possibility of aspiration. The upright position should be maintained for at least 30 to 60 minutes after eating (the longer interval is necessary for esophageal dysphagia) (Gillen, 2016). The location of food placement in the mouth as well as the size, consistency, and temperature of food items are important sensory cues to promote safe swallowing. If the individual has a sensory loss or oral muscular weakness, placing food on the unaffected or least affected side may help improve control over the bolus and its movement to the back of the mouth. If movement of the food to the back of the mouth is the problem, then placement of the bolus at the back of the tongue may be necessary to trigger the swallow (Gillen, 2016). The bolus size also influences swallow. A small bolus will not enter the pharynx as quickly as a large bolus, decreasing the risk of aspiration. However, a large bolus improves movement through the oral cavity in persons with delayed oral transit and also prolongs laryngeal elevation and closure (Gillen, 2016). For persons with decreased oral sensation or the impaired oral movement of food, cold items may improve posterior tongue movements and laryngeal swallow; for other persons, a warm bolus facilitates swallowing (Gillen, 2016). Careful questioning and observation of the conditions that result in optimal intake without evidence of swallowing problems and those associated with apparent problems will help guide eating techniques and feeding strategies. Having said this, a study looking at dysphagia between Parkinson's and dementia patients found that honey-thick foods were more effective than nectar-thick foods in preventing aspiration; the chin-down swallowing posture was least effective (Logemann et al., 2008).

Characteristics of the environment, including assistive personnel and dining partners, are factors that can facilitate or interfere with a safe, efficient swallow and adequate intake. For the first meal or eating or feeding session (and subsequent meals in some cases), a quiet room is preferable to decrease distractions and allow greater concentration on eating. The healthcare provider should sit down to assist with eating, positioning herself or himself and the food tray directly across from the patient in order to maintain the proper posture for the patient and ensure that she or he can see and reach food items and utensils (Gillen, 2016). An unhurried, calm demeanor is important. Conversation should be limited to after a swallow is completed and before the next bite is taken. However, interaction that requires a response from the person eating is necessary to provide information about changes in voice quality as well as to promote a more pleasant social experience.

Diet Modifications

Modifying the texture of the food and fluids consumed is a common response to suspected swallowing problems. Alterations in diet consistency should be tailored to the type of swallowing disorder. An example of levels for food consistency is provided in **Table 17-3**. Foods can be prepared in blenders or food processors to the approved consistency or purchased in the infant-child food section. Attention to seasoning may improve flavor and therefore adherence to and intake of a modified diet.

Thickened fluids frequently present a challenge to adequate hydration. Complaints about the texture, taste, and ability to quench thirst are common. The Dysphagia Diet Task Force has standardized food and fluid textures for the *dysphagia diet* (see **Table 17-4**). Certain fluids have a thicker consistency naturally, whereas others will require thickening to the appropriate consistency with commercial or natural thickeners. Instant potato flakes, instant baby rice cereal, and mashed bananas are natural thickeners, but may not meet special diet requirements and may change the taste of the thickened items. Commercial thickening agents differ with respect to the directions for preparation and the effect of time on consistency. The type and temperature of the fluid to be thickened also affects mixing directions, so it is important to be familiar with the product used by the facility or individual at home.

CLINICAL TIP

Therapeutic diets should be avoided if at all possible, but all factors related to eating and safe swallowing should be considered when instituting a special diet.

Data from Tariz, S. H., Karcic, E., Thomas, D. R., et al. (2001). The use of a no-concentrated-sweets diet in the management of type 2 diabetes in nursing homes. *Journal of the American Dietetic Association, 101*, 1463–1466; Coulston, A. M., Mandelbaum, D., & Reaven, G. M. (1990). Dietary management of nursing home residents with non-insulin-dependent diabetes mellitus. *American Journal of Clinical Nutrition, 51*, 67–71.

TABLE 17-3   Dysphagia Diet According to Viscosity

Level I: Pudding, crushed potato, and ground meat
Level II: Curd-type yogurt, orange juice (3% thickener mixed), cream soup, and thin soup with starch
Level III: Tomato juice; fluid-like yogurt; and thick, fluid rice
Level IV: Water and orange juice

Data from Paik, N. (2014). *Dysphagia*. [Web online article]. Retrieved from http://emedicine.medscape.com/article/2212409-overview

TABLE 17-4   The National Dysphagia Diet

The National Dysphagia Diet (NDD) provides guidelines for progressive diets to be used nationally in the treatment of dysphagia. The following are some examples:

- Dysphagia Pureed (NDD 1): "Pudding-like" consistencies; pureed, no chunks or small pieces; avoid scrambled eggs, cereals with lumps.
- Dysphagia Mechanically Altered (NDD 2): Moist, soft foods; easily formed into a bolus; ground meats; soft, tender vegetables; soft fruit; slightly moistened dry cereal with little texture. No bread or foods such as peas and corn. Avoid skins and seeds.
- Mechanical Soft: Same as the mechanically altered but allows bread, cakes, and rice.
- Dysphagia Advanced (NDD 3): Regular textured foods except those that are very hard, sticky, or crunchy. Avoid hard fruit and vegetables, corn, skins, nuts, and seeds.

Liquid consistencies:

- Spoon thick
- Honey-like
- Nectar-like
- Thin: All beverages such as water, ice, milk, milkshakes, juices, coffee, tea, and sodas

Data from McCallum, S. L. (2003). The national dysphagia diet: Implementation at a regional rehabilitation center and hospital system. *Journal of the American Dietetic Association, 103*(3), 381–384.

Encouraging fluid intake with thickened liquids often requires creativity and persistence. Some facilities allow patients with dysphagia to drink plain water between meals when requiring thickened liquids with meals. There are contradictory beliefs about the likelihood that allowing plain water will lead to aspiration pneumonia (Sura et al., 2012). Oral care appears to be a crucial link in the aspiration to pneumonia process (Gillen, 2016). Frequent oral care to ensure the oral cavity is clear of food particles and to prevent the growth of bacteria is a critical component of liberalized fluid programs and an essential strategy to minimize the risk for pneumonia.

CLINICAL TIP

Older adults who require thickened liquids for a safe swallow often do not get enough fluids due to resistance to the taste or consistency of the thickening agent.

Oral Hygiene

Examination of the relative risk of multiple factors (medical or health status, functional status, dysphagia or gastroesophageal reflux, feeding or mode of nutritional intake, and oral or dental status) in the development of pneumonia in older persons suggests that colonization and host resistance are key contributors (Liantonio, Salzman, & Snyderman, 2014). Oropharyngeal colonization from inadequate oral care, decayed teeth, or periodontal disease is the initial process that can lead to the development of pneumonia. Aspiration of these organisms in liquids, food, or saliva, combined with decreased immunity, increases the risk of development of pneumonia.

Regular cleaning of the teeth or dentures, gums, and tongue and maintaining moisture in the mouth are essential components of an oral hygiene protocol. (See Johnson and Chalmers [2002] for tools and strategies to address various problems in providing oral care.) A soft toothbrush, gauze-covered swabs, or foam Toothettes may be used to scrub the surfaces of the oral cavity after meals. Electric toothbrushes also may be useful tools and, depending on the person's physical and cognitive abilities, may enable the older person with limited hand grasp and movement to more adequately and independently clean the mouth's surfaces. Individuals who receive nonoral feedings also need to have regular oral care to remove debris. The teeth and mouth should be cleaned upon awakening, after meals (or snacks for persons with dysphagia), and before bed. Dentures should be taken out and scrubbed at least daily with a brush; chemical denture cleaner tablets may be used in addition to brushing with soap or toothpaste (Johnson & Chalmers, 2002). Soaking dentures in a solution of white wine vinegar and cold water (a 50:50 solution) will help remove built-up calculus. Denture cups must also be cleaned or replaced regularly. A weekly cleaning and soaking of the denture cup in a diluted hypochlorite solution for an hour followed by thorough washing with soap and water will help sterilize the container (Johnson & Chalmers, 2002) if frequent replacement is not feasible.

Maintaining moist mucous membranes is essential to the health and integrity of the oral cavity. Dry membranes contribute to an increased rate of plaque accumulation and dental and denture plaque serves as a major reservoir for pathogenic organisms in the elderly (Liantonio et al., 2014). Many of the medications prescribed for chronic conditions result in a dry mouth. Limited fluid intake and infrequent oral care, especially for persons who are ordered to have nothing by mouth, contribute to dryness. Meticulous oral care as outlined previously is crucial; however, additional measures may be needed. Saliva substitutes, toothpaste and mouth rinses without alcohol or excessive additives such as in the Biotene range, water or mouthwash in spray bottles to spritz inside the mouth, water-soluble lubricants applied to the tongue and cheeks, and Vaseline or lanolin applied frequently to the lips are among the strategies recommended for combating dry mouth in the physically dependent or cognitively impaired older adult (Johnson & Chalmers, 2002).

Adaptive Equipment

The modification of utensils or use of adaptive equipment is frequently necessary to promote independence in eating and to facilitate safe swallowing. However, careful evaluation of eating is needed for each person to ensure safe and effective tools are used. Using a straw to drink moves a fluid bolus quickly through the mouth and can exacerbate problems with swallowing. Drinking from a cup requires the head to be tilted to empty the glass; this maneuver (hyperextension) can increase the risk of aspiration. Specially designed cups with a cutout for the nose can be purchased or made to prevent the need to tilt the head back. Similarly, shallow bowls on spoons may be helpful in preventing hypertension when eating with a spoon (Gillen, 2016). An ongoing assessment of abilities and problems at mealtime will help ensure that necessary changes to the plan of care are made in a timely manner. Rehabilitation nurses and texts and continuing education programs focusing on swallowing evaluation and feeding techniques are resources for new tools and techniques. Physical, occupational, and speech–language therapists can recommend specific techniques and equipment for safe intake and can help modify available tools. Their expertise and assistance should be sought.

Enteral Feeding

The initiation of tube feedings is a complicated decision made by the patient, healthcare provider, and family or healthcare surrogate. Often prescribed to maintain adequate nutrition and hydration levels and prevent aspiration, persons receiving enteral feedings are still at risk for aspiration (Liantonio et al., 2012) and inadequate nutritional intake. The most appropriate mode and method of administering enteral feeding (e.g., continuous or intermittent, intestinal or gastric) remains controversial (Paik, 2012).

Nasogastric tube. **Nasogastric tube** (NGT) feeding is a commonly used method of enteral feeding for patients with a short-term life expectancy. Insertion of a nasogastric tube is a quick, easy, relatively noninvasive procedure; however, many patients find the tube uncomfortable and pull the tube out. Prolonged use of nasogastric tubes can lead to complications such as lesions to the nasal mucosa, chronic sinusitis, gastroesophageal reflux, and aspiration pneumonia (Paik, 2012).

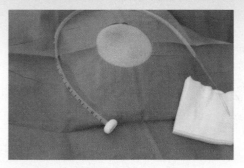 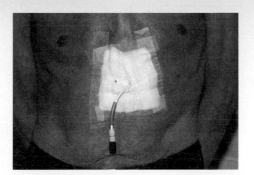

Figure 17-1 PEG tube.
Left: © Barry Slaven, MD, PhD/Medical Images RM; Right: © Dr. P. Marazzi/Science Source

Percutaneous endoscopic gastrostomy. *Percutaneous endoscopic gastrostomy* (PEG) (**Figures 17-1** & **17-2**) requires the invasive insertion of a feeding tube through the anterior abdominal wall, which can be complicated by bleeding, peritonitis or perforation of other abdominal organs, chest infections, insertion site infection, and ease of tube removal (Paik, 2012). PEG has several advantages over surgical gastrostomy, including reduced procedure time, cost, and recovery time, and it requires no general anesthesia. Contraindications for PEG are aspiration pneumonia due to gastroesophageal reflux, significant ascites, and morbid obesity (Paik, 2012). Whether or not to insert a PEG tube can be an ethical and quality-of-life issue. Nearly 50% of patients die within 6 months after PEG insertion, often from insertion complications such as peritonitis or severe wound infections (Wirth et al., 2012).

CLINICAL TIP

Weight loss can be predictive of mortality and is considered clinically significant when there is an unintentional 2% decrease in baseline body weight in 1 month, a > 5% weight loss in 3 months, or a > 10% weight loss in 6 months.

Data from Morley, J. E. (2011a). Assessment of malnutrition in older persons: A focus on the Mini Nutritional Assessment. *Journal of Nutrition, Health, and Aging, 15*(2), 87–90; Kaiser, M. J., Bauer, J. M., Ramsch, C., & MNA-International Group. (2009). Validation of the Mini Nutritional Assessment short-form (MNA-SF); A practical tool for identification of nutritional status. *Journal of Nutrition, Health, and Aging, 13*(9), 782–788.

Attention to positioning during and after a feeding and meticulous oral hygiene are very important in preventing or minimizing the risk for aspiration in persons receiving enteral nutrition. In a literature review on gastrointestinal motility, feeding tube site, and aspiration, Metheny, Schallom, and Edwards (2004) reported that the aspiration risk exists to some extent in all tube-fed patients, depending on gastrointestinal dysmotility patterns and individual patient characteristics. However, regardless of the feeding site, it is ultimately regurgitated gastric contents that are aspirated into the lungs. For this reason, the assessment of greatest interest for tube-fed patients is the evaluation of gastric emptying (p. 131).

Although the need for additional research is indicated, Edwards and Metheny (2000) suggested the early recommendation of McClave et al. (1999) that a residual volume (RV) of 200 cc or greater for nasogastric tubes and 100 cc or greater for gastrostomy tubes, which should raise concerns about intolerance, seems to remain common practice. Further, in their 2008 observation study, Methany, Schallom, Oliver, and Clouse (2008) did not find a consistent correlation between residual volume and aspiration, but did find that patients who were

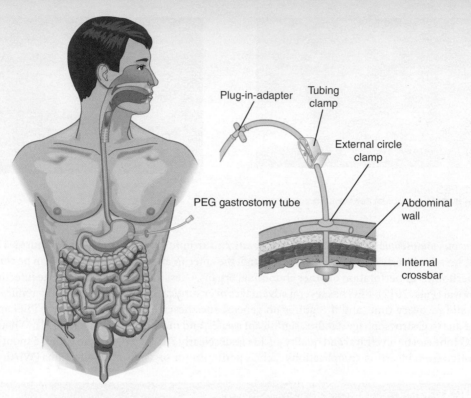

Plug-in-adapter   Tubing clamp

External circle clamp

PEG gastrostomy tube

Abdominal wall

Internal crossbar

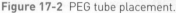

Figure 17-2 PEG tube placement.

categorized as frequent aspirators had a greater incidence of two or more RVs at 200 mL or greater and one or more RVs greater than 250 mL than did the infrequent aspirators. With any evaluation of RVs, it is important to understand that interruptions of tube feedings interfere with the nutritional adequacy of nonoral diets. In actuality, nausea and/or vomiting, absent bowel sounds, abdominal distention, and stool pattern are clues to intolerance that should be evaluated and factored into the decision to continue or halt a tube feeding.

The administration of medications to patients with dysphagia remains a challenge for nurses. If a patient is eating but needs changes in food consistency to promote swallowing, the problem then arises—should medications be crushed? The answer is simple and has been identified as being the best practice in delivering medications to patients with dysphagia. Only medications that have been specifically designed to be crushed or opened (in the case of capsules) may be administered in that way. To crush or open capsules not designed for that purpose alters the pharmacodynamics and pharmacokinetics of the drug and must not be done. If the patient cannot take the medications, the nurse's responsibility is to contact the prescribing practitioner and seek a different medication. To not do so is negligence on the part of the nurse and potentially life-threatening for the patient.

Malnutrition

Prevalence

As described earlier, anorexia of aging is a physiological process that occurs with older age. This physiological anorexia increases the risk of developing malnutrition and weight loss when an older adult develops a physical or psychological illness (Morley, 2013). *Malnutrition* is defined as "the state of being poorly nourished" (Hickson, 2006, p. 4) and can be caused by a lack of nutrients (undernutrition) or an excess of nutrients (overnutrition). For the older adult, the cause is usually a lack of nutrients, or undernutrition. The prevalence of malnutrition in community-dwelling older adults is 15%, increasing to 5% to 44% if the older adult is homebound (Hajjar, Kamel, & Denson, 2004). The prevalence among those living in nursing homes is 30% to 85% (Hajjar et al., 2004; Omran & Morely, 2000), and 20% to 65% if hospitalized (Hajjar et al., 2004).

Two major markers of malnutrition in older adults are sarcopenia and cachexia (Cruz-Jentoft et al., 2010). *Sarcopenia* is defined as "a syndrome of progressive and generalized loss of skeletal muscle mass and strength, which increases the risk of adverse outcomes, such as physical disability, poor quality of life, and even death" (Loreck, Chimakurthi, & Steinle, 2012, p. 20). Diagnosis is confirmed with findings of decreased muscle mass and either decreased muscle strength or decreased physical performance. *Cachexia* is defined as complex metabolic processes associated with an underlying terminal illness (e.g., cancer, end-stage renal disease) and is characterized by loss of muscle mass and fat and anorexia (Morley, 2011b). Cachexia is usually characterized by severe wasting and is frequently associated with inflammation, insulin resistance, and breakdown of muscle protein. Most older adults with cachexia also have sarcopenia, but those with sarcopenia frequently do not have cachexia (Loreck et al., 2012).

Micronutrient Deficiency

Vitamin and mineral supplements are commonly recommended for older adults. However, challenges exist with this strategy including additional costs to the elder, access to the vitamins and minerals, and compliance. Further, in long-term care facilities, micronutrient supplementation may be underutilized secondary to polypharmacy concerns and drug–nutrient reactions.

When caring for frail elders in the community (nursing homes, assisted living facilities, or group homes), oral nutritional supplements may not be the best first approach. *Fortified foods*, or those foods chosen based on their enhancement during processing (with vitamins and minerals) or enhanced with butter or cream during preparation, were found to be the best first approach to improving food intake and health of these elders (Bourdel-Marchasson, 2010).

Vitamin D and calcium are commonly deficient in older adults. Supplementation is a simple and direct method for delivering these micronutrients that do not depend on the elder's appetite. However, only those older adults with an actual deficiency determined via a laboratory blood test should be treated with an oral supplement.

Implications

A lack of food or nutrients can affect nearly every organ system (Hajjar et al., 2004). Malnutrition can lead to delayed wound healing, the development of pressure ulcers, increased susceptibility to infections, functional decline, cognitive decline and depression, delayed recovery from acute illness (Hajjar et al., 2004), difficulty in swallowing, and dehydration (Morley, 2011b). Poor nutritional status also can result in decreased lean body mass; lessened muscular strength and aerobic capacity, which can lead to chronic fatigue; and alterations in gait and balance, increasing the risk of falls and fractures. For many older adults, this sequence of events leads to a deterioration in overall quality of life, causing dependence on others (Morley, 2011b).

CLINICAL TIP

Body mass index (BMI) is a useful measurement for assessing nutritional status and can be calculated using the following formula: $BMI = Weight (kg)/height (m)^2$

Data from Hajjar, R. R., Kamel, H. K., & Denson, K. (2004). Malnutrition in aging. *The Internet Journal of Geriatrics and Gerontology, 1*(1), 1–16.

Factors Influencing Nutritional Risk

Many factors contribute to malnutrition and weight loss in elders. These factors can be classified into three major groups: social, psychological, and biological (see **Table 17-5**).

Social Causes

The most significant social cause of malnutrition and weight loss in older adults is poverty. Affording expensive medications is a common problem for older adults with limited incomes. If insurance does not cover all or most of this expense, older adults are faced with going without medications or reducing their food budgets to afford the prescribed medication. Social isolation, loneliness, and grieving due to the death of family or friends have long been known as important risk factors for malnutrition and weight loss (McIntosh, Shifflet, & Picou, 1989). In a study by Keller, Beck, and Namasivayam (2015), socialization with others resulted in increased food intake at meals. Other social risk factors or causes of malnutrition and weight loss in older adults are their inability to shop, cook, or feed themselves (Keller et al., 2015).

Psychological Causes

Depression is one of the most common treatable causes of weight loss in older adults. Elders suffering from depression can have many symptoms that can lead to weight loss, including weakness (61%), stomach pains (37%), nausea (27%), anorexia (22%), and diarrhea (20%) (Morley, 2011b). Successful treatment of depression has been shown to reverse weight loss in nursing home residents (Morley, 2011b).

Dementia is commonly associated with weight loss. Older adults with dementia often forget or refuse to eat, and feeding can become a time-consuming process. Elders with late-stage dementia may wander excessively, may express

---

TABLE 17-5   Factors Influencing Nutritional Risk in Older Adults

a. Social
  - Isolation
  - Loneliness
  - Poverty
  - Dependency

b. Psychological
  - Depression
  - Anxiety
  - Dementia
  - Bereavement

c. Biological
  - Dentition
  - Loss of taste or smell
  - Gastrointestinal disorders
  - Muscle weakness
  - Dry mouth
  - Olfaction
  - Renal disease
  - Physical disability
  - Infections
  - Chronic obstructive pulmonary disease (COPD)
  - Drug interactions

Reproduced from Loreck, E., Chimakurthi, R., & Steinle, N. I. (2012). Nutritional assessment of the geriatric patient: A comprehensive approach toward evaluating and managing nutrition. *Clinical Geriatrics*, *20*(4), 20–26. www.Consultant360.com.

TABLE 17-6   Medications Associated with Weight Loss

- Digoxin
- Theophylline
- Metformin
- Antibiotics
- Nonsteroidal anti-inflammatory drugs
- Psychotropic drugs: Prozac (fluoxetine), lithium, phenothiazines

Data from Hickson, M. (2006). Malnutrition and ageing. *Postgraduate Medical Journal, 82*, 2–8.

---

paranoid ideation, and may be prescribed psychotropic medications that cause anorexia. Some demented older adults develop apraxia of swallowing and must be reminded to swallow after each mouthful of food (Gillen, 2016).

Biological Causes

Numerous medical conditions can cause malnutrition and weight loss by one or more of the following mechanisms: hypermetabolism, anorexia, swallowing difficulty, or malabsorption (Hajjar et al., 2004). Diseases such as stroke, tremors, or arthritis can affect an older adult's ability to eat or prepare food, thereby leading to decreased food intake. Swallowing disorders (dysphagia) are associated with increased risk of aspiration and food aversion, which may be conscious or subconscious (Gillen, 2016). Infections are another cause of weight loss in older adults, especially those who live in nursing homes. Infections may result in confusion, anorexia, and negative nitrogen balance (Hajjar et al., 2004). Another physical cause is chronic obstructive pulmonary disease (COPD). Older adults with COPD experience a decrease in arterial oxygen tension when eating due to the thermic energy of eating and the brief interruption of respiration with swallowing. They frequently are unable to eat their meals because of dyspnea. Further, their condition is aggravated by hyperventilation and use of accessory muscles, leading to increased metabolism. Hyperthyroidism and Parkinson's disease also cause hypermetabolism, which can lead to weight loss (Hajjar et al., 2004). Finally, several medications are associated with poor appetite and weight loss (see **Table 17-6**).

Assessment

Nutritional risk screening should be integrated into the comprehensive geriatric assessment (Bauer, Kaiser, & Sieber, 2010). Many screening methods are available, including specific clinical screening tools, *anthropometric* and body composition measurements, laboratory tests, a review of clinical data, and examination of an individual's diet history. Each method has its pros and cons, so a combination of assessments may be necessary to provide a more accurate picture of a patient's nutritional status (Loreck et al., 2012).

Clinical Screening Tools

Mini Nutritional Assessment (MNA): The MNA is a simple and reliable tool for assessing nutrition status in older adults. Originally developed by Vellas and Guigoz in 1989 (Guigoz, Vellas, & Garry, 1996), it has become the tool of choice for many healthcare providers. The original MNA is an 18-item questionnaire that takes 10 to 15 minutes to administer. A shortened version (MNA-SF) includes 6 items and takes less than 5 minutes to administer. The questions examine food intake, weight loss, mobility, psychological stress, acute disease incidence, neuropsychological problems, and BMI or calf circumference (Loreck et al., 2012). Calf circumference was provided as an option because BMI can be difficult to assess in older adults. On the MNA-SF, a score between 8 and 11 indicates an increased risk of malnutrition, and a score less than 7 reflects malnutrition (Loreck et al., 2012).

   Instant Nutritional Assessment (INA): The INA is a simple and practical nutrition screening tool that combines three easily obtainable elements: lymphocyte count, albumin, and weight change (referred to as "LAW") (Hajjar et al., 2004). Each item, if used alone, has limited predictive value, but when combined has a high degree of accuracy (Hajjar et al., 2004).

Nutritional Screening Initiative and the DETERMINE Checklist: The DETERMINE checklist was developed by the Nutritional Screening Initiative (NSI), an interdisciplinary multiorganizational effort aimed at introducing nutritional screening into the healthcare system (Detsky et al., 1984). The checklist is self-administered and includes 10 questions about risk factors for malnutrition. Total scores of 6 or higher (highest score is 21) indicate a need for further assessment. The checklist is a screening tool, not a reliable diagnostic tool, but has had some success in promoting public awareness of malnutrition.

Malnutrition Risk Scale (SCALES): The malnutrition risk scale was developed by Morley (1989) as an outpatient screening tool. The acronym SCALES represents the six elements in the tool (**S**adness, **C**holesterol, **A**lbumin, **L**oss of weight, **E**ating problems, and **S**hopping) that cover common known-risk factors for malnutrition, including depression, which has emerged as a major risk factor for malnutrition and mortality. A score of three or higher suggests high risk for malnutrition.

Malnutrition Screening Tool (MST): A quick, valid, and reliable two-item tool developed by Ferguson, Capra, Bauer, & Banks (1999), this free tool can be used by any health professional and does not require any anthropometrical or biochemical measurements. The tool simply asks about unplanned weight loss and poor appetite. If the patient reports weight loss or poor appetite, he or she may be at risk for malnutrition.

Food Expectations—Long Term Care (FoodEx-LTC): FoodEx-LTC is a 28-item, 4-domain instrument developed to measure nursing home-resident food satisfaction (Crogan, Evans, & Velasquez, 2004; Crogan & Evans, 2006). The instrument can be self-administered or administered by an evaluator who reads each item and marks the resident's response. During development and pilot testing of the FoodEx-LTC, internal consistency reliability (Cronbach's alpha) estimates ranged from 0.65, "Exercising Choice" to 0.82, "Providing Food Service." All alpha coefficients were above the 0.50 criterion for a new scale and 3 of 4 scales met the more stringent criterion of 0.70. Two-week test–retest coefficients ranged from 0.79 for "Enjoying Food and Food Service" to 0.88 or "Providing Food Service" and "Exercising Choice."

Other tools are described in **Table 17-7**.

Laboratory Assessments

Laboratory assessment is another component of a comprehensive nutritional assessment (see **Table 17-8**). Even though serum proteins such as *albumin* and *prealbumin* are widely used to assess nutritional status, their levels are affected by non-nutritional factors. Proteins are influenced by cellular processes, including inflammation and renal disease, so their use is limited in definitively establishing nutritional status in older adults (Morley, 2011a). Total lymphocyte count (TLC) also has been used as a marker of nutritional status, but there is limited evidence that low TLC levels reflect malnutrition in older adults (Kuzuya, Kanda, Koike, Suzuki, & Iguchi, 2005). In cross-sectional studies, low total cholesterol (<150 mg/dL) is often seen among individuals with poor nutritional status (Loreck et al., 2012). Two additional studies evaluated the use of *leptin* as a clinical predictor of nutritional status in older adults (Amirkalali et al., 2010; Bouillanne et al., 2007). Leptin levels decrease as malnutrition becomes more pronounced in older adults.

Clinical Data Review

Clinical data specific to nutritional assessment in older adults includes a review of current medications, evaluation of oral and swallowing problems, review of gastrointestinal problems, and a review of psychiatric and neurologic disorders (Bauer et al., 2010).

Diet History Review

The final component of the nutritional assessment is an evaluation of the older adult's diet history. Numerous strategies could be used to complete a *diet history review*. For example, the older adult could be asked to keep a food diary, the healthcare provider could conduct a 24-hour recall, or a questionnaire could be administered to determine the frequency with which foods from various food groups are consumed (Thompson & Subar, 2012).

TABLE 17-7   Other Tools: Anthropometric and Body Composition Measures

Serial Body Weight

Serial body weight is a useful way to identify a change in overall nutritional status. However, body weight can be unreliable if the patient also suffers from congestive heart failure, hepatic disorders, or renal disease (Loreck et al., 2012).

Body Mass Index

Body mass index (BMI) is used to determine body fat levels, with a BMI less than 18.5 kg/m^2 indicating underweight and in increased risk of mortality (Loreck et al., 2012). A BMI of 18.5 to 24.9 kg/m^2 indicates normal weight, 25 to 29.9 kg/m^2 overweight, and greater than 30 kg/m^2 obesity (Loreck et al., 2012). In older adults, BMI may be problematic, in that an inaccurate height may be obtained and BMI does not accurately predict body composition. In this population, inaccurate heights may be due to vertebral collapse, change in posture, or loss of muscle tone. In these cases, height can be estimated by measuring knee height or arm span (Hickson & Frost, 2003).

Triceps Skin Fold

Triceps skin fold (TSF) is reflective of fat stores. It is measured using a skin fold caliper by measuring the mid-point between the acromion process and the olecranon process of the upper arm. The clinician palpates the site to distinguish fat from muscle, grasps a fold of skin approximately 1 cm above the mid-point, and performs three readings. The average of these readings is used. Nutritional depletion is defined as a skin fold measure of less than 11.3 mm in women and less than 4.3 mm in men (Burr & Phillips, 1984).

Mid-Upper Arm Circumference.

Mid-upper arm circumference (MUAC) is a predictor of mortality in older adults living in long-term care facilities (Allard et al., 2004). To determine MUAC, the mid-point of the upper arm is measured with a tape measure placed snugly against the skin. Once the TSF and MUAC are measured, a mid-arm muscle circumference (MAMC), an indicator of lean mass, can be calculated using the following equation MAMC = AC – (TSF × 0.314) (Burr & Phillips, 1984). Older adults are considered nutritionally depleted when their measure falls below the tenth percentile, which are less than 17.2 cm in women and less than 19.6 cm in men.

Bioelectrical Impedance Analysis

Bioelectrical impedance analysis (BIA) is an inexpensive, quick, and noninvasive tool used in clinical practice to estimate fat mass versus lean mass. BIA-enabled devices send a low current through the body to determine the electrical impedance of body tissues, which provides an estimate of total body water. Total body water measures are then plugged into an equation that can determine body composition (Loreck et al., 2012). The ideal percentage body fat for older adults is 27.6% to 34.4% for women and 20.3% to 26.7% for men. Accuracy of BIA can be affected by patient obesity; body position, hydration status, recent consumption of food; ambient air and skin temperature; recent physical activity, and conductance of the examining table (Loreck et al., 2012).

TABLE 17-8   Laboratory Studies Associated with Poor Nutrition

Serum albumin < 3.5 g/dL
Serum prealbumin < 11 mg/dL
Cholesterol < 150 mg/dL
Leptin < 4.0 mcg/L in men, < 6.48 mcg/L in women

Data from Loreck, E., Chimakurthi, R., & Steinle, N. I. (2012). Nutritional assessment of the geriatric patient: A comprehensive approach toward evaluating and managing nutrition. *Clinical Geriatrics, 20*(4), 20–26.

Evidence-Based Strategies to Improve Nutrition

Previous accepted strategies to improve nutrition in older adults included educating them on diet and providing various supplements, including vitamins, minerals, and meal replacements. However, more recent research findings do not support all of these past strategies. For example, in a population-based study of 38,772 older women from the Iowa Women's Health Study (Mursu, Robien, Harnack, Park, & Jacobs, 2011), vitamin and mineral supplementation was associated with increased mortality risk. This association was strongest with supplemental iron. In contrast to these findings, calcium was associated with decreased risk. In short, dietary supplementation should not be routinely recommended, but rather used only to treat symptomatic nutrient deficiency disease.

The consumption of food is always preferable to meal replacements. If this is not possible or realistic, between-meal snacks or liquid caloric supplements can increase energy intake (Morley, 2011b). Maintenance of good oral hygiene, sensible treatment of dysphagia and depression, and decreasing or limiting the number of prescribed and over-the-counter medications also play an important role in enhancing food intake (Morley, 2011b).

CLINICAL TIP

Antioxidant use could be harmful to older women.

Data from Crogan, N. L. (2012). Various vitamin and mineral supplements are observed to increase mortality risk in older women, with the exception of calcium, which decreases risk [Peer commentary on the paper Dietary supplements and mortality rate in older women: The Iowa Women's Health Study, by Mursu et al., (2011). *Archives of Internal Medicine, 171*(18), 1625–1633] *Evidence-Based Nursing*, Mar 22. Advance online publication.

An illustrative tool that could be used to demonstrate what constitutes healthy eating and portion size is the U.S. Department of Agriculture's (USDA's) MyPlate method, which divides a plate into quarters, with one fourth appropriated to grains, one fourth to protein, and the remaining half to fruits and vegetables (see **Figure 17-3**). Older adults should be advised that their nutrient intake might be inadequate if they are not eating close to this food composition.

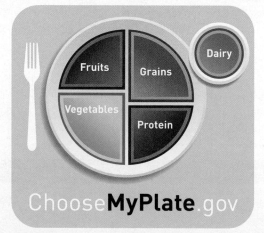

Figure 17-3 USDA's My-Plate Method.

Nutrients found to be essential to older adults are protein and vitamin D. Deficiencies in these nutrients are associated with higher risk of falls in this population (Zoltick et al., 2011). Zoltick et al. examined food intake in 807 men and women, aged 67 to 93 years, from the Framingham Study. Higher protein intake was associated with decreased odds of falling. In those with a weight loss greater than 5% from baseline, higher protein intake significantly decreased fall incidents. The researchers concluded that protein intake might be a modifiable factor for fall prevention in older adults.

A systematic review and meta-analysis of older adults investigated the effectiveness of vitamin D in the prevention of falls and found that vitamin D therapy (200 to 1,000) resulted in 14% fewer falls (Kalyani et al., 2010).

Older adults who reside in nursing homes are especially at risk for malnutrition. Improving the dining experience by offering food choice, select menus, and buffet dining, as well as ice cream parlors, have been successful in increasing food intake and decreasing weight loss (Calkins, & Brush, 2016; Crogan, Dupler, Short, & Heaton, 2013; Heaton, Crogan, Short, & Dupler, 2011).

Finally, it may be necessary to refer the older adult to other healthcare providers after completing a nutritional assessment. A speech–language pathologist can be invaluable in assessing and treating dysphagia and swallowing problems. A registered dietitian can be of value in the assessment and treatment of reversible nutritional issues, such as by determining the adequacy of intake, developing a custom meal plan, making recommendations for increasing oral intake, or developing a plan to initiate nutrition support. A social worker can assist elders and families to obtain access to home-delivered meals, congregate feeding programs, food stamps, and other assistance programs. A referral to a dentist for oral health issues or to a geriatric psychiatrist for mental health issues also may be warranted. An occupational or physical therapist consultation may be of value for older adults with physical limitations. A pharmacist can provide assistance with nutrition-related medication management issues (Loreck et al., 2012). Nutritional assessment and the selection of specific interventions are not just the responsibility of the nurse but, rather, the responsibility of the interdisciplinary team.

The 2015–2020 Dietary Guidelines for Americans

The U.S. Department Health and Human Services (DHHS) and the U.S. Department of Agriculture (USDA) compile recommendations and publish updated dietary guidelines every 5 years. The guidelines published January 11, 2016 (Dietary Guidelines, 2016), fit into the following broad categories:

> Maintain a healthy diet throughout your life
> Eat a variety of nutrient-dense foods, and manage portion sizes
> Limit caloric intake from added sugars and saturated fats, and reduce intake of sodium
> Shift current food and drink choices to healthier alternatives
> Support others in healthy eating

The guidelines pertain to older adults, wherever they reside. An older adult's diet should consist of a variety of vegetables, fruits (preferable whole fruits), grains (half of which should be whole grains), fat-free or low-fat dairy, protein from a variety of sources, and a limited amount of oils. The 2015 guidelines also limit the amount of caffeinated drinks to three to five 8-ounce cups of coffee per day. No other caffeinated drinks are recommended. This may be challenging for older adults who drink tea or soda.

Summary

Malnutrition in older adults is a multifaceted and complex issue. No single tool or clinical marker accurately predicts nutritional status. However, integrating a validated nutrition screening tool with anthropometric and laboratory data, the geriatric nurse or provider can get a more accurate picture of the older adult's nutrition status. When reversible causes of malnutrition are identified, evidence-based approaches should be undertaken, which may require referral to other disciplines.

Clinical Reasoning Exercises

1. Mrs. Jones, an 80-year-old widow living alone in the community, was recently diagnosed with congestive heart failure. Concurrent health problems include osteoarthritis and osteoporosis. During the initial home health visit, the nurse notices that Mrs. Jones is very thin. Upon questioning, Mrs. Jones reports she rarely gets out to buy food. She says she is not a big eater and has neighbors who bring her food. Should this be considered a problem? What additional information is needed for decision making? What evidence can the nurse provide to Mrs. Jones to support a need for further evaluation and treatment of this problem?

2. A 60-year-old African American woman has been admitted to the rehabilitation hospital for treatment following a stroke. Her past medical history includes congestive heart failure, type 2 diabetes mellitus, and hypertension. While obtaining her history, you note that she has difficulty speaking. You suspect she may also suffer from dysphagia. What would be your next step? What referrals may be needed? What nursing interventions may help improve her ability to swallow?

Personal Reflections

1. Have someone feed you an entire meal. What was your interaction like (who talked, what were the topics of conversation)? How did it feel to be fed? Did your pattern for eating or the amount of food and fluid consumed differ from normal?

2. Have you ever cared for a person with dysphagia? Malnutrition? After reading this chapter, reflect on that experience and think about some strategies that may have helped to improve care for that person.

References

Allard, J. P., Aghdassi, E., McArthur, M., McGeer, A., Simor, A., Abdolell, M., . . . & Liu, B. (2004). Nutrition risk factors for the survival in elderly living in Canadian long-term care facilities. *Journal of the American Geriatric Society, 52*(1), 59–65.

American Dietetic Association. (2003). National Dysphagia Diet. *Journal of the American Dietetic Association, 103*(3), 748–765.

Amirkalali, B., Sharifi, F., Fakhrzadeh, H., Mirarefein, M., Ghaderpanahi, M., Badamchizadeh, Z., & Larijani, B. (2010). Low serum leptin serves as a biomarker of malnutrition in elderly patients. *Nutrition Research, 30*(5), 314–319.

Bauer, J. M., Kaiser, M. J., & Sieber, C. C. (2010). Evaluation of nutritional status in older persons: Nutritional screening and assessment. *Current Opinion on Clinical Nutrition Metabolic Care, 13*(1), 8–13.

Bibi, S., Iqbal, A., Ayaz, S., Khan, A., & Matee, S. (2015). The impact of oropharyngeal dysphagia on quality of life in individuals with age over 50 years. *Rawal Medical Journal, 40*(1), 37–40.

Bouillanne, O., Golmard, J. L., Coussieu, C., Noel, M., Durand, D., Piette, F., & Nivet-Antione, V. (2007). Leptin a new biological marker for evaluating malnutrition in elderly patients. *European Journal of Clinical Nutrition, 61*(5), 647–654.

Bourdel-Marchasson, I. (2010). How to improve nutritional support in geriatric institutions. *Journal of the American Medical Directors Association, 11*(1), 13–20.

Burr, M. L., & Phillips, K. M. (1984). Anthropometric norms in the elderly. *British Journal of Nutrition, 51*(2), 165–169.

Calkins, M., & Brush, J. (2016). Honoring individual choice in long-term residential communities when it involves risk: A person-centered approach. *Journal of Gerontological Nursing, 42*(8), 12–17.

Castellanos, V. H., Litchford, M. D., & Campbell, W. W. (2006). Modular protein supplements and their application to long-term care. *Nutrition in Clinical Practice, 21*(5), 485–504.

Coulston, A. M., Mandelbaum, D., & Reaven, G. M. (1990). Dietary management of nursing home residents with non-insulin-dependent diabetes mellitus. *American Journal of Clinical Nutrition, 51*(1), 67–71.

Crogan, N. L. (2012). Various vitamin and mineral supplements are observed to increase mortality risk in older women, with the exception of calcium, which decreases risk (Peer commentary on the paper Dietary supplements and mortality rate in older women: The Iowa Women's Health Study, by Mursu, J., Roblen, K., Harnack, L.J., Park, K., & Jacobs, D. R. Jr. (2011). *Archives of Internal Medicine, 171*[18], 1625–1633). *Evidence-Based Nursing,* March 22 [Epub ahead of print].

Crogan, N., & Evans, B. (2006). The shortened food expectations, long-term care questionnaire: Assessing nursing home residents' satisfaction with food and food service. *Journal of Gerontological Nursing 32*(11), 50–59.

Crogan, N., Evans, B., & Velasquez, D. (2004). Measuring nursing home resident satisfaction with food and food service: Initial testing of the FoodEx-LTC. *Journals of Gerontology: Medical Sciences, 59A*(4), 370–377.

Crogan, N. L., Dupler, A. E., Short, R., & Heaton, G. (2013). Food choice can improve nursing home resident meal service and nutritional status. *Journal of Gerontological Nursing, 39*(5), 38–45.

Cruz-Jentoft, A. J., Baeyens, J. P., Bauer, J. M., Boirie, Y., Caderholm, T., Landi, F., European Working Group on Sarcopenia in Older People. (2010). Sarcopenia: European consensus on definition and diagnosis—Report of the European Working Group on Sarcopenia. *Age and Ageing, 39*(4), 412–423.

Detsky, A. S., Baker, J. P., Mandelson, R. A., Wolman, S. L., Wesson, D. E., & Jeejeebhoy, K. N. (1984). Evaluating the accuracy of nutritional assessment techniques applied to hospitalized patients: Methodology and comparisons. *Journal of Parenteral and Enteral Nutrition, 8*(2), 153–159.

Dietary Guidelines. (2016). Office of Disease Prevention and Health Promotion website. Retrieved from http://health.gov/dietaryguidelines/

Edwards, S. J., & Metheny, N. A. (2000). Measurement of gastric residual volume: State of the science. *MEDSURG Nursing, 9*(3), 125–128.

Ekberg, O., Hamby, S., Woisard, V., Wuttge-Hanning, A., & Ortega, P. (2004). Social and psychological burden of dysphagia: Its impact on diagnosis and treatment. *Dysphagia, 17*(2), 139–146.

Ferguson, M., Capra, S., Bauer, J., & Banks, M. (1999). Development of a valid and reliable malnutrition screening tool for adult acute hospital patients. *Nutrition, 15*(6), 458–464.

Gillen, G. (2016). *Stroke rehabilitation: A function-based approach* (4th ed.). Philadelphia, PA: Mosby.

Guigoz, Y., Vellas, B., & Garry, P. J. (1996). Assessing the elderly: The mini nutritional assessment as part of the geriatric evaluation. *Nutrition Review, 54*(1 Pt 2),S59–S65.

Hajjar, R. R., Kamel, H. K., & Denson, K. (2004). Malnutrition in aging. *The Internet Journal of Geriatrics and Gerontology, 1*(1), 1–16.

Hassan, H. E., & Aboloyoun, A. I. (2014). The value of bedside tests in dysphagia evaluation. *Egyptian Journal of Ear, Nose, Throat and Allied Sciences, 15*(3), 197–203.

Heaton, G., Crogan, N., Short, R., & Dupler, A. (2011). Resident food choice: Evolution of the facility menu using Rate the Food. *Dietary Manager, 20,* 30–34.

Herskowitz, J. (2012). *Do you have a swallowing problem?* Retrieved from http://EzineArticles.com/?expert=Joel _Herskowitz

Hickson, M. (2006). Malnutrition and ageing. *Postgraduate Medical Journal, 82*(963), 2–8.

Hickson, M., & Frost, G. (2003). A comparison of three methods for estimating height in the acutely ill elderly population. *Journal of Human Nutrition & Dietetics, 16*(1), 13–20.

Johnson, V., & Chalmers, J. (2002). *Oral hygiene care for functionally dependent and cognitively impaired older adults: Research dissemination core.* Iowa City, IA: University of Iowa.

Kaiser, M. J., Bauer, J. M., Ramsch, C., & MNA-International Group. (2009). Validation of the Mini Nutritional Assessment short-form (MNA-SF): A practical tool for identification of nutritional status. *Journal of Nutrition, Health & Aging, 13*(9), 782–788.

Kalyani, R. R., Stein, B., Valiyil, R., Manno, R., Maynard, J. W., & Crews, D. C. (2010). Vitamin D treatment for the prevention of falls in older adults: Systematic review and meta-analysis. *Journal of the American Geriatric Society, 58*(7), 1299–1310.

Keller, H., Beck, A., & Namasivayam, A. (2015). Improving food and fluid intake for older adults living in long-term care: A research agenda. *Journal of the American Medical Directors Association, 16*(2), 93–100.

Kuzuya, M., Kanda, S., Koike, T., Suzuki, Y., & Iguchi, A. (2005). Lack of correlation between total lymphocyte count and nutritional status in the elderly. *Clinical Nutrition, 24*(3), 427–432.

Liantonio, J., Salzman, B., & Snyderman, D. (2014). Preventing aspiration pneumonia by addressing three key risk factors: Dysphagia, poor oral hygiene, and medication use. *Annals of Long-Term Care: Clinical Care and Aging, 22*(10), 42–48.

Logemann, J. A., Rademaker, A., Pauloski, B. R., Kelly, A., & Stangl-McBreen, C. (2009). A randomized study comparing the Shaker Exercise with traditional therapy: A preliminary study. *Dysphagia, 24*(4), 403–11.

Logemann, J. A., Gesler, G., Robbins, J., Lindblad, A. S., Brandt, D., Hind, J. A., Gardener, P. J. (2008). A randomized study of three interventions for aspiration of thin liquids in patients with dementia or Parkinson's disease. *Journal of Speech, Language, and Hearing Research, 5*(1), 173–183.

Loreck, E., Chimakurthi, R., & Steinle, N. I. (2012). Nutritional assessment of the geriatric patient: A comprehensive approach toward evaluating and managing nutrition. *Clinical Geriatrics, 20*(4), 20–26.

Mayo Clinic, (2014). Dysphagia. Retrieved from http://www.mayoclinic.org/diseases-conditions/dysphagia/basics/causes/con-20033444

McClave, S. A., Sexton, L. A., Spain, D. A., Adams, J. L., Owens, N. A., Sullins, M. B., Blandford, B. F. & Snider, H. L. (1999). Enteral tube feeding in the intensive care unit: Factors impeding adequate delivery. *Critical Care Medicine, 27*(7), 1252–1256.

McIntosh, W. A., Shifflet, P. A., & Picou, J. S. (1989). "Social" support stressful events, strain, dietary intake, and the elderly. *Medical Care, 27*(2), 140–153.

Metheny, N. A., Schallom, M. E., & Edwards, S. J. (2004). Effect of gastrointestinal motility and feeding tube site on aspiration risk in critically ill patients: A review. *Heart and Lung, 33*(3), 131–145.

Methany, N. A., Schallom, L., Oliver, D. A., & Clouse, R. E. (2008). Gastric residual volume and aspiration in critically ill patients receiving gastric feedings. *American Journal of Critical Care, 17*(6), 512–519.

Morley, J. E. (1989). Death by starvation: A modern American problem? *Journal of the American Geriatric Society, 37*(2), 184–185.

Morley, J. E. (2011a). Assessment of malnutrition in older persons: A focus on the Mini Nutritional Assessment. *Journal of Nutrition, Health, and Aging, 15*(2), 87–90.

Morley, J. E. (2011b). Undernutrition: A major problem in nursing homes. *Journal of the American Medical Directors Association, 12*(4), 243–246.

Morley, J. E. (2013). Pathophysiology of the anorexia of aging. *Current Opinion in Clinical Nutrition and Metabolic Care, 16*(1), 27–32.

Mursu, J., Robien, K., Harnack, L. J., Park, K., & Jacobs, D. R. (2011). Dietary supplements and mortality rate in older women. *Archives of Internal Medicine, 171*(18), 1625–1633.

National Institute on Deafness and Other Communication Disorders. (2010). *Dysphagia.* NIH Pub. No. 13-4307.

Omran, M. L., & Morely, J. E. (2000). Assessment of protein energy malnutrition in older persons, Part 1: History, examination, body composition, and screening tools. *Nutrition, 16*(1), 50–63.

Oropharyngeal dysphagia. (2009). *Mosby's Medical Dictionary* (8th ed.). Retrieved from http://medical-dictionary .thefreedictionary.com/oropharyngeal+dysphagia

Paik, N. (2012, March 26). Dysphagia. Retrieved from http://emedicine.medscape.com/article/324096-overview

Poorjavad, M., & Jalaie, S. (2014). Systematic review on highly qualified screening tests for swallowing disorders following stroke: Validity and reliability issues. *Journal of Research and Medical Sciences, 19*(8), 776–785.

Smith, H. A., & Connolly, M. J. (2003). Evaluation and treatment of dysphagia following stroke. *Topics in Geriatric Rehabilitation, 19*(1), 43–59.

Stroke Research Unit, Queen Elizabeth Hospital, Gateshead. (2001). Collaborative Dysphagia Audit (CODA) Study. Retrieved from http://www.nursingtimes.net/nursing-practice-clinical-research/an-interdisciplinary -approach-to-the-management-of-dysphagia/199842.article

Sura, L., Madhavan, A., Carnaby, G., & Crary, M. A. (2012). Dysphagia in the elderly: Management and nutritional considerations. *Clinical Interventions in Aging, 7,* 287–298.

Swigert, N. (2016). *Use of the Shaker technique for dysphagia treatment.* Retrieved from http://www.speechpathology .com/ask-the-experts/use-shaker-technique-for-dysphagia-742

Tariz, S. H., Karcic, E., Thomas, D. R., Thomson, K., Philpot, C., Chapel, D. L., & Morley, J. E. (2001). The use of a no-concentrated-sweets diet in the management of type 2 diabetes in nursing homes. *Journal of the American Dietetic Association, 101*(12), 1463–1466.

Thompson, F. E., & Subar, A. F. (2012). *Dietary assessment methodology.* Retrieved from https://epi.grants.cancer .gov/diet/adi/thompson_subar_dietary_assessment_methodology.pdf

Udayakumar, N., & Eubanks, S. (2015). Approach to patients with esophageal dysphagia. In Oleynikov, D. (Ed.), *Surgical approaches to esophageal disease* (pp. 483–489). Philadelphia, PA: Elsevier.

Wirth, R., Voss, C., Smoliner, C., Sieber, C. C., Bauer, J. M., & Volkert, D. (2012). Complications and mortality after percutaneous endoscopic gastrostomy in geriatrics: A prospective multicenter observational trial. *Journal of the American Medical Directors Association, 13*(3), 228–233.

Zoltick, E. S., Sahni, S., McLean, R. R., Quach, L., Casey, V. A., & Hannan, M. T. (2011). Dietary protein intake and subsequent falls in older men and women: The Framingham study. *Journal of Nutrition, Health, and Aging, 15*(2), 147–152.

For a full suite of assignments and additional learning activities, see the access code at the front of your book.

CHAPTER 18

Pressure Ulcers

Sandra Higelin

(Competencies 7, 17)

LEARNING OBJECTIVES

At the end of this chapter, the reader will be able to:

> Describe the etiology of pressure ulcers.
> Discuss the implications and relevance of pressure ulcers.
> Classify pressure ulcers using the staging system.
> Identify key components of pressure ulcer prevention and management.
> List the components of assessment of skin and wounds.
> Identify interventions for pressure ulcer prevention and management.
> Describe critical factors in wound management.
> Develop a care plan for potential impaired skin integrity.

KEY TERMS

Avoidable/unavoidable pressure ulcers
   Braden Scale for Pressure Ulcer Risk
   Assessment
Causative factors
Facility acquired pressure ulcers
National Pressure Ulcer Advisory Panel

Pressure injury
Pressure redistribution
Pressure ulcers
Pressure ulcer management
Pressure ulcer risk assessment
Pressure ulcer staging system

Pressure ulcers are now recognized as a significant healthcare threat to patients with restricted mobility or chronic disease and to older patients. A pressure ulcer can cause serious complication, pain, decreased quality of life, increased morbidity and mortality, a significant increase in caregiver time, and an increase in the spending of healthcare dollars. Patients with pressure ulcers have a higher rate of morbidity and mortality. Research indicates that approximately 60,000 patients die each year from complications of pressure ulcers; the most common major complication is infection, which can result in sepsis (Salcido, 2012). It has recently been reported that pressure ulcers affect 2.5 million patients per year. The pressure ulcer cost is 9.1 to 11.6 billion per year in the United States according to the Agency for Healthcare Research and Quality (AHRQ, 2014). Pressure ulcer prevention and management is important to hospitals, skilled nursing facilities, community-based healthcare services, and other community settings. Over the past 20 years there has been a burgeoning of knowledge related to pressure ulcer prevention and management, as well as a significant increase in the types of wound care products and treatment modalities that can be used in the management of pressure ulcers.

CLINICAL TIP

Pressure ulcers result in pain, serious infections, death, and in increased healthcare utilization and costs.

Etiology

"A pressure ulcer is localized injury to the skin and/or underlying tissue usually over a bony prominence, as a result of pressure, or pressure in combination with shear. A number of contributing or confounding factors are also associated with pressure ulcers; the significance of these factors is yet to be elucidated" (National Pressure Ulcer Advisory Panel [NPUAP] & European Pressure Ulcer Advisory Panel [EPUAP], 2014, p. 12). In 2016, the NPUAP proposed that the term *pressure injury* replace the term "pressure ulcer" to better capture injuries with both intact and nonintact skin.

The most common sites for pressure ulcers to occur are the coccyx, sacrum, ischial tuberosity, trochanter, and the calcaneus. These sites have less soft tissue present between the bone and the skin. There are also device-related pressure ulcers that develop as a result of nasal cannulas, urinary catheters, casts, orthotics, and other types of medical equipment or tubing.

The major *causative factor* in pressure ulcer formation is pressure. Several factors are involved to determine what pathological effect pressure has on soft tissue to create ischemia, which results in tissue anoxia and cell death. Depending on the physical health of the individual, pressure ulcers can develop within 1 to 24 hours of the insult and may take up to 7 days to manifest. Factors that influence pressure ulcer development are (1) intensity of pressure, (2) duration of pressure, and (3) tissue tolerance, which is the ability of skin and its supporting structures to endure pressure (Bryant & Nix, 2012).

Shear and friction are also extrinsic causative factors that are involved in pressure ulcer development. Shear is caused by a force, working parallel to the skin that is exerted when gravity is pushing down on the body and there is resistance between the patient and a surface such as a chair or bed. As a result of this resistance, the skin is held in place while the weight of the skeleton pulls the body downward; thus, injury to deeper tissues overlying bony prominences occurs. Friction is resistance to motion in a parallel direction and acts in concert with shear. If friction is the only factor present, the injury to the skin is confined to the epidermis and upper dermal layers of the skin (Bryant & Nix, 2012).

Moisture, usually caused by incontinence, is another extrinsic factor for pressure ulcer development. Moisture alters the resiliency of the epidermis to external forces by weakening the lipid layer of the stratum corneum and collagen. In the presence of urinary or fecal incontinence, the skin's pH is alkalinized and the normal skin flora are altered (Bryant & Nix, 2012).

Intrinsic factors that influence the development of pressure ulcers include advanced age, nutritional deficiency, smoking, medications, and other comorbidities such as chronic obstructive lung disease, cardiac disease, musculoskeletal disorders, renal disease, diabetes, and cognitive impairment. The normal skin changes associated with aging, combined with the effects of illness, contribute to the higher risk of ulcer development in the older population. Skin becomes thinner, has less collagen and moisture, and can lose the ability to protect itself against invading organisms. Blood flow to the dermis is reduced, resulting in fewer nutrients reaching the skin and less waste removal. It is also more susceptible to friction and shear injuries (Bryant & Nix, 2012).

Implications, Prevalence, and Incidents of Pressure Ulcers

Pressure ulcer prevalence is defined as the number of patients with at least one pressure ulcer who exists in a given patient population at a given point in time. Incidence is defined as the number of patients who were initially ulcer free and developed a pressure ulcer within a particular time period in a defined population.

Pressure Ulcer Prevalence in Healthcare Settings

When pressure ulcer care is involved, hospitalizations are longer and more expensive. Acute hospital admissions with a pressure ulcer diagnosis are cited as 0 to 46%. incidence rates are cited as 0 to 12%. When a pressure ulcer is diagnosed, the average hospital stay extends from 5 days to 14 days, with additional costs ranging from $500 to $70,000 per individual pressure ulcer, depending on the medical condition of the patient (NPUAP & EPUAP, 2014). Pressure ulcer prevalence rate in long-term care settings are cited as 4.1% to 32% with incidents rates cited as 1.9% to 59%. In adult patients. 56.5% of patients with pressure ulcers were age 65 or older. Hospital patients with a diagnosis of pressure ulcer are discharged to long-term care facilities at a rate of approximately 54%. In older adults with pressure ulcers, comorbidities such as fluid and electrolyte disorders, nutritional disorders, diabetes, multiple system failure, and dementia are also part of the patient's medical condition (VanGilder, Amlung, Harrison, & Meyer, 2009; Wound, Ostomy and Continence Nurses Society [WOCN], 2010).

A pressure ulcer affects quality and duration of life. Pressure ulcers can be painful, odorous, and disfiguring; social isolation can frequently result. Hospital mortality for patients with pressure ulcers as a secondary diagnosis is approximately 11% and greater than 4% if pressure ulcer is the primary diagnosis. Research further indicates approximately 60,000 patients die each year from pressure ulcer–related complications. These deaths occurred more frequently in patients over 75 years of age. Septicemia was reported in 39.7% of the reported deaths from pressure ulcer complications (Bryant & Nix, 2012).

Pressure ulcer development is considered an indicator for quality of care. The Centers for Medicare and Medicaid Services (CMS) added stage III and stage IV pressure ulcers to the list of reportable Never Events in 2008. Never Events are defined as errors in medical care that are clearly identifiable, preventable, and have serious consequences for patients (Miller, 2009); the costs associated with these Never Events are nonreimbursable by Medicare and Medicaid. In 2004, the CMS addressed the prevention of pressure ulcers in long-term care residents by defining *avoidable* and *unavoidable pressure ulcers*. When pressure ulcers develop during admission and are identified as avoidable, civil monetary penalties can be assessed in the long-term care setting (Black et al., 2011). According to the CMS, *avoidable* means that a resident developed a pressure ulcer when the facility did not evaluate the resident's clinical condition and pressure ulcer risk factors; did not define and implement interventions consistent with the resident's needs, goals, and recognized standards of practice; or did not monitor and evaluate the impact of the intervention or did not revise the interventions as appropriate to the findings of the evaluation. *Unavoidable* means that a resident developed a pressure ulcer even though the facility had appropriately and comprehensively assessed the residents clinical condition and risk factors, implemented appropriate interventions, monitored and evaluated the effectiveness of these interventions, and revised them as indicated by the care plan (CMS, 2004).

Pressure Ulcer Prevention

The overall goal for the prevention of pressure ulcers is to identify persons at risk and initiate early prevention strategies to maintain intact skin, prevent complications, optimize potential for wound healing, and involve the patient and the caregiver in the plan of care. It is also an important goal to implement cost-effective strategies in the plan of care.

Assessment

A complete medical history should be included in the *pressure ulcer risk assessment*. Risk factors for pressure ulcer development include advanced age; immobility; malnutrition; incontinence; diminished level of consciousness; impaired sensation; history of pressure ulcers; multiple comorbidities such as diabetes, chronic obstructive pulmonary disease, renal disease, and arterial/vascular disease; medication history; and previous treatment with steroids, radiation, or chemotherapy.

Risk assessment instruments are utilized to ascertain pressure ulcer risk and should be completed on all patients. The *Braden Scale for Pressure Ulcer Risk Assessment* is the most widely used instrument that determines risk of pressure ulcer development. The scale assesses sensory perception, skin moisture, activity, mobility, nutrition, and friction/shear. Each area is scored on a scale of 1 to 3 or 4, with a possible total score of 23 points—the lower the Braden score, the higher the risk of pressure ulcer development (Braden & Bergstrom, 1987). A Braden score of 16 or less indicates a high risk of pressure ulcer development in the general population, whereas a score of 18 or less is indicative of high risk in older adults or persons with darkly pigmented skin. Subset scores of 2 or less in any one category also places one in a high-risk category even if the patient has an overall score greater than 16 (see **Box 18-1**).

BOX 18-1   Braden Scale for Pressure Ulcer Risk Assessment

Sensory Perception
Ability to respond meaningfully to pressure-related discomfort

1. Completely Limited: Unresponsive (does not moan, flinch, or gasp) to painful stimuli, due to diminished level of consciousness or sedation.

OR

Limited ability to feel pain over most of body surface.

2. Very Limited: Responds only to painful stimuli.

Cannot communicate discomfort except by moaning or restlessness.

OR

Has a sensory impairment, which limits the ability to feel pain or discomfort over half of body.

3. Slightly Limited: Responds to verbal commands but cannot always communicate discomfort or need to be turned.

OR

Has some sensory impairment, which limits ability to feel pain or discomfort in one or two extremities.

4. No Impairment: Responds to verbal commands. Has no sensory deficit that would limit ability to feel or voice pain or discomfort.

Moisture
Degree to which skin is exposed to moisture

1. Constantly Moist: Perspiration, urine, etc. keep skin moist almost constantly. Dampness is detected every time patient is moved or turned.
2. Moist: Skin is often but not always moist.
3. Linen must be changed at least once a shift.
4. Occasionally Moist: Skin is occasionally moist, requiring an extra linen change approximately once a day.
5. Rarely Moist: Skin is usually dry; linen requires changing only at routine intervals.

Activity
Degree of physical activity

1. Bedfast: Confined to bed.
2. Chairfast: Ability to walk is severely limited or nonexistent. Cannot bear own weight and/or must be assisted into chair or wheelchair.
3. Walks Occasionally: Walks occasionally during the day but for very short distances, with or without assistance. Spends majority of each shift in bed or chair.
4. Walks Frequently: Walks outside the room at least twice a day and inside room at least once every 2 hours during waking hours.

Pressure Ulcers

Ability to change and control body position

1. Completely Immobile: Does not make even slight changes in body or extremity position without assistance.
2. Very Limited: Makes occasional slight changes in body or extremity position but unable to make frequent or significant changes independently.
3. Slightly Limited: Makes frequent though slight changes in body or extremity position independently.
4. No Limitations: Makes major and frequent changes in position without assistance.

Nutrition

Usual food intake pattern

1. Very Poor: Never eats a complete meal. Rarely eats more than one third of any food offered. Eats two servings or less of protein (meat or dairy products) per day. Takes fluids poorly. Does not take a liquid dietary supplement.

OR

Is NPO (nothing by mouth) and/or maintained on clear liquids or intravenous for more than 5 days.

2. Probably Inadequate: Rarely eats a complete meal and generally eats only about half of any food offered. Protein intake includes only three servings of meat or dairy products per day. Occasionally will take a dietary supplement.

OR

Receives less than optimum amount of liquid diet or tube feeding.

3. Adequate: Eats over half of most meals. Eats a total of four servings of protein (meat, dairy products) each day. Occasionally will refuse a meal, but will usually take a supplement if offered.

OR

Is on a tube feeding or TPN regimen, which probably meets most of nutritional needs.

4. Excellent: Eats most of every meal. Never refuses a meal. Usually eats a total of four or more servings of meat and dairy products. Occasionally eats between meals. Does not require supplementation.

Friction and Shear

1. Problem: Requires moderate to maximum assistance in moving. Complete lifting without sliding against sheets is impossible. Frequently slides down in bed or chair, requiring frequent repositioning with maximum assistance. Spasticity, contractures, or agitation leads to almost constant friction.
2. Potential Problem: Moves feebly or requires minimum assistance. During a move, skin probably slides to some extent against sheets, chair, restraints, or other devices. Maintains relatively good position in chair or bed most of the time but occasionally slides down.
3. No Apparent Problem: Moves in bed and in chair independently and has sufficient muscle strength to lift up completely during move. Maintains good position in bed or chair at all times.

TOTAL SCORE:

Baseline Braden scores should be determined upon admission to the healthcare facility, and the assessment should be repeated at regular intervals or when the patient's condition changes. Hospitals, long-term care facilities, and community healthcare facilities should implement nursing care policies to determine the frequency of assessment.

CLINICAL TIP

The Braden scale gives a measure of risk of developing pressure ulcers.
Braden score summary:

15 to 18 = At risk

13 to 14 = Moderate risk

10 to 12 = High risk

≤ 9 = Very high risk

The standard of care is to perform accurate and routine skin inspections and assessments. A total-body skin inspection should be completed on admission to the healthcare facility to determine if there are any skin impairments, including reddened areas, rashes, abnormal lesions, abrasions, bruises, skin tears, traumatic injuries, and pressure ulcers. The temperature of the skin should also be assessed. Any area of skin that deviates from what is normal needs to be compared to the adjacent skin, and the findings should be documented. Skin assessment includes the skin inspection, the interpretation of the findings from the inspection, and the synthesis of the inspection information combined with information from the comprehensive assessment of the patient, such as comorbidities, medication history, nutrition, perfusion, and pressure ulcer history.

Evidence-based practice includes nutritional status as part of the total assessment. Assessment of nutritional status is critical to identify the risk of malnutrition, as malnutrition is associated with poor wound healing and overall morbidity and mortality (Demling, 2009). A nutritional assessment should be performed upon entry to a new healthcare setting and whenever there is a change in the individual's condition. A comprehensive nutritional assessment includes:

1. Current weight and usual weight (an actual weight, not a stated weight)
2. History of unintended weight loss or gain
3. Body mass index (BMI)
4. Determining possible protein energy malnutrition
5. Food intake
6. Dental health
7. Oral and gastrointestinal history, including chewing and swallowing difficulties and the ability to feed one's self
8. Medical/surgical history or interventions that influence nutrient intake or absorption of nutrients
9. Drug/nutrient interaction
10. Psychosocial factors affecting food intake
11. Cultural and lifestyle influences on food selection

Laboratory parameters for nutritional status should be evaluated. Serum albumin levels are frequently used to assess nutritional status, but they are a poor indicator of protein status as multiple factors decrease albumin levels even when protein intake is adequate. Factors that affect albumin levels include infection, acute stress, surgery, cortisone excess, dehydration, and kidney disease. Normal albumin levels are approximately 3.5 to 5, which reflects what protein levels were approximately 14 to 21 days prior to the examination. Prealbumin is a more current reflection of protein stores, indicating status for the past 2 to days, though it may be artificially low in the presence of severe inflammation or infection. Normal prealbumin levels range from 18 to 28.

The latest research on serum albumin and nutritional supply in patients with pressure ulcers indicates "the serum albumin level appears to reflect inflammation, wound healing, and disease severity rather than nutrition supply in patients with pressure ulcer" (Sugino et al., 2014, p. 15).

Interventions for the Prevention of Pressure Ulcers

Evidence-based practice indicates the interventions that should be present in a pressure ulcer prevention program include *pressure redistribution* and offloading, maintaining skin health, nutrition and hydration, and patient and family education. Because prevention and treatment interventions overlap, both prevention and treatment strategies are addressed for tissue redistribution in this section.

Tissue Load Management

Tissue load is the distribution of friction, pressure, and shear on the tissue. Pressure redistribution is the ability of a support surface to distribute load over the contact areas of the human body to reduce the overall pressure and avoid areas of focal pressure. Offloading is provided by turning and repositioning the patient. Both pressure redistribution and offloading are necessary activities for the at-risk patient and the patient with existing pressure ulcers while in bed, in a chair, on a gurney, or in the operating room. Support surfaces should be utilized on beds and chairs to redistribute pressure, but they should be used only as adjuncts and do not replace the need for manual turning and repositioning. The type of support surface to be used is determined by the patient's condition, the healthcare setting, the cost, and the availability of product. Properly sized equipment should be used for morbidly obese patients; these are classified by the weight limits of the equipment. The terms and definitions developed by the National Pressure Ulcer Advisory Support Surface Standard Initiative in 2007 should be used when choosing support surfaces (Bryant & Nix, 2012) (see **Table 18-1**).

Many factors affect product choice such as complex comorbidities, patient size, product cost, and user environment. The criteria for use of a support surface are usually defined in the facility's policies and procedures. Table 18-1 illustrates a therapeutic support surface selection guide. When a support surface is indicated by the patient's clinical condition, the physician order is obtained and the facility vendor or product supplier is notified (Oklahoma Foundation for Medical Quality, 2009).

Repositioning reduces the duration and intensity of pressure over a bony. The standard has been turning and repositioning at least every 2 hours; however, evidence for the optimal frequency of repositioning is

TABLE 18-1	Specialty Support Surface Selection Guide						
Therapeutic Support Surface	Prevention At Risk	Trunk Stage I	Trunk Stage II	Multiple Trunk Stage II	Trunk Stage III	Trunk Stage IV	Multiple Trunk Stage III/IV
Mattress Overlay (alternating pressure, self-adjusting mattress)	X	X	X	X			
Low Air Loss			X	X	X	X	
Gel Overlay			X	X	X	X	
Alternating Pressure			X	X	X	X	X
Low Air Loss Bed (total bed system)			X	X	X	X	X
Air Fluidized						X	X

lacking. The current research suggests that repositioning every 4 hours when combined with any pressure redistribution mattress is just as effective for prevention of pressure ulcers (Lyder & Ayello, 2008). The patient's activity and mobility level and overall clinical condition should be considered to determine the frequency of repositioning.

According the current evidence-based practice guidelines developed by NPUAP and EPUAP (2014), when determining repositioning frequency: (1) Consider the pressure redistribution support surface in use when determining the frequency of repositioning. (2) Determine repositioning frequency with consideration to the individual's tissue tolerance, level of activity and mobility, general medical condition, overall treatment objectives, skin condition, and comfort. (3) Establish pressure relief schedules that prescribe the frequency and duration of weight shifts. Teach individuals to do "pressure relief lifts" or other pressure-relieving maneuvers as appropriate. (4) Regularly assess the individual's skin condition and general comfort.

If the individual is not responding as expected to the repositioning regimen, reconsider the frequency and method of repositioning. Frequent assessment of the individual's skin condition will help identify the early signs of pressure damage and, as such the patient's tolerance of the planned repositioning schedule. If changes in skin condition should occur, the repositioning care plan needs to be reevaluated.

The frequency of repositioning must be individualized per the patient's needs and outlined in the patient's plan of care, and the plan of care should be evaluated frequently per the facility's policy and procedures and revised according to changes in the patient's clinical condition. Frequent small position changes can be achieved by using pillows and wedges. To avoid skin surfaces rubbing together, such as at the knees, a pad placed between the legs can be effective (WOCN, 2010).

While the patient is in bed, the head of the bed should be maintained at 30 degrees or below. Use a 30-degree, side-lying position and alternative positions (right, back, left); these techniques will prevent sliding, shearing, and pressure-related injuries. Other methods to minimize friction and shear include the use of dry lubricants, transparent films, foams, or hydrocolloids to bony prominences. Avoid pulling or dragging the patient by using lift sheets and lift equipment for repositioning or transfer activities. Friction and shear are enhanced in the presence of moisture, so the skin should be cleaned and dried as soon as possible after each incontinent episode (WOCN, 2010).

CLINICAL TIP

Patients who use a wheelchair for mobility should be measured and fitted by a qualified therapist or mobility expert to ensure proper fit of the chair. Wheelchairs and other mobility aides can cause pressure injuries if they are not appropriately tailored to the individual's height, weight, build, and body measurements.

For chair-bound patients it is important to redistribute the weight frequently. Pay special attention to the individual's anatomy, postural alignment, and support of the feet. While the patient is sitting in a chair, it is recommended that he or she be repositioned at least every hour with small shifts in position every 15 to 30 minutes. A pressure redistribution cushion should be placed in the chair. When pressure ulcers are present on the sacrococcyx area, sitting should be limited to 3 times a day in periods of 60 minutes or less (WOCN, 2010).

"When choosing a particular position for the individual, it is important to assess whether the pressure is actually relieved or redistributed. Avoid positioning the individual on bony prominences with existing nonblanchable erythema. Nonblanchable erythema is an indication of the early signs of pressure ulcer damage. If an individual is positioned directly onto bony prominences with preexisting nonblanchable erythema, the pressure and/or shearing forces sustained will further occlude blood supply to the skin, thereby worsening the damage and resulting in more severe pressure ulceration" (NPUAP & EPUAP, 2014).

BOX 18-2 Preventing Pressure Ulcers

1. Assess all patients for risk of pressure ulcer development.
2. Identify all risk factors to determine specific interventions.
3. Inspect the skin at least daily and document results.
4. Use mild cleansing agents for bathing, avoiding hot water, harsh soaps, and friction.
5. Moisturize after bathing and minimize environmental factors that lead to dry skin.
6. Avoid massaging bony prominences.
7. Assess for incontinence. Use skin barriers after cleansing, provide absorbent underpads or briefs, and monitor frequently for episodes of incontinence.
8. Use dry lubricants, such as cornstarch, on transfer surfaces (linens) to prevent friction.
9. Assess for compromised nutrition, particularly protein and caloric intake. Consider nutritional supplements and support for patients at risk.
10. Maintain or improve patient's mobility and activity levels.
11. Reposition bed-bound patients at least every 2 hours and chair-bound patients every hour. Patients should be instructed or assisted to shift their positions more frequently (i.e., every 15 minutes for chair-bound patients and at least every hour for bed-bound).
12. Place at-risk patients on pressure-reducing devices. (Donut devices should not be used—they simply displace the pressure and friction to the periphery of the area that is meant to be protected.)
13. Use lifting devices to transfer patients.
14. Pillows or foam wedges should be used to keep bony prominences from direct contact with each other (e.g., knees, ankles).
15. Avoid positioning the patient on the trochanter when lying on his or her side. (Use a 30-degree lateral inclined position.)
16. Elevate the head of the bed to 30 degrees or less. (Shearing injuries can occur at elevations higher than 30 degrees.)
17. Evaluate and document the effectiveness of interventions, and modify the plan of care according to patient response.
18. Provide education to patients, family, and caregivers for the prevention of pressure ulcers.

Maintaining skin health through good skin care is another important intervention for prevention of pressure ulcers. Managing incontinence and cleansing the skin gently at each incontinent episode using a pH-balanced perineal skin cleanser will be more effective for the prevention and treatment of incontinence-associated dermatitis (IAD) than soap and water. Avoid vigorous cleansing as it leads to erosion of the epidermis. Incontinence skin barriers such as creams, ointments, and paste are effective in protecting and maintaining intact skin. The use of briefs to manage incontinence increases the risk of IAD, and a patient with IAD is at higher risk for pressure ulcer development. The use of external containment systems for urine (e.g., condom catheters) and external and internal containment systems for feces should be considered to reduce moisture's effect on the skin. **Box 18-2** provides a summary of strategies to prevent pressure ulcers.

Nutrition

Nutritional deficiencies should be addressed. A dietary consult should be ordered for all patients at moderate to high risk for pressure ulcer development or if there is a change in the patient's condition. Assessment of the adequacy of nutritional intake is essential. Weight should be monitored; a weight loss of more than 5% in 30 days or more than 10% in 180 days is considered significant (NPUAP & EPUAP, 2014). When the patient has a pressure ulcer and is underweight or losing weight, calories need to be enhanced and protein supplementation needs to be provided.

Adequate hydration is essential to maintaining skin health. Dehydration causes skin to become fragile and prone to breakdown; decreases the circulating blood volume; and reduces peripheral blood flow, impairing the delivery of nutrients and oxygen to wounds. Risk factors for dehydration should be assessed in all patients. The risk factors for dehydration include fluid loss, fluid restriction, altered cognition, poor oral intake of food or fluids, functional impairments, dysphagia, medications, incontinence, and acute illness. When a patient is at risk of or has a pressure ulcer, a comprehensive nutritional assessment should be conducted by a registered dietician (RD). The average adult requires 30 to 40 mL/kg of body weight in daily fluid intake. When a patient has a pressure ulcer, additional fluids are required to compensate for losses, including wound exudates, fever, vomiting, or diarrhea. The RD will evaluate the patient's fluid needs based on the patient's clinical condition and make recommendations (Kondracki & Collins, 2009).

Patient and Family Education

Patient and family education in pressure ulcer prevention is very important to help reduce the incidence of pressure ulcers in any care setting. Through education, the patient and family are empowered to participate in the prevention of pressure ulcers.

Documentation of the assessments, interventions, and outcomes is an integral part of the prevention program and should be completed according to the institutions nursing policies for documentation.

The Challenges of Pressure Ulcer Prevention

Pressure ulcer prevention requires an interdisciplinary approach to care. Some parts of pressure ulcer prevention care arestandard for all patients, but nursing care should be tailored to the address the specific risks identified for each person. No individual clinician working alone, regardless of how talented, can prevent all pressure ulcers from developing. Rather, pressure ulcer prevention requires activities among many individuals, including the multiple disciplines and multiple teams involved in developing and implementing the care plan. To accomplish this coordination, high-quality prevention requires an organizational culture and operational practices that promote teamwork and communication, as well as individual expertise. Therefore, improvement in pressure ulcer prevention calls for a system focus to make needed changes.

Pressure Ulcer Prevention Performance Improvement

The Preventing Pressure Ulcers in Hospitals (PUPPI) toolkit was designed to assist hospital staff in implementing effective pressure ulcer prevention practices. The toolkit was developed under a contract with the AHRQ (2014) through the Accelerating Change and Transformation in Organizations and Networks (ACTION) program, with additional support from the Health Services Research and Development Service of the Department of Veterans Affairs. The PUPPI tool consists of several areas: sensory perception, moisture, activity, mobility, nutrition, and friction and shear (Scalzitti, 2015).

The toolkit is designed for multiple uses. "The core document is an implementation guide organized under six major questions intended to be used primarily by the implementation team charged with leading the effort to plan and put the new prevention strategies into practice" (AHRQ, 2014). Because the guide is lengthy, the toolkit includes one-page pressure ulcer prevention implementation highlights to introduce the project to other key players, such as hospital senior management and unit nurse managers. The PUPPI toolkit can be downloaded from the AHRQ Website: http://www.ahrq.gov/professionals/systems/hospital/pressureulcertoolkit/index.html.

CLINICAL TIP

The PUPPI toolkit can be used to prevent pressure ulcers in various settings. The questions in the toolkit also can assist with data gathering and research.

BOX 18-3   Evidence-Based Practice Highlight

Highlights research done to understand if implementation of a pressure ulcer prevention tool decreases incidence of pressure ulcers in nursing home

Scalzitti executed a research project seeking to explore the occurrence of pressure ulcers in nursing homes and determine whether a prevention tool and staff education could reduce the number of pressure ulcers reported. Scalzitti found this two sided approach had a significant impact on reducing the incidence of pressure ulcers in the nursing home environment. Sign into

your database of nursing literature (CINAHL or PubMed, for example) and use the citation below to perform a search for this article. Describe the pressure ulcer prevention tool this researcher used. What kind of staff education did she implement alongside it? How could a nursing home begin incorporating this strategy?

Scalzitti, K. L. (2015). Using education and a prevention protocol tool to decrease the incidence of pressure ulcers in a nursing home. *Evidence-Based Practice Project Reports* (Paper 69). Retrieved from http://scholar.valpo.edu/ebpr/69

Pressure Ulcer Management

Pressure ulcer management includes nursing assessment, accurate staging (classification) of the pressure ulcer, and documentation of the onset and assessed stage. Appropriate interventions and frequent evaluations of the healing progress are implemented with changes made to the plan of care as indicated by changes in the wound.

Classification of Pressure Ulcers

The International Association for Enterostomal Therapy, now known as the WOCN Society, modified the Shea *pressure ulcer staging system*, originally developed in 1975. The *National Pressure Ulcer Advisory Panel* (NPUAP) updated the staging system to provide clarity and accuracy by including more descriptors and defining suspected deep tissue injury and unstageable pressure ulcers (NPUAP, 2016). **Figure 18-1** provide examples of each stage of pressure ulcer. International guidelines released in 2009 added the term *category* and specified that the suspected deep tissue injury and unstageable pressure ulcer are categories used in the United States (see **Box 18-4**) (NPUAP & EPUAP, 2014).

Assessment and Monitoring

Nursing assessment and documentation of pressure ulcers should include onset, location, staging (classification), measurement, exudate description, wound bed characteristics, pain, condition of

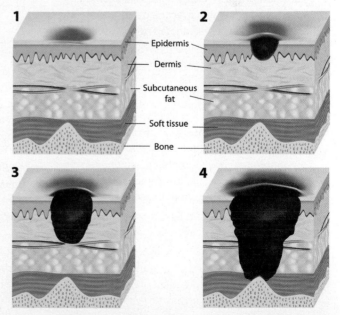

Figure 18-1 Stages of pressure ulcers.
© Alila Sao Mai/Shutterstock

BOX 18-4 International NPUAP-EPUAP Pressure Ulcer Classification System

Category/Stage I: Non-blanchable erythema of intact skin

Intact skin with a localized area of non-blanchable erythema, which may appear differently in darkly pigmented skin. Presence of blanchable erythema or changes in sensation, temperature, or firmness may precede visual changes. Color changes do not include purple or maroon discoloration; these may indicate deep tissue pressure injury.

Further description: The area may be painful, firm, soft, warmer, or cooler compared to adjacent tissue. Category/stage I may be difficult to detect in individuals with dark skin tones. May indicate at-risk persons.

Category/Stage II: Partial-thickness skin loss with exposed dermis

Partial-thickness loss of skin with exposed dermis. The wound bed is viable, pink or red, moist, and may also present as an intact or ruptured serum-filled blister. Adipose (fat) is not visible and deeper tissues are not visible. Granulation tissue, slough and eschar are not present. These injuries commonly result from adverse microclimate and shear in the skin over the pelvis and shear in the heel. This stage should not be used to describe moisture associated skin damage (MASD) including incontinence associated dermatitis (IAD), intertriginous dermatitis (ITD), medical adhesive related skin injury (MARSI), or traumatic wounds (skin tears, burns, abrasions).

Further description: Manifests as a shiny or dry shallow ulcer without slough or bruising. This category/stage should not be used to describe skin tears, tape burns, incontinence-associated dermatitis, maceration, or excoriation.

Category/Stage III: Full-thickness skin loss (fat visible)

Full-thickness loss of skin, in which adipose (fat) is visible in the ulcer and granulation tissue and epibole (rolled wound edges) are often present. Slough and/or eschar may be visible. The depth of tissue damage varies by anatomical location; areas of significant adiposity can develop deep wounds. Undermining and tunneling may occur. Fascia, muscle, tendon, ligament, cartilage and/or bone are not exposed. If slough or eschar obscures the extent of tissue loss this is an Unstageable Pressure Injury.

Further description: The depth of a category/stage III pressure ulcer varies by anatomical location. The bridge of the nose, ear, occiput, and malleolus do not have (adipose) subcutaneous tissue and category/stage III ulcers can be shallow. In contrast, areas of significant adiposity can develop extremely deep category/stage III pressure ulcers. Bone and tendon are not visible or directly palpable.

Category/Stage IV: Full-thickness skin and tissue loss (muscle/bone visible)

Full-thickness skin and tissue loss with exposed or directly palpable fascia, muscle, tendon, ligament, cartilage or bone in the ulcer. Slough and/or eschar may be visible. Epibole (rolled edges), undermining and/or tunneling often occur. Depth varies by anatomical location. If slough or eschar obscures the extent of tissue loss this is an Unstageable Pressure Injury.

Further description: The depth of a category/stage IV pressure ulcer varies by anatomical location. The bridge of the nose, ear, occiput, and malleolus do not have (adipose) subcutaneous tissue, and these ulcers can be shallow. Category/stage IV ulcers can extend into muscle and/or supporting structures, e.g., fascia, tendon, or joint capsule) making osteomyelitis or osteitis likely to occur. Exposed bone or muscle is visible or directly palpable.

Additional Categories for the United States Unstageable/Unclassified: Obscured full-thickness skin and tissue loss

Full-thickness skin and tissue loss in which the extent of tissue damage within the ulcer cannot be confirmed because it is obscured by slough or eschar. If slough or eschar is removed, a Stage 3 or Stage 4 pressure injury will be revealed. Stable eschar (i.e. dry, adherent, intact without erythema or fluctuance) on the heel or ischemic limb should not be softened or removed.

Further description: Until enough slough and/or eschar are removed to expose the base of the wound, the true depth cannot be determined; but it will be either a category/stage III or IV. Stable (dry, adherent, intact without erythema or fluctuance) eschar on the heels serves as "the body's natural (biological) cover" and should not be removed.

Deep Tissue Pressure Injury: Persistent non-blanchable deep red, maroon or purple discoloration

Intact or non-intact skin with localized area of persistent non-blanchable deep red, maroon, purple discoloration or epidermal separation revealing a dark wound bed or blood filled blister. Pain and temperature change often precede skin color changes. Discoloration may appear differently in darkly pigmented skin. This injury results from intense and/or prolonged pressure and shear forces at the bone-muscle interface. The wound may evolve rapidly to reveal the actual extent of tissue injury, or may resolve without tissue loss.

If necrotic tissue, subcutaneous tissue, granulation tissue, fascia, muscle or other underlying structures are visible, this indicates a full thickness pressure injury (Unstageable, Stage 3 or Stage 4). Do not use DTPI to describe vascular, traumatic, neuropathic, or dermatologic conditions.

Further description: The area may be preceded by tissue that is painful, firm, mushy, boggy, warmer, or cooler compared to adjacent tissue. Deep tissue injury may be difficult to detect in individuals with dark skin tones. Evolution may include a thin blister over a dark wound bed. The wound may evolve further and become covered by thin eschar. Evolution may be rapid, exposing additional layers of tissue even with treatment.

Reproduced from National Pressure Ulcer Advisory Panel, European Pressure Ulcer Advisory Panel and Pan Pacific Pressure Injury Alliance. (2014). *Prevention and treatment of pressure ulcers: Quick reference guide*. Emily Haesler (Ed.). Osborne Park, Western Australia: Cambridge Media.

surrounding tissue, and any undermining or tunneling factors. The healing process is described by the Pressure Ulcer Scale for Healing (PUSH) tool, which provides a consistent method of recording the effectiveness of treatment. The scale has three subscales, with a possible total score of 17; the score will trend downward when treatment is effective, and a score of 0 indicates the pressure ulcer has completely healed. Wound assessments should be performed on admission and at least weekly to monitor the healing or deterioration of the pressure ulcer (see **Table 18-2**).

If eschar is present, it must be debrided before staging can occur. The ulcer should be documented as an eschar-covered pressure ulcer. Structures beneath the epidermis and dermis, including muscle, are more susceptible to the effects of ischemia. Pressure ulcers are usually much worse than they appear on the surface; therefore, staging should be to the maximum anatomical depth after necrotic tissue debridement is performed. This is also the case for a deep tissue injury. These types of wounds should be documented as a suspected deep tissue injury, and documentation should indicate that the wound will likely develop into a stage III or stage IV pressure ulcer.

The length, width, and depth of pressure ulcers should be measured and documented with distinctions made between the healed and nonhealed areas of the ulcer.

Photographs are often used to document the occurrence and healing of pressure ulcers. The quantity and characteristics of any exudates and the types of wound bed tissue—necrotic, slough, or granulation—are also documented. The surrounding skin should be assessed for any maceration, induration, crepitus, or injury, including abrasions. Pressure ulcers with undermining or tunnels often lead to further skin breakdown.

CLINICAL TIP

Check your organization's policy for photographing pressure injuries on admission. An evidence-based policy that properly and visually documents wound size and characteristics is important for quality care and may also be used in litigation processes.

TABLE 18-2   PUSH (Pressure Ulcer Scale for Healing)

Length × Width	0 0 cm² 6 3.1–4.0 cm²	1 <0.3 cm² 7 4.1–8.0 cm²	2 0.3–0.6 cm² 8 8.1–12.0 cm²	3 0.7–1.0 cm² 9 12.1–24.0 cm²	4 1.1–2.0 cm² 10 >24.0 cm²	5 2.1–3.0 cm²	Subscore
Exudate Amount	0 None	1 Light	2 Moderate	3 Heavy			Subscore
Tissue Type	0 Closed	1 Epithelial tissue	2 Granulation tissue	3 Slough	4 Necrotic tissue		Subscore

Exudate Amount: Estimate the amount of exudate (drainage) present after removal of the dressing and before applying any topical agent to the ulcer. Estimate the exudate (drainage) as none, light, moderate, or heavy.

Tissue Type: This refers to the types of tissue present in the wound (ulcer) bed. Score as a 4 if there is any necrotic tissue present. Score as a 3 if there is any amount of slough present and necrotic tissue is absent. Score as a 2 if the wound is clean and contains granulation tissue. A superficial wound that is reepithelializing is scored as a 1. When the wound is closed, score as a 0.

4—Necrotic tissue (eschar): Black, brown, or tan tissue that adheres firmly to the wound bed or ulcer edges and may be either firmer or softer than surrounding skin.

3—Slough: Yellow or white tissue that adheres to the ulcer bed in strings or thick clumps or is mucinous.

2—Granulation tissue: Pink or beefy red tissue with a shiny, moist, granular appearance.

1—Epithelial tissue: For superficial ulcers, new pink or shiny tissue (skin) that grows in from the edges or as islands on the ulcer surface.

0—Closed/resurfaced: The wound is completely covered with epithelium (new skin).

Reproduced from National Pressure Ulcer Advisory Panel. (1998). Pressure Ulcer Scale for Healing (PUSH): PUSH Tool 3.0. Retrieved from http://www.npuap.org/resources/educational-and-clinical-resources/push-tool/

Pain related to a pressure ulcer should be assessed. It is also important to identify and document pain relief measures and provide analgesia prior to dressing changes or other interventions.

Reevaluation of the pressure ulcer, the plan of care, and the individual should be done at least every 2 weeks, if there is a significant change in the wound or progress toward closure is not observed.

Treatment Modalities

A central component of pressure ulcer care is wound dressing. The dressing used should be based on the tissue in the wound bed, the condition of the skin around the pressure ulcer, and the desired outcomes (see **Table 18-3**). A clean, moist wound bed is ideal to promote healing. When selecting a dressing, the following guidelines should be considered:

1. Assess pressure ulcers at every dressing change and confirm the appropriateness of the current treatment plan.
2. Follow the manufacturer recommendations, especially regarding the frequency of dressing changes.
3. The care plan should be used to guide the frequency of dressing changes.
4. A dressing that maintains a moist wound bed should be chosen.
5. The dressing should remain in contact with the wound bed and the periwound protected to prevent maceration. Several moisture-retentive dressings are available to maintain a moist wound bed.
6. Dressings should be used to help decrease the bioburden in the wound bed and prevent infection. These include a variety of antimicrobial ointments and silver dressings.
   > Silver-impregnated dressings are used for pressure ulcers that are infected or heavily colonized with bacteria. Most of the wound care products utilized today are impregnated with silver.
7. Secondary dressings are to secure a dressing in place and are selected based upon patient comfort.
   > Gauze dressings are mainly used as secondary dressings. As primary dressings they are labor-intensive and can cause pain when removed if they dry out. Desiccation of viable tissue can occur when gauze dressings dry out and adhere to the wound bed.

TABLE 18-3   Wound Care Product Guide

Types and Examples	Indications	Advantages	Change Frequency
Polymeric Film (Transparent film)	• Superficial, partial-thickness wounds • Wounds with necrosis and slough • Wounds with little or no exudate	• Can visualize the wound • Control gas exchange • Promotes autolytic debridement • Impermeable to contaminates	24–72 hours
Impregnated Nonadherent Dressings	• Abrasions • Burns • Graft donor sites • Skin tears	• Covers, soothes, and protects underlying tissues where exudate is light	Every 8–12 hours
Polyurethane Foam	• Partial- and full-thickness wounds with minimal to moderate exudate May be used as a secondary dressing for wound packing and fillers	• Nonadherent, repels contaminants • Hydrophilic: Absorbs a moderate amount of exudate	1–5 days depending on drainage amount
Hydrogels (Water based sheets or amorphous gel)	• Dry wounds • Burns or radiation necrosis or injuries	• Pain reduction • Rehydrates dry wounds • Promotes autolytic debridement • Fills the dead space	1–5 days depending on drainage amount
Hydrocolloid	• Superficial, partial-thickness wounds • Shallow, full-thickness wounds • Wounds with slough or eschar	• Promotes autolytic debridement • Self-adherent • Protects wounds from contaminants	1–7 days depending on drainage amount
Calcium Alginates (ropes and sheets)	• Partial- and full-thickness wounds • Wounds with slough and necrosis • Wounds with undermining and tunneling	• Fills dead spaces, tunnels, and undermining • Absorbs large amount of drainage • Promotes autolytic debridement • Forms a gel interacting with the drainage	1–4 days depending on the drainage amount

BOX 18-5   Guidelines for Pressure Ulcer Treatments

1. Cleanse the wound with a noncytotoxic cleanser (saline) during each dressing change.
2. If necrotic tissue or slough is present, consider the use of high-pressure irrigation.
3. Debride necrotic tissue.
4. Do not debride dry, black eschar on heels.
5. Perform wound care using topical dressings determined by wound and availability.
6. Choose dressings that provide a moist wound environment, keep the skin surrounding the ulcer dry, control exudates, and eliminate dead space.
7. Reassess the wound with each dressing change to determine whether treatment plan modifications are needed.
8. Identify and manage wound infections.
9. Patients with stage III and IV ulcers that do not respond to conservative therapy may require surgical intervention.

Modified from National Guideline Clearinghouse Guideline for Prevention and Management of Pressure Ulcers. Retrieved from http://www .guideline.gov

TABLE 18-4   Methods of Pressure Ulcer Debridement

Extrinsic	Factors
Sharp	Devitalized tissue is removed with a scalpel, scissors, or other sharp instrument. This is the most rapid form of debridement and can be used for removing areas of thick eschar.
Enzymatic	Topical debriding agents are applied to devitalized tissue areas.
Autolytic	Appropriate for noninfected ulcers only. Synthetic dressings that aid self- digestion of devitalized tissue.
Mechanical	Wet-to-dry dressings, hydrotherapy, and irrigation.

Several biophysical agents are used in the management of pressure ulcers. These include electrical stimulation, phototherapy, ultrasound, hydrotherapy, laser, negative-pressure wound therapy, and hyperbaric oxygen therapy (see **Box 18-5**).

Debridement of devitalized tissue in the wound bed is essential for healing to progress. If necrotic tissue is present, it must be debrided before staging can occur.

The main types of debridement include autolytic, mechanical, enzymatic, and sharp/surgical debridement (refer to **Table 18-4** for a description of these types of debridement). The debridement method utilized should be determined by the condition of the wound. The wound should be assessed for the presence or absence of infection, amount of necrotic tissue, vascularity of the wound, pain tolerance, setting, and availability and access to various debridement methods. A thorough vascular assessment should be performed prior to debridement of lower extremity ulcers. Dry, hard, stable eschar in ischemic limbs should not be debrided. When using an enzymatic debriding ointment on dry eschar, the eschar should be scored or crosshatched prior to applying the ointment. Maintenance debridement on a chronic wound should be performed until the wound bed is covered with granulation tissue. Sharp debridement is performed by clinicians who have been trained in sharp debridement, which would be a wound consultant, a physician, or a physical therapist (Table 18-4). When undermining, tunneling, and extensive necrotic tissue are present in the wound, it may be necessary for a physician to perform surgical debridement (WOCN, 2010).

Critical Factors

There are many critical factors that must be considered in the management of pressure ulcers, including nutrition, pain, infection, and goals of treatment. These factors must be evaluated, and care plans must be implemented to address these factors based on the individual needs of the patient. Nutrition is fundamental for cellular integrity, tissue repair, and tissue regeneration. Wound healing is an anabolic process that requires specific nutrients for the biochemical processes in wound healing. The prevalence of malnutrition in hospitals throughout the United States is between 20% and 50%, and further deterioration in nutritional status often occurs during hospitalization. In addition, malnutrition is associated with increased morbidity of 25% and mortality of 5% in patients with acute or chronic diseases. Undernutrition is often called protein malnutrition, which occurs when intake is inadequate, from poor absorption or metabolism that occurs with chronic illnesses or from acute and traumatic injuries. With malnutrition, the patient experiences severe weight loss, muscle wasting, and loss of adipose tissue. Nutrition screening is essential to identify if the patient is at risk for malnutrition. This screening should be performed by a registered dietician and should be performed on admission and every week (or as often as indicated by the patient's clinical condition). Plasma protein levels are frequently used to determine the patient's protein status. Serum albumin (3.5 to 5.0 normal level) is the most frequently used blood test to evaluate nutritional status. It has a long half-life of 17 to 21 days and is not sensitive to rapid changes in nutritional status. Serum prealbumin (18 to 28 normal range) has a short half-life of 2 days and reflects the decreased intake of protein or calories more rapidly. Serum prealbumin is expected to reflect not only what has been ingested but also what the body has been able to absorb, digest, and metabolize. Serum albumin and prealbumin results may be low even when protein intake is adequate if the patient is suffering from severe inflammation, infection, acute stress, dehydration, and surgery-related cortisone excess. Protein needs are increased after injury and prolonged illness, and a protein deficiency prolongs wound healing time. As much as 100 grams of protein per day can be lost through wound exudate. More calories are also needed to improve healing potential. Nutrients involved in wound healing include protein, arginine, zinc, and vitamins A, B, and C. If dietary intake is inadequate, nutritional support should be used to provide approximately 35 calories/kg per day and 1.5 grams of protein/kg per day. The registered dietician will recommend the calories and protein based on the patient's nutritional status, weight, and other variables (Bryant & Nix, 2012) (see **Box 18-6**).

Wound pain has a negative effect on physiological processes, including oxygenation and infection control, as well as on the quality of life. Undertreatment of patients with chronic wound pain is far too common. If undertreated, wound pain can lead to poor wound healing and increased risk of infection; therefore, assessment of all individuals for pain related to pressure ulcers and their treatment is essential to promote healing. A validated pain scale should be used when assessing pain. The assessment of pain should also include assessment of body language and nonverbal cues. Care delivery should be coordinated with pain medication administration and minimal interruptions while providing patient care. Pressure ulcer pain can be reduced by using nonadherent dressings and maintaining a moist wound bed. Encourage repositioning as a means to reduce pain.

Infection does not usually occur in stage I or II ulcers, as ischemic tissue is more susceptible to the development of infection. The level of bacteria inhibiting wound healing is not always manifested by the clinical signs of infection. Critically colonized or infected pressure ulcers may exhibit signs of infection such as delayed healing, poor or friable granulation tissue, changes in odor or increased exudate, and wound tissue discoloration. Induration also may be present. Culturing of the wound for infection is not recommended if acute signs of infection are not present, because bacteria are present on all wounds and a positive culture would likely result even in the absence of infection. A diagnosis of spreading acute infection should be considered if there is erythema extending from the ulcer edge, induration, new or increasing pain, warmth, or purulent drainage. Crepitus, fluctuance, an increase in size, and discoloration in the surrounding skin also may be signs of acute infection in the wound. There may be systemic signs of infection such as a fever, malaise, lymph node enlargement, confusion, and anorexia. To

BOX 18-6   Laboratory Studies Associated with Poor Nutrition

Serum albumin < 3.5 g/dL
Serum transferrin < 200
Prealbumin < 15 mg/dL

Data from Clark, A.P., & Baldwin, K. (2004). Best practices for care of older adults. *Clinical Nurse Specialist, 18*(6), 288–299.

determine the bacterial bioburden of the pressure ulcer, a tissue biopsy or quantitative swab technique might be performed. Management of infection includes prevention of contamination of the pressure ulcer. Cleansing and debridement of necrotic tissue removes loose debris and planktonic, free-floating bacteria. Debridement can also remove biofilms. Antimicrobials are used to decrease the bacterial bioburden on the wound bed and may slow the rate of biofilm development. Antiseptics can be used for a limited time to control the bacterial bioburden, clean the ulcer, and reduce surrounding inflammation. Topical antimicrobial silver, cadexomer iodine, hypertonic saline, methylene blue/gentian violet–impregnated foams, or medical-grade honey dressings can be used for pressure ulcers infected with multiple organisms. Make sure to assess the patient for allergies to honey, bee products, and bee stings before using honey dressings. Systemic antibiotics are used for patients with clinical evidence of a systemic infection, such as cellulitis, fasciitis, osteomyelitis, and positive blood cultures. Osteomyelitis should be suspected and evaluated if bone is exposed or the ulcer has failed to heal (WOCN, 2010).

Special Populations

The principles of effective wound management must utilize a holistic approach that is individualized to the patient's clinical and psychosocial situation. Effective wound care identifies and intervenes to minimize or abate the underlying etiology, including coexisting contributing factors. Cost effectiveness of the treatment plan also must be taken into account when recommending wound care products and devices. There are special patient populations that can be very complex when developing their wound management care plan. These include obese patients and terminally ill patients. The goals of treatment for these patient populations must be clearly defined.

The obese patient has special skin care needs that need to be evaluated and planned. There are many common problems in the obese patient that interfere with skin integrity. These include pressure ulcers, intertrigo, and IAD. Difficulty with off-loading pressure is a significant problem in the obese patient. Friction, shear, and pressure existing in locations unique to the obese patient compound the problem. As a result, atypical pressure ulcers result from tubes, catheters, and ill-fitting chairs and beds. Pressure within skin folds also can result in pressure ulcers. It is vital that frequent, careful assessments are performed of these atypical areas of potential skin breakdown. Make sure proper interventions are implemented to reduce the risk of skin breakdown as well as to properly manage wounds that are already present. The use of bariatric beds with pressure redistribution mattresses and other appropriate bariatric equipment will reduce the risk of pressure ulcers, promote patient independence, decrease staff workload, help control costs, and improve clinical outcomes (Bryant & Nix, 2012).

> **CLINICAL TIP**
>
> Tubes and catheters burrow into skin folds. Reposition tubes and catheters every 2 hours. Place tubing so that patient does not rest on them. Use tube and catheter holders.

Another special-needs patient is the patient in palliative care or hospice. Palliative care and hospice are associated with the end of a patient's life. The wound management goals for this patient population are relief from distressing symptoms, easing pain, and enhancing the quality of life. Preventing wound deterioration or healing the wound are not realistic goals; instead, the goal in this patient is palliation or maintenance. The focus of wound management in the terminally ill is management of symptoms such as odor, exudate, pain, infection, bleeding, and skin integrity. The wound management care plan should be developed and implemented to encourage comfort and prompt symptom management with consistency between the care provided and consideration of the patient's and the family's goals (NPUAP & EPUAP, 2014).

Emerging Therapies for Pressure Ulcer Prevention and Management

Through continued research new emerging therapies are now available, including but not limited to pressure mapping for appropriate positioning and repositioning, microclimate manipulation, fabrics designed to reduce shear and friction; prophylactic dressings, and electrical stimulation of muscles in individuals with spinal cord injury and chronic wounds, and early assessment of deep tissue injury (see **Figures 18-2, 18-3, and 18-4**).

Pressure Map

A pressure map is a computerized clinical tool for assessing pressure distribution. A thin sensor map is placed on a wheelchair seat or a mattress surface. When the patient sits or lies on the mat, a computer screen displays a map of pressures, using colors, numbers, and a graphic image of the patient.

Microclimate Control

The use of specialized surfaces that come into contact with the skin may be able to alter the microclimate by changing the rate of evaporation of moisture and the rate at which heat dissipates from the skin. These include seating pads and low air loss overlay mattresses.

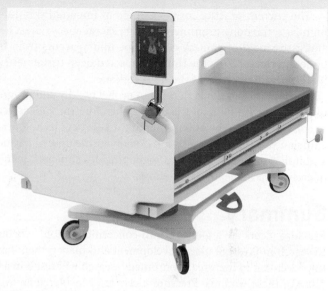

Figure 18-2 Pressure map.
Courtesy of Wellsense

Prophylactic Dressings

Prophylactic dressings are used to protect skin from medical devices such as Foley catheters nasal cannulas, and tracheostomies. These include polyurethane foam dressing to bony prominences (e.g., heels, sacrum) for the prevention of pressure ulcers in anatomical areas frequently subjected to friction and shear.

Electrical Stimulation

Electrical stimulation therapy is the application of a current across a wound. This current has been shown in various models to promote angiogenesis, fibroblast migration promoting granulation, and keratinocyte migration promoting epithelialization.

Infrared Scanning and Imaging

For use in early assessment of suspected deep tissue injury.

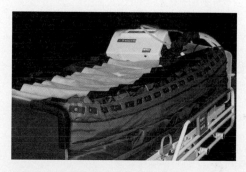

Figure 18-3 Microclimate control.
© R.A. Penne-Casanova/Science Source

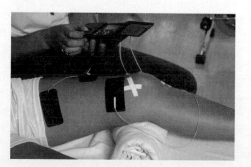

Figure 18-4 Electrical stimulation.
© Carolyn A. McKeone/Science Source

The current practice for assessment of impaired skin integrity is visual inspection of the skin in areas of high risk; the bony prominences (e.g., sacral coccyx area, heels). This assessment includes manual palpation and assessment of pain. A deep tissue injury occurs from the inside out at the point where the muscle and bone interface. So, by the time a suspected deep tissue injury is visible on the skin surface, there already may be significant necrosis of the muscle tissue.

Suspected deep tissue injury can evolve rapidly and progress to unstageable, stage III and stage IV pressure ulcers even with optimal treatment. Therefore early identification and treatment are important to reduce risk of complications. One of the emerging assessment techniques is infrared scanning and imaging, which help the clinician visualize, measure, and document the unseen parities and disparities of metabolic activity, perfusion, and inflammation. This information provides clinicians with an objective, noninvasive and quantitative means of early deep tissue injury diagnosis.

Summary

Pressure ulcers are a global health concern commonly encountered in both hospital and community settings. Research in pressure ulcer development and management has historically been lacking, though there has been improvement in this area. Continued research will result in a better understanding of the etiology and management of these wounds. Pressure ulcers are considered an avoidable, costly complication caused by unrelieved pressure and inappropriate care.

A comprehensive, multidisciplinary plan that includes risk assessment; comprehensive assessment; regular and routine skin assessment; frequent evaluations; collaboration; safe handoffs; continuity of care across all healthcare settings; and patient, family, and staff education is required to appropriately prevent and manage pressure ulcers (see **Case Study 18-1**). A team approach with clear communication (see **Box 18-7**), incorporating all of the described components, is essential to accomplishing good clinical outcomes for pressure ulcer prevention and management.

Case Study 18-1

Peter Douglas is a 77-year-old nursing home resident with congestive heart failure and insulin-dependent diabetes mellitus. He is alert and oriented times three and needs maximum assistance with all mobility needs. He was recently admitted to the nursing home after a 6-week hospitalization for pneumonia and congestive heart failure. When he was admitted to the nursing home, the nurse admitting Mr. Douglas documented that he had a pressure ulcer on his sacrum. She described this pressure ulcer as measuring 3 cm by 5 cm by 0 cm. The wound bed presented with 100% yellow necrotic tissue, a moderate amount of drainage, and a foul odor. He was underweight, and his albumin level was 2. He was admitted to the

nursing home for physical therapy to provide a program to improve strength, balance, and mobility after his long hospital stay. A nutritional consult and a wound consult were ordered by the physician.

Questions:

1. What factors put Mr. Douglas at greater risk of developing pressure ulcers?
2. What factors would delay wound healing for this patient?
3. What stage would you classify this wound?
4. What are the signs and symptoms of an active infection in a wound?
5. What products would you use on this type of wound?

BOX 18-7   Research Highlight

Examination of research done to describe accuracy and quality of nursing documentation of prevalence, risk factors, and prevention of pressure ulcers

Hansen and Fossum examined nursing documentation to analyze the risk factors leading to pressure ulcers and the prevention of pressure ulcers. Their goal was to compare audits of nursing documentation with patient exams in nursing home settings. Sign into your database of nursing literature (CINAHL or PubMed, for example) and use the citation below to perform a search for this article. What were the findings of this study? Why is this important to understanding the prevalence of pressure ulcers?

Hansen, R-L., & Fossum, M. (2016). Nursing documentation of pressure ulcers in nursing homes: Comparison of record content and patient examinations. *Nursing Open, 3*(3), 159–167.

Clinical Reasoning Exercises

1. Of the types of wounds discussed in this chapter, which have you seen the most of in your experience?
2. What information discussed in this chapter can you apply to your daily practice to promote skin integrity and prevent pressure ulcers?
3. What type of risk assessment tool is used at your facility? Is it helpful? Effective?

Personal Reflections

1. Have you ever cared for an older adult with a pressure ulcer? If so, what stage wound did the patient/resident have? What steps might have prevented it? How was it being treated?
2. Visit http://www.consultgerirn.com and review the clinical practice guideline on pressure ulcers. How can you apply this to your practice?
3. Look at the photographs provided in this chapter. How do you think these wounds occurred? What measures can you think of that might have prevented initial breakdown and/or subsequent deterioration of wounds?
4. According to current best practice guidelines, how would you stage a closed, black wound on a person's heel?

References

Agency for Healthcare Research and Quality. (2014). *Preventing pressure ulcers in hospitals.* Rockville, MD: Author. Retrieved from http://www.ahrq.gov/professionals/systems/hospital/pressureulcertoolkit/index.html

Black, J. M., Edsberg, L. E., Baharestani, M. M., Langemo, D., Goldberg, M., McNichol, L., . . . National Pressure Ulcer Advisory Panel. (2011). Pressure ulcers: Avoidable or unavoidable? Results of the national pressure ulcer advisory panel consensus conference. *Ostomy Wound Management, 57*(2), 24–37.

Braden, B., & Bergstrom, N. (1987). A conceptual schema for the study of the etiology of pressure sores. *Rehabilitation Nursing, 12*(1), 8–12, 16.

Bryant, R., & Nix, D. (2012). *Acute and chronic wounds: Current management concepts.* St. Louis, MO: Mosby.

Centers for Medicare and Medicaid Services. (2004). *CMS manual system.* Publication No. 100-07 State Operations. Baltimore, MD: Author.

Demling, R. H. (2009). Nutrition, anabolism, and the wound healing process: An overview. *Eplasty, 9,* e9.

Hansen, R-L., & Fossum, M. (2016). Nursing documentation of pressure ulcers in nursing homes: Comparison of record content and patient examinations. *Nursing Open, 3*(3), 159–167.

Kondracki, N. L., & Collins, N. (2009). The importance of adequate hydration. *Ostomy Wound Management, 55*(12), 16–20.

Lyder, C. H., & Ayello, E. A. (2008). Pressure ulcers: A patient safety issue. In *Patient safety and quality: An evidence-based handbook for nurses* (Agency for Healthcare Research and Quality, Publication No. 08-0043, Vol. 2). Washington, DC: U.S. Government Printing Office.

Miller, A. (2009). Hospital reporting and "Never Events." Retrieved from https://psnet.ahrq.gov/primers/primer/3/never-events

National Pressure Ulcer Advisory Panel. (2016). National Pressure Ulcer Advisory Panel (NPUAP) announces a change in terminology from pressure ulcer to pressure injury and updates the stages of pressure injury. Retrieved from http://www.npuap.org/national-pressure-ulcer-advisory-panel-npuap-announces-a-change-in-terminology-from-pressure-ulcer-to-pressure-injury-and-updates-the-stages-of-pressure-injury/

National Pressure Ulcer Advisory Panel and European Pressure Ulcer Advisory Panel. (2014). *Pressure ulcer prevention and treatment: Clinical practice guideline.* Washington, DC: Author.

Oklahoma Foundation for Medical Quality. (2009). Pressure ulcer prevention and treatment. Retrieved from http://docplayer.net/7338872-S-o-s-toolkit-for-pressure-ulcer-prevention-and-treatment-sav-e-o-kl-a-homa-s-s-k-i-n-a-systems-approach-to-quality-improvement-in-health-care.html

Salcido, R. (2012). Pressure ulcers and wound care. Retrieved from http://emedicine.medscape.com/article/319284-overview

Scalzitti, K. L. (2015). Using education and a prevention protocol tool to decrease the incidence of pressure ulcers in a nursing home. In *Evidence-Based Practice Project Reports* (Paper 69). Retrieved from http://scholar.valpo.edu/ebpr/69

Sugino, H., Hashimoto, I., Tanaka, Y., Ishida, S., Abe, Y., & Nakanishi, H. (2014). Relation between the serum albumin level and nutrition supply in patients with pressure ulcers: Retrospective study in an acute care setting. *Journal of Medical Investigation, 61*(1–2), 15–21.

VanGilder, C., Amlung, S., Harrison, P., & Meyer, S. (2009). Results of the 2008–2009 international pressure ulcer prevalence survey and a 3-year, acute care unit specific analysis. *Ostomy Wound Management, 55*(11), 39–45.

Wound, Ostomy and Continence Nurses Society. (2010). *Clinical practice guidelines for prevention and management of pressure ulcers.* Mount Laurel, NJ: Author. Retrieved from http://guideline.gov/content.aspx?id=23868

For a full suite of assignments and additional learning activities, see the access code at the front of your book.

Unit VI
Leadership and Responsibility

(COMPETENCIES 1, 11–13)

© Creativimage/Venta/Getty

CHAPTER 19

The Gerontological Nurse as Manager and Leader within the Interprofessional Team

Brenda Tyczkowski
Kristen L. Mauk
Deborah Dunn
Dawna S. Fish

(Competencies 1, 11, 13)

LEARNING OBJECTIVES

At the end of this chapter, the reader will be able to:

> Identify characteristics of effective nurse managers and leaders.
> Compare and contrast the roles of nurse manager and leader.
> Compare various leadership styles and strategies.
> Distinguish among multidisciplinary and interdisciplinary or interprofessional teams.
> Describe the roles and educational background of various team members.
> Discuss the challenges and benefits of interdisciplinary geriatric teams.
> Appreciate the unique contributions that the interprofessional geriatric team can make toward helping older adults achieve their maximal levels of independence.
> Describe effective communication strategies.
> Describe the process of delegation, including how it is used in the management of unlicensed assistive personnel.
> Compare various leadership roles available to nurses who care for older adults.
> Analyze the characteristics of the major generations of nurses.
> Recognize the value of professional associations to the nurse manager and leader.
> Evaluate one's own strengths and weaknesses as a future nurse manager or leader.

KEY TERMS

21st-century leadership
Acute care for elders
Behavior theory
Communication

Complexity leadership
Conflict resolution
Culture of safety
Delegation

Emotional intelligence

Employee retention

Geriatric assessment interdisciplinary team

Geriatric assessment team

Geriatric evaluation and management

Geriatric interdisciplinary team training

High-performance work team

Interdisciplinary team

Interprofessional team

Kotter's Change Model

Leaders

Long-term care facility

Multidisciplinary team

Nurse manager

Nurse Manager Leadership Partnership (NMLP) Learning Domain Framework

Palliative care and hospice team

Servant leadership

Standards of care

Transactional leadership

Transformational or charismatic leadership

The nursing profession has changed significantly in the past decade, with advances in technology, knowledge, and healthcare demands. Nursing is a highly skilled profession, with growing opportunities in all healthcare settings. Exciting breakthroughs in medicine occur daily, and with those breakthroughs come greater responsibilities, challenges, and competence requirements for nurses. Nurses are in constant contact with patients, caregivers, family members, and medical staff, and they play a key role in the dynamics of meeting the complex healthcare needs of older adults. In this chapter, the roles and skills of the nurse as manager and leader in settings where care is provided to older adults will be explored.

The Nurse Manager

Over the last decade, the role of the *nurse manager has* evolved from a focus on clinical expertise to one that focuses on the administrative management of a unit (McCallin & Frankson, 2010). Responsibilities now include management and leadership of unit staff, stewardship of organizational resources, and meeting clinical concerns. The span of control has increased significantly, increasing the importance of having nurse managers who are well-prepared to meet the challenges inherent in the role. Today, the role of the nurse manager is complex, ambiguous, and demanding (McCallin & Frankson, 2010).

The nurse manager is sometimes selected for the position based on his or her skill as a clinician. Nurse managers need a wider variety of skills to meet the challenges of healthcare delivery today. Trial and error is not a safe or efficient manner of becoming familiar with the role. Although it is ideal to participate in a formal development program to gain self-understanding, when this is not available, working with an experienced manager in a coaching relationship is helpful.

The *Nurse Manager Leadership Partnership (NMLP) Learning Domain Framework* (American Organization of Nurse Executives [AONE], 2006) (see **Figure 19-1**) describes essential functions of nurse managers and outlines opportunities that may be useful to achieve mastery of these functions. The framework includes three domains: (1) the leader within: creating the leader in yourself; (2) the art of leadership: leading the people; and (3) the science of leadership: managing the business.

The Leader Within: Creating the Leader in Yourself

In domain one, the new leader develops a personal understanding, gaining self-confidence and learning to trust and empower others. Specific tasks included in this domain are: (1) personal and professional accountability; (2) career planning; (3) personal journey disciplines; and (4) optimizing the leader within (AONE, 2006).

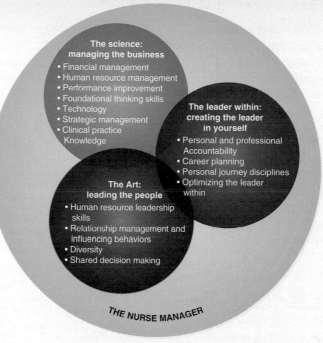

**Nurse manager leadership partnership
learning domain framework**

**The science:
managing the business**
• Financial management
• Human resource management
• Performance improvement
• Foundational thinking skills
• Technology
• Strategic management
• Clinical practice
  Knowledge

**The leader within:
creating the leader
in yourself**
• Personal and professional
  Accountability
• Career planning
• Personal journey disciplines
• Optimizing the leader
  within

**The Art:
leading the people**
• Human resource leadership
  skills
• Relationship management and
  influencing behaviors
• Diversity
• Shared decision making

THE NURSE MANAGER

Figure 19-1 Nurse Manager Leadership Partnership (NMLP) Learning Domain Framework.

A good place to start with gaining this understanding of self is to do a self-assessment. For example, the Center for Creative Leadership (CCL, n.d.) has a variety of tools to provide a baseline self-assessment. These assessments provide focus on areas that may need additional attention as the manager becomes comfortable in the new role.

New managers should set goals for themselves that will lead to growth in the role. Relationships with employees are established, and networks of peers are built. Managers develop an awareness of self, see how their actions affect the unit, and learn to find the style that is comfortable for them and works well for the unit.

The Art of Leadership: Leading the People

In the second domain, the focus is on building and leading effective teams. Specific areas include: (1) human resource leadership skills; (2) relationship management and influencing behaviors; (3) diversity; and (4) shared decision making (AONE, 2006).

Nurse managers use effective communication, conflict resolution skills, and motivation techniques to move the team beyond day-to-day conflicts (see **Case Study 19-1**). Building a *high-performance work team* is critical to providing high-quality patient care. Teams are usually comprised of high, middle, and low performers (Rushing, 2008). High-performing individuals have brilliance and drive, with the ability to propose solutions to problems. Middle performers are supportive of the team, but often lack the knowledge, expertise, or self-confidence to put solutions forward. Low performers place blame on others, fear change, and spread discontentment. Effective nurse managers will recognize the strengths, talents, and skills of each individual on the team and strive to assist each one to become an even better performer.

High performers should be encouraged to bring concerns and solutions forward. The manager can foster this by conducting rounds and interacting with the high performers, soliciting their input and offering praise

Case Study 19–1: Change and Conflict Resolution

LaShundra Keyes, Unit Manager at Jefferson Manor, announces to staff that the facility will be incorporating culture change and person-centered care within the organization. They hope to create a person-centered and homelike environment for the residents. Staff and families will support decisions made by residents regarding their own care, instead of the traditional model, in which staff directs the care and makes many decisions for residents. Resident choice and self-determination will become more meaningful.

As the change begins to take shape, the following barriers emerge:

- *Relationships:* The quality of "staff to staff" and "staff to resident/family" relationships are not adequate to sustain the change.
- *Standards and expectations:* Residents, families, coworkers, and regulators each have different expectations for care provided.
- *Motivation and vision:* Individual staff members do not share the same vision of the responsibility and relationships that need to be maintained to incorporate person-centered care.
- *Workload:* The case-mix and staffing ratios have not changed, yet staff perception is that the tasks to be accomplished have increased.
- *Respect of personhood:* Providing respect of the residents' dignity, individuality, and choice may be in conflict with facility policies designed to promote safety or encourage activity and socialization.
- *Physical environment:* Furnishings brought in by residents may be more homelike, but they also may be impractical for residents with functional or mobility limitations.

Consider the following questions:

1. What proactive measures could the unit manager have put in place to facilitate a smooth transition from the traditional model of care to person-centered care?
2. For each of the barriers, describe at least two measures that could be utilized to foster adaptation to the change.
3. Describe which skills LaShundra will need to utilize that are primarily associated with leadership versus those primarily associated with management, in successfully implementing this change.
4. What other key staff need to be involved in developing plans to move forward with the change? What should their role be?

Data from Corazzini, K., Twersky, J., White, H. K., Buhr, G. T., McConnell, E. S., Weiner, M., & Colón-Emeric, C. S. (2015). Implementing culture change in nursing homes: An adaptive leadership framework. *The Gerontologist, 55*(4), 616–627.

for proposed solutions. To encourage middle performers to become high performers, the manager needs to be visible to them, empowering them by offering support and encouragement. Low performers can be encouraged to become better performers by arranging private meetings where direct and decisive plans for improvement should be described. The plans should be attached to a specific timeline for improvement, with clear consequences for continued low improvement. Follow-up meetings should be scheduled to monitor progress (Rushing, 2008).

The Interdisciplinary Team

The benefit of a geriatric *interdisciplinary team* (IDT), or *interprofessional team*, centers on the ability to deliver patient-centered care, which takes into account the whole person, the context in which they find themselves, and their presenting concerns (see **Table 19-1**). Because the professionals on a geriatric team have advanced

TABLE 19-1   Potential Members of Geriatric IDTs

Discipline	Education/Certification/Licensure	Roles in Gerontology	Web Resource
Audiologist	Master's degree Certificate of clinical competence National examination	Hearing assessment, including audiometric studies, evoked potentials, and other diagnostic procedures, and treatment of hearing loss	American Speech-Language-Hearing Association (ASHA) http://www.asha.org/
Caregiver		Varying degrees of expertise	National Family Caregivers Association http://www.nfcacares.org/ Caregiver Support http://www.agingcare.com/Caregiver-Support
Chaplain (title based on religion: priest, rabbi, parish nurse, minister, etc.)	Education varies depending on requirements of religion and requirements of institution	Provide support to the client/patient, family, and others as it relates to spiritual needs May assist in identifying resources from within congregation for support, visitation, or respite	Association of Professional Chaplains http://www.professionalchaplains.org/ Center for Aging and Spirituality http://www.spirituality4aging.org/
Client/patient	Life experience	Expert in their experience	
Dietician	Bachelor's degree Internship National examination	Assess nutritional status and implementation of a nutritional plan	Gerontological Nutritionists http://www.gndpg.org
Geriatrician	Licensed medical physician with fellowship (2 years) in gerontology after medical internship and residency Board certification	Use knowledge of normal aging as part of assessment Specialize in the diagnosis and treatment of the elderly	The American Geriatric Society http://www.americangeriatrics.org
Advanced practice adult-gerontology Primary Care Nurse Practitioner (AGPCNP) Adult-gerontology Acute Care Nurse Practitioner (AGACNP)	Master's degree as an adult-gerontology nurse practitioner National certification State licensure May also be prepared at the Doctor of Nursing Practice level with same certification and licensure requirements	Provide primary care, including history and physical, chronic disease management **Note:** Adult nurse practitioners, family nurse practitioners, and palliative nursing practitioners also may have a role in geriatrics	Gerontological Advanced Practice Nurses Association http://www.gapna.org

(continues)

TABLE 19-1   Potential Members of Geriatric IDTs (*continued*)

Discipline	Education/Certification/ Licensure	Roles in Gerontology	Web Resource
Advanced practice adult-gerontological Clinical Nurse Specialist (AGCNS)	Master's degree as an adult-gerontology Clinical Nurse Specialist National certification State licensure May also be prepared at the Doctor of Nursing Practice level with same certification and licensure	Provides advanced care for older adults, their families, and significant others in a variety of settings **Note:** Adult health, public, and community CNS may have a role in geriatric care	National Association of Clinical Nurse Specialists http://www .nacns.org National Gerontological Nursing Association https://www.ngna.org
Occupational Therapist	Master's degree as an occupational therapist National certification State licensure Specialty certification in gerontology May also be prepared as a Doctor of Occupational Therapy	Assess and treat functional, sensory, and perceptual deficits that have an impact on ADLs Assess need for assistive devices Assess and treat cognitive deficits Rehabilitative services in geropsychiatrics	American Occupational Therapy Association http://www.aota.org
Physical Therapist	DPT (Doctor of Physical Therapy) transitioning from MPT (Master of Physical Therapy) Licensure examination Specialty certification in gerontology is available State licensure	Assessment of mobility and functional capacity of the elderly Treatment includes rehabilitation, strengthening, mobility, and use of assistive devices	American Physical Therapy Association: Section on Geriatrics http://geriatricspt.org
Pharmacist	Pharm D, 4 years beyond prerequisite 2 years National examination NABPLEX State licensure required Certification available as geriatric pharmacotherapy	Preparation and dispensation of medication Clinical consultation and education for patient and geriatric team	American Society of Consultant Pharmacists V Commission for Certification in Geriatric Pharmacy http://www .ccgp.org/
Physician	Professional doctorate with a degree in allopathic or osteopathic medicine Medical degree with residency and board certification in psychiatry State licensure	Dependent on the area of residency, specialty focus is on the area/disease process as it relate to aging	

Discipline	Education/Certification/ Licensure	Roles in Gerontology	Web Resource
Physician Assistant	Two-year education, usually post-bachelor's degree State licensure	Midlevel practitioner	American Academy of Physician Assistants http://www.aapa.org
Psychiatrist	Medical degree with residency and board certification in psychiatry State Licensure	Geropsychiatry evaluation, treatment, and management of mental health issues faced by the elderly Includes pharmacotherapy evaluation of cognition, and psychotherapy	American Association for Geriatric Psychiatry http://www.aagponline .org
Psychologist	Graduate education, usually at the PhD or PsyD level State licensure	Geropsychology assessment, consultation, intervention, and management of conditions related to adaptation, bereavement, counseling, and treatment for clinical cognitive and behavioral needs	Society of Clinical Geropsychology http:// www.geropsychology.org/
Registered Nurse	Associate degree, diploma, or bachelor's degree National Board examination NCLEX Optional certification in gerontology State licensure	Assessment, planning, providing, coordinating, and evaluating care, which focuses on health, optimal wellness, disease prevention, and advocacy	Hartford Geriatric Nursing Initiative http:// www.hgni.org/ National Gerontological Nursing Association http://www.ngna.org/
Social Worker	Bachelor's degree in social work (LSW) Master's degree in social work (MSW) State licensure	Assist with coping and problem solving as individuals and families adjust and face changes with aging and chronic illness Provide counseling and psychotherapy	National Association of Social Workers http:// www.naswdc.org Geriatric Social Work Initiative http://www .gswi.org/
Speech–Language Pathologist	Master's degree and clinical fellowship (CFY) State licensure	Assessment and treatment of communication disorders, which include speech, language, hearing, swallowing, and cognitive deficits	American Speech-Language-Hearing Association (ASHA) http://www.asha.org/

knowledge of aging, chronic illness, and disease, as well as functional loss prevention, the older adults they treat receive a more comprehensive approach to their care. Satisfaction is increased through the inclusion of the patient or caregiver in the assessment as well as the planning and goal setting. Improvements in quality and continuity of care, better health outcomes, and lower costs are also seen when geriatric IDTs are used (Montagnini et al., 2014).

From a professional standpoint, the benefits include shared values, goals, and responsibilities for the care of older adults. The opportunity to work together and learn from one another has the potential for growth of the team members within the specialty. Another advantage to working in IDTs is the development of new skills in communication, collaboration, negotiation, conflict resolution, and time management as one gains comfort working within the IDT.

The potential for time saving and increased productivity is also part of a team effort. The time saving relates not only to the patient but also to the professional who does not need to wait for consultations, avoids duplication of assessment information, and maintains an understanding of what resources are available within the IDT. An increase in productivity occurs through team meetings, versus individual contacts, with all involved in the assessment or treatment of a patient.

> ### CLINICAL TIP
>
> Older adults are best cared for by an interprofessional team of experts working together.

There are a variety of types of teams providing care for older adults. **Table 19-2** provides an overview of several.

Specific strategies that are useful to foster improved teamwork among all unit staff include establishing a common goal for the team (Vogelsmeier & Scott-Cawiezell, 2011), conducting briefings for staff, and using team huddles to ensure that the lines of communication are open. In order to have effective communication, staff members need to trust the manager. When the manager seeks out staff members' opinions, the staff feel valued and empowered and trust is established (Vogelsmeier & Scott-Cawiezell, 2011).

Conflict is a struggle for power or property or a strong disagreement between people that may lead to an argument. *Conflict resolution* is often an uncomfortable task for new managers, though it is a task that is essential to the functioning of the unit. When faced with conflict, new managers often use avoidance, body language, or unprofessional behaviors. Instead, managers need to recognize that staff are often ill-equipped to deal with conflict too. Rather than addressing this deficit, it is often easier to step in and take care of the problem. Another strategy sometimes employed, usually unsuccessfully, is to direct staff to work out the problems for themselves. Instead, invite staff to participate in the development of ground rules for acceptable and unacceptable behavior on the unit. Staff then need to be provided with education regarding the expectation for dealing with these behaviors (Cohen, 2014). When dealing with conflict, the manager should focus on mutual goals among the team and encourage collaborative decision making to move the team beyond the conflict (Case 19-1).

Relationship management, described in the second domain, includes fostering a *culture of safety* within the unit. In a unit with a blame-free culture, there is an assumption that errors spring up as a result of problems within a system. On the other end of the spectrum is a punitive culture, in which errors are blamed on individuals. When there is a culture of safety, there is middle ground between these two ends of the spectrum, with a balance between them (Hebling & Huwe, 2015).

The composition of teams providing care for older adults may include staff with a wide variety of educational preparation and skill development, ranging from registered nurses (RNs), to certified nursing assistants (CNAs), to unlicensed assistive personnel (UAP), such as medication aides. The RN is responsible for safely delegating care to appropriate members of the team. In 2005, the National Council of State Boards of Nursing (NCSBN) and American Nurses Association (ANA) (2005) issued a joint statement on *delegation*, defining delegation as "the

TABLE 19-2   Types of Geriatric Teams

Type of Team		Features
Acute care for elders	ACE	Inpatient unit, staffed with geriatric specialists.
Geriatric assessment interdisciplinary team	GAIT	Project funded by the University System of Maryland to introduce students to "comprehensive geriatric assessment and the fundamentals of interprofessional collaboration, through both didactic and clinical sessions" (GAIT, n.d.)
Geriatric assessment team	GAT	Geriatric consultation teams vary with the purpose of the consultation and may occur in an in-patient or out-patient setting. The emphasis of the consultation may be on activities of daily living (ADLs), home assessment, and the etiology of the functional changes.
Geriatric evaluation and management	GEM	In-patient unit, staffed with **multidisciplinary team** with geriatric expertise. Includes in-patient rehabilitation unit as well as acute care unit. It includes the following components: specialized environment, patient-centered care, medical review, and interdisciplinary care (Deschodt, Flamaing, Haentjens, Boonen, & Milisen, 2013)
Geriatric interdisciplinary team training	GITT	GITT is a resource of the Hartford Institute for Geriatric Nursing (HIGN). This is a formal initiative, created in 1995, to improve care of older adults by enhancing the interdisciplinary training of health profession students and professionals (HIGN, 2015)
Interdisciplinary team	IDT	Team members from various disciplines working mutually and reciprocally, pooling their knowledge to achieve the common goal of providing high-quality care. Formal structures, such as shared decision making and conflict resolution processes are typically used (Chamberlin-Salaun, Mills, & Usher, 2013)
Multidisciplinary team	MDT	Team members from various disciplines working parallel to each other to provide care. Information is shared, but formal processes are not necessarily used (Chamberlin-Salaun, et al., 2013)
Palliative care and hospice team		Goal is to optimize care of older adults with advanced multiple, chronic, and progressive illness. Emphasis on interdisciplinary care and care coordination (McCormick, 2012). May take place in a variety of settings, ranging from the patient's home, to a nursing home, to an in-patient hospice unit.

process for a nurse to direct another person to perform nursing tasks and activities" (p. 1). Steps to the delegation process include (see **Figure 19-2**): (1) assessment of the patient, the staff, and the context of the situation; (2) communication to provide direction and opportunity for interaction during the completion of the delegated task; (3) surveillance and monitoring to assure compliance with standards of practice, policies, and procedures; and (4) evaluation to consider the effectiveness of the delegation and whether the desired patient outcome was attained (ANA, 2012; NCSBN & ANA, 2005) (see **Case Study 19-2**).

In order to safely delegate a task, the nurse needs to be familiar with the certification, educational preparation, and skill level of the staff member to whom they are delegating a task. Asking questions of the staff member about the task, seeking clarification of their knowledge about the task, or requesting a return demonstration of the task prior to delegating are all good ways of determining if a task can be safely delegated to a specific team member

Delegation Process

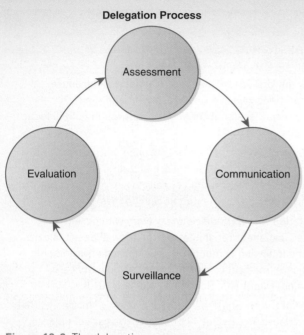

Figure 19-2 The delegation process.

Data from National Council of State Boards of Nursing. (2005b). Working with others: A position paper. Retrieved from https://www.ncsbn.org/Working_with_Others.pdf

(NCSBN, 2005a). **Box 19-1** outlines the "Five Rights of Delegation."

Though the nurse practice acts vary from state to state, RNs should be aware that in most states licensed practical nurses (LPNs) do not independently develop the plan of care, make changes in the plan of care, or perform telephone triage (NCSBN, 2005a). Therefore, these duties may not be delegated to them (Case Study 19-2).

The use of UAP provides an additional delegation challenge for RNs in the long-term care setting. The NCSBN (2005a) found significant variation from state to state with regard to the educational preparation of and roles for UAP. In some states, UAP pass medications, while in others they do not; when states do allow UAP to pass medications, they do receive some training, but this also varies greatly from one state to another. If UAP will be passing medications, the RN is responsible for ensuring that the UAP is competent enough to do so, because it is a complex process that holds the potential for serious complications if not completed safely.

Case Study 19–2: Nursing Management and Delegation

Ms. Brown, RN, is the night charge nurse for an in-patient geriatric rehabilitation unit with 30 beds in a small acute-care hospital. She is making her nightly assignments and finds that she has herself, one LPN, and two CNAs to care for 28 patients with relatively high acuity. Ms. Brown does not feel this staffing is adequate, because the evening charge nurse reported that one of the patients was receiving a blood transfusion and might need to be transferred to intensive care, and another patient was complaining of atypical shortness of breath, so tests were being run to determine the cause. The LPN is experienced, but one of the CNAs is still in orientation to the night shift and has little experience.

Questions:

1. What is Ms. Brown's best course of action?
2. If she feels she needs more help to provide high-quality care to her patients, whom should she contact?
3. What should she do if told no more help is available?
4. What is the most assertive response in this situation?
5. How should Ms. Brown divide assignments between herself and the LPN? Between the CNAs?
6. Is there a certain nursing model of care that might work better than another in this situation?
7. How should Ms. Brown apply the delegation process to this situation?

> **BOX 19-1   The Five Rights of Delegation**
>
> 1. Right task
> 2. Right circumstance
> 3. Right person
> 4. Right direction/communication
> 5. Right supervision
>
> Data from National Council of State Boards of Nursing. (2016). National guidelines for nursing delegation. *Journal of Nursing Regulation, 7*(1), 5–14; National Council of State Boards of Nursing. (2005b). Working with others: A position paper. Retrieved from https://www.ncsbn.org/Working_with_Others.pdf

> **CLINICAL TIP**
>
> Managers handle the day-to-day operations of the unit or facility.

It is the manager's responsibility to provide sufficient resources for care, such as adequate staff members, and to set up systems and policies that foster appropriate delegation. Some nursing functions may not be delegated; these include assessment, planning, evaluation, and nursing judgment (NCSBN, 2005a). The principle of patient safety must be the behind every delegated act.

Another role of the nurse manager, included in the second domain of the NMLP (AONE, 2006), is to provide intentional acknowledgement of the work and contributions of staff to the unit. Staff members need to feel valued and respected by the manager. Specific strategies range from a simple thank you, to providing rewards to celebrate achievements, to nominating staff for awards.

The Science of Leadership: Managing the Business

The third domain in the NMLP focuses on developing effective business practices for the unit. Specific competencies include: (1) financial management; (2) human resource management; (3) performance improvement; (4) foundational thinking skills; (5) technology; (6) strategic management; and (7) clinical practice knowledge (AONE, 2006).

Staff members are being asked to do more, with fewer resources. The manager needs to understand how to provide high-quality care in an efficient manner in their unit. One of the most important aspects of this is having a clear understanding of how staffing decisions impact the financial stability and health of the organization as a whole. Managers need to become familiar with the graphs and reports used within the organization to monitor budgets. To facilitate this, it is helpful for the manager to find someone in the organization to serve as a budget-specific coach.

There are many tasks often specifically associated with the role of nurse manager; outlines some of these tasks. The role and responsibilities charged to the nurse manager are varied and complex, requiring many skills. The nurse manager balances the needs of the patients, unit staff, and the overall organization with the provision of safe, high-quality care. Although many aspects of the manager's role are skill-focused, the effective manager will also exhibit the qualities of a leader.

The Nurse Leader

"Management is doing things right; leadership is doing the right things" (Drucker, n.d.). This implies that there are subtle differences between the roles of managers and leaders. Kotter International's *Change Leadership Model* (n.d.) describes managers as those who "make systems of people and technology work well day after day, week after week, year after year" (p. 1) and *leaders* as those who create the systems that managers manage and changes

BOX 19-2   Comparisons between Managers and Leaders

Managers	Leaders
Administer	Innovate
Ask how and when	Ask what and why
Focus on systems	Focus on people
Do things right	Do the right things
Maintain	Develop
Rely on control	Inspire trust
Short-term perspective	Long-term perspective
Accept status quo	Challenge status quo
Have eye on the bottom line	Have eye on the horizon
Imitate	Originate
Classic "good soldiers"	Own person
A copy	The original

Data from Bennis, W. (1989). *On becoming a leader*. New York, NY: Addison-Wesley.

them in fundamental ways to take advantage of opportunities and to avoid hazards (p. 1). Bennis (1989) provides comparisons between managers and leaders, which appear in **Box 19-2**.

Leadership is the "ability to effectively move a group of people to successfully achieve the mission and vision of the organization" (American Health Care Association and National Center for Assisted Living [AHCA/NCAL], n.d., p. 1). Effective management requires leadership skills, and effective leadership requires management skills. However, leaders tend to be visionaries who focus on the larger picture, whereas managers focus on day-to-day operations. Managers are appointed, but leaders arise from within a group.

The AHCA and NCAL (2009) describes long-term care leaders as the central resource for staff, residents, and families integral to providing high-quality care. **Box 19-3** describes seven major roles and the competencies associated with leaders, which are explored in more depth here.

Leader

The first role described by AHCA and NCAL (2009) is that of leader. The effective leader is able to develop and articulate a clear vision of the future of the organization. To achieve this, the leader must be able to create a mental picture of the vision that can be easily communicated to others. For example, the Healthy People (n.d.) "About Healthy People" is committed to the vision of a "society in which all people live long, healthy lives." This simple, yet descriptive, statement allows a vision of the future to be easily seen. This vision is translated into strategies or processes, which are designed to turn the vision into action. When the vision is successfully conveyed, all members of the organization know how their role fits the vision of the organization (Baker & Orton, 2010).

Merely passing on the vision is not enough. Heuston and Wolf (2011) describe inspiring a shared vision as the "ability to get staff nurses engaged in aligning the vision of their unit to that of the [facility]" (p. 248). To achieve this, they indicate that the nurse leader should encourage others to join in spreading the vision, discuss with staff any potential barriers to this, and solicit their ideas for improvement. Leaders should present changes with enthusiasm and spend time explaining to staff why changes need to occur. Communication about proposed changes should occur early in the process, so staff has time to absorb the changes.

BOX 19-3   Leader Roles and Associated Competencies

Role	Associated Competencies
1. Leader	The leader models, advocates, communicates, and leads in creating systems, processes, and programs all within the focus of the facility/organizational mission and vision.
2. Performance Improvement Catalyst	Acts as a catalyst to systematically analyze and evaluate performance, design and implement strategies, and empower staff toward performance improvement.
3. Interpersonal Relations Facilitator	Models healthy communications, interacts sensitively, and promotes cooperative behaviors.
4. Human Resources Developer	Develops strategies to recruit and retain, coaches, ensures high-quality education/training, and ensures meaningful work to maximize job satisfaction of the facility's human resources.
5. Resource and Finance Manager	Budgets, manages resources, and monitors revenues and expenses to optimize available resources and finances.
6. Standards and Compliance Expert Resource	Is a regulatory (expert) resource, institutes proactive strategies to meet and exceed standards, and ensures meeting ongoing compliance standards and *high standards of care*.
7. Customer Service Advocate	Is continually customer-focused, builds and maintains trust relationships, initiates/seeks satisfaction feedback, and implements/evaluates improvement in customer services.

Modified from American Health Care Association, & National Center for Assisted Living [AHCA/NCAL]. (2009). Leadership excellence. Retrieved from http://www.ahcancal.org/quality_improvement/leadership_excellence/Documents/Section2-RolesAndCompetencies.pdf

BOX 19-4   Kotter's Change Management Model

Phase 1—Creating a climate for change
- Increase urgency
- Build guiding teams
- Get the vision right

Phase 2—Engaging and enabling the whole organization
- Communicate for buy-in
- Enable action
- Create short-term wins

Phase 3—Implementing and sustaining the change
- Do not let up
- Make it stick

Data from Campbell, R. J. (2008). Change management in healthcare. *The Health Care Manager, 27*(1), 23–39.

Utilizing a change management model can help plan for a successful transition through the change process. Kotter's Change Model, described by Campbell (2008), helps leaders generate positive feelings among employees toward the change. It also allows leaders instill feelings of action in employees' hearts, by helping them to envision the problem and identify solutions to the problem (Campbell, 2008). Kotter's Change Model is seen in **Box 19-4**.

Performance Improvement Catalyst

The second role is that of "performance improvement catalyst" (AHCA/NCAL, 2009). Improvements in quality of care have been noted when staff have been empowered, feel engaged in decision making, and are satisfied in their work (Brody, Barnes, Ruble, & Sakowski, 2012). One way that leaders can facilitate these outcomes is through a shared governance structure. This type of structure gives staff nurses control over practice-related decision making. It also holds them accountable for high-quality patient outcomes. Shared governance often includes the development and support of staff-led councils. Brody et al. (2012) found that council members had a greater sense of ownership in the organization and pride in their work. Staff also reported an increase in the meaningfulness of their work and a heightened sense of the impact they had on the organization. Empowerment through staff nurse-led councils also positively affected job satisfaction, trust in management, labor relations, turnover, and commitment to the organization.

Like managers, leaders need to foster a culture of resident safety, in which a commitment to safety permeates the organization. Open discussion of errors, without fear of reprisal, should occur. Process improvements are ongoing, and system issues can be discussed without fear of attack or criticism. In addition, there is an expectation that there will be compliance with established procedures. Common safety-related concerns in the population of frail elders include medication errors, falls, pressure ulcers, and urinary tract infections (Arnetz et al., 2011).

Interpersonal Relations Facilitator

Leaders need to be an interpersonal relations facilitator, according to AHCA and NCAL (2009). Effective leaders "tune in" to the needs of individual employees, recognizing the contributions they make to providing high-quality care. This is accomplished using a guiding and nurturing approach to communication with employees. The use of keen listening skills, soliciting feedback from employees, and eliminating communication barriers facilitate creating an environment in which staff voices are heard (Harvarth et al., 2008). Effective nurse leaders are visible to staff, creating opportunities for one-to-one interaction and holding regular meetings to discuss care issues.

Nursing leaders spend considerable time crafting effective messages, using high-quality care as a cornerstone to convey the need for action (Keys, 2011). They distance themselves from their own emotions, viewing situations objectively and from various perspectives. Leaders must be persistent in keeping a message alive (see **Box 19-5**). Messages must be delivered with presence and confidence in order to be effective.

Nurse leaders must set professional *communication* standards and then role model these standards in their interactions with others. Examples of these standards include responding quickly to staff questions and following up on concerns. Nonverbal messages are also sent to staff when nurse leaders answer call lights, pick up trash, and present a calm demeanor when dealing with others (Heuston & Wolf, 2011).

Human Resources Developer

The next role of the leader described by AHCA and NCAL (2009) is that of human resource developer. *Employee retention* has become even more crucial in the long-term care environment. In 2010, estimates of turnover rates continued to be very high. The rate for RNs was 62.8%, LPNs 43%, and CNAs (55%) (Trinkoff et al., 2013). Turnover of staff has been associated with higher hospitalization rates for infections, declines in ADLs, and problems with physical restraint use, catheter use, pressure ulcers, and pain management (Trinkoff et al., 2013).

Shifting demographics and workforce demands lead to the prediction that additional nurses will be needed. Brody et al. (2012) noted the potential to empower, engage, and satisfy nurses through the formation of staff-led evidence-based practice (EBP) councils. By giving nurses a voice in the implementation of EBP findings, there is potential to improve quality outcomes and reduce turnover.

BOX 19-5   Evidence-Based Practice Highlight

Consistent Assignments

As many organizations move toward delivering person-centered care, one intervention they often include is that of consistent assignments of staff to residents. It is thought that this provides the opportunity for staff and residents to develop a deeper bond and know each other better, thereby improving the delivery of care.

Roberts, Nolet, and Bowers (2015) reviewed 20 original research reports related to consistent assignments in nursing homes, with surprising results. There was little consistency in the definition of "consistent assignment" among the homes in the study. Each operationalized the concept differently, making it difficult to draw conclusions about the impact.

Despite these limitations, consistent assignments resulted in positive resident outcomes in these areas: better hygiene, improved relationships among staff and residents, a decrease in negative behavior, and improvement in care outcomes such as decreased incidence of pressure ulcers, higher satisfaction with care, improved affect, increased participation in social activities, and enhanced choice and control. Staff reported no change in satisfaction, turnover, or absenteeism. At the organizational level, it was difficult to sustain the consistent assignments due to unbalanced workloads and unavailability of staff to cover off-shifts (Roberts et al., 2015, p. 443)

The study concluded that additional study on the topic is needed before conclusions about the benefits of consistent assignments should be drawn.

Food for Thought

1. As a manager and leader, would you undertake consistent assignments as part of a change toward person-centered care? What factors would you consider in this decision?
2. If you do move forward with implementing consistent assignments, what measures would be meaningful in knowing whether this has been a successful change? How will you monitor the change?

Data from Roberts, T., Nolet, K., & Bowers, B. (2015). Consistent assignments of nursing staff to residents in nursing homes: A critical review of conceptual and methodological issues. *The Gerontologist, 55*(3), 434–437.

Although adequate pay is a factor in turnover, employee retention is enhanced when leaders create satisfying work environments. To achieve this, the leader needs to help employees to feel valued, acknowledged, challenged, and engaged in unit decision making (Utley, Anderson, & Atwell, 2011).

These findings were echoed by those of Tourangeau, Cranley, Spence Laschinger, and Pachis (2010), who found that staff turnover was tied to psychological and global empowerment, as well as perceived organizational support. These are all areas over which the leader has the ability to exert influence. When an employee identifies with and feels accepted as a member of a work group, this leads to increased job satisfaction and retention. Sponsoring celebrations and social events are one way to accomplish this. Opportunities for ongoing education also can foster workgroup cohesion. Leaders can foster feelings of personal accomplishment among the staff by recognizing and rewarding employee accomplishments, which is just one method of addressing staff turnover.

Burnout, which is a state of physical, emotional, and psychological exhaustion, also leads to job turnover. Another prevalent cause of burnout is bullying by staff (Allen, Holland, & Reynolds, 2015).

Emotional exhaustion is detrimental to job satisfaction. Finding ways to make sure that staff takes their coffee and meal breaks can prevent emotional exhaustion and boost feelings of satisfaction (Tourangeau et al., 2010). The work environment should also assist employees to find a better quality of work–life balance (Curtis & O'Connell, 2011).

Resource and Financial Manager

An important leader role is that of resource and financial manager (AHCA & NCAL, 2009). In these difficult economic times, the focus in health care has been leaning toward doing more with less. The nurse leader's role is crucial to maintaining a balance between high-quality care and cost-effective care. This is achieved by setting the right goals for the organization and motivating others to achieve the goals (Goetz, Janney, & Ramsey, 2011). As funding cuts continue to occur, it takes thoughtful planning, adequate resources, support, innovation, and strong partnerships among nursing, finance, administration, and medical leaders to bring about achievement of financial goals while maintaining safe and high-quality care (Valentine, Kirby, & Wolf, 2011).

In most healthcare facilities, salary and benefits for nurses and UAP make up the largest portion of the budget, which puts nursing at the center of most budget decisions. Nursing is ultimately responsible for identifying, developing, and implementing plans to meet annual productivity forecasts. These plans are achieved through accountability for outcomes at all levels in the nursing department. Expectations must be clearly communicated to nursing staff, and nurses must know that their role is essential to the provision of high-quality care and to the achievement of financial viability of the entire organization. In order for staff to "buy in" to the financial goals, the nurse leader must be able to clearly articulate not only what needs to be achieved, but why it is important (Goetz et al., 2011).

Progress toward goals must be frequently reviewed with staff, so their contributions may be acknowledged. If goals are not being met, plans are revisited by the nurse leader and alterations to the work plan may be made.

Standards and Compliance Expert Resource

Leaders are responsible for acting as standards and compliance expert resources (AHCA & NCAL, 2009). Although this responsibility is present in many healthcare settings, it is of particular importance in the long-term care and assisted living settings. Health care is highly regulated in these industries, and facilities providing this care undergo frequent regulatory oversight reviews, which can be in the form of survey visits or other monitoring efforts by the state and federal governments. A variety of federal and state regulations are in place to ensure that minimum standards of safe care are provided.

For example, nursing homes must be in compliance with over 180 federal regulations at all times (Centers for Medicare and Medicaid Services [CMS], n.d.). State survey agencies regularly inspect facilities to ensure compliance. Health inspections consist of a review of the care of residents and processes used to give care, how the staff and residents interact, and the overall nursing home environment. The second component of inspections is the fire safety inspection, which ensures compliance with the Life Safety Code standards and the National Fire Protection Agency standards (CMS, n.d.). If the facility does not meet the standards of the health or Life Safety Code inspections, a deficiency citation is issued. This may result in fines or denial of payment for new admissions whose payer source is Medicare or Medicaid until the deficiency has been remedied.

CLINICAL TIP

Leaders see the big picture and compel others to follow their vision.

Leaders need to create a culture of compliance, comprises three components (Abell, 2011). The first is the development and implementation of policies and procedures that reinforce compliance with the regulations. Second, it is important to maintain an awareness of quality-of-care issues, through a rigorous quality compliance program—Abell (2011) points out that "you never want to be in a situation where the government is discovering things before you are" (p. 36). The final component of a culture of compliance is an effective training program, designed to reinforce compliance in areas of potential concern.

Customer Service Advocate

Leaders serve as customer service advocates, according to AHCA and NCAL (2009). The key to customer service is maintaining a proactive, rather than a reactive, position. Anticipating patients' needs instead of waiting for them to arise sets this proactive tone. When you go beyond the expected, providing exceptional care, customer loyalty is built (Basom, 2012). Making regular contact with patients and their family is crucial to building trusting relationships. This allows them the opportunity to express concerns, if there are any. Lack of communication is one of the biggest customer dissatisfiers in health care (Abbott-Shultz, 2010). Making regular rounds to engage with patients and their families is an important task for the leader.

Staff members also need to be on board with a proactive stance toward customer service. Empowering staff to make decisions related to customer service goes a long way in making this happen. A feeling of "family" needs to be established among the patients, families, and staff. By allowing staff to make customer service decisions at the bedside, instead of through the bureaucratic structure of the facility, a quick resolution to concerns can be achieved, which is important to patients and their families.

Keys to customer satisfaction include doing things right the first time, welcoming and encouraging complaints, and apologizing for the issue and for any inconvenience (Abbott-Shultz, 2010). A satisfied patient or family member will be a wonderful advocate for the facility, drawing more potential patients to the organization. On the other hand, a dissatisfied patient can drag an organization down, particularly when that person is spreading concerns out in the community.

Leadership Qualities and Theories
Qualities of Effective Leaders

Although no one can possess every quality of an effective leader, he or she should be able to demonstrate most of them. Effective leaders maintain an awareness of these qualities and strive to grow and gain knowledge in any areas in which they may identify weaknesses.

There are numerous leadership theories that are useful for nurse leaders. Sometimes an organization may embrace a specific theory and expect that all staff use this theory as a basis for relationships and decision making. At other times, a leader may be free to select whatever theory is comfortable for them. This chapter takes a look at some of the more widely used leadership theories.

Transactional Leadership

Transactional leadership has been described as "you scratch my back, I'll scratch yours" (National Research Council [NRC], 2003, p. 110). Leaders and followers exchange economic, political, or physical items of value, which ties them loosely together. Sims (2009) indicates that an individual employee's strengths are identified and a system of rewards and punishments is established by the leader. The ties between the leader and the employee are loose at best, and relationships are superficial. Transactional leaders may exhibit behaviors associated with management-by-exception, where action is taken only after problems occur or mistakes are made. They intervene only when issues are obvious, seeking to maintain the status quo (Gardner, 2010). When transactional leadership is used, control is maintained at the top of the hierarchy (Weberg, 2010).

Behavior Theory

Behavior theory comprises four types of leadership styles (Sims, 2009). Unique behaviors are associated with each style.

The first style is autocratic; it is sometimes known as *authoritarian* style. These leaders make most of the decisions, with little decision-making authority being extended to the followers. The authoritarian leader is generally viewed as aloof or impersonal (Lewin, Lippitt, & White, 1939). Under this style of leadership, efficiency is foremost. These leaders need to be highly confident and competent in their skills.

The second style is bureaucratic leadership. Bureaucratic leaders expect that rules will be followed at all times. They value structure and uniformity. Bureaucratic leaders focus attention on irregularities and mistakes.

Participative, or democratic leaders, allow others to have input into decision making and problem solving. The leader is perceived as objective and focused on facts (Lewin et al., 1939). In this style, the decision-making process is time-consuming and the leader must be willing to give up control over decisions.

Free rein, or laissez-faire, style of leadership centers on the concept that employees are able to set their own goals or tasks, with minimal interference from the leader. These leaders offer little direction or support to employees, appearing indifferent to their needs. Laissez-faire leaders avoid making decisions and often refuse to take sides in disputes (Gardner, 2010).

The final model drawn from behavioral theories is situational leadership. The premise is that there is no one single leadership style that is appropriate for every situation, so a leader needs to draw from several styles, depending on the situation at hand. Situational leaders identify the needs of the job, determine successful ways of dealing with people to meet these needs, and then select a leadership style that will match the needs of the organization with the abilities of the staff. Situational leaders use directing, coaching, supporting, and delegating behaviors to be flexible in the style they select to meet the needs of the organization (Lynch, McCormack, & McCance, 2011).

21st Century Leadership

As we transition from an industrial age to a "sociotechnical age," leaders need to rethink their approach to *21st Century leadership*, adopting new strategies to meet the changing scene in health care (Porter-O'Grady & Malloch, 2009). There is an emerging need for visionary leaders who can facilitate innovation and change within the organization.

Transformational or Charismatic Leadership

The landmark work by the Institute of Medicine (IOM) (National Research Council [NRC], 2003) indicates that transformational leaders "seek to engage individuals in the recognition and pursuit of a commonly held goal—in this case, patient safety" (p. 111). Transformational leaders seek to attain a collective goal for the organization, rather than a series of potentially disjointed goals, as found in translational leadership. Transformational leaders stimulate innovative thinking and transform followers' beliefs. They understand the need for change in the organization and clearly communicate the vision to achieve the change. In doing so, they motivate and empower the followers to commit to the vision (Curtis & O'Connell, 2011). Emphasis is placed on inspirational messages, moral values, individual attention, and intellectual stimulation (Avolio, Walumbwa, & Weber, 2009).

Many transformational leaders display characteristics of *emotional intelligence* (EI). EI is the ability to motivate one's self, control impulses, regulate moods, and to empathize with others. Components include stress management, decision making, interpersonal skills, self-expression, and self-perception. Tyczkowski et al. (2015) found a significant positive relationship between EI and transformational leadership styles of nurse managers. *Transformational or charismatic leadership* has been particularly useful in the long-term care environment. According to Utley et al. (2011), improved resident outcomes, such as a reduction in falls and pressure ulcers, has been shown in institutions with transformative leaders. Employees felt valued and empowered in their work; the work environment was perceived as more positive, resulting in greater job satisfaction. In particular, CNAs were more likely to stay employed at the facility. Residents also reported increased satisfaction with the quality of life. In facilities in which leaders used transformational leadership, effective communication techniques, teamwork, leadership, and quality of care were stressed. Weberg (2010) found that transformational leadership created a healthy work environment. Improved employee satisfaction and reduced staff turnover rates were noted in the acute care setting. **Table 19-3** displays characteristics of transformational leaders.

Servant Leadership

Robert K. Greenleaf, the founder of the servant leadership movement, describes *servant leadership* as "the servant-leader is servant first. . . . It begins with the natural feeling that one wants to serve, to serve first. Then

TABLE 19-3   Characteristics of Transformational Leaders

Inspire a Shared Vision
- Clearly articulate the vision
- Discuss barriers to change and solicit ideas for improvement
- Explain why changes are needed
- Communicate regularly about proposed plans, so changes are not as surprising to staff

Model the Way
- Model enthusiasm and optimism to employees
- Provide frequent feedback and recognition
- Praise good communication and teamwork
- Promote employee independence and empowerment
- Encourage employees to do their best

Challenge the Process
- Challenge the norm when indicated
- Encourage staff development by encouraging creativity, problem solving, and learning
- Acknowledge the importance of employees' knowledge and skills

Enable Others to Act
- Be visible and approachable
- Demonstrate competency and integrity
- Coach and mentor, give staff the tools for the job, but do not do the work for them

Encourage the Heart
- Get to know employees and create feelings of being cared about as a person
- Create opportunities to succeed
- Show concern for employees' needs

Data from Utley, R., Anderson, R., & Atwell, J. (2011). Implementing transformational leadership in long-term care. *Geriatric Nursing, 32*(3), 212–219; Heuston, M. M., & Wolf, G. A. (2011). Transformational leadership skills of successful nurse managers. *Journal of Nursing Administration, 41*(6), 248–251; Schwartz, D. B., Spencer, T., Wilson, B., & Wood, K. (2011). Transformational leadership: Implications for nursing leaders in facilities seeking Magnet® designation. *AORN Journal, 93*(6), 737–748.

conscious choice brings one to aspire to lead. That person is sharply different from one who is leader first, perhaps because of the need to assuage an unusual power drive or to acquire material possessions" (Greenleaf Center for Servant Leadership, n.d., para. 2).

Servant leadership differs from other leadership models, in that the focus is on the leader meeting the needs of the followers before the needs of the leader or the organization are met. In the healthcare setting, the needs of the patients and staff are of utmost importance.

Spears (as cited in Avolio et al., 2009) lists the characteristics of a servant leader as the following (p. 436):

1. Listening
2. Empathy
3. Healing
4. Awareness
5. Persuasion
6. Conceptualization
7. Foresight
8. Stewardship
9. Commitment
10. Building community

Complexity Leadership

Avolio et al. (2009) describe how research has led to the development of complexity theory, which attempts to account for the dynamic state of leadership in a knowledge-driven society. Leadership is viewed as "an interactive system of dynamic, unpredictable agents that interact with each other in complex feedback networks, which can then produce adaptive outcomes such as knowledge dissemination, learning, innovation and further adaptation to change" (Uhl-Bien, Marion, & McKelvey, 2007, p. 299). Complexity leadership roles within a bureaucratic structure include adaptive roles, such as facilitating brainstorming sessions to overcome challenges; administrative roles, such as formal planning; and enabling roles, such as minimizing bureaucratic restraints to enhance follower potential (Avolio et al., 2009). The very nature of *complexity leadership* is that it embraces adaptation and innovation.

Regardless of the leadership model used, the relationship between the nurse leader and his or her followers is important. Followers do not simply follow, but rather leaders and followers are interdependent (Kean & Haycock-Stuart, 2011). Nurse leaders should carefully consider the style that suits their own needs, the needs of the nurses, and the needs of the organization.

Effective Communication

Issues such as working in IDTs, leading a multigenerational workforce, and dealing with shrinking budgets necessitate strong communication skills and effective conflict resolution strategies. Disruptive communication may occur between nurses, between nurses and physicians, or between nurses and other stakeholders, raising the potential of negatively affecting patient safety.

The hierarchal authority structure and sexism in the healthcare environment further complicate the issues (Robinson, Gorman, Slimmer, & Yudkowsky, 2010). In some settings, nurses do not feel supported by the bureaucratic structure of the organization, perceiving that decisions are made at higher levels in the organization and then imposed upon them. They do not feel they have a voice in the organization. In addition, in some environments, there is a perception that female nurses are not on the same level as male members of the IDT. This can be a barrier to effective and collegial communication.

Robinson et al. (2010) asked focus groups comprising nurses and physicians to reflect on effective communication strategies. They found that the need for straightforward and unambiguous communication is paramount. In order to be effective, there needs to be an opportunity to verify what was heard and ask clarifying questions. Visibility and open communication among the leader, subordinates, and colleagues provide this opportunity.

Collaborative problem solving emerged as the next theme. By bringing people together to discuss concerns, a sense of team camaraderie emerged, instead of an "us-versus-them" mindset. This has implications for patient safety. Team members were open to hearing different perspectives and weighing various options. The opinions of others were highly valued and sought after as respect grew among the team members.

> **CLINICAL TIP**
>
> Find out your own leadership style and use your strengths to lead.

Robinson et al. (2010) also found that maintaining a calm and supportive demeanor, even in stressful situations, was integral to effective communication. This included displaying a collegial tone and normal volume of voice. Positive reinforcement, expressed as appreciation, was also part of this strategy.

Establishing a sense of trust and building mutual respect also emerged as a theme. A comfortable rapport among members of the team ensures that even uncomfortable issues can be raised with the knowledge that they will be dealt with in a professional manner.

Developing an authentic understanding of and appreciation for the unique role of each member of the team was the final theme described by Robinson et al. (2010). Each profession experiences unique challenges and brings unique contributions to the team process. When everyone works in isolated silos, instead of in teams, they lose the richness that comes with welcoming others to the table for discussion. By developing an understanding of these varied contributions, each profession will establish a sense of respect for the other.

Gil (2010) describes aspects of communication styles that lead to effective communication by leaders. These include: "listen[ing] to the concerns of stakeholders, maintain[ing] professional integrity, adher[ing] to ethical standards, balanc[ing] stakeholders' interests, and be[ing] aware of the emotional barriers (preconceived opinions and beliefs, prejudices, biases, egos and politics)" (p. 451). Gil also describes four additional key attributes of effective communication. The first is assertiveness, which is the ability to forcefully state your own position, despite opposition from influential others. Leaders need to exhibit strategic influence, which is the ability to build coalitions with influential others, gaining their support and mutually overcoming obstacles. Spending time and energy getting to know influential others is referred to as relationship development. Political awareness is the final area of effective communication, wherein the leader understands who the influential people are and how to work effectively with them.

The role of the nurse leader in the process of establishing effective communication is to facilitate the establishment of a collegial relationship among the team members, whether the team comprises all nurses or is more interdisciplinary. When the nurse leader sets clear expectations for the atmosphere of professionalism, respect, and collegiality, this fosters effective communication and patient safety. The nurse leader should serve as a role model for effective communication and promote opportunities for ongoing education about effective communication strategies. Patient safety and quality care can flourish in an environment in which the leader actively pursues establishing effective communication among the team.

Nursing Leadership Roles in Caring for Older Adults

Nurses who work with older adults show a strong motivation to provide high-quality care (Dwyer, 2011). Geriatric nursing is considered a specialty area, as the care needs of older adults are complex. Because care for older adults is provided in a variety of settings, the range of leadership roles available to nurses is extensive. Though not an exhaustive list, the most common leadership roles (see **Table 19-4**) are discussed.

TABLE 19-4 Nursing Leadership Roles, Responsibilities, and Skills	
Role Title and Major Responsibilities	**Skills Needed**
Executive • Often hold dual licensure as Nursing Home Administrator (NHA) • Exert influence over policy development and quality of care for older adults • Responsible for budget for entire operation • Regulatory compliance for all departments	• Communication • Relationship management • Leadership • Professionalism • Knowledge of the healthcare environment • Business skills (per Healthcare Leadership Alliance (HLA) and described in VanDriel, Bellack, and O'Neil (2012)
Director of Nurses • Hiring and staff evaluations • Staffing • Oversight of all nursing care • Policy development • Nursing budget • Regulatory compliance	• Human resource management • Budgeting • Communication • Leadership • Business skills • Change agent

(continues)

TABLE 19-4   Nursing Leadership Roles, Responsibilities, and Skills (*continued*)

Role Title and Major Responsibilities	Skills Needed
Charge Nurse • Resource person for staff nurses • Role model • Mentor • Change agent (per Wojciechowski, Ritze-Cullen, and Tyrrell [2011]) • Responsible for day-to-day concerns at the unit level • Ensure that the unit operates efficiently and effectively	• Communication • Supervision • Delegation • Conflict management • Team building (per Wojciechowski et al., [2011])
Staff Nurse • Supervise care that has been delegated to paraprofessionals, such as licensed practical nurses (LPNs) and certified nursing assistants (CNAs)	• Strong clinical skills • Decision making • Delegation • Supervision • Critical thinking • Communication
Gerontological Nurse Practitioner (GNP) • GNPs are "advanced practice nurses with specialized education in the diagnosis, treatment, and management of acute and chronic conditions often found among older adults and generally associated with aging" (Gerontological Advanced Practice Nurses Association [GAPNA], 2003, p. 2). • In the nursing home setting, regulatory visits to examine residents may alternate between the physician and the GNP (CMS, 2011). • Take call to cover routine care needs, in concert with attending physician	• Advanced physical examination skills • Prescribing authority
Clinical Nurse Leader • Not yet widely used in settings outside of acute care • Focus is on enhancing safety • Provides direct clinical leadership, usually at the unit-level • Ensure that care delivery is safe, is evidence-based, and achieves high-quality outcomes (Reid & Dennison, 2011).	• Clinical expertise • Knowledge of quality improvement processes • Familiar with EBP concepts
Registered Nurse Assessment Coordinator (RNAC) • The Minimum Data Set (MDS) is a standardized, primary screening and assessment tool, used in Medicare and/or Medicaid–certified long-term care facilities (CMS, 2012) • A RN must conduct or coordinate completion of the MDS. The RNAC often has special training to complete this process. • Note that a similar assessment (Outcome and Assessment Information Set [OASIS]) is completed by the RN in the home care setting.	• In-depth knowledge of physical, psychological, and psychosocial aspects of care • Familiarity with state and federal regulations covering nursing home care • Ability to generate and update plans of care based on individual residents' needs • Knowledge of the connection between the MDS and payment for services

As the population of older adults in need of healthcare services continues to climb, the need for an adequate supply of nurses prepared to meet their complex and specialized needs will increase as well. Maintaining a stable staff is important and retention of staff is essential. The workforce is made up of nurses from several generations, each with unique views, attributes, and concerns. **Table 19-5** summarizes these differences.

Generational differences may lead to misunderstandings and conflicts surrounding communication styles, values, problem-solving methods, and work ethics. If left unresolved, the organization may see absenteeism, interpersonal conflict, communication breakdown, and turnover (Stanley, 2010). Strategies regarding differences of multigenerational workforces include (Stanley, 2010):

> Emphasize core nursing values
> Maintain accountability with institutional standards and goals
> Provide opportunities for nurse to voice concerns, opinions, contributions to ideas
> Leaders should be open, flexible, approachable, and motivational

TABLE 19-5   Multigenerational Workforce Attributes

Veterans (Silent Generation/ Traditionalist) Born before 1945	Baby Boomers Born 1946–1964	Generation Y (Millennials) Born 1981–1999	Generation X Born 1965–1980
Loyal, work for one organization their entire career	Loyal and very committed, optimistic, independent, goal-oriented, competitive Deep-seated idealism	Competent with technology	Experienced a rapid changing society, values technological literacy
Value professional image, respect for authority, dedicated, sacrifice, hardworking, and emphasize on honor	Equate work with personal fulfilment and self-worth	Multitaskers	Likes to have fun, less emphasis on work and more on family
Consider work a privilege	Strong work ethic Value interpersonal communication	Confident, optimistic, creative, open minded, achievement-oriented, diverse	Values independence, informality, diversity, challenge, creativity, responsibility
Slow to change work habits	Suspicious of people in authority	Wish to be part of the decision-making process	Short-term employment
Avoids conflict in the workplace	Motivated by responsibility, perks, encouragement, and challenges	Community service, group membership important, sociable	Focus on outcomes rather than processes

Data from Weston, M. (2006). Integrating generational perspectives in nursing. *OJIN: The Online Journal of Issues in Nursing, 11*(2), Manuscript 1; Cordinez, J. A. (2002). Recruitment, retention, and management of generation X: A focus on nursing professionals. *Journal of Healthcare Management, 47*(4), 237–249; Stanley, D. (2010). Multigenerational workforce issues and their implications for leadership in nursing. *Journal of Nursing Management, 18*(17), 846–852. Weingarten, R. M. (2009) Four generations, one workplace: A gen X-Y staff nurse's view of team building in the emergency department. *Journal of Emergency Nursing, 35*(1), 27–30; Duchscher, J.E., & Cowan, L. (2004) Multigenerational nurses in the workplace. *The Journal of Nursing Administration, 34*(11), 495–501; Gursory, D., Maier, T. A., & Chi, C. G. (2008). Generational differences: An examination of work values and generational gaps in the hospitality workforce. *International Journal of Hospitality Management, 27*(3), 448–458.

> Maintain respect for all employees
> Avoid stereotyping
> Create a supportive environment

To deal with these differences, several strategies should be used (Stanley, 2010). Core nursing values that transcend the generations, such as high-quality care, respect, and ethical decision making, should be emphasized. The mission and values of the organization also should be reinforced. Each employee should be held to the same standards as described in the goals, policies, and procedures in the organization. Opportunities should be made available for nurses to have a voice in the organization.

Leaders need to be open, flexible, and approachable. Hahn (2011) suggests that leaders conduct a self-assessment of their own managerial style and generational cohort; this can help with achieving a greater understanding of their own values, in relation to those of the nurses in their unit. Efforts must be made to deal with conflict and differences through dialogue and solutions that retain respect for all employees.

In summary, nurses from all generations should be given the opportunity to make contributions to the organization that recognize and celebrate their unique perspectives, insights, and views. Engaging nurses from all generations will improve retention and facilitate high-quality care.

Professional Associations

Knowledge about professional associations will assist in providing high-quality care to patients and offers the latest information in gerontology for staff and the community (**Figure 19-3**). There are many organizations for the gerontological nurse manager or leader. A few of the more common associations pertaining to this field are presented in **Table 19-6**.

All of the associations provide useful education and have Websites that are easily accessed. Information provided by the associations ranges from certification examinations, continuing education, standards of care, best practices, and political updates (important legislation affecting long-term care) to research and publications. The gerontological nurse as manager and leader can use information from these Websites to provide the latest information to staff, improve care for residents, and empower caregivers in a variety of settings.

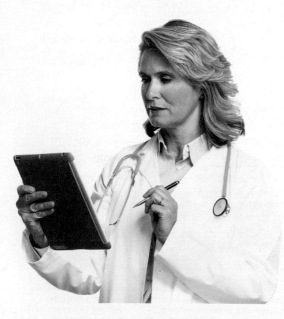

Figure 19-3 Nurse managers and leaders have the ability to positively influence the care of older adults.
© kurhan/Shutterstock

Summary

In conclusion, both nurse managers and nurse leaders are needed in gerontological nursing. Although managers focus on direction of the details of a unit, leaders are visionaries who see the larger picture. Both must develop good communication skills and healthy interpersonal relationships. Specific strategies discussed in this chapter can be used to assist staff in feeling engaged in the operations of the unit or organization, to foster recruitment and retention, develop strong IDTs, and ultimately to result in safe care and better health outcomes for patients and residents. Developing sound management strategies requires the desire to change and maintain a constant state of self-reflection (see **Case Study 19-3**).

TABLE 19-6   Professional Organizations to Assist Gerontological Nurse Managers and Leaders

Organization	Website	Purpose and/Benefits
Coalition of Geriatric Nursing Organizations (2015)	http://www .hartfordign .org/advocacy /cgno/	Represents 28,700 geriatric nurses seeking to improve the health care of older adults across care settings
National Gerontological Nursing Association (NGNA, 2015)	http://ngna.org	Dedicated to the clinical care of older adults across diverse care settings; membership benefits include: • *Geriatric Nursing* journal • Reduced rates to attend the annual NGNA convention • Continuing education • Bimonthly newsletter: *SIGN (Supporting Innovations in Gerontological Nursing)* • NGNA local chapter • Fellows program • Discounted certification examinations through a cooperative arrangement between NGNA and the American Nurses Credentialing Center (ANCC)
The National Association of Directors of Nursing Administration in Long Term Care (NADONA/LTC, 2015) Membership is in both the United States and Canada.	http://www .nadona.org	An advocate and educational organization for directors of nursing (DONs), assistant directors of nursing (ADONs), and RNs in long-term care Mentor system that allows directors to speak with a veteran DON in administration Education, including conferences both regional and national, and other professional materials A quarterly journal that provides continuing education units (CEUs Scholarships for all educational stages) Fellows program Director of nursing certification program
The American Association for Long Term Care Nursing (AALTCN, 2015)	http://aaltcn.org	Promotes the importance of and advances excellence in practice for the entire nursing department of long-term care facilities • Comprehensive association Website • Monthly e-newsletters, current news, and education articles • Discounts on numerous certification programs, position statements, core competencies • Clinical education and toolkits • Opportunities for networking and sharing of resources • Tuition discounts to Chamberlain College • Representation on national committees and with national initiatives

(continues)

TABLE 19-6 **Professional Organizations to Assist Gerontological Nurse Managers and Leaders (*continued*)**

Organization	Website	Purpose and/Benefits
The American Association of Nurse Assessment Coordinators (AANAC, 2015)	http://www .aanac.org	Not-for-profit professional association that provides access to accurate and timely information on clinical assessment, regulatory requirements, reimbursement, computer automation, research, and the law • Discounts on education and certification opportunities, webinars, conference registration • Updates on CMS regulations and requirements • Regular communication in the form of emails, e-newsletters, articles, and discussion feeds • 24/7/365 advice from peers and experts in a members-only online forum/community setting • Networking

The American Health Care Association (AHCA, 2015)	http://ahcancal .org	Not-for-profit group of state health organizations advocating for high-quality care and services for frail, elderly, and disabled Americans, providing care to about 1 million individuals in 12,000 not-for-profit and member facilities. Membership is through state affiliates and open to vendors and providers.
		• Preferred Products and Services Program
		• Long Term Care Career Center
		• Numerous publications
		• Awards program
		  • Volunteers of the Year
		  • ID/DD Hero of the Year
		  • Not for Profit Program of the Year

Leading Age (2015a, b)	(http://www .leadingage.org/)	An association of not-for-profit organizations dedicated to making America a better place to grow old. Leading Age work is focused on advocacy, leadership development, applied research and promotion of effective services, home health, hospice, community services, senior housing, assisted living residences, continuing care communities, nursing homes, as well as technology solution for seniors, children, and others with special needs, expanding the world of possibilities for aging. • Insurance program • Publications such as *Leading Age,* weekly newsletters • Serves as a hub for articles, analyses and information about legislative and political action related to services for aging • The facts on aging services • Consumer information • Discounts on national and international conferences • Access to members-only sections on the Website • Buyers guide • Innovations fund • Provides a link to other services and programs

Organization	Website	Purpose and/Benefits
The National Association of Health Care Assistants (NAHCA, 2015)	http://www.nahcacares.org/	Advocates for CNAs to elevate their profession and performance while promoting high-quality patient and resident care Various levels of membership that include: • Association pin • Educational opportunities • Newsletter • Resource page • Coaching • Scholarship program for higher education
The American Medical Directors Association (AMDA, 2015a, 2015b)	http://www.amda.com	The Society for Post-Acute and Long-Term Care Medicine (AMDA) is a professional association of medical directors, attending physicians, and others practicing in the long-term care continuum to promote excellent patient care. • Educational programs • Discounts on conference and core curriculum • Print and online resources, including *Caring for the Ages, Journal of the American Medical Directors Association*, and AMDA Reports • Exclusive member rates and members-only access • Access to clinical tools and practice guidance • Networking
American Assisted Living Nurses Association (AALNA, 2015a, 2015b)	http://www.alnursing.org/	Associations represents assisted living nurses and promotes safe practice in assisted living. • Members only access to resources and services • Subscription to the *Geriatric Nursing Journal* • Subscription to three assisted living newsletters • Discount on the AALNA national conference registration fee • Discount on the Assisted Living Nurse Certification Examination • Discount on CEUs and educational materials • Discount on Long Term Care Insurance from PCALIC • Free membership to EM Alliance • State chapters

Nurse managers and leaders of today are faced with unique challenges related to multigenerational staffing patterns. Professional organizations can be excellent resources to provide support and information to those in management positions. Gerontological nurses should choose the most appropriate professional organization(s) in which to be active. As nursing leaders in the specialty of gerontology (see **Case Study 19-4**), they can also contribute to advancing the mission and services of their organization through scholarly activities and political activism.

Case Study 19-3: Standards of Care and Disciplinary Policies

Mr. Gonzalez, RN, is the charge nurse on the evening shift of the skilled care unit at a **long-term care facility**. The day shift nurses have complained to Mr. Gonzalez that the evening shift CNAs have not been showering the residents as scheduled. They tell him that family members of the residents have complained about poor hygiene of their loved ones.

Questions:

1. What is the first step Mr. Gonzalez should take in resolving this situation?
2. To which staff members should he speak?
3. What immediate steps must be put in place to remedy this situation?
4. If no action is taken by Mr. Gonzalez and the complaints are true, what could happen?
5. Who has responsibility in this situation for the quality of patient care?

Case Study 19-4: Leadership, Vision, and Staffing

Mrs. Petty, RN, BSN, is the director of nursing (DON) for the assisted living portion of a for-profit healthcare facility. One of her jobs is to hire an assistant director of nursing (ADON), a new position created to help the DON with the growing number of residents in the facility.

Questions:

1. What qualifications should Mrs. Petty look for in an assistant director of nursing?
2. Describe the ideal candidate for this position. What types of experience, background, and education would be expected in this position?
3. Where does the ADON position fall in the organizational structure of this facility?
4. Where does the DON position fall in the organizational chart?

Clinical Reasoning Exercises

1. Examine the organizational chart of a facility where you work or have your clinical experiences. Analyze the hierarchical levels in comparison to the discussion of leadership roles in this chapter
2. Follow a nurse manager for a day. Make a list of duties that you observe and what skills seem important.
3. Map out your own personal strategic plan for your career goals. Set goals for 1 year, 5 years, and 10 years.
4. Make a list of your own strengths and weaknesses as a manager or leader. Determine which of your weaknesses you wish to improve upon and how you will accomplish this.
5. Think of a nurse whom you admire as a good role model of a leader or manager. Write down the qualities you have observed in this person. Compare them to the list in Table 19-2.

Personal Reflections

1. Where do you presently see yourself in the hierarchy of management in nursing? Where do you want to be in 5 years? In 10 years? What is your ultimate goal related to advancement in your nursing career? Do you have a plan to accomplish this?

2. Is management an avenue you have considered? What are your personal strengths and weaknesses with regard to the qualities of leaders and managers discussed in this chapter?

3. Do you see yourself more as a leader or as a manager? What leadership styles fit your personality the best? How do you feel about delegating tasks to other nurses and UAP? What skills do you feel you need to develop in order to be comfortable in a charge nurse position?

4. To which nursing organizations do you belong? Have you ever considered applying for a leadership position? Why or why not?

5. Which of the organizations discussed at the end of this chapter would be most appropriate for you to become involved in to help you reach your goals?

References

Abbott-Shultz, B. (2010, October). Engaging families: Enhancing the relationship among residents, their families, and your community. *Long Term Living Magazine, 36*–39.

Abell, T. (2011, May). Creating a compliance/QA culture: Training to achieve corporate compliance and quality assurance. *Long Term Living Magazine, 36*–37.

Allen, B. C., Holland, P., & Reynolds, R. (2015). The effect of bullying on burnout in nurses: The moderating role of psychological detachment. *Journal of Advanced Nursing, 71*(2), 381–390.

American Assisted Living Nurses Association. (2015a). Individual membership. Retrieved from https://www.alnursing.org/membership/individual/

American Assisted Living Nurses Association. (2015b). About AALNA. Retrieved from https://www.alnursing.org/about/

American Association for Long Term Care Nursing. (2015). Member benefits. Retrieved from http://www.aaltcn.org/nursing-membership-benefits.htm

American Association of Nurse Assessment Coordinators. (2015). Benefits of membership. Retrieved from http://www.aanac.org/Membership-Benefits/Benefits-of-Membership

American Health Care Association. (2015). AHCA membership. Retrieved from http://www.ahcancal.org/about_ahca/ahca_membership/Pages/default.aspx

American Health Care Association & National Center for Assisted Living. (n.d.). NCAL's guiding principles for leadership. Retrieved from http://www.ahcancal.org/ncal/about/Documents/GPLeadership.pdf

American Health Care Association, & National Center for Assisted Living. (2009). Leadership excellence. Retrieved from http://www.ahcancal.org/quality_improvement/leadership_excellence/Documents/Section2-RolesAndCompetencies.pdf

American Medical Directors Association. (2015a). Mission, value statements, and history. Retrieved from http://www.paltc.org/about-amda

American Medical Directors Association. (2015b). Benefits of AMDA membership. Retrieved from http://www.amda.com/membership/benefits.cfm

American Nurses Association. (2012). Principles for delegation by registered nurses to unlicensed assistive personnel (UAP). Retrieved from http://www.nursingworld.org/MainMenuCategories/ThePracticeof ProfessionalNursing/NursingStandards/ANAPrinciples/PrinciplesofDelegation.pdf.aspx

American Organization of Nurse Executives. (2006). Nurse manager leadership domain framework (NMLP). Retrieved from http://www.aone.org/resources/Nurse%20Manager%20Leadership%20Domain%20Framework

Arnetz, J. E., Zhdanova, L. S., Elsouhag, D., Lichtenberg, P., Luborsky, M. R., & Arnetz, B. B. (2011). Organizational climate determinants of resident safety culture in nursing homes. *The Gerontologist, 51,* 739–749.

Avolio, B. J., Walumbwa, F. O., & Weber, T. J. (2009). Leadership: Current theories, research and future directions. *Annual Review of Psychology, 60,* 421–449.

Baker, E. L., & Orton, S. N. (2010). Practicing management and leadership: Vision, strategy, operations and tactics. *Journal of Public Health Management Practice, 16*(5), 470–471.

Basom, J. (2012, February). Proactive customer service: strong customer service sends positive message to residents, families and the community at large. *Long Term Living Magazine,* 28–29.

Bennis, W. (1989). *On becoming a leader.* New York, NY: Addison-Wesley.

Brody, A. A., Barnes, K., Ruble, C., & Sakowski, J. (2012). Evidence-based practice councils: Potential path to staff nurse empowerment and leadership growth. *Journal of Nursing Administration, 42*(1), 28–33.

Campbell, R. J. (2008). Change management in healthcare. *The Health Care Manager, 27*(1), 23–39.

Center for Creative Leadership. (n.d.). About CCL. Retrieved from http://www.ccl.org/leadership/about/index.aspx

Centers for Medicare and Medicaid Services. (n.d.). Nursing home compare. Retrieved from http://www.medicare.gov/NursingHomeCompare/search.aspx

Centers for Medicare and Medicaid Services (2011). State operations manual. Retrieved from http://www.cms.gov/Regulations-and-Guidance/Guidance/Manuals/downloads/som107ap_pp_guidelines_ltcf.pdf

Centers for Medicare and Medicaid Services. (2012). Minimum Data Set (MDS). Retrieved from https://www.cms.gov/Research-Statistics-Data-and-Systems/Files-for-Order/IdentifiableDataFiles/LongTermCareMinimumDataSetMDS.html

Chamberlin-Salaun, J., Mills, J., & Usher, K. (2013). Terminology used to describe health care teams: An integrative review of the literature. *Journal of Multidisciplinary Healthcare, 6,* 65–74.

Cohen, S. (2014). Resolving conflict by setting ground rules. *Nursing Management, 45*(5), 17–21.

Corazzini, K., Twersky, J., White, H. K., Buhr, G. T., McConnell, E. S., Weiner, M., & Colón-Emeric, C. S. (2015). Implementing culture change in nursing homes: An adaptive leadership framework. *The Gerontologist, 55*(4), 616–627.

Cordinez, J. A. (2002). Recruitment, retention, and management of generation X: A focus on nursing professionals. *Journal of Healthcare Management, 47*(4), 237–249.

Curtis, E., & O'Connell, R. (2011). Essential leadership skills for motivating and developing staff. *Nursing Management, 18*(5), 32–35.

Deschodt, M., Flamaing, J., Haentjens, P., Boonen, S., & Milisen, K. (2013). Impact of geriatric consultation teams on clinical outcome in acute hospitals: A systematic review and meta-analysis. *BioMed Central Medicine, 11,* 48. Retrieved from http://bmcmedicine.biomedcentral.com/articles/10.1186/1741-7015-11-48.

Drucker, P. (n.d.). *Peter F. Drucker quotes.* Retrieved from http://thinkexist.com/quotes/peter_f._drucker/

Duchscher, J. E., & Cowan, L. (2004). Multigenerational nurses in the workplace. *The Journal of Nursing Administration, 34*(11), 495–501.

Dwyer, D. (2011). Experiences of registered nurses as managers and leaders in residential aged care facilities: A systematic review. *International Journal of Evidence-Based Healthcare, 9*(4), 388–402.

Gardner, B. (2010). Improve RN retention through transformational leadership styles. *Nursing Management, 41*(8), 8–12.

Geriatric assessment interdisciplinary team. (n.d.). Retrieved from https://www.umaryland.edu/gerontology/education-and-training/geriatric-assessment-interdisciplinary-team/

Geriatric interdisciplinary team. Retrieved from http://hartfordign.org/education/gitt/

Gerontological Advanced Practice Nurses Association. (2003). Position statement: Clinical practice of gerontological nurse practitioners. Retrieved from http://enp-network.s3.amazonaws.com/Gulf_Coast_GNP/pdf/Clinical%20Practice%20of%20GNP_2003.pdf

Gil, N. A. (2010). Language as a resource in project management: A case study and a conceptual framework. *IEEE Transactions on Engineering Management, 57*(3), 450–462.

Goetz, K., Janney, M., & Ramsey, K. (2011). When nursing takes ownership of financial outcomes: Achieving exceptional financial performance through leadership, strategy, and execution. *Nursing Economic$, 29*(4): 173–182.

Greenleaf Center for Servant Leadership. (n.d.). What is servant leadership? Retrieved from http://www.greenleaf.org/whatissl/

Gursory D., Maier T. A., & Chi C. G. (2008) Generational differences: An examination of work values and generational gaps in the hospitality workforce. *International Journal of Hospitality Management, 27*(3), 448–458.

Hahn, J. A. (2011). Managing multiple generations: Scenarios from the workplace. *Nursing Forum, 46*(3), 119–127.

Hartford Institute for Geriatric Nursing (2015). Coalition of nursing organizations. Retrieved from http://www.hartfordign.org/advocacy/cgno/

Harvarth, T. A., Swafford, K., Smith, K., Miller, L. L., Volpin, M., Sexson, K., . . . Young, H. A. (2008). Enhancing nursing leadership in long-term care: A review of the literature. *Research in Gerontological Nursing, 1*(3), 187–196.

Healthy People. (n.d.). About Healthy People. Retrieved from http://www.healthypeople.gov/2020/about/default.aspx

Hebling, N. L., & Huwe, J. (2015). Finding the balance for a culture of safety. *Nursing, 45*(12), 65–68.

Heuston, M. M., & Wolf, G. A. (2011). Transformational leadership skills of successful nurse managers. *Journal of Nursing Administration, 41*(6), 248–251.

Kean, S., & Haycock-Stuart, E. (2011). Understanding the relationship between followers and leaders. *Nursing Management, 18*(8), 31–35.

Keys, Y. (2011). Perspectives on executive relationships. *Journal of Nursing Administration, 41*(9), 347–349.

Kotter International. (n.d.). Change leadership. Retrieved from http://www.kotterinternational.com/our-principles/change-leadership

Leading Age. (2015a). Member services. Retrieved from https://annualmeeting.leadingage.org/member_services.aspx

Leading Age. (2015b). Home page. Retrieved from http://www.leadingage.org/

Lewin, K., Lippitt, R., & White, R. K. (1939). Patterns of aggressive behavior in experimentally created "social climates." *Journal of Social Psychology, 10,* 271–298.

Lynch, B. M., McCormack, B., & McCance, T. (2011). Development of a model of situational leadership in residential care for older people. *Journal of Nursing Management, 19*(8), 1058–1069.

McCallin, A. M., & Frankson, C. (2010). The role of the charge nurse manager: A descriptive exploratory study. *Journal of Nursing Management, 18*(3), 319–325.

McCormick, W. C. (2012). Report of the geriatrics-hospice and palliative medicine work group: American Geriatrics Society and American Academy of Hospice and Palliative Medicine leadership collaboration. *Journal of the American Geriatrics Society, 60*(3), 583–587.

Montagnini, M., Kaiser, R. M., Clark, P. G., Dodd, M. A., Goodwin, C., Periyakoil, V. S., . . . Supiano, K. (2014). Position statement on interdisciplinary team training in geriatrics: An essential component of quality health care for older adults. *Journal of the American Geriatrics Society, 62*(5), 961–965.

National Association of Directors of Nursing Administration in Long Term Care. (2015). Benefits of membership. Retrieved from http://www.nadona.org/benefits-of-membership/

The National Association of Health Care Assistants. (2015). Mission. Retrieved from http://www.nahcacareforce.org/mission

National Council of State Boards of Nursing. (2005a). Practical nurse scope of practice white paper. Retrieved from https://www.ncsbn.org/Final_11_05_Practical_Nurse_Scope_Practice_White_Paper.pdf

National Council of State Boards of Nursing. (2005b). Working with others: A position paper. Retrieved from https://www.ncsbn.org/Working_with_Others.pdf

National Council of State Boards of Nursing. (2016). National guidelines for nursing delegation. *Journal of Nursing Regulation, 7*(1), 5–14

National Council of State Boards of Nursing & the American Nurses Association. (2005). Joint statement on delegation. Retrieved from https://www.ncsbn.org/Delegation_joint_statement_NCSBN-ANA.pdf

National Gerontological Nursing Association. (2015). NGNA membership. Retrieved from https://www.ngna.org/membership

National Research Council. (2003). Transformational leadership and evidence-based management. In *Keeping patients safe: Transforming the work environment of nurses* (pp. 108–161). Washington, DC: The National Academies Press. Retrieved from http://books.nap.edu/openbook.php?record_id=10851&page=108

Porter-O'Grady, T., & Malloch, K. (2009). Leaders of innovation: Transforming postindustrial healthcare. *Journal of Nursing Administration, 39*(6), 245–248.

Reid, K. B., & Dennison, P. (2011). The clinical nurse leader (CNL): Point-of-care safety clinician. *OJIN: The Online Journal of Issues in Nursing, 16*(3), Manuscript 4.

Richmond, P. A., Book, K., Hicks, M., Pimpinella, A., & Jenner, C. A. (2009). C.O.M.E. be a nurse manager. *Nursing Management, 40*(2), 52–54.

Roberts, T., Nolet, K., & Bowers, B. (2015). Consistent assignments of nursing staff to residents in nursing homes: A critical review of conceptual and methodological issues. *The Gerontologist, 55*(3), 434–437.

Robinson, F. P., Gorman, G., Slimmer, L. W., & Yudkowsky, R. (2010). Perceptions of effective and ineffective nurse-physician communication in hospitals. *Nursing Forum, 45*(3), 206–216.

Rushing, J. (2008). Transforming staff through leadership excellence. *Nursing Management, 39*(8), 8–10.

Schwartz, D. B., Spencer, T., Wilson, B., & Wood, K. (2011). Transformational leadership: Implications for nursing leaders in facilities seeking Magnet® designation. *AORN Journal, 93*(6), 737–748.

Sims , J. M. (2009). Styles and qualities of effective leaders. *Dimensions of Critical Care Nursing, 28*(6), 272–274.

Stanley, D. (2010). Multigenerational workforce issues and their implications for leadership in nursing. *Journal of Nursing Management, 18*(17), 846–852.

Tourangeau, A., Cranley, L., Spence Laschinger, H. K., & Pachis, J. (2010). Relationships among leadership practices, work environments, staff communication and outcomes in long-term care. *Journal of Nursing Management, 18*(7), 1060–1072.

Trinkoff, A. M., Han, K., Storr, C. L., Lerner, N., Johantgen, M., & Gartrell, K. (2013). Turnover, staffing, skill mix and resident outcomes in a national sample of US nursing homes. *Journal of Nursing Administration, 43*(12), 630–636.

Tyczkowski, B. L., Vandenhouten, C., Reilly, J., Bansal, G., Kubsch, S. M., & Jakkola, R. (2015). Emotional intelligence (EI) and nursing leadership styles among nurse managers. *Nursing Administration Quarterly, 39*(2), 172–180.

Uhl-Bien, M., Marion, R., & McKelvey, B. (2007). Complexity leadership theory: Shifting leadership from the industrial age to the knowledge age. *The Leadership Quarterly, 18*(4), 298–318.

Utley, R., Anderson, R., & Atwell, J. (2011). Implementing transformational leadership in long-term care. *Geriatric Nursing, 32*(3), 212–219.

Valentine , N. M., Kirby, K. K., & Wolf, K. M. (2011). The CNO/CFO partnership: Navigating the changing landscape. *Nursing Economic$, 29*(4), 201–210.

VanDriel, M. K., Bellack, J. P., & O'Neil, E. (2012). Nurses in the C-Suite: Leadership beyond chief nurse. *Nursing Administration Quarterly, 36*(1), 5–11.

Vogelsmeier, A., & Scott-Cawiezell, J. (2011). Achieving quality improvement in the nursing home: Influence of nursing leadership on communication and teamwork. *Journal of Nursing Care Quarterly, 26*(3), 236–242.

Weberg, D. (2010). Transformational leadership and staff retention: An evidence review with implications for healthcare systems. *Nursing Administration Quarterly, 34*(3), 246–258.

Weingarten, R. M. (2009). Four generations, one workplace: A gen X-Y staff nurse's view of team building in the emergency department. *Journal of Emergency Nursing, 35*(1), 27–30.

Weston, M. (2006). Integrating generational perspectives in nursing. *OJIN: The Online Journal of Issues in Nursing, 11*(2), Manuscript 1.

Wojciechowski, E., Ritze-Cullen, N., & Tyrrell, S. (2011). Understanding the learning needs of the charge nurse. *Journal for Nurses in Staff Development, 27*(4), E10–E17.

For a full suite of assignments and additional learning activities, see the access code at the front of your book.

CHAPTER 20

Ethical and Legal Principles and Issues

Janice Edelstein
Carolyn A. Laabs

(Competencies 1, 11, 12, 13)

LEARNING OBJECTIVES

At the end of this chapter, the reader will be able to:

> Recognize key ethical constructs as they relate to the care of geriatric patients.
> Translate concepts of ethics to their implications in the care of geriatric patients.
> Relate the influence of personal values, attitudes, and expectations about aging on care of older adults and their families and extended families.
> Analyze the impact of fiscal, sociocultural, and medico-legal factors on decision making in the care of geriatric patients.
> Formulate strategies for facilitating appropriate levels of autonomy and supporting the right to self-determination decisions in the care of geriatric patients.

KEY TERMS

Advance directives	Ethics of care
Advocacy	Failure to rescue
Autonomy	Fidelity
Beneficence	Fiduciary
Codes of ethics	Informed consent
Competence	Guardianship
Confidentiality	Justice
Conflict	Malpractice
Conflict of interest	Moral courage
Dilemma	Moral dilemma
Duty	Moral distress

Moral principles	Power of attorney
Moral sensitivity	Quality of life
Moral uncertainty	Sanctity of life
Negligence	Standard of care
Nonmaleficence	Values
Patient rights	Veracity
Physician orders for life-sustaining treatment	

As the population ages and healthcare technology advances, the need for nurses to be skilled in the ethical care of older adults grows. The *ethics of care* in the geriatric population can be complex and can present many challenges to decision-makers. Continual development of skills in ethical decision making is required for competence in geriatric care.

As with all nursing specialties, geriatric care concerns matters of compassion, equity, fairness, dignity, and confidentiality. Moreover, nursing practice requires mindfulness of a person's autonomy, particularly as it pertains to the physical ability and mental capacity to be self-governing, which may change with aging and disease. In the care of the geriatric population, it is impossible not to be faced with issues regarding patients' ability to care for themselves and live independently safely. Independence in the community requires an appropriate level of self-sufficiency in the management of activities of daily living (ADL), use of medication, mobility and transportation, and maintenance and operation of a home (self-care, pet care, meals, housekeeping, shopping, banking, etc.). Besides self-sufficiency, finances, health literacy, personal preferences, and choices are all factors that have a direct impact on a patient's understanding of and adherence to a plan of care for the promotion of safety, health, and well-being. When health and safety become an issue, extended healthcare services are necessary (see **Figure 20-1**).

The exercise of autonomy may be further challenged by the effects of aging and chronic disease on cognitive functioning and thus on decision making. The ability to make decisions related to such things as advance directives, informed consent, and refusal of treatment depends on mental functioning that is unimpaired and appropriate to the task. Choices can be difficult and call for assessment of decision-making capacity, consideration of patient preferences, and determinations of what may be in the patient's best interest. The difficulty of making personal choices can be compounded further by societal pressures associated with the cost and availability of technologic developments and devices, participation in genetic testing and research, options for organ and tissue donation and transplantation, allocation of resources to the aged, and care at the end of life. Advances in healthcare science and technology have raised legal and ethical concerns that the elderly and their families should discuss, preferably before issues arise. As pointed out by Burkhardt and Nathaniel (2008), dilemmas may occur with the use of technology in making healthcare decisions. Legal documents of advance directives, such as a *power of attorney* for health care ordinarily requested by healthcare agencies, can be helpful when the patient lacks decision-making capacity yet important treatment decisions need to be made.

Treatment decisions should not be made without consideration of ethical principles. Ethical principles are fundamental propositions pertaining to the moral practices, beliefs, and standards of individuals and groups. Derived from our beliefs and *values*, ethical principles find their foundation in philosophy, religion, and culture and find their expression in personal and familial choices and expectations. Ethical principles inform decision making and guide professional behavior.

Ethical decision making is driven by our moral reasoning, and our judgments about right, wrong, good, and bad and are influenced by our beliefs about what types of behavior or conditions in life are desirable or valuable. Such beliefs and judgments define our character and are expressed in our decisions and actions. Professional

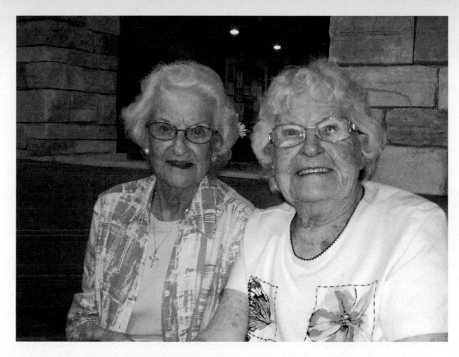

Figure 20-1 Supporting the autonomy of competent older adults is an important component of the ethical code for nurses.
Photo courtesy of Amy Paige

codes of ethics and standards of practice serve to further inform decision making and ethical action. It is the hallmark of a profession to have a code of ethics, and, since 1950, American nurses have had such a code, revising it periodically, most recently in 2015. This corresponds to marking 2015 as the "Year of Ethics" by the American Nurses Association (ANA) (Jones, 2015) (see **Box 20-1**).

   Although ethical principles, professional codes, and standards can guide decision making, changes in our social networks, awareness of our global community, diversity among cultures, and advances in science, medicine, and technology, have created increasingly complex ethical conflicts and moral dilemmas. Thus, decision making may not always be easy and nurses must have a clear understanding of their own values and a strategy for decision making as a care provider. As noted by Vicki D. Lachman, *moral courage* is "the ability of not being afraid to stand up for one's core values and ethical obligations" (Jones, 2015, p. 16). According to Chinn and Kramer (2008), values clarification and values analysis are important components in making moral and ethical decisions and can assist in the decision-making process. In that process it is important to recognize that nurses' personal beliefs and values may differ from those of the patients, the organization within which they work, or even the norms of society. This may create situations of moral conflict.

Conflict and Dilemma

A *conflict* is a situation in which there are opposing or incompatible needs, views, or demands. Three types of moral conflict in nursing are moral distress, moral uncertainty, and moral dilemma (Jameton, 1984). *Moral distress* occurs when a person believes he or she knows the right thing to do but is limited in doing so by organizational or societal constraints. *Moral uncertainty is* the state in which a person is unsure what the moral problem is or which moral principles or values apply. A *moral dilemma* arises when two or more moral principles apply that

BOX 20-1   Provisions of the American Nurses Association Code of Ethics for Nurses (2015)

1. The nurse practices with compassion and respect for the inherent dignity, worth, and unique attributes of every person.
2. The nurse's primary commitment is to the patient, whether an individual, family, group, community, or population.
3. The nurse promotes, advocates for, and protects the rights, health, and safety of the patient.
4. The nurse has authority, accountability, and responsibility for nursing practice; makes decisions; and takes action consistent with the obligation to promote health and to provide optimal care.
5. The nurse owes the same duties to self as to others, including the responsibility to promote health and safety, preserve wholeness of character and integrity, maintain competence, and continue personal and professional growth.
6. The nurse, through individual and collective effort, establishes, maintains, and improves the ethical environment of the work setting and conditions of employment that are conducive to safe, quality health care.
7. The nurse, in all roles and settings, advances the profession through research and scholarly inquiry, professional standards development, and the generation of both nursing and health policy.
8. The nurse collaborates with other health professionals and the public to protect human rights, promote health diplomacy, and reduce health disparities.
9. The profession of nursing, collectively through its professional organizations, must articulate nursing values, maintain the integrity of the profession, and integrate principles of social justice into nursing and health policy.

Reproduced from American Nurses Association. (2015). *Code of ethics for nurses with interpretive statements*. Silver Spring MD: Author.

support mutually inconsistent actions. A true *dilemma* occurs when it appears there are no morally acceptable options. An important component of ethical behavior is *moral sensitivity*, or the ability to identify a moral problem and how our decisions and actions may affect others (Rest, 1994).

Nursing, by its nature, is a moral enterprise, and value conflicts are inevitable in a society in which there are multiple points of view. Some conflicts rise to the level of dilemmas. **Case Study 20-1** provides one example. Some conflicts are resolved through dialogue, others through legislation, and others by agreement regarding basic rights. In any case, opposing values should be discussed openly and respectfully. Healthcare organizations often utilize ethics committees, who can offer advice to help resolve conflicts and dilemmas. Nurses with geriatric expertise may be asked to serve on an ethics committee as a healthcare representative.

Moral Principles and the Nurse–Patient Relationship

Moral principles are incorporated into professional *codes of ethics*, organizational value statements, and position statements published by professional groups, such as the ANA. Fowler (2015) states that the nurse's code of ethics "functions as a general guide for the profession's members and as a social contract with the public whom it serves" (p. xiii). The *Code of Ethics for Nurses with Interpretive Statements* (ANA, 2015) forms the cornerstone of all nursing practice. A nurse's understanding of moral principles and the code of ethics facilitates decision making in daily practice and in professional relationships, in particular, the nurse–patient relationship.

The professional–patient relationship is *fiduciary* in nature. The term *fiduciary* is derived from the Latin word *fidere*, to trust. Fiduciaries hold something in trust for another. In the case of health care, the nurse holds in trust

Case Study 20-1

Mr. Bowen is 74 years old. He has been very healthy and active, working as a farmer. He had a right-sided cerebrovascular accident 14 days ago and currently has moderate leg weakness, significant arm weakness, slurred speech, and mild difficulty swallowing. He is expected to recover the ability to ambulate with a cane, though return of arm function is guarded. His ability to speak and swallow will likely improve, but he may require a special diet to prevent aspiration.

Mr. Bowen has decided to stop eating, stating that he does not want to live as an invalid. His family is very distressed and wants the nursing staff to force him to eat. The staff cannot imagine why he has made this choice, given that his prognosis is so good. He has been evaluated for depression and an antidepressant has been ordered, which he refuses to take, along with all other medication for his newly diagnosed cardiovascular disease. Mr. Bowen is oriented to time, place, and person. Prior to this decision to refuse to eat, his decision-making capacity had never been questioned. Some of the staff support his decision and others do not. Discussion with the family reveals that Mr. Bowen has frequently made deriding remarks about persons with disability, including remarks such as, "If I ever

end up that way, just take me out behind the barn and shoot me." The psychologist comments that Mr. Bowen is clinically depressed and that part of his depression is related to the areas of the brain that are affected by the stroke, which prevents him from returning to work on the farm. The psychologist strongly believes that if the depression were resolved, Mr. Bowen would most likely change his opinion.

Questions:

1. What is the ethical dilemma?
2. What ethical principles apply in this case study?
3. Does Mr. Bowen have the right to refuse to eat and take medications when he clearly is not in an end-of-life situation?
4. How does the team resolve the situation when his depression is so evident and he refuses treatment for it?
5. As the nurse, how would you approach and direct the care for Mr. Bowen?
6. What elements (provisions) from the code of ethics come to mind as you prepare to care for Mr. Bowen?
7. Can you apply theory related to the concept of grief to the care of Mr. Bowen?

the health and well-being of the patient. This is due to the fact of the patient's illness and infirmity, lack of medical knowledge and expertise, and dependence on healthcare professionals to gain access to services, all creating a state of vulnerability for the patient (Pellegrino & Thomasma, 1981). This is especially true among the elderly, who may lack independence and decision-making capacity and experience not only the physical effects of illness, infirmity, and aging but also the existential effects as one approaches the end of life. Because patients must place their trust in the nurse and in fact sometimes must place their very lives into the hands of nurses, the focus of the nurse's decision making must always be on the benefit or the good of the patient (principle of beneficence).

Beneficence and Nonmaleficence

Doing good (*beneficence*) and avoiding harm (*nonmaleficence*) are integral to health care. Nurses must always act to promote the good of patients, and never act, or fail to act, such that harm results. Consider the situation of a busy understaffed medical unit where a nurse, due to the demands of a heavy workload, does only a cursory assessment on rounds. One new admission is an elderly woman who, after a recent crisis with heart failure, is having her medication adjusted. Significantly deconditioned, she has spent the last couple of weeks in her recliner. Near the end of the shift she suddenly complains of severe chest pain and anxiety. An emergent work-up determines that she has a deep vein thrombosis with pulmonary embolism, a life-threatening situation. Is this an example of harm possibly due to the nurse's inadequate assessment of risk factors and lack of attention to risk reduction? It is clear from the *Code of Ethics* that a nurse must never act with the intent of ending the life of the patient. However, consider the ethical dimensions of failure to rescue or failure to act and how an unsafe environment of understaffing, for example, can contribute to the potential for harm.

Quality and patient safety are major concerns when providing care to older adults. *Failure to rescue* is one measure of the effectiveness of healthcare facilities in rescuing a patient from a complication versus preventing one. Data are collected by measuring the number of deaths occurring out of discharges with potential complications as defined under failure to rescue (pneumonia, deep vein thrombosis/pulmonary embolism, sepsis, acute renal failure, shock/cardiac arrest, gastrointestinal hemorrhage/acute ulcer). There are many reasons for failure to rescue, ranging from issues as simple as educational background, inexperience, and lack of knowledge to the more complex such as attitudes toward work, staffing patterns, and resource allocation (See **Case Study 20-2**.) Due to the fiduciary nature of the nurse–patient relationship, patients place their trust in nurses that they always will act beneficently toward them and never act or fail to act in a manner that would be maleficent. In this way, they serve as patient advocates.

Advocacy, Confidentiality, Fidelity, and Veracity

The term *advocate* comes from the Latin word *advocare* to call, to voice, or to plead the case for another. Provision 3 of the *Code of Ethics* describes the meaning of *advocacy* in nursing as protecting the rights, health, and safety of the patient. To be the voice of the patient and to advocate for the patient, the nurse, holding in trust the good of the patient, must not only avoid harm but also do good by respecting the patient's right to confidentiality and acting with fidelity and veracity.

In healthcare settings, patients share a good deal of personal information not only with nurses but also, for example, with physicians, therapists, and insurance providers. That information is disclosed in confidence, in full trust, that it will not be disclosed to others without the patient's permission. *Confidentiality*, maintaining privacy of information, not only is an expectation of ethics but also is protected under the law in the Health Insurance Portability and Accountability Act (HIPAA). Ethics requires that nurses, as advocates for patients

---

Case Study 20-2

Mr. Jacobs, a young-acting 72-year-old obese man, was admitted following a motorcycle accident in which he broke his femur. He is 24 hours postoperative and requested pain medications at 0400. The medications were given and the nurse glanced in the room 2 hours later and noted he appeared to be sleeping. At 0700, the nurse on the next shift enters the room and turns on the light to see the patient cyanotic and difficult to arouse. Aggressive stimulation and oxygen revived him. Discussion with the patient revealed a history of sleep apnea that appeared to have been worsened by the effects of the pain medication.

Questions:

1. Was this a near miss or failure to rescue?
2. Did the night shift nurse adhere to principles of beneficence and nonmaleficence?
3. What should the nurse have done differently? Consider a decision tree for your answers.

and out of respect for them, educate patients about their rights under HIPAA, protect patient privacy, and share information with others only as permitted by the patient or required by law.

By maintaining patient confidentiality, nurses demonstrate fidelity toward them. *Fidelity* refers to keeping promises or being true to another—being faithful to established agreements, commitments, and responsibilities (Ellis & Hartley, 2012). Fidelity is particularly important in the care of geriatric patients because of the amount of trust they place in the healthcare system and in the nurses who care for them. Fidelity is also important in relationships with team members and the organization with which the nurse works. The team and the organization need to be able to trust the nurse to keep promises and honor relationships with them. Trust is earned, and fidelity is demonstrated in daily work and the relationships therein.

Trust depends on truthfulness; thus, *veracity*, or truth-telling, is an essential moral principle in the nurse–patient relationship. Failure to be truthful impairs trust and reliability (Ellis & Hartley, 2012). However, sometimes being truthful may cause conflict and distress, such as when breaking bad news. However, although the truth may be brutal, the telling of it does not have to be (Jonsen, Siegler, & Winslade, 2002, p. 62). There is a difference between saying, "You had a stroke and you will probably never walk again," and "You had a stroke and, while you cannot walk, we are here for you and will work with you to regain as much function as possible." Nurses should always be about the work of caring, and, even in situations of helplessness, hope remains despite its change in focus. Truthfulness is grounded in beneficence toward and respect for the patient as a person deserving of the truth. To lie would be an injustice.

Justice and Autonomy

Justice refers to fairness, equitableness, and appropriateness of an action or situation given what is due or owed to persons. For example, patients have a right to expect nurses to be competent practitioners and nurses have a *duty* to maintain competence. Anything less would be an injustice to the patient, not to mention the harm that could result.

Distributive justice considers the just distribution of scarce resources, a situation that can create challenges in health care at all levels and raise many questions. For example, donated organs are in short supply. At what age, if ever, should patients no longer be eligible for transplants? The home care nurse has many patients and not much time. How should the nurse decide which patients to see and how much time to spend with them? There are a limited number of beds available on the rehabilitation unit and many patients who could benefit from services. How should transfers be decided? What should be the role of government? The Medicare Prospective Payment System requires strict accounting for where its dollars go in post-acute care, leading to a redistribution of services and a limitation of access to home health, outpatient, and rehabilitation services for the geriatric population. Is care of geriatric patients being seen as a burden? Are age-related biases influencing resource allocation? Is the distribution of services fair, equitable, and appropriate given what is due or owed to persons?

According to Provision 1 of the *Code of Ethics*, what is owed to every person is respect for their inherent dignity, worth, unique attributes, and human rights. One of those rights is *autonomy*, the right to self-governance, to make one's own choices and decisions. Evidence of respect for autonomy is found in care that considers the patient's lifestyle, culture, value system, and religious beliefs. Such respect does not necessarily mean that the nurse condones those beliefs or choices, but rather that the nurse respects the patient as an autonomous person who has the right to determine what will be done to the patient's own person.

Informed Consent

A practical application of the principles of autonomy, beneficence, nonmaleficence, and justice is the *informed consent* process. Informed consent means that the person clearly understands the choices offered. In exercising the right to self-determination, the patient has a right to be given accurate, complete, and understandable information in a manner that allows the person to make a prudent decision on his or her own behalf. To be a truly autonomous decision it must be truly informed and truly voluntary. The elements of informed consent can be found in **Box 20-2**.

Problems develop when one no longer has the capacity to make healthcare decisions. Nurses should involve patients in the planning of their own health care to the extent that they are able to participate. But what do we do when the patient is confused and refusing care that is necessary for both comfort and health? Do we perform that care against the person's will, documenting that clarity of thought was limited? We do. Under our ethical standards, we are equally obligated to provide the best care under the circumstances (ANA, 2010a). Each state has laws indicating who is designated as a decision-maker in the event a person becomes confused, unconscious, or considered incompetent to make informed decisions. Organizational guidelines are established in line with these laws to guide staff in management of such situations. If a physician determines a person is no longer competent for such decision making, it should be noted in writing with an explanation of the probable cause and its likely duration.

Just as the decision to accept treatment must be truly autonomous, so too must be the decision to forego treatment. Particularly among the elderly, autonomy may be limited by cognitive deficits that impair clarity of thought and the ability to make decisions. A growing concern today related to self-determination is self-neglect in older adults, creating a dilemma to care (Mauk, 2011). Thus, assessing the decision-making capacity of patients is critically important and the elements of this can be found in **Box 20-3**.

It is the responsibility of the nurse, as patient advocate, to assess the patient's decisional capacity and ensure the patient's consent to or refusal of treatment is truly informed. All too often nurses discover that patients do

---

BOX 20-2   Elements of Informed Consent

1. Adequate disclosure of information
   a. Disease process (diagnosis in understandable terms)
   b. Prognosis
   c. Nature and purpose of proposed treatment or procedure
   d. Potential benefits and risks of proposed treatment or procedure
   e. Reasonable alternative treatments or procedures and their potential benefits and risks
   f. Likely effect of no treatment or procedure

2. Decisional capacity of the patient
3. Patient comprehension of the information
4. Voluntariness of the patient (free from coercion or undue influence)
5. Consent of the patient

Data from Grisso, T., & Appelbaum, P. S. (1998). *Assessing competence to consent to treatment: A guide for physicians and other health professionals.* New York, NY: Oxford University Press.

BOX 20-3   Clinical Assessment of Decision-Making Capacity

Ability to understand relevant information
1. Ability to appreciate the current situation and its consequences
2. Ability to reason or manipulate information rationally
3. Ability to communicate a choice

If the patient demonstrates satisfactory response in all four areas, the patient is said to be "decisional."

Data from Appelbaum, P. S., & Grisso, T. (1988). Assessing patients' capacities to consent to treatment. *The New England Journal of Medicine, 319*, 1635–1638.

BOX 20-4 Ways to Facilitate Autonomy	
• Encourage completion of advance directives • Provide patient-centered care • Provide appropriate education and training to patients and their family • Ensure consents and refusals are truly informed • Support and educate patients about their rights	• Stay informed of regulatory guidelines and laws related to the elderly • Provide feedback to legislators developing laws that affect the elderly • Know how to assist patients to access resources and navigate insurance and the healthcare system

not really understand why they are doing something that was prescribed by a healthcare provider. We often err by assuming they understood and provided consent because they were participating (Aveyard, 2005). Care should be taken that nurses do not abuse their power in their fiduciary relationship by persuading patients either to comply with treatment they do not want or to refuse treatment they ordinarily would accept. Any influencing factors such as "pain, depression, psychiatric illness, or effects of medications, can affect this decision-making capacity"; [furthermore] "decisions should not be made under duress or under great stress" (Guido, 2010, p. 525).

The elderly are often overwhelmed by the multiple choices they must make regarding health insurance, prescription coverage, healthcare access, and disability support. Decisions regarding living arrangements, transportation, and support services also stress resources and potentially limit autonomy. Elderly patients may need support from healthcare professionals to be assertive regarding their needs and expectations. Healthcare professionals across the continuum of care should actively include elders in decision making and care planning, as long as they are able to participate. Healthcare professionals are in a unique position to be able to direct elders to community resources and to educate and support them should they appeal the system. Feedback to regulatory bodies regarding patient needs by patients and healthcare professionals alike provides opportunities for changing regulations. Ways that nurses can facilitate autonomy in elder patients can be found in **Box 20-4**.

> **CLINICAL TIP**
>
> Nurses are expected to maintain clinical competence and adhere to applicable *standards of care*, or the degree of care that can be expected of a reasonably prudent person of the same profession in a similar situation (Peterson & Kopishke, 2010).

Quality and Sanctity of Life

Issues of justice and access to care are reminders that many decisions regarding self-determination and autonomy are related to *quality of life*, or one's personal perception of conditions of life and the degree of acceptability of such conditions, and to *sanctity of life*, or the ultimate value of life itself as sacred and inviolable and the right to live.

Quality of life is a perception based on personal values and beliefs. Views on quality of life are widely variable and likely to change when circumstances differ. They are influenced by emotional, physical, economic, and social needs. Quality of life is enhanced, for example, by prevention and management of chronic disease through preventive care, support for healthy lifestyle choices, education, and home evaluations to reduce risk of injury. Nurses are responsible for creatively thinking about and problem-solving situations that limit functional status and safety to support quality of life and independent living (**Box 20-5**). However, even the best nurse cannot prevent

---

BOX 20-5　Evidence-Based Practice Highlight

The authors provide an overview of the international literature on ethical considerations in the field of assistive technology (AT) related mainly to older adults (especially those with dementia) who live in the community. AT is generally considered useful in terms of promoting independence (as with assistive devices or monitoring), but ethical aspects are not commonly studied. A systematic literature review on the topic of AT and ethics yielded 46 papers that met the inclusion criteria. The authors found three major themes: (1) personal living environment, (2) the outside world, and (3) the design of AT devices. The evidence revealed that there was not much ethical debate surrounding the use of AT with older adults living at home; instead, most discussions centered around the concepts of autonomy and the right of elderly persons to be have self-determination. The authors noted there was a lack of clarity in concepts and assumptions in the literature, and more research is needed to shed light on different ethical aspects of the use of AT.

Data from Zwijsen, S. A., Niemeijer, A. R., & Hertogh, C. M. P. (2011). Ethics of using assistive technology in the care for community-dwelling elderly people: An overview of the literature. *Aging & Mental Health, 15*(4), 419–427.

---

injury or reduce risk of complications in those who continue to make unhealthy choices or fail to heed health or safety recommendations (Hoeman & Duchene, 2002). Some quality-of-life decisions are made in direct relation to the perceived burden being placed on others, whereas other decisions are related to the perceived indignity and emotional burden associated with problems such as incontinence and dependency.

Sanctity of life supports the belief that all human life is of value and that this value is not based on how functional, useful, effective or pleasant a person's life may seem, but rather that human life is holy, sacred, and of such value that it should never be violated. A patient can express personal perspectives on quality and sanctity of life in an advance directive document. Still, conflicts in health care are rife with issues related to value judgments of quality and sanctity of life, especially when it comes to care at the end of life. The ANA (2015) addresses this in the *Code of Ethics* in that that nurses should practice with compassion and respect for the inherent dignity, [and] worth of every person (p. 1) and should provide interventions to relieve pain and other symptoms in the dying patient that are consistent with good palliative care practice standards but may not act with the intent of ending the life of the patient (p. 3).

Patient Rights

Patient rights direct actions on ethical issues in the care of geriatric populations. The concept of rights forms the basis of many of our laws and is indeed the basis for the foundation of the U.S. Constitution. Rights are considered basic to human life, and each person is entitled to them on a legal, moral, or ethical basis (Ellis & Hartley, 2012; Beauchamp & Childress, 2013). Over the last several decades, considerable effort has been put into defining patients' rights. These rights are defined by organizational values, accreditation standards, professional codes, and legislative guidelines. The American Hospital Association has published a document addressing patient rights and hospital responsibility, entitled The *Patient Care Partnership: Understanding Expectations, Rights and Responsibilities,* in an effort to define these rights and to hold hospitals and patients accountable to them. This document is available in plain language and has been translated into multiple languages at http://www.aha.org/advocacy-issues/communicatingpts/pt-care-partnership.shtml.

Rights also evolve as values within a cultural or social group change. The right to decide what can and cannot be done to a person evolved as a legal definition due to a malpractice lawsuit in 1957 (Quallich, 2004). The right to effective pain management has evolved due to changes in perception and studies assessing the impact of poor pain management on outcomes. This is supported by The Joint Commission, which identifies pain assessment and effective pain management as a right and is part of the survey and accreditation process. As pointed out by Horgas and Yoon (2008), older adults have a high prevalence of pain due to the increase in chronic conditions. Thus, the concern for pain in older adult care is important.

CLINICAL TIP

Malpractice occurs when there is a deviation from the standard of the care and harm occurs to the patient.

Advance Directives and Living Wills

The most fundamental patient right is the right to decide. The Patient Self-Determination Act of 1990 was enacted to reduce the risk that life would be shortened or prolonged against the wishes of the individual. Following the belief that each person has a fundamental right to decide (autonomy), this law requires that patients are provided the opportunity to express their preferences regarding life-saving or life-sustaining care on entering any healthcare service, including hospitals, long-term care centers, and home care agencies. The law also requires that adequate information be supplied to the patient so that he or she can make informed decisions regarding self-determination.

Decisions regarding life-saving or life-sustaining care are recorded in legal documents known as advance directives. *Advance directives* describe actions to be taken in a situation in which the patient is no longer able to provide informed consent. Living wills are alternative documents that direct preferences for end-of-life care issues, providing an "if . . . then. . ." plan. They often include what type of care to provide and whether resuscitation measures should be taken. The "if" condition (e.g., If I am terminally ill and not expected to recover, . . .) must be confirmed by a physician (Ellis & Hartley, 2012). Laws vary from state to state regarding living wills, and some require two physicians to agree to the status of the patient before enacting directives. In states where living wills have been enacted into law, healthcare providers who do not agree with a patient's directives must remove themselves from the case (Ellis & Hartley, 2012). Remember that living wills are equally as likely to indicate that resuscitation efforts be limited as they are that all possible efforts be taken. Similar to advanced directives is the *physician orders for life-sustaining treatment* (POLST), which is intended for those who do not want to be resuscitated in an emergency (Guido, 2010). Not all states recognize a POLST at this time, but it is suggested that both advance directives and a POLST should be completed. This also allows an opportunity for one's wishes to be discussed in advance. However, not only should a patient's preferences be discussed, but they also must be recorded. In a study supported by the Agency for Healthcare Research and Quality (HS17621), Yung, Walling, & Min (2010) reported the lack of documentation in electronic health records even though patient preferences were identified in advance. This supports the need for up-to-date information in charting, especially when medical conditions change.

Durable Power of Attorney

A durable power of attorney for health care is a legal document designating an alternative decision maker in the event the person is incapacitated. This document supersedes all other general legal designations for decision-makers. In other words, a patient may designate a close friend with durable power of attorney, superseding the designation of immediate family members in decision making in a situation in which the patient is incapacitated. The reasoning behind having a proxy appointment is that the person's wishes have been discussed with the proxy prior to incapacitation (Mitty & Ramsey, 2008). If there is no designated proxy, a living will provides direction to the decision-maker. The use of a durable power of attorney can decrease conflicts between family members and allows the designated decision-maker to perform in roles negotiated in advance with the patient (Ellis & Hartley, 2012).

The absence of a living will or "do not resuscitate" order requires that all possible efforts at resuscitation should be initiated. Care of the incapacitated person is greatly simplified by an advance directive or living will. However, the issues of paternalism and boundary violations can cause ethical conflicts in the pursuit of such directives if not handled empathetically. It is imperative that information be supplied in an ethically appropriate manner for each patient because the manner in which alternatives are discussed greatly influences choices made (Elliot & Hartley, 2012). Cultural values influence decisions made, as well as the way in which decisions are made. Whereas one family may see the decision as solely up to the individual involved, others may feel it is a family decision because of duty, compassion, or the concern of those ultimately assuming the burden of care. The nurse supports the preferences of the patient in resolving self-determination issues (**Box 20-6**).

Competence

Competency refers to one's mental clarity and appropriateness for decision making based on a mental status examination (Vogel, 2010). *Competence* must be present for persons to exercise autonomy and their right to decide. Inherent in autonomy is the right to choose, the right to be informed, and the right to refuse treatment, including whether to participate in research. Loss of competence due to impaired memory or sensory function significantly affects one's ability to make such informed decisions. There is a difference between being declared legally incompetent and situations in which there is evidence of impaired competence that may be transient due to health problems or side effects of medications. Legal competence is determined by the court, and if a person is deemed legally incompetent, a legal guardian may be appointed.

BOX 20-6   Recommended Reading

American Nurses Association (ANA). (2008). Some nurses still need end-of-life education. Retrieved from http://ana.nursingworld.org/MainMenuCategories/EthicsStandards/Resources/IssuesUpdate/UpdateArchive/IssuesUpdateSpring2001/EndofLifeEducation.aspx

Anthony, J. S. (2007). Self-advocacy in health care: Decision-making among elderly African Americans. *Journal of Cultural Diversity, 17*(2), 88–97.

Beauchamp, T. L., & Childress, J. F. (2009). *Principles of biomedical ethics* (6th ed.). New York, NY: Oxford University Press.

Butts, J. B., & Rich, K. L. (2008). *Nursing ethics across the curriculum and into practice* (2nd ed.). Sudbury, MA: Jones & Bartlett.

Dauwerse, L., Van der Dam, S., & Abma, Y. (2012). Morality in the mundane: Specific needs for ethics support in elderly care. *Nursing Ethics, 19*(1), 91–103.

Dunbar, B. (2011). Ethical perspectives of sustaining residential autonomy: A cultural transformation best practice. *Nursing Administration Quarterly, 28*(2), 126.

Joint Commission. (2007). *"What did the doctor say?": Improving health literacy to protect patient safety.* Oakbrook Terrace, IL: Author.

Winterstein, T. B. (2012). Nurses' experiences of the encounter with elder neglect. *Journal of Nursing Scholarship, 44*(1), 55–62.

Guardianship

Legal *guardianship* or conservatorship is the legal appointment of a person to make decisions on behalf of a person who has been found by the court to be incapable of making his or her own decisions. Guardianship is the most restrictive and gives the guardian full custody over the person, whereas a limited guardianship sets out specific activities and decisions to be assigned to the guardian. Conservatorship gives the guardian authority regarding financial issues, but not medical decisions. **Box 20-7** provides some general background on sources of law.

Assisted Suicide

Another ethical issue of self-determination and autonomy is that of assisted suicide. In most states, intentionally aiding a person in death is considered a crime of manslaughter. The ANA published a position statement on assisted suicide in 1994 that still applies today, stating that it is a violation of the *Code of Ethics for Nurses*. Instead, it suggests that nurses focus on providing competent, comprehensive, and compassionate end-of-life care (**Box 20-8**).

BOX 20-7   Sources of Law

- **Constitutional law** is the supreme law in the United States and takes precedence over state and local laws. These laws govern federal and state governments, corporations, and society and guarantee individual rights such as privacy, freedom of speech, and the right to equal protection.
- **Statutory laws** are ones enacted by federal, state, and local legislation and may include such things as reporting abuse or communicable disease.

- **Administrative laws** include ones that originate from administrative agencies, including state boards of nursing that enforce the state's nurse practice act.
- **Common law**, sometimes called **case law**, is based on prior decisions of the court and provides historical references that may be used during argument of a case in court or during settlement negotiations.

BOX 20-8   Research Highlight

Using the Moral Distress Scale, a team of researchers assessed hundreds of nurses and their feelings of conflict in situations where they understood an ethical action they should take, but were inhibited from following through with that action. Sign into your database of nursing literature (CINAHL or PubMed, for example) and use the citation below to perform a search for this article. What does this study tell us about moral distress in nurses caring for geriatric end-of-life patients?

Piers, R. D., Van den Eynde, M., Steeman, E., Vlerisck, P., Benoit, D. D., & Van Den Noortgate, N. J. (2012). End-of-life care of the geriatric patient and nurses' moral distress. *American Medical Directors Association, 13*, 80e7–80e13.

Oregon enacted the Death with Dignity Act in 1997 to allow terminally ill residents of Oregon to use voluntary self-administration of lethal medications to end their lives. These medications are expressly prescribed by physicians for this purpose. The law applies only to mentally competent adults who must:

> Provide written documentation of their intentions
> Be diagnosed as terminally ill
> Participate in a prescribed waiting period
> Take the prescribed medication themselves—medications must be taken orally

The Death with Dignity Act specifically disallows lethal injection, mercy killing, or active euthanasia and protects those who participate in the process from liability and criminal prosecution (Oregon Department of Human Services, 1997). There were many concerns that outsiders would flock to Oregon to take advantage of the law, but that has not happened (Oregon Department of Human Services, 2007). Guido (2010) reports that 341 people have died under the law, citing reasons for their choice as "loss of autonomy, decreasing ability to participate in activities that made life enjoyable, and loss of dignity" (p. 187).

Ethics in Practice

Despite efforts to live by moral principles and under the guidance of a code of ethics, ethical conflicts remain in nursing practice. Conflict situations can create challenges to one's character. They raise profound questions such as, "Who am I? What am I doing? What am I becoming as a result of what I am doing?" These are questions of moral integrity.

The *Code of Ethics* recognizes the vital importance of a nurse's moral integrity. "Nurses have a right and a duty to act according to their personal and professional values and to accept compromise only if reaching a compromise preserves the nurse's moral integrity and does not jeopardize the dignity or well-being of the nurse or others" (pp. 20–21). Patients, too, recognize the critical importance of a nurse's moral integrity because patients, in their vulnerability, must be able to trust nurses to be the kind of person who will do the right thing even when no one is looking and even when it might be unpopular. Situations of medical error and conflicts of interest are two examples.

Medical Errors

Because of the increased awareness regarding the frequency and cost of medical mistakes, as reported in *Preventing Medication Errors: Quality Chasm Series* (2007), considerable effort has been put into reducing mistakes and improving patient safety. As noted in the Institute of Medicine (2007) report, *Informing the Future: Critical Issues in Health,* "the average hospital patient can expect to be subjected to at least one medication error per day" (p. 14). Consider the potential number of errors in long-term care in which multiple treatments and medications are part of care and the potential harm. Nurses can become more proactive in preventing medical errors by recognizing and reporting the multiple areas in which system failures may occur. Designing prevention strategies, rather than responding to mistakes, must be a priority in care delivery (see **Case Study 20-3**). Systems or other financial gains create conflict between professional integrity and self-interest. Nurses should facilitate resolution of conflicts by disclosing potential or actual conflicts of interest or withdraw from participation in care or processes that are causing the conflict (ANA, 2010a).

CLINICAL TIP

Negligence is deviation of accepted practice, a wrongful act, or failure to act by a healthcare professional, usually due to lack of knowledge or skill or poor judgment in application of the knowledge and skill (Bulau, 2011).

Case Study 20-3

Jane is a junior-level baccalaureate nursing student who is doing her clinical rotation in a long-term care facility. She is assigned to care for a resident who occupies a double room, 111-2. The resident assigned to Jane is named Iva Wittacker, and Iva's roommate is Ida Wallace. Both residents are elderly women and have the same initials. While passing out medications, Jane asks the nursing assistant to identify Ms. Wittacker because the residents do not wear armbands, Ms. Wittacker's picture is missing from the medication book, and Jane has not cared for this resident in the past. The certified nursing assistant (CNA) points to a white-haired woman in room 111. Jane administers the medications to the resident, and then her roommate enters the room and asks where her pills are. Jane asks the woman's name and she states she is Iva Wittacker. Jane realizes that she has administered medications to the wrong resident.

Questions:

1. What should Jane do immediately in this situation?
2. What could and should have been done to prevent such an error from occurring?
3. Who is responsible for Jane's mistake? What about accountability of the facility, the CNA, and/or the clinical instructor?
4. What are the ethical and legal implications in this situation?
5. Discuss what might happen if this mistake occurred in the facility where you are practicing.

Conflict of Interest

A *conflict of interest* arises in situations in which a person who has a duty to act for the benefit of another exploits that relationship for some kind of personal benefit. Due to the moral nature of nursing and the fiduciary nature of the nurse–patient relationship, the potential for conflicts of interest can exist. For example, a nurse case manager is responsible for helping patients find assisted living facilities. The nurse's spouse owns an assisted living facility and the more patients enrolled in that facility the more the nurse and spouse profit financially. The expectation is, as it says in Provision 2 of the *Code of Ethics*, that the nurse's primary commitment is to the patient (p. 5) and, so, the referral should be made to the facility that could best meet the needs of the patient, not the one that could best meet the needs of the nurse. The problem with situations of conflict of interest, or even the appearance of a conflict, is that it damages trust in the professional–patient relationship because it raises questions about the real motives of the professional. That is why the *Code of Ethics* advises that "any conflict of interest situation, whether perceived or actual, should be disclosed to all relevant parties and, if indicated, nurses should withdraw, without prejudice, from further participation" (p. 6).

Reporting errors and disclosing conflicts of interest takes courage, honesty, and humility, virtues that describe a person's character and whose actions preserve moral integrity. Not to be confused with conflict of interest but still a threat to moral integrity, is conflict of conscience, which is referred to in the *Code of Ethics* as "conscientious objection" (p. 21). Fowler (2015) explains that, "In nursing, conscientious objection [is] the refusal to participate in some aspect of patient care on moral or religious grounds" (p. 87). Some examples that are particularly pertinent in geriatrics may be participation in certain situations of withholding or withdrawal of nutrition and hydration, withdrawal of life-sustaining treatment, forced medication, use of restraints, and assisted suicide. The *Code of Ethics* has consistently maintained that a nurse has a duty to self and a right and duty to preserve moral integrity. "Conscientious objection permits nurses to preserve their integrity in the face of a clinical activity or situation to which they have moral objections to participation" (Fowler, p. 88).

Summary

As trusted professionals, nurses must continue to respect the worth, dignity, and rights of the elderly as they provide care that meets their patients' comprehensive needs across the lifespan continuum. Nursing's fundamental commitment to the uniqueness of the person creates opportunities for participation in planning and directing care with patients, their families, and the community. Nursing's vigilance in advocating for dignified, just, and humane care establishes a standard that can be appreciated by all. It is not through rules and regulations that ethical care delivery is created—it is through the actions of every nurse in every day of practice.

Understanding the uniqueness of the geriatric population as it relates to age-related changes, psychosocial pressures, spiritual needs, and adapting to change provides the nurse with multiple ethical challenges as one prepares for the end of the lifespan. The *Scope and Standards of Practice* (ANA, 2010b) in nursing identifies the code of ethics as the framework of practice, "regardless of the practice setting, role, and provides guidance for the future" (p. 26). Providing respectful care that puts the patient's safety and welfare first helps us avoid situations that can result in failure to rescue, abuse of power, exploitation, and over-involvement (Ellis & Hartley, 2012). Developing a framework for ethical decision making provides a foundation for discussion when dilemmas present themselves, smoothing the way for integrity-saving compromise. The nurse's conscientious effort to follow professional ethical standards in daily practices supports the quality of care we all strive to provide and experience.

Clinical Reasoning Exercises

1. Are your patients truly informed about their care? Ask five patients why they are taking the medications they are prescribed and evaluate their responses.

2. Mrs. Gomez is confused and at times combative. Her family regularly visits and is actively involved in her care. She has been agitated and wandering the unit for the last several days and has not had a bowel movement for 6 days. She is constantly complaining of stomach pain and refuses all oral or rectal medications to facilitate bowel emptying. Her bowel sounds are diminished, and a hard mass, suspected to be stool, can be felt in the descending colon. Will you restrain her and give her an enema to prevent further complications?

3. Mrs. S. has been transferred from the hospital to your rehabilitation center. The family is trying to understand the severity of her right-sided CVA, along with Mrs. S's concern for her change in body image. How will you approach the family about her care and the role of the rehabilitation center?

4. You answer the phone, and a woman, indicating she is the daughter of your patient, asks you about her status. How will you respond considering confidentiality and privacy issues?

5. You observe a CNA undressing an elderly woman and restraining her hands. The woman has been crying and yelling out for much of the night and is obviously confused. She leaves the woman naked on the stripped bed and walks out of the room, closing the door behind her and commenting as she passes you, "There, let her wet herself all night, I am done with her." As the nurse in charge, how would you handle this situation?

Personal Reflections

1. As you prepare to care for older adults, what values, conflicts, or ethical dilemmas do you anticipate you will face?
2. Assess your feelings about the right to die and assisted suicide. Do you agree with the ANA's stand on this issue? How would you respond in the event that an elderly patient asks "please help me die" when death is not near?
3. An elderly person is becoming unsafe living alone and has been identified as being at risk for serious injury. During admission to an alternative living setting, the person appears oriented and appropriate. Furthermore, the person expresses disagreement with the recommendations for this admission. How would you respond in this situation?

References

American Nurses Association. (2010a). *Position statement: The nurse's role in ethics and human rights—Protecting and promoting individual worth, dignity, and human rights in practice settings.* Retrieved from http://www.nursingworld.org/MainMenuCategories/Policy-Advocacy/Positions-and-Resolutions/ANAPosition Statements/Position-Statements-Alphabetically/NursesRole-EthicsHumanRights-PositionStatement.pdf

American Nurses Association. (2010b). *Scope and standards of practice* (2nd ed.). Silver Spring, MD: Nursebooks.org.

American Nurses Association. (2015). *Code of ethics for nurses with interpretive statements.* Silver Spring MD: Author.

Appelbaum, P. S., & Grisso, T. (1988). Assessing patients' capacities to consent to treatment. *The New England Journal of Medicine, 319,* 1635–1638.

Aveyard, H. (2005). Informed consent prior to nursing care procedures. *Nursing Ethics, 12*(1), 19–29.

Beauchamp, T. L., & Childress, J. F. (2013). *Principles of biomedical ethics* (7th ed.). New York, NY: Oxford University Press.

Bulau J. M. (2011). Liability for negligence and error in judgment. *Journal of Legal Nurse Consulting, 22*(3), 28–29.

Burkhardt, M. A., & Nathaniel A. K. (2008). *Ethics and issues in contemporary nursing* (3rd ed.). New York, NY: Delmar Cengage Learning.

Chinn, P. L., & Kramer, M. K. (2008). *Integrated theory and knowledge development in nursing* (7th ed.). St. Louis, MO: Mosby.

Fowler, M. (2015). *Guide to the code of ethics for Nurses with interpretive statement* (2nd ed.). Silver Spring, MD: American Nurses Association.

Grisso, T., & Appelbaum, P. S. (1998). *Assessing competence to consent to treatment: A guide for physicians and other health professionals.* New York, NY: Oxford University Press.

Guido, G. W. (2010). *Legal and ethical issues in nursing* (5th ed.). Upper Saddle River, NJ: Pearson.

Hoeman, S. P., & Duchene, P. M. (2002). Ethical matters in rehabilitation. In S. P. Hoeman (Ed.), *Rehabilitation nursing process, application, and outcomes* (3rd ed., pp. 28–35), St. Louis, MO: Mosby.

Horgas, A. L., & Yoon, S. L. (2008). Pain management. In E. Capezuti, D. Zwicker, M. Mezey, & T. Fulmer (Eds.), *Evidence-based geriatric nursing protocols for best practice* (3rd ed., pp. 199–222). New York, NY: Springer.

Institute of Medicine. (2007). *Informing the future: Critical issues in health* (4th ed.). Washington, DC: National Academies Press.

Jameton, A. (1984). *Nursing practice: The ethical issues.* Upper Saddle River, NJ: Prentice-Hall.

Jones, J. (2015). Walk forward with a strong ethical agenda. *The American Nurse, 47*(4): 16.

Jonsen, A. R., Siegler, M., & Winslade, W. J. (2002). *Clinical ethics: A practical approach to ethical decisions in clinical medicine* (5th ed.). New York, NY: McGraw Hill.

Lachman, V. D. (2009). Practical use of the nursing code of ethics. I. *MEDSURG Nursing, 18*(1), 55–57.

Mauk, K. L. (2011). Ethical perspective on self-neglect among older adults. *Rehabilitation Nursing, 36*(2), 60–65.

McEwen, M., & Wills, E. M. (2002). *Theoretical basis for nursing.* Philadelphia, PA: Lippincott, Williams, & Wilkins.

Oregon Department of Human Services. (2007). Oregon's Death with Dignity Act—2007. Retrieved from https://public.health.oregon.gov/ProviderPartnerResources/EvaluationResearch/DeathwithDignityAct/Documents/year10.pdf

Pellegrino, E. D., & Thomasma, D. C. (1981). *A philosophical basis of medical practice: Toward a philosophy and ethic of the healing professions.* New York, NY: Oxford University Press.

Peterson, A. M. & Kopishke, L. (2010). Legal nurse consulting principles. London, England: Taylor & Francis.

Piers, R. D., Van den Eynde, M., Steeman, E., Vlerick, P., Benoit, D., & Van Den Noortgate, N. J. (2012). End-of-life care of the geriatric patient and nurses' moral distress. *Journal of American Medical Directors Association, 13*, 80.e7–80.e13.

Quallich, S. A. (2004). The practice of informed consent. *Urologic Nursing, 24*(6), 513–515.

Rest, J. R. (1994). Theory and research. In J. R. Rest & D. Narvaez (Eds.), *Moral development in the professions: Psychology and applied ethics* (pp. 1–26). Hillsdale, NJ: Lawrence Erlbaum Associates.

Vogel, T. M. (2010). Legal and financial issues related to health care for older people. In R. H. Robnett & W. C. Chop (Eds.), *Gerontology for the health care professional* (2nd ed., pp. 285–314). Sudbury, MA: Jones & Bartlett.

Yung, V. Y., Walling, A. M., & Min, L. (2010). Elder's preferences for end-of-life are not captured by documentation in their medical records. *Journal of Palliative Medicine, 13*(7), 861–867.

Zwijsen, S. A., Niemeijer, A. R., & Hertogh, C. M. P. (2011). Ethics of using assistive technology in the care for community-dwelling elderly people: An overview of the literature. *Aging & Mental Health, 15*(4), 419–427.

For a full suite of assignments and additional learning activities, see the access code at the front of your book.

Unit VII
Information and Health Care Technologies

(COMPETENCIES 5, 18)

CHAPTER 21   TECHNOLOGY AND CARE
OF OLDER ADULTS (COMPETENCIES 5, 18)

Technology and Care of Older Adults

Linda L. Pierce
Victoria Steiner

(Competencies 5, 18)

LEARNING OBJECTIVES

At the end of this chapter, the reader will be able to:

> Identify assistive technology and methods for teaching older adults about its use.
> Recognize common applications of assistive technology to enhance older adults' functioning, independence, and safety.
> Describe Internet and Web approaches for assistive technology, including learning activities, health information, and healthcare services that can be used in caring for older adults and their families, along with teaching strategies for its access.
> Discuss new assistive technologies.

KEY TERMS

Assistive devices

Assistive technologies

Augmentative and alternative communication

Emergency response system

Environmental controls

Home health care

Internet

Nursing informatics

Smart home

World Wide Web

This century reflects a time of change for nursing and the way nurses deliver health care to the population over the age of 65 years. Americans are living longer, and this age cohort will increase from 35.9 million in 2003 to 44.7 million in 2013 and then to about 82.3 million by the year 2040, which is twice their number in 2000 (Administration on Aging [AOA], 2014). Most of these individuals expect to have an active life in the community well into their seventh decade. Improved health care for acute illnesses and diseases helps these individuals live longer, but it also increases their chances of chronic conditions accompanied by increased disability (American Association of Retired Persons [AARP] Public Policy Institute, 2009; Ladika & Ladika, 2016). Nurses, as well as family members, friends, and neighbors, who are caring for older adults must advocate for and use new ways to provide care to these adults that promotes their quality of life. Examples of these new care strategies include (1) the electronic medical record (EMR), which is a digital version of a person's chart. The EMR contains all the medical and health–related history from a provider that can be used for diagnosis and treatment (Agency for Healthcare Research and Quality [AHRQ], 2016), and (2) electronic intensive care units (eICUs), in which state-of-the art video cameras, microphones, alarms, and other tools connect the sickest people in the eICU, no matter where they are located, with medical providers and specialists from remote sites miles away for treatment (Khan, 2014). The purpose of this chapter is to provide information about the integration of nursing care with the latest *assistive technologies* that support the care of older adults, as well as to describe several new technologies.

Introduction to Assistive Technology

The growing population of older adults will change many aspects of health care. One change will be an increase in the number of people who experience a disabling condition. As individuals age or become disabled, mental and physical changes may influence their ability to live as independently and productively as they would wish. A lessening or loss of strength, balance, visual and auditory acuity, cognitive processing, and/or memory may affect the way they are able to function at home.

Assistive technology (AT) devices are mechanical aids that substitute for or enhance the function of some physical or mental ability that is impaired (Kelker, 1997; National Institute of Standards and Technology, 2011; Spillman, 2004). The term **assistive technology** encompasses a broad range of devices, from "low tech" (e.g., pencil grips, splints, paper stabilizers) to "high tech" (e.g., computers, voice synthesizers, Braille readers). These devices include the entire range of supportive tools and equipment, from adapted spoons to wheelchairs to computer systems for environment control.

As a tool for living, the primary purpose of AT is to bridge the gap between an older person's declining capabilities and the unchanging environmental demands of home and community (Gitlin, 1998; National Institute of Standards and Technology, 2011; Spillman, 2004). The use of *assistive devices* may enable independent performance, increase safety, reduce risk of injury, improve balance and mobility, improve communication, and limit complications of an illness or disability. These devices are not just for those who are disabled or have functional limitations. Assistive devices also can help individuals who are aging and who may benefit from using them to promote safety and reduce the risk of injury. Individuals experiencing age-related changes or functional decline also may benefit from equipment and devices that enable independent performance and prevent disability.

In 1995, Norburn et al. found that a large number of older adults practice some form of self-care, even in the absence of reported disability. Their study determined the "extent to which self-care coping strategies, defined as modifying the environment, changing behavior, and/or using special equipment and devices, are employed by older adults at all levels of functioning in order to maintain a viable and independent social life without the need for institutional care" (Norburn et al., 1995, p. S101). More than 75% of the subjects made behavioral changes in their daily routines (e.g., doing things more slowly) during the year before the survey. About 42% of the subjects reported using assistive devices, and almost one third had modified their built environment.

More recently, Matthews, Beach, de Bruin, Mecca, & Schulz (2010) studied intelligent systems (in the areas of driving, home management, personal care, and mobility and manipulation) capable of learning how individuals manage their daily activities, determining when they need help and providing cognitive and physical assistance when indicated. They found that older respondents to their national, Web-based survey were moderately supportive of using technology to reduce dependence on others. However, they preferred to "interact with a person when a human could accomplish a task as well as the technology" (p. 8). Factors considered very important in deciding to use intelligent AT included how safe it would be to use, its cost, how adequately it could meet one's needs, and its impact on privacy.

Assistive Device Use

Living at home can be made easier with the use of assistive devices. The increased independence afforded individuals who use these devices may ultimately result in their being able to remain in their homes for longer periods with reduced concerns for safety. Many of these devices are inexpensive and easy to obtain, but the general population's knowledge of them is poor. Consequently, individuals who are aging or disabled may not be living their lives to their fullest potential.

There is no evidence to suggest that older adults use AT and devices less than young adults, but it is not known whether there is greater reluctance among the elderly to use high-technology versus low-technology solutions. A number of research and service programs have evaluated the willingness of older adults to use high technology, such as computer-based systems to increase communication, and social integration and smart house arrangements to increase safety and function (Gitlin, Schemm, Landsberg, & Burgh, 1996; Johnson, Davenport, & Mann, 2007; Mann, Belchior, Tomita, & Kemp, 2007; Matthews et al., 2010; Tomita, Mann, Stanton, Tomita, & Sundar, 2007). A *smart home* is an environment constructed with various technological applications and devices that are directed by a central control unit to assist the residents in performing daily activities.

Johnson et al. (2007) gathered input from potential smart home users in an effort to develop more beneficial and usable applications. Many older adults felt that these technologies were for others or that they could use them in the future. Individuals also expressed concern that if they relied on technology to do tasks for them, they would lose abilities, but were willing to use technology for things they were unable to do themselves. Users were most favorable regarding applications that were related to their type of impairment. For example, individuals with mobility impairments liked smart door applications, which allowed them to answer the door and enter the house hands-free. Older adults were also willing to receive assistance from smart technology if it enabled them to remain independent and stay in their home.

The probability of engaging in self-care practices and the type of strategy employed vary with levels of impairment. Older adults with moderate levels of impairment rely more on special equipment and assistive devices, whereas those with slight functional impairments tend to change their behavior (Norburn et al., 1995). "Of importance is the consistent finding that device use has a dual outcome: At the same time that a device promotes independence, it appears to also raise concerns about social stigma, feelings of embarrassment, and issues related to personal identity and self-definition" (Gitlin, 1998, p. 154). There is no stigma involved in the use of developmentally appropriate equipment or tools for children (e.g., jumbo crayons), so why should equipment and device use in older adults be seen as a response to disability (e.g., wide Dr. Grip pens)?

Mann, Hurren, and Tomita (1993) studied assistive device use by interviewing 157 noninstitutionalized older persons in their homes. Study participants were not selected randomly, however, but were individuals who were recently or currently receiving services from a human service agency, hospital, or nursing home. The researchers used the definition of an assistive device provided in the Technology-Related Assistance for Individuals with Disabilities Act of 1988: "Any item, piece of equipment, or product system, whether acquired commercially off the shelf, modified, or customized that is used to increase, maintain, or improve functional capabilities of individuals with disabilities" (U.S. Congress, 1988). They found that subjects owned a mean of 13.7 devices and used 10.8 of the devices. Older persons with multiple impairments that included physical impairments used the greatest number of devices. Subjects also expressed a need for additional equipment and devices.

Another study by Mann, Hurren, and Tomita (1995) examined the need for and current use of assistive devices by home-based older adults with arthritis. Subjects were assigned to a moderate or a severe arthritis group based on the impact arthritis had on their activities. Subjects in the severe arthritis group had more chronic diseases, a higher level of pain, and a lower level of independence in self-care activities than subjects in the moderate group. Both groups reported using a high number of assistive devices (about 10 per person) and expressed the need for additional devices, such as reachers, magnifiers, jar openers, grab bars, and hearing aids. Generally, there was a high rate of satisfaction with the equipment and devices used.

More recently, Kraskowsky and Finlayson (2001) reported usage rates from 47% to 82% of equipment and devices prescribed. Mann, Goodall, Justiss, and Tomita (2002) found that study participants owned a mean of 14.2 assistive devices, used 84.8% of the devices, and were satisfied with 84.2% of the devices they owned. Mann, Llanes, Justiss, and Tomita (2004) looked at the value older individuals themselves place on their equipment and devices by interviewing 1,016 home-based frail older adults in western New York and northern Florida, specifically asking them what they considered their "most important" assistive device and why. Although "importance" is a general construct, it embodies the perception of "usefulness" and impact on ability to do tasks and participate in activities. Not considering the number of users, the top five most important equipment and devices were eyeglasses, canes, wheelchairs, walkers, and telephones. Controlling for the number of people using the device, the top five most important devices were oxygen tanks, dentures, 3-in-1 commodes, computers, and wheelchairs.

Pressler and Ferraro (2010) used three waves of data from a nationally representative sample of older adults to examine how assistive devices are adopted by persons facing activities of daily living (ADLs) disability. Their results indicated that incident disability is the precursor of assistive device adoption. More specifically, although baseline levels of disability result in adoption of assistive devices, incident disability leads to additional assistive device use. They also found that lower body disability, advanced age, and obesity are consistent predictors of the number of assistive devices used. Based on their study, Pressler and Ferraro recommend that healthcare providers and caregivers be aware of an increase in lower body disability and facilitate the use of assistive devices to effectively bridge the gap between impairment and function.

Mann, Ottenbacher, Frass, Tomita, and Granger (1999) studied the effectiveness of assistive devices and environmental modifications in maintaining independence and reducing home care costs. Researchers assigned 104 frail older adults recently referred to *home health care* to either a treatment group or a control group. Individuals in the treatment group received a functional assessment, a home assessment, and any necessary equipment and/ or assistive devices and environmental interventions. The control group received usual care services. The frail older adults in the study experienced functional decline over time, but the control group declined significantly more. Costs related to hospitalization and nursing home stays were more than three times higher for the control group. In a study of community-dwelling older adults with one or more limitations in ADLs, Hoenig, Taylor, and Sloan (2003) found that the use of AT was associated with the use of fewer hours of personal assistance. These studies provide strong evidence that appropriate and necessary equipment or devices can slow the rate of functional decline and reduce health-related costs.

CLINICAL TIP

Assistive technologies provide a possible solution to promote independence among the very old.

The fastest growing sector of the population are those individuals over 85 years, and they pose a particular challenge because they have high rates of comorbidity and cognitive impairment AOA, 2014). Assistive technologies are one possible solution to promote independence in these oldest old individuals, but these are often underutilized in routine care (Robinson et al., 2013). A UK cohort study of 851 older adults, 85 year old, showed that over 80% of participants did not use common, low-cost assistive technologies. This study also concluded that although the evidence base evaluating the effectiveness of assistive technologies in caring for the oldest old is increasing, it is difficult to determine their effectiveness in this age group because the oldest old are often excluded from research trials (Davies et al., 2010). The use of AT in people over 85 years with dementia also raises ethical dilemmas; it is critical for healthcare practitioners to assess an individual's mental capacity and his or her ability to make decisions about future care before such devices can be employed (Robinson et al., 2013). A core issue in decision making around the use of AT, such as tracking devices, is the balance between an individual with dementia's right to independence and the caregivers' duty to minimize harm (Robinson et al., 2007).

Based on the literature, a number of conclusions can be drawn. Although studies have shown varied results, a consistent finding is that older adults are willing to use assistive devices. Studies have also concluded that some individuals, particularly those who are less impaired, might be more likely to modify their behaviors than use equipment or devices for assistance. Unfortunately, the definition of assistive devices varies across studies, as do the characteristics of the individuals studied; for example, Mann et al. (1999) tended to seek older adult subjects who were impaired or at risk for needing assistive devices. Regardless of the study, however, researchers have stated that older adults are lacking adequate information about AT that could improve quality of life.

Evaluating the Use of Assistive Technology

Use of AT is a type of health behavior among older adults to maintain their independence and enable them to live at home. This type of technology offers the potential of increasing independence and quality of life for older individuals, as well as reducing health-related costs. From the viewpoints of the national health economy and the quality of life of older adults and caregivers, it is important to understand who does not use devices and why they do not.

A study by Mann et al. (2002) sought to identify those types of equipment and devices with a higher frequency of nonuse and the reasons given by older adults for not using them. Based on the Rehabilitation Engineering Research Center on Aging Consumer Assessments Study, 1,056 subjects reported use or nonuse of assistive devices. Of these subjects, 873 identified reasons for not using or being dissatisfied with certain equipment and devices. The devices were grouped into categories based on the type of impairment they addressed (hearing, vision, cognition, and musculoskeletal/neuromotor). Study participants owned the largest number of equipment and devices in the musculoskeletal/neuromotor category, such as canes. Equipment and devices in the hearing impairment category were rated lowest by participants in terms of satisfaction. Almost half of all reasons listed for not using certain assistive devices related to perceived lack of need.

The purpose of a study by Tomita, Mann, Frass, and Stanton (2004) was to identify predictors of the use of assistive devices that address physical impairments among cognitively intact, physically frail older adults living at home. Interviewers who visited the subjects' homes identified equipment and devices in use. White elders who live alone in the South, are physically disabled, take more medications, and are less depressed tend to use more equipment and devices to address physical impairments than nonwhite elders who are living with someone in the northern United States and who have less severity of physical disability, take fewer medications, and are more depressed. Among all the variables, physical disability was the most significant predictor of use. Consistent with findings from previous studies, income, education, and marital status were not associated with their use. In addition, age and gender were not significant.

Kraskowsky and Finlayson (2001) compared 14 studies of factors influencing use of assistive devices by older adults. They found that use of them decreased over time. The primary reason for nonuse was lack of fit among the device, the person, and the person's environment. They suggested a range of factors to consider when prescribing AT to older adults, including personal (patient) factors, the equipment and device's fit with the patient's environment, and intervention-related factors. Creating a positive expectation for the use of the equipment or device, when it is introduced, can influence the patient factor. Knowing what to expect in the patient's environment when prescribing an assistive device can influence its fit within the environment. Increasing the frequency and duration of education on the assistive device can also positively influence use.

A careful evaluation of older adults is an important step in determining their need for assistive devices and equipment to enhance and maintain independence and quality of life (Kraskowsky & Finlayson, 2001). The evaluation may occur during acute care, in-patient rehabilitation, home care, or outpatient visits (Roelands, Van Oost, Depoorter, & Buysse, 2002) by any interdisciplinary team (IDT) member (i.e., nurse, physician, therapist,

---

BOX 21-1   Guidelines for Introducing Technology and Teaching the Elderly about Its Use

- The use of technology must be perceived as needed and meaningful, and must be linked to the lifestyle of the person.
- Cautions and disbelief in one's capability may be an obstacle in accepting new technology and must be considered when creating the learning environment.
- A generous amount of time, as well as repeated short training sessions, should be allowed.
- More stress should be placed on the practical application of the device than on its technical features.
- Only selective, central facts should be presented.

- Mnemonics and cues will favorably affect self-efficacy in handling new products.
- Training sessions should be held in the home or natural meeting places of the elderly.
- The instructor should be well known by the elderly or introduced well in advance of the training.
- The attitudes of the instructors toward the aged must be positive and realistic.

Data from Idaho Assistive Technology Project. (1995). Assistive technology and older adults. Information Sheet #25. Retrieved from http://www.idahoat.org/

---

dietitian, or social worker). Typically, an occupational therapist determines whether the equipment is appropriate for older adults and their environment and educates them and their caregivers on use and care of assistive devices. However, all team members have a responsibility for evaluation and follow-up, as needed. Appropriate fit between the person's ability, the demands of the environment, and each piece of equipment or device is essential to successful task performance.

Assistive devices and equipment are typically first introduced in the hospital, outpatient, or home care setting, primarily to enhance independence in self-care. During in-patient rehabilitation, an older adult will receive an average of eight pieces of equipment and/or devices to use in the home for mobility, dressing, seating, bathing, grooming, and feeding. Those with a functional impairment living in the community report having an average of 14 pieces of equipment and/or devices in the home, including those for hearing and vision (Gitlin et al., 1996; Mann et al., 2002). With shortened hospital stays and briefer exposure to occupational and physical therapy, the need for efficient and effective instruction in assistive device use becomes that much more important for nurses. Teaching an elderly person to use technology should not be limited to the person alone, but should include caregivers and other family members. Education must be sensitive to any physical, cognitive, psychological, and environmental factors that affect the elderly person. When introducing technology to the elderly and teaching them to use it, several guidelines can be employed (see **Box 21-1**).

Common Applications of Assistive Technology

The following are common applications for AT (Kelker, 1997): (1) position and mobility, (2) environmental access and control, (3) self-care, (4) sensory impairment, (5) cognitive impairment, (6) social interaction and recreation, and (7) computer-related technology.

Position and Mobility

Older adults may need assistance with their positions for seating so they can effectively participate in activities and interact with others. Generally, nurses or therapists try to achieve an upright, forward-facing position for the individual by using padding, structured chairs, straps, supports, or restraints to hold the body in a stable and comfortable manner (Hoeman, Liszner, Alverzo, 2008; Kelker, 1997). Examples of equipment used for different types of positioning are walkers, floor sitters, chair inserts, wheelchairs, straps, traps, and standing aids. Conversely, older adults whose physical impairments limit their mobility may need a device to help them get around or participate in activities. Mobility devices include self-propelled walkers, manual or powered wheelchairs, and powered recreational vehicles such as bikes and scooters.

Environmental Access and Control

Access to shopping centers, places of business, schools, recreation, and transportation is possible because of AT modifications. This kind of AT includes modifications to buildings, rooms, or other facilities that allow people with physical impairments to use ramps and door openers to enter, allow people with visual disabilities to follow Braille directions and move more freely within a facility, and allow people of short stature or people who use wheelchairs to reach pay phones or operate elevators (Kelker, 1997).

Once inside a building, various types of *environmental controls*, including remote control switches and special adaptations of on/off switches to make them accessible (e.g., Velcro attachments, pointer sticks), can promote independent use of equipment by an older adult. Robotic arms and other environmental control systems turn lights on and off, open doors, and operate appliances. For example, X-10 is an electronic environmental control that allows individuals to control lights, heating, and cooling, as well as just about any electrical piece of equipment, such as curtains, garage doors, and gates. Basic installation is very easy for lamps and plug-in items. The minimum requirements are one control unit and one control module. No wiring is required. First, the control unit is plugged in, then the lamp to be controlled is plugged into a module, and finally the module is plugged into an outlet. There are also several types of modules and switches available to replace existing wall switches (X-10, 2005).

X-10 could be considered the father of home automation, and today a number of other technologies exist, all of which can be used in a "smart home" system. A person's residence can have appliances, lighting, heating, air conditioning, televisions, computers, entertainment audio and video systems, security systems, and camera systems that are capable of communicating with one another and can be controlled remotely by a time schedule, from any room in the home, as well as remotely from any location in the world by telephone or internet (Smart-HomeUSA, 2016). If memory and mobility issues are a problem, voice controls and speech recognition modules can act as solutions. For example, the VoiceIR Environmental Voice Controller provides users with hands-free control over dozens of household electronics, as well as garage doors, lighting, etc. (Broadened Horizons, 2011).

Self-Care

Assistive devices for self-care include such items as robotics, electric feeders, adapted utensils, specially designed toilet seats, and aids for tooth brushing, washing, dressing, and grooming. An *emergency response system* (ERS) can increase the safety of an individual who requires assistance with self-care activities. The most common ERS is the telephone-based personal emergency response system (PERS), which consists of the subscriber wearing a small help button as a necklace or wristband and a home communicator that is connected to a residential phone line (Mihailidis & Lee, 2007). In the event of an emergency, the subscriber presses the help button and is connected to a live emergency response center, which arranges for appropriate help, such as calling paramedics or the person's family. Mihailidis, Cockburn, Longley, and Boger (2008) found that home monitoring technologies would be acceptable to older adults if they allowed the participants to remain in their homes and age in place.

Remote health monitoring devices also have been developed that measure and track various physiological parameters, such as pulse, skin temperature, and blood pressure (Mihailidis & Lee, 2007). These systems are less commonly found in the home, but are growing in demand despite their restrictions. They require the user to wear the device at all times and/or to manually take the required measurements and enter the data into the system, which then automatically transmits to an evaluation and emergency service station.

Many of the PERS and physiological-based monitoring systems are inappropriate, obtrusive, and difficult for an older adult to operate. These systems require effort from the person, sometimes long training times for the person to learn how to use the required features, and they become ineffective during more serious emergency situations, such as if the person has a stroke (Mihailidis & Lee, 2007). As a result, new systems are being developed that do not require manual interaction from the user and that use nonphysiologic measures to determine health parameters. For example, the FitBit is a wearable health monitoring device that tracks daily activities and can be a helpful piece of AT equipment for a variety of health-related needs. It allows users to monitor the number of steps they take, the amount of exercise they do, the calories they burn, and the quantity and quality of their sleep. When the wearer is within 15 feet of its wireless base station, the FitBit automatically offloads data and statistics go to an online or mobile user profile (FitBit, 2016).

Studies have shown that a decline in an older adult's ability to complete ADLs is a strong indicator of declining health and may increase the likelihood of an emergency situation occurring (Mihailidis & Lee, 2007). Several researchers are developing systems that can monitor ADLs in the home. These systems use simple switches, sensors, and transducers located at various places in the user's environment and attached to various objects to detect which tasks are being completed.

Sensory Impairment

Older adults may experience impairment in their speech, hearing, or sight. Approximately one in six Americans will experience a communication disorder to some degree in his or her lifetime. For those individuals, the basic components of communication (sensing, interpreting, and responding to people and things in the environment) can be extremely challenging (National Institute on Deafness and Other Communication Disorders (NIDCD), 2009–2011). The term *augmentative and alternative communication* (AAC) refers to all forms of communication that enhance or supplement speech and writing, either temporarily or permanently. AAC can both enhance (augmentative) and replace (alternative) conventional forms of expression for people who cannot communicate through speech, writing, or gestures. AAC devices offer dynamic displays (i.e., electronic displays that change with user input) and synthesized (computer-generated) and digitalized (recorded) speech, and are accessible through many input modalities, including touch screen, keyboard, and infrared headpointers (Dickerson, Stone, Panchura, & Usiak, 2002).

The goal of AAC is to encourage and support the development of communicative competence so people can participate as fully as possible in home and community environments, and improve the efficiency and use of communication aids. Selecting the communication methods that are best for an individual is not as simple as getting a prescription for eyeglasses (American Speech-Language-Hearing Association [ASHA], 2002). Language is complex, and individuals learn to use it every day. Indeed, developing the best communication system for a person with a severe speech and language problem requires evaluation by many specialists (ASHA, 2002; Speech-Language and Audiology Canada, 2015), all of whom may not have offices in the same building or even in the same city. Communication boards, which use pictures as symbols for words, may need to be made. Vocabulary to meet the needs of a wide range of communication disorder situations must be selected. Equipment may need to be ordered and paid for. Health plans or other third-party payers may need to be contacted. Once all the parts of the communication plan are in place, the user must learn to operate each part of the system effectively and efficiently. Professionals (e.g., nurses, therapists) need to help the user and his or her communication partners learn a variety of skills and strategies, which might include the meaning of certain hand shapes and how to make them, starting and stopping a piece of electronic equipment at a desired word or picture, ways to get a person's attention, ways to help a communication partner understand a message, and increasing the rate of communication (ASHA, 2002; Speech-Language and Audiology Canada, 2015). Without effort by the user, professional help, ongoing practice, and support from friends, family, and colleagues, the promises of augmentative communication may not be realized.

Much of the time, individuals are expected to learn through listening. Hearing impairments can interfere with an older adult's speaking, reading, and ability to follow directions. Assistive devices to help with hearing and auditory processing problems include hearing aids, personal FM units, Phonic Ear devices, or closed caption TV.

Vision is also a major learning mode. General methods for assisting with vision problems include increasing contrast, utilizing stronger stimuli, and making use of tactile and auditory assistive devices. Devices that assist with vision include screen readers, screen enlargers, magnifiers, large-type books, taped books, Braillers, light boxes, high-contrast materials, and scanners.

Cognitive Impairment

Commonly available devices can help augment the memory of an individual with a cognitive disability. Early work on memory aids investigated the application of commonplace technologies, such as clocks and calendars (Wilson, 1984). These technologies are inexpensive, easy to use, and have no social stigma that might otherwise be attached to "rehabilitation" devices. However, these devices have limitations in the amount of information that can be stored and how information can be presented to the user. More importantly, written lists and calendars provide no prompting to the user as to when he or she needs to perform a task.

People who have problems remembering a sequence of tasks can also use audio recordings. A task can be broken down into its component steps, and a recording can be created outlining these steps. This recording can be used to guide the person through work and can be repeated until the task is done. Some AT interventions seek to provide support with planning and problem solving as well as memory. The Planning and Execution Assistant and Training (PEAT) System uses artificial intelligence to automatically generate daily plans and re-plans in response to unexpected events (LoPresti, Simpson, Kirsch, Schreckenghost, & Hayashi, 2008).

Social Interaction and Recreation

Older adults still want to have fun and interact socially with others. AT can help them to participate in all sorts of interactive recreational activities with friends (Kelker, 1997; Reed, 2011). Some adapted recreational activities include drawing software, computer games, computer simulations, painting with a head or mouth wand, adapted puzzles, or online computer games. Free lifetime park passes are available from the United States National Park Service to people with disabilities, and discounted passes are available for adults aged 62 years and older (U.S. National Park Service, 2012).

Computer-Based Assistive Technology

Some older adults may require special devices that provide access to computers. Controllable anatomical movements such as eye blinks, head or neck movements, or mouth movements may be used to operate equipment that provides access to the computer. Once a controllable anatomical site has been determined, decisions can be made about input devices, including switches, alternative keyboards, mouse, trackball, touch window, speech recognition, and head pointers (Hoeman et al., 2008; Kelker, 1997).

Computers are an important type of AT because they open up so many exciting possibilities for writing, speaking, finding information, or controlling an individual's environment. Software can provide the tools for written expression, calculation, reading, basic reasoning, and higher level thinking skills. The computer also can be used to access a wide variety of databases.

Many examples of the assistive devices mentioned earlier can be found on the AbleData Website (http://www.abledata.com). AbleData is a federally funded project whose primary mission is to provide information on AT, including all types of adaptive equipment and assistive devices, available from domestic and international sources to consumers, organizations, professionals, and caregivers within the United States. The database contains detailed descriptions of each product, including price and company information. The database also contains information on noncommercial prototypes, customized and one-of-a-kind products, and do-it-yourself designs.

BOX 21-2   Ten of the Best Applications for Older Adults

Read2Go: Read2Go is an accessible ebook reader that makes reading Bookshare titles easy. Bookshare is the world's largest accessible online library for people with print disabilities with over 345,000 titles.

Dragon Dictation: This voice-recognition application allows users to dictate text or email messages and see them instantly, including tweets or status updates for Facebook.

Voice Reading: Excellent for those who get tired reading long emails or Web content; the application will read aloud any text shared from other applications, URLs, or even text files.

EyeReader: This application acts as a magnifying glass. By holding their iPhone in front of a book or newspaper users get a clear picture of the text with a light to help brighten it.

Vouchercloud: This application, from one of the original money-saving coupon Websites, offers on-the-go discount vouchers.

Idealo: An application that allows cost-conscious shoppers to scan the barcode on a product and search for the cheapest place to buy it online.

Mint Bills: Users can streamline their bill pay and view all of their accounts in one place with this mobile application.

Pill Reminder Pro: Users can enter in the name of their pill, dosage, frequency, and what time(s) of day it is taken, and PillReminder will alert them when it is time to take their pill(s).

Blood Pressure Monitor—Family Lite: Practical and easy to use, this application helps keep track of a users' blood pressure and provides a weight health monitor.

Lumosity Mobile: This application features games designed by neuroscientists to enhance memory and cognitive speed.

Mobile applications began appearing in 2008 and have transformed the delivery of many of these common applications for AT. Mobile applications are computer programs designed to run on mobile devices such as smartphones and tablet computers (Wikipedia, 2016). Older adults can use them to make life more convenient, more fun, and safer. **Box 21-2** contains a selection of the best applications for seniors (most of them are iOS for an iPhone or iPad, some of them are Android applications).

The Internet and the World Wide Web

The *Internet* is not just about data; it is an international community of people who share information, interact, and communicate. From the point of view of its users, the Internet as an AT is a vast collection of resources that includes people, information, and multimedia. The Internet is best characterized as the biggest labyrinth of computer networks on earth (Dictionary.com, 2016a; Merriam-Webster Dictionary, 2016a).

A computer network is a data communications system comprising hardware and software that transmit data from one computer to another. In part, a computer network includes a physical infrastructure of hardware, such as wires, cables, fiberoptic lines, undersea cables, and satellites. The other part of a network is the software to keep it running. Computer networks can connect to other computer networks to produce an even bigger computer network. Thus, the Internet is a set of connected computer networks. In contrast, the *World Wide Web* (WWW or Web) is not a network. The Web is not the Internet itself, nor is it a proprietary system such as America Online. Instead, the Web is a system of clients (Web browsers) and servers that use the Internet to exchange data (Dictionary.com, 2016b; Merriam-Webster Dictionary, 2016b).

BOX 21-3   Varied Examples of Web-Based Applications for Older Adults

AARP:
http://www.aarp.org

Adaptive and assistive technology:
http://www.rehabtool.com

BrainBashers games and puzzles:
http://www.brainbashers.com/CataList, the
official catalog of LISTSERV lists:
http://www.lsoft.com/catalist.html

ElderWeb:
http://www.elderweb.com

Free greeting cards:
 http://www.123greetings.com/

Healthfinder:
http://www.healthfinder.gov

Learn the Net:
http://www.learnthenet.com/index.php/index.html

National Library of Medicine:
https://www.nlm.nih.gov/

SeniorNet:
http://www.seniornet.org/

The Internet and the World Wide Web are evolving into an environment for collaboration, content exchange, mentorship, and creative endeavors (see **Box 21-3**). This virtual environment is becoming an accessible place for the building of intellectual assets, in which knowledge can be effectively identified, distributed, and shared. Nursing professionals are joining this growing evolution in a number of different ways. Many nurses work hard to shape at least some of the Internet and World Wide Web into a milieu for active participation that serves to inform, educate, and advocate for older adults and their caregivers, such as family members, friends, and neighbors. Some nurses may specialize in *nursing informatics*.

Nursing Informatics

Nursing informatics is a 21st-century science with great potential for improving the quality, safety, and efficiency of health care. About 25 years ago, Kathryn Hannah proposed a simple definition for nursing informatics: She said that nursing informatics encompasses the use of information technologies in relation to any functions that are within the sphere of nursing and that are carried out by nurses in the performance of their practice (Ball & Hannah, 1988).

Later, Graves and Corcoran (1989) presented a more complex definition of nursing informatics. They argued that "nursing informatics is a combination of computer science, information science, and nursing science, designed to assist in the management and processing of nursing data, information, and knowledge to support the practice of nursing and the delivery of nursing care" (p. 227). The American Nurses Association (ANA, 1994) modified the Graves and Corcoran definition when it developed the *Scope and Practice for Nursing Informatics* and distinguished between practice and theory (see recommended readings in **Box 21-4**). The ANA more recently defined nursing informatics as "a specialty that integrates nursing science, computer science, and information science to manage and communicate data, information, and knowledge in nursing practice . . . to support patients, nurses, and other providers in their decision-making . . . using information structures, information processes and information technology" (ANA, 2001, p. 46).

The *Scope and Standards of Nursing Informatics Practice* (now known as *Nursing Informatics: Scope and Standards of Practice*) is a professional guideline and an essential reference for nurses that emphasizes competencies and functional areas (ANA, 2001, 2008, 2014). It articulates the essentials of nursing informatics, including the who, what, when, where, and how of its practice for both specialists and generalists. This booklet, revised by the American Nursing Informatics Association (http://www.ania.org) in 2014, builds upon historical knowledge and includes new, state-of-the-science material for the specialty. Although nursing informatics is a growing area of specialization, all nurses can employ basic information technology in their practice.

BOX 21-4   Recommended Readings

American Nurses Association. (2014). *Nursing informatics: Scope and standards of practice* (2nd ed.). Washington, DC: Author.

Chellen, S. (2015). *Essential guide to the internet for health professionals.* New York, NY: Routledge.

Hart, T. A., Chaparro, B. S., & Halcomb, C. G. (2008). Evaluating websites for older adults: Adherence to "senior-friendly" guidelines and end-user performance. *Behaviour & Information Technology, 27*(3), 191–199.

McGonigle, D., & Mastrian, K. (2015). *Nursing informatics and the foundation of knowledge.* Burlington, MA: Jones & Bartlett Learning.

Moritz, E. (Ed.). (2014). *Assistive technologies for the interaction of the elderly.* New York, NY: Springer.

Teel, A. (2011). *Alone and invisible no more: How grassroots community action and 21st century technologies can empower elders to stay in their homes and lead healthier, happier lives.* White River Junction, VT: Chelsea Green Publishing.

Thede, L. (2013). *Informatics and nursing: Opportunities and challenges.* Philadelphia, PA: Lippincott Williams & Wilkins.

Using the Web

Smith (2014) in a report on older adults and technology usage by the Pew Research Center found that that 59% of American seniors 65 years and older go online. In addition, among older adults who use the Internet, 46% of them use social networking sites such as Facebook. Smith also noted that 77% of the seniors own cell phones, with 18% owning SmartPhones. Of these older adults, 27% own a tablet (e.g., iPad), an e-book reader, or both (Smith, 2014). Whereas Keenan (2009) found no gender differences in frequency of Internet use, Smith (2014) noted few gender differences in Internet use (65% men; 55% women).

Computer ownership also has increased among older adults; 60% of these adults currently report having a personal computer at home. Additionally, fewer than 1 in 10 older adults without access to the Internet from home or from work say that they sometimes access the Internet from another place such as a friend's, neighbor's, or relative's home or the public library (Keenan, 2009). Among seniors who use the Internet, 71% report that they go online nearly every day and 11% note that they go online three to five times a week (Smith, 2014). Of older adults who use the Internet, 42% said they had done so for more than 10 years (Keenan, 2009) (see **Figure 21-1**).

Researchers have found that Web use by older adults enhances self-esteem and increases a sense of productivity and accomplishment, as well as increases their social interaction (Erickson & Johnson, 2011; Hogeboom, McDermott, Perrin, Osman, & Bell-Ellison, 2010; Kautzmann, 1990; McComish, Peura, & Richeson, 2010; Post, 1996; Purnell & Sullivan-Schroyer, 1997). For seniors, social networking sites such as Facebook or Twitter provide connection with family and friends. Among these older adults, 81% use such a site to socialize with others on a daily or near-daily basis (Smith, 2014). Web use also meets older adults' needs for personal control, mental stimulation, and fun (Gatto & Tak, 2008; McConatha, McConatha, & Dermigny, 1994; Weisman, 1983). They are passive and active participants who primarily use email, watch videos, buy products, make travel reservations, and search for financial or healthcare information (Keenan, 2009; Pew Internet and American Life Project, 2010; Smith, 2014). Now that the Baby Boomer generation, most of whom are already computer-literate, is becoming the Medicare generation, older adult Web use will soar. Therefore, gearing access to and design of Websites toward this older population becomes an important task.

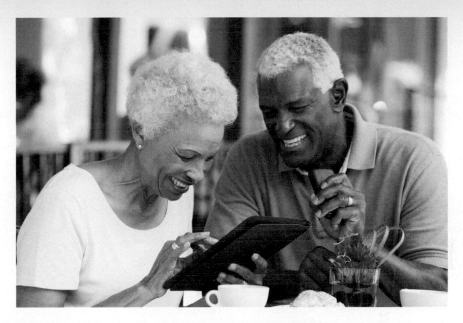

Figure 21-1 Older adults obtain many benefits from computer use, including social interactions, mental stimulation, and health information exploration.
© Monkey Business Images/Shutterstock

Website Design

Designers for Websites sometimes fail to recognize older adults or their caregivers, who also may be elderly, as potential user groups for their technology. Industry only recently has begun adapting access to hardware and designing software that makes accommodations for the needs of older adults (Reuben et al., 2004). This age group has specific abilities and performance attributes that need to be addressed to coincide with several life changes. Functional limitations related to visual, hearing, and mobility changes are common among older adults as a result of bodily changes secondary to the aging process. These changes may lower their ability to use the Web (Reuben et al., 2004; Smith, 2014). After age 65, a large proportion of this population begins to demonstrate significant visual acuity deficits. In addition, beyond age 65, one in four older adults is affected by hearing loss and some of them may develop essential benign tremor that may impair their fine motor skills (Reuben et al., 2004). Increasing font size to at least 18 points or using computer magnification screens compensates for decreased visual acuity, using the tab key or a touch screen attached to a monitor eliminates the need to have fine motor skills to move the cursor, and using external speakers or headphones for increased amplification can compensate for sensory and mobility impairments.

Historically, older adults have been slower in using the computer, traveled to fewer Web pages, and spent more time selecting targets for tasks than younger users (Chaparro, Bohan, Fernandez, Choi, & Kattel, 1999; Czaja & Sharit, 1998; Liao, Groff, Chaparro, Chaparro, & Stumpfhauser, 2000; Smith, 2014). Many groups and researchers have developed comprehensive sets of guidelines to improve Web design and thus, usability and accessibility for older adults (e.g., Web Content Accessibility Guidelines and Web Accessibility Initiative from the World Wide Web Consortium [2012] and the government-instituted U.S. Section 508 Guidelines [General Service Administration (GSA), 2015]) (see **Case Study 21-1**). The National Institute on Aging (NIA) and the National Library of Medicine (NLM) advanced the preceding guidelines one step further by developing specifications that are even more geared to the older adult Web user. They published *Making Your Web Site Senior Friendly: A Checklist*, consisting of 25 empirically based guidelines for Websites targeting these users (NIA & NLM, 2002), that still

Case Study 21-1

Roscoe Brown is a 73-year-old man who recently had a stroke that resulted in left hemiparesis. He was admitted to an acute care hospital where he was diagnosed with a right middle cerebral artery thrombosis. After a course of medication, the thrombosis dissolved and Mr. Brown demonstrated neurological gains. He has been transferred to the rehabilitation unit and has been assigned to your team. He can walk 50 feet with some assistance, his speech is slow and his words are slurred, but his short-term memory is intact. He owns his home and has $75,000 in a savings account that he is saving for a "rainy day." Just prior to his stroke, your team learned that Mr. Brown was the primary caregiver for his wife, Verna, who has senile dementia. The Browns have no children. Mr. Brown expressed a desire to get home as soon as possible so that he can once again care for his wife.

Questions:

Assuming Mr. Brown is able to be discharged home and care for his wife:

1. What Websites would you use to help in identifying community resources for Mr. and Mrs. Brown?
2. Discuss the community resources suggested to Mr. Brown.
3. What Websites might be helpful for Mr. Brown in terms of education and social support for (a) stroke and (b) dementia?
4. What assistive devices might you suggest for Mr. Brown? Where did you find information about this equipment and/or devices, and, if appropriate, how would you teach Mr. Brown about their use?

Assuming Mr. Brown is unable to return home and care for his wife:

1. Discuss home care and/or placement options for both Mr. and Mrs. Brown, including Web-based information about these options.

---

contains current valuable information. Research in aging, cognition, human factors, and print materials led to the development of these guidelines that cover three areas of design: (1) designing readable text, (2) increasing memory and comprehension of Web content, and (3) increasing the ease of navigation. These guidelines for Website design may result in greater accessibility of Web-based information for older adults, leading to a future willingness to explore the Web and increased enthusiasm toward technology (see **Box 21-5**).

Teaching about Accessing Websites and Using Apps

People use computers to access Websites, and many Websites are also accessed via applications on tablets and smartphones. To begin teaching older adults and/or their caregivers how to access these Websites via a computer, tablet, or smartphone, the nurse needs to be knowledgeable about the capacity of the learner. These adults must (1) be oriented; (2) have an attention span and be capable of short-term memory; (3) not be agitated, combative, or destructive; and (4) be able to respond to one-step commands and make choices. Individuals with severe motor disability must be able to raise an eyebrow, puff with the mouth, tap with a finger or foot, or talk to make selections. Adaptive or assistive devices can be used to expedite the learning process. In 1991, McNeely identified eight useful factors affecting teaching–learning outcomes for Web-based instruction and older adults. Each factor is still applicable in the 21st century and is described in the following list (McNeely, 1991):

> The rate of presentation of information needs to be individualized. Older adults need training that is self-paced and includes ways to ask questions. Enough time needs to be given to perform the task.
> All new information needs to be presented in a highly organized manner. Initially, the task and end goals need to be introduced. Then, parts should be identified and each related to the preceding step(s) and

BOX 21-5   The Internet and the World Wide Web "Senior-Friendly" Guidelines for Web Page Construction

Phrasing: Use the active voice.

Scrolling: Avoid automatically scrolling text and provide a scrolling icon.

Mouse: Use single clicks to access information.

Lettering: Use uppercase and lowercase for body text and reserve all capitals for headlines.

Justification: Use left-justified text.

Style: Use positive phrasing and present information in a clear manner without need for inferences.

Menus: Use pull-down and cascading menus sparingly.

Simplicity: Use simple language for text; provide a glossary for technical terms.

Typeface: Use a sans serif typeface that is not condensed.

Color: Avoid using yellow, blue, and green in proximity to each other.

Backgrounds: Use light text on dark backgrounds or vice versa; avoid patterns.

Consistent layout: Use a standard page design, and provide the same navigation on each page.

Organization: Use a standard format; break lengthy documents into short sections.

Navigation: Use explicit step-by-step navigation procedures—simple and straightforward.

Help and information: Offer a tutorial on the Website or offer contact information.

Icons and buttons: Use large buttons; incorporate text with an icon when possible.

Text alternatives: Provide text alternatives for all other media types.

Illustrations and photos: Use text-relevant images only.

Type weight: Use medium or boldface type.

Type size: Use 16- point type for body text with a capacity for enlarging.

Font: Use Arial, Tahoma, or Verdana fonts

Site maps: Use a site map to show how the site is organized.

Hyperlinks: Use icons with text as hyperlinks.

Animation, video, and audio: Use short segments to reduce download time.

Backward/forward navigation: Use buttons such as "previous" and "next" for reviewing text.

Physical spacing: Use double spacing in body text.

Data from National Institute on Aging. (2016). *Making your website senior friendly.* Retrieved from https://www.nia.nih.gov/health/publication /making-your-website-senior-friendly

---

to the whole. Visual displays should be simple and demonstrate only important information. Relevant information is presented and social chatter is avoided to help prevent the older adult from getting distracted.

> Older adults need to feel that they can practice as much as they like without slowing the pace of the instruction. Thus, older and younger adults need separate training sessions. This will also prevent a situation in which older adults would hesitate to ask questions around younger people for fear of embarrassment.

> There needs to be an opportunity for practice because it not only improves learning and mastery, but also has a direct influence on older adults' attitude. Unlimited trials need to be given. Cognitive support through use of software is important because it offers nonthreatening and repetitive tutoring that does not judge a person's mistakes.

> Web use that is interesting and personally meaningful to the older adult has been related to a positive attitude change. Older adults should dictate what they need and want from the Web. People perform best when the task is relevant to their lives.
> Teaching older adults about Web usage needs to be done in a comfortable environment. A calm, patient, unhurried, sensitive, interested, and knowledgeable instructor can decrease situational stress and promote a climate of acceptance and reassurance.
> Step-by-step graphic instructions or even video demonstration (i.e., YouTube) rather than relying on manuals provided by vendors are helpful in teaching older adults. Use concrete language as often as possible, because it is absorbed more readily and efficiently than abstract information. Printing a hard copy of their work is beneficial. Seeing work in print may increase enthusiasm and a sense of productivity and provide stimulus for further participation.
> Supportive verbal feedback may improve the older adult's performance. This should be done right after an activity. Interactive feedback via Web-based instruction may stimulate learning.

Learning Activities

Many adults participate in Web-based learning activities that lead to increased interaction and shared learning. They use the Web to create their own letters and use email, greeting cards, and posters in addition to playing word and board games and participating in music and art activities. In fact, Keenan (2009) and Malcolm et al. (2001) found that most older adults primarily used the Internet for email, but that they also used readers and tablets for game playing and reading newspapers, magazines, and books (Smith, 2014). Email letters provide an opportunity to reconnect with old friends and distant family; it also can be used to resolve a billing question with a cable company, find out about services at a local volunteer organization, track down old classmates, or request information from a national organization. And it would be impossible to overstate the satisfaction older adults can feel when they are called "the coolest grandparent in the world" because they have sent an email, e-greeting card, or poster to a grandchild.

Online games and activities can be a fun way to engage the older person's mind when no one else is around. For example, Garfield (http://www.garfield.com) is an interactive Website that can be used by all ages to play games, create electronic cards, or build their own comic strip. Angry Birds (https://www.angrybirds.com/) is also an example of fun gameplay for use on computers, tablets, and smartphones. Jigzone (http://www.jigzone.com) is a jigsaw puzzle site containing hundreds of picture puzzle shapes with a controlled level of difficulty. There are also several joke Websites (see **Box 21-6**) that are fun and easy to use.

At Websites such as http://www.live365.com/genres/40s or http://fiftiesweb.com/1950s-and-1960s-music/ or by searching and using a variety of free applications for tablets and smartphones, older adults can find the words to some of those common songs they knew as young adults. An application such as Spotify allows multiple downloads of music the person chooses for a small fee to join. The music can be downloaded to a phone or tablet for repeated enjoyment. The Web fulfills older adults' needs for fun and mental stimulation.

BOX 21-6   Web Exploration

Visit these Websites to find some humor for the day:

- http://www.jokes.com
- http://www.joke-of-the-day.com
- http://www.cleanjokes4u.com
- http://www.jokesclean.com

Check out more about technology and aging from the Center for Aging Services Technologies: http://www.leadingage.org/center-aging-services-technologies or http://www.leadingage.org/center-aging-services-technologies/resources

Research has explored the degree to which brain fitness training can combat the cognitive decline associated with the normal course of aging (Ball et al., 2002). Unlike other online brain games (Sudoku, crossword puzzles), comprehensive training programs target specific cognitive functions such as working memory, processing speed, and fluid intelligence and present users with specific cognitive tasks in a form that is intensive, repeatable, adaptive, and highly targeted. For a fee, Lumosity.com and Dakim.com offer brain-training exercises.

Health Information

The emphasis on early discharge and the movement of care from in-patient settings to the home mandates the development of electronic information systems to augment and extend services. The use of information searching on the Web is a promising tool for older adults and their caregivers. Nurses can use the Web to discover evidence about practice interventions from valid and reliable research and apply Melnyk and Fineout-Overholt's (2015) critical steps in the evidence-based process (see **Box 21-7**).

Traditional sources of evidence, such as peer-reviewed journals and books, can be found through electronic searches. The following serve as four examples:

1. The Cumulative Index to Nursing and Allied Health Literature (CINAHL) index began in 1955 and contains an extensive listing of nursing publications plus additional materials, such as evidence-based care sheets and quick lessons that provide concise overviews of diseases and conditions, with an outline of the most effective treatment options. (Grove, Burns, & Gray, 2013). The CINAHL database is available at https://www.ebscohost.com/academic/cinahl-plus-with-full-text.
2. Clinical Practice Guidelines from the Institute of Medicine are designed to enhance clinician and patient decisions about appropriate health care for specific clinical circumstances (Graham, Mancher, Wolman, Greenfield, & Steinberg, 2011).

BOX 21-7 Melnyk and Fineout-Overholt's Seven Critical Steps of the Evidence-Based Practice Process

1. Develop a spirit of inquiry
2. Ask the burning clinical questions (PICOT components):
   P: Patient population of interest
   I: Intervention or issue of interest
   C: Comparison of interest
   O: Outcome expected of interest
   T: Time it takes for the intervention to achieve the outcome(s)
3. Seek and collect the most relevant and best evidence.
4. Critically appraise the evidence:
   What were the study results?
   Are the study results valid (were sound scientific methods used)?
   Will the study findings facilitate care?
5. Integrate the best evidence: Can the study evidence be incorporated into the clinician's practice, given the clinician's expertise, the clinical resources available, and the patient's preferences?
6. Evaluate the outcomes or the effectiveness of the evidence-based interventions for a particular patient or care situation.
7. Communicate/disseminate the outcomes of the evidence-based practice (EBP) change(s) and decision.

Data from Melnyk, B. M., & Fineout-Overholt, E. (2015). *Evidence-based practice in nursing & healthcare: A guide to best practice* (3rd ed.). Philadelphia, PA: Lippincott Williams & Wilkins.

3. The Medical Literature Analysis and Retrieval System Online (MEDLINE) is the bibliographic database covering the fields of medicine, nursing, dentistry, veterinary medicine, the healthcare system, and the preclinical sciences from the NLM (U.S. National Library of Medicine, 2015); PubMed compiles millions of citations from biomedical literature via MEDLINE and is available http://www.ncbi.nlm.nih.gov/pubmed/

4. The National Guideline Clearinghouse houses summaries of evidence-based clinical practice guidelines and related documents (National Guideline Clearinghouse, 2015). A condensed version of the guideline and a link to the full clinical practice guideline are available at http://www.guideline.gov

In searching for information, it is important to document where the search was done (e.g., CINAHL or MEDLINE), as well as keywords/standardized subject headings (e.g., MeSH or CINAHL), and limiters (e.g., date range, language, or any other limiting criteria used). In addition, it is best to keep track of terms when searching the Internet or other nonlibrary resources. This enables anyone to re-create the search. The uncovered evidence from these searches and from other sources, plus expert opinions and the older adult's values and preferences, can then be applied when working with older adults (Melnyk & Fineout-Overholt, 2015).

Gies (2011a, 2011b) completed an EBP project in which she assessed problems of caregivers of persons with Alzheimer's disease (AD) and developed gender-specific, Web-based educational modules to address their problems. In the future, Gies suggests that incorporating these modules into an open-access Website accessible by computer or tablet has the potential to not only support caregivers, but to also serve as a resource for nurses and other professionals.

Thus, information provided on the Web can help inform and educate nurses and others about acute illnesses, chronic conditions, and health promotion, as well as resource availability. The following are just some of the resources available:

> As previously mentioned, the AbleData Web site (http://www.abledata.com/) can be used to locate companies that sell particular assistive devices.

> The National Institutes of Health and the U.S. NLM currently maintain several Websites designed to provide accurate health information to consumers. MEDLINEplus (http://www.nlm.nih.gov/medlineplus/) has sections in English and Spanish on health topics, medications, physicians, and medical terminology that are easy to use and understand. Information on this site can be accessed through alphabetical menus, buttons, and the search window. There is also a site from the National Institutes of Health (http://nihseniorhealth.gov) just for older adults that contains information on age-related health topics, remedies, and help for caregivers.

> The Department of Health and Human Services (http://www.dhhs.gov) is a comprehensive source on health information, diseases, and aging, and contains a resource locator.

> A nationwide locator service, Eldercare Locator (http://www.eldercare.gov/Eldercare.NET/Public/Index.aspx), helps people find local services that are provided to older adults. Users simply enter their state and ZIP code, and the Eldercare Locator will link to information, referral services, and their state and area agencies on aging.

These resources all help consumers identify appropriate information and services in the area where they reside.

Healthcare Services

Beyond information searches, the Internet has other applications. For many years, traditional face-to-face support groups facilitated by nurses and other professionals have been used extensively with positive outcomes for persons and their family members dealing with chronic diseases and long-term illnesses (Broadhead & Kaplan, 1991). Web-based support groups managed by professional providers, including nurses, are gaining credibility, as positive outcomes are obtained (Brajdottir, 2008; Larkin, 2000) (see **Box 21-8**).

BOX 21-8   Research Highlight

Aim: This descriptive study examined the problems and successes that a sample of 73 adult caregivers new to the role expressed in the first year of caring for stroke survivors.

Method: Bimonthly, trained telephone interviewers asked the participants open-ended questions to elicit their experience in caregiving. Data were collected from May 2002 to December 2005. Guided by Friedemann's framework of systemic organization, the data were analyzed using Colaizzi's method of content analysis.

Results: There were 2,455 problems and 2,687 successes reported. Three themes emerged from the problems: (1) being frustrated in day-to-day situations (system maintenance in Friedemann's terms), (2) feeling inadequate and turning to others for help (coherence), and (3) struggling and looking for "normal" in caring (system maintenance vs. change). Three themes were attributed to the successes: (1) making it through and striving for independence (system maintenance), (2) doing things together and seeing accomplishments

in the other (coherence), and (3) reaching a new sense of normal and finding balance in life (individuation and system maintenance).

Application to practice: These findings provided an in-depth, theory-based description of the experience of being a new caregiver and helped increase understanding of how caring can be a difficult, yet rewarding experience. Knowledge of the changes over time allows healthcare professionals to tailor their interventions, understanding, and support. Nurses should be aware that caregivers of stroke survivors may experience common frustrations and challenges in the caring role and that the successes reported in this study may be enhanced by nursing interventions to promote positive family adjustment to the poststroke experience.

Modified from Pierce, L., Steiner, V., Govoni, A., Thompson, T., & Friedemann, M. (2007). Two sides to the caregiving story. *Topics in Stroke Rehabilitation, 14*(2), 13–20. Available at http://www.tandfonline.com/doi/abs/10.1310/tsr1402-13.

Emotional and social support are gained by the participants in these Internet-based groups, in addition to information about best treatments, doctors, medical centers, and more (Marziali, Damianakis, & Donahue, 2006; Marziali & Donahue, 2006; Veggeberg, 1996). According to White and Dorman (2000) and Northouse and Peters-Golden (1993), members of Internet support groups share experiences and opinions that often include helping persons cope with body changes or providing encouragement to other group members, such as helping persons work through healthcare problems. For instance, international, national, and local organizations and medical centers offer group discussion. The Wellness Community (TWC) is a nonprofit organization dedicated to providing support to individuals dealing with cancer (Wellness Community, 2007). In 2002, in collaboration with the University of California at San Francisco and Stanford University, TWC established an online support group for those individuals. One can join at https://www.cancerexperienceregistry.org/

Researchers at the University of Toledo in Ohio tested Caring~Web, a restricted Website geared toward providing education and support services for caregivers of persons with stroke (Pierce, Steiner, Khuder, Govoni, & Horn, 2009) (see **Box 21-9**). The caregiver users positively rated the Website's appearance and usability and reported they on average spent 1 to 2 hours at the Website each week (Pierce & Steiner, 2013).

Some other Websites are interactive and include monitoring devices that enable the person to send temperature, blood pressure, glucose levels, and other health data to healthcare providers electronically. Televisual Websites allow healthcare providers to conduct virtual house calls with older adults (Spry Foundation, 2005). For example, Brennan et al. (2001) demonstrated the effectiveness of computer-mediated information and support services for patients recovering from coronary artery bypass graft surgery, and McKay, Glasgow, Feil, Boles,

BOX 21-9   Research Highlight

Aim: The purpose of this randomized controlled trial was to examine if carers of stroke survivors who participate in the Web-based intervention, Caring~Web©, would have higher well-being than non-Web users. A secondary aim was to explore whether those survivors whose carers participated in Caring~Web would use fewer healthcare services.

Method: A randomized, two-group, repeated measures design was used. Subjects were recruited from four rehabilitation centers in Ohio or Michigan from which first-time stroke survivors were discharged to home. Of 144 carers screened, 103 carers of these survivors who were novice Internet users were assigned to a Web or non-Web user group. Caring~Web was a Web-based intervention of education and support provided to the Web-user group for 1 year. A bimonthly telephone survey collected data on all carers' well-being (perceived depression, life satisfaction) and survivors' healthcare service use (self-reported provider and emergency department visits, hospital readmissions, nursing home placement). Seventy-three subjects completed the study.

Results: No statistical differences were found between the groups in carers' well-being or in the number of provider visits for survivors. There were significant differences in emergency department visits (p = 0.001) and hospital readmissions (p = 0.0005) related to the health of survivors. Because only three subjects reported that the stroke survivor became a nursing home resident, statistical analysis of nursing home placement was not possible. However, in the Web-user group, only one survivor was placed in a nursing home after 7.5 months. In the non-Web-user group, two survivors became residents between months 2 and 4.

Applications to practice: This Web-based intervention helped new carers make informed decisions about healthcare needs of stroke survivors, thus, reducing service use and its associated costs. Healthcare providers could use Caring~Web for their carers of stroke survivors' after rehabilitation treatment.

Modified from Pierce, L., Steiner, V., Khuder, S., Govoni, A., & Horn, L. (2009). The effect of a web-based stroke intervention on carers' well-being and survivors' use of healthcare services. *Disability and Rehabilitation, 31*(20), 1676–1684. Available at http://www.tandfonline.com/doi/full/10.1080/09638280902751972.

and Barrera (2002) suggested that Web-based information and support interventions exert a positive impact on health-promoting behaviors of patients with type 2 diabetes. Further, tablets and their applications can generate voice for people unable to speak (Callison, 2012). The device can be preprogramed to ask and answer questions by pushing a button, such as when asked, "How are you?" the response is a computer generated voice that says "I'm not feeling well, thank you."

New Technologies

New technologies are being developed and used to facilitate EBP, enhance education, and improve older adults' quality of life. A number of companies and organizations are testing computer-based technologies that have the potential to provide help for people dealing with chronic illness and disability. The practical application of these technologies may be especially important for older adults and their caregivers living in community settings.

Gerontechnology is designing technology and environments for independent living and social participation of older adults with the aim of compressing morbidity and increasing vitality in the lifespan, as well as improving quality of life. Older adults want to remain independent, and gerontechnology experts analyze how technology can help them. Based on this analysis, companies and/or organizations create products for the elderly (Bouma & Graafmans, 1992; Graafmans, Taipale, & Charness, 1998; Harrington & Harrington, 2000) that may be affordable for some older adults and their family caregivers. For instance, what if a smartphone or tablet could detect abnormal cells circulating in the blood or warn a person of an impending heart attack? Beyond reading email and surfing the Web, companies are already looking for ways to transform these devices into sensors that could help adults take better control of their health by not only tracking blood pressure and monitoring blood sugar, but also hearing heartbeats and charting heart activity (Topol, 2012).

Another example of utilizing existing technology in novel ways involves using a global positioning system (GPS) device, the same as the kinds that have become common in cars, to help locate someone with dementia who has wandered from home. The GPS Shoe, manufactured by a New Jersey company, hides a miniature locator in the heel of one shoe and counterweighs the other shoe, so they feel balanced (Span, 2011). A family member sets a perimeter, so that the wearer of the shoe can freely move around the environment, house, yard, or a familiar immediate neighborhood. If that perimeter is broken, Google Maps pops up on the family member's computer, tablet, or smartphone to show where the wandering person has gone, so that the authorities can be informed and the person retrieved (Span, 2011). Of course, other devices that can detect when a person falls and inform family members or emergency response teams also help older adults stay in their independent home environments and facilitate continued socialization (Mattke et al., 2010).

Robotic Assistance

Two factors suggest that now is the time to establish mobile robots in the home-care arena. First, the technology is available to develop robots that exhibit the necessary power, reliability, and level of competence. Second, now more than ever, there is a need for cost-effective solutions to maintain older adults in home settings. Researchers, scientists, and designers are partnering to create new technology to help older adults live independently throughout their lives.

The Oregon Center for Aging and Technology, part of Portland's Oregon Health & Science University and in partnership with Intel Corporation, is testing technology in their metro area (Abrahms, 2012). Designed for people showing signs of cognitive decline, family members can now contact aging parents or grandparents and check up on them by remotely controlling Celia the Robot. Celia is a large white robot with a video screen that works like Skype, in that the family member can remotely text, talk, and see the aging person, making it simple to share experiences. Family members can direct Celia through installed software on their computer and move the robot to different rooms so relatives can "visit." The program, run by Dr. Jeffrey Kaye, hypothesized that Celia would be too intrusive, but they found that the participants (care recipients) loved the family contact and that it reduced isolation, as long as they could turn off the video screen for privacy purposes (Abrahms, 2012).

In a federally supported study, researchers from the University of Pittsburgh, University of Michigan, and Carnegie Mellon University (2005) are collaborating to produce a personal robotic assistant for older adults, called Nursebot. The goal of this project is to develop mobile personal service robots—autonomous mobile robots that "live" in the private home of a chronically ill person—that assist older adults suffering from chronic disorders in their everyday life. The robot provides a research platform on which to test out a range of ideas for assisting these adults, such as the following (University of Pittsburgh, University of Michigan, & Carnagie-Mellon University, 2005):

> *Intelligent reminding:* Many older adults have to give up independent living because of memory loss. They forget to visit the restroom, to take medicine, to drink, or to see the doctor. One project explores the effectiveness of a robotic reminder, which follows people around so they cannot become lost.
> *Telepresence:* Professional caregivers can use the robot to establish a "telepresence" and interact directly with remote care recipients. This makes many doctor visits unnecessary.

> *Data collection and surveillance:* Robots can be used for a wide range of emergency conditions that can be avoided with systematic data collection (e.g., certain types of heart failures).
> *Mobile manipulation:* A semi-intelligent mobile manipulator integrates robotic strength with a person's senses and intellect. This mobile manipulation can overcome barriers in handling objects (e.g., refrigerator, laundry, and microwave) that currently force older adults to move into assisted-living facilities. This technology could be used for any person dealing with function problems, such as arthritis, as the main reason for giving up independent living.
> *Social interaction deprivation:* This affects a huge number of elderly people who are forced to live alone. This project seeks to explore whether robots can take over certain social functions for these older adults.

Testing is under way at a retirement community with a Nursebot named Pearl. This project could change the way health care is delivered to an ever-growing contingent of older adults, while significantly advancing the state of the art for mobile service robotics and human–robot interaction (Jajeh, 2005; University of Pittsburgh, University of Michigan, & Carnagie-Mellon University, 2005). Nursebot Pearl has the potential to help the elderly with daily tasks, provide companionship, and even help them to remotely communicate with physicians and caregivers. Positive feedback was reported in 2011 (INDEX, 2011).

Sensor-Based Monitoring

The Medical Automation Research Center (MARC) at the University of Virginia has developed and is testing technological solutions for in-home distance monitoring of the functional abilities of older adults. The goal of this system is to enable older adults with disabilities to remain in their own homes for as long as possible. The system is composed of unobtrusive and low-cost sensors (no cameras or microphones) that detect movement and pressure. There is a data logging and communications module, in addition to an integrated data management system, linked to the Internet. Using the appropriate data analysis tools, important observations about ADLs can be made from the data generated by the monitored person. These observations may yield early indicators of the onset of a disease or a sudden change of activity (or inactivity) that can indicate an accident. Although the system is not meant as an emergency prompt system, the caregiver may receive alerts over the Internet or urgent notifications over the phone in case of such sudden accident-indicating changes. Additionally, there is a potential for information about sickness or accidents to be transmitted immediately to a service provider (MARC, 2005).

In a 4-month pilot project, MARC's health status monitoring system was evaluated in regard to the functional independence and quality of life of 13 older adult caregivers in a home care setting (Alwan et al., 2006). Strain and burden of the informal caregivers and workloads of 16 professional caregivers also were examined. As expected, there was no change in their premonitoring and postmonitoring functional independence assessment scores, due to the short period of the project. However, results did show that there was an increase in quality of life of these monitored older adults that could be attributed to improved quality of care and/or to increased sense of security, due to the use of the monitoring technology. For these monitored adults, their caregivers had reduced levels of strain, but there was no change in their level of burden. The professional caregivers experienced no change in their workload assessment score after monitoring, indicating that the technology did not add to their workloads. Based on these results, the researchers suggested further testing with larger sample sizes and over longer periods of time (Alwan et al., 2006).

Recently, the Massachusetts Institute of Technology Age Lab tested a monitoring system that uses the same software NASA used to communicate with astronauts in space to see if it could improve older adults' medication adherence and food habits (Abrahms, 2012). They installed a videoconference and touch-screen computer system in the older adult's kitchen. This system sends data instantly to the family's computer, and they can log on to see if their relative took their medications and leave messages, upload photos, or have a video chat. They found that videoconferencing helped the relative take medications on time and encouraged good eating habits, as well as provided socialization (Abrahms, 2012).

Intel's Assistance Program

The Alzheimer's Association and Intel Corporation have formed a consortium to spur development of technologies for the home to help support the care of older adults. This group grew out of several separate and ongoing efforts. In 2001, the Alzheimer's Association convened a group of caregivers as well as experts from diverse disciplines, including bioengineering, robotics, artificial intelligence, communications, systems design, software engineering, medicine, nursing, biology, economics, finance, and business. Around the same time, Intel funded and conducted research on the ways in which computing and communications technologies could support the daily health and wellness needs of people of all ages in their homes and everyday lives. An example of Intel's technology is a wireless "sensor network" made up of thousands of small sensing devices that could someday be embedded throughout the home to monitor important behavioral tendencies, such as sleep and eating patterns. It could also send prompts to a person, such as reminders to take medication (Intel News Release, 2003).

Continuing this work, the Alzheimer's Association and Intel Corporation, in partnership with Agilent Technologies, worked with university professors at the Florida Institute of Technology to develop a portable caregiver support system called PocketBuddy (Rhine, 2005). This system would issue audio and text messages to caregivers that could include medication information, appointment reminders, and automated checklists for daily support. Imbedded information could contain the location of important documents and emergency contact names. The creators project that family and friends might access information about the person with AD and their caregivers via a Web log, a "Buddy Blog," linked to a PocketPC. This technology could bridge time and space barriers that separate these individuals. A study is under way to test and validate the use and acceptance of this technology (Rhine, 2005).

Another example is the Cognitive Orthosis for Activities in the Home (COACH) prototype of an intelligent supportive environment (Mihailidis, 2007). The COACH is being developed by the Alzheimer's Disease Association of Canada and Intel Corporation, in collaboration with researchers at the University of Toronto and several other universities, to assist people with dementia to complete ADLs with less dependence on a caregiver. The COACH represents one of the first clinically tested supportive devices to use artificial intelligence techniques. Using a personal (desktop) computer and a single video camera to unobtrusively track a user during an ADL, this device provides prerecorded (visual or video) prompts when necessary (Mihailidis, 2007). In pilot studies, two successive prototypes of the COACH system have been trialed with subjects who had moderate to severe dementia based around the ADL of handwashing (Mihailidis, Barbenel, & Fernie, 2004; Mihailidis, Boger, Canido, & Hoey, 2007). These trials showed that the number of steps in handwashing that the subjects were able to complete without assistance from the caregiver increased noticeably when the device was present (Mihailidis et al., 2004; Mihailidis et al., 2007). Planned future studies will examine, for example, (1) a new color tracking system that is able to track the position of both hands of the person with dementia, the position of task objects (e.g., soap and towel), and the interaction between them; and (2) a new system that implements algorithms, which allow for good decision making under conditions of uncertainty (Mihailidis, 2007).

Summary

Today's technologies provide many opportunities for older adults to maintain their independence and stay connected to the world even when functional limitations are present. Nurses should be aware of the latest trends in technology, the use of computers among the older adult population, and how assistive devices help promote autonomy for this cohort. In addition, nurses can use the strategies suggested in this chapter to enhance learning and teaching with older adults and their families by incorporating technology into the care of both well and ill elderly.

Clinical Reasoning Exercises

1. If someone stopped you on the street and demanded to know your definition of the Internet and World Wide Web, what would you say? Define the Internet in your own words. How is the Web different from the Internet? Discuss your findings with another student nurse in one of your clinical groups.

2. Explore the Websites of the American Stroke Association (http://www.americanstroke.org) and the National Stroke Association (http://www.stroke.org). What are differences and similarities between these Websites? Discuss your findings with another student nurse in one of your clinical groups.

3. Discuss with students in your clinical group at least two factors affecting teaching—learning outcomes for Web-based instruction and older adults.

4. Describe an assistive device to students in your clinical group, and tell how you would teach the patient and/or caregiver about its use when discharging a patient to a home setting.

5. How can information be located about the AT and assistive devices currently available for consumers' use?

Personal Reflections

1. Do you know an older adult who is a novice computer user? Interview this person, asking how his or her life has changed (what is better and/or worse) since becoming a user. Think about how these changes may affect his or her quality of life.

2. How do you feel about older adults becoming part of the technology revolution? Do you think they are using the computer and World Wide Web more often? Do you know any older adults who use iPods, iPhones, mp3 players, PDAs, flash drives, or other gadgets used by the younger population today? How is their use the same as or different from use by your generation?

References

Abrahms, S. (2012). Independent living for the aging is possible with new technology. *AARP Bulletin.* Retrieved from http://www.aarp.org/technology/innovations/info-04-2012/living-laboratories-aging-place.html

Administration on Aging, Administration for Community Living, U.S. Department of Health and Human Services. (2014). A profile of older Americans: 2014. Retrieved from http://www.aoa.acl.gov/aging_statistics/profile/2014/docs/2014-Profile.pdf

Agency for Healthcare Research and Quality. (2016). Electronic medical records systems. Retrieved from https://healthit.ahrq.gov/key-topics/electronic-medical-record-systems

Alwan, M., Mack, D., Dalal, S., Kell, S., Turner, B., & Felder, R. (2006). Impact of passive in-home health status monitoring technology in home health: Outcome pilot. Retrieved from http://citeseerx.ist.psu.edu/viewdoc/summary?doi=10.1.1.156.6734

American Association of Retired Persons Public Policy Institute. (2009). Chronic conditions among older Americans. In *Chronic care: A call to action for health reform.* Retrieved from http://assets.aarp.org/rgcenter/health/beyond_50_hcr_conditions.pdf

American Nurses Association. (1994). *The scope and practice for nursing informatics.* Washington, DC: Author.

American Nurses Association. (2001). *Scope and standards of nursing informatics practice.* Washington, DC: Author.

American Nurses Association. (2008). *Nursing informatics: Scope and standards of practice.* Washington, DC: Author.

American Nurses Association. (2014). *Nursing informatics: Scope and standards of practice* (2nd ed.). Washington, DC: Author.

American Speech-Language-Hearing Association. (2002). *Augmentative and alternative communication: Knowledge and skills for service delivery.* Retrieved from http://www.asha.org/policy/PS2005-00113/

Ball, M., & Hannah, K. (1988). What is informatics and what does it mean to nursing? In M. Ball, K. Hannah, U. Gerdin Jelger, & H. Peterson (Eds.), *Nursing informatics: Where caring and technology meet* (pp. 81–87). New York, NY: Springer Verlag.

Ball, K., Berch, D. B., Helmers, K. F., Jobe, J. B., Leveck, M. D., Marsiske, M., . . . Willis, S. (2002). Effects of cognitive training interventions with older adults: A randomized controlled trial. *Journal of the American Medical Association, 288*(18), 2271–2281.

Bouma, H., & Graafmans, J. (Eds.). (1992). *Gerontechnology.* Washington, DC: IOS Press.

Brajdottir, H. (2008). Computer-mediated support group intervention for parents. *Journal of Nursing Scholarship, 40*(1), 32–38.

Brennan, P. F., Moore, S. M., Bjornsdottir, G., Jones, J., Visovsky, C., & Rogers, M. (2001). HeartCare: An Internet-based information and support system for patient home recovery after coronary artery bypass graft (CABG) surgery. *Journal of Advanced Nursing, 35*(5), 699–708.

Broadened Horizons. (2011). Products. Retrieved from http://www.broadenedhorizons.com/voiceir

Broadhead, W., & Kaplan, W. (1991). Social support and the cancer patient: Implications for future research and clinical care. *Cancer, 67*(3), 794–799.

Callison, J. (April 7, 2012). iPad helps brain-injured woman express herself. *USA Today.* Retrieved from http://www.usatoday.com/news/health/story/2012-04-07/ipad-brain-injury/54107314/1

Chaparro, A., Bohan, M., Fernandez, J., Choi, S., & Kattel, B. (1999). The impact of age on computer input device use: Psychophysical and physiological measures. *International Journal of Industrial Ergonomics, 24*(5), 503–513.

Czaja, S., & Sharit, J. (1998). Age differences in attitudes toward computers. *Journal of Gerontology, 53B*(5), 329–340.

Davies, K., Collerton, J. C., Jagger, C., Bond, J., Barker, S. A. H., Edwards, J., Hughes, J., . . . Robinson, L. (2010). Engaging the oldest old in research: Lessons from the Newcastle 85+ study. *BMC Geriatrics, 10*(64), 1–9.

Dickerson, S. S., Stone, V. I., Panchura, C., & Usiak, D. J. (2002). The meaning of communication: Experiences with augmentative communication devices. *Rehabilitation Nursing, 27*(6), 215–221.

Dictionary.com. (2016a). Internet. Retrieved from http://dictionary.reference.com/browse/internet?s=t

Dictionary.com. (2016b). World Wide Web. Retrieved from http://dictionary.reference.com/browse/world-wide-web?s=t

Encarta World English Dictionary. (2007). Assistive technology.

Erickson, J., & Johnson, G. (2011). Internet use and psychological wellness during late adulthood. *Canadian Journal on Aging, 30*(2), 197–209.

FitBit. (2016). Products. Retrieved from https://www.fitbit.com/

Gatto, S., & Tak, S. (2008). Computer, internet, and e-mail use among older adults: Benefits and barriers. *Educational Gerontology, 34*(9), 800–811.

General Service Administration. (2015). U.S. section 508 standards. Retrieved from https://www.gsa.gov/portal/content/105254

Gies, C. (2011a). *Developing gender-specific web-based educational modules for caregivers of persons with Alzheimer's disease* (Unpublished doctoral evidence-based project). The University of Toledo, Toledo, Ohio.

Gies, C. (2011b). Developing gender-specific web-based education modules for caregivers of persons with Alzheimer's disease. *Western Journal of Nursing Research, 33*(8), 110–111.

Gitlin, L. (1998). The role of social science research in understanding technology use among older adults. In M. G. Ory & G. H. DeFriese (Eds.), *Self-care in later life* (pp. 142–169). New York, NY: Springer.

Gitlin, L., Schemm, R., Landsberg, L., & Burgh, D. (1996). Factors predicting assistive device use in the home by older people following rehabilitation. *Journal of Aging and Health, 8*(4), 554–575.

Graafmans, J., Taipale, V., & Charness, N. (1998). *Gerontechnology: A sustainable investment in the future.* Washington, DC: IOS Press.

Graham, R., Mancher, M., Wolman, D., Greenfield, S., & Steinberg, E. (Eds). (2011). *Institute of Medicine (US) committee on standards for developing trustworthy clinical practice guidelines.* Washington, DC: National Academies Press.

Graves, J., & Corcoran, S. (1989). The study of nursing informatics. *Image: Journal of Nursing Scholarship, 21*(4), 227–231.

Grove, S., Burns, N., & Gray, J. (2013). *The practice of nursing research: Appraisal, synthesis, and generation of evidence* (7th ed.). St. Louis, MO: Saunders.

Harrington, T., & Harrington, M. (2000). *Gerontechnology why and how.* Maastricht, The Netherlands: Shaker Publishing B.V.

Hoeman, S., Liszner, K., & Alverzo, J. (2008). Functional mobility with activities of daily living. In S. Hoeman (Ed.), *Rehabilitation nursing: Prevention, intervention, and outcomes* (4th ed., pp. 200–257). St. Louis, MO: Mosby.

Hoenig, H., Taylor, D. H., & Sloan, F. A. (2003). Does assistive technology substitute for personal assistance among the disabled elderly? *American Journal of Public Health, 93*(2), 330–337.

Hogeboom, D., McDermott, R., Perrin, K., Osman, H., & Bell-Ellison, B. (2010). Internet use and social networking among middle aged and older adults. *Educational Gerontology, 36*(2), 93–111.

Idaho Assistive Technology Project. (1995). Assistive technology and older adults. Information Sheet #25. Retrieved from http://www.idahoat.org/

INDEX. (2011). Nursebot: Personal mobile robotic assistants for the elderly. Retrieved from https://designto improvelife.dk/nursebot-personal-mobile-robotic-assistants-for-the-elderly/

Intel News Release. (2003). The Alzheimer's Association, Intel team up to expand home care technology research. Retrieved from http://www.intel.com/pressroom/archive/releases/2003/20030724corp.htm

Jajeh, D. (2005). Robot nurse escorts and schmoozes the elderly.

Johnson, J. L., Davenport, R., & Mann, W. C. (2007). Consumer feedback on smart home applications. *Topics in Geriatric Rehabilitation, 23*(1), 60–72.

Khan, A. (2014, October). What it's like inside an eICU. *U.S. News and World Report.* Retrieved from http://health.usnews.com/health-news/patient-advice/articles/2014/10/24/what-its-like-inside-an-eicu

Kautzmann, L. (1990). Introducing computers to the elderly. *Physical and Occupational Therapy in Geriatrics, 9*(1), 27–36.

Keenan, T. (2009). Internet use among midlife and older adults: An AARP bulletin poll. Retrieved from http://assets.aarp.org/rgcenter/general/bulletin_internet_09.pdf

Kelker, K. (Ed.). (1997). *Family guide to assistive technology.* Retrieved from http://www.pluk.org/Pubs/PLUK_ATguide_269K.pdf

Kraskowsky, L. H., & Finlayson, M. (2001). Factors affecting older adults' use of adaptive equipment: Review of the literature. *American Journal of Occupational Therapy, 55*(3), 303–310.

Laditka, J. N., & Laditka, S. B. (2016). Associations of multiple chronic health conditions with active life expectancy in the United States. *Disability and Rehabilitation, 38*(4), 354–361.

Larkin, M. (2000). Online support groups gaining credibility. *Lancet, 355*(9217), 1834.

Liao, C., Groff, L., Chaparro, A., Chaparro, B., & Stumpfhauser, L. (2000). A comparison of Web site usage between young adults and the elderly. *Proceedings of the IEA 2000/HGES 2000 Congress.* San Diego, CA: Human Factors and Ergonomics Society.

LoPresti, E. F., Simpson, R. C., Kirsch, N., Schreckenghost, D., & Hayashi, S. (2008). Distributed cognitive aid with scheduling and interactive task guidance. *Journal of Rehabilitation Research and Development, 45*(4), 505–522.

Malcolm, M., Mann, W., Tomita, M., Fraas, L., Stanton, K., & Gitlin, L. (2001). Computer and internet use in physically frail elders. *Physical and Occupational Therapy in Geriatrics, 19*(3), 15–32.

Mann, W., Hurren, D., & Tomita, M. (1993). Comparison of assistive device use and needs of home-based older persons, with different impairments. *American Journal of Occupational Therapy, 47*(11), 980–987.

Mann, W., Hurren, D., & Tomita, M. (1995). Assistive devices used by home-based elderly persons with arthritis. *American Journal of Occupational Therapy, 49*(8), 810–820.

Mann, W., Goodall, S., Justiss, M., & Tomita, M. (2002). Dissatisfaction and nonuse of assistive devices among frail elders. *Assistive Technology, 14*(2), 130–139.

Mann, W., Belchior, P., Tomita, M. R., & Kemp, B. J. (2007). Older adults' perception and use of PDAs, home automation system, and home health monitoring system. *Topics in Geriatric Rehabilitation, 23*(1), 35–46.

Mann, W., Llanes, C., Justiss, M. D., & Tomita, M. (2004). Frail older adults' self-report of their most important assistive devices. *OTJR: Occupation, Participation, and Health, 24*(1), 4–12.

Mann, W., Ottenbacher, K. J., Fraas, L., Tomita, M., & Granger, C. V. (1999). Effectiveness of assistive technology and environmental interventions in maintaining independence and reducing home care costs for the frail elderly. *Archives of Family Medicine, 8,* 210–217.

Marziali, E., & Donahue, P. (2006). Caring for others: Internet video-conferencing group intervention for family caregivers of older adults with neurodegenerative disease. *The Gerontologist, 46*(3), 398–403.

Marziali, E., Damianakis, T., & Donahue, P. (2006). Internet-based clinical services: Virtual support groups for family caregivers. *Journal of Technology in Human Services, 24*(2–3), 39–54.

Matthews, J. T., Beach, S. R., de Bruin, W. B., Mecca, L. P., & Schulz, R. (2010). Preferences and concerns for quality of life technology among older adults and persons with disabilities: National survey results. *Technology and Disability, 22*(1–2), 5–15.

Mattke, S., Klautzer, L., Mengistu, T., Garnett, J., Hu, J., & Wu, H. (2010). *Health and well-being in the home: A global analysis of needs, expectations, and priorities for home health care technology.* Pittsburgh, PA: Rand Corporation.

McComish, H., Peura, C., & Richeson, N. (2010). Computer and internet engagement for older adults. *Activities Directors' Quarterly for Alzheimer's & Other Dementia Patients, 11*(3), 43–46.

McConatha, D., McConatha, J., & Dermigny, R. (1994). The use of interactive computer services to enhance the quality of life for long-term care residents. *The Gerontologist, 34,* 553–556.

McKay, H. G., Glasgow, R. E., Feil, E. G., Boles, S. M., & Barrera, M. M. (2002). Internet-based diabetes self-management and support: Initial outcomes from the Diabetes Network Project. *Rehabilitation Psychology, 47*(1), 31–48.

McNeely, E. (1991). Computer-assisted instruction and the older-adult learner. *Educational Gerontology, 17,* 229–237.

Medical Automation Research Center. (2005). Smart in-home monitoring system.

Melnyk, B. M., & Fineout-Overholt, E. (2015). *Evidence-based practice in nursing & healthcare: A guide to best practice* (3rd ed.). Philadelphia, PA: Lippincott Williams & Wilkins.

Merriam-Webster Dictionary. (2016a). Internet. Retrieved from http://www.merriam-webster.com/dictionary/internet

Merriam-Webster Dictionary. (2016b). World Wide Web. Retrieved from http://www.merriam-webster.com/dictionary/world%20wide%20web

Mihailidis, A. (2007). Intelligent supportive environments for older adults (COACH project).

Mihailidis, A., & Lee, T. (2007). Intelligent emergency response and fall detection system.

Mihailidis, A., Barbenel, J., & Fernie, G. (2004). The efficacy of an intelligent cognitive orthosis to facilitate hand-washing by persons with moderate-to-severe dementia. *Neuropsychological Rehabilitation, 14*(1/2), 135–171.

Mihailidis, A., Boger, J., Canido, M., & Hoey, J. (2007). The use of an intelligent prompting system for people with dementia: A case study. *ACM Interactions, 14*(4), 34–37.

Mihailidis, A., Cockburn, A., Longley, C., & Boger, J. (2008). The acceptability of home monitoring technology among community-dwelling older adults and baby boomers. *Assistive Technology, 20,* 1–12.

National Guideline Clearinghouse. (2010). About NGC. Retrieved from http://www.guideline.gov/help-and-about/

National Guideline Clearinghouse. (2015). Home page. Retrieved from http://www.guideline.gov

National Institute on Aging & National Library of Medicine. (2002). Making your Web site senior friendly. Retrieved from http://www.nlm.nih.gov/pubs/staffpubs/od/ocpl/agingchecklist.html

National Institute of Standards and Technology. (2011). What is assistive technology?

National Institute on Aging. (2016). *Making your website senior friendly.* Retrieved from https://www.nia.nih.gov/health/publication/making-your-website-senior-friendly

National Institute on Deafness and Other Communication Disorders. (2009–2011). Strategic plan. Retrieved from https://www.nidcd.nih.gov/about/strategic-plan/2012-2016

Norburn, J., Bernard, S. L., Konrad, T. R., Woomert, A., DeFriese, G. H., Kalsbeek, W. D., . . . Ory, M. G. (1995). Self-care and assistance from others in coping with functional status limitations among a national sample of older adults. *Journals of Gerontology: Series B, Psychological Sciences and Social Sciences, 50*(2), S101–S109.

Northouse, L., & Peters-Golden, H. (1993). Cancer and the family: Strategies to assist spouses. *Seminars in Oncology Nursing, 9*(2), 74–82.

Pew Internet and American Life Project. (2004). *Demographics: Older Americans and the Internet.* Retrieved from http://www.pewinternet.org/2004/03/28/older-americans-and-the-internet/

Pew Internet and American Life Project. (2010). *Generations 2010.* Retrieved from http://www.pewinternet.org/Reports/2010/Generations-2010.aspx

Pierce, L., & Steiner, V. (2013). Usage and design evaluation by family caregivers of a stroke intervention website. *Journal of Neuroscience Nursing, 45*(5), 254–261.

Pierce, L., Steiner, V., Govoni, A., Thompson, T., & Friedemann, M. (2007). Two sides to the caregiving story. *Topics in Stroke Rehabilitation, 14*(2), 13–20.

Pierce, L., Steiner, V., Khuder, S., Govoni, A., & Horn, L. (2009). The effect of a web-based stroke intervention on carers' well-being and survivors' use of healthcare services. *Disability and Rehabilitation, 31*(20), 1676–1684.

Post, J. (1996). Internet resources on aging: Seniors on the Net. *The Gerontologist, 36,* 565–569.

Pressler, K. A., & Ferraro, K. F. (2010). Assistive device use as a dynamic acquisition process in later life. *The Gerontologist, 50*(3), 371–381.

Purnell, M., & Sullivan-Schroyer, P. (1997). Nursing home residents using computers: The Winchester houses experience. *Generations, 21*(3), 61–62.

Reed, K. (2011). Health maintenance and management of therapeutic regimens. In C. Jacelon (Ed.), *The specialty practice of rehabilitation nursing* (6th ed., pp. 77–101). Glenview, IL: Association of Rehabilitation Nurses.

Reuben, D., Herr, K., Pacala, J., Pollock, B., Potter, J., & Semla, T. (2004). *Geriatrics at your fingertips.* Malden, MA: Blackwell.

Rhine, K. (2005). *A pocketful of help for Alzheimer's sufferers and caregivers.* Retrieved from http://www.eurekalert.org/pub_releases/2005-12/fiot-apo121305.php

Robinson, L., Gibson, G., Kingston, A., Newton, L., Pritchard, G., Finch, T., & Brittain, K. (2013). Assistive technologies in caring for the oldest old: a review of current practice and future directions. *Aging Health, 9*(4), 365–375.

Robinson, L., Hutchings, D., Corner, L., Finch, T., Hughes, J., Brittain, K., & Bond, J. (2007). Balancing rights and risks: Conflicting perspectives in the management of wandering in dementia. *Health, Risk, & Society, 9*(4), 389–406.

Roelands, M., Van Oost, P., Depoorter, A., & Buysse, A. (2002). A social-cognitive model to predict the use of assistive devices for mobility and self-care in elderly people. *The Gerontologist, 42*(10), 39–50.

Smith, A. (2014). *Pew Research Report: Older adults and technology use.* Washington, DC: Pew Research Center.

SmartHomeUSA. (2016). What is a smart home? Retrieved from http://www.smarthomeusa.com/smarthome/

Span, P. (2011). A shoe for wanderers. *New York Times.* Retrieved from http://newoldage.blogs.nytimes.com/2011/10/14/a-shoe-for-wanderers/

Speech-Language and Audiology Canada. (2015). The role of speech-language pathologists with respect to augmentative and alternative communication (AAC). Retrieved from http://www.sac-oac.ca/sites/default/files/resources/aac_position-paper_en.pdf

Spillman, B. C. (2004). Changes in elderly disability rates and the implications for health care utilization and cost. *Milbank Quarterly, 82*(1), 157–194.

Spry Foundation. (2005). *Computer-based technology and caregiving of older adults.* Retrieved from http://www.spry.org/pdf/CBTCOA_English.pdf

Tomita, M., Mann, W. C., Fraas, L. F., & Stanton, K. M. (2004). Predictors of the use of assistive devices that address physical impairments among community-based frail elders. *Journal of Applied Gerontology, 23*(2), 141–155.

Tomita, M. R., Mann, W. C., Stanton, K., Tomita, A. D., & Sundar, V. (2007). Use of currently available smart home technology by frail elders: Process and outcomes. *Topics in Geriatric Rehabilitation, 23*(1), 24–34.

Topol, E. (2012). *The creative destruction of medicine: How the digital revolution will create better health care.* New York, NY: Basic Books.

University of Pittsburgh, University of Michigan, & Carnegie Mellon University. (2005). *Nursebot project.* Retrieved from http://www.cs.cmu.edu/~flo/

U.S. Congress. (1988). *Technology-Related Assistance for Individuals with Disabilities Act of 1988.* Retrieved from http://www.resnaprojects.org/nattap/library/laws/techact88.htm

U.S. National Library of Medicine. (2010). MEDLINE fact sheet. Retrieved from http://www.nlm.nih.gov/pubs/factsheets/medline.html

U.S. National Park Service. (2012). *America the beautiful: The national parks and federal recreational lands pass series.* Retrieved from http://www.nps.gov/findapark/passes.htm

Veggeberg, S. (1996). Online health and healing. *Molecular Medicine Today, 2*(8), 315.

Weisman, S. (1983). Computer games for the frail elderly. *The Gerontologist, 23*(4), 361–363.

Wellness Community. (2007). Home page.

White, M., & Dorman, S. (2000). Online support for caregivers: Analysis of an internet alzheimer mailgroup. *Computers in Nursing, 18*(4), 168–176.

Wikipedia. (2016). Mobile app. Retrieved from https://en.wikipedia.org/wiki/Mobile_app

Wilson, B. A. (1984). Memory training in practice. In B. Wilson & M. Moffat (Eds.), *Clinical management of memory problems.* Rockville, MD: Aspen Systems Corporation.

World Wide Web Consortium. (2012). *Web content accessibility guidelines.* Retrieved from http://www.w3.org/WAI/intro/wcag

X-10. (2005). Home page. Retrieved from http://www.x10.com

For a full suite of assignments and additional learning activities, see the access code at the front of your book.

Unit VIII
Gerontological Care Issues

CHAPTER 27   END-OF-LIFE CARE
(COMPETENCIES 11, 16)

CHAPTER 28   CARE TRANSITIONS, SYSTEM
MODELS, AND HEALTH POLICY IN AGING
(COMPETENCIES 4, 5, 8, 10, 14)

CHAPTER 22

Culture and Spirituality

Kristen L. Mauk
MaryAnne Shannon
Linda Hassler

(Competencies 8, 10, 13, 18, 19)

LEARNING OBJECTIVES

At the end of this chapter, the reader will be able to:

> Recognize the importance of providing culturally sensitive care to older adults in a world of changing demographics.
> Discuss the importance of assessing health literacy and usage of translation services.
> List components of a cultural questionnaire.
> Discuss various interventions to provide culturally aware care to elders from culturally diverse groups.
> Differentiate between religiosity and spirituality.
> Identify strategies in conducting a spiritual assessment with the older client.
> Apply knowledge of various religions to give spiritually sensitive nursing care.

KEY TERMS

Acculturation	Cultural sensitivity
African Americans	Culturally competent
American Indians	Culture
Asian Americans	Ethnogeriatrics
Assimilation	European Americans
Continuity theory	Health disparities
Core values	Health–illness continuum
Cultural awareness	Hispanic Americans
Cultural competence	Holistic
Cultural congruence	Immigrants

Interpretation	Spiritual assessment
Limited English proficiency	Spiritual baseline assessment
Medical anthropology	Spiritual resources
Minority	Spiritual well-being
Myth	Spirituality
Native Americans	Spiritually thriving
Non-Hispanic White	Transcultural
Older adults	Translation
Religiosity	Vietnamese

The demographics of our world are changing. The numbers of older adults is increasing, not just in the United States, but across most countries in the world. The Pew Research Center (2016) stated that "By 2055, the U.S. will not have a single racial or ethnic majority" (para 2). This is largely due to immigration, a hot topic in the political arena of the 2016 U.S. Presidential election. Asians will replace Latinos as the largest immigration group to the United States. The results of these demographic shifts have enormous impact on the education of nursing students, and nurses to prepare them to provide culturally and spiritually sensitive care to diverse older adults.

The purpose of this chapter is to explore culture and spirituality, including what it means to provide sensitive care in these areas to older clients. This chapter prepares the nurse to envision culture and spirituality as two essential client-centered factors to be considered when assessing, planning, implementing, and evaluating nursing care with older clients.

Culture and Cultural Awareness, Sensitivity, and Competence

There is a growing body of literature that proposes that patients whose *culture* is taken into consideration have better outcomes than those whose culture is not. The Institute of Medicine (2003) stated that nursing education needs to support the development of patient-centered care that identifies, respects, and addresses differences in patients' values, preferences, and expressed needs. The Centers for Disease Control and Prevention (2011) indicated that healthcare organizations continue to need to eliminate *health disparities*; to accomplish this goal, nurses will need to be prepared to function in a global environment, in partnership with other healthcare disciplines. Calvillo et al. (2009) developed a series of cultural competency guidelines for nurses that apply to a variety of healthcare settings, to patients across the health–illness continuum, and to patients across the lifespan.

Although it is unrealistic to expect a nursing student to be proficient in working with every category and subgroup of minority older persons, it is possible to develop levels of awareness, skills, and sensitivity that can be applied to interactions with ethnic minority older persons and their families (Campinha-Bacote, 2011). This chapter challenges nursing students and nurses to develop *cultural awareness*, *sensitivity*, and *competence*.

Campinha-Bacote (2011) stated that "cultural competence is viewed as an expansion of patient-centered care. More specifically, cultural competence can be seen as a necessary set of skills for nurses to attain in order to render effective patient-centered care" (p. 1). These are skills that can be taught and learned in nursing to provide more person-centered care for diverse populations.

Cultural Diversity in the United States

For many years, America had been called "the melting pot," wherein people would melt (blend) together into one culture, assimilating into the mainstream culture of their new home. They would adopt the values, beliefs, behaviors,

TABLE 22-1	Statistics on Immigrants				
Continent of Origin	1820–1849	1850–1899	1900–1949	1950–1999	2000–2011
Africa	152	2,203	30,395	596,598	955,409
Asia	210	357,015	750,741	7,152,188	4,319,624
Europe	1,891,894	15,592,768	16,035,248	5,383,656	1,535,750
North and Central America	92,094	1,129,118	3,498,453	12,351,111	5,101,287
Oceania	6	19,931	51,378	173,193	77,564
Other America	18	7,440	25,411	82,939	23
South America	2,424	9,557	127,868	1,573,100	1,026,978
Not specified	109,864	102,396	35,046	347,251	223,961

Data from U.S. Department of Homeland Security. (2011). Available at http://www.dhs.gov/sites/default/files/publications/immigration-statistics/yearbook/2011/ois_yb_2011.pdf

and attitudes of the majority culture. Recently, America has been called a "tossed salad." Many cultures are still coming together, but they are keeping their unique identities. The millennial generation of the United States is the most diverse generation in recent history, with 43% of this group being nonwhite (Pew Research Center, 2016). Such new groups experience some majority-culture *assimilation* but keep the group affiliations, traditions, and values of their original culture. Due to these changes, there is a need in nursing to both accept and appreciate the differences among people. In this way, nurses can better understand and care for their patients (Spector, 2009).

According to the U.S. Department of Homeland Security (2011), when statistics were first gathered in 1820, there were 8,385 people who immigrated to the United States, as compared to 2011, when there were 1,062,040 immigrants, an 89% increase in 191 years. **Table 22-1** shows the number of legal, permanent resident *immigrants* into the United States over the past 191 years. It is interesting to note how the pattern of immigration has changed. From 18 20 to 1949, the continent of origin was mainly Europe, though there were fluctuations in the regional immigration patterns (e.g., Western Europe vs. Eastern Europe). Starting in 1950, there was an increase in the number of immigrants from Latin America (which includes Mexico, much of the Caribbean, and Central and South America). **Figure 22-1** shows the age distribution of the foreign born as a percentage of the total foreign-born population for the United States from 1870 to 2010.

Characteristics of the Five Major Ethnic Groups in the United States

The five major ethnic groups in the United States will be discussed here: *European Americans*, *African Americans*, *Hispanic Americans*, *Asian Americans*, and *Native Americans*. Some basic health and religious beliefs of each group will be explored. Brief summaries of culturally sensitive nursing research to promote health in each ethnic group are also discussed in this section (**Table 22-2**).

European Americans

Currently, European Americans constitute the majority of the population in the United States. This demographic is changing, however, and by the year 2050, European Americans will no longer be the prevalent cultural group (Pew Research Center, 2016). The majority of European Americans describe themselves as Christian (Pew Research Center, 2016). Within this sect, European Americans include the two major Christian denominations: Catholics and Protestants. Protestant denominations further fracture into, among others, Lutherans (Scandinavian Americans),

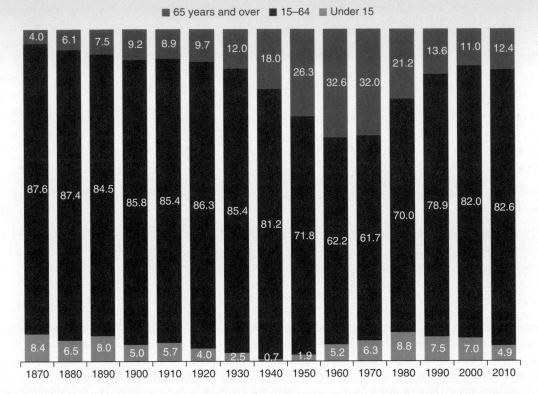

FIGURE 22-1 Age Distribution of the Foreign Born as a Percentage of the Total Foreign-Born Population, for the United States: 1870 to 2010.

Data from Migration Policy Institute. (2011). Retrieved from http://www.migrationinformation.org/datahub/charts/age.shtml; Gibson, C. J., and Lennon, E. (1999). US Census Bureau Population Division Working Paper No. 29: Historical census statistics on the foreign-born population of the United States: 1850 to 1990. Retrieved from https://www.census.gov/population/www/documentation/twps0029/twps0029.html

TABLE 22-2 Place of Death by Race and Ethnicity

Place	Non-Hispanic White	Non-Hispanic Black	Hispanic	American Indian or Alaskan Native	Asian or Pacific Islander
Inpatient hospital	31.1%	38.2%	41.1%	40.5%	43.6%
Nursing home/long-term care facility	28.4%	18.8%	15.8%	19.4%	17.2%
Residence	24.3%	21.3%	28.4%	26.5%	24.4%
Other	16.2%	21.7%	14.8%	13.5%	14.8%

Note: *Other* refers to outpatient or emergency department, including dead on arrival, inpatient hospice facilities, and all other places and unknown. Reference population: These data refer to the resident population.

National Vital Statistics System. Mortality public use files, 2009, as printed in *Older Americans 2012*, page 154.

Reproduced from Federal Interagency Forum on Aging-Related Statistics. (2012). *Older Americans 2012: Key indicators of well-being.* Washington, DC: US Government Printing Office. Retrieved from https://agingstats.gov/docs/PastReports/2012/OA2012.pdf

Presbyterians (German Americans), Methodists (Scottish Americans), and Episcopalians (Anglo Americans). Of note is that these sects are not hard-and-fast rules; many Irish and Italian Americans are not Catholics, but Protestants; likewise many German and Anglo Americans are Catholic. Furthermore, many of these churches, upon movement to the United States, split off from their parent churches and evolved into nondenominational Christian churches (Kelley, Small, & Tripp-Reimer, 2004). European Americans are less likely to turn to religion or *spirituality* as coping or problem-solving mechanisms. European males tend to be more extroverted and open than other cultural groups (Eap et al., 2008). European Americans tend to rely on science to explain health and illness, rather than one's communion with God. European Americans also are more likely to turn to the government as the responsible caretaker for the infirm and elderly (Walker, Lester, & Joe, 2006).

> ### CLINICAL TIP
>
> European Americans value the healthcare system and tend to rely on science to explain health and illness.

European Americans generally do not have as close ties to their extended families as other cultural groups within the United States. European Americans tend to be individualistic when it comes to health care, often presenting a stoic attitude about illness, so as not to "be a burden" on others. This is represented by the value system of European Americans as "doers." Upon reaching retirement, European Americans can lose their sense of self-worth (Giger & Davidhizar, 2004). European Americans are more accepting of the paternalistic nature of the healthcare system, are generally more trusting of authority, and therefore tend to follow the advice of healthcare providers to engage in more physical and mental activity than other cultural groups within the United States (Njoku, Jason, & Torres Harding, 2005). The U.S. healthcare system is primarily designed to meet the needs of European Americans.

Crespo and Arbesman's (2003) analysis of the differences in factors associated with obesity in different cultural and ethnic groups is an excellent way to emphasize the importance of cultural assessments when providing nursing care. The prevalence of obesity is higher among African American (35%) and Hispanic (33%) women than among European American women (22%). In African Americans and Hispanics, obesity is associated with poverty: It may not be safe to walk or run for exercise in poorer neighborhoods, and there may not be affordable gyms nearby. Poverty is associated with higher fat diets, as higher fat foods are less expensive. In African Americans and Hispanics with higher education and higher income levels, obesity levels are similar to European Americans. On the other hand, obesity in European Americans is associated with higher income and less education, or truly a disease of excess living. In all groups, increased time watching television is associated with obesity. Thus, when intervening with older adults who are obese, it is important to identify specific factors that are contributing to obesity, and make culturally sensitive recommendations to exercise more, reduce fat and calorie intake, and watch television less.

African Americans

As seen in Chapter 2, African Americans make up the second-largest *minority* population in the United States, only recently being overtaken by Hispanics. Currently, 12.6% of the U.S. population are Black (Agency for Healthcare Research and Quality [AHRQ], 2016). They are a diverse population totaling 39.9 million with the following origins: U.S.-born Blacks (36.2 million), foreign-born Blacks (3.8 million), Jamaican (682,000), Haitian (586,000), Nigerian (226,000), Dominican (166,000), Hispanic Blacks (3.2 million) (AHRQ, 2016). In 2010, the top health conditions included hypertension, obesity and overweight, and diabetes. The leading causes of death are consistently the same as other groups with cardiovascular disease, cancer, and stroke being the top three, followed by diabetes among Blacks (AHRQ, 2016).

African Americans' religions vary as much as European Americans, but most African Americans are Protestant (Baptist, Pentecostal, and others). A fair number of African Americans are Muslim, or followers of Islam. It is therefore of vital importance not to generalize about any particular culture, but to inquire about religious beliefs and practices instead of making assumptions (Holt et al., 2016).

CLINICAL TIP

African Americans tend not to want to put their older relatives in nursing homes, rather choosing to care for them at home.

The role of religion and spirituality plays an important part in the African American health and wellness belief system. Often, African Americans equate good luck, good fortune, and good health with "being right with God." Therefore, disease and illness can be thought of as being in disfavor with God, and incurring His wrath. Likewise, African Americans believe they have less control over their health and well-being than God, and illness and disease are part of "God's plan" (Walker et al., 2006). This is, however, an oversimplification of a much more complex locus of control discussion that is beyond the scope of this chapter.

Despite the systematic destruction of the family unit by 200 years of slavery in the United States, African Americans have much closer ties to their extended families compared to other cultural groups within the United States. African Americans tend to rely on their close family ties or close neighbors when in need of support rather than turning inward, as with other cultural groups. Along with slavery, other historical injustices, such as segregation and economic disparity, have influenced African Americans' distrust of authority. African Americans are particularly distrustful of healthcare personnel because of discrimination in medical care and because most authority figures in health care are not African Americans. Wallace et al. (2007) found that the "Tuskegee Syphilis Study continues to influence the relationship of the African American patient and the biomedical community" (p. 722). A study of older, community-dwelling African Americans identified the following categories of coping strategies for chronic health conditions: dealing with it, engaging in life, exercising, seeking information, relying on God, changing dietary patterns, medicating, self-monitoring, and self-advocacy (Loeb, 2006).

The impact of racism toward African Americans has long been considered one of the factors that contributes to decreased longevity and increased chronic illnesses (see **Table 22-3**). Moody-Ayers, Stewart, Covinsky, and Inouye (2005) studied the prevalence and correlates of perceived societal racism in African American adults age 50 or older with type 2 diabetes mellitus. The investigators found that 92% of the sample experienced social racism, which correlated with fair or poor health. The investigators caution healthcare providers that day-to-day societal racism may affect patients' trust in healthcare providers, adherence to medical advice, and self-management of chronic health problems.

Hispanic Americans

Hispanic Americans have recently become the second largest population demographic in the United States, and as a result of immigration and higher-than-average birth rates, the number of Hispanic Americans (people of Latin descent) is projected to make up 29% of the United States population by the year 2050 (Passel & Cohn, 2008; Supple & Small, 2006). It is for these reasons, and others, that it is important for healthcare providers to understand the needs of this population and find ways to meet those needs.

CLINICAL TIP

Hispanic Americans often use folk remedies before traditional Western medicine.

Most Hispanic Americans place high value on family, religion, and community. Hispanic cultures emphasize family interdependence over independence. For this population, self-care is not as important as receiving care in recovery from illness. An individual who becomes ill will turn to the family first before seeking outside health care. Often those of Hispanic culture will first seek the use of homeopathic remedies in conjunction with religious

TABLE 22-3 Percentage of People Age 65 and Over Who Reported Having Selected Chronic Health Conditions, by Sex, 2007–2008

	Heart Disease	Hypertension	Stroke	Asthma	Chronic Bronchitis or Emphysema	Any Cancer	Diabetes	Arthritis
				Percent				
Total	31.9	55.7	8.8	10.4	9.0	22.5	18.6	49.5
Men	38.2	53.1	8.7	8.9	8.6	23.9	19.5	42.2
Women	27.1	57.6	8.9	11.5	9.2	21.4	17.9	54.9
Non-Hispanic White	33.7	54.3	8.7	10.2	9.7	24.8	16.4	50.6
Non-Hispanic Black	27.2	71.1	10.8	11.3	5.9	13.3	29.7	52.2
Hispanic	23.8	53.1	7.7	10.9	6.2	12.4	27.3	42.1

Note: Data are based on a 2-year average from 2007–2008.
Reproduced from Federal Interagency Forum on Aging-Related Statistics. (2010). *Older Americans 2010: Key indicators of well-being.* Federal Interagency Forum on Aging-Related Statistics. Washington, DC: U.S. Government Printing Office; Data from Centers for Disease Control and Prevention, National Center for Health Statistics, National Health Interview Survey.

artifacts before engaging a healthcare professional. Additionally, direct disagreement with a healthcare provider is uncommon; the usual response to a decision that the patient or the family disagrees with is silence and non-compliance. Other Hispanic Americans may choose not to seek health care because they, like members of other cultures and religions, think their affliction is a punishment for sins. However, a growing number of Hispanic Americans do not seek health care because they do not have access to health care. This could be because they lack health insurance, have communication difficulties, or fear legal ramifications for residing in the country illegally (Gonzalez & Kuipers, 2004; Padilla & Villalobos, 2007).

Most Hispanic Americans are Catholic, but as with most cultures, the role that religion plays in health practices varies greatly from person to person. Those Hispanic Americans who have experienced *acculturation* to the United States generally accept the scientific theory of health and illness, although many subscribe to a more naturalistic approach. This approach in the Hispanic American culture strives to achieve a balance between "hot" and "cold" within the body. Illnesses are categorized as either hot or cold and treated with the reciprocal type of substance, found in either medicine or food (Gonzalez & Kuipers, 2004).

Diabetes and heart disease are two health problems that have an increased prevalence and mortality in Hispanic Americans. Whittemore (2007) conducted a systematic review of the literature to identify culturally competent interventions for Hispanic adults with type 2 diabetes. In reviewing 11 studies, Whittemore found that providing educational sessions and written materials in both English and Spanish, employing bilingual Hispanic staff, including family members in an informal atmosphere in healthcare encounters, incorporating cultural traditions in interventions, developing culturally relevant program literature, and providing fact sheets about risks and potential poor outcomes of chronic conditions such as diabetes will increase the effectiveness of interventions.

Asian Americans

Often, immigrants from China, India, the Philippines, Vietnam, Korea, and the Middle East are grouped together as Asian Americans (**Table 22-4**). However, to do so not only is a gross oversimplification, but also does an injustice to the

TABLE 22-4 Asian American Information at a Glance

	Asian Indians (third largest)	Chinese (largest sub-group)	Filipino (second largest)	Japanese	Korean (fastest growing sub-group)	Pakistani	Vietnamese
Abuse *statistics from APIIDV and NAPAWF	Spousal abuse private between husband and wife; in-law emotional abuse; 36–65% women report abuse	Coin rubbing may look like abuse; women more tolerant; "do not tell"—certain times "may be justified"; 18–22% women report abuse	Vulnerable group—WWII veterans, esp.; sexual exploitation; spousal abuse ignored; 20–31% women report abuse	Human trafficking for sex work, domestic servitude, hotel work, agricultural labor, sweatshop factories; 32.9% women report abuse;** Moxibustion: resultant bruising may look like abuse	Coin rubbing may look like abuse. 30–60% women report abuse	Domestic violence not explicitly prohibited, considered "a private family matter"	Family violence related to "thinking too much"; healing coin rubbing (superficial abrasions) may appear as abuse; 30–47% women report abuse
Advance directives	Aggressive intervention; unlikely to use AD; talking may make reality	Reluctance due to karma; lack of information; don't want to burden children	May avoid conversation as this may bring on death; approach gradually; may be resistive	More open as death is natural process; approach with courteous respect	Involve family members; discussing death may bring sadness and depression; unlikely to have written documents	May be reluctant to discuss as this may make it a reality; withholding food is forbidden in Islam	Death is natural phase, make concrete preparations but not AD due to lack of knowledge
Alcohol	15–20% abuse; whiskey popular; prohibited some areas	Lower rates	Tuba (philippin beer) and hard liquor; Islam forbids alcohol	2% population	Moderate risk of abuse	Rare according to Islamic laws	Abuse related to "thinking too much"
Decision makers	Men and family; mother-in-law has special status; Youngest son takes care of elders	Husband, son, or physician; Father head of family; filial piety—oldest son	Husband; may have surrogate decision maker	"Master of the home": husband or oldest adult son; family consulted before medical decisions made	Men have more status; more concern over men's illness	Older women may defer to their sons or daughters; family may want to shield the patient from negative diagnosis: ask patient if family can make decisions for patient; do not use word cancer; males make decisions	Oldest male

Dementia	Lower rates of Alzheimer's and vascular dementia: 1.8–3.6%	Vascular	Very small amount	Vascular higher in men; undiagnosed and untreated; 1.8–5.4%	Noted	Al-Harim (severely debilitated or demented elderly); fourth major health problem	Natural part of aging and the life cycle
End of Life/Dying	Family-centered decision; do not tell elder poor prognosis; die at home. Move to floor—family wash body and wrap in red cloth. Belief in resurrection; may want to return to India to die	Bad luck to talk about death: Karma; surgery may be avoided as it disrupts life cycle; want patient alert till time of death. Bathe after death, three grains of rice on tongue for journey to next life, may not visit friends for 30–100 days. Buddhist: stay with body for 3 days and pray; won't show emotion; believe in euthanasia	Tell family first of poor prognosis as they may wish to spare elder suffering; "Last Rites"; resistant to stop life support. Family washes body before transport	Defer decisions to children/oldest son; concept of shiata go ni: it cannot be helped; family may not tell of poor prognosis; commit suicide with terminal illness	Prefer to die at home or return to Korea to die; death is a virtue; burial. Descendants visit ancestors' tombs on Korean Thanksgiving Day; inform family of poor prognosis first, they may/may not tell elder; may chant or burn incense; wash body of deceased	Focus spiritually on preparing soul for life after death; withholding food is forbidden in Islam; same-sex caregiver dealing with dead body. Extensive death rituals: ceremonies, washing body, positioning on left or right side towards Mecca (Southeast in North America), recitation of the Holy Qur'an by fakirs (holy men). Never give up hope; inform family of poor prognosis before elder; resistance to postmortem exam; burial within 24 hours linked to prayer timing	Sudden Unexpected Nocturnal Death Syndrome: nightmare or attack of evil spirits, press the life of terrified victim; hospital strangers at death may be viewed as negative for a "Bad Death"; withdrawal of life support may be viewed as causing or speeding up death; palliative care more acceptable. Cultural difference in truth telling about death: may cause elder to lose hope, lack of respect, upsetting, may bring death sooner

(continues)

TABLE 22-4 Asian American Information at a Glance (continued)

	Asian Indians (third largest)	Chinese (largest sub-group)	Filipino (second largest)	Japanese	Korean (fastest growing sub-group)	Pakistani	Vietnamese
Family system	Men play major role; decisions by family; men arrange marriages	Family and society over individual; different between rural and urban areas; may wash patient in hospital; may never leave patient alone	Respect and love for parents and elders; group harmony; loyalty; family reunification and elders with children; adherence to health practice related to desire to participate in family group; core value kapwa: shared identity, interacting as equals; extended family membership; females stay with patient in hospital.	Provide physical care to patient; individuals less important than family	Family collectivity; clearly divided family roles; blood relatives important; children of mixed ethnicity are undesirable to elders; believe family and friends over medical practitioner; education important; self-esteem tied to identification with family; males more status; family stay in hospital	Marriages between first cousins; family important to identity; extended families live in one home	Eldest male head of family; if adults work, elders take care of grandchildren and cook
Folk lore/ Folk healers Indigenous Health beliefs	Ayurvedic medicine: knowledge of life; holistic, balance, natural remedies; spiritual; body, mind, senses, soul; Karma: law of behavior and consequence; Mangalsutra: sacred thread around neck	Illness results from imbalance of yin/yang; vital energy; organs associated with illness: lung (worry), gallbladder/ liver (anger), heart (happy), kidney (fear), spleen (desire); acupuncture	Timbang: principles of balance, range of hot/cold beliefs; prevention and curing; elders use dual systems; rice porridge during illness; may refuse oxygen because it means serious illness; bowel movement means good health; for	Kampo: strives to restore energy flow; herbs, acupuncture; acupressure; massage; moxibustion: burning a cone or cylinder of downy or woolly material; shiatsu: healing massage; green or Chinese teas remedy; ginger, sake, eggs help	Hanbang or hanyak: balance between um (yin) and yang and balance of fire, earth, metal, water, wood; use of acupuncture, herbs, moxibustion, and cupping; may alternate	Traditional folk medicine first, then Western medicine when disease is intolerable; Unani: therapy based on humeral theory of Hippocrates; three body states: health, disease, neutral state: six primary factors: air, food/beverage, movement/rest, sleep/wake, eat/	Opium or backache remedies used to cope with accultura-tion stress; speaking of vomiting or bowels not common and uncomfortable; don't touch head; holistic concept of health; illness as suffering has value as a cata-lyst for change and development; herbal medicines; coining (coin rubbing);

[women] or chest [men]: consult astrologist; apply poultices; folk medicine; home remedies prior to physician; food for hot and cold illnesses; water and cumin for indigestion; black pepper and licorice to protect health; combine with Western medicine; yoga, meditation, prayer to achieve balance; may not wear gown worn by another; nod = no, shake = yes; woman with a red dot on forehead are married; spirituality, fashion

[may cause skin irritations]; Cupping (vacuum on skin); Coining (hot coins on skin); moxibustion [burn mugwart burn near skin]; herbology; meditation; blood work will cause weakness; licorice to protect health; combine with Western medicine; yoga, meditation, prayer to achieve balance; may not wear gown worn by another; dyspnea and vomiting treat with soup and liquids; ginseng for anemia, colic, depression, indigestion, impotence, rheumatisms; exorcism; good luck articles worn; aromatherapy; rice teas treat diarrheas; congee [rice porridge] to help recover from illness

stomach ache: toast, uncooked rice, add water, drink liquid. **Illness theories:** Mystical: retribution from ancestors for unfilled obligations; *Bangungot*: nightmares after heavy meal result in death; *Personalistic:* Social punishment or retribution by supernatural beings, such as *Mankukulam* [sorcerer]; wears anting ant ng [a amulet or talisman] for protection; Naturalistic: nature events, stress, incompatible food, drugs, infection. Same sex care provider; aromatherapy; once illness effects functional capacity, then seek medical treatment; may not perform IADLs as part of living with family; rest after surgery is important

during a cold; don't want to look for something bad, so no screenings

between Eastern medicine and Western medicine; shamans remove evil spirits; illness is interruption of flow of life energy: lack of control of food, physical exertion, blood, elements; spiritual causes of illness; may not trust patent medications; traditional Korean medicine aimed at relieving symptoms and not treating underlying condition; natural ways of improving health; fatalistic; vomiting and bowel issues embarrassing and not discussed

evacuate; emotions; *hakim: unani* practitioner; certain hot/cold foods promote recovery from certain illnesses; do not believe in self-care during illness

cupping; *moxibustion* (therapeutic burning); accupuncture Vietnamese three models of health. 1. *Am-Duong* – illness imbalance of yin and yang, clear by acupuncture; 2. *Than kinh suy nhuoc*: neuroses or illness of nerves; *Than kinhthac loan*: psychosis or turmoil of nerves; for "weak nerves," prescribe nerve tonic or tranquilizer; 3. Supernatural interventions: *Ten deities*: protection; humoral imbalance from Ayurvedic medicine: five basic elements [ether, wind, water, earth, fire] are upset; ritual ceremonies to deal with spirits and pay homage; practitioners of "black magic." Hmong *Shamar* [leader and healer] can communicate with spirits; spirit illness and soul loss a factor in illness; Laotians Chinese Taoist, healing Lao-tsu and his priests; spirit influence; accumulated merits

(continues)

TABLE 22-4 Asian American Information at a Glance (continued)

	Asian Indians (third largest)	Chinese (largest sub-group)	Filipino (second largest)	Japanese	Korean (fastest growing sub-group)	Pakistani	Vietnamese
Folk lore/ Folk healers Indigenous Health beliefs (cont.)							in life; 12 souls relate to 12 parts of body; *hwen:* illness created by malevolent ancestors in one part of body or soul; *Dia:* hereditary illness; *Tsiang:* ceremonies by grand master priests, other priests, or spirit mediums for supernatural illness; Eastern and herbal remedies
Health Disparities	Tuberculosi, malaria, and CAD rates higher; 1:8 have breast cancer; high risk for osteoporosis; insulin resistance; Lathyrism: paralysis from eating plant; diarrheas related to intestinal parasites; HIV; Chikungunya viral dengue hemmorrhaggic fever; bacterial meningitis; hepatitis A, B, C, & E	"Model minority" (all Asians are affluent and healthy) myth; Increased rates of cancers of the breast, colon and prostate; hepatitis B and associated liver cancer; tuberculosis; naso-pharyngeal cancer; lower smoking rates; thalassemia and glucose 6 dehydrogenase deficiency; CVD; COPD; malaria; poor air quality and pollution; Less likely to get mammograms	HTN, CHD, DM (3X), Lower rates of cancer and cancer survival of women; higher rates of gout in men; tuberculosis; HIV; hepatitis B; vitamin A and iron deficiency;	Longest life expectancy in world; risk of most diseases lower than for other elders; lower heart disease, CAD, and strokes; cancer; diabetes higher in America; Higher type II diabetes	Low risk for obesity; moderate risk for adjustment problems; High risk for Type II diabetes (4x risk); HTN; CVD; hepatitis B carriers; malaria; cirrhosis of liver; tuberculosis; oxygen means a life-threatening illness, so patients may not want to use; acupressure and massage; sensitive to cold feelings; air and water pollution concern in Korea	High risk for coronary heart disease and DM; oral sub-mucous fibrosis (from *paan*/ chewing tobacco); women risk for dyslipidemia; tuberculosis; HTN; higher risk breast cancer; asking questions about sex may be insult to widow	High risk for osteoporosis and HTN; high total cholesterol; obesity; cigarette smoking; seizures; men have high risk of cancer of nasopharnx, liver, stomach; women have high risk for cancer of the cervix, stomach, thyroid; insulin resistance; hepatitis B; Agent Orange exposure; chewing *betel nut quid* (stimulant/ narcotic) causes oral squamous cell cancer in women; low participation in screening programs

Historical Events	1908: Alienation of Land Act in India forced immigration; 1947: M. Gandhi lead non-violent protests for independence; 1980s: Family Reunification laws	1941: Japan invaded, many war crimes committed; post WWII immigration to United States; 1945: U.S. War Bride Act; Southeast Asia: Chinese refugees	1930s: *Pinoys*—overt racism, discrimination, oppressive farm management practices; WWII: war brides; 1965: Family Reunification Act, health professions, veterans; 1970s: refugees from Marcos regime; 1990: amendment to Naturalization Act, WWII veterans; negative attitudes may be passed on by generations	Hawaiian sugar industry; internment during WWII; Japanese wives of U.S. servicemen	1948: war, split to North and South; Hawaiian sugar industry; 1950: Korean War, war orphans sent to United States; 1965: Immigration Act; elders are "followers of children"	1947: Pakistan separated from India; 1971: Bangladesh separated from Pakistan	1975: Vietnam War, refugees left country; boat people. Cambodia: genocide—Po. Pot and Khmer Rouge; killing fields; 1987: Ameras an Homecoming Act; 1996 – Welfare Reform Act: funds withheld for elders
Languages	LEP: English Hindu Gujarati Punjabi Bengali Urdu Marathi Oriya Kannada Tamil Maylayalam	LEP: English Mandarin Yue (Cantonese) Wu (Shanghainese) Minbei (Fuzhou) Minnan (Hokkien—Taiwanese) Xiang Gan Hakka Many dialects	English Over 170 languages: Pilipino Tagalog "Tag-lish" (combo of Tagalog and English) Cebuano Ilocano Ilonggo Bicolano Waray Kampangan Pangasinanes Ask if medical interpreter needed	English Japanese dialects: Okinawan	Korean LEP: English	Urdu Punjabi Pashto Saraiki Sindhi Kashmiri Balochi English; Same sex professional interpreters (for modesty)	Vietnamese Hmong Mong English
Living arrangements	Financially dependent on children who they followed; grandparents raise grandchildren	Sickly live with son	Multigenerational households	Elderly cared for in their homes; close family network	Children provide physical care to elders	Elderly cared for at home and shown great respect; extended family members live together in a family home	Extended families; polygamous; elders as "followers of children"

(continues)

TABLE 22-4 Asian American Information at a Glance (continued)

	Asian Indians (third largest)	Chinese (largest sub-group)	Filipino (second largest)	Japanese	Korean (fastest growing sub-group)	Pakistani	Vietnamese
Long-Term Care (Overall: 1.5% of long term care population are Asian/Pacific Islanders)	Elderly cared for in home	Reluctance: filial piety	Children take care of elders in their home	Reluctance due to filial piety, unless dementia; care for in home of adult children; retirement homes increasing	Seen as last resort; financial support lacking; adult children guilt; women take care of elder in home; extended family criticize family decision	Elderly cared for in home; extended families live together in one home	Demented elderly cared for by sons in home; LTC only when sanctioned by entire extended family
Mental Health	Due to possession of the evil eye; stigma; high suicide rate; may complain vague symptoms when depressed; lower levels of people (castes) believe they did bad things in former life	Depression; 3x suicide rate women (hanging); Buddhist believe shame family; medications; underdiagnosed and undertreated; psychosomatic and hypochondriac for emotional distress or attention; psychotherapy for seriously mental ill only; lower does of psychiatric medications	Situational depression; headache, loss of appetite, sleeplessness, fatigue, low energy; medication preferred over talk therapy; psychiatry perceived for affluent; mental problems result of witchcraft or demons; shameful; stigma	Stigma; avoid shame to family name (hazukashii); shame a powerful driver; shaming family is devastating; social stigma; no therapy; problems caused by own behavior; suicide a major problem; kamikaze: honorable suicide; physical problems instead of stress complaints	Hwabyung: fire illness results from failure to keep emotions from being expressed, especially in women; suicide rates are high; depression; stress of adaption; caregiver stress and guilt;	Stigma; may describe illness in physical terms; anxiety and depression high; pir or fakir (holymen) will visit shrines and tombs to prevent and cure physical and mental illness	Horrific life events during Vietnam War; refugee migration lead to depression, loss, and trauma (PTSD); elderly at higher risk due to above; PruitChiit/ KiitChraen: thinking too much; sadness, depression related to killing fields events; severe headaches and dizziness may lead to family violence; "weak nerves" cause anxiety, depression, mental deterioration; social stigma; may be due to lack of spiritual harmony—ancestors coming back to visit. Vision loss related to conversion hysteria from wartime experience

Nutrition	Ramadan (fasting from sunrise to set); fasting by women improves welfare of family; often vegetarians; no beef or pork; risk of malnutrition; eat rice, beans, chicken, nuts, vegetables, fish, coconut; eat with fingers; overweight gives stature.	Hot and cold foods: must have proper balance to maintain health; Risk for malnutrition and anemia; eat rice, vegetables, seafood, tofu, soy sauce; high-sodium meals; tea is the main drink; burned rice is bad luck; lactose intolerant; use of chopsticks	Arbularyo (herbalist) has special treatment; skills with liquid infusion and dietary measures; use of salty condiments, pork fat, and coconut milk; being overweight is a sign of wealth; many lactose intolerant; roasted pig, sausage, chicken; dog meat a delicacy	Rice, vegetables, fruit, noodle, tofu, and seafood (raw and cooked); high sodium; low obesity rates.	Rice, vegetables, meat, and fruit as dessert; diet high in salt; preserved foods; lactose intolerant; "hot" and "cold" foods to restore balance; kimchi: pickled cabbage; hot liquids preferred	Poor nutrition; foods high in saturated fat; halal: lawful or sanctified meat; all forms of pork forbidden; withholding food is forbidden in Islam; wheat flatbread, lentils, vegetables; at mealtime, express gratitude and be serious; sweet foods not common; fish, red meat, certain fruits not with dairy; Ramadan fast sunrise to sunset; anemia in women	Rice, meats, vegetables, French bread, noodles; soft, warm foods for ill patients; iced drinks not accepted; lactose intolerance
Organ donation/ Transplants/ Autopsy	Not common	Resistant (keeping body whole after death); rare	May be difficult due to religious beliefs (resurrection) and that body parts should be buried	Not favored, as there is an importance of dying intact; body should be clean and orifices be blocked with cotton or gauze; assisted suicide legalized in Japan (1995) for severe pain or impending death; cremation; practice Buddhist rituals after death: wetting lips with water, flowers, incense, and candle on table, a knife or the body to drive away evil spirits; head facing north or west, towards the realm of Buddha.	Not commonly accepted	Subject of great debate in Muslim faith; some feel it mutilates the body and shows disrespect to a gift from Allah	Less likely because donors would be reborn without their vital organs in the next life (reincarnation); Vietnamese may be more willing for barter of medical care or monetary awards

(continues)

TABLE 22-4 Asian American Information at a Glance (continued)

	Asian Indians (third largest)	Chinese (largest sub-group)	Filipino (second largest)	Japanese	Korean (fastest growing sub-group)	Pakistani	Vietnamese
Pain	Stoic; Hinduism believes that suffering is positive and leads to spirituality; fear drug abuse and addiction	Not readily expressed; offer pain medication frequently as it is impolite to accept something first time it is offered	Physical or emotional pain is challenge to ones spirituality; "will of God"; prefer IV or oral to IM	Belief ub tolerating pain and not expressing discomfort; may refuse pain medication; oral medications preferred	Men may not express; pain medication accepted	Not comfortable expressing pain; ask specific questions to determine pain; Islam prohibits narcotics; pain relievers may not be utilized on religious holidays	Tolerant of pain; smile or appear happy to cover pain; warm compresses are acceptable
Religion	Hinduism Islam Sikhism Buddhism Jainism Christianity Rites are preformed at death; Sikhs don't cut hair; black, white, blue are colors of death and funeral	Confucianism (achieve harmony); Buddhism (dignity); Taoism (the way: selflessness, cleanliness, emotional calm, conformity); Christianity; Islam; Ancestor worship; numbers are of great significance: 4,7 = unlucky; 8,6,2 = lucky; People's Republic of China's official religion is atheism	Catholic Protestant Aglipay Muslims (Mindanao and Sulu regions); Mysticism; church affiliation may encourage health promotion; importance of prayer, church affiliation, spiritual fellowship and faith; God as "divine physician"; religious jewelry to promote healing; babaylan: practitioner uses prayers and rituals, herbal plants, and massage manipulation for health and wellness; prayer and spiritual counseling part of treatment plan; "Soul Loss" due to shock, fear, or desire, requires prayer or exorcism	Shintoism: belief in Kami (spirit gods); Buddhism: code of ethics, harmony with themselves, universe, and society for good health; Confucianism: importance of family and social order; Christianity; may combine religious customs; many agnostic	Buddhist; Christian (Protestant, Catholic); churches/ temples play important role; Korean church ties; 50% do not claim a religious affiliation; fatalistic; luck or past doings create illness; shamans remove evil spirit or promote spiritual healing	Islam; Christianity; Hinduism; spiritual peace part of health; disease a direct punishment from God; wear taawiz: amulet with holy Qur'an verses; sickness is a test from God; avoid complaining about sickness; illness is for atonement of sins; may wear taawiz or topi (religious cap); Ramadan: self-purification by a fast from eating, drinking, smoking, or sex sunrise to sunset (not applicable to children, pregnant women, or Al-Harim (severely debilitated or demented elderly); at sunset,	Buddhist; Cambodians: Theravada Buddhism; in United States, Catholic; Delays in obtaining relief from illness may be a Buddhist stoic response to religious awakening; tiendietes: errant spirit ancestors not properly venerated by descendants with worship or offerings and cause mental illness; spirit mediums and sorcerers deal with spirits; Buddhist priests and monks give amulets and medicines for physical ailments or do exorcism for spiritual ailments; spirit world can influence health; placing rice, coins, or jewels in

Religion (cont.)				fast is broken with prayers and *iftar* (meal), then visit with friends and family; *Namaz*: obligatory prayers five times per day; facing Mecca, after washing themselves; Fridays go to *masjid* (mosque or church) offer special prayers; *Wudu*: ceremonial washing before prayers	mouth of deceased to help travel after death; Last Rites for Catholics; Buddhists: death ritual last 3 days; include praying and burning incense
Respect	Same sex caregivers; patient is passive; direct eye contact from women to men limited; remove shoes before entering home; physical contact limited; older person has high respect	*Li*: proper way, control of emotions, restraint, obedience to authority, conforming, and "face" are highly valued and important; authority and elders; filial piety: protect elders from poor prognosis; may hesitate to ask questions as not to appear disrespectful or inconvenient; proper title and name; older adults called auntie and uncle; direct eye	Address by Mr/Mrs/Miss; with permission *Lola* (grandma) or *Lolo* (grandpa): protect elders from external forces; respect for elders and authority; children should be taught to care for elders and take care of aging parents; firm handshake and greet elder first; ask to repeat instructions as a sign of respect (instead of asking if they understand); healthcare provider respected and may not be questioned or challenged; sit at eye level; keep personal	*Filial piety*: taking care of one's own parents; courtesy and thoughtfulness; great respect for elders and authority; introduce self to elder first; children provide physical care to elderly; may call by title	Proper title and bow; filial piety; same sex provider; respect for authority; no direct eye contact or physical contact; silence; modesty; use both hands when giving object; silence	May not make direct compliment as this may bring attention to evil spirits; proper titles; no eye contact; large area of personal space; elders highly respected

(continues)

TABLE 22-4 Asian American Information at a Glance *(continued)*

	Asian Indians (third largest)	Chinese (largest sub-group)	Filipino (second largest)	Japanese	Korean (fastest growing sub-group)	Pakistani	Vietnamese
Respect *(cont.)*		contact avoided; no head touching; no winking	space; covering mouth = shyness or embarrassment; don't want to be burden so won't seek health care; saving face is important				
Utilization of Health Care	Surgery only on auspicious days	Language barriers, geography, economic barriers	Lack of health insurance; lack of mobility; LEP; adherence to own cultural health beliefs	Medical problems, not mental illness	Decreased due to LEP, unfamiliar systems and food in hospitals; utilize "Korean" hospitals in United States, which are unlicensed private homes	Lack of health insurance (50%)	Buddhists may avoid hospitals where "lost souls gather"; souls of dead people linger and may create havoc upon living as they have no place to rest

*NAPAWF: National Asian Pacific American Women's Forum http://napawf.org

*APIIDV: Asian and Pacific Islander Institute on Domestic Violence http://www.apiidv.org/violence/ethnic-specific-information.php

**The Yomiuri Shimbun 2012. (Tokyo): One-third of married Japanese women are victims of domestic abuse.

http://www.standard.net/stories/2012/05/02/one-third-married-japanese-women-are-victims-domestic-abuse

The Rise of Asian Americans video: http://www.pewsocialtrends.org/2012/06/19/video-the-rise-of-asian-americans/

ancient histories of these cultures, with recorded history going back 10,000 years (Spector, 2009). The majority of Asian Americans in the United States are Chinese Americans, and this section will briefly cover health and religious practices of the Chinese culture.

Most Asian Americans' health beliefs and practices follow the same trajectory as those of other cultures within the United States—that is, the more acculturated to Western traditions, the more they move toward the scientific theory of health and illness. Asian culture places high value on personal relationships, connections, and "face" (Eap et al., 2008).

Hsiung and Ferrans (2007) identified four Chinese American groups in the acculturation continuum: the most traditional and least acculturated elderly immigrants, less acculturated elderly immigrants of working class, bi-acculturated professionals, and Chinese Americans born and raised in the United States. The most traditional and least acculturated elderly Asian Americans may still practice holistic (naturalistic) medicine and may incorporate this as an adjunct to allopathic (Western) medicine. Some of these herbal supplements may have undesired effects when combined with prescribed medications; therefore, it is vital that all complementary medicine and treatment be taken into consideration in directing care for individuals (Giger & Davidhizar, 2004).

CLINICAL TIP

There are many subgroups of Asian Americans, each with a unique set of cultural norms.

Chinese cultural beliefs are influenced by forms of Buddhism, Confucianism, and Taoism, but it should be noted that many persons in China do not claim any religion or say that they are atheists. The majority of historical influence in religion and culture comes from Confucianism. Confucianism stresses accommodation and avoids confrontation; it heavily influences health beliefs and practices. Confucianism follows a naturalistic perspective, defining health and illness as a balance between the individual and the world around the individual. Individuals are a component of the universe, and it is believed that the individual should strive to be in harmony with the universe in which he or she lives. The basic concept of Chinese medicine is that all things, including the body, are composed of opposing forces called yin and yang. Health is said to depend on the balance of these forces. Chinese medicine focuses on maintaining the yin–yang balance to maintain health and prevent illness. If the balance between yin and yang is broken, it is essential to restore this balance to bring about health. To regain balance, the belief is that the balance between the internal body organs and the external elements of earth, fire, water, wood, and metal must be adjusted.

Treatment to regain balance may involve the following (Xu & Chang, 2004):

> Acupuncture
> Moxibustion (the burning of herbal leaves on or near the body)
> Cupping (the use of warmed glass jars to create suction on certain points of the body)
> Massage
> Herbal remedies
> Movement and concentration exercises (such as Tai Chi)

Some elderly Chinese patients may forgo life-sustaining treatment because of the principle of *ren*. Ren is considered the golden rule of Chinese decision making, and is embodied in Confucius's axiom, "Do not do to others what you do not want done to yourself" (Hsiung & Ferrans, 2007, p. 135).

Two nursing studies of health promotion interventions to prevent breast and cervical cancer among Asian Americans confirm that nurses need to modify interventions for subgroups of Asian Americans, because the strongest correlations were within the specific subgroups of Chinese, Filipino, Korean, Japanese, or *Vietnamese* decent; however, there were no correlations with Asian Americans when lumped together in a single group (Kim, Ashing-Giwa, Singer, & Tejero, 2006; Lee-Lin & Menon, 2005). These studies show how important it is to not lump together people who may look alike to the European American, when the differences among diverse Asian cultures may be even greater than the differences between European American culture and all Asian cultures.

Native Americans

There are about 500 different *Native American* tribes within the United States, and nearly half of these 2.4 million people reside in the western part of the country due to forced migration. The two predominant tribes are the Cherokee and the Navajo, each with more than a quarter million people (Spector, 2009). *American Indians* did not immigrate to the United States; therefore, the process of acculturation does not apply. In fact, many American Indians' culture is insulated from the rest of the country, either literally (by way of land reservation) or in other ways, such as linguistically. For example, the majority of Navajo people speak both English and Navajo, but many speak Navajo alone and require an interpreter when interacting with someone who does not speak Navajo (Hanley, 2004).

CLINICAL TIP

Native Americans often have a closed, close-knit community. Nurses working with Native American groups will need to earn their trust. The help of a key informant (or key person within the tribe) is often required.

Like other cultures throughout the world, Native Americans follow a naturalistic approach to health and illness, believing that health is a balance of the mind, body, and spirit, and illness occurs when there is an imbalance or disharmony with nature (Abbott, 2010). Native American religion is centered on legends of sacred spirits that take many forms, some human and some animal. Native American health beliefs and practices are blended with religion, thus carrying a magic facet as well as holistic and naturalistic approaches (Hanley, 2004).

Native Americans have a shorter lifespan than other groups, with an average lifespan of 72.3 years (Abbott, 2010). Their health disparities include alcoholism, diabetes, tuberculosis, homicide, and suicide. The prevalence of these conditions among Native Americans point to the lack of effective programs to reduce alcohol consumption among those Native American individuals who are at high risk of alcoholism. There continues to be a pressing need for culturally sensitive interventions to address major health problems in Native Americans. Poor glycemic control is considered a risk factor for diabetes and heart disease. In a review of cardiovascular research in Native Americans, Eschiti (2005) found only one study, conducted by nurses; the existing research of other disciplines relies on only a few tribes of the more than 500 tribes in the United States; and very little intervention research. Eschiti recommended that studies focus on the establishment of trust with providers as well as those working in governmental agencies by involving tribal members in all aspects of program design, implementation, and evaluation. Miller and Clements (2006) also call for active partnerships between healthcare providers and tribal communities to identify the extent of elder abuse and effective treatment measures that are sensitive and responsive to tribal cultures and conditions in order to assist Native Americans in their desire to care for and honor their elders.

English Language Proficiency

According to the Migration Policy Institute (Pandya, Batalova, & McHugh, 2011), the number of *Limited English Proficiency* (LEP) persons is steadily increasing (see **Table 22-5**) as the number of foreign-born immigrants increases. In 1990, 6.1% of the total U.S. population had LEP; in 2000, the LEP share was 8.1%; and in 2010, the number has grown to 8.7%. The highest states in the country with LEP individuals were California (27%) and Texas (13.3%).

TABLE 22-5   English Proficiency According to the U.S. Census Bureau, American Community Survey (2010)

- Speak only English 79.4%
- Speak language other than English 20.6%
- Speak English "very well" 11.9%
- Speak English less than "very well" (LEP) 8.7%

Data from U.S. Census Bureau. (2010). American Community Survey.

In the Hispanic population, English is not spoken in 12% of Puerto Rican homes, 14% of Mexican American, 15% of other Hispanic, and 33% of Cuban homes. Between 28% and 54% of Hispanics are linguistically isolated (Mutchler and Brailler, 1999). The top 10 languages spoken by LEP individuals in 2010 were Spanish (65%), Chinese (6.1%), Vietnamese (3.3%), Korean (2.5%), Tagalog (1.9%), Russian (1.7%), French Creole and Arabic (1.3% each), and Portuguese, Portuguese Creole, or African languages (1.1% each).

In order to meet the needs of immigrants with LEP, policies have been put into place for *translation* services for all patients at the bedside. Healthcare organizations have an obligation to provide LEP patients, and patients with disabilities, with a meaningful access to care through effective communication free of charge. It is important to note that is **not** appropriate to ask a family member, especially a child, to interpret your healthcare activities. Asking a nontrained interpreter can lead to risk management issues and litigation. The U.S. Department of Health and Human Services Office for Civil Rights considers inadequate *interpretation* as a form of discrimination.

There are four different types of translation services, as follows:

1. *In-person interpreters:* Each facility should have trained interpreters in languages that are common to their demographic area. Typically, trained interpreters complete 45 hours of training in order to be certified.
2. *Sign language interpreters:* For those who are deaf or hard of hearing utilizing American Sign Language (ASL).
3. *Over the phone interpretation:* For this type of service, the nurse would call a toll-free number, give the facility identification number, state which language is needed, and then be connected via phone to the interpreter.
4. *MARTI (my accessible real-time trusted interpreter) video remote interpretation:* For deaf, hard of hearing, and over 150 languages. The television monitor provides an on-screen interpreter (see **Figure 22-2**) (for more information, visit http://www.languageaccessnetwork.com).

Culture and Nursing Care History

The *Transcultural* Nursing Society (TCNS) was organized in 1974 (see **Figure 22-3**) and has as its mission to enhance the "quality of culturally congruent, competent, and equitable care that results in improved health and wellbeing for people worldwide" (Transcultural Nursing Society, 2016, p. 1). The Society has developed standards for cultural competence in nursing practice as seen in **Box 22-1**.

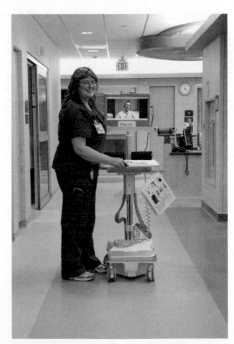

Figure 22-2 Technological advances such as MARTI may assist when interpretation/translation is needed.
Courtesy of Bryan Health

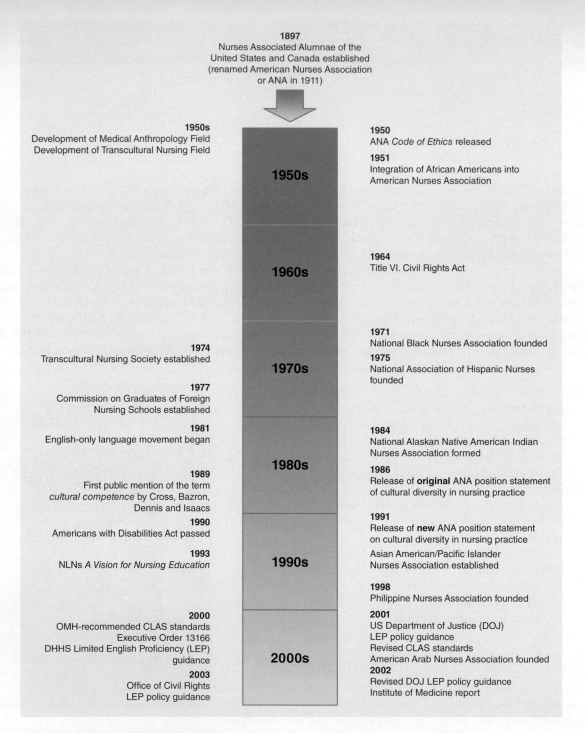

Figure 22-3 Transcultural nursing.
Reproduced from Office of Minority Health, U.S. Department of Health & Human Services.

BOX 22-1   Standards for Cultural Competence in Nursing

Standard 1. Social Justice

Standard 2. Critical Reflection

Standard 3. Knowledge of Cultures

Standard 4. Culturally Competent Practice

Standard 5. Cultural Competence in Healthcare Systems and Organizations

Standard 6. Patient Advocacy and Empowerment

Standard 7. Multicultural Workforce

Standard 8. Education and Training in Culturally Competent Care

Standard 9. Cross Cultural Communication

Standard 10. Cross Cultural Leadership

Standard 11. Policy Development

Standard 12. Evidence-Based Practice and Research

Data from Douglas, M.K., Pierce, J.U., Rosenkoetter, M., Pacquiao, D., Callister, L.C., Hattar-Pollara, M., Lauderdale, J., Milstead, J., Nardi, D., & Purnell, L. (2011). Standards of practice for culturally competent nursing care: 2011 update. *Journal of Transcultural Nursing, 22*(4), 317–333.

Knowledge of Cultures, Standard No. 3 states, "Nurses shall gain an understanding of the perspectives, traditions, values, practices, and family systems of culturally diverse individuals, families, communities, and populations for whom they care, as well as a knowledge of the complex variables that affect the achievement of health and wellbeing" (Transcultural Nursing Society, 2011, p. 1).

Gerontological nurses need to be culturally aware, which is a dynamic, lifelong learning process. Understanding the process for assessing cultural patterns and factors that influence individual and group differences is critical in preventing overgeneralization and stereotyping. Leininger (1999) believed that all nurses should be *culturally competent*. The following are essential in order to provide culturally competent, evidence-based care for *older adults*, otherwise known as *ethnogeriatrics* (Transcultural Nursing Society, 2011):

A. Awareness of one's personal biases through critical self-reflection
B. Understanding of:
  1. Culturally diverse health-related values, beliefs, and behaviors
  2. Disease incidence, prevalence, or mortality rates
  3. Population-specific treatment outcomes
  4. Individuals, families, communities, and populations for whom they care
C. Skills in working with culturally diverse populations

Assessment of Culture

"The goal of a cultural assessment is to obtain accurate information from the patient that will allow the nurse to formulate a mutually acceptable and culturally relevant treatment plan for each patient problem" (Campinha-Bacote, 2011, para 10). The culturally aware nurse should ensure the assessment tool being utilized has been researched in the cultural population as a reliable and valid instrument (**Box 22-2**). One tool to assess cultural needs was developed by Arthur Kleinman, Leon Eisenberg, and Byron Good (1978). They developed eight questions to recognize and validate patients' conceptions, explanations, and expectations of their own illness experiences, many of which are based on cultural beliefs. This patient illness narrative is also termed the "Explanatory Model of Illness."

The Transcultural Assessment Model developed by Giger and Davidhizar (2002) is a tool to "assess cultural values of patients about health and disease behaviors and their effects" (Karabudak, Tas, & Basbakkal, 2013, p. 342). This model examines six cultural dimensions: Communication, space, social organizations, time, environmental control, and biological variations. By using these categories as a guide, the nurse can gain insight into the specific cultural practices and beliefs of the patient.

BOX 22-2   Questions to Validate Illness Experiences

1. What do you call the problem?
2. What do you think has caused the problem?
3. Why do you think it started when it did?
4. What do you think the sickness does? How does it work?
5. How severe is the sickness? Will it have a short or long course?
6. What kind of treatment do you think you (or your loved one) should receive? What are the most important results you hope to receive from this treatment?
7. What are the chief problems the sickness has caused?
8. What do you fear most about the sickness?
9. What do you want most from your work with me?

Another questionnaire that can be utilized is from the SCAN Health Plan (2012) Website and is aptly called D-I-V-E-R-S-E: A Mnemonic for Patient Encounters. This mnemonic can assist the nursing student in developing a personalized care plan based on aspects of cultural diversity. After it is completed, it should be placed on the patient chart for future reference.

Other tools for cultural assessment have been developed by various authors. Berlin and Fowkes (1982) using the mnemonic, LEARN:

Listen

Explain

Acknowledge

Recommend

Negotiate

Similarly, Levin, Like, and Gottlieb (2000) used the word ETHNIC to cue cultural assessment of:

Explanation

Treatment

Healers

Negotiate

Intervention

Collaboration

Although there are a variety of tools available for cultural assessment, geriatric nurses should choose one that best fits their population and reflects the needs of the older adult within that group.

Developing Cultural Skills

A key strategy for achieving *cultural congruence* and *cultural competence* is to learn about different cultural and religious preferences, customs, and restrictions and then use this knowledge in planning and providing care. This involves developing cultural skill, defined as is "the ability to collect relevant cultural data regarding the patient's presenting problem" (Campinha-Bacote, 2011, para 5). The culturally competent nurse knows how to take data obtained from the patient and use this information to provide culturally sensitive and relevant care.

In the journal *Minority Nurse*, ElGindy (2004) has written guides to meeting the special dietary needs of those of several faiths, including Jewish, Muslim, Hindu, and Buddhist. When an elder is in the hospital or extended care facility, encourage the family to bring in favorite foods from home, unless there are dietary restrictions that prevent this. Encourage the family to eat together. Hostler (1999) found that bringing in food promoted both

> **BOX 22-3**   Aging Elders Specific Cultural Websites
>
> - National Asian Pacific Center on Aging: http://www.napca.org/
> - National Caucus and Center on Black Aged: http://www.ncba-aged.org/
> - National Center for Native Hawaiian Elders: http://manoa.hawaii.edu/hakupuna/
> - National Hispanic Council on Aging: http://www.nhcoa.org/
> - National Indian Council on Aging and Alaska Native Elders: http://nicoa.org/

recovery and family integrity in hospitalized children, and it is likely bringing in food for elders will also promote recovery. Again, remember that food preferences within a cultural group, even within families, vary greatly.

Economic diversity is also great among elders. Some are barely getting by, whereas others are among the wealthiest in society. Ensuring that all have adequate food, shelter, and health care has always been a societal problem. The effects of age also differ. Some 60-year-olds who have lived with chronic illness may be frail and disabled, though the majority of persons at this age are active, productive, and independent. Likewise, 80 year olds are frail, yet a growing number are still active, productive, and independent. The key for nurses is to assess each individual's level of activity, health status, and heritage and plan care accordingly, rather than relying simply on age in planning care.

Another aspect of diversity is in religion and faith practices. Again, the elderly are a very diverse group. Some have practiced only one faith for their entire lives, whereas others may have made many changes in a lifelong spiritual quest. Faith communities provide a great deal of support for some elderly. These communities are active in promoting health for elders and in overcoming health disparities.

Health care for elders is also diverse. Those who are wealthy, well educated, and used to having power have access to the best care. Those who are poor, poorly educated, and used to living on the margins of society suffer from health disparities and often have poor access to care.

Box 22-3 lists Websites that offer more information for aging elders in specific cultures. **Table 22-6** provides general guidelines to promote a better understanding of a cultural group, but remember that the members of a culture are not necessarily homogenous. Always ask the patient/family if you have any questions that pertain to providing culturally congruent care (see **Figure 22-4**).

Spirituality and Religion

When the nurse addresses the client in a *holistic* way, attention needs to be directed to assess the mind, the body, and the spirit (Anderson, 2007). Viewing all three of these components individually and recognizing that they are in dynamic relation with one another is an important responsibility for all nurses, regardless of their nursing role in relation to client care. As with the body and mind, the spirit is recognized to be a universal, intrinsic, and integrated basic human component of the patient's being, transcending socioeconomic status, race, gender, culture, and age (Taylor, 2002). Even though attention to the spirit should occur in the care of all clients, this chapter will focus on the role of the nurse in addressing the needs of the older client.

Spirituality encompasses but is not limited to religiosity (Barnum, 2011; Touhy & Jett, 2014). Spirituality is highly personal, whereas religions involves organizational ties (Barnum, 2011). Our spirit incorporates our sense of identity and our understanding about our place and status in the world (Thompson, 2007). Demonstrations of the spirit are reflective of the individual's perception of quality and meaning of life and can be explicit or implicit in nature. In the literature, spirituality has been associated with a variety of terms (beliefs, faith, morals, values, ethics, standards, symbols, rituals, culture, religion, balance, nature, connectedness, centeredness, homeostasis, mystic, resiliency, transcendence, hope, well-being, God, deity, etc.). Some clients report that their spirituality is fully in the context

TABLE 22-6 Comparison of Cultural Groups

	American Indian	Hispanic and Latino	African American	Native Hawaiian/Pacific Islanders
Abuse incidence and type – if noted (White 77%)(NCEA % of all cases)	0.6% Neglect; financial	10.5%	21.2%	0.7% Spousal and child, ignored
Advance directives	Develop trust relationship before asking	Involve family; Trust physician; Complex	Less likely; God is ultimately in charge	Reluctant
Decision makers	Clan leaders, matriarchs, patriarchs, religious or medicine	Nuclear and extended family, fictive kin (non-relatives), friends, church members	Loved one; fictive kin: long-standing family relationships	*Ohana*: family
Dementia deaths (White 25.4%) (Health, US 2011)	11.4% Rare	15% Lower rates	19.7% Vascular dementia; higher rates	8.9% Guam Parkinsonism dementia (*lytico-bodig*); lower rates
Education (all older adults: 76.5% high school; 20.2% bachelor's or higher)	All ages: 77% high school 13% bachelor's 4.5% advanced degree; doing rather than talking	All ages: 60.9% high school 12.6% bachelor's or higher; Cubans: higher levels	Older adults: 44% high school; 7% bachelor's or higher	All ages: 85.3% high school 49.7% bachelor's or higher
End of Life/Dying	Death natural part of life; home care; family may not visit – spiritually bad for living & dying; death rituals: dressing and positioning body, burning herbs and grasses, funerals and burials	Protect from cancer dx; more likely to use heroic measures; *El Dia de Los Muertos* (Day of Dead) celebrate and honor lives; *dicos* – sayings about God; hospice less likely; die at home	Death rates higher till crossover; reluctant to participate due to mistrust; certain diseases and prognosis withheld	Keep at home; hospice; home care; *Ohana*: family stay at side of sick; *uwe*: death chant, wailing to express grief; money and cards given at funerals

Family system	Extended; mixed tribal heritage; many single-parent homes	Live with children; *familismo*; fictive kin (*compadres*)	Dependant care from children, grandchildren, or fictive kin; many raising grandchildren	Importance of group; multi-generational; value society; revere elders; defer to judgment of adult children; men live alone
Folk lore/folk healers	558 tribes/nations; allopathic medicine, but "healer" used first; chanting to promote healing and remove evil; do not cut hair	Over-the-counter; home remedies; *curanderos* (general practitioners); *yerbistas* (herbalists) *sobadores* (massage); *empacho*: locked bowels	Herb and root doctors; *conjurer*: place a hex or ward off evil; spiritual healers; natural illness—physical cause; occult illness—supernatural forces/evil spirits; spiritual illness—willful violation of sacred beliefs or sin	*Kahuna lapaʻau*: priest heals with medicines; tattoos denote significant achievement in rank; illness is seen as curse; *noni* plant to heal bowel problems and menstrual cramps; *lokani triangle*: physical body, environment, relationships with others, mental and emotional states; *poi*: taro root used for illness; talking about illness hastens death
Functional status	Assess if they have ever performed ADLs first; self-care limitations and health-related mobility problems	More disabilities; dear of admitting one's dependence; report greater activity limitations; needed more help with personal and routine activities, and more used of assistive devices for walking; women appeared to be higher than for men (IHE1)	Higher rates of walking difficulties and higher rates of activity limitation	Higher levels of physical limitation

(continues)

TABLE 22-6 Comparison of Cultural Groups (*continued*)

	American Indian	Hispanic and Latino	African American	Native Hawaiian/Pacific Islanders
Health disparities	Diabetes; heart disease; gallbladder disease; poor survival rates with all types of cancer; low incidence of brain cancer; kidney disease; liver disease: tuberculosis; rheumatoid arthritis; hearing and vision problems	Border medications; complimentary and alternative medicine; heart disease; cancer; cerebrovascular disease; respiratory disease; increased hip fractures specifically in Mexican Americans	Diabetes; prostate cancer; HTN; blindness: specifically glaucoma; John Henryism: making it because of sheer determinism against overwhelming odds	Obesity; diabetes and lower extremity infections; HTN; tuberculosis death; rheumatic fever and heart disease; Women: high rates of HIV; Simoan men: cancer; rehab less likely; *Vog*: respiratory disease from volcano smoke
Historical Events	Indian Self Determination and education Act 1975; Indian Health Service	1910: Mexican revolution; 1940: Mexicans for labor (Cesar Chavez); 1996: welfare reform; Puerto Rico: overcrowding; Cuba: Fidel Castro, Bay of Pigs, Mariel Boatlift	Exploitation: South—legalized discrimination, North—covert discrimination; suspicious of healthcare providers (see Tuskegee Experiment)	Distrust: confiscated land, mistreated; harbor resentment towards Whites
Languages	106 Indian dialects; Indian sign language; LEP	Spanish; LEP	English	English; Hawaiian; Pidgin
Life expectancy (Whites: 78.9 years)	72.6 years	81.3 years; Centenarians by 2050 = 19%	75 years; Shorter "Crossover Phenomenon" (Reversal in average life expectancy after age 80)	68.3 years; Lowest
Long-Term Care	No provision in Indian Health Service; 12 tribally run nursing homes, but are a long distances for most families; social adult day care (ADC) centers	Less likely; Cultural Aversion Hypothesis: myth of aversion to LTC and "they take care of own"	Less likely; remain at home with support of family, church-paid home caregivers; higher over age 85	Half the rate of White elders; last resort

Mental Health	Increased rate of major depression—Indian Depression Scale is highest Apache tribe with 1.5x suicide rate; "bad spirits"	Depression (woman); GDS less valid	Depression usually not treated	Decreased suicide rate; many homeless; drug abuse
Nutrition	Food expression of taking care of people; high fat, high sugar, processed food, corn	*Tapas*: snacks; *sobremesa*: sitting after meal and talking; wine with meals; coffee important with meals: *café con leche* (coffee with milk), *café solo* (coffee without milk), or *café cortado* (coffee with some milk); *churros*: twisted donut sprinkled with sugar or dunked in hot chocolate; large lunch; *arroz*: rice with meals; *chimichangas*: large, deep-fried burritos; spices in food and drinks	"Soul food": during slavery, had to cook with leftovers; okra, collard greens, black-eyed peas and sweet potato; pigs feet, chicken livers, beef neck bones and chitterlings (cleaned pig intestines); fried fish and chicken; corn as cornbread and grits	Rice; *musubi*: Spam, rice, and seaweed wrap; bar-b-que; meats; macaroni salad; soda
Organ transplant need and donations (White: 45% need; 68.2% donors)	Do not desire; ESRD possibly; 1% need; 0.4% donors.	18% need; 13.4% donors: deceased donors; mistrust of the medical profession; religious acceptance concern; perceptions of inequity in the distribution of donated organs; women more likely than men	Largest group in need of transplants: 29%; 14% donors	0.5% need; 0.2% donors; deceased donors

(continues)

TABLE 22-6 Comparison of Cultural Groups (continued)

	American Indian	Hispanic and Latino	African American	Native Hawaiian/Pacific Islanders
Pain	Withstand the pain: survival	Stoic; folk beliefs and non-drug; do not understand scales	Higher pain intensity	Stoic; use massage, relaxation, and prayer
Religion	Indian spiritual beliefs and Christianity	*Espiritismo* (Puerto Rican): belief that good/evil spirits can affect well-being; *santeros* (Cuban faith healers)	Protestant, Catholic, Muslim; Part of life fabric; Church community plays important role	Catholic, LDS, Baptist, Pentacostal; Worship god and goddesses, nature, human spirit; Mana: spiritual essence of protection
Respect	Listening; calmness; slow down; nondirect eye contact; may be guarded; modesty and privacy; obtain permission	Early attention to build rapport; use titles and last name	Titles: Mr/Mrs	Revere elders: *filial piety*; indirect communication; negative not expressed; females: *Aunties*
Utilization of health care (White: 11.7% uninsured)	29.2% uninsured; Indian Health Service; LEP concern; cautious of nontribal health care	30.7% uninsured; LEP concern	20.8% uninsured	17.4% uninsured

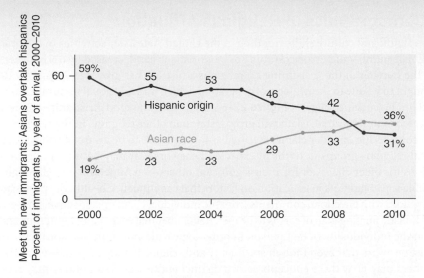

Meet the new immigrants: Asians overtake hispanics
Percent of immigrants, by year of arrival, 2000–2010

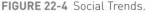

FIGURE 22-4 Social Trends.

Reproduced from Pew Research Center. (2012). The rise of Asian Americans. Washington, DC: Pew Research Center. Retrieved from http://www.pewsocialtrends.org/2012/06/19/the-rise-of-asian-americans/.

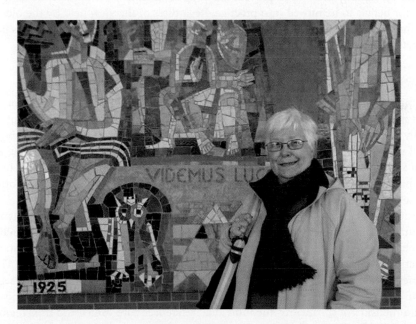

Figure 22-5 Nurses should be sensitive to spiritual and cultural differences among families.

of dogmatic guidelines affiliated with a specific formal religious group. For these clients, the terms *religiosity* and spirituality may appear to be synonymous. However, the nurse must be cautious against stereotyping and accepting the common *myth* that the practices proposed by one religious sect are perceived and practiced the same way by each group member, because complex variations in adherence to religious practices can actually range from excessively strict compliance for some to being lax or even nonexistent for others (Barnum, 2011). For this reason, the nurse should be open and respond in a nonstereotypic manner when questioning religious preference notations in the patient's chart or seeing a religious symbol on the patient's bedside stand (Miller, 2009) (see **Figure 22-5**).

Changing Demographics in Religious Affiliation

Not only are there significant culture shifts trending in the United States, but activities in the practice of religion are also changing. The number of persons claiming to be Christians has decreased by 6% between 2007 and 2014 to 71%, whereas the number of those claiming no religious affiliation has grown to 23% (Pew Research Center, 2016). This is thought to be due to the Millennial generation, which is nearly equal in number to the Baby Boomers, but tend to claim no specific religion. **Figure 22-6** shows that although Christianity will remain the largest religion in the United States, by 2050, Islam will grow faster than other religions in the world.

It is helpful in considering an older client's spirituality for the nurse to be aware of some practices and rituals outlined by formal religious groups in terms of expected behaviors that may have an impact on health and/or healthcare decisions for older clients or for their significant others (see Appendix A). Although such resources can serve as valuable starting points in education on factors that can influence health, the professional nurse must supplement such guides with anecdotal comments from the individual client's perspective if the goal for designing an individualized holistic nursing plan of care is to be met. Remember that each patient is unique and it is the nurse's role to learn about the individuality of that person in order to provide culturally and spiritually competent care.

The nurse must be aware that even though spirituality and religiosity may be perceived as the same by some elderly clients, others may view these concepts as two distinct entities, and still others may report that neither plays any role in their health or their healthcare decision making. This refutes a set of commonly held myths that all people need spirituality as a way to provide meaning for their lives, and that spirituality must be tied to a formal religion for beliefs to be moved into practice. Regardless of the view held by the older client, it is the responsibility of the nurse to take the direction provided by the client and respect that client's point of reference for his or her spirituality.

Three Dimensions of Spirituality

The purpose of this chapter is to explore the dynamic and complex nature of spirituality for consideration in planning holistic nursing care; thus, it is important to consider all dimensions of the concept perceived by the older client. Shelly and Miller, in their book *Called to Care: A Christian Worldview for Nursing* (2006), caution that "the spiritual world is not neutral" (p. 97). By putting this term in full context, the nurse will gain a better understanding of spirituality in view of (1) the client's relationship with himself or herself (intrapersonal), (2) the client's relationship with others (interpersonal), and (3) the client's relationship with another higher entity greater than himself or herself (transpersonal).

In the first spiritual dimension, the focus is on the individual and how that individual feels about and relates to himself as a human being. This first dimension of a person's spirituality consists of uniquely wrapped inner *core values* and beliefs that provide "meanings" that the individual holds to be true and just. It is through the individual's reflection on these "meanings" that the person gains a sense of self and purpose (Thompson, 2007). The nurse is witness to the status of this first dimension in assessing how the client addresses personal needs and cares for "self."

In the second dimension of spirituality, the individual references core values and uses them as standards to guide behaviors and relationships with other people. These contacts can be personal (e.g., the client provides attention and respect to others during conversations with them) or impersonal (e.g., observing how the client chooses to treat property that belongs to someone else). It is the individual alone who decides which standards to apply in dealings with other people.

In the third dimension of spirituality, the view is broadened to focus on the relationship between the individual and a greater entity or power (God, Deity, Allah, Mother-Earth, Nature, etc.), a higher other. Again, tied back to the inner core of the individual's values and beliefs, this third dimension relies strongly on the individual's faith and confidence in self within the context of a "bigger picture" that transcends life on earth as we know it, viewing life purpose in an even larger context (Koenig, 2006).

Projected Change in Global Population

With the exception of Buddhists, all of the major religious groups are expected to increase in number by 2050. But some will not keep pace with global population growth, and, as a result, are expected to make up a smaller percentage of the world's population in 2050 than they did in 2010.

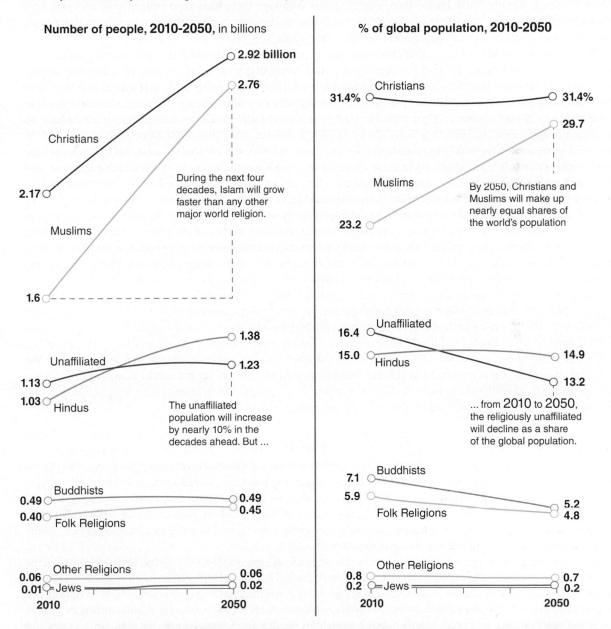

Figure 22-6 Project Change in Global Population.

Reproduced from Pew Research Center. (2015). The future of world religions: Population growth projections, 2010–2050. Washington, DC: Pew Research Center. Retrieved from http://www.pewforum.org/2015/04/02/religious-projections-2010-2050/

The Role of Spirituality for Some Older Clients

Even if one chooses to view spiritual development as universal and lifelong, the process remains unique for each individual (Miller, 2009). The interpretation of the "age factor" in the study of religion and spirituality has proven to be difficult for researchers, who cite the need for more longitudinal research studies on the topic (Atchley, 2009; Carson & Koenig, 2008; Dalby, 2006, Koenig, 2006). Although there have been many hypotheses proposed that address religion in later life (Moberg, 2001), there is no evidence to support the common myth that people become more spiritual and/or religious as they age (Dalby, 2006).

It has been suggested, however, that elders may use their existing spirituality differently in old age than they did in their youth (Krause, 2011). The sociological frame using a type of *continuity theory* is one way to help the nurse understand the relationship some elders have with their spirituality and/or religious practices over time (Moberg, 2001). When spirituality of the older client is viewed within a historic context, the nurse needs to consider the amount of time accrued with advancing age, and the role developmental life experiences have on the normal aging process. With this focus, the nurse recognizes that older clients are more likely to have had (a) more life experiences, especially in relation to different types and intensities of loss (Krause, 2011), (b) more time for introspective reflection in efforts to make meaning of those life experiences in relation to life purpose, and (c) that they most likely had an early life experience with religion and/or spiritually during a period of time in our society where the religious spirit of the individual was highly valued, accepted, and expected (Moberg, 2001).

Individuals who have had success utilizing their spirituality to cope with difficult times in the past are apt to attempt to access these *spiritual resources* when confronted with difficulties in their present (Shannon & Hassler, 2014). Beyond these historic factors, the nurse must understand that the older client's present health/illness status may also influence how the older client implicitly and/or explicitly engages with spirituality. There is a growing amount of evidence that spirituality and health are closely related (Puchalski, 2014). Older clients are likely to attach profound meanings to their illness states (Atchley, 2009), but there is little evidence in the literature to support the myth that elders seek out religious/spiritual supports more often at times of reported loss of control over their health. Even if spiritual resources are not utilized by elders more often during difficult times, Krause (2011) suggests that clients (and their family members) may approach spiritual resources differently as they see the elder move along the *health–illness continuum*—during times of wellness, illness, and at end-of-life. For example, if a client practice is found to have no scientific evidence indicating that it would harm or put the client at risk for harm, then the nurse must demonstrate spiritual competence in remaining open and nonjudgmental toward including that spiritual practice into the client's plan of care (Miller, 2009).

Spirituality and the Nursing Profession

Not only does the profession of nursing have a strong foundation for spiritual care giving (Barnum, 2011; Beckman, Harges, Sorge, & Salmon, 2007), but the essence of nursing practice also has a strong spiritual component not related to doctrine or dogma (Mauk & Schmidt, 2004). The practice of nursing centers on caring for and caring about the holistic well-being of others. In the infancy of our profession, nurse training was tightly linked to religion, as it was provided by members of a religious group who viewed nursing as a "call to service." Many Christian nursing programs view nursing as ministry.

Over the years, the importance of the nurse facilitating a client's *spiritual well-being* has been addressed in the work of many nurse theorists (Nightingale, Henderson, Watson, Neuman, Orem, etc.), as well as many supportive theorists from other disciplines. It has also been suggested that spiritual nursing care is not merely an option, but a responsibility for all nurses (Beckman et al., 2007), with mandates for assessing the client's spirituality noted in both organizational and professional nursing guidelines (health agency/organizational standards, codes and guidelines, professional nursing codes for ethical practice, Joint Commission on Accreditation of Healthcare Standards, nursing care specialty competencies such as those noted in the American Holistic Nurses Association, the Oncology Nursing Society, etc.).

In efforts to maintain a holistic nursing practice and follow mandates to address the spiritual needs of clients, it is essential for the nurse to make time to first assess his or her own personal attitudes, values, and beliefs regarding spirituality. It is only in becoming self-aware of his or her own spirituality that the nurse is able to make a conscious effort to be accepting of other points of view and to work to refrain from the dangers of becoming spiritual-centric in nursing practice (Myers, 2009). In addition to determining how spirituality is incorporated into practice, it is essential to consider how spirituality can assist in building personal strength and resiliency for both the client and the nurse.

Spirituality and the Nursing Process

If the nurse is expected to take an active role in nursing care with older clients, it is essential that he or she assembles accurate, current information and documents all data to present a complete picture of the older client. Although some feel that client spirituality is a personal topic best left for discussions between clients and their chaplains, others report that nurses are in the best position for this conversation with clients at admission and throughout the course of nursing care (O'Brien, 2008).

When nurses employ successful observational and interview techniques with the older client (client-directed communication, developing trust, use of appropriate timing and concern for readiness to share, active listening, providing a comfortable and private setting for discussions, control over resources to maximize vocal and written information in consideration for the normal sensory changes with advancing age, use of valid and reliable assessment tools and documentation formats, etc.) in efforts to obtain client admission information on the status of the body, mind, and spirit, two important messages are relayed to the older client. The first message is that the human spirit is an important part of the client's health, and the second message is that the nurse is available and interested in helping the client work to improve his health status.

Hussey (2009) noted that although spiritual caregiving is individualized, some nursing roles are universal when it comes to caring for older clients (roles of assessor, friend, advocate, caregiver, case manager, and researcher). The nursing role in this process is supported by professional and agency mandates that recognize spirituality as an important component of client care that help to guide best practice for nursing.

Assessment and Nursing Diagnosis

When one considers the dynamic nature of the health–illness continuum (Neuman, 1990), it is easy to see that in addition to obtaining the first *spiritual assessment* upon admission, there is an essential need for the nurse to re-assess the spiritual status of the client at various points during the care experience. As with all other categories of client assessment, it is important that a systematic approach be utilized for conducting the spiritual assessment (Miller, 2009). The literature provides a variety of tools for the nurse to use when conducting a spiritual evaluation of the older client (forms based on care competencies, spiritual inventories, and spiritual assessments), noting that there is no one standardized "best" tool to date that can be used for conducting a spiritual assessment (Eliopoulos, 2013). Admission resources for the nurse should include a set of agency-determined tools for screening and history taking, as well as a form to address the next level, which calls for a more detailed and focused spiritual assessment. Information obtained from the *spiritual baseline assessment* should be placed in the client's record so that a baseline data set for comparison purposes is available whenever a spiritual re-assessment is conducted.

CLINICAL TIP

One simple question to ask patients that introduces the topic of spirituality without being threatening or judgmental is: Where do you see yourself on your spiritual journey?

As a part of the assessment process, it is essential for the nurse be alert to any changes in client behavior that may signal spiritual distress, spiritual risk, or the client's need for a more focused spiritual re-assessment

(Mauk & Schmidt, 2004). Because of this, on-going evaluation is best accomplished by the nurse who has strong client observational and communication skills. A good knowledge base in these areas helps the nurse become aware of subtle client behaviors that can signal early client difficulties: identifying what the older client does and/or says, as well as what he does not do and/or does not say, over the course of daily nurse–client contacts. Chapter 6 provides additional information on conducting a comprehensive assessment of the older adult, including a spiritual component.

To insure a consistent and speedy referral process, it is to everyone's benefit to have a written agency-supported referral procedure in place before any client spiritual screenings or spiritual assessments begin. If the older client can read and is provided an easy-to-understand, large-print form to complete with the nurse as a part of his spiritual assessment, both client and nurse are more apt to complete the form and begin spiritual dialogue. If a form is given to the client to complete independent of the nurse, it is important for the nurse to verify that it was indeed the older client who supplied the information contained in that form (as some family members complete such forms without the client's knowledge).

First-level spiritual screening questions (see **Box 22-4**) can be those where the client provides a yes/no response to a simple set of five close-ended questions asked by the nursing professional. Following client direction (based on responses to these first level questions), the nurse can choose to conduct a second level screening utilizing five open-ended questions aimed at clarifying or expanding this part of the spiritual intake process (see **Box 22-5**).

BOX 22-4   Spiritual Screening Tools Level 1

FIVE **FIRST-LEVEL** SPIRITUAL SCREENING QUESTIONS FOR THE NURSE TO ASK THE OLDER CLIENT:

1. "Do you see yourself as a spiritual person at this time?"
2. "Do you have any spiritual/religious behaviors or practices that are important to you at this time?"
3. "Do you associate with a religious or spiritual community or group at this time?"
4. "Does your spirituality play any role in helping you to understand your health or illness condition(s) at this time?"
5. "Is there anything here that you see would get in the way of having your personal spiritual needs met?"

Modified from Mauk, K., & Schmidt, N. (2004). *Spiritual care in nursing practice* (p. 213). Philadelphia, PA: Lippincott Williams & Wilkins.

BOX 22-5   Spiritual Screening Tools Level 2

FIVE **SECOND-LEVEL** SPIRITUAL SCREENING QUESTIONS FOR THE NURSE TO ASK THE OLDER CLIENT:

1. "One of our jobs to help you while you are here is to keep you comfortable. I am hoping that you can share information about what things are meaningful in your life so I can try to help you access those while you are here with us?"
2. "Life can be difficult at times, and we all cope with our difficulties in different ways. Please tell me what strategies you use to help you to understand and make sense about your current health situation."
3. "If faith is a part of your life, how does your faith fit for you right now?"
4. "Do you feel that your present health situation has created any disturbance in your core values or belief system?"
5. "How are your energy reserves holding up when you consider your health status at the present time?"

Modified from O'Brien, M. (2008). *Spirituality in nursing: Standing on holy ground* (p. 111). Sudbury, MA: Jones & Bartlett Learning.

TABLE 22-7   Example of Data from Spiritual Assessment

Date	No Spiritual Need Identified 0	Identified Spiritual Need Diagnosis	Spiritual Continuum Client Perceived Need Level (low) 1	(medium) 2	(high) 3	Signature
		Loss of spiritual integrity				

Narrative:

SAMPLE SPIRITUAL CONTINUUM ENTRY

Date	No Spiritual Issues Identified 0	Identified Spiritual Issues Diagnosis	Client Perceived Spiritual Continuum Level (low) 1	(medium) 2	(high) 3	Signature
04/23/12		Loss of spiritual integrity		X		Jane Doe, RN

Narrative:

S. "My doctor said he was very hopeful that the stem cell treatment would help put me in remission. I prayed hard for the last few months that this would buy me a little more time so I can hold on to see my son one more time. Today I found out that there has been no change in my bloodwork levels as I had hoped, and the doctor said there is little more he can do but keep me comfortable. He said that he is confused by my lack of progress. I don't blame him but do feel that God is no longer listening to my prayers. so I will be alone at the end. I have been a faithful and religious person all my life, but this lack of progress is really wearing down my faith."

O. Labwork on 04/23/12 post–stem cell treatment shows continued deterioration of client's health state. Physician put client on palliative list today after talking with him about his active cancer status. Rates physical pain level at 2 (scale 0–10) and spiritual integrity need at 2 (scale 0–3).
Refused to see pastor at regularly scheduled visit this afternoon.

A. Client reports loss of spiritual integrity at level 2 during spiritual assessment today.

P. Reassess client needs when wife arrives during afternoon shift, later this evening. Contact hospital chaplain with current spiritual assessment results. Provide active listening with client during dressing change this evening and then reassess for planning using spiritual continuum form.

The client's response to two sets of screening questions will inform the nurse if questions for a spiritual history need to be obtained and/or if a more detailed and focused spiritual assessment needs to be completed for the client's chart.

Data obtained from the spiritual assessment process can be placed in a large-print spiritual continuum form, which will support on-going communication between the nurse and the older client for re-assessments of spiritual status over time (see **Table 22-7**). This continuum form has a quantifiable score card determined by the older client with a range from zero to three. A perceived score of zero represents that the older client either does not identify with spirituality or perceive any spiritual need at that assessment point in time. If a spiritual need is expressed by the older client, the need is identified and reported to the nurse, who works with the client in determining an appropriate nursing diagnosis for its communication to other members of the client's health team (see **Case Study 22-1**).

Case Study 22-1

Seventy-year-old Mr. Hutt has attended the local Presbyterian church regularly since he was 14 years old. He has maintained his spiritual strength through his religious participation over the years, and has worked his way up to church elder. When admitted he said that one of his proudest accomplishments is that he and his wife raised four sons who actively practice their Presbyterian faith.

When he was admitted after a stroke to the long-term-care (LTC) facility 6 months ago, he noted on his initial spiritual assessment form that "attending Sunday services was most important to him," ranking that as his no. 1 "personal strength factor." Together, he and his wife have regularly attended Sunday services at the LTC chapel, until a couple of months ago. It was at that time that Mr. Hutt told his wife that she should go to the services alone because he was just too tired and would rather read his Bible alone in his room at that time. This Sunday you are assigned to work on Mr. Hutt's LTC wing. You acknowledged Mr. Hutt's wife before she entered the chapel for Sunday service, and she told you Mr. Hutt wanted to stay in his room again today. She said that she has tried everything to get him to join her at Sunday again, but he refuses. When you go in to see Mr. Hutt later in the day, he tells you "I thought we had a merciful God, but He hasn't shown me much mercy in the last couple months. It has been 6 months since my stroke, and I expected to be out of here by now. I guess I probably have to do more suffering yet for all the bad things I have done in my lifetime—that is, if He is even listening to my prayers anymore."

Questions:

1. What would be your nursing diagnosis for Mr. Hutt at this time?
2. What signs and symptoms provide the evidence to support your diagnosis?
3. What would be the goal you would identify with Mr. Hutt to improve his present state?
4. What spiritual care intervention options are available for the nurse to assist Mr. Hutt at this time?
5. What other words and/or behaviors would be important for the nurse to be alert to when working with Mr. Hutt?
6. What would be the nurse's response if Mr. Hutt refuses to participate in any activities intended to assist in his spiritual recovery?
7. What nonverbal behaviors by the nurse would communicate a nonjudgmental response to Mr. Hutt's vocal expressions of despair?
8. Should the nurse work to incorporate Mrs. Hutt in activities intended for improving Mr. Hutt's spiritual status? What might be some positive factors for involving her? What might be some negative factors if she were involved?
9. What other contributing factors (besides the slower than expected stroke progress) may be affecting Mr. Hutt's spirituality strength?

After identification of the spiritual need via the documented nursing diagnosis, the client determines the level of need at that time, using a scale of 1 to 3 (1 identifying a low spiritual need level, 2 identifying a medium spiritual need level, or 3, which recognizes a high spiritual need level). By reviewing this large-print continuum form with the older client over the course of his stay, the nurse can seek clarification from the client directly as to his status over time, as well as identify any emerging needs that can be addressed early in the process. The goal for the older client who values spirituality is that his spirit will serve as an inner resource to provide hope and faith in times of need while giving an inner serenity and resilience to promote health (Wold, 2012).

It is important to consider putting nursing interventions in place to help support older clients who are "*spiritually thriving*" at assessment (spiritual continuum score of 0), as well as for those who report they are in spiritual need (spiritual continuum score of 1, 2, or 3). Determining the level of a spiritual need is based upon the client's perception, but would be reflected in the client who reports that he is unable to forgive himself or others for perceived failures. He may also report or demonstrate a low spiritual reserve or a low self-esteem and feelings of being immobilized, apathetic, hopeless, worthless, depressed, or a bother to others—all disturbances that can threaten his meanings of life (Atchley, 2009). Early case finding may result in an "at risk" nursing diagnosis for losing spiritual integrity, with these older clients expressing guilt, fear, anxiety, or frustration directly related to their spiritual self.

Planning

Once the initial assessment and diagnosis segments of the nursing process are completed, the nurse works with the older client (and a significant other of the elder's choosing if indicated) to begin a plan intended to shift the client toward the "spiritually thriving" category on the spirituality continuum. In addition to providing a list of the older client's strengths and needs, at that point, spiritual resource building can serve to empower the older client in decision making if he is able. If it is determined that the older client has limited capacity at this time, a significant other (family member, client advocate, etc.) may assist the nurse in the planning process if the client allows for such.

It is important in this phase of the nursing care plan that spiritual resource banks (activity ideas, support agencies and Websites, spirituality tools, "people" contacts, etc.) be identified and individualized. The nurse needs to work with the client (or his representative) on his care planning by incorporating his desired practices as long as there is evidence to support that these would not put the client at a health risk. In addition to incorporating this written plan as a part of the client's formal record, providing start and reevaluation dates next to each activity and linking each with the name of the responsible planning team member will foster good communication among all those who have a vested interest in the health of the older client.

Nursing Interventions

Nursing interventions are as unique as the individuals receiving and providing them (Carson & Koenig, 2008). In the planning process, the client may report a desire to use environmental supports (e.g., time out of the facility to sit outside in nature) to strengthen his or her inner spiritual core. With the guidance of the older client (or his or her planning representative), nurse interventions could include a variety of activities to assist the client to gain a better sense of self in this first dimension of spirituality (use of music, sounds of nature, journaling, aroma therapy, painting, deep breathing exercises, hygiene care, visit from a barber or hairdresser, quiet time, pictures or symbols that have spiritual meaning for the older client, prayer, animal therapy, meditation, humor therapy, guided imagery exercises, deep breathing activities, exercise therapy, etc.).

To focus on the second dimension of spirituality (relationship with others), the nurse may wish to consider interventions that include scheduling visits with the older client's family and friends in ways that would strengthen energy levels. If there are few or no visitors for the older client, with client approval the nurse can make a referral to a volunteer or friendly visitor program. If the client is able, the nurse may suggest that the older client considers participation in group activities in which clients are able to share their feelings with others in similar life situations (common, shared practices as a part of spiritual caregiving). In addition, the nurse may choose to provide a personal spiritual care strategy by scheduling a 10-minute visit with the older client in which the nurse could utilize therapeutic communication skills (e.g., active listening, nonverbal tools of appropriate touch, and silence) to support a "connectedness" that can help provide feelings of worth and value for the withdrawn or isolated elder (Touhy & Jett, 2014).

Efforts to strengthen the third dimension of spirituality for the older client start with the nurse's demonstrated respect for the client and the client' values, beliefs, and privacy. Nursing interventions to support this dimension can be achieved by gaining contact (through nurse referrals) with the client's preferred spiritual advisor/coach if one is identified. This procedural example of spiritual care by the nurse refers out the patient contact but keeps the nurse actively involved through support of such visits by scheduling daily routines. The nurse can help maintain these contacts through indirect involvement with mailings, television, telephone, radio or emailing services.

The nurse also can suggest some supplemental options via referrals to a social worker, parish nurse, activity director, or pastoral care service group at the client's agency of choice. This culturalistic type of nursing intervention incorporates what the nurse knows of the client's spiritual history, taking client direction and finding adaptations for the environment or an activity to fit the client situation (e.g., arranging for a client's reactivation into prayer contacts/groups, arranging wheelchair Tai Chi sessions for a man who no longer can attend his stand up Tai Chi program, etc.). This type of spiritual nursing care can provide a renewed spiritual energy for the older client, providing greater reflection of him or her in a larger life context (Koenig, 2006).

Evaluation

Evaluation is the nursing action that sets the stage for ongoing reassessment (formative evaluation) through a review of both goal achievement and the client plan of care (Mauk & Schmidt, 2004). As with all interventions aimed at strengthening the mind, body, or spirit of the older client, it is important for the nurse to work closely with the client to monitor the impact of the intervention strategies employed. This process requires a focus on both the desired outcomes (summative evaluation) from the plan as well as the unexpected outcomes that occurred with the process. By incorporating the use of the spiritual continuum grid as a part of the ongoing evaluation process, the client and nurse can share a visual display of spiritual progress or regression over time. Including the older client (or his representative) as a member of the planning team reinforces client empowerment in selected care decisions, which in itself can work to strengthen the older client's spiritual core (Moberg, 2001).

Summary

If the nurse is to practice in a holistic way with older clients, it is important to recognize that a complete client picture must be obtained through the careful utilization of nursing assessments. Although culture (see **Box 22-6**) and spirituality have different meanings for members in our society, it is reflective of the individual client's core values and beliefs and therefore can play an important role in health and healthcare decision making for our healthcare clients. For this reason, the professional nurse must recognize the value of conducting cultural assessments, spiritual screening, spiritual health histories, and focused spiritual assessments for all clients in the nurse's care, identifying spiritual strengths and planning with the client to meet any spiritual needs that have an impact on health. **Boxes 22-7** and **22-8** provide additional resources for nurses seeking to incorporate cultural and spiritual awareness into their practice.

BOX 22-6   Research Highlight

Gunn and Davis examined cultural practices and the use of healing plants among elderly African American women in the rural south. The researchers aimed to use what they learned to help practitioners provide culturally competent care to this population. Sign into your database of nursing literature (CINAHL or PubMed, for example) and use the citation below to perform a search for this article. What did this research team find?

Gunn, J., & Davis, S. (2011). Beliefs, meanings, and practices of healing with botanicals recalled by elder African American women in the Mississippi Delta. *Online Journal of Cultural Competence in Nursing and Healthcare, 1*(1), 37–49.

BOX 22-7   Recommended Readings

Artifacts of Cultural Change Tool:
http://paculturechangecoalition.org/Resources
/Articles/Cms%20-%20Culture%20Change%20
Artifact%20Tool%20Explanation.Pdf

Stages of Change:
http://www.context.org/iclib/ic09/gilman1/

Culture of Medicine:

Taylor, J. S. (2003). Confronting "culture" in
medicine's "culture of no culture." *Academic
Medicine, 78*(6), 555–559. Retrieved from
http://journals.lww.com/academicmedicine
/Fulltext/2003/06000/Confronting__Culture__in
_Medicine_s__Culture_of_No.3.aspx

Stuart, B., Cherry. C., & Stuart, J. (2011).
Pocket guide to culturally sensitive health care.
Philadelphia, PA: FA Davis.

Yeo, G. (2000). Ethnogeriatrics: Overview,
Introduction. In V. S. Periyakoil (Ed.),
eCampus-Geriatrics [online]. Stanford, CA: Author.
Retrieved from
https://geriatrics.stanford.edu/wp-content
/uploads/2016/08/ethnogeriatric_introduction.pdf

BOX 22-8   Websites

Center for Minority Veterans:
http://www.va.gov/centerforminorityveterans

Center for Spirituality and Aging:
 http://www.spiritualityandaging.org

Cultural Competence Project:
http://www.ojccnh.org/project/index.shtml

Culturally Competent Nursing Care: A
Cornerstone for Caring:
 https://ccnm.thinkculturalhealth.hhs.gov/

Developing Nurses Cultural Competencies,
Train-the-Trainer program:
https://www.ncbi.nlm.nih.gov/pmc/articles
/PMC2690913/
DiversityRX: http://www.diversityrx.org

John Hartford Institute for Geriatric Nursing
(HIGN) Assessment of Spirituality in Older
Adults—FICA Spiritual History Tool:
https://consultgeri.org/try-this/specialty-practice
/issue-sp5

Standards for Accreditation Programs (n.d.).
Spiritual assessment:
http://www.jointcommission.org
/AccrediationPrograms/HomeCare/Standards

Madeleine Leininger, Transcultural nursing
and leader in transcultural nursing education,
administration, and practice:
http://www.madeleine-leininger.com/en/index
.shtml

Medical Anthropology:
http://www.medanthro.net

Network of Multicultural Aging:
http://www.asaging.org/noma/

Online Journal of Cultural Competence:
http://www.ojccnh.org/

Quality Improvement in our Nation's Nursing
Homes:
http://www.cms.gov/Medicare
/Provider-Enrollment-and-Certification
/CertificationandComplianc/Downloads/2012
-Nursing-Home-Action-Plan.pdf

Registry of Interpreters for the Deaf:
http://rid.org/

Stanford School of Medicine, ecampus Geriatrics,
Health and Healthcare of Multi-Cultural Older
Adults:
https://geriatrics.stanford.edu/ethnomed.html

National Adult Protective Services Association:
http://www.napsa-now.org/

Transcultural Care Associates:
http://www.transculturalcare.net/

Transcultural Nursing Society:
http://www.tcns.org

Transitions of Care:
https://www.jointcommission.org/assets/1/18/
Hot_Topics_Transitions_of_Care.pdf

Clinical Reasoning Exercises

1. Explore one of the common cultural groups served in your area. Discuss your findings with another student nurse in your clinical groups. How is this culture different from your own?

2. Interview *your* family. What is your family background, nationality, and religion? How does your family's heritage affect health practices for health maintenance, health protection, and health restoration? What year did your family first come to America? Share with the class.

3. Utilizing the Transcultural Nursing Society's Standards of Practice for Culturally Competent Nursing Care—Standard 3, do one of the following:

    a. Generate and/or provide staff education modules on the general principles of culturally competent care.

    b. Generate and/or provide staff education modules focusing on increasing specific knowledge of the most common cultural groups served.

    c. As a group of student nurses on a clinical unit or in a clinical agency, establish journal clubs/staff in-service sessions to review current literature about the most common cultural groups served to ensure evidence-based practice (EBP).

    d. As a group of student nurses on a clinical unit or in a clinical agency, generate monthly cultural awareness activities for you and your colleagues that promote cultural competence (i.e., culturally diverse speakers, media, ethnic food).

    e. As a student nurse working with colleagues and a science librarian (if available), gain information literacy skills in order to access electronic sources to gain current knowledge of cultures and cultural assessment tools (diversity Websites, cross-cultural health care case studies) as well as multimedia sources and professional webinars.

Personal Reflections

1. What role does spirituality play in your life?

2. It is important that nurses assess spirituality for themselves before they can be successful assessing this domain with their clients. Think about your answers to each of the following questions:
    - How would I describe my spirituality?
    - How would I describe the dynamic interaction of my physical, social, mental, and spiritual selves?
    - What formal and informal organizations have helped me develop my spirituality over time?
    - What factors have contributed to my "spiritual" status today?
    - How much do I value my own spirituality?
    - How much do I value the spirituality of others?
    - How comfortable am I speaking about the topic of spirituality with others? What resources can I use to assist in helping me discuss spirituality with others?
    - What role does my spiritual self-play in my professional practice of nursing?
    - What behaviors do I utilize to strengthen my spiritual reserve?
    - What tools do I utilize to measure my spiritual strength?

3. As the nurse, what would you do or say to the following older adult clients? On what factors do you base your response?

1. Client asks to hold your hand and pray aloud with him before he goes down for surgery.
2. Client's nutritionist from home provides a smelly bark tea for the client to drink each evening in the hospital. The tea was approved by the client's physician; however, storage is a problem because of its bad smell in the kitchen on the floor.
3. Native American client asks if he can have his traditional healer "smudge" his patient room. Because smudging involves burning sage, cedar, and other herbs in the room, you are unsure if this can be done in the hospital setting.
4. Catholic client asks to keep his rosary pinned to his hospital gown while on the floor.
5. Client asks to switch bed positions in the two-patient room so that he can face east instead of staying in his assigned bed that faces west.
6. The client is due for gallstone removal and asks if she can keep the gallstones that are retrieved from her surgery to make a set of "worry beads" to help in her meditation practice.

References

Abbott, K. (2010). Culture, values, and beliefs affecting native american health. Retrieved from http://www.augie .edu/pub/aas/AAS_KarlaAbbott_NativeAmericanHealth_2010-03-24.pdf

Agency for Healthcare Research and Quality. (2016). Chartbook on health care for blacks. Content last reviewed June 2016. Retrieved from http://www.ahrq.gov/research/findings/nhqrdr/chartbooks/blackhealth/index.htm

American Geriatrics Society. (2009). Retrieved from http://www.americangeriatrics.org/files/documents/2009 _Guideline.pdf

Anderson, M. (2007). *Caring for older adults holistically* (4th ed.). Philadelphia, PA: F.A. Davis.

Atchley, R. (2009). *Spirituality and aging.* Baltimore, MD: The John Hopkins Press.

Barnum, B. S. (2011). *Spirituality in nursing: The challenges of complexity.* New York, NY: Springer.

Beckman, S., Harges, S., Sorge, C., & Salmon, B. (2007). Five strategies that heighten nurses' awareness of spirituality to impact client care. *Holistic Nursing Practice, 21*(3), 135–139.

Berlin, E., & Fowkes, W. (1982). A teaching framework for cross-cultural health care. *The Western Journal of Medicine, 139*(6), 934–938.

Calvillo, E., Clark, L., Ballantyne, J. E., Pacquiao, D., Purnell, L. D., & Villarruel, A. M. (2009). Cultural competency in baccalaureate nursing education. *Journal of Transcultural Nursing, 20*(2), 137–145.

Campinha-Bacote, J. (2011). Delivering patient-centered care in the midst of a cultural conflict: The role of cultural competence. *OJIN: The Online Journal of Issues in Nursing, 16*(2), Manuscript 5.

Carson, V., & Koenig, H. (Eds.). (2008). *Spiritual dimensions of nursing practice.* Conshohocken, PA: Templeton Foundation Press.

Centers for Disease Control and Prevention. (2011). CDC Health Disparities and Inequalities Report, United States, 2011. Retrieved from http://www.cdc.gov/mmwr/pdf/other/su6001.pdf

Centers for Disease Control and Prevention, National Center for Health Statistics. (n.d.). National Health Interview Survey. Atlanta, GA: Author.

Crespo, C. J., & Arbesman, J. (2003). Obesity in the United States: A worrisome epidemic. *Physician and Sports Medicine, 31*(11), 23–28.

Cultural Competence Project. (2012). *Online Journal of Cultural Competence in Nursing.* Retrieved from http:// www.ojccnh.org/project/about.shtml

Dalby, P. (2006). Is there a process of spiritual change or development associated with aging? A critical review of the research. *Aging & Mental Health, 10*(1), 4–12.

Douglas, M.K., Pierce, J.U., Rosenkoetter, M., Pacquiao, D., Callister, L.C., Hattar-Pollara, M., Lauderdale, J., Milstead, J., Nardi, D., & Purnell, L. (2011). Standards of practice for culturally competent nursing care: 2011 update. *Journal of Transcultural Nursing, 22*(4), 317–333.

Eap, S., DeGarmo, D. S., Kawakami, A., Hara, S. N., Hall, G. C. N., & Teten, A. L. (2008). Culture and personality among European American and Asian American Men. *Journal of Cross-Cultural Psychology, 39*(5), 630–643.

ElGindy, G. (2004, Fall). We are what we eat: Cultural competence and dietary needs. *Minority Nurse,* 54–55.

Eliopoulos, C. (2013). Spirituality. In *C. Eliopoulos' gerontological nursing* (8th ed., pp. 150–158). Philadelphia, PA: Lippincott-Raven.

Eschiti, V. S. (2005). Cardiovascular disease research in Native Americans. *Journal of Cardiovascular Nursing, 20*(3), 155–161.

Gibson, C. J., & Lennon, E. (1999). *Historical census statistics on the foreign-born population of the United States: 1850 to 1990.* U.S. Bureau of the Census, Working Paper No. 29. Washington, DC: US Government Printing Office. Retrieved from https://www.census.gov/population/www/documentation/twps0029/twps0029.html

Giger, J. N., & Davidhizar, R. (2002). The Giger and Davidhizar Transcultural Assessment Model. *Journal of Transcultural Nursing, 13*(3), 185–188, discussion 200, 201.

Giger, J. N., & Davidhizar, R. E. (2004). *Transcultural nursing assessment and intervention* (4th ed.). St. Louis, MO: Mosby.

Giger, J., Davidhizar, R. E., Purnell, L., Harden, J. T., Phillips, J., & Strickland, O. (2007). American Academy of Nursing expert panel report: Developing cultural competence to eliminate disparities in ethnic minorities and other vulnerable populations. *Journal of Transcultural Nursing, 17,* 95–102.

Gonzalez, T., & Kuipers, J. (2004). Hispanic-Americans. In J. N. Giger & R. E. Davidhizar (Eds.), *Transcultural nursing assessment and intervention* (4th ed., pp. 221–253). St. Louis, MO: Mosby.

Gunn, J., & Davis, S. (2011). Beliefs, meanings, and practices of healing with botanicals recalled by elder African American women in the Mississippi Delta. *Online Journal of Cultural Competence in Nursing and Healthcare, 1*(1), 37–49

Hanley, C. (2004). Navajos. In J. N. Giger & R. E. Davidhizar (Eds.), *Transcultural nursing assessment and intervention* (4th ed., pp. 255–277). St. Louis, MO: Mosby.

Healthy People 2020. (2012). About Healthy People 2020. Retrieved from http://healthypeople.gov/2020/

Holt, C. L., Wang, M. Q., Clark, E. M., Williams, B. R., & Schulz, E. (2013). Religious involvement and physical and emotional functioning among African Americans: The mediating role of religious support. *Psychology & Health, 28*(3), 267–283.

Hostler, S. L. (1999). Pediatric family-centered rehabilitation. *Journal of Head Trauma Rehabilitation, 14*(4), 384–351.

Hsiung, Y., & Ferrans, C. (2007). Recognizing Chinese Americans cultural needs in making end-of-life treatment decisions. *Journal of Hospice and Palliative Nursing, 9*(3), 132–140.

Hussey, T. (2009). Nursing and spirituality. *Nursing Philosophy, 10*(2), 71–80.

Institute of Medicine (2003). *Health professions education: A bridge to quality.* Washington, DC: National Academies Press. Retrieved from https://www.nap.edu/read/10681/chapter/1

Karabudak, S., Tas, F., & Basbakkal, Z. (2013). Giger and Davidhizar's Transcultural Assessment Model: A case study in Turkey. *Health Sciences Journal, 7*(3), 342–345.

Kelley, L. S., Small, C. C., & Tripp-Reimer, T. (2004). Appalachians. In J. N. Giger & R. E. Davidhizar (Eds.), *Transcultural nursing assessment and intervention* (4th ed., pp. 279–299). St. Louis, MO: Mosby.

Kim, J., Ashing-Giwa, K. T., Singer, M. K., & Tejero, J. S. (2006). Breast cancer among Asian-Americans: Is acculturation related to health-related quality of life? *Oncology Nursing Forum, 33*(6), E90–E99.

Kleinman, A., Eisenberg, L., & Good, B. (1978). Culture, illness and care. *Annals of Internal Medicine, 88*(2), 251–258.

Koenig, H. (2006). Religion, spirituality and aging. *Aging and Mental Health, 10*(1), 1–3.

Krause, N. (2011). Age stereotypes. In K. W. Schaie & S. L. Willis (Eds.), *Handbook of the psychology of aging* (7th ed., pp. 249–262). San Diego, CA: Elsevier.

Lee-Lin , F., & Menon, U. (2005). Breast and cervical cancer screening practices and interventions among Chinese, Japanese, and Vietnamese Americans. *Oncology Nursing Forum, 32*(5), 995–1003.

Leininger, M. (1999). What is transcultural nursing and culturally competent care? *Journal of Transcultural Nursing, 13*(3), 189–192.

Levin, S., Like, R., & Gottlieb, J. (2000). *ETHNIC: A framework for culturally competent clinical practice.* New Brunswick, NJ: Department of Family Medicine, UMDNJ-Robert Wood Johnson Medical School.

Loeb, S. J. (2006). African-American older adults coping with chronic health conditions. *Journal of Transcultural Nursing, 17*(2), 139–147.

Mauk, K., & Schmidt, N. (2004). *Spiritual care in nursing practice.* Philadelphia, PA: Lippincott Williams & Wilkins.

Migration Policy Institute. (2011). Immigrant profiles. Retrieved from http://www.migrationpolicy.org/topics /immigrant-profiles-demographics

Miller, C. (2009). *Nursing for wellness in older adults* (5th ed.). Philadelphia, PA: Lippincott Williams & Wilkins.

Miller, R. I., & Clements, P. T. (2006). Fresh tears over old griefs: Expanding the forensic nursing research agenda with Native American elders. *Journal of Forensic Nursing, 2*(3), 147–153.

Moberg, D. (Ed.). (2001). *Aging and spirituality: Spiritual dimensions of aging theory, research, practice and policy.* New York, NY: Haworth Pastoral Press.

Moody-Ayers, S. Y., Stewart, A. L., Covinsky, K. E., & Inouye, S. K. (2005). Prevalence and correlates of perceived societal racism in older African-American adults with type 2 diabetes mellitus. *Journal of the American Geriatrics Society, 53*(12), 2202–2208.

Mutchler, J. E., & Brailler, S. (1999). English language proficiency among older adults in the United States. *The Gerontologist, 39*(3), 310–319.

Myers, J. (2009). Spiritual calling. *Nursing Standard, 23*(40), 22.

National Center for Health Statistics. (2012). *Health, United States 2011: With special feature on socioeconomic status and health.* Hyattsville, MD: Centers for Disease Control and Prevention. Retrieved from http://www .cdc.gov/nchs/data/hus/hus11.pdf#024

Neuman, B. (1990). Health as a continuum based on the Neuman Systems Model. *Nursing Science Quarterly, 3*(2), 129.

Njoku, M. G. C., Jason, L. A., & Torres-Harding, S. R. (2005). The relationships among coping styles and fatigue in an ethnically diverse sample. *Ethnicity and Health, 10*(4), 263–278.

O'Brien, M. (2008). *Spirituality in nursing: Standing on holy ground* (3rd ed.). Sudbury, MA: Jones & Bartlett Learning.

Padilla, Y. C., & Villalobos, G. (2007). Cultural responses to health among Hispanic American women and their families. *Family and Community Health, 30*(18), S24–S33.

Pandya, C., Batalova, J., & McHugh, M. (2011). *Limiting English proficient individuals in the United States: Number, share, growth, and linguistic diversity.* Washington, DC: Migration Policy Institute. Retrieved from http://www .migrationpolicy.org/research/limited-english-proficient-individuals-united-states-number-share-growth-and-linguistic

Passel, J. S., & Cohn, D. (2008). U.S. population projections 2005–2050. Pew Research Center. Retrieved from http://pewhispanic.org/files/reports/85.pdf

Pew Research Center. (2016). 10 Demographic trends that are shaping the US and the world. Retrieved from http:// www.pewresearch.org/fact-tank/2016/03/31/10-demographic-trends-that-are-shaping-the-u-s-and-the-world/

Puchalski, C. M. (2014). The FICA Spiritual history tool #274. *Journal of Palliative Medicine, 17*(1), 105–106.

SCAN Health Plan. (2012). D-I-V-E-R-S-E: A mnemonic for patient encounters. Retrieved from http://www .scanhealthplan.com/provider-tools/benefits-resources/multi-cultural-resources/communication/diverse/?

Shannon, M. P., & Hassler, L. J. (2014). Culture and spirituality. In K. L. Mauk, *Gerontological nursing: Competencies for care* (pp. 735–791). Sudbury, MA: Jones & Bartlett Learning.

Shelly, J. A., & Miller, A. B. (2006). *Called to care: A Christian worldview for nursing* (2nd ed., Rev. and expanded). Downers Grove, IL: IVP Academic/InterVarsity Press.

Spector, R. (2009). *Cultural diversity in health and illness* (7th ed.). Upper Saddle River, NJ: Prentice Hall.

Supple, A. J., & Small, S. A. (2006). The influence of parental support, knowledge, and authoritative parenting on Hmong and European American adolescent development. *Journal of Family Issues, 27*(9), 1214–1232.

Taylor, E. (2002). *Spiritual care: Nursing theory, research and practice.* Upper Saddle River, NJ: Prentice Hall.

Thompson, S. (2007). Spirituality and old age. *Illness, Crisis, & Loss, 15*(2), 167–178.

Touhy, T., & Jett, K. (2014). *Ebersole & Hess's toward healthy aging: Human needs and nursing response* (7th ed.). St. Louis, MO: Mosby.

Transcultural Nursing Society. (2011). Standards of practice. Retrieved from http://www.tcns.org/TCNStandardsofPractice.html

Transcultural Nursing Society. (2016). Transcultural nursing. Retrieved from http://www.tcns.org

U.S. Department of Homeland Security. (2011). *Yearbook of immigration statistics: 2011.* Retrieved from http://www.dhs.gov/files/statistics/publications/LPR11.shtm

Walker, R. L., Lester, D., & Joe, S. (2006). Lay theories of suicide: An examination of culturally relevant suicide beliefs and attributions among African Americans and European Americans. *Journal of Black Psychology, 32*(3), 320–334.

Wallace M. W. J., Weiner. J. S., Pekmezaris, R., Almendral, A., Cosiquien, R., Auerbach, C., & Whittemore, R. (2007). Culturally competent interventions for Hispanic adults with type 2 diabetes: A systematic review. *Journal of Transcultural Nursing, 18*(2), 157–166.

Wold, G. (2012). *Basic geriatric nursing* (5th ed.). St. Louis, MO: Mosby.

Wolf-Klein, G. (2007). Physician cultural sensitivity in African American advance planning: A pilot study. *Journal of Palliative Care, 10*(3), 721–727.

Xu, J. Q., Kochanek, K. D., Murphy, S. L., & Tejada-Vera B. (2010). *Deaths: Final data for 2007.* National vital statistics reports (Vol. 58, No. 19). Hyattsville, MD: National Center for Health Statistics.

Xu, Y., & Chang, K. (2004). Chinese Americans. In J. N. Giger & R. E. Davidhizar (Eds.), *Transcultural nursing assessment and intervention* (4th ed., pp. 407–427). St. Louis, MO: Mosby.

Yeo, G. (2000). Ethnogeriatrics: Overview, introduction. In V. S. Periyakoil (Ed.), *eCampus-Geriatrics* [online]. Stanford, CA: Author. Retrieved from https://geriatrics.stanford.edu/wp-content/uploads/2016/08/ethnogeriatric_introduction.pdf

Appendix A

Baha'i

Abortion	Forbidden
Artificial insemination	No specific dictate
Autopsy	Acceptable if medical or legal need
Birth control	Individual can choose best family planning method
Blood and blood products	No restrictions
Diet	Alcohol and drugs forbidden
Euthanasia	Destruction of life not allowed
Healing beliefs	Harmony between religion and science
Healing practices	Pray
Medications	No vaccine restrictions; medications acceptable with prescriptions
Organ donations	No restrictions
Right-to-die issues	Forbidden
Surgical procedures	No restrictions
Visitors	Community members assist and support

Buddhist Churches of America	
Abortion	Dependent on condition of patient
Artificial insemination	Acceptable
Autopsy	Individual choice
Birth control	Individual choice
Blood and blood products	Acceptable
Diet	Restricted food combinations
Euthanasia	Allowed
Healing beliefs	Do not believe in healing through faith
Healing practices	No restrictions
Medications	No vaccine or any medication restrictions
Organ donations	Considered act of mercy; all means can be taken if hope for recovery
Right-to-die issues	With hope, all means encouraged
Surgical procedures	Acceptable except for extremes
Visitors	Family and community assist and support
Roman Catholics	
Abortion	Prohibited
Artificial insemination	Illicit, even between husband and wife
Autopsy	Permissible
Birth control	Natural rhythm method is only option acceptable
Blood and blood products	Permissible
Diet	No restrictions except during Lenten season before Easter (holy week fast and abstain from meat)
Euthanasia	Direct life-ending procedures prohibited
Healing beliefs	Many within religious belief system
Healing practices	Sacrament and anointing of the sick/dying, use of candles and religious articles, laying of hands
Medications	No vaccine restrictions; medications may be taken if benefit outweighs risks
Organ donations	Acceptable
Right-to-die issues	Obligation to take ordinary (but not extraordinary) means to prolong life
Surgical procedures	Acceptable except for abortion and sterilization
Visitors	Family, friends, priest, deacons, lay ministers assist and support

(*continues*)

Appendix A   (*continued*)

Christian Science

Abortion	Incompatible with faith
Artificial insemination	Unusual
Autopsy	Unusual but family can decide to do so
Birth control	Individual choice
Blood and blood products	Ordinarily not used
Diet	Generally no restrictions except abstain from alcohol and tobacco and some abstain from tea and coffee
Euthanasia	Forbidden
Healing beliefs	Looks at physical and moral healing
Healing practices	Full-time healing ministers, active practice of spiritual healing
Medications	No vaccine restrictions that comply with laws; no medication restrictions
Organ donations	Individual choice
Right-to-die issues	Unlikely to seek medical help to prolong life
Surgical procedures	No medical ones practiced
Visitors	Family, friends, Christian Science community and healers, Christian Science nurses assist and support

Church of Jesus Christ of Latter Day Saints

Abortion	Forbidden
Artificial insemination	Acceptable between husband and wife

Church of Jesus Christ of Latter Day Saints

Autopsy	Permitted with consent by next of kin
Birth control	Forbidden
Blood and blood products	No restrictions
Diet	Alcohol, tea (except herbal), coffee, and tobacco are forbidden; fasting (24 hours without food or drink) is required once a month
Euthanasia	Forbidden
Healing beliefs	Power of God can bring healing
Healing practices	Anointing with oils, sealing, prayer, and laying-on of hands
Medications	No restrictions for vaccines, prescribed medications, or folk medicine use
Organ donations	Permitted
Right-to-die issues	If death is inevitable, promote a peaceful and dignified death
Surgical procedures	Individual choice
Visitors	Family, friends, Church members (especially Elder & Sister), and the Relief Society assist and support

Hinduism	
Abortion	No policy
Artificial insemination	No restrictions
Autopsy	Acceptable
Birth control	All types are acceptable
Blood and blood products	Acceptable
Diet	Eating of meat is forbidden
Euthanasia	Forbidden
Healing beliefs	Some believe in faith healing
Healing practices	Traditional faith healing system
Medications	Vaccines and all medication uses are acceptable
Organ donations	Acceptable
Right-to-die issues	No restrictions as death is viewed as one step toward nirvana
Surgical procedures	With an amputation, view is that this happened due to sins from an earlier life
Visitors	Family, friends, and priest assist and support
Islam	
Abortion	Acceptable
Artificial insemination	Permitted between husband and wife
Autopsy	Permitted for medical and legal purposes
Birth control	Acceptable
Blood and blood products	No restrictions
Diet	Alcohol and pork prohibited
Euthanasia	Forbidden
Healing beliefs	Faith healing is generally not acceptable
Healing practices	Some use herbal remedies and faith healing
Medications	Vaccines and all prescribed and folk medicines are acceptable
Organ donations	Acceptable
Right-to-die issues	Attempts to shorten life is prohibited
Surgical procedures	Most permitted
Visitors	Family and friends assist and support

(continues)

Appendix A (*continued*)

Jehovah's Witnesses	
Abortion	Forbidden
Artificial insemination	Forbidden
Autopsy	Acceptable if required by law
Birth control	Sterilization forbidden but all other methods are of the individual's choice
Blood and blood products	Forbidden
Diet	Abstain from tobacco; moderate use of alcohol accepted
Euthanasia	Forbidden
Healing beliefs	Faith healing is forbidden
Healing practices	Use of scriptures to comfort and lead to spiritual and mental healing
Medications	Vaccines and all other medications not derived from blood products are accepted
Organ donations	Forbidden
Right-to-die issues	Individual choice
Surgical procedures	Not opposed but administration of blood strictly prohibited
Visitors	Family and friends assist and support; congregation members and Elders pray for the sick person
Judaism	
Abortion	Therapeutic permitted by all groups; some groups accept abortion on demand
Artificial insemination	Permitted
Autopsy	Permitted under certain circumstances; all body parts must be buried together
Birth control	Permitted for all groups except Orthodox Jews
Blood and blood products	Acceptable
Diet	Variability among groups, when kosher rules followed, milk and meat products cannot be mixed or served on the same plates; predatory fowl and shellfish, as well as all pork products, are forbidden; many will request only kosher products
Euthanasia	Prohibited
Healing beliefs	Medical care is an expectation
Healing practices	Prayers for the sick
Medications	Vaccines and all medications are accepted
Organ donations	Complex issue; some groups do accept this based on situation
Right-to-die issues	Right to die with dignity; if death inevitable, no new procedures but continue with present ones

Surgical procedures	Most allowed
Visitors	Family, friends, rabbi, and many community members and services to assist and support

Mennonite

Abortion	Therapeutic is acceptable
Artificial insemination	Individual conscience for husband and wife
Autopsy	Acceptable
Birth control	Acceptable
Blood and blood products	Acceptable
Diet	No restrictions
Euthanasia	Not condoned
Healing beliefs	Part of God's work
Healing practices	Prayers and anointing with oils
Medications	Vaccines and all other medications allowed
Organ donations	No restrictions
Right-to-die issues	Forbidden as "life must continue at all costs"
Surgical procedures	No restrictions
Visitors	Family, friends, and community assist and support

Seventh-day Adventists

Abortion	Therapeutic is acceptable
Artificial insemination	Acceptable between husband and wife
Autopsy	Acceptable
Birth control	Individual choice
Blood and blood products	No restrictions
Diet	Vegetarian diet is encouraged
Euthanasia	Not practiced
Healing beliefs	Divine healing
Healing practices	Prayers and anointing with oils; opposes use of hypnotism
Medications	Vaccines and all medications are acceptable
Organ donations	Acceptable
Right-to-die issues	Follow the ethic of prolonging life
Surgical procedures	No restrictions
Visitors	Pastor and elders pray and anoint the sick person; because there is a SDA world-wide health system of both hospitals and clinics, some clients will seek care only from these facilities

(continues)

Appendix A   (*continued*)

Unitarian/Universalist Church	
Abortion	Acceptable
Artificial insemination	Acceptable
Autopsy	Recommended
Birth control	Acceptable
Blood and blood products	No restrictions
Diet	No restrictions
Euthanasia	Favor nonaction; acceptable to withdraw treatment if death imminent
Healing beliefs	Sees faith healing as superstitious
Healing practices	Use of science to facilitate healing
Medications	No restrictions
Organ donations	Acceptable
Right-to-die issues	Favor the right to die with dignity
Surgical procedures	No restrictions
Visitors	Family, friends, and church members assist and support

Modified from Spector, R. (2009). Selected religion responses to health events. In *Cultural diversity in health and illness* (7th ed., pp. 120–125). Upper Saddle River, NJ: Prentice Hall.

For a full suite of assignments and additional learning activities, see the access code at the front of your book.

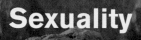

CHAPTER 23

Sexuality

Donald D. Kautz
Elizabeth R. Van Horn

(Competencies 8, 18)

This chapter addresses sexual issues in providing holistic nursing care for older adults. A basic human need of people of all ages is intimacy with others. Loneliness, loss, and lack of meaningful social relationships have been addressed in other chapters in this text. This chapter is designed to assist the nurse in enhancing romantic intimacy and sexual function in older adults. Individuals over 50 are a very diverse group, especially related to romantic intimacy and sexual expression; therefore, a variety of strategies may be helpful in addressing their unique needs.

Despite decades of research showing that older adults want to discuss intimacy and sexual concerns (Mola, 2015; Minkin, 2016), these needs continue to be ignored or inadequately addressed by healthcare professionals, for several reasons. Often sex is not seen as a priority for either the patient or the provider, and sexual concerns have not traditionally been addressed in healthcare encounters. As nurses, we rarely see any consequences to not addressing sexual concerns. One reason for this is that *sexuality* is seen as separate from healthcare issues, rather than integral to quality of life. Anxiety and fear of embarrassment prevent patients and nurses from addressing sexual concerns. Further, nurses may fear that they may not have the expert knowledge or resources to assist patients to overcome sexual problems.

Despite these barriers, most sexual concerns that result from aging or chronic health problems are within the realm of nursing practice (Mola, 2015; Song et al., 2011; Steinke et al, 2013). By failing to address the underlying health issues that lead to sexual problems, nurses may contribute to a patient's ongoing sexual dysfunction. For example, urge or stress incontinence in women may lead to vaginal infections and *dyspareunia*, or painful intercourse; in addition, the woman or her partner may be inhibited by any unpleasant odors associated with the condition (Garrett & Tomlin, 2015). Hospital nurses should routinely ask about this type of incontinence when a patient is admitted, especially for women over 50, to address this common problem and any related sexual concerns.

Other conditions, including acute respiratory infections, abdominal surgery, and mobility limitations following surgery, also may lead to temporary urge or stress incontinence; therefore, nurses should educate patients about this possibility and treat or refer those with problems. For example, sending a patient home with a long-term indwelling Foley catheter will certainly interfere with sexual intercourse. Teaching a woman to tape the catheter to her abdomen and wear a t-shirt to prevent the catheter from rubbing during intercourse or to wear crotchless underwear are effective and safe strategies to keep the catheter out of the way and intact. Men with an indwelling catheter can fold the catheter back over an erect penis and then apply a condom. Partners report not being able to feel the catheter during intercourse, and ejaculation will occur unimpeded around the catheter. Both of these techniques have been recommended for decades, and they are not thought to increase the chances of urinary tract infection (Rye & Murphy, 2015). Nurses can teach clients who are discharged with catheters these effective and safe techniques for maintaining sexual function.

CLINICAL TIP

Reassure older patients with urinary catheters that this does not prohibit them from having sexual intercourse with their partner. Teaching in this area is essential.

In addition to addressing existing health conditions, most health promotion strategies have the potential to have a positive impact on sexual relationships and sexual function. Smoking cessation, limiting fat in the diet, losing weight, and exercising all may reverse the sexual changes that occur as a result of aging (Mola, 2015; Santoro, 2015). Helping patients understand that heightened intimacy and regained sexual function may result from these lifestyle changes may be important motivators for them to make the changes needed.

Romantic Relationships in the Elderly

Elders differ greatly in their romantic relationships. Some older adults have been in the same romantic relationship for 50 years and have developed a profoundly deep relationship. (See **Box 23-1**, in which Tim, an 81-year-old man, and Teresa, a 79-year-old woman, discuss how they feel about their 50-year relationship.) In contrast, some people become involved in a romantic relationship for the first time after retiring. Research on social relationships in older adults supports that many are actively seeking partners and using technology as an aid. Davis and Fingerman (2015), studied over 4,000 dating profiles from online dating websites of adults aged 18 to over 90.

BOX 23-1 Tim and Teresa

Tim (81): "I think she feels about me just about the same way I feel about her. I'm sure I come first in her life, and I'm sure she's first in my life. It's always been that way. She was the girl that I wanted. I got her and I still want her. Both of us try to please each other. One of the most important things in a marriage is a connection. That if you do [have a connection] show your relationship in love and with expressions of love. We say it every day, two or three times. I love you."

Teresa (79): "I couldn't live without him. I like to know where he is every minute. I like to touch him, I like him by me in bed. I like him. I just like him. Tim married for keeps and so did I. We're always together, and most of the time either holding hands or he has his arm around me or I have my hand on his knee. And there's not just one, it's not just Teresa, and it's not just Tim, its Teresa and Tim."

Reproduced from Kautz, D. D. (1995). The maturing of sexual intimacy in chronically ill, older adult couples. (Doctoral dissertation, University of Kentucky). *Dissertation Abstracts International* (UMI Order #PUZ9527436), p. 55.

Many over the age of 60 years, and some in their 90s, were seeking partners. The study also found that older adults are more positive in their profiles, focus less on "self" and focus more on connectedness and relationships to others than younger adults.

Diversity abounds in older adults' sexual and social relationships. Some older adults have been married many times and others not at all. Some have had dozens of partners over their lifetime; others have had only a few, or one, and still others none. Some were nuns and priests or celibate for other reasons, who then gave up being celibate in order to be in a romantic relationship. Others became nuns or priests or otherwise became celibate after being married when younger. May–December relationships also occur, and an older adult may have a partner who is 30 or even 40 years younger.

As in all populations, diversity in sexual orientation also occurs in older adults. Some older adults have been gay or straight their entire lives; others are bisexual and were in gay or lesbian relationships when younger, then later married and had children. The opposite is true as well. Nurses need to remain nonjudgmental of those who are transgender or questioning their gender. There is ample evidence that lesbian, gay, bisexual, and transgender (LGBT) individuals experience discrimination from healthcare providers (American Geriatrics Society [AGS], 2015). AGS has published a position statement to address their vision of care of (LGBT) older adults and specific steps to be taken to ensure they receive the care they need.

As a society, we continually strive to come to terms with the diversity of romantic relationships. As nurses, remaining nonjudgmental will ensure that our care includes and is respectful of those who are most important to our patients, regardless of whether we believe their romantic relationships to be healthy or morally or politically correct. Indeed, excluding a patient's loved ones during illness may potentiate complications or hasten death, whereas including them can promote recovery. Even though gay marriage is now legal in all 50 states, straight couples and gay couples may not pursue legal marriage due to family, personal, or social constraints. When assessing family status, nurses should ask, "Whom should I call?" rather than asking specifically about marital status. Unfortunately, those who are most important to our patients may stay away out of fear or unease when the partner is admitted to a healthcare facility. Nurses have a unique opportunity to be welcoming to those individuals our patients love.

The loss of one's romantic partner is common for older adults, through divorce or death. However, the sexual loss is overlooked by most of society. Research on grieving rarely addresses how people adjust to the loss of sex after losing a lifelong romantic partner and what we as health professionals can do to assist them in coping with and overcoming their loss. Of course, not all experience grief; the last years of a long-term relationship may have been sexless due to physical issues or problems in the relationship. Nevertheless, nurses need to assess for the loss of intimacy and sex, acknowledge the loss, and listen to our patients as they express emotions of grief.

Sexual Development in Older Adults

Contrary to other forms of development, adults continue to develop sexually throughout their lives. Chronic illnesses have the potential to affect sexual function, and those who are older who continue to have sex have to adapt to many changes. Many adults who are now over 65 were raised not to talk about sex, and they may not talk with their partners about their sexual desires or preferences. They may see this silence as a way of protecting their partner, even though the silence results in loss of intimacy.

The oldest among us have lived through several sexual revolutions. The first was in the roaring 20s, when women gained the right to vote and with it a great deal of sexual freedom. The second came shortly after World War II, when Kinsey published *Sexuality in the Human Male* in 1948 and *Sexuality in the Human Female* in 1952. The third was in the 1960s and early 1970s, with the advent of the birth control pill and legalization of abortion. A fourth revolution occurred with the discovery of the human immunodeficiency virus (HIV), which led to the promotion of safe sex and the use of condoms (see **Box 23-2**). Some might argue that another sexual revolution is occurring now for older adults due to the advent of better treatments for *erectile dysfunction* (ED) and vaginal dryness.

BOX 23-2   Research on Older Adults with Human Immunodeficiency Virus Infection

- People over 50 account for 30% of the people living with HIV, largely due to the success of anti-HIV drugs (highly active antiretroviral therapy [HAART]), which increase the quality of life and life expectancy of those with HIV.
- Heterosexual sex is the dominant mode of HIV transmission in older adults.
- African American and Hispanic women report higher levels of risk-taking behaviors.
- The poor make up a disproportionate number of those with HIV.
- Elders may not reveal risky behaviors that are socially unacceptable.
- Depression is undertreated in older adults with HIV infection.
- Comorbid conditions (heart disease, arthritis, hypertension, diabetes), normal aging, and age-related changes in drug absorption and distribution may increase adverse drug reactions, drug interactions, and mortality among those with HIV.

Nursing strategies:
- Identify those at risk and provide referrals, social support, and educational materials.
- Target HIV prevention efforts to older adults.
- Increase public education to reduce HIV stigma, homophobia, and ageism in health care.
- Promote more qualitative and quantitative research on elders and HIV.

Data from Center for Disease Control and Prevention. (2015). HIV surveillance report, 2014. Vol 26. Retrieved from http://www.cdc.gov/hiv/library/reports/surveillance/.

Triphasic Human Response and Changes with Aging

Kaplan (1990), building on early work by Masters and Johnson, identified a *triphasic model of human sexual response*. The three phases are desire, excitement, and orgasm. The desire phase includes the sensations that move one to seek sexual pleasure. Sexual desire is probably stimulated by endorphins; pleasure centers are stimulated by sex, whereas pain inhibits sexual desire. Love is a powerful stimulus to sexual desire. The second phase, sexual excitement, primarily occurs due to myotonia, or increased muscle tone, and vasodilation of the genital blood vessels. In men, the penis becomes erect; in women, the vagina becomes lubricated, the clitoris and vagina become longer and wider, and the labia minora extend outward. Sexual excitement is controlled by the sympathetic nervous system, and fear will inhibit sexual excitement. The orgasm phase is a climactic release of the genital vasodilation and myotonia of the excitement phase. Orgasm is an automatic spinal reflex response. Typically sexual problems can be classified as desire, excitement, or orgasm phase disorders, or combinations of the three.

Changes in sexual response have for decades been considered normal consequences of aging. Desire may or may not change with aging; levels of desire may remain the same throughout life (see **Box 23-3**). However, both men and women experience changes in excitement with age. Achieving an erection may require more direct stimulation and take longer, and the erection may be softer. Ejaculation may not be as forceful and may not occur with every sexual encounter. Vaginal lubrication is often decreased, and women find the need for more direct stimulation. Orgasms for women include uterine contractions, and changes in the uterus may change the way an orgasm feels.

Elders differ greatly in their response to these changes. Some couples adapt by increased genital fondling and caressing, taking more time, and paying more attention to each other's needs. In this way, sex may be better than when they were younger. Other couples may welcome an end to sex. Still others may transcend the need for sex and actually become closer.

If an elder abstains from sex for months to years when in a sexless relationship or due to loss of a sexual partner, desire will eventually decrease. This loss of sexual desire has been thought to be permanent; however, anecdotal reports suggest that when a person who has not been involved in a sexual relationship for many years meets a new partner, desire will return. In these cases, some individuals regain erectile function and vaginal lubrication after several weeks of manual or oral genital stimulation. Still others may seek help from their healthcare provider for medical treatment to improve sexual function (Minkin, 2016).

Vaginal Dryness and Erectile Dysfunction (ED)

The decreased ability of a man to achieve and maintain an erection and the decreased ability for a woman to achieve vaginal lubrication have, for decades, been considered normal consequences of aging (Katsiki, Wierzbicki, & Mikhailidis, 2015). As with most changes associated with aging, changes in sexual function may begin as early as age 40 and occur in almost every adult by age 80. The English Longitudinal Study of Ageing (ELSA) conducted by Lee and colleagues (2016) studied 6,201 individuals 50 to 90 years of age and found that 31% of men in the 80 to 90 age bracket still have sex and masturbate and 60% of men ages 70 to 80 have sex or masturbate. The numbers are lower in women, with 14% of women between 80 and 90 and 34% between 70 and 80 regularly engaging in sex or masturbation. Of the women and men who were sexually active, 32% of women reported difficulty becoming sexually aroused and 27% reported difficulty achieving orgasm. Of the men, 39% reported ED. These findings are similar to those in earlier studies in the United States. Yet some have estimated that less than 50% of men and women seek treatment for sexual issues, due to embarrassment or because they are not bothered by the problems; in addition, many do not discuss the issue with their partners (Barnett, Robleda-Gomez, & Pachana, 2012).

BOX 23-3   Harry and Alice Kautz

Harry (1920–2009) and Alice (1920–2008) were classmates in high school in the rural town of Custer, South Dakota, where they both graduated in 1938. Alice held various jobs and during WWII moved to Denver, where she became a nurse. She married Morris Lang and had three children while living in rural Colorado, until Morris died of cancer in May, 1957. Harry worked his way through engineering school at the School of Mines in South Dakota and remained a bachelor while working in a variety of engineering jobs in Florida, New York, West Virginia, Michigan, and Colorado. When Alice's brother told Harry that his old classmate and friend, Alice, was a widow, they began to correspond. After a courtship of only a few months, in December 1957, Harry married Alice, taking on a ready-made family with three small children. When they married, both were 37 years old, devoted to their family, and enjoyed camping and other outdoor activities.

When their son Don got married in 1983, Harry's advice was, "To be successful in marriage, it is important to show your love, every day, whether you are feeling that love or not."

After Harry retired in his early 60s and they moved to Sun City, Arizona, Harry began to drink every day. Alice said that his interest in sex waned. However, they still were very active socially together, especially through their church and social clubs.

When they were 75, Alice told her son Don that at 75, life was better than ever. They had moved into a new condo in the retirement community, where they were both very active. She said "All of my clothes fit" and "Harry had quit drinking and has a renewed interest in sex." They continued to be active in their church, where Alice adopted the nickname "Bad Alice" because she was a constant flirt.

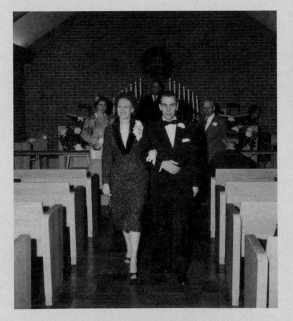

Alice and Harry's wedding in 1957 when they were both 37 years old

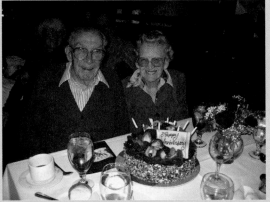

Harry and Alice in 2007 celebrating their 50th wedding anniversary when they were both 87 years old

Due to health problems in their mid-80s, Harry and Alice moved into an independent living community, where they celebrated their 50th wedding anniversary in December 2007.

Shortly after their 50th anniversary, Alice was diagnosed with metastatic breast cancer. In the last months, Alice was cared for by hospice. Because of his dementia, the hospice nurse asked Harry who Alice was. He responded, "That's my Alice." When asked who she was to him, he responded, "She is the world to me." Alice died at home, with Harry by her side. The hospice nurse, who was there for her death, said that Harry's goodbye to Alice after she died was very tender. Harry was moved to an Alzheimer's unit, where he died the next year.

ED and vaginal dryness are also associated with diabetes, heart disease, hypertension, and arthritis (Mola, 2015, Santoro, 2015). Current recommendations for the therapeutic management of ED and vaginal dryness include stopping smoking; limiting drinking alcohol to moderate amounts; increasing exercise; and reducing obesity, especially abdominal fat. Physiologically, smoking, obesity, and a sedentary lifestyle increase atherosclerosis in genital blood vessels, and evidence supports that these lifestyle changes aid in reversing this process. Vaginal dryness in women is the physiologic correlate of ED in men, and thus it is possible that the same illnesses and lifestyle habits may be correlated with vaginal dryness.

The introduction of sildenafil (Viagra) in 1998, followed by vardenafil (Levitra), tadalafil (Cialis), and avanafil (Stendra), have changed the norms for sexual dysfunction. The constant barrage of ads in print media, on television, and through the Internet imply that ED is common, almost expected, and the norm is to seek treatment. Twenty years ago, ED and vaginal dryness may have been a private matter for a couple; however, it is now literally impossible for couples to escape these ads, which has led to what some call the "Viagra revolution," "Viagra Mindset," or biomedicalization of sex (Gledhill & Schweitzer, 2014). These marketing campaigns pressure men and women who otherwise might not have considered treatment or not thought the problem was important, to seek treatment. The audience for these ads is plentiful, because an estimated 61% of men over 70 years of age report ED and 61% of men age 40 to 69 have ED, yet 72% have never received treatment (Wagle et al., 2012). There are also ads for nutritional supplements and natural remedies for ED.

Other treatments for ED include axillary applied external testosterone (Axiron), testosterone pellet implants (Testopel), ED vacuums, alprostadil penile injections (Caverject) or intraurethral suppositories (Muse), penile implants, or vascular reconstruction surgery (Katsiki et al., 2015). Men and their partners who want to effectively treat ED are encouraged to go to their healthcare provider together, discuss the options, and then work together to integrate the treatments into their sexual activities.

Vaginal dryness is a common problem in postmenopausal women due to changes in estrogen levels and does not improve without treatment (Santoro, 2015). Current treatments for vaginal dryness include oral estrogen hormone therapy, skin patches, topical creams, gels and sprays, and vaginal estrogen therapy. Specific vaginal treatments include a vaginal estrogen ring (Estring), a soft flexible ring inserted into the vagina and replaced every 3 months, vaginal estrogen tablets (Vagifem) inserted regularly into the vagina with a disposable applicator, and vaginal estrogen cream (Estrace, Premarin) inserted with an applicator into the vagina regularly (Santoro, 2015). Although there are no medications for women that are direct corollaries of Viagra, Levitra, Cialis, and Stendra, multiple ads target women regarding treatments to relieve vaginal dryness and increase sexual desire with hormonal medications and nutritional or natural supplements.

The use of a sexual lubricant can effectively aid with both ED and vaginal dryness (Palacios, Mejie, & Neyro, 2015). A variety of types of lubricants are commonly available at most larger chain drug stores. Lubricants can be purchased in single-use packets, bottles, or pump dispensers that facilitate use if impaired hand function or paraparesis interferes with opening packets or bottles. Many websites provide information on the types and brands of lubricants.

Although studies have examined the effectiveness of Viagra in improving both erectile function and quality of life in men, little is known about couples' experiences with these medications. Men receive the prescription for Viagra, but it is possible that women may be the ones taking the medication. Researchers have studied the effectiveness of Viagra in women (Barnett et al., 2012) and found it is effective in relieving vaginal dryness. However, most women with vaginal dryness also have a decrease in sexual desire, and for this Viagra is not helpful. It is also unclear whether couples use lubricants during intercourse to help the man achieve an erection through stimulation or to assist the woman to overcome vaginal dryness. Finally, the differences in views and experiences of men and women are unknown. Most studies of Viagra have examined only the men taking it, not their partners. Barnett and colleagues (2012) point out that "Viagra is the little blue pill with big repercussions" (p. 84). Some women may encourage their husbands to take Viagra, others may find it a "bother," and still others may experience several detrimental effects, including unwanted changes in their sexual relationship, tension, communication difficulties, fears of infidelity, and, in some cases, vaginal trauma. The authors point out that nurses and physicians need to ask women if their partners take Viagra, and if so, do they have any concerns or need treatment for vaginal dryness.

CLINICAL TIP

Any male beginning Viagra for the first time should be seen by an eye doctor to rule out factors associated with blindness that may occur in some men who use this product.

Clinical literature has long recommended that maintaining a healthy lifestyle will lead to more satisfying sexual relationships. Many reputable websites, maintained by healthcare organizations and providers, including the Mayo Clinic and Dr. Dean Ornish, and self-help groups such as the Diabetes and Heart Associations, advocate healthy behaviors as a first step in overcoming problems with erections and vaginal dryness. Books such as *Sex After 60: Tips for Enjoying a Healthy and Happy Sex Life Into Your 60s* (Viljoen, 2012) and *Sex in the Golden Years: The Best Sex Ever* (Billett & Seiden, 2008) recommend aerobic exercise, a low-fat diet, and stopping smoking as ways to improve sexual performance for both men and women. Nurses can focus patient education on the adoption of healthy behaviors as one step in overcoming sexual dysfunction. Because both ED and vaginal dryness may be early signs of hypertension, heart disease, dementia, or diabetes (Mola, 2015; Santoro, 2015), all patients should be advised to see their primary healthcare provider for problems with ED or vaginal dryness to ensure there are no underlying problems and to explore all treatment options.

One approach to adopting healthy behaviors to prevent or alleviate sexual dysfunction is the popular South Beach Diet (Agatston & Signorile 2009). One of the diet's claims to fame is the loss of abdominal fat first. A waist size of over 40 inches in either men or women has been associated with ED and vaginal dryness, respectively. Loss of abdominal fat, when combined with exercise, is an effective treatment for ED in men and vaginal dryness in women (Mola, 2015; Santoro, 2015). Similarly, adopting a Mediterranean diet, which also decreases abdominal fat, has been shown to increase erectile ability (Mola, 2015).

Promoting Sexual Function in Community-Dwelling Elders

Nurses can have a tremendous impact in assisting elders who reside in the community and wish to maintain sexual function despite a myriad of health problems and physical limitations due to aging. Those who wish to maintain an active sex life will need to learn to overcome and compensate for the changes. Articles have been written by nurses to assist clients to overcome sexual problems due to heart disease and stroke (Steinke et al., 2013), incontinence (Garrett & Tomlin, 2015), diabetes (Raper, 2013), and cancer (Anderson, 2013) and how to treat lack of desire, vaginal dryness, anorgasmia, and pain in women (Albaugh, 2014). Whatever the underlying cause(s), the three major obstacles to *sexual intimacy* that elders need to overcome are fatigue, pain, and mobility limitations. These obstacles may occur for either men or women, and for either one partner or both. However, there are practical ways to help overcome these problems.

Fatigue and Pain

Overcoming fatigue and pain is essential to feeling desire and having the stamina to give and receive pleasure. The specifics of fatigue and pain are addressed in detail elsewhere in this text. One common way to overcome fatigue is to plan for sex when rested, which is often in the morning. Another key factor is to plan one's activities to save some time and energy for pleasure.

Pain is a hallmark of aging. Arthritis and other chronic illnesses have a chronic pain component that lasts until death. Most pain management strategies leave some residual pain, which may interfere with sexual desire and sexual excitement. The irritability, fatigue, and depression that accompany chronic pain also can have an impact on a couple's sexual relationship. Recommendations include planning for sex at a time when the pain is at its lowest level, often mid-morning for those with rheumatoid arthritis, or when pain medications have their peak action. Incorporating massage, a hot bath for chronic arthritic pain, cold packs for acute inflammation, or using an electric massager or vibrator may relax sore muscles, relieve stiffened joints, and, when done with a partner, stimulate sexual excitement. Women may focus the water jets from a hot tub on their clitoris, and both men and women may use the vibrator for sexual stimulation. Anecdotal reports from those with arthritis suggest that the relaxing effects of these pain relief strategies and orgasm actually relieve chronic pain for many hours. This effect is thought to be due to endorphin release during the relaxing treatment and sexual stimulation.

Mobility Limitations

To adapt to mobility limitations from disease and disability, some elders need to adopt new positions for lovemaking. **Box 23-4** lists resources that provide suggestions for comfortable positions, as well as additional information about sex and intimacy with specific chronic illnesses. **Figure 23-1** provides examples of positions for intercourse

---

BOX 23-4 **Resources for Information and Comfortable Positions for Intercourse**

- COPD and Sex. Available from http://www.webmd.com/lung/copd/features/copd-sex
- Sex and Arthritis. Available from: http://www.orthop.washington.edu
- Sex and Cancer (several articles by American Cancer Society). Available from: http://www.cancer.org
- Sex After Stroke. Available from: http://www.strokeassociation.org
- Intimacy and Diabetes. Available from: http://www.netdoctor.co.uk

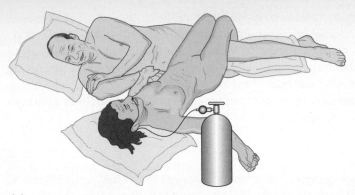

(a)

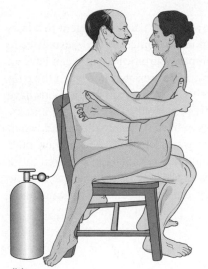

(b)

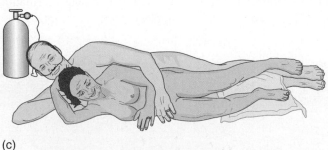

(c)

Figure 23-1 These positions may be used by men and women when either or both have limited endurance, chronic obstructive pulmonary disease (COPD), hip or knee replacement, or stroke. Those with gastroesophageal reflux disease may find sitting in a chair will not exacerbate their symptoms.

when adapting to chronic illness or disability. **Box 23-5** lists reputable sex education websites where couples can obtain educational materials and products to enhance sexual intimacy.

Promoting Romantic and Sexual Relationships in Long-Term Care Facilities

Intimacy and sex among elders residing in long-term care facilities is rarely addressed in the literature. Barriers exist in virtually all facilities, including lack of privacy and door locks, lack of queen size beds, and the literal lack of opportunities for romance. Inability to leave a facility overnight without risk of "losing the bed" prevents couples who have had long-term relationships from spending even one night outside of the facility. Although it is important for staff to ensure safety and protect patients from sexual abuse, policies and environmental design have the unintended consequence of preventing intimacy. Studies confirm that staff continue to be uncomfortable with residents' sexual behavior (Doll, 2013; Lester et al., 2016). A timeless story of love in a nursing home, *The Notebook* by Nicholas Sparks (1999), shows what is possible if nursing staff respect the rights and privacy of those who have entrusted them with the last years of their lives. Some staff may actually promote romance and sex in long-term care, but they may not reveal these efforts for fear of reprisal.

Scott (2015) addresses how complicated sex in the nursing home is and provides resources and practical recommendations in the June 2015 issue of the AARP Bulletin. Doll (2013) provides guidelines for sex in the nursing home, taking into account the issues of what to do if a resident is cognitively impaired, the health needs of the residents, and how to aid

---

BOX 23-5   Web Links: Sex Education Websites

The following are a few professional websites that are highly recommended by the authors for older people to obtain sex education materials. Reassure older adults these are legitimate sex education websites and are not "porno sites."

- http://www.womenshealth.org (a forum for women's health)

- http://www.webmd.com (erectile dysfunction health center)
- http://marriage.about.com (intimacy and sexuality information for couples)
- http://www.sexsmartfilms.com (includes videos for those with disability and the elderly)

---

the staff in ensuring the privacy of the couple is maintained (Roelofs, Luijkx, & Embregts, 2015). Salladay (2016) examines the ethical issue of sexual relations in nursing homes. The author notes that staff, nursing students, and nursing instructors are often untrained and may be confused about patient and resident rights related to sexual relations within a nursing home, including those who have dementia. She offers recommendations for sexual discussions to help staff, students, faculty, and residents.

Additional resources for healthcare providers include the video *Freedom of Sexual Expression: Dementia and Resident Rights in Long-Term Care Facilities,* developed by the Hebrew Home for the Aged, a facility that is nationally known for its policies promoting intimacy between residents. Their current policies can be obtained at http://www.hebrewhome.org. This film and many others on a wide range of topics on aging, including intimacy and sexuality, are available through Terra Nova Films, http://www.terranova.org.

Evidence-based practice guidelines that balance safety with the lifelong need for intimacy are needed. The need to be touched and held by a loved one, and the need to feel loved, not just cared for, does not diminish with age or with physical or cognitive impairment (Heath, 2011). Nurses are in a key position to enhance couples' abilities to give and receive love with each other, whether through physical, emotional, or sexual expression.

Extinguishing Sexually Inappropriate Behavior

Unfortunately, nursing staff may sometimes be confronted with an older adult, either a man or a woman, who displays sexually inappropriate behavior. Most of the incidents reported involve men, but women may display these behaviors as well. Sexually inappropriate behaviors include inappropriate language, gestures, requests for personal care, or inappropriate behaviors such as exposing one's self, masturbating in public places, or touching or groping others. All of these behaviors constitute sexual harassment and are not to be tolerated. These behaviors may reflect a power issue, a loss of inhibition due to cognitive impairment, or a combination of factors. The behaviors make it difficult or impossible to care for the patient exhibiting them.

In each of these examples, the goal is to extinguish the behavior while maintaining the dignity of the patient. Nursing staff need to confront the patient calmly and firmly, saying, "This behavior is inappropriate, interferes with me doing my job, and will not be tolerated." Laughing it off, reacting violently, or showing anger are all likely to encourage the behavior. Saying, "Oh, Mr. Smith, you wouldn't know what to do even if you could," although meant light-heartedly, is demeaning and may encourage the patient to try the behavior with someone else. Communication among staff regarding patterns of inappropriate behavior is important. This promotes monitoring and prevents surprise and embarrassment by unsuspecting care providers. One quadriplegic client told the authors he had rubbed the breasts of every nursing staff member on the unit with his upper arm when they were leaning over him to assist in dressing. He had continued this behavior for weeks because the staff had not communicated with each other about his behavior, therefore, they did not know it was a pattern. After identification of the problem, two nursing staff firmly and compassionately confronted him together and the behavior ended. Confronting him led several staff to talk with him about his fears of dating and being seen as unattractive, which was the underlying motive that drove his behavior.

CLINICAL TIP

Communicate with staff regularly about best practice in handling residents who may exhibit inappropriate sexual behavior.

Although extinguishing sexually inappropriate behavior is necessary to care for older adults, there is some "good news" about this behavior because it is an indicator of recovery in a client who has been too ill to think or worry about his or her sexuality. It may be an expression of power or anger, both of which are expressions of independence. Interest in sexuality can aid in the rehabilitation process. After confronting a patient and ensuring that the client is not going to act out again, the nurse can initiate discussions about recovery and how to take an active role in that process.

Confronting cognitively impaired clients who act out may be effective in extinguishing the behavior. If this strategy does not work, other strategies may extinguish the behavior. If a client has a habit of inappropriately touching staff during a bath or bed-to-chair transfer, put a washcloth in the client's hand during the bath, or place the patient's hand on the armrest to assist in the transfer. Approach a client from the weaker side, which will both protect the staff member and discourage the client from acting out. Another strategy is to encourage appropriate behaviors and ignore inappropriate behaviors. In rehabilitative settings, rewarding appropriate behaviors can be included as a part of a behavioral modification program. If possible, get a client's family involved in extinguishing the behavior. Do not assume that the behavior is a premorbid or lifelong behavior, and try not to feed into perceptions of the client as a "dirty old man."

Another strategy is to avoid using language the client may misinterpret as sexual. Nurses typically say, "I am your nurse today," or "I am going to take care of you," both of which may be misinterpreted as flirting. Instead say, "I am going to work with you" or "I am going to assist you," which sound much more businesslike. Joller and colleagues (2013) outline pharmacologic therapies that may be necessary when sexually inappropriate behaviors continue, despite the interventions provided here.

Addressing Masturbation in Public

Masturbation is self-limiting and has no known harmful effects. It does not spread sexually transmitted diseases, and it can be performed with minimal cognitive and hand function. The comedian Phyllis Diller has been quoted as saying that another advantage is "You don't have to get dressed up." However, masturbation is appropriate only in private. Public masturbation is best extinguished using the strategies described previously for sexually inappropriate behaviors. The goal is to allow privacy, yet not draw undue attention. If "privacy" signs are necessary, keep them visible, yet inconspicuous. Try to provide privacy even if clients' rooms are only semi-private, such as by giving the client some private time or drawing the curtain if available. Clients using sex toys or explicit materials should do so in private and store them in a private space, away from public view.

Display of sexually explicit materials is a problem that is ignored in the nursing literature. Nursing staff may need to set limits with patients or establish policies regarding posters, jokes, magazines, or cards on display on the patient's room wall or on dressers or over-bed tables. Staff need to recognize that although having these materials is the patient's choice, openly displaying them is a form of sexual harassment. A good guideline to follow is materials with a PG-13 rating, such as the *Sports Illustrated* swimsuit issue, are acceptable, but those with naked bodies are not. Guidelines or policies to limit sexually explicit materials apply equally to men and women, regardless of the patient's sexual orientation. In addition to pictures, cards that overtly encourage sexual relationships with patients or nursing staff are also inappropriate. If a patient has displayed these materials, calmly tell the patient why they are inappropriate and encourage the patient or family to remove them. Use respect when approaching a patient about offensive material, remembering it is the patient's home too, especially in a long-term care setting. Try a compassionate approach first, focusing on your feelings. Keep the confrontation one-on-one if possible.

Occasionally, nursing staff who visit patients in their homes may encounter sexually explicit materials on display. Tell patients you cannot work with them in the rooms in which the materials are displayed. Negotiate with the patient for the materials to be removed or to establish one room of the house in which treatment can occur where there are no explicit materials on display.

Summary

This chapter has addressed a wide variety of areas related to sexuality and intimacy in older adults. The goal is to promote intimacy when appropriate by assisting older adults to overcome the effects of age and chronic illness (see **Box 23-6**).

BOX 23-6   Evidence-Based Practice Highlight

A documentary film on HIV was developed to increase awareness and encourage protective behavior change related to HIV for older adults of racial or ethnic minorities. The authors found that clinicians and older adults who watched the film had increased knowledge, and they encouraged healthcare providers to implement HIV prevention action steps with their patients.

Data from Ebor, M., Murray, A., Gaul, Z., & Sutton, M. (2015). HIV awareness and knowledge among viewers of a documentary film about HIV among racial- or ethnic-minority older adults. *Health & Social Work, 40*(3), 217–234.

Clinical Reasoning Exercises

1. You are caring for an older man with dementia who keeps wandering into the rooms of female residents in the long-term care facility. What are strategies to manage this behavior and ensure the safety and privacy of the residents?
2. What have you read about HIV and AIDS among the older adult population? Do you think this is a real problem? Why or why not?
3. An older client in an assisted living facility asks you to buy him a pornographic magazine because he cannot drive to the store and get one for himself. What is your response and why?

Personal Reflections

1. If an older patient was having problems dealing with sexuality after a life-changing event, how could you assist him or her?
2. What is your comfort level with discussing sexual information with patients? How could you become more comfortable with this important aspect of nursing?
3. What resources are available in your area for older persons or those with disabilities who may need additional information and counseling about sexuality after an event such as a stroke or heart attack?

References

Agatston, A., & Signorile, J. (2009). *The South Beach diet supercharged: Faster weight loss and better health for life.* New York, NY: St. Martin's Press.

Albaugh, J. (2014). Female sexual dysfunction. *International Journal of Urology Nursing, 8*(1), 38–43.

American Geriatrics Society Ethics Committee. (2015). American Geriatrics Society care of lesbian, gay, bisexual, and transgender older adults position statement. *Journal of the American Geriatrics Society, 63,* 423–426.

Anderson, J. L. (2013). Acknowledging female sexual dysfunction in women with cancer. *Clinical Journal of Oncology Nursing, 17*(3), 233–235.

Barnett, Z. L., Robleda-Gomez, S., & Pachana, N. A. (2012). Viagra: The little blue pill with big repercussions. *Aging & Mental Health, 16,* 84–88.

Billett, J. L., & Seiden, O. J. (2008). *Sex in the golden years: The best sex ever.* Parker, CO: Books To Believe In.

Center for Disease Control and Prevention (CDC). (2014). HIV surveillance report, 2014, vol 26. November 2015. Retrieved from http://www.cdc.gov/hiv/library/reports/surveillance/

Davis, E. M., & Fingerman, K. L. (2015). Digital dating: Online profile content of older and younger adults. *The Journals of Gerontology Series B: Psychological Sciences and Social Sciences,* Oxford University Press.

Doll, G. M. (2013). Sexuality in nursing homes: Practice and policy. *Journal of Gerontological Nursing, 39*(7), 30–37.

Ebor, M., Murray, A., Gaul, Z., & Sutton, M. (2015). HIV awareness and knowledge among viewers of a documentary film about HIV among racial- or ethic-minority older adults. *Health & Social Work, 40*(3), 217–234.

Garrett, D., & Tomlin, K. (2015) Incontinence and sexuality in later life. *Nursing of Older People, 27*(6), 26–29.

Gledhill, S., & Schweitzer, R. D. (2014). Sexual desire, erectile dysfunction and the biomedicalization of sex in older heterosexual men. *Journal of Advanced Nursing, 70*(4), 894–903.

Heath, H. (2011). Older people in care homes: Sexuality and intimate relationships. *Nursing Older People, 23*(6), 14–20.

Joller, P., Gupta, N., Seitz, D. P., Christopher, F., Gibson, M., & Gill, S. S. (2013). Approach to inappropriate sexual behaviour in people with dementia. *Canadian Family Physician, 59,* 255–260.

Kaplan, H. S. (1990). Sex, intimacy, and the aging process. *Journal of the American Academy of Psychoanalysis, 18,* 185–205.

Katsiki, N., Wierzbicki, A. S., & Mikhailidis, D. P. (2015). Erectile dysfunction and coronary heart disease. *Current Opinion in Cardiology 4,* 416–421.

Kautz, D. D. (1995). *The maturing of sexual intimacy in chronically ill, older adult couples.* (Doctoral dissertation, University of Kentucky). *Dissertation Abstracts International* (UMI Order no. PUZ9527436).

Lee, D. M., Nazroo, J., O'Conner, D. B., Blake, M., & Pendleton, N. (2016). Sexual health and well-being among older men and women in England: Findings from the English Longitudinal Study of Ageing. *Archives of Sexual Behavior, 45,* 133–144.

Lester, P. E., Kohen, I., Stefanacci, R. G., & Feuerman, M. (2016). Sex in nursing homes: A survey of nursing home policies governing resident sexual activity. *Journal of the American Medical Directors Association, 17*(1), 71–74.

Minkin, M. J. (2016). Sexual health and relationships after age 60. *Maturitas, 83,* 27–32.

Mola, J. R. (2015). Erectile dysfunction in the older adult male. *Urologic Nursing, 35*(2), 87–93.

Palacios, S., Mejia, A., & Neyro, J. L. (2015). Treatment of the genitourinary syndrome of menopause. *Climacteric, 18*(Suppl. 1), 23–29.

Raper, M. (2013). Sexual dysfunction: Reflections on a neglected area of diabetes care. *Practice Nursing, 24*(10), 505–509.

Roelofs, T. S. M., Luijkx, K. G., & Embregts, P. J. C. M. (2015). Intimacy and sexuality of nursing home residents with dementia: A systematic review. *International Psychogeriatrics, 27*(3), 367–384.

Rye, J., & Murphy, M. P. (2015). Physical healthcare patterns and nursing interventions. In C. Lehman (Ed). *The specialty practice of rehabilitation nursing: A core curriculum* (7th ed) (pp. 353–401). Chicago, IL: Association of Rehabilitation Nurses.

Salladay, S. A. (2016). Christian ethics: Sex in the nursing home. *Journal of Christian Nursing, 33*(1), 13.

Santoro, N. (2015). Perimenopause: From research to practice. *Journal of Women's Health, 25*(4), 332–339.

Scott, P. S. (2015). Sex in the nursing home. *AARP Bulletin, 56*(5), 10, 12–13.

Song, H., Oh, H., Kim, H., & Seo, W. (2011). Effects of a sexual rehabilitation program on stroke patients and their spouses. *NeuroRehabilitation, 28,* 143–150.

Sparks, N. (1999). *The notebook.* New York, NY: Warner Books.

Steinke, E. E., Jaarsma, T., Barnason, S. A., Byrne, M., Doherty, S., Dougherty, C. M. . . . Moser, D. K. (2013). Sexual counseling for individuals with cardiovascular disease and their partners: A consensus document from the American Heart Association and the ESC Council on Cardiovascular Nursing and Allied Professions (CCNAP). *Circulation, 128,* 2075–2096.

Viljoen, P. O. (2012). *Sex after 60: Tips for enjoying a healthy and happy sex life into your 60s.* Amazon Digital Services.

Wagle, K. C., Carrejo, M. H., & Tan, R. S. (2012). The implications of increasing age on erectile dysfunction. *American Journal of Men's Health, 6*(4), 273–279.

For a full suite of assignments and additional learning activities, see the access code at the front of your book.

CHAPTER 24

Elder Abuse and Mistreatment

Kristen L. Mauk
Stefanie Benton

(Competencies 3, 4, 6, 15, 17)

LEARNING OBJECTIVES

At the end of this chapter, the reader will be able to:

> Distinguish between elder abuse and self-neglect.
> Describe several categories of the mistreatment of older adults.
> Recognize risk factors for elder abuse.
> Identify characteristics of perpetrators of mistreatment.
> Recognize signs that an older adult is being mistreated.
> Describe evidence-based screening for elder abuse.
> Discuss strategies to prevent the mistreatment of older adults.
> Synthesize interventions in various cases of abuse.

KEY TERMS

Abandonment	Financial exploitation
Assault	Financial or material exploitation
Caregiver burden	Physical abuse
Chemical restraint	Psychological or emotional abuse
Direct physical abuse	Psychological or emotional neglect
Elder abuse	Respite care
Elder mistreatment	Self-neglect
Emotional neglect	Sexual abuse
Financial abuse	Violation of personal rights

Elder abuse is "a single, or repeated act, or lack of appropriate action, occurring within any relationship where there is an expectation of trust which causes harm or distress to an older person" (World Health Organization [WHO], 2016, para. 1). Elder abuse is also defined as "any form of mistreatment that results in harm or loss to an older person" (National Committee for the Prevention of Elder Abuse, 2008). It is connected with a wide variety of adverse health outcomes. There is evidence of risk of greater mortality (Baker et al., 2009; Lachs, Williams, O'Brien, Pillemer, & Charlson, 1998); higher dependence in performance of activities of daily living (ADL) (Cohen, 2008); and increased dementia, delusions, and depression (Cooper et al., 2006; Cooper, Manela, Katona, & Livingston, 2008; Dyer, Pavlik, Murphy, & Hyman, 2000; Pillemer & Suitor, 1992). Other findings suggest that older women who have experienced abuse are likely to report to their physicians with fatigue, headache, myalgias, depression, anxiety, and gastrointestinal disorders, as well as with gynecological issues and physical injuries.

Elder abuse or mistreatment is an often-underestimated problem. Statistics on abuse of older adults may not be reliable, due to underreporting or a lack of scientific evidence. There is no national reporting system, so statistics may be based on varying definitions of abuse. The Administration on Aging suggests that hundreds of thousands of older adults are victims of some type of abuse each year (U.S. Administration on Aging, 2014). Combined with the fact that older adults may be hesitant to report abuse because of fear of reprisal, the American system of gathering data and reporting abuse is woefully inadequate. The statistics that are available are outdated.

Data from the 1990s estimated that 5% to 10% of older adults experienced abuse (Pritchard, 1995), which translates to 1 to 2 million people (Frost & Willette, 1994; Thobaben, 1996). In 2010 the National Center on Elder Abuse (2010) cited that 1 in 10 older adults experiences some form of abuse, but fewer than 1 in 5 report it. Fulmer (2012) cited that "elder abuse and neglect is a serious and prevalent problem that is estimated to affect 700,000 to 1.2 million older adults annually in this country" (p. 1). There is a wide variation across sources as to the extent of elder mistreatment or abuse, and much of our information is outdated.

CLINICAL TIP

The National Center on Elder Abuse (2010, p. 1) reminds us that "elder abuse is an under recognized problem with devastating and even life threatening consequences."

For the purposes of this discussion, elder abuse will be defined simply as "the mistreatment of an older adult that threatens his or her health or safety" (Hildreth, 2011, p. 568). There are several types of elder abuse that will be discussed in this chapter. Prevention, identification, and intervention strategies will also be reviewed.

Types of Elder Abuse

Elder mistreatment may be classified into several different categories. These include neglect; *financial exploitation*; and emotional, physical, or *sexual abuse* (Daly, 2011). Some authors include violation of personal rights as another category of abuse. Neglect of older adults and financial exploitation seem to be the two most commonly reported types of mistreatment (Fulmer & Greenberg, 2012). Several types of abuse may be present at once, and abuse or neglect tends to be recurring (Quinn & Tomita, 1986). Abuse is often ongoing, may be eventually tolerated by the person being mistreated, and can have long-lasting negative consequences on health and emotional well-being (McGarry & Simpson, 2011).

Sengstock and Barrett (1992) distinguished six types of abuse or neglect in their seminal work; these distinctions are still applicable today because they distinguish between degrees of abuse or neglect and can be helpful in providing specificity to reporting and documentation. These include psychological or emotional neglect, psychological or emotional abuse, violation of personal rights, financial abuse, physical neglect, and direct abuse or neglect. These are discussed in the next section.

Psychological or Emotional Neglect

Psychological or emotional neglect may be present when a person receives good or adequate physical care, but is socially isolated. The older adult in such a situation may stay in his or her room, have decreased socialization with others outside of the home, and express little purpose for living. This may present as a type of "failure to thrive" in older adults.

Psychological or Emotional Abuse

Sometimes preceded by psychological or emotional neglect, *psychological or emotional abuse* shows a greater degree of severity of mistreatment. This type of abuse includes verbal or nonverbal insults, such as hurtful things said or done to damage the person's self-esteem. Humiliation, intimidation, and harassment fall into this category (Fulmer & Greenberg, 2012). Common *assaults* in this category of abuse include telling the older person that he is a burden and threatening to send him to a nursing home.

Violation of Personal Rights

Ignoring the rights of an older person who is capable of decision making can be considered a *violation of personal rights*. Healthcare facilities may be guilty of this type of mistreatment. For example, addressing questions to a younger adult about the older adult in his presence or making wrong assumptions that an older adult is not mentally competent are common violations. In long-term-care settings, not allowing persons to marry or assuming lack of competence if a person answers too slowly are other examples. Within families, if a relative goes into Grandma's purse or on her cellphone to retrieve information without permission, this is also a violation of personal rights.

Financial Abuse

Financial abuse is one of the most common types of mistreatment and may be easier to quantify than other forms of abuse. Also referred to as material abuse, *financial abuse* can include stealing money or property, making the person feel obligated to the abuser in some way in order to obtain goods or possessions, or borrowing money and not repaying it.

Another avenue leading to financial abuse of older adults on a larger scale is mail fraud. This may occur through attractive fliers and brochures that promise prizes or the chance to win large amounts of money over time. Such "contests" frequently target susceptible older people with limited means. They may win small items that lead them to think they are more likely to win big prizes, so they send money to remain in the contest. Older adults who fall prey to this misleading advertising may spend thousands of dollars for little return, much like more traditional gambling.

A study by MetLife (2012b) estimated that over one million older adults are victims of financial abuse. The same study estimated that $2.6 billion was lost annually in the United States to this type of abuse. The most common characteristics of victims included white, frail, ages 70 to 89 years, cognitively impaired, isolated, and trusting. About 55% of financial abuse cases were due to exploitation from family members (MetLife, 2012b). In a later examination of the data, women were twice as likely as men to experience financial abuse. These women tended to be between the ages of 80 and 89, live alone, and require some type of assistance for health problems. Sixty percent of perpetrators were men between the ages of 30 and 59 (MetLife, 2012a). Financial abuse appeared to be worse during the holidays as a result of friends and family members taking advantage of older adults. Financial exploitation can have negative effects on an older adult, including credit problems, depression, and loss of independence (MetLife, 2012b).

Physical Neglect

Physical neglect is not providing what the older adult needs, such as glasses, dentures, medications, food, or adaptive equipment. Though stopping short of direct physical abuse, signs of this type of neglect could be insect or vermin bites, overgrown toenails, overuse of restraints, pressure ulcers, malnutrition, and poor hygiene.

It should be noted that some older adults engage in self-neglect, so care should be taken to complete a thorough assessment of the living situation. Self-neglect among older adults is a difficult problem to manage, particularly when a competent elder chooses to live in this way.

Self-Neglect

Self-neglect is defined as the inability to provide basic needs for one's self (Dyer, Goodwin, Pickens-Pace, Burnett, & Kelly, 2007) and is associated with poor nutrition and functional decline (Reyes-Ortiz, 2006). Persons who do not maintain a socially acceptable level of self-care would be considered to be engaging in self-neglect (Gibbons, Lauder, & Ludwick, 2006). Signs of self-neglect may include inadequate physical hygiene, poor diet, missing medical appointments, medication mismanagement, and lack of follow-up with prescribed medical care (Mauk, 2011).

Although gerontological nurses strive to uphold the autonomy and independence of older adults, "dilemmas result when people's poor health behaviors put them or others at risk for negative consequences" (Mauk, 2011, p. 64). Careful assessment is needed if self-neglect is suspected, as reporting such a case to adult protective services could eventually result in an older adult being forcibly removed from his or her place of residence. An "interdisciplinary team of professionals should be consulted and decisions should be made that are in the ultimate best interest of the older adult" (Mauk, 2011, p. 64) when self-neglect is serious enough to produce negative health outcomes.

Direct Abuse

This is the most obvious type of mistreatment seen in older adults. *Direct physical abuse* involves the use of physical force to purposefully inflict pain or harm to another. Direct abuse includes assault and aggressive violence such as hitting, kicking, biting, punching, pushing, shoving, burning, restraining, overmedicating, and slapping. Sexual assault and rape are also included in this category. Female victims are more likely to experience significant injury, especially if the abuser is a male.

Case Studies

Within this section of the chapter are several case studies to test your knowledge related to assessment of elder mistreatment. Look at each situation and see if you can correctly distinguish the type of elder abuse as described in this section.

Case Study 24 – 1

You are working in the emergency room. A 65-year-old woman comes in with bruises to her inner thighs and small burns on her the bottom of her feet. Her major complaint is abdominal pain. She is 5 feet, 7 inches and weighs 100 pounds. She has no teeth. She is accompanied by her son, a 40-year-old man who appears unkempt and belligerent, and he does not want you to examine his mother without him in the room. What is your best course of action? What is your initial impression of this situation? What interventions should be taken?

Case Study 24-2

You are working in your backyard and hear yelling from the house next door. You hear a woman screaming and glass breaking. All you know about your neighbors is that their mother, 80 years old, has Alzheimer's disease and they have recently brought her to live with them. A few minutes later you see the old woman running outside in her underwear with a middle-aged woman chasing after her. What is your best course of action? What is your initial impression of this situation? What interventions should be taken?

Case Study 24-3

You are living in a small suburban neighborhood. You notice that the younger couple from down the street frequently visit the older man who lives across the street from you. They seem to be taking care of him, mowing his lawn and driving him to the doctors. When you take cookies over to this gentleman, he tells you that the neighbors down the street charge him a lot of money to look after him, but he has nobody else to do it. Upon questioning him further, he confesses that they have threatened to stop helping him if he doesn't give them $1,000 each week for their troubles. He is perplexed but does not know what else to do. He says he now feels scared of them. What is your best course of action? What is your initial impression of this situation? What interventions should be taken?

Case Study 24-4

You come from a large family of 7 children and 30 grandchildren. Your elderly parents do not have much money, but one of their children, your brother, seems to always be borrowing money from them. You learn, rather by accident through another sibling, that your mom and dad cosigned a loan for your brother and he defaulted. Now your mom and dad are in financial trouble but do not want the rest of the family to know. What is your best course of action? What is your initial impression of this situation? What interventions should be taken?

Case Study 24-5

A woman is admitted to the emergency room where you are working. She has large bruises across her left shoulder, abdomen, and chest to her right hip. Her face has some cuts and bruises. She states that she was in a car accident. The accident report states she was wearing her seatbelt. What is your best course of action? What is your initial impression of this situation? What interventions should be taken?

Case Study 24-6

You are working at an underserved clinic where an 81-year-old man comes in for treatment of a cough that has lingered for weeks. The man seems quiet and withdrawn. He is accompanied by his wife, who is 15 years younger than he is, and who displays loud, aggressive behavior, speaking rudely to the staff. During your assessment, you find that the man appears malnourished, underweight, and dehydrated. He is reluctant to answer any questions about his living situation at home with his wife and he cowers when she is in the room. What is your best course of action? What is your initial impression of this situation? What interventions should be taken?

Risk Factors of Victims

With an estimated 700,000 to 1.2 million elderly adult victims annually, it is essential to understand the risk factors of both the victim and the perpetrator. The U.S. Census Bureau's national population projects that 25% of the entire U.S. population will be retired between the years 2011 and 2029 (Bond & Butler, 2013). With an increase in older adults, the potential for abuse also proliferates. Though every victim is different, studies have shown that certain risk factors appear more frequently in victims (see **Table 24-1**). The most significant risk factor is related to psychiatric illness or psychological problems with a high functional dependency component. Victims also tend to be female over the age of 75 years, and the majority are in poor physical health. Ethnicity is a consideration, and studies have shown that African Americans have an increased probability of financial exploitation, and nonwhite elderly adults are more likely to be at risk for overall maltreatment, and the risk of physical and sexual abuse is higher in Canadian Aboriginals. The likelihood of abuse or neglect increases if the older adult demonstrates aggressive behavior or resists care. Abuse and neglect of an older adult may escalate when there is significant *caregiver burden* or stress, and if the social support system for the caregiver is poor. There also appears to be a link between family disharmonies with conflicted relationships and elder maltreatment. Most victims live with others versus living alone. Interestingly, abuse and neglect in the elderly appear to be executed more frequently by females versus males, which is not the case in child abuse or *physical abuse* in general (Johannesen & LoGiudice, 2016). Table 24-1 lists risk factors associated with being a victim of elder abuse or neglect.

Older persons who are substance abusers, who experience depression or loneliness, and have a lack of social support are also at risk (Fulmer & Greenberg, 2012; Hildreth, 2011; MetLife, 2012a). Persons who have memory problems or physical disabilities and those who are socially isolated are at increased risk. More specifically,

TABLE 24-1   General Risk Factors for Elder Abuse or Mistreatment (Victim)

- Psychiatric illness/psychological problems
- Poor physical health or frailty
- Behavior (provocative/aggressive/resists care)
- Cognitive impairment
- Older than 75 years
- Female
- Ethnicity
- Low Income
- Trauma or past abuse
- Personality traits

Data from Johannesen, M., & LoGiudice, D. (2016). Elder abuse: A systematic review of risk factors in community-dwelling elders. *Age and Ageing, 45*(1), 1–7.

TABLE 24-2 General Risk Factors for Elder Abuse or Mistreatment (Perpetrator)
• Low social support
• Caregiving burden or stress
• Family disharmony; poor or conflicted relationship
• Living with elder adult
• Psychiatric illness or psychological problems
• Personality traits

Data from Johannesen, M., & LoGiudice, D. (2016). Elder abuse: A systematic review of risk factors in community-dwelling elders. *Age and Ageing, 45*(1), 1–7.

"lower levels of global cognitive function, MMSE, episodic memory, and perceptual speed are associated with an increased risk of elder abuse" (Dong, Simon, Rajan, & Evans, 2011, p. 209). Zhang et al. (2011), in the *Journal of Elder Abuse and Neglect*, stated that some studies indicate that an older person's mental, physical, and cognitive impairments are related to neglect both in the community and in institutions. According to Rosen, Pillemer, and Lachs (2008), resident-to-resident aggression is "negative and aggressive physical, sexual, or verbal interactions between long-term care residents that in a community setting would likely be construed as unwelcome and have high potential to cause physical or psychological distress to the recipient" (p. 1398).

Characteristics of Perpetrators of Elder Abuse

One of the most popular older theories used to explain elder abuse is the caregiver stress model, which stated that elders who become abused have created extreme levels of stress on their caregiver, resulting in an intolerable burden, which leads to mistreatment. Wilson (1992) summarized caregiver stress theory by stating that the hypothesis is that "elders' physical, emotional, and financial dependency needs create an unfair and inescapable relationship with the caregiver" (p. 69), which leads to abuse. Other research, however, suggested that "the dependency of the victim may simply be a catalyst for abuse in a caretaker who cannot cope effectively" (Barnett, Miller-Perrin, & Perrin, 1997, p. 26).

Some common characteristics of those who mistreat older adults have emerged through several studies in the 1990s and more recently (see **Table 24-2**). Maladaptive personality characteristics, anxiety, a history of family violence, inability of the caregiver to meet the demands of the elder, and lack of knowledge have all been associated with abusers (Buckwalter, Campbell, Gerdner, & Garand, 1996; Fulmer & Greenberg, 2012; Saveman, Hallberg, & Norberg, 1996; Wierucka & Goodridge, 1996). The perpetrator is often someone who knows the victim and on whom the victim may be dependent. Nurses must be alert to the fact that "children, family members, friends, and formal caregivers are prospective perpetrators of elder abuse" (Stark, 2011, p. 431).

Prevention of Abuse or Mistreatment

The best prevention is education, so education about elder abuse should be a priority. Laws regarding elder abuse are not standard from state to state, and the magnitude of elder abuse is not fully realized due to few population-based studies. All gerontological nurses, social workers, healthcare workers, law enforcement workers, and the general public should be educated about the signs and symptoms, screening, identifying, reporting, and support services for the elderly abused and the abuser (see **Table 24-3**).

Communities should look at developing outreach programs that involve elders, *respite care*, and education. Families and friends need to understand and realize how important it is to give support to caregivers and help them with rest on a regular basis.

TABLE 24-3   Nursing Interventions in the Prevention of Elder Abuse

- Establish a trusting relationship with the elder.
- Know about community resources and be able to appropriately refer people for help.
- Strengthen social supports and networking of older adults.
- Encourage regular respite for the caregiver.
- Identify and refer to appropriate caregiver support groups.
- Identify caregivers who are at high risk to be abusers and target interventions to prevent stress from caregiver burden.
- Interview the patient and family or caregiver to find out normal patterns for stress management.
- Identify possible scenarios and facilitate strategies to cope with those.
- Observe family interactions, dynamics, and body language.
- Encourage single older adults to remain involved and connected to society.
- Be aware of risk factors and contributing factors.
- Perform thorough physical assessments and carefully document findings, including appearance, nutritional state, skin condition, mental attitude and awareness, and need for aids to enhance sensory perception.
- If abuse is suspected, interview caregivers and other possible informants separately to confirm or refute suspicions.
- Know the reporting laws for your own state.
- Encourage the older person to let a trusted person know where valuable papers are stored.

TABLE 24-4   Suggestions for Older Adults to Reduce the Potential for Abuse

- Stay active—keep involved in social activities.
- Have access to a telephone and use of it in private.
- Store important contact information in two separate places (e.g., in a cellphone and a phone directory).
- Maintain contact with family and friends.
- Know your financial situation and when to expect deposits and automatic withdrawals.
- Have a secure, private place where your important files are kept.
- Have a family member or friends visit regularly and unannounced.
- Have an emergency safety plan if you are concerned about potential abuse.
- Let a trusted person know where you are going if you are traveling or visiting out of town.

CLINICAL TIP

Family members, friends, and caregivers are potential perpetrators of elder mistreatment, so nurses should be alert advocates for vulnerable elders.

Community education is necessary for everyone to realize how important and valuable it is to plan financially for one's own care in his or her "golden years." Older adults can be taught to decrease their risk of being victimized (Canadian Network for the Prevention of Elder Abuse [CNPEA], 2016) (see **Table 24-4**). Remaining involved and engaged in the community, participating in outside interests, and maintaining connections with family and friends can help provide older adults with a buffer against the potential for abuse.

Gerontological nurses have a great opportunity to educate representatives, senators, and other policymakers on the issues of elderly abuse, encouraging them to make legislative changes that can have an impact on effective services for the elderly and their caregivers (Stark, 2011).

Assessment and Screening

Screening for abuse is imperative to prevent further harm and to advocate for patients' overall well-being. It is important to interview the patient alone because a relative or caregiver could be the abuser, and the victim may be tentative to disclose neglect or abuse when the caregiver is nearby. Furthermore, the healthcare provider may expose disparities amid the patient's accounts of events of any suspected injury to those of the caregiver's explanation. All elderly adults should be screened for abuse at least once or twice annually. Although not all victims will exhibit the same behavioral, emotional, psychological, and/or physical patterns, certain criteria should alert the healthcare practitioner to assess the patient further. Conditions include but are not limited to the following:

> Pain: New onset or increasing
> Depression: New onset or increasing
> Delirium: New onset or increasing
> Deviations in social network: New or decreased circle of network
> Change in behavior: Now withdrawn/angry/tearful
> Sudden fluctuations in financial circumstances: Decreased or increased spending
> Variation in personal hygiene, dress, and/or appearance
> Drastic difference in weight

TABLE 24-5   Diseases and Conditions That Mimic Abuse in Older Persons

Abuse Mimicked	Condition
Blunt force trauma/contusion	• Allergic reactions • Bleeding disorder secondary to medications • Cushing syndrome • Fixed drug eruption • Fracture from osteoporosis or Paget disease of bone • Fragile photo-aged skin • Senile purpura • Steroid purpura • Subdural hematoma secondary to a fall or coagulopathy • Thrombocytopenia
Burns and scalds	• Contact dermatitis • Stevens-Johnson syndrome from medications • Toxic epidermal necrolysis
Chemical restraint	• Iatrogenic polypharmacy or drug–drug interactions • Increased drug levels secondary to decreased renal clearance
Neglect	• Constipation from medications or hypercalcemia • Dehydration secondary to medications • Diabetes mellitus • Fecal impaction • Poor wound healing • Urinary tract infection (in women) • Vaginitis
Sexual assault	• Cystocele, uterine prolapse • Decreased anal sphincter function

Reproduced from Hoover, R. M., and Polson, M. (2014). Detecting elder abuse and neglect: Assessment and intervention. *American Family Physician, 89*(6), 453–460.

Over the last several decades, many screening tools have been developed to improve assessment and screening for abuse. Most screening tools are similar in format and structure and focus on key questions, such as safety in the home or if the patient is feeling threatened, abused, and/or neglected. Nonverbal behavior is taken into consideration and guides the more direct questions: "Has anyone hurt you?" or "Tell me about these bruises/cuts/skin tears." Given that older adults have a higher likelihood of depression and/or dementia, a formal assessment of cognition and mood, performed by either the primary care physician or a mental health professional, neurologist, or geriatrician is necessary to provide the patient with a holistic assessment (Lachs & Pillemer, 2015).

In 2015, the *New England Journal of Medicine* published a guideline for physicians on the five most common types of abuse manifestations and how to properly screen and assess each category.

Regardless of what tool is chosen to screen for elder abuse or mistreatment, it is important that facilities adopt some type of consistent measure to assess for this common problem. Some organizations have a few specific questions about abuse built into their admitting documentation. Those facilities providing care to older adults are responsible for ensuring that this issue is not overlooked. Gerontological nurses can help facilitate the use of appropriate screening tools and share information with their peers and administrators.

Recognizing the Signs and Symptoms of Elder Abuse or Mistreatment

Distinguishing among key terms related to abuse is important. Here are some key definitions:

> Abrasion: The rubbing or scraping of the surface layer of cells or tissue from an area of the skin or mucous membrane
> Contusion: Bruise; an injury transmitted through unbroken skin to underlying tissue causing rupture of small blood vessels and escape of blood into the tissue, with resulting discoloration
> Cut: A wound made by something sharp
> Erythema: Abnormal redness of the skin due to capillary congestion (as in inflammation)
> Hematoma: A mass of usually clotted blood that forms in a tissue, organ, or body space as a result of a broken blood vessel
> Laceration: A torn and ragged wound

It is also important to differentiate among illness, accidental injury, or manifestations of disease and actual abuse (see **Table 24-6**). Physical signs of abuse are universal and are not segregated by age. Every victim can suffer the same injuries; however, the older adult may be more fragile and suffer greater consequences. Physical signs and symptoms include, but are not limited to, bruising (especially in various stages of healing), lacerations, abrasions, fractured bones, chipped or missing teeth, ligature marks on wrists and ankles, bite marks, finger marks (especially around neck or upper arms), edema around orbits with or without bruising, missing toes or fingers, torn ear cartridge, traumatic alopecia, and stab wounds and burn marks. Sexual assault victims may or may not have any visible injuries. A (former or currently) sexually active female adult may not have any lacerations, abrasions, tears, bleeding, bruising, or redness and inflammation or tenderness and pain of the vagina, labia majora, labia minora, fossa navicularis, posterior fourchette or injury to hymen or cervix. It is estimated that less than 50% of female victims will have genital injuries. If an injury does present itself, it is most frequently located at the posterior fourchette, perineum, fossa navicularis, vagina, labia majora and minora, urethral orifice, clitoris, hymen and cervix, respectively. The most frequently found injuries are abrasions and tears, bruising, redness, and inflammation (Jina et al., 2015). A male victim will generally not exhibit injuries to the shaft of the penis or his testicles unless an object was inserted into his urethra or his testicles were injured via squeezing, ligature, or blunt trauma. An injury to the testicles is a medical emergency and requires immediate medical attention. In both female and male victims, injury to the anus is more common if the victim was sodomized. In a study published in 2015, 56.3% of anal injuries were at the sphincter, with redness and inflammation, bruising, swelling and tyre sign (perianal swelling in the form of a ring), tenderness, and pain being most prevalent (Jina et al., 2015).

TABLE 24-6   Recognizing Potential Markers for Elderly Abuse

Physical condition and quality of care

- Documented but untreated injuries
- Undocumented injuries and fractures
- Multiple, untreated, or undocumented pressure sores
- Medical orders not followed
- Poor oral care, poor hygiene, and lack of cleanliness of resident (e.g., unchanged adult diapers, untrimmed fingernails and toenails)
- Malnourished residents who have no documentation for low weight
- Bruising on nonambulatory residents; bruising in unusual locations
- Family has statements and facts concerning poor care
- Level of care for residents with nonattentive family members

Facility characteristics

- Unchanged linens
- Strong odors (urine, feces)
- Trashcans that have not been emptied
- Food issues (cafeteria smells at all hours; food left on trays)
- Past problems

Inconsistencies between

- Medical records, statements made by staff members, or what is viewed by investigator
- Statements given by different groups
- The reported time of death and condition of the body

Staff behaviors

- Staff members who follow the investigator too closely
- Lack of knowledge or concern about a resident
- Evasiveness, both unintended and purposeful, verbal and nonverbal
- Facility's unwillingness to release medical records

Reproduced from National Institute of Justice. (2008). Potential markers for elder mistreatment. Retrieved from http://www.nij.gov/topics/crime/elder-abuse/pages/potential-markers.aspx

CLINICAL TIP

Remember: *No injury does not translate to no assault!* If the victim states she or he has been assaulted, she or he **has** been assaulted.

Neglect is concomitant to physical abuse, so the physical signs of neglect are similar to the physical signs and symptoms of abuse. Neglect also can include poor nutrition and hydration, sleep disturbances, increased susceptibility to new infections or illnesses, or an exacerbation of a preexisting health condition. Furthermore, the victim will exhibit a mood change and depression and anxiety are now present or increased (CDC, 2015a).

CLINICAL TIP

Bruises of various colors may indicate injury over time and is a red flag for possible abuse.

CLINICAL TIP

The injury observed should match the description of what happened; otherwise, suspect abuse or neglect.

Treatment and Reporting

Treatment of the results of abuse or neglect will be specific depending on the extent and type of injury. **Table 24-7** gives some guidance about reporting elder abuse and how to respond if abuse is suspected. A clinical practice guideline summary and resources are provided in **Box 24-1** and **Box 24-2**.

Facilities should also specify a Sexual Assault Treatment Plan. Such a plan includes:

> Medical interventions (e.g., sutures, laboratory tests, X-rays)
> Collection of physical evidence (e.g., swabs of bite wounds, bloody or torn clothing)

TABLE 24-7   The Three Rs in Detecting and Reporting Elderly Abuse
RECOGNIZE
• Risk factors: Older age, dementia, depression, isolation, caregiver strain.
• Types of abuse: Physical, sexual, emotional, financial exploitation, neglect, and *abandonment*.
• Signs and symptoms: Signs of physical harm (e.g., bruising), agitation, withdrawn behavior, underuse or overuse of medications, malnutrition, dehydration, unkempt appearance, poor living conditions, sudden changes in financial matters, unmet needs despite financial ability to provide.
• Never ignore an older adult's report of abuse.
RESPOND
• Perform a thorough assessment.
• If abuse is suspected, follow facility protocol.
• Meet with care team or social worker for further guidance.
• Check state laws regarding mandatory reporting and how to handle if adult is competent and able to report abuse, but does not wish to report it.
REPORT
• The care team or social worker will meet with patient/abuse reporter regarding intent to report.
• The type of abuse will determine which departments will be involved and notified of the case (e.g., adult protective service, law enforcement).
• After intent to report has been made, follow up according to facility policy.
• Provide accurate and detailed documentation.
• Provide assistance for nonmedical personnel in reporting abuse by referring them to abuse hotlines, which can be found on National Center on Elder Abuse Website.
• Refer to local adult protective agencies and/or ombudsman programs.

BOX 24-1   Web Resources

MetLife Study of Elder Financial Abuse:
https://www.metlife.com/mmi/research/elder
-financial-abuse.html#key%20findings

National Center on Elder Abuse:
https://ncea.acl.gov/

The National Center on Elder Abuse/
Administration on Aging:
https://aoa.acl.gov/AoA_Programs/Elder_Rights
/NCEA/index.aspx

BOX 24-2   Clinical Practice Guidelines: Elder Abuse Prevention

Guideline Category

- Diagnosis
- Evaluation
- Management
- Prevention
- Risk Assessment
- Screening

Guideline Objective(s)

To facilitate healthcare professionals to assess older persons in domestic and institutional settings who are at risk of elder abuse and to recommend interventions to reduce the incidence of mistreatment

Interventions and Practices Considered

1. Perform cognitive assessment screen, such as Mini-Mental State Examination (MMSE).
2. Ask brief screening questions such as, "How are things at home?" and "Do you feel safe at home?"
3. If elder abuse is suspected:
   - Proceed with assessment.

- Evaluate risk factors for abuse (e.g., Indicators of Abuse Screen, Geriatric Depression Scale).
- Obtain a patient history, using the appropriate agency or institutional history form.
- Conduct a physical assessment, using the appropriate agency or institutional physical assessment form.
- Interview significant other persons who are present with the patient.
- Follow the agency or institution reporting policy and procedure. If a crime has been committed, notify local law enforcement.

4. Implement interventions and services
   - Abuse protection support
   - Respite care
   - Additional support for other less frequent concerns

Reproduced from Daly, J. M. (2011). Evidence-based practice guideline: Elder abuse prevention. *Journal of Gerontological Nursing, 37*(11), 11–17. Reproduced with permission of SLACK Incorporated.

> Evaluate risk factor for possible human immunodeficiency virus (HIV) exposure; if perpetrator can be tested, it is the recommended first step. If perpetrator cannot be tested, postexposure prophylaxis with a 28-day course of zidovudine within 72 hours of assault is advised.

> Medications for adults, as an empiric antimicrobial regimen for chlamydia, gonorrhea, and trichomonas
   - Ceftriaxone intramuscularly in a single dose *OR* cefixime orally in a single dose
     PLUS
   - Metronidazole orally in a single dose
     PLUS
   - Azithromycin orally in a single dose *OR* doxycycline orally twice daily for 7 days
   (CDC Sexual Assault, 2015b)

Each state has provisions on reporting elder abuse (see **Table 24-8**). There are reporting exemptions that protect the victim's information. Such situations include when there is a legal privilege between attorney–client, clergy–penitent or victim–(community-based) advocate. It is the victim's privilege, and only the victim can waive it (NCall, n.d.a).

Additionally, the victim must meet specific guidelines for the abuse to require mandatory reporting; otherwise, the reporter is breaching victim's confidentiality. When specific guidelines are not met, the victim must give written and informed consent (NCall, n.d.b).

The following states designated that certain persons are *required* to report to adult protective services (Table 24-8).

Reporting elder abuse is an obligation of healthcare providers. Elderly adults, by the nature of their increased health problems, visit hospitals and doctors' offices frequently. This means that healthcare providers, and especially nurses, have a greater opportunity than others to recognize when elder abuse may be occurring.

TABLE 24-8   Mandatory Reporting States with Specific Legislation

Alabama	Kentucky	Oklahoma
Alaska	Louisiana	Oregon
Arizona	Maine	Pennsylvania
Arkansas	Maryland	Rhode Island
California	Massachusetts	South Carolina
Colorado	Michigan	South Dakota
Connecticut	Minnesota	Tennessee
Delaware	Mississippi	Texas
District of Columbia	Missouri	Utah
Florida	Montana	Vermont
Georgia	Nebraska	Virginia
Hawaii	Nevada	Washington
Idaho	New Hampshire	West Virginia
Illinois	New Mexico	Wisconsin
Indiana	North Carolina	Wyoming
Iowa	Ohio	
Kansas		

Data from New York County District Attorney's Office & NAPSA Elder Financial Exploitation Advisory Board. (2013). 2013 Nationwide survey of mandatory reporting requirements for elderly and/or vulnerable persons. Retrieved from http://www.napsa-now.org/wp-content/uploads/2014/11/Mandatory-Reporting-Chart-Updated-FINAL.pdf

For cases that occur in institutions, often the agency that licenses the residential facility is the State Department of Health. It is the gerontological nurse's responsibility to know the appropriate course of action in the state in which he or she practices. Proper follow-through, with adequate security protection for the abuse victim and the abuse reporter and with appropriate interventions, must be in place.

Sometimes healthcare providers do not report abuse because of fear of repercussion, especially if the investigation turns out to be negative. To combat this fear, geriatric nurses need to become very knowledgeable and comfortable with the laws in their state and adult protective services regulations. A person will likely not get into trouble for reporting suspicions of abuse. In fact, there will be greater blame for failure to report if the scenario turns out to be real. Forty-four states have a provision for penalties for failure to report elder abuse. Iowa is the only state that has mandatory education for reporters.

The gerontological nurse also should work in collaboration with other members of the healthcare team, notably physicians, social workers, chaplains, and psychiatrists, to help determine whether elder abuse is present. Interviews with the victim and the possible offender should be done separately. Benefits of the care team include support during difficult decisions; reduction of duplicity, burnout, and workload; improved safety for the victims; and earlier intervention (Brandt, Dyer, Heisler, Otto, & Thomas, 2007). The team should meet with victim and the reporter, notifying him or her of the intent to report.

The nurse's core responsibility is to report suspected elder abuse, not to confirm the abuse. The nurse does not need to analyze the intention of the abuser. The nurse's role is to protect the rights of older adults, treating them with dignity and respect, while providing appropriate care.

Summary

All gerontological nurses should be educated in the prevention, detection, and treatment of elder abuse. Content on this topic should be included in all basic nursing programs. Better mechanisms are needed for reporting abuse and neglect of older adults. Nurses should be aware of the reporting laws for the state in which they reside and practice.

Elder abuse occurs across many socioeconomics groups and settings. Older adults, particularly those with dementia, are often marginalized and stripped of their dignity in today's society. This is our duty, our obligation, and our privilege as gerontological nurses to protect the treasure of our older generation and value all that they have to offer us. The responsibility rests with all of us. The gerontological nurse can lead the way.

Clinical Reasoning Exercises

1. Have you ever worked with a patient, resident, or older adult living in the community who was a victim of mistreatment or abuse? If so, what type of mistreatment was it?
2. Using the case studies presented in this chapter, identify the various types of elder abuse.
3. What type of abuse do you think is most prevalent in the areas where you live and work? Why?
4. Of the risk factors for elder abuse identified in this chapter, which are the ones that you have seen the most in older adults in the clinical setting? In the community? In long-term care?
5. Find the phone number and Website for adult protective services for your state. Browse the Website.

Personal Reflections

1. What is one strategy that you could use from this chapter to prevent elder abuse or mistreatment in the patient or resident population where you work?
2. How do you feel when you hear about abuse of older adults in the media?
3. If you recognized financial abuse of an older parent or grandparent occurring in your family, what action would you take?
4. What are the laws regarding reporting suspected abuse in the state in which you live?

References

Baker, M. W., LaCroix, A. Z., Wu, C., Cochrane, B. B., Wallace, R., & Woods, N. F. (2009). Mortality risk associated with physical and verbal abuse in women aged 50 to 79. *Journal of the American Geriatrics Society, 57*(10), 1799–1809.

Barnett, O. W., Miller-Perrin, C. L., & Perrin, R. D. (1997). *Family violence across the lifespan.* Thousand Oaks, CA: Sage.

Bond, M. C., & Butler, K. B. (2013). Elder abuse and neglect. *Clinics in Geriatric Medicine, 29*(1), 257–273.

Brandt, B., Dyer, C. B., Heisler, C. J., Otto, J. M., & Thomas, R. W. (2007) *Elder abuse detection and intervention: A collaborative approach,* New York, NY: Springer.

Buckwalter, S. C., Campbell, J., Gerdner, L. A., & Garand, L. (1996). Elder mistreatment among rural family caregivers of persons with Alzheimer's disease and related disorders. *Journal of Family Nursing 2*(3), 249–265.

Canadian Network for the Prevention of Elder Abuse. (2016). Prevention. Retrieved from http://www.cnpea.ca/en/what-is-elder-abuse/prevention

Centers for Disease Control and Prevention. (2015a). Elder abuse: Consequences. Retrieved from http://www .cdc.gov/violenceprevention/elderabuse/consequences.html

Centers for Disease Control and Prevention. (2015b). Sexual assault and abuse and STDs. Retrieved from http:// www.cdc.gov/std/tg2015/sexual-assault.htm

Cohen, M. (2008). Research assessment of elder neglect and its risk factors in a hospital setting. *Internal Medicine Journal, 38*(9), 704–707.

Cooper, C., Katona, C., Finne-Soveri, H., Topinkova, E., Carpenter, G. I., & Livingston, G. (2006). Indicators of elder abuse: A crossnational comparison of psychiatric morbidity and other determinants in the Ad-HOC study. *American Journal of Geriatric Psychiatry, 14*(6), 489–497.

Cooper, C., Mandela, M., Katona, C., & Livingston, G. (2008). Screening for elder abuse in dementia in the LASER-AD study: Prevalence, correlates and validation of instruments. *International Journal of Geriatric Psychiatry, 23*(3), 283–288.

Daly, J. M. (2010). *Elder abuse prevention.* Retrieved from http://m2.wyanokecdn.com/fc2950712fe18a26caf6c92f937b8c4e .pdf

Daly, J. M. (2011). Evidence-based practice guideline: Elder abuse prevention. *Journal of Gerontological Nursing, 37*(11), 11–17.

Decalmer, P., & Glendenning, F. (Eds.). (1993). *The mistreatment of elderly people.* London, UK: Sage.

Dong, X., Simon, M., Rajan, K., & Evans, D. A. (2011). Association of cognitive function and risk for elder abuse in a community-dwelling population. *Dementia & Geriatric Cognitive Disorders, 32*(3), 209–215.

Dyer, C. B., Pavlik, V. N., Murphy, K. P., & Hyman, D. J. (2000). The high prevalence of depression and dementia in elder abuse or neglect. *Journal of the American Geriatrics Society, 48*(2), 205–208.

Dyer, C. B., Goodwin, J. S., Pickens-Pace, S., Burnett, J., & Kelly, P. A. (2007). Self-neglect among the elderly: A model based on more than 500 patients seen by a geriatric medicine team. *American Journal of Public Health, 97*(9), 1671–1676.

Frost, M. H., & Willette, K. (1994). Risk for abuse/neglect: Documentation of assessment data and diagnoses. *Journal of Gerontological Nursing, 29*(8), 37–45.

Fulmer, T. (2012). *Elder mistreatment assessment.* Retrieved from https://consultgeri.org/try-this/general -assessment/issue-15.pdf

Fulmer, T., & Greenberg, S. (2012). *Elder mistreatment and abuse.* Retrieved from https://consultgeri.org /geriatric-topics/elder-mistreatment-and-abuse

Gibbons, S., Lauder, W., & Ludwick, R. (2006). Self-neglect: A proposed new NANDA diagnosis. *International Journal of Nursing Terminologies and Classifications, 17*(1), 10–18.

Hildreth, C. J. (2011). Elder abuse. *Journal of the American Medical Association, 306*(5), 568.

Hoover, R. M., and Polson, M. (2014). Detecting Elder Abuse and Neglect: Assessment and Intervention. *American Family Physician, 89*(6), 453–460.

Jina, R., Jewkes, R., Vetten, L., Christofides, N., Sigsworth, R., & Loots, L. (2015). Genito-anal injury patterns and associated factors in rape survivors in an urban province of South Africa: A cross-sectional study. *BMC Womens Health, 27*(15), 29.

Johannesen, M., & LoGiudice, D. (2016). Elder abuse: A systematic review of risk factors in community-dwelling elders. *Age and Ageing, 45*(1), 1–7.

Lachs, M. S., & Pillemer, K. A. (2015). Elder abuse. *The New England Journal of Medicine, 373*(20), 1947–1956.

Lachs, M. S., Williams, C. S., O'Brien, S., Pillemer, K. A., & Charleson, M. E. (1998). The mortality of elder mistreatment. *Journal of the American Medical Society, 280*(5), 428–432.

Mauk, K. L. (2011). Ethical perspectives on self-neglect among older adults. *Rehabilitation Nursing, 36*(2), 60–65.

McGarry J., & Simpson, C. (2011). Domestic abuse and older women: Exploring the opportunities for service development and care delivery. *Journal of Adult Protection, 13*(6), 294–301.

MetLife. (2012a). *The MetLife study of elder financial abuse.* Retrieved from https://www.metlife.com/mmi /research/elder-financial-abuse.html#keyfindings

MetLife. (2012b). *Broken trust: Elders, family, & finances.* Retrieved from http://www.metlife.com/mmi/research /broken-trust-elder-abuse.html#findings

National Center on Elder Abuse. (n.d.). Identifying elder abuse: Tools, techniques, and guidelines for screening and assessment. Retrieved from http://www.ncea.aoa.gov/main_site/library/cane/CANE_Series/CANE_EA _Assessment2.aspx

National Center on Elder Abuse. (2010). Why should I care about elder abuse? Retrieved from http://www.ncea .aoa.gov/ncearoot/Main_Site/pdf/publication/NCEA_WhatIsAbuse-2010.pdf

National Committee for the Prevention of Elder Abuse. (2008). What is elder abuse? Retrieved from http://www .preventelderabuse.org/elderabuse/

National Institute of Justice. (2008). Potential markers for elder mistreatment. Retrieved from http://www.nij .gov/topics/crime/elder-abuse/pages/potential-markers.aspx

National Research Council. (2003). Elder mistreatment: Abuse, neglect and exploitation in an aging America. Retrieved from http://www.nap.edu/openbook.php?isbn=0309084342

NCall. (n.d.a). Mandatory reporting. Retrieved from http://www.ncall.us/content/mr

NCall. (n.d.b). Respecting elders, protecting elders: Untangling the mystery of what sexual assault advocates need to know about the mandatory reporting of elder abuse. Retrieved from http://www.ncall.us/category/tags /mandatory-reporting

New York County District Attorney's Office & National Pension Scheme Authority Elder Financial Exploitation Advisory Board. (2013). 2013 Nationwide survey of mandatory reporting requirements for elderly and/or vulnerable persons. Retrieved from http://www.napsa-now.org/wp-content/uploads/2014/11/Mandatory -Reporting-Chart-Updated-FINAL.pdf

Pillemer, K. A., & Suitor, J. J. (1992). Violence and violent feelings: What causes them among family caregivers? *Journal of Gerontology: Social Sciences, 47*(4), 165–172.

Pritchard, J. (1995). *The abuse of older people: A training manual for detection and prevention.* London, UK: Jessica Kingsley.

Pritchard, J. (1996). Darkness visible . . . elder abuse. *Nursing Times, 92*(42), 26–31.

Quinn, M. J., & Tomita, S. K. (1986). *Elder abuse and neglect.* New York, NY: Springer.

Reyes-Ortiz, C. A. (2006). Self-neglect as a geriatric syndrome. *Journal of the American Geriatrics Society, 54*(12), 1945–1975.

Rosen, T., Pillemer, K., & Lachs, M. (2008). Resident-to-resident aggression in long-term care facilities: An understudied problem. *Aggression and Violent Behavior, 13*(2), 77–87.

Saveman, B., Hallberg, I. R., & Norberg, A. (1996). Narratives by district nurses about elder abuse within families. *Clinical Nursing Research, 5,* 220–236.

Sengstock, M. C., & Barrett, S. A. (1992). Abuse and neglect of the elderly in family settings. In J. Campbell & J. Humphreys (Eds.), *Nursing care of the survivors of family violence* (pp. 173–208). St. Louis, MO: Mosby.

Stark, S. W. (2011). Blind, deaf, and dumb: Why elder abuse goes unidentified. *Nursing Clinics of North America, 46*(4), 431–436.

Thobaben, M. (1996). Beyond physical care: Elder abuse and neglect. *Home Care Provider, 5,* 267–269.

Tomlin, S. K. (1989). *Abuse of elderly people: An unnecessary and preventable problem.* London, UK: British Geriatrics Society.

U.S. Administration on Aging. (2010). Older American's Act. Retrieved from http://www.aoa.acl.gov/AoA _programs/OAA/index.aspx

U.S. Administration on Aging. (2014). What is elder abuse? Retrieved from http://www.aoa .acl.gov/aoa_programs /elder_rights/ea_prevention/whatisea.aspx

Wierucka, C., & Goodridge, D. (1996). Vulnerable in a safe place: Institutional elder abuse. *Canadian Journal of Nursing Administration, 9*(3), 82–104.

Wilson, J. S. (1992). Granny dumping: A case of caregiver stress or a problem relative? *Home Healthcare Nurse, 10*(3), 69–70.

World Health Organization. (2016). Elder abuse. Retrieved from http://www.who.int/ageing/projects/elder_abuse/en/

Zhang, Z., Schiamberg, L. B., Oehmke, J., Barboza, G. E., Griffore, R. J., Post, L. A., . . . & Mastin, T. (2011). Neglect of older adults in Michigan nursing homes. *Journal of Elder Abuse and Neglect, 23*(1), 58–74.

For a full suite of assignments and additional learning activities, see the access code at the front of your book.

CHAPTER 25

Pain Management and Alternative Health Modalities

Carole A. Pepa

(Competencies 8, 9, 12, 15, 18)

LEARNING OBJECTIVES

At the end of this chapter, the reader will be able to

> Describe pain in relation to duration and types.
> Explain the difference in management between the types of pain.
> Describe how to perform a pain assessment.
> Explain the benefits and challenges of the most common types of pain assessment instruments.
> Explain how to overcome the barriers to pain management.
> Explain the pathophysiology and management differences between neuropathic and nociceptive pain.
> Explain the World Health Organization pain ladder.
> Describe the difference among complementary, alternative, and integrative health.
> Explain the pros and cons of using natural products.
> Discuss mind–body therapies and how they might be used.
> Discuss the state of evidence for complementary health approaches.
> Explain the difference between naturopathic and homeopathic medicines.
> Compare Ayurvedic medicine principles with traditional Chinese medicine principles.

KEY TERMS

Acupuncture	Ceiling effect
Acute pain	Chiropractic practice
Addiction	Chronic (persistent) pain
Adjuvant	Cupping
Ayurveda	Curative treatment
Breakthrough pain	Dosha

Homeopathy	Qi (chi)
Integrative health care	Qigong
Massage therapy	Relaxation techniques
Meditation	Tai Chi
Meridians	Tolerance
Mind–body medicine	Traditional Chinese Medicine
Moxibustion	Visceral pain
Natural products	Whole medical systems
Naturopathic medicine	Yang
Neuropathic	Yin
Nociceptive	

As most nurses are aware, the population of older adults is increasing globally, and by the year 2030, adults over the age of 65 years will make up 20% of the U.S. population (Centers for Disease Control and Prevention [CDC], 2013). With aging comes both joys and health concerns. The prevalence of pain increases with age (Lynch, 2015), and the burden of disease and disability is greatest for the elderly.

Currently, the Joint Commission (Baker, 2016) has estimated that over 76 million people in the United States have acute and chronic pain. In addition, it is estimated that between 18% and 57% of nonistitutionalized older adults in the United States experience chronic pain (Institute of Medicine [IMO], 2011). Although estimates are difficult to validate because of underreporting and inconsistent definitions, it is evident that as the older population increases, so will the number of persons experiencing pain.

This phenomenon will create a challenge for nurses and other healthcare providers. Pain affects the pathophysiological, social, psychological, and quality dimensions of life; it is also subjective and personal. The challenge for nurses and other healthcare providers is to assess and treat the pain through the perspective of the older adult patient. Unfortunately, healthcare professionals, including nurses, tend to underestimate the existence of pain in the elderly. One of the reasons for inadequate management of pain is the lack of understanding of what pain is: a personal phenomenon that cannot be experienced by any other individual in the exact same way.

Unfortunately, some elderly persons will not accurately report pain because they do not want to be perceived as complainers, they feel it is inevitable, they fear more diagnostic tests and medicines, and they fear losing their independence (American Geriatrics Society [AGS], 2009). Therefore, pain is undiagnosed and undertreated in the elderly population. Subsequently, pain that is unrelieved can affect the elder's well-being in more ways than the discomfort experienced. Additional possible consequences of persistent pain are listed in **Box 25-1**.

Descriptions of Pain
Duration of Pain

There are two distinct categories of pain in relation to duration: *acute pain* and *persistent (chronic) pain*. The acute phase of pain persists for a relatively short time, usually hours to days. It is perceived as a temporary sensory experience and can be of benefit because it signals the body that it is not in homeostatic balance. However, when severe, it can have negative physiological and pathophysiological effects. Acute pain can be secondary to tissue damage, illness, trauma, surgery, or any other painful medical procedure. The acute pain phase intensity will most often terminate after the cause of the pain has been identified and managed (AGS, 2009).

BOX 25-1   Potential Consequences of Persistent Pain in the Elderly

- Poorer quality of life
- Worse self-reported health
- Functional impairment
- Falls
- Depression
- Decreased appetite
- Impaired sleep
- Social isolation
- Limitation or inability to perform activities of daily living

Data from Gagliese, L. (2009). Pain and aging: Emergence of a new subfield of pain research. *The Journal of Pain, 10*(4), 343–353; Malec, M., & Shega, J.W. (2015). Pain management in the elderly. *Medical Clinics of North America, 99,* 337–350.

Persistent (chronic) pain continues for a prolonged period time and may or may not be associated with a specific disease process (AGS, 2009, p. 1331). The terms "persistent pain" and "chronic pain" may be used interchangeably in the literature, but the term "persistent pain" is a more current term and has fewer negative connotations (AGS, 2009). The duration of persistent pain is usually greater than 3 months and is multidimensional in nature. It disrupts sleep, socialization, appetite, and the ability to perform activities of normal living. It may be *nociceptive*, *neuropathic*, or both. Common sources of chronic pain in the elderly can include injury, malignant conditions, and musculoskeletal disorders (e.g., arthritis, degenerative spine disorders). The goal in managing pain is different depending on the category of pain. In acute pain, the focus is on treating the cause of the pain, whereas in chronic pain, the emphasis is on reducing pain, improving function, and limiting the possibility for disability.

Types of Pain

The three major components of the nervous system that cause the sensation and perception of pain are the (1) afferent (reception), (2) central nervous system (perception), and (3) efferent pathways (reaction). The type of pain an individual experiences is controlled by the location of the sensitized nerve fibers. A description of different types of pain is included in **Table 25-1**.

Mechanism of Pain

Knowledge of the pathways of pain may help in understanding how to best manage pain. The sensation of nociceptive pain is processed through four pathways: (1) transduction, (2) transmission, (3) perception, and (4) modulation (Rodriguez, 2015).

Transduction begins when noxious stimuli (e.g., broken radius) activate nociceptors. These receptors then convert the stimuli into an electrical current (action potential) by transduction (Rodriguez, 2015). Transmission is the movement of the action potentials from the site of noxious stimulus to the dorsal horn at the base of the brain by way of dorsal root ganglion. It only takes microseconds for the signal to be conducted from the injury to the brain (Rodriguez, 2015). In the third phase, when pain is perceived, neurotransmitters are released from nociceptor endings in the brain and trigger signals to the dorsal horn neurons (Rodriguez, 2015). Through ascending nociceptive pathways, the signal is transmitted from the dorsal horn neurons to the higher axes of the brain, where it is perceived as pain (Rodriguez, 2015). The final process of the pain pathway is modulation. Modulation is the inhibitory pathway that descends from the brain to the periphery. A release of norepinephrine, serotonin, and other substances bind to and inhibit the nociceptors; this limits the pain response (Rodriguez, 2015).

Neuropathic pain is a more complex clinical situation (Dimitroulas, Duarte, Behura, Kitas, & Raphael, 2014). Unlike nociceptive pain, which is protective, neuropathic pain is not protective and does not always require a stimulus (D'Arcy, 2014). Neuropathic pain indicates pathophysiological changes in peripheral and central nervous

TABLE 25-1   Types of Pain

Type	Definition	Additional Information
Nociceptive pain 1. Somatic pain 2. *Visceral pain*	Caused by tissue injury. Originates in the muscles, joints, connective tissues, and bones and usually manifests as dull, throbbing, or aching. Originates in the internal organs and may manifest as a squeezing or deep ache (Faull & Blankley, 2015).	Responds to traditional pain interventions, such as analgesics, and nonpharmacological methods Include arthritis (bone and joint), and **myofascial** (muscle) pain. Includes pain from gallstones, appendicitis, and pancreatitis
Neuropathic pain	Caused by a pathophysiological dysfunction of the nervous system and described as a burning, numbness, or tingling sensation that feels electrically charged, like a shock.	Does not respond well to traditional interventions such as nonsteroidal antiinflammatory drugs (NSAIDs) or opioids and requires combination therapy with adjuvant medications such as anticonvulsants, antidepressants, and antiarrhythmic drugs. Examples include phantom limb pain and postherpetic neuralgia
Breakthrough pain	Increases above the level of pain addressed by the prescribed analgesic and includes end-of-dose failure and incident pain (Pain Types, 2015).	Reported by many with persistent pain
Incident pain	Triggered by specific activity such as physical therapy.	Treated by medicating with an analgesic before the activity
Allodynia	Felt as painful although nonpainful stimulus and normal-appearing tissue.	Common in neuropathic pain conditions. Example is an older adult who feels discomfort with bed sheets resting on legs or feet (Pain Types, 2015).

systems (Blumstein & Barkley, 2015). The following mechanisms can modify the nervous system and contribute to neuropathic pain:

> Atypical nerve redevelopment (causing a production of makeshift release of impulses leading to a perception of pain)
> Amplified communication of membrane sodium channels (causing a decrease in the threshold of stimulation)
> Temporary loss of inhibition on modulating processes (may lead to a decrease in perceived threshold of pain and perceived increase in the pain experience)
> Reduced availability of μ-opioid peptide receptors (Rodriguez, 2015, p. 341).

These different mechanisms can cause various symptoms that make diagnosis and treatment difficult.

Assessment of Pain
Occurrence of Pain

The elderly experience with pain can be atypical and complex. Several conditions may be present simultaneously, which makes assessment and treatment more challenging. Pain may be present when not normally expected and absent when normally expected to be present. Therefore, the most important aspect of pain management is a comprehensive assessment including a thorough history and physical examination as well as a review of laboratory and diagnostic results. These assessments are especially important for older persons because effective pain management often depends on the appropriate treatment of underlying disease or illness. An assessment should also include the following:

> Location of the pain
> Effect of pain on activities of daily living (ADL) and physical function
> Level of pain at rest and during activity
> Provoking and precipitating factors
> Medication usage, effectiveness, and adverse effects
> Quality of pain (in the individual's words: achy, hurting)
> Radiation of pain—does it extend beyond the site?
> Severity of the pain (intensity, 0 to 10 scale)
> Pain-related symptoms
> Timing (constant, occasional)

CLINICAL TIP

A comprehensive assessment is the most important aspect for successful pain management.

Because pain is a subjective experience, self-report is the most reliable and accurate information (Tracy & Morrison, 2013. Many physical assessment books recommend using the mnemonic PQRST to assist in remembering how to ask questions regarding pain. The mnemonic may differ from text to text, but the meaning is similar. The P stands for the place of the pain (location); Q, quality of the pain (stabbing, aching, dull, etc.); R, radiation (does the pain go anywhere?); S, severity of the pain (influence of pain on ADLs and responses to medications); and T, the timing (duration, frequency, how long the pain lasts) (MacSorley et al., 2014).

CLINICAL TIP

Age-related changes place the elderly at increased risk of pain-related complications.

Types of Instruments

Although there are several instruments to assess for pain, the distinction between assessment and measurement in pain is not clearly defined. The application of measurement usually refers to a specific aspect for pain, such as intensity, whereas the assessment aspect encompasses the entire pain experience.

Selection of the appropriate pain assessment tools in the elderly population, although difficult, is necessary for diagnostic efforts, proper pain management, and evaluation of efficacy in treatment modalities. Different types of measurements assess pain through different lenses. It is important that the elderly are able to respond to and use the instrument that will best provide an accurate assessment of their pain intensity. Issues such as cognition, psychological limitations, culture, and communication disorders may affect the older person's ability to use any one particular instrument to rate pain. **Table 25-2** describes different types of instruments used to measure pain. Every assessment instrument has strengths and weaknesses, but consideration should be given to the following two factors: the instrument needs to meet the cognitive and sensory needs of the individual, and the instrument must have proven reliability and validity (**Figure 25-1**).

TABLE 25-2   Examples of Measures of Pain

Numeric Rating Scales	Utilizes numbers to quantify the intensity of the pain experience for the person. Scale ranges from 0 to 10, with 0 indicating no pain; 5 represents moderate pain; and 10 represents the worst pain ever experienced. This scale may also be color coded, with blue (0) representing no pain and increasing to red (10).
Visual Rating Scales	Have pictures of human anatomy to help the person explain the intensity and location of the pain experienced. Wong Baker FACES Pain Scales is one of the most popular. The scale range is 0 to 5 and is helpful for elderly individuals who sometimes may not have the cognitive or verbal ability to explain how they are feeling.
Verbal Descriptor Rating Scales	Uses word descriptors to help describe pain levels. The individual is asked questions and responds verbally using descriptors such as mild, moderate, severe, no pain, a lot of pain, discomforting, distressing, horrible, and excruciating. Each term has a preestablished meaning to most individuals.
McGill Pain Questionnaire (MPQ) long or short form	Assesses quality and intensity of pain associated especially with sensory and affective qualities. Both forms are multidimensional and have 15 words that describe 11 sensory and 4 emotional descriptors that are each rated on a 4-point scales ranging from 0 for not affected to 3 for severely affected by the pain experience. The SF MPQ-2 assesses major symptoms of both neuropathic and nonneuropathic pain.
Pain Assessment in Advanced Dementia (PAINAD)	Evaluates items related to breathing, body posturing, facial grimacing, increased vocalization, agitation, and consolability. These behavioral factors assist in the scoring of 0 to 10 for pain intensity and quality of control for individuals with advanced dementia who cannot self report pain.
Checklist for Nonverbal Pain Indicator (CNPI)	Includes six pain behavioral items commonly observed in older adults: Breathing, posturing, facial grimacing, nonverbal vocalizations, and wincing. Each item is scored at rest and on movement, with a range of 0 to 6 points for each situation, but there is no interpretation of total score. Trending of the score may help interpret the efficacy of pain interventions over time. Can be reviewed at http://www.Kentuckyonehealth.org/documents/Nursing/CNPI.pdf
Pain Assessment Checklist for Seniors with Limited Ability to Communicate (PACSLAC)	Consists of 60 items organized into 4 categories: Facial expressions, activity/body movement, social/personality/mood indicators, and physiological indicators/sleeping changes/eating/vocal behavior, Each item is scored as present or absent. Can be reviewed at http://www.geriatricpain.org/Content/Assessment/Impaired/Pages/PACSLAC.aspx.
Behavioral Pain Scale (BPS)	Uses facial expression, upper limb movement, and mechanical ventilator compliance to determine pain. Each component is scored on a scale of 1 to 4. A score of 5 or higher indicates pain. This can be used with noncommunicative critically ill patients.
Critical-Care Pain Observation Tool (CPOT)	Uses four behavioral categories associated with pain: Facial expression, body movements, muscle tension, ventilator compliance, or vocalization. Each component is scored 0 to 2. A score of 3 or above represents pain (Reardon, Anger, Szumita, 2015).

0	1	2	3	4	5	6	7	8	9	10
No Pain					Moderate Pain					Worst Pain

Figure 25-1 Example of a simple pain scale.

BOX 25-2   Possible Signs of Pain in Cognitively Impaired and Nonverbal Patients

- Elevated blood pressure
- Tachycardia
- Tachypnea
- Dilated pupils
- Retention of secretions
- Muscle spasms
- Delayed gastric and bowel function
- Grimacing
- Moaning

- Agitation
- Restlessness
- Sweating
- Withdrawal movements when repositioning
- Guarded posturing
- Social avoidance behavior
- Fatigue
- Anorexia

CLINICAL TIP

Either a visual or numerical rating scale will measure the intensity of pain.

Challenges for the Impaired Elderly

The cognitively impaired and the nonverbal elderly patients require instruments different from others because their behavior is different. Instead of complaining about pain, the individuals most often exhibit visible physiological and behavioral signs of distress. Some signs of pain in cognitively impaired and nonverbal patients are listed in **Box 25-2**.

Barriers to Appropriate Management

There can be many types of barriers impeding the process for accurate assessment and appropriate management of pain in the elderly. Even though there is no clear understanding on age-associated changes in pain perception, elderly individuals and their caregivers, as well as healthcare providers, often believe that pain is a normal part of aging. The barriers to why pain in the elderly goes undiagnosed and untreated can be divided into three major sources (1) healthcare provider, (2) system, (3) patient and caregiver (AGS, 2009). Some barriers to adequate pain management are listed in **Box 25-3**.

CLINICAL TIP

Barriers to why the elderly go undiagnosed and untreated can be divided into three major sources: healthcare provider, healthcare system, and patient and caregiver barriers.

BOX 25-3   Barriers to Pain Management in the Elderly

Healthcare Provider Barriers

- Lack of education regarding pain assessment and management
- Lack of education on the cultural beliefs about pain
- Concern regarding regulatory scrutiny about prescriptions
- Fear of opioid-related side effects
- Assumption that pain is part of the aging process and cannot be managed
- Lack of ability to assess pain in the cognitively impaired

Healthcare System Barriers

- Cost
- Time
- Cultural bias regarding opioid use
- Concern about pain medication overuse

Patient and Caregiver Barriers

- Fear of medication side effects
- Concerns related to addition
- Concerns that by discussing pain, they will be perceived as a "bad patient"
- Belief that pain is incurable and/or part of the aging process
- Seek *curative treatment* rather than palliative approaches
- Concerns that pain signifies disease progression

Data from Barriers to effective pain management. (2015). Retrieved from www.geriatricpain.org/Content/Education/Clinical/Documents/Barriers.pdf; Fitzcharles, M., Lussier, D., & Shir, Y. (2010). Management of chronic arthritis pain in the elderly. *Drugs & Aging, 27*, 471–490.

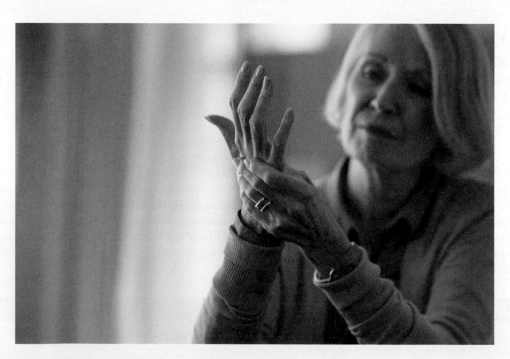

Figure 25-2 Musculoskeletal pain is common among older adults.
© Amble Design/Shutterstock

Cultural Considerations

Because pain is both a physical and emotional experience, adequate pain management also requires knowledge of cultural and ethnic beliefs about illness and pain. However, many healthcare providers feel unprepared to render culturally responsive approaches to assessment and treatment of pain and find management of pain in ethnically diverse patients challenging (Booker, Pasero, & Herr, 2015). Chapter 22 provides insights into culture and spirituality to assist the nurse in understanding the role these may play in an elder's perception of illness.

Misconceptions and Facts

Unfortunately, many healthcare providers, as well as the elderly and their family members, think pain is a natural occurrence of aging and chronic disease. This is one of several misconceptions about pain. In fact, pain in the elderly requires aggressive assessment, diagnosis, and management similar to that in younger individuals. Another misconception is that aging causes decreased pain sensitivity and perception when, in fact, research is conflicting regarding age-associated changes in pain perception, sensitivity, and tolerance (Kaye, Baluch, & Scott, 2010). As a result of this misconception, elderly patients may experience needless suffering and undertreatment of pain and its underlying cause(s) (American Pain Society [APS], 2008). Other myths about pain are listed in **Box 25-4**. Given the high prevalence of pain in the elderly population, pain should be assessed and monitored on a regular basis. To that end, the Joint Commission (Baker, 2016) has identified requirements that should be included in an organization's policies. These requirements are listed in **Box 25-5**.

Pain Management

Team Approach

An interdisciplinary team (IDT) is often the optimal approach to pain management. The team usually consists of the medical providers, nursing staff, physical and occupational therapists, psychologists, nutritionists, the patient and caregiver, and a social worker. The physician or nurse practitioner oversees the individual's medical management, prescribes medications, and monitors for changes in medical status. Nurses in the hospital, home, long-term care facility, clinic, or community setting have a key role in assessment, medication administration, evaluation, and patient education on appropriate use of medications and nonpharmacological treatments. The physical therapist assesses functional mobility and biomechanic abnormalities that may be contributing to pain and recommends therapeutic interventions to help improve strength, balance, and function. The occupational therapist works with the patient to reduce pain associated with the ADLs. Depression is often associated with chronic pain, so a psychologist is able to work with the patient on cognitive strategies to manage pain. Patients with pain may be overweight or undernourished, in which case the nutritional specialist can educate patients on appropriate dietary selections and requirements. The pharmacist in the hospital or community monitors patient medication usage and can identify potential drug–drug interactions that can interfere with treatment. The patient's spiritual counselor can help the patient understand the meaning of pain and support treatment recommendations. Ultimately, the pain management plan needs to address the patient's goals. The patient and family are essential members of the pain management team.

Pain management strategies do not differ significantly based on patient age; however, there are some general considerations when treating pain in older adults. Just as patients are reluctant to report pain, similar biases may exist related to treatment. Patients may perceive pain as normal or expected as one grows older and be reluctant to seek treatment. Older adults may be reluctant to take additional medications, so the treatment approach should include both pharmacological and nonpharmacological interventions (see **Box 25-6**). The key to success is to maximize patient participation in management of the treatment plan.

Pharmacological Modalities

Pharmacological therapy can be safe and effective, but before prescribing medications it is important to address the individual's cultural beliefs about medication usage. For example, it is not uncommon to encounter older

BOX 25-4   Common Myths about Pain in the Elderly

Myth: Pain is an unavoidable part of growing old.

Reality: Although pain is common after age 65 because of the prevalence of painful diseases in that age group, it is not inevitable. More importantly, it does not have to be tolerated; pain can be treated.

Myth: Patients with dementia are unable to report their pain.

Reality: Persons with dementia may be able to self-report pain. In addition, several pain rating scales have reliability and validity established for patients with dementia.

Myth: Pain is mostly an emotional or psychological problem.

Reality: There are physical reasons for pain. However, pain can cause emotional responses that can worsen a person's perception of pain. Pain is a physical and emotional response to stimuli.

Myth: Doctors and nurses are the true experts about pain.

Reality: The patient is the expert in his or her pain. Because pain is objective, it is best explained by the person who is experiencing it. When the older person cannot report pain because of physical or cognitive impairments, then those closest to the patient should be consulted.

Myth: It is important to be stoic about pain.

Reality: Being stoic prevents healthcare providers from identifying and treating the cause of the pain. Older adults who "don't want to be a bother" should be educated that reporting pain is the only way to treat it. Older adults should realize that they have a right to have the pain treated and that by reporting it, they are not complaining or a bother.

Myth: Painful conditions cause the same amount and type of pain in all people

Reality: Pain perception is affected by many factors such as previous injury and experiences, stress, fatigue, and emotions. Therefore, two people can respond differently to the same noxious stimuli.

Myth: Not much can be done to relieve the pain in nursing home residents

Reality: Chronic pain management often requires a multimodal approach including both pharmacological and nonpharmacological strategies. Finding the best therapeutic regimen for an individual may take several trials to find the most effective strategies.

Modified from Mary Ersek, PhD, RN. (n.d.). Common myths about pain — and the reality. Retrieved from www.geriatricpain.org/Content /Education/Clinician/Pages/PainMyths.aspx. Reprinted by permission of Mary Ersek, PhD, RN.

BOX 25-5   The Joint Commission Recommendations for Pain Policies

1. The hospital conducts a comprehensive pain assessment that is consistent with its scope of care, treatment, and the patient's condition.
2. The hospital uses methods to assess pain that are consistent with the patient's age, condition, and ability to understand.
3. The hospital reassesses and responds to the patient's pain, based on its reassessment criteria.
   a. The hospital either treats the patient's pain or refers the patient for treatment.

Note: Treatment strategies may include pharmacological and nonpharmacological approaches (Baker, 2016, para 4).

Reproduced from Baker, D.W. (2016). Joint Commission statement on pain management. Retrieved from https://www.jointcommission .org/topics/pain_management.aspx.

BOX 25-6   Examine These Resources on Pain

Resources on Pain

American Academy of Pain Management:
https://www.aapainmanage.org/

American Academy of Pain Medicine:
http://www.painmed.org

American Pain Society:
http://www.ampainsoc.org

American Geriatrics Society:
http://www.americangeriatrics.org

Geriatric Pain:
http://www.geriatricpain.org

Health Topics A-Z:
https://nccih.nih.gov/health/atoz.htm

Herbs at a Glance:
https://nccih.nih.gov/health/herbsataglance.htm

The Homoeopathic Pharmacopoeia of the United States:
http://www.hpus.com/

Information for Consumers on Using Dietary Supplements:
http://www.fda.gov/food/dietarysupplements/usingdietarysupplements/default.htm

National Institutes of Health Senior Health:
http://nihseniorhealth.gov

Pain:
https://nccih.nih.gov/health/pain

adults who are reluctant to use pain medication for fear of *addiction*. They may recount a story from their own past or that of a relative or friend who experienced problems with pain medications, or they may express concern after hearing media accounts about pain medication abuse. It is useful to explain the difference between addiction and *tolerance* as well as how the medications work. It is not uncommon for an older adult to follow a cultural pain remedy, so it is important to assess all therapeutic approaches a patient could be using. In addition, concern over expense may prevent an older patient from filling a prescription or taking it as ordered. This is an area that should be explored with the patient and the family. The World Health Organization (WHO) has identified a three-step pain ladder for pain relief **Figure 25-3**. Although it was originally created as a guide for treating pain in cancer patients, it is now an accepted guide for choosing analgesics for relief of pain with any diagnosis (Malec & Shega, 2015). Step 1 corresponds to mild intensity level pain (1 to 3 rating on scale) and suggests the use of acetaminophen or NSAIDs or both with or without adjuvant agents. Step 2 is for patients with moderate intensity pain (4 to 6 rating on scale). This step recommends adding a weak opioid alone or in combination with a nonopioid (such as used in Step 1), with or without an *adjuvant* agent. An example would be codeine with acetaminophen. Step 3, for patients with severe pain (7 to 10 on a rating scale), suggests the use of a strong opioid, with or without an adjuvant agent. Examples would be morphine, oxycodone, and hydromorphone. When using the WHO pain ladder, patients with episodic (acute) pain, such as postsurgical pain, would start higher on the ladder and progress down the ladder, whereas a patient with persistent pain would begin at Step 1 and progress up the ladder. The WHO pain ladder provides a guide for pain management, but the nurse still has to perform frequent and thorough assessments to determine if the pharmacological interventions match the patient's pain level.

In steps two and three of the WHO pain ladder, an adjuvant drug may be added to the opioid to enhance the analgesic effects of the other medications. Examples of some of the adjuvant drugs that may be used to treat pain include, but are not limited to the following (Kaye et al., 2010, p. 185):

Antidepressants

Anticonvulsants

Local anesthetics

Corticosteroids

Baclofen

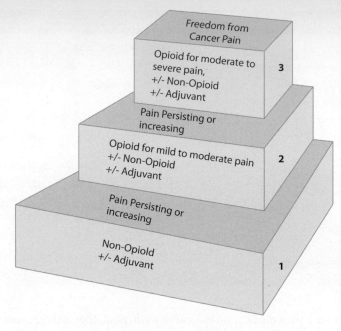

Figure 25-3 Who Pain Ladder.
Reproduced from WHO. (2016). WHO's cancer pain ladder for adults. Retrieved from www.who.int/cancer/palliative/painladder/en/

Muscle relaxants

Neuroleptics

Topical creams and gels

Table 25-3 lists some of the commonly used medications with side effects and concerns in acute, persistent, and end-of-life pain relief. This table is not an endorsement of any therapeutic agent, nor is it intended to reflect a hierarchy of treatment. Similarly, it is not meant to be an exhaustive listing.

Regardless of the medication prescribed as part of the pain management regimen, the nurse must be alert for side effects. The normal physiological changes in aging may have an effect on how the medications work and intensify the side effects. **Table 25-4** describes some of the common pharmacological concerns and physiological changes associated with normal aging.

In response to concerns about the misuse of opioids, the CDC has issued guidelines for prescribing opioids for chronic pain. Although opioids are the therapies of choice when the benefits outweigh the risks, these guidelines established that nonpharmacological and nonopioid therapies are preferred for chronic pain when they are as efficacious (Dowell, Haegerich, & Chou, 2016). The inclusion of nonpharmacological therapies emphasizes the need for nurses to be knowledgeable about nonpharmalological therapies to both assess and teach about their safety and effectiveness.

Nonpharmacological Modalities

The use of healthcare approaches developed outside mainstream Western or conventional medicine is becoming more common in the United States. According to the National Center for Complementary and Integrative Health (NCCIH) (2015a), more than 30% of adults and 12% of the children use these modalities. To reflect this trend, the National Center for Complementary and Alternative Medicine (NCCAM) was renamed the National Center for Complementary and Integrative Medicine in December 2014.

TABLE 25-3 Common Pain Medications Used in the Elderly

Medication	Alerts
Acetaminophen	1. Insignificant antiinflammatory or antiplatelet effects. 2. Maximum doses for elderly preferred = 3 grams/24 hours; otherwise 4 grams/24 hours. 3. Lower doses for those with liver disease or those who drink more than 3 alcoholic drinks/day. 4. Caution taken when taking analgesics that contain acetaminophen (e.g., Vicodin). The maximum dose includes **all** acetaminophen ingested. 5. Leading cause of acute liver failure in the United States.
Nonsteroidal antiinflammatory drugs (NSAIDS)	1. Use with extreme caution or rarely or for limited periods in elderly. 2. High risk for older adults for gastrointestinal bleeding and other gastrointestinal symptoms such as dyspepsia and abdominal pain. 3. Inhibits platelet aggregation. 4. Cardiovascular effects include fluid retention which could worsen hypertension, congestive heart failure, cerebrovascular accident, or myocardial infarction. 5. Renal systems contribute to water and sodium retention, decreased blood flow, electrolyte imbalances. 6. Has a *ceiling effect* in which increasing the dose beyond a certain point does not increase the analgesic effect, but only increases risks.
All opioids	1. Ask about previous opioid experiences. 2. Patients with persistent pain may require ongoing *titration* to find an effective dose. 3. Should include measures to combat constipation when opioids started. 4. Older adults may be more sensitive to opioid effects.
Weak Opioids Tramadol	1. Metabolized in the hepatic system; excreted through the renal system. 2. Side effects: Constipation, nausea, appetite loss, drowsiness, dizziness, falls.
Hydrocodone	1. Metabolized in hepatic system; excreted through the renal system. 2. If combined with acetaminophen may increase liver toxicity. 3. Side effects: Constipation, anxiety, dry mouth, headache.
Codeine	1. Metabolized in hepatic system; excreted through renal system. 2. Suppresses cough reflex. 3. Side effects: Constipation, nausea, appetite loss, drowsiness, dizziness, sweating, falls.
Strong Opioids Morphine	1. Metabolized in liver; excreted through kidneys. 2. Side effects: Constipation, nausea, vomiting, appetite loss, confusion, hypotension; respiratory depression rare. 3. Medication for breakthrough pain may be needed with sustain-released morphine. 4. Liquid may be used for those who cannot swallow.

(continues)

TABLE 25-3   Common Pain Medications Used in the Elderly (*continued*)

Medication	Alerts
Hydromorphone	1. Metabolized in the liver; excreted through the renal system. 2. Side effects: Confusion, sedation, hypotension, constipation. 3. Suppresses cough reflex. 4. Considered safer in renal insufficiency.
Oxycodone	1. Metabolized in the liver and excreted through the renal system. 2. Side effects: Constipation, dizziness, drowsiness, heartburn, nausea, vomiting.
Methadone	1. Metabolized in the liver and excreted through feces, so safer in renal failure. 2. Side effects: Constipation, dizziness, dry mouth, headache, sweating, nausea. 3. Long half-life. 4. Useful in neuropathic pain.
Fentanyl	1. Metabolized in the liver and excreted through the renal system. 2. Can be used in morphine allergy. 3. Side effects: Anxiety, confusion, constipation, headache, indigestion, nausea. 4. Not appropriate for opioid-naïve patients.
Adjuvant drugs Tricyclic antidepressants (nortriptyline, desipramine)	1. Significant risk of adverse effects in older adults. 2. Anticholinergic effects.
Other antidepressants Duloxetine	1. Side effects: Seizures, dizziness, insomnia, decreased appetite, constipation. 2. Multiple drug–drug interactions.
Venlafaxine	1. Side effects: Seizures, increased heart rate and blood pressure
Anticonvulsants Carbamazepine	1. Multiple drug–drug interactions 2. Use with caution in older men with benign prostatic hyperplasia or increased intraocular pressure. 3. Side effects: Ataxia, drowsiness, increased blood pressure.
Gabapentin	1. Side effects: Sedation, ataxia, edema. 2. Use cautiously in renal insufficiency. 3. Multiple drug–drug interactions.
Pregabalin	1. Use cautiously in renal impairment. 2. Side effects: Dizziness, drowsiness, ataxia, dry mouth.

Data from American Geriatrics Society Panel on the Pharmacological Management of Persistent Pain in Older Persons. (2009). Pharmacological management of persistent pain in older persons. *Journal of the American Geriatrics Society, 57,*1331–1346; Malec, M., & Shega, J. W. (2015). Pain management in the elderly. *Medical Clinics of North America, 99,* 337–350; Tracy, B., & Morrison, R. S. (2013). Pain management in older adults. *Clinical Therapeutics, 35,*1659–1668.

What Is Complementary, Alternative, or Integrative Health?

According to NCCIH, complementary therapies are "non-mainstream practice used together with conventional medicine" (NCCIH, 2015a, para 3). Alternative medicine, on the other hand, refers to "non-mainstream practice that is used in place of conventional medicine" (NCCIH, 2015a, para 3). *Integrative health care* is defined as a

TABLE 25-4	Normal Physiological Changes in the Elderly and Effect on Drug Clearance	
System	**Change**	**Effect on Medication**
Hepatic	Decrease in liver mass by 1%/year after age 50 Decrease in blood flow and portal blood velocity after age 65 Decline in demethylation	Drug half-life may be prolonged May require dosage changes in benzodiazepines
Renal	Loss of nephrons Decreased renal plasma flow Decreased glomerular filtration rate (GFR)	Decreased drug clearance leading to a buildup in metabolites Increased risk of nephrotoxicity related to decrease thirst and volume depletion Medications (e.g., NSAIDS) more likely to damage kidneys
Brain and central nervous system changes	Pain perception is often altered	May lead to under treatment because pain is not decreased
Gastrointestinal	Passage through esophagus and colon may be slowed Decrease in gastric acid	May affect absorption and metabolism of some medications May increase opioid-related bowel dysmotility
Body composition	Decrease in total water and lean mass Increase in body fat Decrease in basal metabolic rate	Water-soluble medications are less efficiently distributed Lipophilic medication (e.g., lidocaine, fentanyl) have an increased volume of absorption so may have a prolonged effect.

Data from American Geriatrics Society Panel on the Pharmacological Management of Persistent Pain in Older Persons (AGS). (2009). Pharmacological management of persistant pain in older persons. *Journal of the American Geriatrics Society, 57*, 1331–1346; Kaye, A.D., Baluch, A., & Scott, J. T. (2010). Pain management in the elderly population: A review. *The Ochsner Journal, 10*(3), 179–187; Tracy, B., & Morrison, R. S. (2013). Pain management in older adults. *Clinical Therapeutics, 35*(11), 1659–1668.

"comprehensive, often interdisciplinary approach to treatment, prevention, and health promotion that brings together complimentary and conventional therapies" (National Institutes of Health [NIH], 2014, para 3). The name change reflects the trend that true alternative medicine is rarely used today, and integrative health care is seen more commonly in hospitals, hospices, and military health facilities in the United States. In addition, NCCIH uses the term "complementary health approaches" (CHA) to refer to modalities and products of nonmainstream origin; the term CAM, used to refer to a group of diverse healthcare systems, products, and practices, is no longer used (NCCIH, 2015a, para 9).

The widespread use of CHA therapies requires healthcare providers to be knowledgeable about these modalities and to educate clients and patients about the safety of their use. See **Table 25-5** for a list of the most commonly used CAM therapies.

Types of Complementary Health Approaches

Previously, the NCCAM had classified complementary and alternative medicine (CAM) into broad categories: (1) *natural products*, (2) manipulative and body-based practices, (3) *mind–body medicine*, (4) *whole medical systems*,

TABLE 25-5 Ten Most Common CHAs among Adults: 2012	
Approach	Percent
Dietary supplements other than vitamins and minerals	17.7
Deep breathing	10.9
Yoga, Tai Chi, Qi Gong	10.1
Chiropractic or osteopathic manipulation	8.4
Meditation	8.0
Massage	6.9
Special diets	3.0
Homeopathy	2.2
Progressive relaxation	2.1
Guided imagery	1.7

Data from National Center for Complementary and Integrative Health. (2016). Complementary, alternative, or integrative health: What's in a name? Retrieved from https://nccih.nih.gov/health/integrative-health

and (5) energy systems (Trail-Maban, Mao, & Bawel-Brinkley, 2013). Currently, the NCCIH addresses two primary CHAs: (1) natural products and (2) mind–body practice. Whole medical systems are classified under "Other" (NIH Senior Health, 2016).

Natural Products

This CHA includes botanicals (herbs), vitamins, minerals, fatty acids, proteins, prebiotics and probiotics, whole diets, and functional foods. Vegetarian, macrobiotic, Atkins, Pritikin, Ornish, Mediterranean, and Zone are examples of whole diets included under natural products. Whole diet therapies may be used to prevent or treat health conditions; for example, the Mediterranean diet has been suggested as possibly decreasing body inflammation and, therefore, decreasing pain. Other diets may not provide all the micronutrients an individual may need. As part of a thorough assessment, nurses should include questions about the patient's whole diet practices.

Dietary supplements are also included in this category. According to Clarke, Black, Stussman, Bames, & Nahin (2015), fish oil supplements and glucosamine, chondroitin, or a combination of both were the two most common nonvitamin, nonmineral dietary supplements used in the past 30 days. Methylsulfonylmethane is used to control pain in osteoarthritis. Nahin, Boinau, Khalsa, and Stussman (2016) reviewed the evidence for this CHA and found that although the methylsulfonylmethane group experienced statistically significant improvement, the difference between placebo and treatment groups was small. S-Adenosylmethionine (SAMe) is another dietary supplement used to improve pain and function in osteoarthritis of the knee. Nahin et al. (2016) reviewed one randomized control study comparing SAMe with celecoxib. There were no differences between the two groups, but the sample size was small. In addition, those taking SAMe had fewer side effects than the participants taking celecoxib (p. 1299).

Table 25-6 lists other commonly used natural supplements. Uses and contraindications for these products are also included.

Because this category includes natural products, individuals, particularly the elderly, may have the mistaken belief that there are no side effects or concerns in using these products. However, caution must be taken in using these products with certain prescribed medications. The ingredients listed on the labels of dietary supplements may be long and printed in a font size difficult for the older adult to read easily. Consequently, ingredients with the potential for interactions with medications could be overlooked.

TABLE 25-6   Commonly Used Natural Products

Name	Action and Use	Contraindications and Side Effects
Fish oil/omega 3	Health benefits unclear. May decrease risk of coronary heart disease. Evidence mixed, with two randomized studies on benefits on severe headache and migraine pain (Nahin et al., 2016).	None
Glucosamine/ chondroitin	Efficacy in relieving pain of osteoarthritis was mixed in patients examined. Doses and definitions varied among reviewed studies (Nahin et al., 2016).	Mild gastrointestinal distress
Probiotics or prebiotics	There is some evidence that probiotics may be helpful for acute diarrhea, antibiotic-associated diarrhea, and atopic eczema (a skin condition most commonly seen in infants) (NCCIH, 2016).	Long-term safety unknown
Melatonin	Studies suggest that melatonin may help with certain sleep disorders, such as jet lag, delayed sleep phase disorder (DSPD) (a disruption of the body's biological clock in which a person's sleep–wake timing cycle is delayed by 3–6 hours), sleep problems related to shift work, and some sleep disorders in children. It has also been shown to be helpful for a sleep disorder that causes changes in blind peoples' sleep and wake times.	None
Coenzyme Q10	Improved heart function and well-being in patients diagnosed with heart failure according to research reviews published in 2007 and 2009. A 2013 meta-analysis also found an association between taking CoQ10 and improved heart function. Some studies suggest that CoQ10 is associated with blood pressure control, but the findings are limited, a 2009 systematic review showed. A 2010 review described research showing that CoQ10 may help ease the myopathy (muscle weakness) sometimes associated with taking statins. However, the findings are not definite (NCCIH, 2016).	Insomnia, increased liver enzymes, rashes, nausea, upper abdominal pain, dizziness, sensitivity to light, irritability, headaches, heartburn, and fatigue. CoQ10 also decreases the effect of warfarin (NCCIH, 2016)
Valerian, valerian root	Sedative and sleep aid.	Should not be used with alcohol, sedatives, or antianxiety medication. Should not be used by mothers breastfeeding Side effects: Mild headache or upset stomach (Zauderer & Davis, 2012)

(continues)

TABLE 25-6   Commonly Used Natural Products (*continued*)

Name	Action and Use	Contraindications and Side Effects
Kava (*Piper methysticum*)	Anxiety, stress, restlessness, insomnia.	Contraindicated in individuals with liver disease or depression (Zauderer & Davis, 2012) Side effects: Drowsiness, involuntary muscle movement, hepatic toxicity. The U.S. Food and Drug Administration (FDA) has issued a warning that using kava supplements have been linked to a risk of liver damage
Saw palmetto	Symptoms related to benign prostatic hyperplasia.	Mild gastrointestinal upset No reported drug interactions
Capsaicin	Used topically to relieve pain from neuralgias, osteoarthritis, rheumatoid arthritis, back pain, nerve pain.	Stinging or burning sensation when initially applied
Yohimbe	Impotence.	**Not recommended by FDA** Side effects with tricyclic antidepressants: Hypertension, renal failure, seizures, hypotension, tachycardia, dizziness
Comfrey	Gastritis, gastrointestinal ulcers, rheumatism, bronchitis, internal bleeding, diarrhea, sprains and pulled ligaments.	**Identified by FDA as a possible health hazard** Side effects: Liver toxicity
Ephedrine alkaloids (ephedra, ma huang, Chinese ephedra)	**Should not be used.** Previously used for energy.	**FDA has limited amount in dietary supplements, but may be found in imported foodstuffs such as teas** Side effects: Nervousness, dizziness, heart attack, stroke, seizures, death
Echinacea purpurea (Echinacea)	Antiinfective; stimulates immune response. Uses: Treatment and prevention of coughs, colds, flu, and bronchitis; wounds and burns; fevers.	May interfere with immunosuppressant drugs; contraindicated in diseases related to immune response, multiple sclerosis, tuberculosis, acquired immunodeficiency syndrome, and autoimmune diseases Should not be used for more than 8-week intervals or immune system may be depressed Allergic reactions

Name	Action and Use	Contraindications and Side Effects
Panax ginseng (Asian ginseng) *Panax quinquefolius* (American ginseng)	Uses: Improve physical and mental stamina, treatment of diabetes, sedative, aphrodisiac, increase immune response, increase appetite	May decrease effectiveness of warfarin; may interfere with monoamine oxidase inhibitors; may have hypoglycemic effects; caffeine may increase herb effect; use with caution with estrogen; may increase risk of bleeding if used with antiplatelet herbs; may prolong QT interval if used with bitter orange; may interfere with immunosuppressant therapy. Side effects: Agitation, insomnia, tachycardia, depression, hypertension (Deglin & Vallerand, 2007)
Gingko biloba (Gingko) Standardized: 24% flavonoid glycosides 6% terpenelactones	Uses: symptomatic relief of organic brain dysfunction; intermittent claudication; vertigo and tinnitus (vascular origin); sexual dysfunction; improve peripheral circulation.	Use with caution if individuals are on anticoagulant or antiplatelet therapy or have diabetes Contraindicated if individuals have bleeding disorders or increased blood sugars Side effects: headache, dizziness, GI disturbances
Garlic	Vasodilator, antiplatelet properties Uses: hypertension, lowering cholesterol.	May increase bleeding; not as effective in lowering cholesterol as other medications Side effects: body and breath odor, heartburn, upset stomach, allergic reactions
Glucosamine	May stimulate cartilage growth. Use: Osteoarthritis.	Contraindicated if shellfish allergy is present May interfere with glucose regulation in diabetics (Deglin & Vallerand, 2007).
St. John's wort (*Hypericum perforatum*)	Antidepressant; when used topically, may have antiviral, antiinflammatory, antibacterial activity. Uses: Mild to moderate depression.	Alcohol and other antidepressives may increase central nervous system side effects. Side effects: Dizziness, restlessness, sleep disturbance, hypertension, bloating, abdominal pain, (Deglin & Vallerand, 2007).

(continues)

TABLE 25-6   Commonly Used Natural Products (*continued*)

Name	Action and Use	Contraindications and Side Effects
Peppermint	Muscle relaxant, particularly in the digestive tract; reduces inflammation in nasal passages. Uses: Irritable bowel syndrome, nausea and vomiting, congestion related to colds and allergies.	May cause choking feeling if applied to chest or nostrils of a child under 5. May intensify symptoms in hiatal hernia; avoid large doses if pregnant because it can relax uterine muscles. Side effects: None identified (Supplements: Peppermint, n.d.)
Ginger supplements	Inhibit platelets, prostaglandins; improve digestion, appetite; may be hypoglycemic. Uses: Nausea and vomiting; joint pain.	Use with caution in patients with bleeding tendencies or on anticoagulant therapy or with diabetics
Soy supplements	Lowers total cholesterol and low-density lipoprotein (LDL).	Side effects: Heartburn. Controversy that isoflavones, a component of soy, are phytoestrogens, a weak estrogen, and may increase cancer risk; other evidence supports that soy may protect against breast cancer (Henkel, 2000)

Although most herbal medications are safe when used as recommended, the concern is that many older adults do not tell their nurse practitioners, physicians, or other healthcare providers about the botanicals they are taking. This increases the possibility of drug interactions (Sackett, Carter, & Stanton, 2014). It is important for healthcare providers to ask their patients what CHAs they are using because the patient may not come forward with that information initially (Sackett et al., 2014). In addition, many safety concerns and drug interactions are under-researched in the elderly. Consumers should be cautioned when using herbal remedies to buy only reputable products, because the FDA does not regulate herbal manufacturing.

Mind–Body Practices

Mind–body practices focus on the interactions among the brain, body, mind, and behavior (NCCIH, 2016). They include a large and diverse group of approaches that are practiced or taught by trained practitioners or teachers (NCCIH, 2015a, para 14) (see **Box 25-7**). These practices are not new; some are rooted in traditional medical systems, and others have been practiced in the United States for over 150 years. Both chiropractic care and massage were reported to be among the 10 most-used CHA therapies (Clarke et al., 2015).

Chiropractic and Osteopathic Manipulation

Chiropractic practice is considered a holistic approach to health. It is thought to provide benefit by helping place the body in proper alignment. Many third-party payers for healthcare provide some reimbursement for chiropractic care. According to Stussman, Black, Barnes, Clarke, & Nahin (2015), more of those who used

BOX 25-7 Practices Included in the Mind and Body Category

- Yoga
- Chiropractic and osteopathic manipulation
- Meditation
- Massage therapy
- Acupuncture
- Relaxation techniques (breathing exercises, guided imagery, progressive muscle relaxation, self-hypnosis)
- Tai Chi/Qi gong
- Healing touch
- Hypnotherapy
- Movement therapies (Feldenkrais method, Alexander technique, Pilates, Rolfing, Trager psychophysical integration)

Data from National Center for Complementary and Integrative Health. (2015a). *Complementary, alternative, or integrative health: What's in a name.* Retrieved from https://nccih.nih.gov/health/integrative-health

spinal manipulation in 2012 did so to treat a specific health condition rather than for general wellness. In an evidence-based evaluation of complementary approaches, Nahin et al. (2016), found that randomized control trials investigating spinal manipulation for relief of back pain had mixed results. A review of articles by Bryans et al. (2011) supported the use of chiropractic care to improve migraine and cervicogenic headaches. However, based on the evidence, the authors could not make a recommendation for the use of spinal manipulation for tension-type headaches (Bryans et al., 2011).

Massage therapy

Massage therapy dates back thousands of years. It includes various techniques that involve the manipulation of soft tissue through pressure and movement. Many individuals use massage therapy to increase relaxation and reduce stress, recover from muscle stress and strain, heal injuries, and relieve pain (see **Box 25-8**). Satisfaction with massage treatments is very high. A Cochrane review by Hillier, Louw, Morris, Uwimana, and Statham (2010) reported that there is some evidence to support the use of massage therapy to improve quality of life for persons living with human immunodeficiency/acquired immunodeficiency syndrome (HIV/AIDS), especially when combined with other stress management modalities. In addition, research studies have supported the use of massage in a variety of situations (Cutshall et al., 2010; Drackley et al., 2012; Nahin et al., 2016; Shengelia, Parker, Ballin, George,& Reid, 2013; Yuan, Matsutani, & Marques, 2015). Although massage is considered a low-risk intervention, it is contraindicated under several circumstances, including deep vein thrombosis, burns, skin infections, eczema, open wounds, bone fractures, and advanced osteoporosis.

Meditation

Meditation has a long history of use for increasing calmness and physical relaxation, improving psychological balance, coping with illness, and enhancing overall health and well-being (NCCIH, 2016a) Although there are many forms of meditation, all share the following characteristics: (1) a quiet location with minimal distractions, (2) a specific, comfortable posture, (3) a focus of attention, and (4) an open attitude (NCCIH, 2016a, para 5). Evidence has supported that meditation may help control pain (Sorrell, 2015; Zeidan et al., 2016) blood pressure (Nyklicek, Mommersteeg, Van Beugen, Ramakers, & Van Boxtel 2013), and depression, anxiety, and loneliness (Sorrell, 2015).

Yoga

The practice of yoga, which has its roots in India, integrates physical, mental, and spiritual health so that the individual can be in harmony with the universe. There are different schools of yoga, and each has a different focus, but basically yoga combines disciplined breathing, defined gestures, and specific postures (asanas) to achieve a sense of harmony. Although some studies have supported the benefits of yoga for a wide variety of

BOX 25-8   Research Highlight

Aim: The purpose of this research was to determine whether postoperative massage could reduce pain and anxiety more effectively than a control intervention for patients undergoing colorectal surgery. Blood pressure, heart rate, and opioid use postoperative were also measured.

Methods: In this randomized control study carried out at a large Midwestern medical center, patients undergoing colorectal surgery were randomized to a massage group or control group. Interventions were initiated on day 2 and day 3 postoperatively. The massage group received an integrative massage provided by a certified massage therapist with hospital experience for 20 minutes. Before the massage, the therapist provided a quick assessment, and the massage was individualized based on the assessment and patient preferences. Patients were instructed to relax for 20 minutes and quiet time was provided with dim lights and either the relaxation channel on the television or soft music playing. After the session, patients were again assessed, and vital signs were recorded. The control group engaged in a 20-minute conversation with the massage therapist about conversational topics after a quick assessment (children, grandchildren, summer activities; medical topics were not discussed). Quiet time was then provided; patients were offered the relaxation channel on the television or soft music, and dim light. After the session, the patient was assessed again and vital signs were taken. Patients reported measures of pain, anxiety, tension, relaxation, and overall satisfaction before and after interventions. A nurse or personal care assistant collected the surveys and took vital signs.

Findings: A total of 127 participants were engaged in the study. Data were analyzed using nonparametric measures, which was consistent with the level of data. Significance was set at $p = 0.05$. On day 2, the massage group had significantly less pain, anxiety, and tension, a significant change in relaxation from before the massage. Systolic blood pressure and respiratory rates also improved. On day 2 the control group also saw a significant decrease in tension and significant improvement in relaxation, blood pressure, and respiratory rate. Although both groups showed statistically significant changes in indicators, the degree of change was less in the control group. On day 3 the massage group again showed significant changes in the indicators, and although the control group was more relaxed and had a decrease in blood pressure and respiratory rate, the change was less than the massage group. There was no difference in oral opioid use between the two groups.

Application to Practice: Massage did help the participants to feel less anxiety, tension, and pain. Interestingly, the control group also had a decrease in these indicators. Perhaps having an opportunity to relax in a quiet environment added to the decrease in tension and anxiety in the stressful hospital environment. As a result of the feedback from this study, a practice change occurred, and all patients at the medical center are offered massage therapy. The program is also spreading to other hospitals. Although many hospitals may not have the resources of a large medical center, providing a relaxation channel on the television and providing an opportunity for quiet time may produce similar outcomes for patients.

Reproduced from Dreyer, N. E., Curshall, S. M., Huebner, M., Foss, D. M., Bauer, B. A., & Cima, R. R. (2015). Effect of massage therapy on pain, anxiety, relaxation, and tension after colorectal surgery: A randomized study. *Complementary Therapies in Clinical Practice, 21*(3),154–159. Copyright 2015, with permission from Elsevier.

medical conditions and a wide variety of ages (Nahin et al., 2016; Okonta, 2012; Shengelia et al., 2013; Tilbrook et al., 2011), an integrative review by Li and Goldsmith (2012) indicated mixed results and a need for additional research with larger sample sizes.

Tai Chi and Qigong

Tai Chi is an ancient Chinese martial art. Although it can be used as a method of self-defense, it is practiced by many to combine gentle exercise, meditation, and deep breathing. The movements in Tai Chi are "circular and rhythmic, and each of the postures moves slowly into the next posture following the sequence of form" (Field, 2011, p. 141). A review of 43 articles supported that Tai Chi improved quality of life for participants, but to the same degree as other low- to moderate-intensity activities (Jimenez, Melendez, & Albers, 2012). However Jimenez et al. (2012) indicated that many of the studies reviewed had methodological weaknesses in their designs, and that more rigorous research should be conducted in this area. In their review, Shengelia et al. (2013) identified that Tai Chi could be used by patients with osteoarthritis, and evidence supported short-term effects for pain, stiffness, and quality of life. Nahin et al. (2016) also identified support for Tai Chi in the relief of fibromyalgia and osteoarthritis of the knee. *Qigong* is a traditional Chinese medicine practice that uses physical activity and meditation to encourage the free flow of energy (qi) through the body (Overcash, Will, & Lipetz, 2013, p. 654). Qi gong refers to exercises that improve health and increase a sense of harmony by manipulating qi (vital energy) through movement and meditation. Studies support the effectiveness of qigong in reducing depression (Overcash et al., 2013;) and blood pressure (Park et al., 2014). Although the studies demonstrated effectiveness of qigong, the sample sizes were small. Continued research in this area is needed.

Relaxation Techniques

Relaxation techniques include several practices (see Table 25-6), but the goal of all is to produce the body's natural relaxation response (NCCIH, 2016b, para 4). Relaxation techniques have been known to reduce anxiety before medical procedures, nausea caused by chemotherapy, and blood pressure on a short-term basis. Relaxation techniques also may be useful in managing pain during labor (NCCIH, 2016b).

Acupuncture

Although *acupuncture* is a mind–body CHA, it is also an integral part of TCM. It will be discussed under TCM in this chapter.

Other CHAs

Pet assisted therapy and music therapy are both interventions that have been considered to relieve stress and increase feelings of well being. Neither therapy is listed under the mind–body approaches, and limited information about music therapy is listed on the NCCIH Website. Pet therapy is not listed on the NCCIH Website. One reason for this paucity of information could be the lack of evidence to support these approaches.

Whole Medical Systems

Whole medical systems are "complete systems of diagnosis and practice" (Rosenzweig, n.d., para 1). Examples include homeopathic medicine, naturopathic medicine, Ayurvedic medicine, and TCM.

Homeopathy

Homeopathy originated with German physician Dr. Samuel Hahnemann's natural law of "like cures like" or the Principle of Similars (Teixeira, 2011). According to homeopathic theory, when a person's vital force or self-healing response is out of balance, health problems will develop. Homeopathy is the art and the science of healing the sick by using substances capable of causing the same symptoms and conditions when administered to healthy people (Homoeopathic Pharmacopoeia of the United States [HPUS],). Homeopathic remedies are derived from substances that come from plants, minerals, or animals. They are prepared by diluting certain substances and then gradually increasing the dilution until no actual measurement of the original substance exists. Although there are no active ingredients in a homeopathic solution, it helps the body to begin to heal itself by using its own defense mechanisms. Homeopathic remedies are recognized and regulated by the FDA, but the agency does not evaluate the remedies for effectiveness or safety. Remedies are also listed in the *Homoeopathic Pharmacopoeia of the United States.*

Homeopathy has been used to treat a variety of illnesses. The use of homeopathy has been controversial because some of the key concepts are inconsistent with fundamental concepts of chemistry and physics (NCCIH, 2015b). Current evidence does not support the use of homeopathy in treating illness (NCCIH, 2015b). Some homeopathic products have been promoted as substitutes for conventional immunizations, but according to the NCCIH, supportive data for this substitution are lacking (NCCIH, 2015b). The NCCIH supports the CDC recommendation for immunizations (NCCIH, 2015b).

Naturopathic Medicine

Naturopathic medicine focuses on keeping the person healthy as well as treating diseases. According to the American Association of Naturopathic Physicians (AANP), the "practice of naturopathic medicine includes modern and traditional, scientific, and empirical methods" (AANP, 2011a, para 1). Principles of naturopathy include "(a) the healing power of nature, (b) identification of the cause and treatment of disease, (c) the concept of 'do no harm,' (d) doctor as teacher, (e) treatment of the whole person, and (f) prevention" (AANP, 2011a, para 2). It encompasses a variety of healing practices, clinical and laboratory diagnostic testing, nutrition, herbs, naturopathic physical medical, including manipulation, public health measures, counseling, minor surgery, homeopathy, acupuncture, prescription medication, intravenous and injection therapy, and natural childbirth (AANP, 2011a, para 3). In naturopathy, if the body is supported and barriers to cure are removed, the body will heal itself. There are minimal risks to naturopathic medicine, but natural healing takes longer than traditional allopathic medicine. Therefore, symptoms may last longer before they are eradicated. Also, qualifications of naturopathy practitioners may vary, so patients should be informed to check the credentials of the practitioners before choosing this CHA. Only 17 states require licensing for neuropathic practitioners. A licensed naturopathic physician (ND) has attended a 4-year graduate-level naturopathic medical school and has passed an extensive postdoctoral board examination (NPLEX) to receive a license (AANP, 2011b).

Traditional medical systems of non-Western cultures are also included under this category of CAM. Ayurveda and TCM are examples of these systems.

Ayurveda

Ayurveda dates back over 2,000 years and is rooted in the ancient Hindu medical texts called Vedas. Sanskrit for "knowledge or science of life," Ayurveda is a comprehensive system that encompasses the body, mind, and consciousness connection and seeks to restore a person's harmony or balance. It emphasizes prevention and encourages maintaining health. Ayurveda "mainly focuses on the use of diet, natural plant-derived medicines, and massage" (Datta-Mitra & Ahmed, 2015, p. 690). According to Ayurveda, five elements make up all things: (1) space or ether, (2) air, (3) fire, (4) water, and (5) earth. These elements are not static, but rather are always in flux. In addition to the five elements, Ayurveda identifies three types of energy, or *doshas*: (1) *vata* is the energy of movements and comes from ether and air, (2) *pitta* is the energy of digestion and comes from fire and water, and (3) *kapha* comes from water and earth and is the energy of lubrication and structure, which keeps the cellular body together (Sharma, Chandola, Singh, & Basisht, 2007). In Ayurvedic medicine, each person has a unique energy pattern. Disease is caused by an imbalance in the body, or disorder. Diagnosis is made through symptomatology rather than through traditional laboratory diagnostics, with the goal of treatment to bring the body into balance. Evidence for the effectiveness of Ayurvedic treatments is unsatisfactory; more well-planned trials are needed (Kessler, Pinders, Michalsen, & Cramer, 2015). One of the biggest concerns about herbal treatments in Ayurvedic medicine is safety. "Sometimes minerals, including sulfur, lead, arsenic, mercury, copper, and gold, are added to formulations with the popular belief that the heavy metals are essential" to the body (Datta-Mitra & Ahmed, 2015, p. 690. The ingestion of these heavy metals can cause poisoning (Datta-Mitra & Ahmed, 2015).

Traditional Chinese Medicine

Traditional Chinese medicine dates back in written form to 200 B.C. Korea, Japan, and Vietnam all have medical systems based on the traditional medical systems in China. TCM consists of six primary branches: (1) acupuncture, (2) herbal medicine, (3) massage, (4) exercise (such as Tai Chi), (5) dietary therapy, and (6) lifestyle modifications (Smith & Bauer, 2012). According to TCM, the body is a balance of two opposing forces: yin and yang. *Yin* represents the cold, slow, darkness, or passive principle, usually considered the female aspect. *Yang*, on the other hand, simulates fire and is the hot, excited, active principle, usually considered the male aspect. In this tradition of medicine, health is balance. Disease is seen as an imbalance between yin and yang; this imbalance impedes the flow of vital energy (*qi* or *chi*) and blood along pathways called meridians (Smith & Bauer, 2012). The four principle diagnostic methods of TCM (*sizhen*) are (1) observation, (2) auscultation and olfaction, (3) interrogation, and (4) palpation. In palpation, the reading of the pulse if the most important (He, 2015). *Bagang* (eight principles) are important principles of treatment in TCM. These principles are *yin and yang*, exterior and interior, and cold and heat (He, 2015). A correct analysis of *bagang* will result in a correct diagnosis. TCM emphasized "curing illnesses that have not yet happened rather than curing illness" (He, 2015, p. 823). Clinical treatment focuses on Chinese herbal medicines along with acupuncture and *moxibustion*, Tui na (traditional Chinese massage), and qigong (He, 2015). Safety of Chinese herbal medicines is a concern because they are not tested for safety as they are considered supplements. Some of the herbal products have been reported to be contaminated with drugs, toxins, or heavy metals (NCCIH, 2013, para 8). In addition, some of the herbs may interact with a patient's prescribed medication.

Acupuncture

Acupuncture is an integral part of TCM; it promotes the flow of qi through pathways in the body called *meridians*. There are 14 major meridians used in acupuncture; each meridian consists of an internal pathway, which often connects with an internal organ, and a corresponding external pathway. A total of 361 regular acupuncture points fall on the external pathways of the 14 meridians. An additional 40 acupuncture points fall outside the meridians (Lee, LaRiccia, & Newberg, 2004). Based on patient history and a physical examination, the acupuncturist determines which points on the external pathway of a meridian to stimulate and for how long (Lee et al., 2004). Very thin, solid, metallic needles are inserted at the appropriate acupuncture point to increase the circulation of qi and to bring the body back into balance. Nothing in Western medicine compares to the meridians in TCM.

Although acupuncture originated in China more than 2,000 years ago, it did not become well known in the United States until 1971, when a *New York Times* reporter wrote about how acupuncture eased his pain postoperatively (White & Ernst, 2004). It is practiced by health professionals certified and licensed in each state. Although acupuncture is more readily available in the United States, particularly for the treatment of pain, the evidence of treatment efficacy is mixed. After a review of 11 randomized control trials (RTCs) and four systematic reviews, Shengelia et al. (2013) concluded that acupuncture is a safe intervention for patients with osteoarthritis of the knee. Treatment effects, however, varied depending on the type of control group used. In a Cochrane review, Paley, Johnson, Tashani, and Bagnall (2015) reviewed five RTCs that investigated acupuncture for cancer pain in adults. Their conclusion was that none of the studies in the review were big enough to produce reliable results. Although none of the studies reported adverse events, the evidence was insufficient to support acupuncture in relieving pain in cancer patients.

Cupping

Cupping is a traditional Chinese medical treatment that has been used for thousands years. It nearly disappeared from Western medicine during the late 20th century, but interest has been renewed in recent years. During the 2016 Olympics, several swimmers displayed bluish circular hematomas over their upper shoulder area; this led the announcers to explain the art of cupping. Dry cupping is performed by placing a cup made of thick glass, bamboo, or earthenware with a rolled rim to create an air-tight contact with the intact skin to create a vacuum effect (Rozenfeld & Kalichman, 2016). Rozenfeld and Kalichman (2016) described how negative pressure is created by heating the air, then allowing it to cool and contract while in contact with the skin (p. 174). The air is heated by swabbing the inside the cup with alcohol or by placing a cotton ball soaked in alcohol inside the cup, lighting it, and placing the cup over the skin as the flame is extinguished. A manual hand pump can also be used to create the vacuum (Rozenfeld & Kalichman, 2016). The exact physiological mechanisms of cupping are unknown, but there are several theories. Cupping increases the circulation surrounding the treatment area, reduces pain, induces deep relaxation, and stimulates the immune system (Rozenfeld & Kalichman, 2016). Cupping is considered safe when applied by an experienced practitioner. Although evidence tends to support cupping to treat various musculoskeletal conditions, more research using strong methodologies must be conducted.

Moxibustion

Moxibustion is another TCM therapy with roots over 2000 years ago; it is used with acupuncture to treat disease (Lim, Huang, & Zhao, 2015). In moxibustion, ignited moxa floss is used to apply heat to certain points or parts of the body. According to Lim et al. (2015), interest in moxibustion has increased as an inexpensive and accessible therapy for health promotion and maintenance and disease prevention (p. 142). However, there is little evidence to support the efficacy of moxibustion.

Nursing Interventions

When performing assessments, nurses must ask patients about their use of CHA as well as prescribed medications for relief of pain. These questions should be phrased in a nonjudgmental manner and should also be phrased to cover the variety of modalities. Patients may not acknowledge they are taking herbal medicines but may identify that they are taking natural products. This is particularly important when patients are on prescribed medications for blood thinning, blood pressure, depression, anxiety, or insomnia. Good communication skills are a key to a thorough assessment of CHA use. Integrated health care may be the best model of care for an older adult. To facilitate this model, the nurse is challenged to implement evidence-based protocols into the clinical setting (Trail-Maban et al., 2013). This includes a knowledge of both CHA and traditional pain therapies to best meet the needs of the older population with acute, persistent, or end-of-life pain.

Summary

Pain management will continue to be a focus of care as the population over 65 years of age continues to increase and present with chronic illnesses that produce pain (see **Box 25-9**). Good pain management relies on good assessment

BOX 25-9 Evidence-Based Practice Application

Pain management for older adults in a long-term care facility is a problem worldwide. To address this clinical problem, an evidence-based pain protocol was initiated in two long-term care facilities in Canada. Before beginning the project, a review of literature determined that using a multifaceted implementation approach was needed instead of a passive dissemination approach. Two advanced practice nurses, a clinical nurse specialist (CNS) and a nurse practitioner (NP), were chosen as change champions to implement the pain protocol. This project was evidence based on several levels. The pain protocol was based on research. Research was used to determine that the NP and CNS were the best choices to serve as change champions because of their relationships and professional status on the units, and the implementation approach was also research based. The project process and data collection were well explained by the authors. Although several barriers were faced during the project implementation, the role of the advanced practice nurse as change agent was supported.

Data from Kaasalaimen, S., Ploeg, J., Donald, F., Coker, E., Brazil, K., Martin-Misener, R., Dicenso, A., & Hadjistavropoulos, T. (2015). Positioning clinical nurse specialists and nurse practitioners as change champions to implement a pain protocol in long-term care. *Pain Management Nursing, 16*(2), 78–88.

BOX 25-10 Recommended Reading

Ellison, D., White, D., & Cisneros, F. (2015). Aging population. *Nursing Clinics of North America, 50*(1), 185–213.

Johnson, J. R., Crespin, D. J., Griffin, K. H., Finch, M. D., Rivard, R. L., Baechler, C. J., & Dusek, J. A. (2014). The effectiveness of integrative medicine interventions on pain and anxiety in cardiovascular inpatients: A practice-based research evaluation. *BMC Complementary and Alternative Medicine, 14,* 486–495.

McCartney, C. J. L., & Nelligan, K. (2014). Postoperative pain management after total knee arthroplasty in elderly patients: Treatment options. *Drugs & Aging, 31*(2), 83–91.

Spilman, S. K., Baumhover, L. A., Lillegraven, C. L., Lederhaas, G., Sahr, S. M., Schirmer, L. L., . . . & Swegle, J. R. (2014). Infrequent assessment of pain in elderly trauma patients. *Journal of Trauma Nursing, 21*(5), 229–235.

so emphasis will be on how to accurately assess for pain and then develop a plan of care that will comfort the patient and reduce the pain. Knowledge of pain medications will be essential so a good match between the type and duration of pain and medication can be made (see **Box 25-10**). Nonpharmaceutical approaches will receive more attention as the trend away from opioids for chronic pain continues. Nurses are in the perfect position to educate about nonpharmaceutical therapies and engage in research to provide additional evidence for the most promising CHAs. This chapter has presented information about pain, pharmaceutical interventions to reduce pain, and CHAs that may reduce pain and increase well-being without medication (**Case Study 25-1**).

Case Study 25–1

Mr. Walters is an 85-year-old widower who lives alone. He was active and had been walking every night except for the last 6 weeks, when his knees began to bother him. He fell last week while trying to get to the bathroom. He hit his elbow, fractured his wrist, and bruised his ribs and knees. During your interview, he tells you this is not the first time he has fallen, but it is the first time he has injured himself. For the most part, Mr. Walters is healthy, with the exception of hypertension, enlarged prostate, mild diabetes controlled with oral medications, controlled atrial fibrillation, and some osteoarthritis in his knees. In addition to the oral hypoglycemic, Mr. Walters is taking furosemide 40 mg each morning, Lanoxin 0.125 mg daily, enteric-coated aspirin daily, enalapril 25 mg twice a day, gingko biloba, *Panax ginseng*, capsaicin to his knees and back, and glucosamine twice a day.

Mr. Walters states the pain now is terrible and nothing seems to help. He rates his pain at a 10.

Mr Walters states, "You don't believe me." In addition, he reports with movement the pain feels like a knife is stabbing him. He reports his knees have been acting up recently along with some numbness to his feet that seems to be worse at night. The doctor gave him some pills, but he states, "I'm afraid to take them because I don't want to get hooked on drugs." He reports not sleeping well.

1. What kind of pain does Mr Walters have? Does he have more than one?
2. Why is Mr Walters' new pain so severe? Is there anything in his current condition that would give an indication of why the pain intensity is so high?
3. How have Mr Walters' comorbidities affected his current pain complaint?
4. How has his pain affected his ability to function? What recommendations would you make?

Clinical Reasoning Exercises

1. Access the NCCIH Website (https://www.nccih.nih.gov) and explore one of the CHAs listed. Review the information presented from the perspective of a consumer with no medical knowledge. What is the reading level? Is the material easy to understand? What would you add and why? What would you delete and why? Is any evidence supporting the CHA presented? Where would you go for additional information if you wanted to explore the therapy further before engaging in it?
2. Visit a pain management clinic and explore the modalities the provider uses to reduce/control a patient's pain. Does the clinic use an integrative health approach? Are both pharmaceutical and nonpharmaceutical therapies used? Are any CHAs used? How are they received by patients? If a CHA is used, who instructs the patient about the therapy?
3. In a group, critique research articles exploring the efficacy of a CHA modality with research reports on clinical trials of allopathic medicines or interventions. Compare the levels of evidence of each report.
4. In a group, discuss three reasons pain management is an important part of patient care for the elderly?
5. Discuss the reasons pain can be more difficult to manage in the elderly population.
6. What are the major principles associated with the use of pharmacotherapy for the elderly?

Personal Reflection Exercises

1. Think about what CHA therapies you have used personally. If you have not used any, think about one therapy you think you may want to try. Why did you use CHA or why would you use CHA? Think about patients you have had who used CHA. What was your reaction to the information? Have you changed your mind about CHA since reading the chapter? Did the patients use CHA for the same reasons you did or thought you may?

2. Have you ever been in pain? Have you ever had postoperative pain? Joint pain? Muscular pain? Nerve pain? What did those types of pain feel like and how were they different or alike? Think about a family member or patient you may have worked with who had chronic pain. How did they handle it? What nonpharmacological strategies did they use to cope? If you had to care for a patient or family member with severe pain, what suggestions would you offer for pain management? What would be the most difficult part for you to personally cope with in this situation?

References

American Association of Naturopathic Physicians. (2011a). Definition of naturopathic medicine. Retrieved from http://www.naturopathic.org/content.asp?contentid=59

American Association of Naturopathic Physicians. (2011b). Professional education. Retrieved from http://www.naturopathic.org/education

American Geriatrics Society Panel. . .Persons.(AGS). (2009). Pharmacological management of persistant pain in older persons. *Journal of the American Geriatrics Society, 57,* 1331–1346.

American Pain Society. (2008). *Principles of analgesic use in the treatment of acute pain and cancer pain.* Glenview, IL: Author.

Baker, D. W. (2016). Joint commission statement on pain management. Retrieved from https://www.jointcommission.org/topics/pain_management.aspx; https://www.researchgate.net/publication/6294729_Barriers_to_effective_pain_management

Blumstein, B., & Barkley, T. W. (2015). Neuropathic pain management: A reference for the clinical nurse. *MEDSURG Nursing, 24*(6), 381–389, 438.

Booker, S., Pasero, C., & Herr, K. A. (2015). Practice recommendations for pain assessment by self-report with African American older adults. *Geriatric Nursing, 36*(1), 67–74.

Bryans, R., Descarreaux, M., Duranleau, M., Marcoux, H., Potter, B., Ruegg, R., . . . White, E. (2011). Evidence-based guidelines for the chiropractic treatment of adults with headache. *Journal of Manipulative and Physiological Treatments, 34*(5), 274–289.

Centers for Disease Control and Prevention. (2013). *The state of aging and health in America 2013.* Atlanta, GA: Author.

Cherkin, D. C., Sherman, K. J., Deyo, R. A., & Shekelle, P. G. (2003). A review of the evidence for the effectiveness, safety, and cost of acupuncture, massage therapy, and spinal manipulation for back pain. *Annals of Internal Medicine, 138*(11), 898–906.

Clarke, T. C., Black, L. I., Stussman, B. J., Barnes, P. M., & Nahin, R. L. (2015). Trends in the use of complementary health approaches among adults: United States, 2002–2012. National Health Statistics Reports, 79, Hyattsville, MD: National Center for Health Statistics.

Committee on Advancing Pain Research, Care, and Education. (2011). *Relieving pain in America: A blueprint for transforming prevention, care, education, and research.* Washington, DC: Institute of Medicine.

Cutshall, S. M., Wentworth, L. J., Engen, D., Sundt, T. M., Kelly, R. F., & Bauer, B. A. (2010). Effect of massage therapy on pain, anxiety, and tension in cardiac surgical patients: A pilot study. *Complementary Therapies in Clinical Practice, 16*(2), 92–95.

D'Arcy, Y. (2014). Living with the nightmare of neuropathic pain. *Nursing2014, 44*(6), 38–45.

Datta-Mitra, A., & Ahmed, O. (2015). Ayurvedic medicine use and lead poisoning in a child: A continued concern in the United States. *Clinical Pediatrics, 54*(7), 690–692.

Deglin, J. H., & Vallerand, A. H. (2007). *Davis's drug guide for nurses* (10th ed.). Philadelphia, PA: F.A. Davis.

Dimitroulas, T., Duarte, R. V., Behura, A., Kitas, G. D., & Raphael, J. H. (2014). Neuropathic pain in osteoarthritis: A review of pathophysiological mechanisms and implications for treatment. *Seminars in Arthritis and Rheumatism, 44*(2), 145–154.

Dowell, D., Haegerich, T. M., Chou, R. (2016). CDC guideline for prescribing opioids for chronic pain—United States. *JAMA, 315*(15), 1624–1645.

Drackley, N. L., Degnim, A. C., Jakub, J. W., Cutshall, S. M., Thomley, B. S., Brodt, J. K., . . . Boughey, J. C. (2012). Effect of massage therapy for postsurgical mastectomy recipients. *Clinical Journal of Oncology Nursing 16*(2), 121–124.

Dreyer, N. E., Curshall, S. M., Huebner, M., Foss, D. M., Lovely, J. K., Bauer, B. A., & Cima, R. R. (2015). Effect of massage therapy on pain, anxiety, relaxation, and tension after colorectal surgery: A randomized study. *Complementary Therapies in Clinical Practice, 21*(3), 154–159.

Faull, C., & Blankley, K. (2015). *Palliative Care*. Oxford, England: Oxford Press.

Field, T. (2011). Tai Chi research review. *Complementary Therapies in Clinical Practice, 17*(3), 141–146.

Fitzbarles, M., Lussier, D., & Shir, Y. (2010). Management of chronic arthritis pain in the elderly. *Drugs & Aging, 27*(6), 471–490.

Gagliese, L. (2009). Pain and aging: Emergence of a new subfield of pain research. *The Journal of Pain, 10*(4), 343–353.

Geriatric Pain. (n.d.). Common myths about pain. Retrieved from http://www.geriatricpain.org/Content /Education/Clinician/Pages/PainMyths.aspx

He, K. (2015). Traditional Chinese and Thai medicine in a comparative perspective. *Complementary Therapies in Medicine, 23*(6), 821–826.

Henkel, J. (2000). The soy health claim. *FDA Consumer, 17*.

Hillier, S. L., Louw, Q., Morris, L., Uwimana, J., & Statham, S. (2010). Massage therapy for people with HIV/AIDS. *Cochrane Database of Systematic Reviews, 1*: C0007502.

Homoeopathic Pharmacopoeia of the United States. (2016). What is homeopathy? Retrieved from http://www .hpus.com/what-is-homeopathy.php

Institute of Medicine. (2011). *The Future of Nursing: Leading Change, Advancing Health*. Washington, DC: The National Academies Press.

Jimenez, P. J., Melendez, A., & Albers, U. (2012). Psychological effects of Tai Chi Chuan. *Archives of Gerontology and Geriatrics, 55,* 460–467.

Kaasalaimen, S., Ploeg, J., Donald, F., Coker, E., Brazil, K., Martin-Misener, R., . . . Hadjistavropoulos, T. (2015). Positioning clinical nurse specialists and nurse practitioners as change champions to implement a pain protocol in long-term care. *Pain Management Nursing, 16*(2), 78–88.

Kaye, A. D., Baluch, A., & Scott, J. T. (2010). Pain management in the elderly population: A review. *The Ochsner Journal, 10*(3), 179–187.

Kessler, C. S., Pinders, L., Michalsen, A., & Cramer, H. (2015). Ayurvedic interventions for osteoarthritis: A systematic review and meta-analysis. *Rheumatology International, 35*(2), 211–232.

Lee, B. Y., LaRiccia, P. J., & Newberg, A. B. (2004). Acupuncture in theory and practice, Part I: Theoretical basis and physiologic effects. *Hospital Physician, 40*(4), 11–18.

Li, A. W., & Goldsmith, C. W. (2012). The effects of yoga on anxiety and stress. *Alternative Medicine Review, 17*(1), 21–35.

Lim, M. Y., Huang, J., & Zhao, B. (2015). Standardisation of moxibustion: Challenges and future development. *Acupuncture Medicine, 33,* 142–147.

Lynch, M. E. (2015). What is latest in pain mechanisms and management? *Canadian Journal of Psychiatry, 60*(4), 157–159.

MacSorley, R., White, J., Connerly, V. H., Walker, J. T., Lofton, S., Ragland, G., . . . Robertson, A. (2014). Pain assessment and management strategies for elderly patients. *Home Healthcare Nurse, 32*(5), 272–285.

Malec, M., & Shega, J. W. (2015). Pain management in the elderly. *Medical Clinics of North America, 99*(2), 337–350.

Nahin, R. L., Boineau, R., Khalsa, P. S., Stussman, B. J., & Weber, W. J. (2016). Evidence-based evaluation of complementary health approaches for pain management in the United States. *Mayo Clinic Proceedings, 91*(9), 1292–1306.

National Center for Complementary and Integrative Health. (2013). *Traditional Chinese medicine.* Retrieved from https://nccih.nih.gov/health/whatiscam/chinesemed.htm

National Center for Complementary and Integrative Health. (2015a). *Complementary, alternative, or integrative health: What's in a name.* Retrieved from https://nccih.nih.gov/health/integrative-health

National Center for Complementary and Integrative Health. (2015b). *Homeopathy.* Retrieved from https://nccih.nih.gov/health/homeopathy

National Center for Complementary and Integrative Health. (2016a). *Meditation.* Retrieved from https://nccih.nih.gov/health/meditation/overview.htm

National Center for Complementary and Integrative Health. (2016b). *Relaxation techniques for health.* Retrieved from https://nccih.nih.gov/health/stress/relaxation.htm

National Institutes of Health. (2014). NIH complementary and integrative health agency gets new name. Retrieved from https://nccih.nih.gov/news/press/12172014

National Institutes of Health Senior Health. (2016). Other complementary approaches. Retrieved from https://nihseniorhealth.gov/complementaryhealthapproaches/whatarecomplementaryhealthapproaches/01.html

Nyklicek, I., Mommersteeg, P. M. C., Van Beugen, S., Ramakers, C., & Van Boxtel, G. J. (2013). Mindfulness-based stress reduction and physiological activity during acute stress: A randomized controlled trial. *Health Psychology, 32*(10), 1110–1113.

Okonta, N. R. (2012). Does yoga reduce blood pressure in patients with hypertension? An integrative review. *Holistic Nursing Practice, 26*(3), 137–141.

Overcash, J., Will, K. M., & Lipetz, D. W. (2013). The benefits of medical qigong in patients with cancer: A descriptive pilot study. *Clinical Journal of Oncology Nursing, 17*(6), 654–658.

Paley, C. A., Johnson, M. I., Tashani, O. A., & Bagnall, A. M. (2015). Acupuncture for cancer pain in adults. *Cochrane Database of Systematic Reviews,* 10: CD007753.

Park, J. E., Hong, S., Lee, M., Park, T., Kang, K., Jung, H., . . . Choi, S, M. (2014). Randomized, controlled trial of qigong for treatment of prehypertension and mild essential hypertension. *Alternative Therapies in Health Medicine, 20*(4), 21–30.

Reardon, D. P., Anger, K. E., & Szumita, P. M. (2015). Pathophysiology, assessment and management of pain in critically ill adults. *American Journal of Health-Systems Pharmacists, 72,* 1531–1543.

Rodriguez, L. (2015). Pathophysiology of pain: Implications for perioperative nursing. *AORN Journal, 101,* 338–344.

Rozenfeld, E., & Kalichman, L. (2016). New is the well-forgotten old: The use of dry cupping in musculoskeletal medicine. *Journal of Bodywork & Movement Therapies, 20*(1), 173–178.

Rozenzweig, S. (n.d.). Whole medical systems. Retrieved from http://www.merckmanuals.com/home/special-subjects/complementary-and-alternative-medicine-cam/whole-medical-systems

Sackett, K., Carter, M., & Stanton, M. (2014). Elders' use of folk medicine and complementary and alternative therapies: An integrative review with implications for case managers. *Professional Case Management, 19*(3), 113–123.

Sharma, H., Chandola, H. M., Singh, G., & Basisht, G. (2007). Utilization of Ayurveda in health care: An approach for prevention, health promotion, and treatment of disease, Part I. Ayurveda, the science of life. *Journal of Alternative and Complementary Medicine, 13,* 1011–1019.

Shengelia, R., Parker, S. J., Ballin, M., George, T., Reid, M. C. (2013). Complementary therapies for osteoarthritis: Are they effective? *Pain Management Nursing, 14,* e275–e288.

Smith, M. E., & Bauer, W. S. (2012). Traditional Chinese medicine for cancer-related symptoms. *Seminars in Oncology Nursing, 28,* 64–74.

Sorrell, J. M. (2015). Meditation for older adults: A new look at an ancient intervention for mental health. *Journal of Psychosocial Nursing and Mental Health Services, 53*(5), 15–19.

Stussman, B. J., Black, L. I., Barnes, P. M., Clarke, T. C., & Nahin, R. L. (2015). Wellness-related use of common complementary health approaches among adults: United States, 2012. National Health Statistics Reports, 85, Hyattsville, MD: National Center for Health Statistics.

Teixeira, M. Z. (2011). New homeopathic medicines: Use of modern drugs according to the principle of similitude. *Homeopathy, 100*(4), 244–252.

Tilbrook, H. E., Hewitt, C. E., Kang'ombe, A. R., Chaung, L. H., Jayakody, S., Aplin, J. D., . . . Watt, I. (2011). Yoga for chronic low back pain: A randomized trial. *Annals of Internal Medicine, 155*(9), 569–578.

Tracy, B., & Morrison, R. S. (2013). Pain management in older adults. *Clinical Therapeutics, 35*(11), 1659–1668.

Trail-Maban, T., Mao, C., & Bawel-Brinkley, K. (2013). Complementary and Alternative medicine: Nurses' attitudes and knowledge. *Pain Management Nursing, 14,* 277–286.

What is homeopathy? (2016). Retrieved from http://www.hpus.com/what-is-homeopathy.php

White, A., & Ernst, E. (2004). A brief history of acupuncture. *Rheumatology, 43*(5), 662–663.

Yuan, S. L. K., Matsutanu, L. A., & Marques, A. P. (2015). Effectiveness of different styles of massage therapy in fibromyalgia: A systematic review and meta-analysis. *Manual Therapy, 20*(2), 257–264.

Zauderer, C., & Davis, W. (2012). Treating post partum depression and anxiety naturally. *Holistic Nursing Practice, 26*(4), 203–209.

Zeidan, F., Alder-Neal, A. L., Wells, R. E., Stangnaro, E., May, L. M., Eisenach, J. C., . . . Coghill, R. C. (2016). Mindfulness meditation-based pain relief is mediated by endogenous opioids. *Journal of Neuroscience, 36*(11), 3391–3397.

For a full suite of assignments and additional learning activities, see the access code at the front of your book.

Disaster Preparation, Response, and Recovery

Elaine Miller
Sharon Farra

(Competencies 14, 17)

LEARNING OBJECTIVES

At the end of this chapter, the reader will be able to:

> Define terminology such as disaster, emergency preparedness, disaster risk reduction, types of disasters, evacuation, and triage.
> Describe the essential elements associated with disaster preparation, response and recovery pertaining to the older adult, primary family caregiver, and healthcare provider of the older adult.
> Identify the special considerations associated with working with an older adult during disaster preparation, response, and recovery.
> List major resources at the international, national, regional, and local levels that can assist in a disaster situation.
> Review major lessons learned from past disasters that illustrate the needs of disabled and chronically ill older adults.

KEY TERMS

Disaster	Emergency preparedness
Disaster recovery	Evacuation
Disaster response	Triage

A *disaster* is a natural or man-made event that requires resources outside of the local community to respond to the event [World Health Organization [WHO], 2005]. Unfortunately, disasters are increasing at an alarming rate. In the United States last year alone, there were 47 federally declared major disasters that caused widespread destruction resulting in morbidity and mortality to citizens and in particular older adults (65 years and older) (Centers for

Disease Control and Prevention [CDC], 2012; Dolan & Messen, 2012; Joint Commission, 2013). Worldwide in 2014, there were 317 catastrophic events resulting in 8,186 deaths with over 107,000,000 affected (International Federation of the Red Cross and Red Crescent Societies [IFRC], 2015). Given older adults' higher incidence of multiple chronic diseases, normal aging changes, and other factors, they are more vulnerable to complications and death during a disaster (Al-rousan, Rubenstein, & Wallance, 2014; Banks, 2013; Evans, 2010). Data from Hurricane Katrina further indicate that 70% of disaster-related fatalities were elderly, with many healthcare workers inadequately prepared to care for and evacuate older adults (Banks, 2013; Evans, 2010). One horrific result from this disaster was the abandonment of many older adults, which continues to be a problem (Banks, 2013; Khorram-Manesh et al., 2013).

As a result of their numerous functional limitations, the elderly have higher vulnerability to the effects of a disaster. Preparation and training of the elderly, their families, and healthcare workers are critical in mitigating the negative effects of disasters (mortality and morbidity) in the elderly population (Banks, 2013; CDC, 2012). According to the WHO, an international priority is for emergency response teams to be trained and prepared to support, protect, and help foster maximum health and functionality of especially frail elderly assisting while aiding in a swift recovery from a disaster (Hutton, 2008). In the United States, the number of adults 65 and older accounts for 13% of the population and is projected to be 20% in 2050 (88.5 million) (U.S. Census Bureau, 2012).

Central to the preparation of the elderly, their family caregivers, and healthcare providers is framing a disaster within the context of disaster preparation, response, and recovery. Emergencies and disasters can strike suddenly without warning, demanding all older adults, family members, and healthcare providers to be well acquainted with disaster preparation, response, and recovery. According to Al-rousan et al. (2014) in a convenience sample of 1,304 U.S. adults 50 and older, less than 25% reported having a disaster plan and only 4.9% reported any healthcare provider discussing disaster preparation with them. Study results further indicated almost 40% of the participants reported having one or more limitations in activities of daily living (ADLs), 14.3% had one or more instrumental activities of daily living (IADLs), and 25% did not have access to a car if an emergency occurred.

Vulnerability in Disasters

The elderly are the most vulnerable to harm resulting from the disaster and tend to experience greater and longer disruption from the event than other age groups (Aldrich & Benson, 2008). With aging, older adults are more at risk for multiple chronic conditions, mortality, and poor functional status and tend to require more coordinated and complex disease management (Freid, Bernstein, & Bush, 2012).

Physical Impairments

In many instances, frail older adults have physical and cognitive impairments or limitations that may call for individualized strategies in response to disasters. Assistance with ADLs and IADLs may be needed at different levels of support. Some persons may need help meeting basic physiological needs, including eating, toileting, grooming, and bathing. Other, more independent elders may need help only with their medications, shopping and preparing meals, transportation, or management of finances. Examples of common needs of frail elderly include help with both bowel and/or bladder incontinence and mobility challenges such as use of walkers and canes (**Figure 26-1**). There is a higher prevalence of chronic illness in older adults, including heart disease, diabetes, chronic pulmonary disease, cancers, and musculoskeletal diseases (e.g., arthritis). These diseases need to be managed and may require medications, special diet, and monitoring of blood sugar, blood pressure, and weight. Some individuals may require oxygen supplementation or positive pressure support. These needs must be planned for and addressed by the nurse during all phases of the disaster cycle.

Cognitive and Emotional Considerations

Many elders may have a hard time processing information or verbalizing their thoughts due to cognitive impairments. They may have difficulty articulating their needs and understanding problems and knowing how to solve them. With aging there are increasing rates of dementia, Parkinson's disease, depression, anxiety, and stroke that occur within the older population. The cognitive effects of these illnesses cover a broad spectrum of impairment ranging from mild memory loss to confusion and total disorientation. In addition, stroke survivors and some elders with Parkinson's disease and other diseases may have cognitive impairment. Lack of impulse control, the potential for wandering, and combativeness may potentially be seen during disasters and negatively affect elders. These risks need to be planned for and responded to during disasters. In some cases, confusion in older adults may result from an acute delirium resulting in disordered thinking and reduced awareness. Acute onset of confusion requires immediate medical treatment. Sensory impairments such as low vision and impaired hearing may further affect the elder's ability to prepare and respond to disaster. Plus, depression can influence an older adult's memory and impair ability to respond to challenges posed by a disaster situation. Other common reactions of older adults during a disaster may be fear of losing independence or being sent to a nursing home; withdrawal and isolation, irritability, anger, or suspicion; fearing loss of independence; irritability; anger; and suspicion.

Need for Assistive Devices

With aging and the increased prevalence of chronic disease, the resultant physical changes may affect an older adult's mobility. Assistive

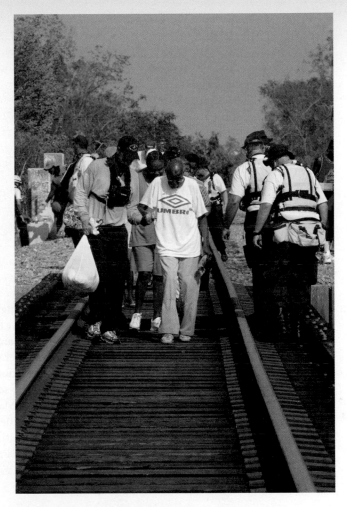

Figure 26-1 New Orleans, LA. Hurricane Katrina.
Photo by Jocelyn Augustino/FEMA

devices, including wheelchairs, walkers, and canes, may be needed, but can be challenging to use in the uncertain environments associated with disasters. The use of bath bars, shower benches, and/or special toilet seats may be needed in shelters to accommodate mobility needs. Along with these assistive devices, declining vision and hearing may necessitate the use of eyeglasses and hearing aids. It is important that both the elder and family are taught to bring assistive devices and equipment with them during evacuation. Spare glasses, extra hearing aid batteries, and hygiene products such as incontinence products should be included in the disaster kit.

Given that many older adults are at greater risk for dehydration, maintaining an adequate fluid intake is important and some may need to be reminded to drink fluids to avert dehydration. In the normal day-to-day routine, frail elders and their caregivers often must balance ADLs, medical care, physical assistance, and social support to ensure their safety. Moreover, stressors associated with a disaster may dramatically increase their needs. During a disaster situation, responders must address the unique needs and challenges of this older population and strive to replicate the community-based coordinated caregiving systems necessary for protecting their health and safety (Dyer et al., 2008a). Predisaster planning is critical for elders and their families. Personal preparedness includes teaching the older adult and the family the importance of bringing medical histories, medications, mobility aids,

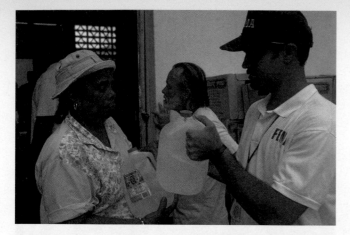

Figure 26-2 Hurricane Maryland, Virgin Islands, FEMA News, 9/2/1995.
Photo by FEMA News

and other needed equipment with them during evacuation. The nurse can assist the older adult in preparing medical histories, a list of healthcare providers, medications lists, and assistive devices required (e.g., hearing aids, glasses, walker, braces, wheelchair). These documents can be electronic, handwritten, or virtual. Shelters are open access and need to meet all community member needs; thus, planning must consider the cognitive and physical challenges of the frail elderly.

Other Challenges to the Elderly

In addition to those already discussed, the elderly face many other challenges. For instance, they may have communication difficulties (e.g., hearing loss, vision loss, difficulty expressing their thoughts clearly). Moreover, the elder may not speak English and may be unable to access emergency information in languages other than English or may have other barriers to receiving information. Cell phone or TV reception may not be available in rural or certain other areas affecting the ability of individuals to receive important notifications during a disaster situation. Also, there may be difficulty obtaining transportation for older adults especially in rural areas or those with limited resources (**Figure 26-2**). In many counties, there may be a widespread, long-term power outage, and the emergency services personnel may not consider this a county emergency and may not provide shelter for vulnerable adults. Moreover, the elderly may be reluctant to leave their home, especially if they have a pet. Because the Red Cross does not allow pets in shelters, this may contribute to a failure of the older adult to evacuate. All of these difficulties could lead to higher morbidity and mortality rates of older adults during disaster situations. Therefore, placing a major emphasis on consistent education and planning before the emergency event are essential to problem solving, addressing these challenges ahead of time, and creating feasible and timely solutions.

Preparation Including Your Plan in a Disaster Situation

Emergency preparedness is defined by the U.S. Department of Homeland Security (DHS) as "a continuous cycle of planning, organizing, training, equipping, exercising, evaluating, and taking corrective action in an effort to ensure effective coordination during incident response" (DHS, 2015, Para 1). There are basic considerations or guiding principles for older adults, family members, and healthcare providers working with elderly and their significant others. Disaster preparation is more complex for older adults and persons with chronic illnesses and disabling conditions (Owens, Stidham, & Owens, 2013). Research further suggests that advanced preparation and evacuation during a disaster leads to better health outcomes. In particular during disaster situations, older adults experience additional risks such as exposure to disease and injury (Cherry & Trainer, 2008), medication separation (Howe, Victor, & Price, 2008), and loss of access to healthcare records (Uscher-Pines et al, 2009).

When preparing for any disaster, three steps are central to preparedness for older adults (American Red Cross [ARC] & Federal Emergency Management Agency [FEMA], 2004; Goundar, 2011; Independent Living Resource Center of San Francisco [ILRCSF], 2012). As part of this process, keep in the forefront of your thinking how vision, hearing, mobility, cognitive, and/or emotional impairments may affect your preparation and outcomes.

1. Make a Disaster Kit of Emergency Supplies

Preparing a disaster kit with emergency supplies is essential and highly recommended by disaster experts (ARC, n.d.; FEMA, 2004; Goundar, 2011; ILRCSF, 2012). For safety and comfort, disaster supplies need to be ready and in one place prior to an actual disaster. Assemble enough supplies to last at least 3 days and place in easy-to-carry containers (e.g., backpack) with an identification tag containing your name and contact information of primary significant others. Label all equipment such as wheelchairs, canes, and walkers with your name, address, phone number, and names and contact information of significant others. If the elder has impaired vision, take into consideration actions such as marking emergency supplies with large print, fluorescent tape, or Braille. Elders also may want to consider preparing two kits, one containing what is needed to stay where they are on their own for a period and the second prepared for if they need to leave their home. Review **Box 26-1**, which lists essential disaster kit supplies that always should be ready to go.

Make sure you keep the disaster kit up to date; review contents at least once every 6 months. Also, review your checklist and plan at least every 6 months and replace all batteries every 12 months. The kit described in

---

BOX 26-1   Emergency Supplies Checklist

A recommended basic checklist of emergency supplies includes the following:

- Water: 1 gallon per person per day for at least 3 days for drinking and sanitation
- Food: At least a 3-day supply of nonperishable food and a can opener if kit contains canned food
- Medications and treatments that the elder takes on a regular basis—at least a week's supply and a copy of the prescriptions as well as treatment information
- If the elder wears contact lenses, cleaning supplies and a storage case
- If the elder wears glasses, uses a wheelchair, or uses oxygen, extra supplies for these
- Battery-operated or hand-crank radio and National Oceanic and Atmospheric Administration weather radio with a tone alert and extra batteries for each
- Flashlight and batteries, high powered if vision is impaired
- First aid kit and whistle to signal for help
- Dust mask if air is contaminated; plastic sheeting and duct tape to shelter in place
- Moist towelettes, incontinence products if needed, garbage bags and plastic ties for personal sanitation
- Wrench or pliers to turn off utilities
- Pet food, extra water, and supplies for pet or service animal

- Local maps
- Extra copies of important papers, such as medical records, medical insurance information, Medicaid and Medicare cards, Social Security number, will, deed, banking information, and operating manuals for lifesaving equipment, all in a plastic bag or waterproof container
- If in a cold climate, appropriate supplies in vehicle

Data from American Red Cross (ARC). (n.d.). *Disaster preparedness: For Seniors by Seniors.* Retrieved from http://www.redcross.org/images /MEDIA_CustomProductCatalog/m4640086 _Disaster_Preparedness_for_Srs-English .revised_7-09.pdf; Federal Emergency Management Agency. (2004). Are you ready? An in-depth guide to citizen preparedness.Retrieved from https://www.fema.gov/pdf/areyouready /areyouready_full.pdf; Goundar, R. (2011). Preparing makes sense for older Americans, Retrieved from http://www.fema.gov/media -library-data/1392389833272-75460345 a2f4adcc5418a1da7cb25eef /2014_PrinterFriendly _ OlderAmericans.pdf; Independent Living Resource Center of San Francisco. (2012). Tips for people with hearing impairments. Retrieved from http://www.ilrcsf.org/wp-content/uploads/2012/08 /Hearing-Impaired.pdf

Box 26-1 should be easily transportable for the purposes of evacuation. Additional items can be stored at home for the kit prepared for sheltering in place. For the kit for sheltering in place, include extra water and food supplies, along with incontinence products, hearing aid batteries, and other items that may be needed to sustain health for a period longer than 3 days.

2. Make a Plan

It is imperative that individuals know their community disaster plans, escape routes, and designated meeting places (ARC, n.d.; ARC & FEMA, 2004). Families need to have their own communication plan and carry information in their wallet, as well as select an out-of-town contact person as part of this plan. It is further recommended that older adults post emergency phone numbers near their telephones; there should be a specific detailed plan for those with disabilities and pets or service animals. Plus, it may be wise for elders to think ahead about utilities, smoke alarms, carbon monoxide alarms (if working correctly), and insurance coverage (adequate for flood damage, etc.).

In addition, elders and their family need to be knowledgeable of their community warning system during disaster and their local neighborhood emergency teams and fire departments, along with how to contact them and what they can realistically offer in an emergency situation. Moreover, elders should determine if they plan to shelter in place versus stay at home and what they need to do if there is a need to evacuate and where they will go—what is feasible?

Given that elders have already gathered essential documents and supplies in the event of a disaster, these items need to be kept in watertight containers and readily accessible. For elders, this may mean next to their bedside stand or a major exit door in their home. Determining this location and making significant others aware of where these things are located are very important. Furthermore, elders should consider creating their own personal support network, especially if they need assistance during a disaster. It is important to make sure this support system is aware of the plan and have a key to the elder's home and knows where the elder's emergency supplies are kept. Practicing this plan with those who have agreed to be part of the elder's personal support network is strongly suggested (Goundar, 2011).

3. Be Informed

What are the most likely hazards or disaster situations in your community? For more information on the types of emergencies possible, visit http://www.ready.gov or call 1-800-BE-READY (ARC, n.d.; FEMA, 2004). Once this information is obtained, it is important to adapt it to the elder's personal circumstances and make every effort to follow instructions given by local authorities. Plus, the older adult needs to know about the local community's warning system and how the residents are notified of a potential disaster. Moreover, the older adult must be aware of the neighborhood emergency response team and how to locate and then access it. Do not make assumptions regarding what is available in disaster situations, and regularly check (at least every 6 months) for changes in these essential community resources.

Disaster Response

Disaster response includes the mobilization of manpower and resources to meet the needs of those affected by disaster events, including saving lives, protecting property and the environment, and meeting basic human needs (DHS, 2013) (**Figure 26-3**). The work that is done in preparing for disasters will aid in disaster response, but

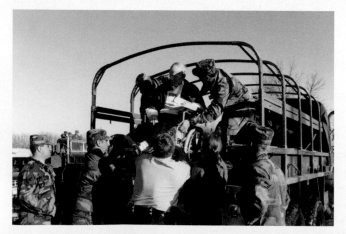

Figure 26-3 Dave Saville, FEMA News, Minnesota, MN Flooding (1997)
Photo by Dave Saville/FEMA News

caring for the older adult in response to disasters is complex. The onset of an event may be abrupt or develop over time. For example, those in the path of a hurricane may have time to evacuate but an explosive event usually occurs without warning. In either case, citizens may be asked to evacuate. Due to a multitude of factors the elderly are at risk during times of evacuation. Mobility concerns, poverty, social isolation, and cognitive difficulties may affect the elders' ability to leave their home.

Evacuation

Evacuation is the moving of people away from potential or actual hazards to a place of safety to reduce morbidity and mortality (Nunes, Roberson, & Zamudio, n.d.). In analyzing census data and hazards spatial data, Zimmerman, Restrepo, Nagorsky, & Culpen (2009) found that older adults tend to live in disproportionately high numbers in areas prone to natural hazards such as hurricanes. Living in these areas puts the elderly at higher risk for evacuation. Unfortunately, many older adults are unable or unwilling to heed evacuation warnings. Elders may decide not to leave their homes and possessions (Dostal, 2015; Smith & McCarthy, 2009). Sensory impairments may prevent the elderly from receiving notice of evacuation. Physical, mental, cognitive, and socioeconomic circumstance may work together to prevent the homebound older adult from evacuation. During the events related to the landfall of Hurricane Katrina, there were circumstances in which residents of nursing homes were abandoned in their facilities and died (AARP, 2006). The Centers for Medicaid and Medicare Services (2013) now requires that these facilities have plans in place for the evacuation of their residents (**Box 26-2**).

CLINICAL TIP

Older adults may be reluctant to leave their home in the event of needed evacuation. Examine factors that might prevent the elderly from receiving a notice or physical issues that would prevent evacuation without assistance.

Triage and Ongoing Risk Assessment

In a mass casualty incident, triage methods will be used to prioritize care for all immediate survivors of a disasters. *Triage* is defined as sorting and assigning priority to disaster survivors when resources are limited, with the goal of doing the most good for the most survivors (Swienton, 2013). Systems such as MASS (Move, Assess, Sort, and Send) are used to sort initial victims. These triage systems are algorithm based and usually rely on color coding or tagging of survivors based on their need for care and likelihood of survival. Two commonly used systems include START (Simple Triage and Rapid Treatment) and SALT (Sort, Assess, Lifesaving Interventions, and Treat/Transport) triage (**Figure 26-4**).

BOX 26-2   Evidence-Based Practice

Emergency planning requires the development of evacuation and sheltering plans. Unfortunately, there has been little research documenting how to best do that, which prevents the development of evidence-based best practices for locating, communicating with, transporting, sheltering, and ensuring the safe recovery of those with medical dependencies. The authors suggest that further fact finding beyond survey research is needed to develop solutions to fill these gaps.

Data from Risoe, P., Schlegelmilch, J., & Paturas, J. (2013). Evacuation and sheltering of people with medical dependencies: Knowledge gaps and barriers to national preparedness. *Homeland Security Affairs* 9(2), 2013. Available at https://www.hsaj.org/articles/234

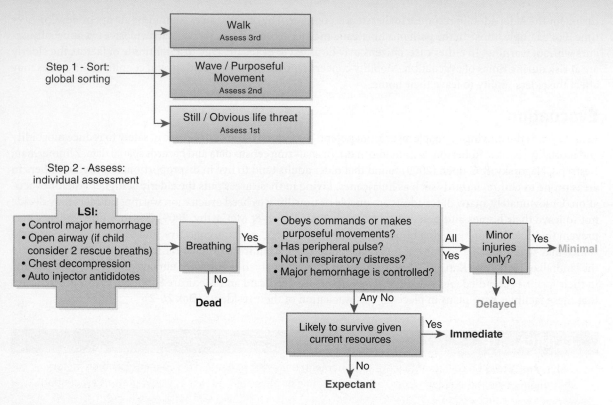

Figure 26-4 SALT Triage

Reproduced from Lerner E. B., Schwartz R. B., Coule P. L., Weinstein, E. S., Crone, D. C., & Hunt, R. C. (2008). Mass casualty triage: An evaluation of the data and development of a proposed national guideline. *Disaster Medicine and Public Health Preparedness, 2*(Supp1), S25–234.

Neither of these systems includes criteria for assessment based on the age of the survivor. The prioritization of care is based solely on key indicators such as respiratory rate and effort. Common categories of triage include immediate, delayed, minimal, and expectant. Those with immediate injuries are highest priority, requiring fast care to avoid decompensation or death. Individuals with delayed injuries are unlikely to decompensate quickly and can wait for care. Minimal injuries may require care at an ambulatory care center or home treatment. Meanwhile, those with expectant injuries have wounds that are not compatible with life given current resources (Lerner et al., 2008).

CLINICAL TIP

Triage is a way to prioritize care in mass casualty situations. Two common systems to use are START and SALT.

Triage also occurs within the hospital systems. Those arriving at the hospital are evaluated based on their condition for priority of admission and treatment. The triage position may be performed by a hospitalist or a nurse. The focus is on optimal utilization of the hospital resources such as operating rooms, bed space, intensive care beds, and other resources that may be limited. There are no standardized methods for hospital allocation of resources with each institution using its own processes. It should be noted that the elderly may be triaged to lower priority due to preexisting conditions and risks (Abrohneim, Arquilla, & Gambale, 2009). In addition, always

SWiFT level	Explanation	Postdisaster Actions
1	Cannot perform at least one basic activity of daily living (ADL: Eating, bathing, dressing, toileting, walking, continence) without assistance	Transfer to a location that can provide skilled or personal care, such as an assisted living facility, nursing home, hospital, or shelter
2	Trouble with instrumental activities of daily living (IADLs: Finances, benefits management, accessing resources)	Connect to a local agency services case manager
3	Minimal assistance with ADLs and IADLs	Connect to a rescue organizations such as the Red Cross

Reproduced from Dyer, C. B., Regev, M., Burnett, J., Festa, N., & Bloyd, B. (2008). SWiFT: A rapid triage tool for vulnerable elders in disaster situations. *Disaster Medicine and Public Health Preparedness, 2*, S45–S50.

Exhibit 26-1 SWiFT Seniors Without Families Triage (Tool).

assess the older adult for safety and health need priorities even in a disaster situation, taking into consideration normal and abnormal aging changes (refer to previous chapters).

The effects of a disaster on the elderly within a community will vary widely based on their risks. The frail elderly with multiple chronic illnesses living in social isolation and poverty are at highest risk, but even healthy older adults may lack the physiologic reserves and therefore be at higher risk during a disaster (Ahronheim et al., 2009). All of those who come to the hospital will not need emergent care. Many homebound older adults, those who require daily care and those who are dependent on equipment and other resources, may come to the emergency department for assistance. The Seniors Without Family Triage (SWiFT) Level Tool can be used after a disaster to determine the level of care needed for these elder survivors (See **Exhibits 26-1** and **26-2**).

Diagnostic Challenges of the Elderly

There is great variability in the physical and cognitive functioning of elders. If the baseline functional status is unknown, it may make it difficult to determine the effects of disasters. New onset of confusion, changes, and physiologic status may be attributed to preexisting conditions when in actuality they are due to the effects of the event. In addition, chronic illness and comorbidities may make it difficult to discern patterns of significant responses (Ahronheim et al., 2009; Filiberto et al., 2011). Unfortunately, there is a dearth of trained gerontology specialists in the United States (American Geriatrics Society, 2009), which may cause difficulties for assessment and treatment of the elder following disasters.

Soft Care Areas

Many people will report to area hospitals, even if they are uninjured. Hospitals are viewed as havens and sources of all types of care. It has been suggested that acute care facilities develop "soft care" areas where elders who do not require skilled, acute care may stay until transferred to shelters or alternative care sites. The loss of community services may result in the need for alternative care sites. These areas could provide refuge for those with functional or cognitive impairments, or both, who have disrupted home care. Abrohneim et al. (2009) describe soft care areas as "Secure place in the hospital staffed to treat medically stable, but frail elderly vulnerable adults, who cannot be safely discharged from the emergency department in a timely manner, but who need psychosocial support and medical oversight" (p. 32). They could be in an unoccupied unit or area of the hospital while maintaining communication with the emergency department and pharmacy. It is further suggested that the area be staffed by individuals trained in geriatric care.

Current date:		Worker's name:	
Name:		DOB:	
DO YOU HAVE FAMILY OR FRIENDS WITH YOU HERE? ☐ Y ☐ N **Confirmed?** ☐ Y ☐ N			

Level 1: <u>**Health/Mental Health Priority**</u>
 	
GOES TO SOCIAL WORK BOOTH IN MEDICAL CLINIC
	A. Do you have any of the following medical problems:
	  ☐ Y ☐ N Diabetes
	  ☐ Y ☐ N Heart disease
	  ☐ Y ☐ N High blood pressure
	  ☐ Y ☐ N Memory
	  ☐ Other
	Note:
	
	B. Do you take medicine?
	  ☐ Y ☐ N
	
	Do you have your medicine?
	  ☐ Y ☐ N
	If "No," treat as Level 1
		C. Do you need someone to help you with:
		  ☐ Y ☐ N Walking
		  ☐ Y ☐ N Eating
		  ☐ Y ☐ N Bathing
		  ☐ Y ☐ N Dressing
		  ☐ Y ☐ N Toileting
		  ☐ Y ☐ N Medication administration
		
		Any checks, treat as Level 1
		Do you use something to help you get around:
		☐ Cane
		☐ Walker
		☐ Wheel chair
		☐ Bath Bench

D. Where are you right now? **If senior cannot or does not answer correctly treat as Level 1**	**E.** Name 3 ordinary items and have them repeat them; for example, "apple, table, penny."	**F.** What year is it? **If senior cannot/ does not answer correctly treat as Level 1**	**G.** Ask them to repeat the three items you previously mentioned. **If more than one item is missed, treat as Level 1.**

Level 2: <u>**Case Management Needs**</u> **IS REFERRED TO A CASE MANAGER**	**A.** Ask them what their major need is right now.	**B**. Do you have a plan for where you will go when you leave here? ☐ Yes ☐ No

		C. *Income/Entitlements*
		
		Are you on:
		  ☐ Y ☐ N Medicare
		  ☐ Y ☐ N Medicaid
		  ☐ Y ☐ N SSI
		  ☐ Y ☐ N Social Security
		  ☐ Y ☐ N Food Stamps
		  ☐ Y ☐ N VA Benefits
		  ☐ Y ☐ N Section 8 housing funds
		
		Do you have your documents?
		  ☐ Yes ☐ No

Level 3: Only <u>**needs to be**</u> <u>**linked to family**</u> <u>**or friends**</u> **DIRECTED TO RED CROSS VOLUNTEER**	**A.** *Family* Do you need help to find your family/ friends? ☐ Yes ☐ No	**B.** Names: Relationship: Location:
		WHERE IS THE SENIOR LOCATED?

Exhibit 26-2 SWiFT Screening Tool.
Reproduced from Dyer, C.B., Regev, M., Burnett, J., Festa, N., & Bloyd, B. (2008). SWiFT—A rapid triage tool for vulnerable elders in disaster situations. *Disaster Medicine and Public Health Preparedness*, 2, S45–S50.

Case Study 26-1

You are working in the emergency department of a large hospital. Your area has been hit by a large tornado. There are mass casualties. There are reports that an extended care facility in close proximity to the hospital has been hit. Survivors begin to arrive. You begin to assess a 78-year-old woman with a history of congestive heart failure and chronic lung disease; she is having moderate difficulty breathing and has small laceration on her forehead. The bleeding is controlled. She is a widow with no children from the extended care facility. What are your patient's risk factors? At what level would you triage her care? Applying the SWiFT assessment, where would the best placement for this patient be?

Sheltering

Shelters should be able to assist most elders with their care. In compliance with the American Disabilities Act, shelters should be accessible to all individuals. Shelters will be able to assist individuals by providing functional need support. This includes providing help with activities of daily living, oxygen therapy, wound care, etc. (FEMA, 2010). If care is beyond the capabilities of the shelter, in some cases medical shelters may be available. Extended care facilities do not evacuate their clients to shelters; they are required to have their own plans for displaced residents (CMS, 2013). The movement of individuals out of their home environment is stressful for everyone, but may be especially difficult for elders. Besides evacuation, citizens may be asked to shelter in place. For example, in events such as chemical or radiation exposures residents may be asked to stay in their homes. This situation may be particularly difficult for elders who are relying on others for care and resources (**Case Study 26-1**).

Psychological Support

Elders may have sustained many losses throughout their life. Death of loved ones, loss of physical capabilities, role changes, and reduced income are related to an increased risk of psychological trauma following a disaster (AARP, 2006). Plus, they may be reluctant to ask for assistance, which also increases their vulnerability. It is always important to assess psychological needs and provide support to older adults involved in disaster or emergency events. As already mentioned, disaster situations may affect mental health (e.g., depression, anxiety) of older adults and individualized assessment is essential. Several screening instruments exist, but are not specific to assessment following a disaster situation. The Screening Questionnaire for Disaster Mental Health (SQD) is a 12-item assessment tool and serves as an excellent starting point, especially for individuals experiencing depression and posttraumatic stress disorder (PTSD) following a disaster situation (Fujii, Kato, & Maeda, 2008). The SQD is also listed on the National Institutes of Health website as a valuable resource (see http://www.ncbi.nlm.nih.gov/pubmed/18762732).

Ethical Challenges

There is an ethical obligation for healthcare providers and agencies to plan for disasters and emergent events. Past experience demonstrates that a lack of planning results in a loss of life. In these stressful times it is important to remember that the elder still has the right to self-determination and patient wishes must be respected. Access to hospice and palliative care need to be available. According to Abrohneim et al. (2009), when resources are limited there is a risk that age discrimination may occur. Remember that chronologic age is not an indicator of overall wellness and decisions must be made fairly. During times of disaster, crisis standards of care may be implemented. Liability and malpractice concerns exist. It is important that nurses follow the laws of their state, which vary widely. Your employer and state board of nursing are resources to assist with these questions.

Disaster Recovery

Disaster recovery includes the mobilization of resources to assist communities affected by a disaster to return to a state of normality (DHS, 2013) (See **Boxes 26-3** and **26-4**). Important needs to be considered during recovery include the following (Dyer et al, 2008b):

BOX 26-3   Research Highlight

In many instances, disasters lead to catastrophic losses that can devastate communities, requiring them to rebuild their homes or relocate. Unfortunately, there is a limited knowledge pertaining to the long-term psychological consequences among disaster survivors. The purpose of this study was to examine the predictors of psychological outcomes for a convenience sample of 219 residents from disaster-affected communities in south Louisiana. The study sample consisted of current coastal residents who had severe property damage from the 2005 Hurricanes Katrina and Rita and exposure to the 2010 British Petroleum Deepwater Horizon oil spill and were compared to a control group of noncoastal residents who had not experienced the 2005 and 2010 disaster situations. The concepts measured were storm exposure and stressors, religiosity, perceived social support, and mental health outcomes. Results indicate that those who had a religious affiliation tended to be at a lower risk for PTSD following the disaster. Disaster survivors who had a lower income and were coastal fisherman experienced more depressive symptoms associated with loss of their ability to work, but their perceived social support appeared to also

have a protective effect for all mental health outcomes. The study findings further indicate that individuals with low income, limited social support, and high levels of no prior religious affiliation were at greater risk for mental health problems (e.g., PTSD, depression). Major clinical implications suggested by the findings are that healthcare professionals must do the following:

* Consider the disaster survivor's psychological reactions in both short and long term (5 years and longer after the event)
* Assess the disaster survivor's specific perceived sources of social support
* Consider the disaster survivor's perceptions of threat, safety, and basic human needs
* Determine and implement age-appropriate and timely interventions that consider the survivor's perceived needs and concerns
* Partner with available community resources to maximize the potential for positive outcomes

Modified from Cherry, K. E., Sampson, L., Nezat, P., Cacamo, A., Marcks, L. D., & Galea, S. (2015). Long-term psychological outcomes in older adults after disaster: Relationships to religiosity and social support. *Aging and Mental Health, 19*(5) 430–443.

BOX 26-4   Resource list

American Red Cross: Nursing Students
http://www.redcross.org/support/volunteer/nurses/students

Federal Emergency Management Agency: Are you ready? An in-depth guide to preparedness

http://www.fema.gov/media-library/assets/documents/7877

Recommendations for Best Practices in Management of Elderly Disaster Victims
https://www.bcm.edu/pdf/bestpractices.pdf

> Finding appropriate temporary and permanent housing
> Reestablishing public benefits and services
> Linkages with physical and mental health services as needed (acute and long-term)
> Acquire needed resources such as medications, durable medical equipment, clothing, and household supplies
> Assist with transportation needs
> Family reunification

It should be further recognized that individual factors such as psychosocial aspects of recovery assistance and loss of treasured possessions can create great stress for those who survive and should be considered in the recovery process (Tuohy, 2010).

Clinical Reasoning Exercises

1. Explore the American Red Cross Student Nursing Pages http://www.redcross.org/support/volunteer/nurses/students

2. Review opportunities for your participation in this volunteer organization. Discuss areas of interest with another student nurse in one of your clinical groups.

Personal Reflections

Have you assisted a patient in a wheelchair to the bathroom? Was it difficult? Consider the difficulties of caring for this patient in the Astrodome. Would there be the equipment you need? Would there be privacy for you and the patient? How would you meet the needs of your patient with limited resources?

References

AARP (2006). *We can do better: Lessons learned for protecting older persons in disasters.* Retrieved from http://assets.aarp.org/rgcenter/il/better.pdf

Aldrich, N., & Benson, W. F. (2008). Disaster preparedness and the chronic needs of vulnerable older adults. *Prep Chronic Disease, 5*(1), A27.

Ahronheim, J. C., Arquilla, B., Greene, R. G. (2009). *Elderly population in disasters: Hospital guidelines for geriatric preparedness.* New York, NY: New York City Department of Health and Mental Hygiene.

Al-rousan, T., Rubenstein, L. M., & Wallace, R. B. (2014). Preparedness for national disasters among older U.S. adults: A national survey. *American Journal of Public Health, 104*: 506–511.

American Geriatrics Society (2009). Geriatrics Workforce Policies Studies Center. Retrieved from http://www.americangeriatrics.org/advocacy_public_policy/gwps/gwps_faqs/id:3190

American Red Cross (ARC). (n.d.). *Disaster preparedness: For Seniors by Seniors.* Retrieved from http://www.redcross.org/images/MEDIA_CustomProductCatalog/m4640086_Disaster_Preparedness_for_Srs-English.revised_7-09.pdf

Banks, L. (2013). Caring for elderly adults during disasters: Improving health outcomes and recovery. *Southern Medical Assocation, 106* (1), 94–98.

Baylor College of Medicine, & American Medical Association. (2006). *Recommendations for best practices in the management of elderly disaster victims*. Retrieved from https://www.bcm.edu/pdf/bestpractices.pdf

Centers for Disease Control and Prevention (CDC). (2012). *Identifying vulnerable older adults and legal options for increasing their protection during all-hazards emergencies: A cross-sector guide for states and communities*. Atlanta, Ga: U.S. Department of Health and Human Services.

Cherry, K. E., Sampson, L., Nezat, P., Cacamo, A., Marcks, L. D., & Galea, S. (2015). Long-term psychological outcomes in older adults after disaster: Relationships to religiosity and social support. *Aging and Mental Health, 19*(5) 430–443.

Cherry, R. A., & Trainer, M. (2008). The current crisis in emergency care the impact of disaster preparedness. *MC Emergency Medicine, 8*, 7.

Dolan, G., & Messen, D. (2012). Social vulnerability: An emergency manager's planning tool. *Journal of Emergency Management,* January/February, 161–169.

Dostal, P. J. (2015). Vulnerability of urban homebound older adults in disasters: A survey of evacuation preparedness. *Disaster Medicine and Public Health Preparedness, 9*, 301–306. doi:10.1017/dmp.2015.50.

Dyer, C. B., Festa, N., Cloyd, B., Regev, M., Schwartzberg, J. G., James, J., & Dix, M. (2008a). Recommendations for best practices in the management of elderly disaster victims. Houston: AARP.

Dyer, C. B., Regev, M., Burnett, J., Festa, N., & Bloyd, B. (2008b). SWiFT: A rapid triage tool for vulnerable elders in disaster situations. *Disaster Medicine and Public Health Preparedness, 2*, S45–S50.

Evans, J. (2010). Mapping the vulnerability of older persons to disasters. *International Journal of Older People Nursing, 5*, 63–70.

Federal Emergency Management Agency. (2004). Are you ready? An indepth guide to citizen preparedness. Retrieved from https://www.fema.gov/pdf/areyouready/areyouready_full.pdf

Federal Emergency Management Agency. (2010). *Guidance on planning for integration of functional needs support services in general population shelters*. Retrieved from http://www.fema.gov/pdf/about/odic/fnss_guidance.pdf

Filiberto, D., Wethington, E., Pillemer, K., Wells, N. M., Wysocki, M., & Parise, J. T. (2011). Older people and climate change: Vulnerability and health effects. Retrieved from http://www.asaging.org/blog/older-people-and-climate-change-vulnerability-and-health-effects

Freid, V. M., Bernstein, A. B., & Bush, M. (2012). Multiple chronic conditions among adults aged 45 and over: Trends over the past 10 years. NCHS Data Brief 100. Hyattsville, MD: National Center for Health Statistics.

Fujii, S., Kato, H., & Maeda, K. (2008). The simple interview-format screening measure for disaster mental health: An instrument new developed after the 1995 Great Hanshin Earthquake in Japan—the Screening Questionnaire for Disaster Mental Health (SQD). *Kobe Journal of Medical Science, 53*(6), 375–385.

Goundar, R. (2011). Preparing makes sense for older Americans, Retrieved from http://www.fema.gov/media-library-data/1392389833272-75460345a2f4adcc5418a1da7cb25eef/2014_PrinterFriendly_OlderAmericans.pdf

Howe, E., Victor, D., & Price, E. (2008). Chief complaints, diagnoses, and medications prescribed seven weeks post Katrina in New Orleans. *Posthospital and Disaster Medicne, 23* (1), 41–47.

Hutton D. (2008). *Older people in emergencies: Considerations for action and policy development*. Geneva: World Health Organization.

Independent Living Resource Center of San Francisco. (2012). Tips for people with hearing impairments. Retrieved from http://www.ilrcsf.org/wp-content/uploads/2012/08/Hearing-Impaired.pdf

International Federation of the Red Cross and Red Crescent Societies. (2015). World disaster report. Retrieved from http://ifrc-media.org/interactive/wp-content/uploads/2015/09/1293600-World-Disasters-Report-2015_en.pdf

Khorram-Manesh, A., Angthong, C., Pangma, A., Sulannakarn, S., Burivong, R., Jarayabhand, R., & Ortenwall, P. (2013). Hospital evacuation: Learning from the past? *British Journal of Medicine and Medical Research, 4*(1), 395–415.

Lerner, E. B., Schwartz, R. B., Coule, P. L., Weinstein, E. S., Crone, D. C., & Hunt, R. C. (2008). Mass casualty triage: An evaluation of the data and development of proposed national guideline. *Disaster Medicine and Public Health Preparedness, 2*(Supp1), S25–S34

Nunes, N., Roberson, K., & Zamudio, A. (n.d.). The MEND Guide: Comprehensive guide for planning mass evacuations in natural disasters (pilot document). Retrieved from http://www.globalcccmcluster.org/system/files/publications/MEND_download.pdf

Owens, J., Stidham, A., & Owens, E.L., (2013). Disaster evacuation for persons with special needs: A content of information on YouTube. *Applied Nursing Research, 26(4), 273–275.*

Smith, S. K., & McCarthy, C. (2009). Fleeing the storm(s): An examination of evacuation behavior during Florida's 2004 hurricane season. *Demography 46*(1), 127–145.

Swienton, R. (2013). *Basic disaster life support* (3rd ed). New York, NY: National Disaster Life Support Foundation.

The Joint Commission. (2013). *Emergency management.* Retrieved from http://www.jointcommission.org/emergency_management.aspx

Tuohy, R. J. (2010). Post-disaster recovery of older adults. *GNS Science Report,* April.

U.S. Census Bureau. (2012). Population projections. Retrieved from http://www.census.gov/population/projections/

Uscher-Pines, L., Hausman, A., DiMara, P., Heake, G., & Hagan, M. (2009). Disaster preparedness of households with special needs in Southeastern Pennsylvania. *American Journal of Preventive Medicine, 37*(3), 227–230.

U.S. Department of Health and Human Services (DHHS); Centers for Medicaid and Medicare Services (CMS). (2013). *Emergency preparedness checklist recommended tool for effective health care facility planning.* Retrieved from https://docs.google.com/document/d/1-Yzw16ItonGwdWos4vbT3kf3wWFekqsUUCqR7SNAhqQ/edit

U.S. Department of Homeland Security. (2013). *National response framework* (2nd ed). Washington D.C.: Federal Emergency Management Agency. Retrieved from https://www.fema.gov/media-library-data/20130726-1914-25045-1246/final_national_response_framework_20130501.pdf

U.S. Department of Homeland Security (DHS). (2015). *Plan and prepare for disasters.* Retrieved from http://www.dhs.gov/topic/plan-and-prepare-disasters

World Health Organization (WHO). (2005). *Disasters and emergencies: Definitions.* Retrieved from http://www.who./disasters/repo/7656.pdf

Zimmerman, R., Restrepo, C. E., Nagorsky, B., & Culpen, A. M. (2009). Vulnerability of the elderly during natural hazard events. Nonpublished Research Reports. Paper 44. Retrieved from http://research.create.usc.edu/nonpublished_reports/44 Retrieved from http://create.usc.edu/sites/default/files/publications/vulnerabilityoftheelderlyduringnaturalhazardevents.pdf

For a full suite of assignments and additional learning activities, see the access code at the front of your book.

CHAPTER 27

End-of-Life Care

Patricia Warring
Luana S. Krieger-Blake

(Competencies 11, 16)

LEARNING OBJECTIVES

At the end of this chapter, the reader will be able to:

> Identify historical influences and attitudes toward death and dying.
> Recognize the choices of older adults and their families in directing their end-of-life care, as well as the nurse's role in support and implementation of the patient's choice of care.
> Compare curative care, hospice care, and palliative care.
> Examine the goals and objectives of curative, palliative, and hospice care at end of life.
> Discuss the nurse's role at end of life using the preceding concepts of care.
> Describe the nurse's role as a member of an interdisciplinary team focused on end-of-life care.
> Identify the fundamentals of pain and other symptom management.
> Discuss death in a contemporary multicultural society.
> Identify cultural traditions at end of life.
> Recognize the importance of spirituality at end of life.
> Describe some effects of grief and mourning on the elderly.
> Recognize caregiver and compassion fatigue.
> Describe ethical and legal issues common at end of life.
> Recognize several aspects of care contributing to a "good death."

KEY TERMS

Addiction

Advance directives

Allow natural death

Communicating bad news

Complementary therapies

Curative and acute care

Dependence	Moral injury
Do not resuscitate	Mourning
End of life	Palliative care
Five Wishes	Physician Orders for Life-Sustaining
Good death	Treatment
Grief	SUPPORT study
Hope	Symptom management
Hospice care	Therapeutic (healing) touch
Interdisciplinary group/team	Tolerance

Woody Allen once said, "It's not that I'm afraid to die, I just don't want to be there when it happens" (Allen, 1976, Act 1). "By excluding death from our life we cannot live a full life, and by admitting death into our life we enlarge and enrich it." This statement, written by a victim of the Holocaust, describes the powerful role that death has in human life (Hillesum, 1996, p. 155).

Reality tells us that every person will die. In 2013, less than 14% of U.S. citizens died suddenly, either from accidents, influenza and pneumonia, or intentional self-harm; the vast majority of Americans died after dealing with prolonged illness (Centers for Disease Control and Prevention [CDC], 2016).

The accumulation of experiences throughout a person's lifetime helps clearly define the way he or she wishes to experience his or her own end of life. Familial and cultural factors, along with life events, often provide defining moments that influence a person's choices when facing the end of life and a death that will come sooner rather than later. Anthropologist Margaret Mead was quoted as saying, "When a person is born we rejoice, and when they're married we jubilate, but when they die we try to pretend nothing happened."

This chapter deals with the nurse's role in assisting a patient and family to identify the options for meeting end-of-life needs. It promotes the role of the nurse as a member of a team of professionals who focus on care and treatment of issues specific to the elderly as their health declines. It also offers practical assistance for nurses as they deal with various aspects of end-of-life care.

Historically, education about end-of-life issues and medical needs has been lacking. Initiatives including those by Last Acts and those encouraged by the Robert Wood Johnson Foundation, such as Education in Palliative and End-of-Life Care (EPEC), End-of-Life Nursing Education Consortium (ELNEC), and Center to Advance Palliative Care (CAPC), are in place to address the need for additional information and research in this area.

One of the most demanding roles nurses undertake is that of caring for patients near the end of life. Nurses provide the most direct care for patients and families and also help the family provide care that is competent, comprehensive, and compassionate. Therefore, nurses "must take the lead in integrating palliative and end-of-life care into the daily practice of every nurse, making it a core competency for all nurses who care for people with actual or potentially life-limiting illnesses. . . . . Nurses must advocate for and deliver this quality care—regardless of specialty" (Rushton, Spencer, & Johanson, 2004, p. 34).

Caring for dying patients and their families is a common component of the nurse's role, yet it can be particularly distressing for nursing students because very little classroom or clinical time is spent in this area. It has been suggested that because of the inherent richness in working with these patients, clinical rotations should be structured appropriately to include end-of-life experiences (Allchin, 2006). Partnering with local hospices and/ or palliative care programs to provide educational opportunities and hands-on care of the dying would benefit the student by providing a relevant life experience.

Historical Attitudes Toward Death and Dying

With the advent of ever-increasing modern technology, especially following World War II, dying in the United States underwent a multitude of changes. In years past, Americans frequently lived in multigenerational homes, often in rural settings where living and dying experiences occurred commonly on the farms. Children were exposed to life and death issues as a matter of fact and grew to be adults having some experience of death before experiencing the death of someone close to them. As the ability to cure illnesses and to prolong life developed, technology took death to the hospital—to the sophistication of machines, antibiotics, chemotherapy, surgery, and such—and away from the comforts of home and family.

The role of nursing has changed along with the evolution of technology in administering end-of-life care in this country. For the most part, nurses shared the focus toward cure prevalent in the hospital setting. Training to care for the dying patient is often linked to the technical aspects of care and the physical preparation of the body after death (Krisman-Scott, 2003). A research and literature review performed by Benoliel for the period 1900 to 1960 revealed only 21 articles for nurses about caring for the dying patient: "There was little evidence that care of the dying was ever a major concern of nurses in this country" (Quint, 1967, p. 11).

As a result of the changes in our attitudes toward death and dying over time, some have said that the United States is a death-denying society. Kerry Crammer, MD, said, "In the Orient, dying is a requirement. In Europe, dying is inevitable. In America, dying appears to be an option" (Lewis, 2001, p. 24).

This death-denying attitude has created very expensive medical care. Spending on behalf of Medicare beneficiaries in their last year of life is five to six times as much as for other beneficiaries. Medicare expenditures are not distributed evenly across the last 12 months of life, but accelerate rapidly in the last few months. Hospice saved in Medicare costs for some number of years, but now, on average, shows no cost savings (Hogan, Lunney, Gabel, & Lynn, 2001). A recent study by Arcadia Healthcare Solutions found that "spending on people who die in the hospital is about seven times that on people who die at home," according to Dr. Richard Parker, chief medical officer at Arcadia. The study further indicated where people died and how much the final month of care cost, as follows (Kodjak, 2016):

> 42% of patients died at home: $ 4,760
> 40% of patients died in the hospital: $ 43,379
> 7% of patients died in hospice care: $ 17,845
> 7% of patients died in a nursing facility: $ 21,221
> 5% of patients died in the ER: $ 7,969

Even though the expense of medical care at *end of life* is great, it does not necessarily follow that the needs of the elderly terminally ill are being met. The *SUPPORT study* (the Study to Understand Prognosis and Preferences for Outcomes and Risks of Treatment) conducted between 1989 and 1994 reported that nurses often were the first to recognize the impending death of a patient (Sheehan & Schirm, 2003). It also revealed that our healthcare system does not meet either the needs of patients with advanced chronic illnesses or the needs of dying, terminally ill patients (Quaglietti, Blum, & Ellis, 2004). Nor does the care we have come to accept meet the wishes of many Americans who are terminally ill. The National Hospice and Palliative Care Organization (NHPCO) reports that a great majority of Americans say their wish is to die at home, but of the 2.4 million Americans who die each year, less than 25% actually die at home. In comparison, of the estimated 1.7million patients who received hospice care in 2014, almost 67% died at home (NHPCO, 2016).

Recently, dying is beginning to be seen in a newer, more realistic light. Ira Byock (2012), a leading palliative care physician and advocate for improving care at end of life, has linked dying to an ongoing potential for growth. "Dying represents more than a set of problems to be solved; it represents an extraordinary opportunity—an opportunity for review, for restitution, for amends, for exploration, for development, for insight. In short, it is an opportunity for growth" (Kinzbrunner, Weinreb, & Policzer, 2002, p. 259). Instead of growing up, growing old, and dying, Dr. Byock suggests we grow up, grow old, and grow on. "Growing on takes place for both the terminally ill aged and their families. And although patients and their families will universally find growth-producing deaths as important and positive, it may not be easy. Indeed there are typically many obstacles that must be overcome if the process of death is to unfold in a productive manner" (McKinnon & Miller, 2002, pp. 259–270).

Nurses have the opportunity and ability to influence the process of death by virtue of their proximity to patients and families. Nurses spend more time with patients and their families at end of life than any other member of the healthcare team (Ferrell, Grant, & Virani, 1999). Families and patients look to the nurse for support, education, and guidance at this difficult time, yet little education is provided to prepare nurses for this unique type of care. Nurses face end-of-life situations in almost all practice settings, including hospitals, hospices, long-term care facilities, home care, prisons, and clinics, but many remain uncomfortable providing care. Because of the importance of end-of-life care, nursing education is beginning to focus on care at this stage of life (Hospice and Palliative Nurses Association [HPNA], 2004b).

The focus of care at end of life should center on living with terminal illness—with medical care, support, and interventions geared toward quality of life and comfort, rather than on prolonging suffering or the dying process—if that is what the patient wants. In determining the wishes of patients for end-of-life care, their physical, emotional, psychosocial, and spiritual needs must all be addressed. The cumulative nature of these aspects of a person's life will have an impact on the choices they make at this important time. See **Box 27-1** for an instructor-led exercise to guide reflection on death and dying.

BOX 27-1   Death and Dying: A Simulation Exercise

This is a very effective guided reflection, with the facilitator reading the scenario and the participants listening, actively taking part with their responses to the slips of paper and subsequent instructions. The element of surprise is effective if the participants do not know the scenario before beginning the exercise. This exercise often provokes emotional responses, which can then be discussed and processed to incorporate into the learning experience.

Supplies: One packet of 12 slips of paper for each participant

Writing utensil

Overhead transparency of questions for class or small group discussion (optional)

Instructions: Slips of paper can be premarked with the following four topics (three slips for each topic):

- A person who is very dear to you
- A thing you own that you regard as very special
- An activity in which you enjoy participating
- A personal attribute or role of which you are proud

Verbal instruction by facilitator:

Write one item per topic on each slip of paper.

Arrange the 12 slips of paper in front of you so that you can see all of them.

Get into a comfortable position; take a deep relaxing breath.

Listen without comment and follow the instructions given to you while I describe some happenings, some situations, and some people.

(Facilitator should develop the scenario carefully, allowing time for awakening all the senses.)

1. You are at your doctor's office; you hear the diagnosis—cancer.

    Please select and tear up three slips of paper. (Allow time [15 to 30 seconds] for selection and tearing . . . brief pause . . . facilitator or assistant may want to physically collect the papers and deposit them in a wastebasket for greater effect.)

2. You are back at home—who is there? Who do you want to be there? What do you say? What do you want to hear?

    Please tear up another three slips of paper. (Provide another appropriate-length pause. Collect and discard.)

3. It is now 2 months later. You are aware your symptoms are worsening and you are feeling weaker. Where are you? What is your lifestyle? What do you continue to do? What can you do? Tear up another two slips of paper. (Provide appropriate time between each phrase for reflection and for choices of paper to be discarded.)

4. Now, it is 4 months later—you are undeniably ill. The pain has increased considerably. Where are you? Who stays with you? Who visits you? Who are the people you want around you? Tear up another two slips of paper (discard).

5. Six months have now passed, and you find that even the smallest activity of daily living takes most of your energy. How do you feel about yourself? Where are you? Who is with you? Turn over the last two slips of paper in front of you.

    I will take one of them at random.

    (Facilitator takes one of the remaining slips from each participant and tears and discards.)

6. Facilitator says only: Tear up your last slip of paper . . . you have died.

Discussion and reflection:
May be discussed in small groups in the class setting.

Personal reflection:

- What issues arose for you from each scenario? Fears? Concerns?
- What were the easiest things to give up? Most difficult?
- What emotional reactions did you have with each scenario?
- What did you think/feel/experience when one of the slips was randomly taken from you?
- Did you anticipate the content of the last scenario?
- What were your thoughts/feelings/reactions to tearing up the last slip of paper?

Reflection in reference to the elderly:

- What different issues would arise for the elderly population? Fears? Concerns? (e.g., caregiving issues, financial concerns, being alone, lack of support, physical limitations)
- Might an elderly person have a harder or easier time giving up things in the four categories on the slips of paper? Why or why not for each category?
- Would the emotional responses of an elderly person be different from your own for each scenario? Why or why not?

First used by Hospice of Bloomington in April 1986, provided by Rev. Dick Lentz from St. Vincent's Hospice, Indianapolis, IN; adapted for use with VNA Hospice of Porter County; further adapted for use in this book.

Communication about End of Life

Talking about Death and Dying

Talking about death and dying is often difficult for both nurses and patients. If the nurse does not respond in a way that encourages discussion, that discussion will likely not take place and death will become the "elephant in the room"—something unavoidable and yet taboo (Griffie, Nelson-Marten, & Muchka, 2004).

> ### CLINICAL TIP
>
> If you are unsure about a patient's preference for end of life care or arrangements, ask him.

The Patient Protection and Affordable Care Act of 2010 addresses some aspects of end-of-life care, but lacks in making services for the dying a priority (Storey, 2016). Widely publicized misconceptions of the Act had many people concerned about "death panels" and "rationing" of health care, so it was omitted from the final version (Medscape, 2016). However, a physician's survey found about 95% of those responding favored Medicare's new provision for payment for helping patients with advance care planning (American Academy of Hospice and Palliative Medicine [AAHPM], 2016.) Since then, the proposal has been included in the Medicare physician fee schedule for 2016, and does allow for voluntary end-of-life counseling (Lowes, 2016). Even so, almost half of the physicians indicated they were not sure what to say to patients during end-of-life conversations (AAHPM, 2016).

Perhaps the easiest method of learning about a person's preferences is for the nurse, physician, or caregiver to simply ask the person. Unfortunately, these conversations are often not held because of fear—the elderly person's fear of being perceived as giving up, the family's fear of not wanting the elderly person to think he or she is wished to be dead, or perhaps the care provider's fear of not knowing what to say or how to discuss bad news. The societal attitudes about denying death are certainly a factor in whether these conversations are held. In hospice circles, it has been implied that most people would rather talk to their children about drugs and sex than to their elderly parents about terminal illness. There are resources designed to assist with these conversations, because not having the conversation may prohibit an individual from having the type of care wanted, simply because the person and the caregivers are not aware of the options.

Communicating Bad News

The EPEC Project, supported by the American Medical Association and the Robert Wood Johnson Foundation (Emanuel, von Gunten, & Ferris, 1999), as well as ELNEC, view the communication of bad news as an essential skill for physicians. It is also an essential skill for nurses and other interdisciplinary team members who interact with the patients and families.

EPEC Project Module 2 presents a 6-step approach to *communicating bad news* (Emanuel et al., 1999):

1. *Get started:* Plan what to say, confirm medical facts, create a conducive environment, determine who else the patient would like present, and allocate adequate time.
2. *Find out what the patient knows:* Assess his or her ability to comprehend bad news.
3. *Find out how much the patient wants to know:* Recognize and support patient preference to decline information and to designate someone else to communicate on his or her behalf; accommodate cultural, religious, and socioeconomic influences.

4. *Share information:* Say it, then stop. Pause frequently, check for understanding, and use silence and body language; avoid vagueness, jargon, and euphemisms.
5. *Respond to feelings:* Expect affective, cognitive, and fight–flight responses; be prepared for strong emotions and a broad range of reactions. Give time to react; listen, and encourage description of feelings. Use nonverbal communication of touch and eye contact.
6. *Plan/follow-up:* Provide additional tests, symptom treatment, and referrals as needed. Discuss potential sources of support; assess the safety of the patient and home supports before he or she leaves. Repeat the news at future visits.

Advance Directives

The Patient Self-Determination Act (PSDA), a federal law, requires healthcare providers to routinely provide information about *advance directives*. There are several nationally recognized advance directives to help an individual identify personal wishes in a legal manner and share that information with the people around them, including medical personnel. Durable power of attorney, living will, appointment of healthcare representative, *do not resuscitate* (DNR), and life-prolonging procedures declarations are all legally recognized documents for indicating one's healthcare wishes. Additionally, *Five Wishes* (Towey, 2005), *allow natural death* (AND), and the *Physician Orders for Life-Sustaining Treatment* (POLST) are three more recent options for stating end-of-life care wishes.

Five Wishes is a movement that encourages people to provide more specific instructions than those offered by a living will, including one's wishes in five categories:

> The person chosen to make decisions when the individual can no longer make them for himself or herself—a durable power of attorney for health care
> The kind of treatment the person wants or does not want—a living will
> How comfortable the person wants to be
> How the person wants to be treated by others
> What the person wants his or her loved ones to know

The Five Wishes documents are legal in 42 U.S. states and the District of Columbia, and can be used as attachments to other documents, showing intent in the remainder of states (Aging with Dignity, 2015).

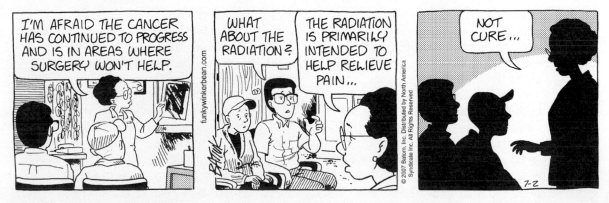

An AND order is considered a more descriptive and more positive order than a DNR. Its focus is on allowing death as nature takes its course at the end of an illness. Do not resuscitate implies taking something away, or not doing something for the patient (i.e., resuscitation), and can be viewed as a harsh and insensitive statement of medical care that promotes a feeling of abandonment by patients and families alike. In contrast, AND provides for comfort measures so that even with the withdrawal of artificially supplied nutrition and hydration, the dying process would occur as comfortably as possible (Meyer, 2001).

The POLST paradigm differs from an advance directive in that it is designed to instruct emergency personnel on what actions to take while the patient is still at home—before emergency treatment is given. It has segments concerning cardiopulmonary resuscitation (CPR), medical interventions, antibiotics, and artificially administered nutrition (Morrow, 2012). It was developed for seriously ill persons receiving treatments that were inconsistent with their stated wishes and designed to honor the person's end-of-life treatment preferences even when transferred from one care setting to another (Center for Ethics in Health Care, Oregon Health & Science University, 2008). Although not recognized in every state, promotion of the paradigm is becoming more prevalent as its value is more widely demonstrated. It is a doctor's order, once signed by the physician.

CLINICAL TIP

There are several types of advance directives, each of which the nurse should be knowledgeable.

Advance directives also can be crafted for specific and personal concerns (e.g., for ongoing care for dependents or a pet). All advance directives should include a periodic review to ensure clarity and reflect changing needs and concerns. Any documents relating to health care should be discussed and shared with physicians, family members, or decision-makers and placed in the medical records held by each of the patient's physicians (see **Case Study 27-1**).

Case Study 27–1: Family Disagreement with Advance Directives

Mary is 78 years old, just home from the acute care hospital and the rehabilitation unit at a local extended care facility for treatment of a cerebrovascular accident (CVA). She has come home with a feeding tube, placed at the urging of the hospital staff when she was unable to take solid foods. Mary's daughter, Sue, is the POA/HCR (power of attorney/healthcare representative)—the only remaining child, because her sibling died 2 years previously. Mary was widowed about 10 years ago.

Sue had been distraught when she received the call from Mary's neighbor and found that her mother had called 9-1-1. When Sue arrived at the hospital, Mary was in the emergency department, and was subsequently transferred to the intensive care unit (ICU). Mary was minimally responsive and therefore unable to speak, not able to make her needs and wishes known. Intravenous nutrition and hydration were implemented. Although Mary had an advance directive, indicating no use of tubes, her daughter Sue acquiesced to the physician's statement that "Starving to death is an awful way to die. . . . I wouldn't want that for MY mother," and agreed to placement of a gastrostomy tube for feeding.

Mary survived and underwent a few weeks of rehabilitation therapy. She regained some abilities—but not the ability to speak or swallow without significant aspiration. Sue noted that Mary seemed very angry, sullen, and withdrawn. Sue was able to ascertain that Mary was very angry with her for the placement of the feeding tube against her wishes. Sue's attempts to explain the rationale for the placement did not lessen Mary's anger. Sue was able to learn that Mary wanted the tube removed, and she contacted the primary physician to facilitate this. The physician contacted the visiting nurse agency seeking an evaluation of the situation and Mary's frame of mind, and requested objective assistance in helping determine a future plan of care for his patient.

Questions:

1. As the evaluating nurse, what information would you want to reference?
2. How would you attempt to obtain input from Mary?
3. How would you respond to Sue's strong statements of guilt for having had the tube placed in spite of Mary's advance directive?
4. What would you begin to look for in evaluating appropriateness for hospice care?

Suggested Actions Responses

The evaluating nurse asked to see Mary's advance directive and found it to be the typical state-approved document, but with some additional clauses that Mary had deemed important as part of her instructions to her family. In actuality, Mary had indicated three specific provisions that mirrored her perceptions of quality of life—the ability to smoke a cigarette, the ability to pet her dog, and meaningful verbal communication.

The evaluating nurse communicated directly with Mary using statements and questions that she could acknowledge with a yes/no nod of the head. The nurse decided, with Mary's nodded approval, to use the provisions of her advance directive to evaluate Mary's quality of life and generate discussion about her end-of-life wishes. Mary agreed that she was unable to communicate in a meaningful way with her family. Her little dog was placed on her lap, and she was unable to pet it or caress it behind its ears. Her daughter lit a cigarette for her, and she was unable to puff on it. The nurse confirmed with Mary that this was a fair assessment of her wishes.

The nurse asked if Mary wanted to hear about the hospice option, and with an affirmative nod in response, explained the goals of comfort and dignity as nature took its course with her remaining life. The nurse further explained how Mary's illness might progress without the feeding tube, and Mary nodded her understanding. Mary indicated she wanted hospice care and confirmed, in her daughter's presence and with her daughter's tearful apology for her hasty decision in the hospital, that hospice was her choice for end-of-life care.

For Personal Reflection

How could this uncomfortable scenario have been avoided for Mary and Sue?

Options for End-of-Life Care
Curative and Acute Care

Curative, life-prolonging, and *acute care* options focus on cure. Despite the findings of the SUPPORT study, some patients, families, and cultures choose the life-prolonging focus of care of a hospital death (see **Case Study 27-2**). Many of these deaths will take place in an ICU setting, with tubes, vents, and devices

Case Study 27–2: Hospital Death

Despite studies showing that the majority of people would prefer to die outside the hospital setting, some individuals find comfort in a more structured environment. Death in the hospital need not be a terrible or frightening event, as evidenced in this case study.

Jake is a 90-year-old man, diagnosed with end-stage dementia. He has been living in the home of his daughter and son-in-law, who are retired and in their 60s. His daughter is a power of attorney–healthcare representative. He has a living will in which he indicates an intentional nondecision about artificially supplied nutrition and hydration. In the past 2 years, he has become progressively weaker, unable to ambulate, unable to carry on a meaningful conversation, and increasingly incontinent of bowel and bladder. He was admitted to the hospital with dehydration and lethargy. A hydration intravenous solution has been started at 75 cc/hr. The physician has mentioned the possibility of a gastrostomy tube (G-tube) for feedings if the family so wishes. The certified nursing assistant (CNA) reports Jake moaned when she turned him during his bath, and he did not arouse when she attempted to feed him his breakfast.

You are the nurse caring for this patient. The daughter is in a quandary, stating, "I don't think Dad would want a tube in his stomach, but he never told me that for sure. My brother thinks we should do it so Dad doesn't starve to death. I tried to feed him his oatmeal this morning, but he seemed to choke. He's been coughing when he eats for a couple of months now." Your physical assessment reveals crackles throughout the lung fields, respiratory rate of 44 breaths per minute, edema to lower extremities, decreased level of consciousness, an irregular apical pulse, and a blood pressure of 76/48 mm Hg.

Questions:

1. What active symptoms affect the decision making for Jake?
2. What quality-of-life issues might also be involved in the decision making?
3. How would you help Jake's daughter understand the benefits and burdens of tube feedings?
4. How would your hospital-based team address the son's differing opinion?
5. What treatment would be appropriate for Jake's pain? His shortness of breath? The crackles in his lungs?

Suggested Actions/Responses

- Jake's symptoms clearly indicate an end-of-life process. You notify the physician of the family's quandary and request permission to set a family meeting for discussion of all the issues, including his terminal status.
- In answering the daughter's questions about G-tubes, you explain to her that sometimes a G-tube may be beneficial when the outcome is uncertain—for example, when there is potential for recovery as in a car accident or after a CVA. Dementia is a progressive disease, with little hope for improvement and with an expectation of terminality. When fluids are added to a failing body, the burdens may outweigh the benefits. These burdens might include increased congestion, edema, and nausea.
- The hospital social worker and/or chaplain might explore Jake's son's fears and feelings about Jake's end-of-life status. Quality-of-life issues might also be discussed to ascertain the importance of this family's cultural background in their decision making.
- Jake's nonverbal cues of pain must be addressed. Because patients' with dementia

are often unable to report pain or its location, it is important for the nurse to observe behavior and treat appropriately. Because Jake is having difficulty swallowing, oral medications are not feasible. A low-dose opioid by intravenous or subcutaneous route would be appropriate.

- The low-dose opioid initiated for pain would also help with his shortness of breath; supplemental oxygen also may be of benefit. Lowering or discontinuing the intravenous rate could improve the congestion and edema. The addition of hyoscine could also be helpful.

to do everything possible to preserve life. It is important that judgments not be made about these choices, but to note that other choices exist as well. Options for non–life-prolonging care at end of life are available and focus on comfort rather than cure.

Hospice Care

Hospice care provides one option for non–life-prolonging care and has the following philosophy. Hospice provides care and support for persons in the last phases of incurable disease (and their families) so they may live as fully and comfortably as possible. Hospice recognizes dying as part of the normal process of living and focuses on maintaining the quality of remaining life. Hospice affirms life and neither hastens nor postpones death. Hospice exists in the hope and belief that through appropriate care, and the promotion of a caring community sensitive to their needs, individuals and their families may be free to attain a degree of mental and spiritual satisfaction in preparation for death (NHPCO, 2016b, para. 1).

Hospice care originated to provide comfort and dignity at end of life. Eligibility for hospice services is based on a life expectancy of 6 months or less, if an illness runs its normal course. Services are available as long as a patient is considered to be terminally ill, even though it may be longer than 6 months. Hospice utilizes a team approach to address the physical, emotional, social, and spiritual needs of the patient and (see **Figure 27-1**) family. Hospice care is discussed in more detail later in this chapter.

CLINICAL TIP

Hospice care is generally for those with 6 months or less until end of life, while palliative care may be covered for those with life-limiting illnesses that may be two years or thereabouts from end of life.

Palliative Care

Palliative care evolved from the hospice movement in the 1960s and 1970s. It assists increasing numbers of people who experience chronic, debilitating, and life-limiting illnesses and can be practiced in a variety of settings, including hospitals, outpatient settings, community home health programs, and hospices (National Consensus Project for Quality Palliative Care [NCP], 2009).

Palliative care refers to the comprehensive management of the physical, psychological, social, spiritual, and existential needs of patients. It is especially suited to the care of people with incurable, progressive illnesses (Quaglietti et al., 2004). According to the *Clinical Practice Guidelines for Quality Palliative Care* (NCP, 2009),

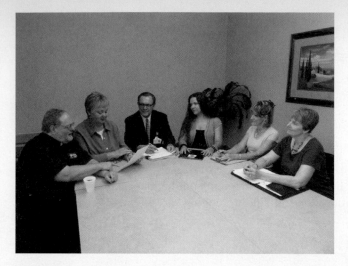

Figure 27-1 The interdisciplinary hospice team meets to discuss patient cases.

palliative care has become an area of special expertise within medicine, nursing, social work, pharmacy, chaplaincy, rehabilitation, and other disciplines. The goal of palliative care is to achieve the best possible quality of life for patients and their families. Control of pain, other symptoms, and psychological, social, and spiritual problems is paramount (Box 27-5). Palliative care has been found to not only promote improved quality of life, but to prolong life itself.

The Choice of End-of-Life Care

It can be very difficult for a patient and family to choose one of these options for care. A practical suggestion that may help the patient and/or family in weighing the choices is to encourage a frank discussion with the physician, which would include several important questions: What is the expected outcome if I do treatment option #1? What is the expected outcome if I do treatment option #2? What is the expected outcome if I do neither of these, and choose comfort care? Weighing the answers to each of these questions may help the individual make an informed choice, based on the differences between the expected outcomes and the individual's own philosophy about how to experience his or her end of life.

End-of-Life Hospice Care

Cicely Saunders, a nurse, social worker, and physician, started St. Christopher's Hospice in London in 1967. She incorporated a variety of team members to work together to help with the problems of care at end of life. The success of her type of care prompted expansion of hospice services to other parts of the world. Hospice care has existed in the United States since 1974, brought to the United States by Florence Wald of Yale University (Storey, 1996) (see **Case Study 27-3**).

The U.S. government, recognizing the cost-effectiveness of hospice care, incorporated hospice benefits into the Medicare program in 1983. Credentialing agencies require that hospices provide all of the mandated services in order to be licensed and/or certified by Medicare and Medicaid and to be recognized by other insurers and some states. Reimbursement to provider agencies is contingent upon this certification (Centers for Medicare and Medicaid Services [CMS], 2012). Hospices are paid per day of service, the rate dependent on the level of care received by the patient. In 2016, CMS initiated a higher payment rate for the first 60 days of hospice care, and a lower rate for days after day 60. A hospice may also receive a "service intensity add-on" rate for the last 7 days of a patient's life (CMS, 2016a).

According to the CMS *Conditions of Participation and Standards,* hospice services include, but are not limited to (CMS, 2016b):

> Nursing services and coordination of care
> Physical therapy, occupational therapy, or speech–language pathology services
> Medical social services
> Home health aide and homemaker services
> Physician services/medical director

Case Study 27-3: Options for End-of-Life Care

Hospice care is appropriate when the plan of care shifts from cure to comfort. This case study exemplifies this process.

Dee is a 72-year-old woman with advanced chronic obstructive pulmonary disease (COPD) and a history of congestive heart failure (CHF). She has been a patient with a home care agency, receiving nursing and physical therapy services for the past 6 weeks. Dee has been unable to maintain the rigors of physical therapy due to her poor lung status. She is oxygen and steroid dependent and homebound. Dee is dependent on her husband, Jay, also age 72, for all aspects of her care. He is in need of a knee replacement, but is unable to receive one due to his caregiving role. Until several years ago, Dee and Jay enjoyed socialization with friends and neighbors, going out to dinner, playing golf and cards, and attending her church on a regular basis. They have a supportive adult daughter who works, lives about 15 miles away, is attentive, and visits nearly every day. Their son lives out of state, calls frequently, and visits on occasion.

Dee voiced to her home care nurse the desire not to return to the hospital. "It doesn't do any good. I'm tired of living this way. Can't we do something at home?" In response to Dee's inquiry, the home care nurse indicates the possibility of hospice care at home because hospice is appropriate for any end-stage illness and because Dee's prognosis was determined to be 6 months or less by her attending physician (according to the National Hospice Organization's guidelines for noncancer diagnoses). For end-stage lung disease, these symptoms include dyspnea at rest, poor response to bronchodilator therapy, and other debilitating symptoms such as decreased functional activity, fatigue, and cough. Dee has had multiple hospitalizations for these symptoms without significant improvement in her overall condition. Her appetite is fair to poor; constipation has been a problem; she is short of breath with any exertion; and has crackles to bilateral bases, with frequent complaints of mid-back pain. She has pedal edema; her hands and feet are cyanotic. Her current medications include an angiotensin-converting enzyme (ACE) inhibitor, furosemide 40 mg/day, prednisone 5 mg/day, and O_2 2 L/min by nasal cannula. Jay reports Dee is forgetful and cries "at the drop of a hat." Dee is admitted to hospice care at home.

Questions:

1. As the admitting nurse, what are your recommendations after this initial assessment?
2. Which team members should be a part of Dee's care plan?
3. How can we determine Dee's goals for her end of life?
4. Evaluate Dee's emotional status; how does it affect her daily functioning? How does it affect her relationship with her husband? How can other team members assist with these issues?
5. What impact do Dee's spiritual life/beliefs have on her condition and functional ability?
6. How might we offer Jay assistance in meeting the physical care needs of Dee?
7. What can be done for Dee's shortness of breath?
8. What should be done for Dee's complaint of constipation?
9. How might one address Dee's back pain?

Suggested Actions and Responses

- The easiest way to determine a patient or family's goals is simply to ask them! Dee is in physical distress, so that is foremost on her mind. Addressing her physical needs first will allow her to be able to identify and concentrate on other goals as her comfort is increased.

(continues)

Case Study 27-3: Options for End-of-Life Care (continued)

- Based on physical and psycho-social-spiritual assessment, Dee and Jay are offered the services of the whole hospice team. They know their individualized plan of care is under the direction of Dee's attending physician and managed by the interdisciplinary team, which includes the services of a hospice-skilled medical director Although apparently overwhelmed by the admission process, Dee and Jay initially agreed to a nurse, social worker, and home health aide (HHA), and decide to consider a volunteer and chaplain.
- The primary nurse first attends to physical symptoms, because that is often the overwhelming need. Dee's shortness of breath is her primary complaint; after consultation with the attending physician, the nurse received orders to initiate liquid morphine 5 mg every 4 hours as needed. The nurse instructed and demonstrated the use of morphine to Dee and Jay, because he will be responsible for administration of medications.
- Depending on the underlying pathology of Dee's back pain, the liquid morphine also may help this complaint. A nonsteroidal antiinflammatory drug (NSAID) was ordered for possible bone pain.
- Adding opioids contributes to additional constipation, so a stool softener/laxative was ordered on a scheduled basis.
- Because activities of daily living (ADLs) are an increasing problem, and in light of Jay's knee pain, hospice can assist with the physical care needs by interventions of an HHA as needed. Stand-by assistance to full bed-bath is available depending on Dee's condition on a given day.
- The social worker often accompanies the admitting nurse for the admission process. This enables the family to be exposed to the "team" from the very beginning, as well as allowing the social worker to hear the patient/family "story" as an aid to assessment. Initial assessment reveals Dee is somewhat tearful in describing her physical decline and realization that her illness is life-ending. However, she is adamant about staying at home, avoiding rehospitalization, and voices several times that she is "tired, not able to fight this anymore. I want to be comfortable. I want Jay to have help."
- When Dee's symptoms indicated she was near death, and when Jay could no longer physically provide her care, she was transferred to the hospice center for the last week of her life. She received around-the-clock symptom management and physical care, allowing Jay to change roles from that of caregiver to husband.

> Counseling services (including dietary, pastoral, bereavement, and other) relative to the terminally ill individual and adjustment to his or her death
> Short-term in-patient care
> Medical appliances and supplies
> Medications and biologicals

See **Box 27-2** for a description of the hospice team.

Focus on Symptoms

Among the nurse's primary responsibilities as a member of any interdisciplinary team is to coordinate the patient's care and to assist with *symptom management*. Patients and families want to know what to expect as they transition through the end of-life process. Nurses must be informed to guide the patient and family and answer questions as they arise. The remainder of this chapter will provide practical assistance with managing the variety of symptoms frequently encountered at end of life.

BOX 27-2   Hospice Team

The *interdisciplinary group or team* (IDG/IDT) provides or supervises the care and services offered by the hospice, including ongoing assessment of each of the patient, caregiver, family's needs. Its members consist of (CMS, 2012):

- Doctor of medicine or osteopathy
- Registered nurse—coordinates the plan of care for each patient
- Social worker
- Pastoral or other counselor
- Other team members who also are required include:

- Volunteers with training appropriate to their tasks—must contribute at least 5% of all staff hours
- Clergy/spiritual support and counseling
- Additional counseling (dietary, bereavement)

Centers for Medicare and Medicaid Services. (2012). Hospice payment system. Retrieved from http://www.cms.gov/Outreach-and -Education/Medicare-Learning-Network -MLN/MLNProducts/downloads/hospice_pay _sys_fs.pdf

Complementary therapies are not required but are often provided to enhance the patient and family care with services such as massage, healing touch, music therapy, pet therapy, and others. Many of these additional therapies are provided by volunteers skilled in these particular areas.

Physical, Nonpain Symptoms

Respiratory

Dyspnea is a distressing difficulty in breathing. It is a symptom, not a sign. A patient may have difficulty breathing and have no abnormal physical signs. Dyspnea, like pain, is whatever the patient perceives it to be. Episodic shortness of breath is sometimes due to hyperventilation. Any patient with dyspnea is prone to episodes of anxiety or panic. Patients have described this complex, subjective, and distressing phenomena as a feeling of suffocation, which often severely impedes their quality of life. The goal of treatment for terminal dyspnea is to relieve the perception of suffocation or breathlessness (Brennan & Mazanec, 2011).

Opioid therapy is used to treat shortness of breath, as morphine reduces the inappropriate and excessive respiratory drive. A low dose is usually very effective—liquid morphine 2.5 to 5 mg orally every 4 hours is a good starting dose. It also may be given subcutaneously at one-third the oral dose if the patient is unable to swallow. It reduces inappropriate tachypnea (rapid breathing) and overventilation of the large airways (dead space). It does not cause carbon dioxide retention and can reduce cyanosis by slowing ventilation and making breathing more efficient. Morphine does not depress respirations when used judiciously and titrated appropriately. For patients who do not tolerate morphine, other opioids such as oxycodone and hydromorphone can be used (McKinnis, 2002).

Anxiety can be precipitated by the fear of suffocation, which worsens the perception of dyspnea, creating a vicious cycle. Antianxiety agents, such as lorazepam 0.5 to 2 mg every 4 to 6 hours as needed, will help with restlessness and thus often decrease respiratory effort. It can be given orally, sublingually, bucally, or rectally (McKinnis, 2002).

Oxygen may not be effective if hypoxemia is not the cause of dyspnea, but may have a placebo effect and decrease the individual's anxiety. Oxygen should be started at 2 L/min by nasal cannula and can be increased to 4 L/min by nasal cannula if needed.

Other helpful and practical techniques might include:

> Head of the bed elevated 30 to 45 degrees
> Cool, humidified air

> Relaxation techniques
> Fan at bedside or ceiling fan

Excess secretions, resulting from fluid overload from artificial hydration or from increasing inability to swallow secretions, allow a buildup in large airways and cause a rattling sound. This rattle may be more distressing to the family at bedside than uncomfortable for the patient. Scopolamine transdermally or subcutaneously or hyoscyamine sublingually may be helpful in treating this condition (McKinnis, 2002).

Gastrointestinal

Constipation results from a variety of causes for persons at end of life. Nonmedical causes include inactivity and decrease in food and fluid intake. Exercise contributes to bowel motility, but persons with life-ending illnesses are often incapacitated by their disease processes. Medications used to control pain almost always have a constipating effect. Rather than withholding opioids, the constipating side effects of the medications must be treated. A combination softener and stimulant should be used, because use of a softener alone could lead to a soft impaction. Legend indicates that Dr. Cicely Saunders (mother of the modern hospice movement) gave a lecture in which every fourth slide read, "Nothing matters more than the bowels!" (Levi, 1991).

   Nausea/vomiting, while common at end of life, may have multiple causes that may or may not be reversible. If a reversible cause is identified, appropriate measures should be taken. The VOMIT acronym is helpful in identifying the causes of vomiting and in choosing the appropriate treatment to address the underlying etiology (Enclara Health Hospice Pharmacy Services, 2011).

   V = Vestibular

> Receptors involved: Cholinergic, histaminic
> Anticholinergic, antihistaminic medication such as scopolamine patches and promethazine are helpful

   O = Obstruction of bowel, due to constipation

> Receptors involved: Cholinergic, histaminic, 5HT3
> Medications that affect the myenteric plexus, such as senna, are helpful

   M = Mobility of the upper gut (lack of)

> Receptors involved: Cholinergic, histaminic, 5HT3
> Prokinetic drugs that stimulate the 5HT receptors, such as metoclopramide, are helpful

   I = Infection and inflammation

> Receptors involved: Cholinergic, histaminic, 5HT3
> Anticholinergic and antihistaminic agents are helpful

   T = Toxins stimulating the chemoreceptor trigger zone (opioids)

> Receptors involved: Dopamine, 5HT3
> Antidopaminergic and 5HT3-antagonists are useful. Examples include prochlorperazine, haloperidol, and ondansetron

   Nonpharmacological measures to help control nausea and vomiting include providing fresh air; loosening clothing; using a cool, damp cloth on the skin; relaxation and visualization techniques; deep breathing; improving oral care; eating small, frequent meals; serving cold food; and discouraging family from wearing strong perfume or deodorants.

Anxiety, Delirium, and Terminal Restlessness

Anxiety, a psychological and physiological state of distress, is characterized by physical, emotional, mental, and behavioral components. At end of life it can be caused by a variety of factors, including loss of control, loss of self-esteem, and loss of independence, which can be very distressing to a person who has previously been autonomous. A change in environment for the dying person may add to the anxiety. These changes may be large—as in a family caregiver, a place of care, or meeting new professional staff—or small, such as a change of bed or medication. Treatment for anxiety includes relieving physical symptoms that may be present, such as pain or shortness of breath. The simple presence of someone the dying person trusts can be very reassuring. Antianxiety medications also may be used in conjunction with these interventions (Wright, 2002).

Delirium is an acute, fluctuating cognitive disturbance, characterized by changes in mental status over a short period of time. It occurs in the last hours to days of life in a large percentage of dying patients. Delirium is especially devastating to family and friends because it can stand in the way of meaningful conversations and goodbyes. The most common physical causes may include dyspnea, pain, constipation, or urinary retention, all of which can be treated. Other causes may include medication reactions, dehydration, hypoxia, anemia, infection, and metabolic and multisystem failure (renal failure, liver failure, hypercalcemia, hyponatremia, or hypoglycemia). Delirium at end of life is often referred to as terminal restlessness, occurring in approximately 25% to 85% of terminally ill patients at time of death (Brajtman, 2005).

Environmental comfort can be provided by reducing stimuli; reorientation, if possible; having familiar persons at the bedside; and interdisciplinary team members providing emotional, social, and spiritual support. Music therapy, *therapeutic/healing touch*, and nonmedical nursing interventions should be considered. Antianxiety medications, used cautiously, also may be helpful.

Uncontrolled restlessness may require pharmacological treatment options, including palliative/terminal sedation. Terminal sedation can be defined as the monitored use of medications to relieve the intractable suffering of imminently dying patients, which persists despite the use of usual multidisciplinary therapies (HPNA, 2003). It is designed to induce unconsciousness, but not death. Before initiating sedation, various factors must be considered and thoroughly discussed, demonstrating informed consent and documentation (Salacz & Wiseman, 2004):

> Review plans for use of artificial hydration and nutrition, including wishes for continuation or stoppage
> Confirm any specific goals to be met prior to implementation of plan (e.g., visitors)
> Confirm patient and family wishes for spiritual support
> Ensure a peaceful and quiet setting, anticipating few interruptions
> Review medication and treatment orders with physician
> Confirm that a DNR order is written

Nutrition and Hydration

Declining appetite is a natural occurrence in the process of dying. This concept is one of the most difficult for caregivers to embrace, because our society tends to equate love with provision of food. When end of life nears, the body is less active and requires less nourishment. From the patient's perspective, food does not taste the same, so favorite foods may no longer provide comfort; appetite is easily satisfied by bites of food rather than regular portions. Caregivers should be encouraged to offer small amounts of a variety of foods. When a patient clenches his or her teeth to negate feeding attempts, it may be his or her way of exerting control.

The attempt to artificially hydrate may be detrimental to comfort, because the failing body may not be able to process the added fluids, contributing to fluid overload (see **Box 27-3**). In this case, thirst may be satisfied by providing small amounts of oral fluids, Popsicles, or ice chips. Dry mouth may be successfully managed with meticulous mouth care (Kinzbrunner, 2002).

BOX 27-3   Evidence-Based Practice

Patients with advanced illness often experience a natural decline in appetite, a loss of interest in eating and drinking, and weight loss. Most patients at the end of life will be unable to take food and fluid by mouth or will simply stop eating. This can be particularly distressing to family and caregivers, who may be concerned that the patient is hungry or starving. They also may perceive that dehydration can result in troublesome symptoms such as thirst, dry mouth, headache, delirium, nausea, vomiting, and abdominal cramps.

Artificial hydration and nutrition (AHN) interventions were developed to provide short-term support for patients who were acutely ill, and are often used to provide sustenance until recovery or to meet therapeutic goals of prolonging life. There are very few studies examining the efficacy of ANH in meeting these goals.

An important goal of hospice and palliative care is to minimize suffering and discomfort. When ANH is used in a terminally ill person, evidence suggests these measures are seldom effective in preventing suffering. ANH is a medical intervention that should be evaluated for each individual utilizing evidence-based practices reflecting the benefits and burdens, the clinical circumstances, and the overall goals of care. (See bullet points that follow.)

Possible side effects of ANH exist for patients with advanced illness. Studies have shown that tube feeding does not appear to prolong life, and complications from tube placement may increase mortality in certain populations. Furthermore, artificially delivered nutrition does not protect against aspiration and, in some patient populations, may actually increase the risk of aspiration and its complications. Tube feedings are associated with increased infections, fluid overload, and skin excoriation around the tube. Since many tube-fed patients are not offered food even if they are able to eat, they may be deprived of human contact and the pleasure of eating.

ANH may lead to life-threatening fluid overload complications with regard to edema, increased secretions, ascites, and pleural effusions. Research has shown that artificial nutrition and nutritional supplements do not enhance frail elder strength and physical function. Finally, therapies such as ANH that require the use of tubes increase the likelihood that the patient will be restrained. Physical restraints are distressing and often increase patient agitation and skin breakdown.

Evidence to consider in the evaluation of ANH for use in hospice should:

- Support education of patient and family about the dying process and its effects on nutrition and fluid status.
- Teach caregivers to enhance the patient's comfort by providing frequent oral and skin care, effective and timely symptom management, and psychospiritual support.
- Support caregivers in coping with feelings of helplessness, loss, and fear.
- Recognize that in certain situations, ANH may be clinically beneficial. It may help with reversal of myoclonus and opioid toxicity. It also might be beneficial in functional patients with mechanical blockage of the mouth, esophagus, stomach, or bowel.
- A time-limited trial may be helpful for evaluation of efficacy; it can be stopped if the desired results are not achieved.
- Artificial nutrition and hydration may have symbolic importance and be related to the religion or culture of the patient and family. This importance should not be overlooked.
- Encourage nurses to collaborate with speech therapists, nutritionists, and other healthcare providers to identify and implement strategies that enable caregivers to provide oral nutrition and fluids safely and effectively as an alternative to ANH. Alternatives may include adaptations such as fluid thickeners,

teaching swallowing techniques, and positioning.

- Acknowledge and support the legal and moral right of competent patients to refuse unwanted treatment, including ANH.
- Promote early discussions about the goals of care and treatment choices, including the expected benefits and burdens of possible end-of-life interventions before starting treatment, refusal, or withdrawal.
- Encourage policies that guide a decision-making process for resolving disagreements

about care among patients, families, surrogates, and healthcare team members.
- Support research on the outcomes of ANH in hospice and palliative care patients.

Modified from Hospice and Palliative Nurses Association. (2016). HPNA position statement: Artificial nutrition and hydration in advanced illness. Retrieved from http://www.hpna.advancing expertcare.org/wp-content/uploads/2015/08 /Artificial-Nutrition-and-Hydration-in-Advanced -Illness.pdf

Physical Pain Symptoms
Relevant Issues for the Elderly

Albert Schweitzer said, "We all must die. But if I can save him from days of torture, that is what I feel is my great and ever new privilege. Pain is a more terrible lord of mankind than even death himself" (1961, p. 62). (See **Boxes 27-4** and **27-5**).

Pain in the elderly is particularly problematic.

CLINICAL TIP

"Unrelieved pain can contribute to unnecessary suffering, as evidenced by sleep disturbance, hopelessness, loss of control, and impaired social interactions. Pain may actually hasten death by increasing physiological stress, decreasing mobility, contributing to pneumonia and thromboemboli" (HPNA, 2004a, p. 62).

BOX 27-4   Research Highlight

Symptoms experienced by patients with metastatic cancer can be severe and treatment is intensive. Temel, Greer, Muzikansky, Gallagher, Admane, and Jackson studied the experience of patients with metastatic non-small cell lung cancer, which presents particularly difficult symptoms and rigorous treatment. The researchers sought to determine whether utilizing palliative care upon diagnosis, along with oncological care, made an impact on quality of life for this patient population. Sign into your database of nursing literature (CINAHL or PubMed, for example) and use the

citation below to perform a search for this article. What was the conclusion of this study? What do these findings tell us about caring for patients in this population and for those facing a similar diagnosis?

Temel, J. S., Greer, J. A., Muzikansky, A., Gallagher, E. R., Admane, A., Jackson, V. A., Dahlin, C. M., Blinderman, C. D., Jacobsen, J., Pirl, W. F., Billings, J. A., & Lynch, T. J. (2010). Early palliative care for patients with metastatic non-small-cell lung cancer. *New England Journal of Medicine, 363*(8), 733–742.

> **BOX 27-5   Research Highlight: Suffering in Terminally Ill Patients with Dementia**
>
> Aminoff and Adunsky studied the experience of patients with terminal dementia. The researchers followed patients from their initial admission to a care center through end of life, observing their level of suffering during that time frame. Sign into your database of nursing literature (CINAHL or PubMed, for example) and use the citation below to perform a search for this article. What did Aminoff and Adunsky find? On the basis of the discussion included in the article, what can a caregiver do to help support patients with terminal dementia?
>
> Aminoff, B. Z., & Adunsky, A. (2004). Dying dementia patients: Too much suffering, too little palliation. *American Journal of Alzheimer's Disease and Other Dementias, 19*(4), 243–247.

Underreporting of pain is common, because the elderly learn to expect chronic pain and accept it as part of growing older. They may minimize pain to avoid diagnostic testing or to protect families or themselves against a poor prognosis. They may also use softening words, such as discomfort, soreness, or aching, instead of the word "pain." In addition, healthcare providers may tend to underestimate and undertreat pain in this population, for fear of promoting addiction to pain medications.

Research has shown that approximately 25% to 50% of community-dwelling elders have significant chronic pain, and between 45% and 80% of nursing home residents have undertreated, substantial pain. The pain of those in nursing homes is generally "underappreciated, underreported, and undertreated" (Ferrell, 1991, p. 2).

Additionally, McCaffery and Pasero (1999) identify that there are many misconceptions about pain in the elderly:

> Pain is a natural outcome of growing old.
> Pain perception or sensitivity decreases with age.
> If an elderly person does not report pain, he or she does not have pain.
> If an elderly patient appears to be asleep or otherwise distracted, he or she does not have pain.
> Potential side effects of opioids make them too dangerous to use to relieve pain in the elderly.
> Patients with Alzheimer's disease and others with cognitive impairments do not have pain, and their reports of pain are most likely invalid (see Box 27-5).

It is important that nurses recognize the many facets of pain in older dying adults. The plan of care should be guided by consideration of physical, psychological, and social aspects of pain. This interdisciplinary plan should evolve over time, in response to the patient's changing needs (Gibson & Schroder, 2001).

To successfully treat pain, the nurse must be able to assess the pain of the individual. "Pain is whatever the experiencing person says it is, existing whenever he says it does" (McCaffery, 1968, p. 95). However, individuals may require assistance in describing their pain. A specialized pain scale for advanced dementia is shown in **Table 27-1**.

Treatment of pain in the elderly is very effective when based on a basic understanding of origins of pain and a systemic approach to treatment. Different types of pain require different treatments (see **Case Study 27-4**). Sometimes a combination of pain medication and adjuvants (such as antidepressants or anticonvulsants) can be more therapeutic than each used alone.

TABLE 27-1   Pain Assessment in Advanced Dementia (PAINAD) Scale

Item	0	1	2
Breathing independent of vocalization	Normal	Occasional labored breathing Short period of hyperventilation	Noisy labored breathing Long period of hyperventilation Cheyne-Stokes respiration
Negative vocalization	None	Occasional moan or groan Low-level speech with a negative or disapproving quality	Repeated trouble calling out Loud moaning or groaning crying
Facial expression	Smiling or inexpressive	Sad Frightened Frowning	Facial grimacing
Body language	Relaxed	Tense Distressed pacing Fidgeting	Rigid Fist clenched Knees pulled up Pulling or pushing away Striking out
Consolability	No need to console	Distracted or reassured by voice or touch	Unable to console, distract or reassure

Reproduced from Warden, V., Hurley, A. C., & Volicer, V. (2003). Development in psychometric evaluation of the Pain Assessment in Advanced Dementia (PAINAD) Scale. *Journal of the American Medical Director Association, 4*(1), 9–15, Copyright 2003, with permission from Elsevier.

Pharmacological interventions remain the first line of treatment for unrelieved pain. Opioids are needed when pain does not respond to nonopioids alone. Some clinicians and patients avoid opioids due to fear *of addiction*. Nurses need to be able to understand and explain to patients and families the differences among addiction, *tolerance*, and physical *dependence*. Fear of addiction should not be a factor in pain control (see **Box 27-6**).

Guidelines for Treatment of Pain in the Older Population

Older adults may experience many different types of pain (**Table 27-2**), often at the same time. Because they may have lived with pain over many years, older adults may be reluctant to report new pain. The nurse must use appropriate assessment skills to get an accurate picture of the person's pain (see Table 27-1).

> As in all patient populations, it is important to assess the type of pain being treated: somatic, visceral, neuropathic, or a combination. The type of pain determines the appropriate medication to use.
> A systematic approach should be utilized in the treatment of pain. The WHO recommends a step approach (Lipman, 2006):
> Step 1: Mild pain (1 to 3 on a 0 to 10 scale, with 0 being no pain and 10 being the worst imaginable pain). Acetaminophen and NSAIDs are the recommended medications for this step. Acetaminophen should be dosed at 4,000 mg/day or less. An adjuvant may also be used.

Case Study 27–4: Use of Medications for Treatment of Pain

Jane is an 84-year-old woman, diagnosed with breast cancer 2 years ago, now with metastases to the bone and lung. She has refused any further active treatment (i.e., chemotherapy and radiation) and has asked her healthcare representative daughter Patty to help her talk to her oncologist about her wishes. After this discussion, the patient, daughter, and physician have agreed upon a hospice evaluation.

Upon evaluation and subsequent admission to hospice services, the patient's most pressing need was adequate pain control. Previously, she had tried scheduled Tylenol without relief—her pain rated at 8 on a scale of 0 to 10. Her oncologist then prescribed hydrocodone 7.5/750 mg, 1 or 2 tabs every 4 hours as needed, which lowered her pain acuity to a 6.

Questions:

1. As the admitting hospice nurse, you recognize that 8 on the pain scale greatly impairs Jane's quality of life. Using the World Health Organization (WHO) step approach, what would be your plan of intervention?
2. Knowing that Jane probably has two types of pain due to the metastases, what adjuvant might you consider for the bone pain?
3. Looking to the future, what other comfort issues might Jane face as her lung metastasis affects her life?
4. How could you help Jane reach her goal of selected activities (e.g., shopping, lunch, church)?

Possible Solutions

The hospice nurse recognized that the maximum dose of Tylenol would be exceeded by the hydrocodone combination, and so short-acting morphine was initiated in place of hydrocodone. Using a conversion chart comparing the two medications, the nurse calculated the amount of morphine that could safely be given every 4 hours. Jane received "around the clock pain medication for her around the clock pain," to keep the pain from getting out of control. The starting dose was at a conservative starting point of 5 mg every 4 hours. The daughter was instructed to call hospice if the patient's pain was not managed at this dose. She was also educated that Jane may be sleepy for 24 to 48 hours until her body adjusted to the new medication, and this would be a temporary side effect and not an adverse reaction. The nurse made plans to visit daily until the pain was controlled.

Twenty-four hours later, Jane reported, "It's better; I'm at a 5 most of the time." Asking Jane about her acceptable level of pain, she indicated, "If I could just get it to a 2, I could do the things I would like to do." The dose was then taken to 10 mg every 4 hours. After 48 hours, Jane reported, "You know, I think I could do a little shopping today and have some lunch with my daughter—of course she will have to drive." The hospice nurse then calculated the therapeutic amount of morphine used in 24 hours, which was 60 mg. The 60 mg was divided by 2, as long-acting morphine lasts for 12 hours. The therapeutic dose would be 30 mg of extended-release morphine every 12 hours. A breakthrough dose of 10 mg (one third of the 12-hour dose) immediate-release morphine is available for as-needed use in case pain occurs between the 12-hour doses during Jane's shopping trip.

At this point, an adjuvant might be considered for bone pain—possibly decadron, 2 to 4 mg daily—because steroids are helpful for the inflammation of bone pain. At this time in Jane's life, steroids are appropriate for use because her life expectancy is weeks or months rather than years, and long-term side effects are less of an issue.

If Jane experiences shortness of breath related to lung metastasis, the morphine and decadron are both helpful in alleviating this symptom.

A variety of interventions can improve the quality of Jane's life, allowing her the flexibility and freedom to continue some favorite activities.

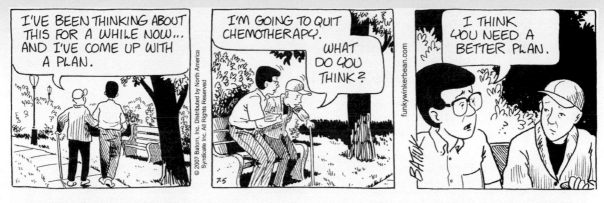

BOX 27-6	Definitions
Tolerance	Drug effect increases with ongoing exposure, may require dose up-titration
Physical dependence	Withdrawal syndromes with administration of antagonist, abrupt discontinuation or significant dose reduction of a drug
Addiction	Maladaptive behavior frequently concurrent with mental illness, with inability to control use of a drug, continued use despite harm, craving
Pseudo-addiction	Drug-seeking behavior similar to addiction but due to inadequately controlled pain

Reproduced from Bodke S., & Ligon, K., (2016). Definitions table. In *Hospice and palliative medicine handbook: A clinical guide* (p. 197). Retrieved from http://www.hpmhandbook.com.

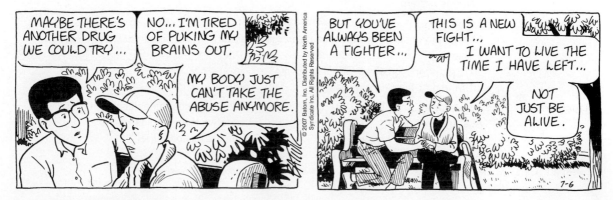

TABLE 27-2 Types of Pain

	Nociceptive Pain	Neuropathic Pain
Site of injury	Peripheral pain receptors Includes somatic and visceral injury	Damaged, dysfunctional or injured nerve fibers Includes peripheral and/or central injury
Typical duration	Acute Protective, leads to reflex withdrawal	Often chronic complex pain state Pain extends beyond expected healing time
If prolonged	Becomes nonprotective and may lead to chronic pain	Becomes an ongoing response with chronic pain
Examples	Somatic: Burn, fracture, cut Visceral: Bowel obstruction, myocardial infarction	Peripheral neuropathy, complex regional pain, phantom limb pain
Transduction-transmission	Direct stimulation of intact nociceptors, transmitted along normal nerves	Disordered transmission along dysfunctional peripheral or central nerves Multiple theories Chronic pain tracts develop unrelated to original injury
Etiology	Somatic Structural damage to skin, muscle, tendon, joint capsule, fasciae, or bone due to tissue disruption, including chemical and thermal injury From stimulation of the somatic nervous system Visceral Injury to internal organs due to swelling, ischemia, inflammation, mechanical pressure or stretch From stimulation of the autonomic nervous system	Neuronal damage or death as a result of compression, transaction, infiltration, ischemia, metabolic injury, drugs Nerve damage with autonomic changes: Complex regional pain syndrome Nerve damage without autonomic changes: Postherpetic neuralgia, diabetic neuropathy, trigeminal neuralgia Central pain: Phantom limb pain, poststroke thalamic pain syndrome, spinal cord injury pain
Descriptors	Somatic Sharp pain in specific, well-localized area Visceral Diffuse, poorly localized, deep ache with cramping or burning, can radiate	Burning, cold, tingling, numbness, shooting, stabbing, electrical, itching
Management	Antiinflammatory: NSAID, steroids Acetaminophen Opioids Adjuvants rarely needed	Adjuvants/coanalgesics, often more effective than opioids Opioids (second line)

Reproduced from Bodke S., & Ligon, K. (2016). *Hospice and palliative medicine handbook: A clinical guide* (p. 210). Retrieved from www.hpmhandbook.com.

> Step 2: Moderate pain (4 to 6 on a 0 to 0 scale). Low-dose, short-acting opioids, in combination with acetaminophen and NSAIDs, are recommended in this step. Combination medications have a ceiling dose because of the nonopioid components of acetaminophen and NSAIDs. Opioid-naïve patients should be started at this level. If pain is uncontrolled with this combination, they may require a move to step 3. Adjuvants also may be used.

> Step 3: Severe pain (7 to 10 on a 0 to 10 scale). Opioids used at this step are not used in combination with Tylenol or NSAIDs, so there is no ceiling for dosing at this level. This allows for the use of higher doses of these opioids as the disease progresses. Nonopioids and adjuvants also may be used at this step.

> Oral medication is the route of choice and is well-tolerated in the geriatric population. However, other routes are acceptable when the patient is unable to swallow at the end of life. These routes may include sublingual, subcutaneous, intravenous, rectal, or topical, depending on the medication.

> To avoid possible adverse drug reactions, it is often recommended to prescribe half the dose usually prescribed to a younger person. However, even though the advice of "start low and go slow" is common, it may create the risk of undertreatment of pain. It is important to treat the individual and not the "geriatric population" (Perley & Dahlin, 2007).

> A study of opioid titration in people with cancer found that older persons required lower doses to achieve comfort. Opioid effects (including dose escalation, number of opioids, and route of administration) did not differ among age groups (Mercadante, Ferrera, Villari, & Casuccio, 2006).

> Special considerations for the geriatric population:

> Acetaminophen is recommended for long-term use because it is well tolerated in the older population. It is especially therapeutic for musculoskeletal pain, a common source of pain in the older adult. Doses higher than 4,000 mg per day should be avoided. Be aware that acetaminophen may be in combination with other medications, and toxic dose ranges may be reached quickly in a person who is moving toward end of life.

> NSAIDs are also useful in the treatment of pain. Older adults with a history of ulcer disease or congestive heart failure are more vulnerable to the side effects of these medications, however. In the palliative setting, the risk-to-benefit ratio helps determine the plan of care, and if prognosis is days-to-weeks, a trial of NSAIDs is acceptable.

> Opioids are an acceptable option for older persons with moderate to severe pain (see **Box 27-7**). It is best to start with a short half-life agonist (e.g., morphine, hydromorphone, oxycodone) because they are generally easier to titrate than the longer half-life agonists (e.g., fentanyl patch, methadone).

> Morphine is considered the gold standard and is the most commonly used opioid due to its cost and various routes of administration. The elderly population may develop sedation or confusion due to the metabolites of morphine after several days of use. If this happens, it might be wise to change to another opioid. (Remember, however, the patient may be drowsy or sleepy because the pain is controlled and the patient is finally able to rest.) This side effect should subside in 48 hours. Assessment continues to be very important. Long-acting morphine should be used only after a several-day trial of short-acting morphine. Morphine is also therapeutic in the treatment of shortness of breath.

> Opioids other than morphine also may be used (e.g., oxycodone, transdermal fentanyl) using the same principle of a short-acting trial before initiation of a long-acting formulation.

> Opioids are constipating, so implementing a concurrent bowel program is essential. A stimulant and stool softener combination is recommended at the onset of opioid therapy (Derby & O'Mahoney, 2006).

Loss and Grief

The elderly are confronted with a variety of losses in many aspects of their lives, not just with the death of a spouse, family members, or long-time friends. Loss of bodily function occurs as illness becomes more prevalent. Loss of support systems occurs as companions die. Loss of independence is a factor as one's physical abilities wane, including loss

BOX 27-7 Research Highlight: Hospice Patients Live Longer

Aim: Some healthcare providers perceive that symptom control in hospice patients, especially the use of opioids and sedatives, may cause patients to die sooner than they otherwise might. Some evidence has suggested, however, that the lives of some patients might be extended through the use of hospice care. This study evaluated the effect of hospice care on elevating the longevity of terminally ill patients.

Method: In this retrospective cohort study, an innovative prospective and retrospective case-control method and Medicare administrative data were used to measure time until death starting from dates narrowly defined within the data. Multiple regression models were used to evaluate the difference of survival periods of terminal illness for patients using hospices and those who did not.

Findings: The survival period was significantly longer for the hospice cohort than for the nonhospice cohort for those patients with congestive heart failure, lung cancer, and pancreatic cancer, and longer—but not statistically significant—for those with colon cancer.

Application to practice: Hospice may, indeed, have a positive impact on patients' longevity, or at least not hasten death. For certain well-defined terminally ill populations, patients who choose hospice care live an average of 29 days longer than similar patients who do not choose hospice. This pattern persisted over four of the six disease categories studied. The findings are important in helping to dispel the myth that hospice care hastens a patient's death. Some factors that may contribute to this longevity may include avoidance of the risks of overtreatment, improved monitoring and treatment, and that the psychosocial supports inherent in hospice care may tend to prolong life. Additional research would clarify the applicability of these findings to other patients and diseases, but nurses can ensure patients and families that the use of hospice is not associated with hastening death.

Reproduced from Connor, S. R., Pyenson, B., Fitch, K., Spence, C., & Iwasaki, K. (2007). Comparing hospice and nonhospice patient survival among patients who die within a three year window. *Journal of Pain and Symptom Management, 33*(3), 238–242.

of mobility, inability to make decisions, and limited access to various other support systems. Not only are the bodily functions lost, but the realization of never regaining these functions is particularly difficult. Primary losses are the loss of people close to them—spouses, children, parents, or siblings. Secondary losses are those resulting from the primary loss—companionship, roles the deceased assumed in the relationship (e.g., bill payer, cook), and independence.

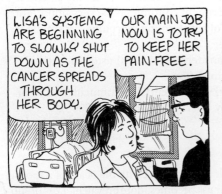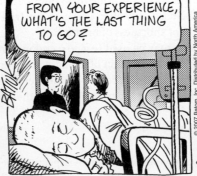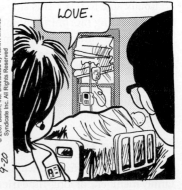

Although the terms *grief* and *mourning are* frequently used interchangeably, each does have a specific meaning. *Grief is* the natural and normal response to loss of any kind and is experienced psychologically, behaviorally, socially, and physically. It involves many changes over time (Rando, 1993). *Mourning* is the cultural and/or public display of grief through one's behaviors. These include accepting the reality of the loss, reacting to the separation and finding ways to channel the reactions, handling the unfinished business, and transferring the attachment to the deceased from physical presence to symbolic interaction. It seeks to accommodate the loss by integrating its realities into ongoing life (Rando, 1993). Alan Wolfelt (2001) distinguishes mourning as the shared social response to grief—grief gone public.

In this author's experience with hospice bereavement support, the practical application of this information suggests a concept that seems logical and is acceptable to people who are mourning: The goal of grieving is not to "get over it" as our society encourages, but rather to figure out how to go on living without the loved one actively present in one's life—learning to better cope with the changes that occur.

Wolfelt (2016a) suggests the following six needs of mourning:

> Acknowledge/accept the reality of the death
> Embrace the pain of the loss
> Remember the person who died
> Develop a new self-identity
> Search for meaning
> Receive support from others

Wolfelt's needs of mourning present some challenges for the elderly because of the limits they may experience physically and emotionally due to chronic or other illnesses. However, it is still important to emphasize reasonable versus unreasonable expectations—grievous loss will produce strong grief, and mourners must be allowed to experience the full dimensions of their unique grief process.

There are patterns to grief that help describe and show progression in the mourning process, regardless of age. Knowing patterns exist is sometimes comforting, but individualized responses must be acknowledged and affirmed. A reasonable goal is to find a personal balance in each of the aspects of grief patterns—physical aspects such as eating and sleeping and emotional aspects such as tears and stoicism, to name a few—as the mourner attempts to incorporate the loss into his or her daily life patterns.

The mourning process has been characterized by stages or phases (see **Box 27-8**). Although it is tempting to consider it as a neat and tidy progression, the concept of overlapping, retrogressing, and recurring jumbles of feelings and responses is more realistic. Phases include the period of numbness occurring at the time of the loss, which provides some emotional protection for a brief time. The period of yearning for the loved one's return tends to deny the permanence of the loss for a time and may include feelings of anger about a variety of aspects of the loss (e.g., anger at the medical profession, at the person who died, and/or at God). The phase of disorganization and despair is one of difficulty in functioning in the environment, in which the mourner begins to do the "figuring out" of how to function in each area of disarray. The phase of reorganized behavior is when one pulls life back together, and in which a new "normal" might be identified (Parkes & Bowlby in Worden, 1991).

There is no timetable for grief; this is one of the individualized differences in the grief/mourning process. Stages, commonly identified as denial, anger, bargaining, depression, and acceptance, are not meant to present a linear progression, but rather to help frame and identify the feelings associated with the adjustments.

A brief review of the risk factors for complicated mourning provides special insight into the vulnerabilities of the elderly, especially in light of the secondary losses noted earlier. According to Rando (1993), there are seven high-risk factors in two categories that might predispose a person to complicated mourning.

Factors associated with the specific death:

> Sudden, unexpected (traumatic, violent, random)
> Overly lengthy illness (multidimensional stresses including anger, ambivalence, guilt, problems obtaining health care)

BOX 27-8   Gone from My Sight: The Dying Experience

Summary of Guidelines for Impending Death

Recognizing that although each person approaches death in his or her own way, some identified patterns assist in the recognition of end-stage status, noted in common language for ease of comprehension by patients and families.

One to 3 months

- Withdrawal from the world and people
- Decreased food intake
- Increase in sleep
- Going inside of self
- Less communication

One to 2 weeks

Mental changes

- Disorientation
- Agitation
- Talking with the unseen
- Confusion
- Picking at clothes

Physical changes

- Decreased blood pressure
- Pulse increase or decrease
- Color change (pale, bluish)
- Increased perspiration

- Respiration irregularities
- Congestion
- Sleeping but responding
- Complaints of body being tired and heavy
- Not eating, taking little fluid
- Body temperature hot/cold

Days or hours

- Intensification of 1- to 2-week signs
- Surge of energy
- Decrease in blood pressure
- Eyes glassy, tearing, half open
- Irregular breathing
- Restlessness or no activity
- Purplish or blotchy knees, feet, hands
- Pulse weak and hard to find
- Decreased urine output
- May wet or stool the bed

Minutes

- "Fish out of water" breathing
- Cannot be awakened

Reproduced from Karnes, B. (1986). Summary of guidelines. In *Gone from my sight: The dying experience* (pp.12–13). Depoe Bay, OR: B.K. Books. Copyright 1986, Barbara Karnes, RN, P.O. Box 189, Depoe Bay, OR, 97341.

> Loss of a child, including adult children
> Perception of the death as preventable (lack of closure, attempt to regain control, search for reasons and meaning)

Antecedent and subsequent variables:

> Markedly angry, ambivalent, or dependent relationship
> Unaccommodated losses, stresses, or mental health problems
> Perception of lack of social support

Mourners must be given the opportunity to process the aspects of their grief, but in a context that is helpful to them. Nurses, who are likely to frequently encounter grieving patients, can facilitate the mourning process by being aware of the aspects of grief and mourning, and by advocacy with the people who surround the mourner. Alan Wolfelt (2016b) suggests a Mourner's Bill of Rights to help mourners sift out the unacceptable advice they are often given. This includes the right to:

> Experience unique grief, without the pressure of "shoulds/shouldn'ts"
> Talk about grief, or be silent as needed
> Feel a multitude of emotions, without feeling judgment
> Tolerate physical and emotional limits and fatigue
> Experience sudden surges of grief/"griefbursts"

> Use rituals
> Embrace spirituality or not
> Search for meaning, recognizing some questions may not have answers
> Treasure memories
> Move toward grief and healing; avoid people who are intolerant of your grief
> Recognize that "grief is a process, not an event"

Other ways nurses can help include active listening without judging the mourner; having compassion and allowing the expression of feelings without criticizing; allowing the mourner to identify his or her own feelings without saying, "I know how you feel;" and offering presence over time (Wolfelt, 2012).

Frequently, when an elderly person experiences the death of a spouse of long standing, the life expectancy of the remaining spouse may be shortened because of the inability to reconcile the needs of mourning, the complications of grief, and the lack of physical and emotional reserves to make the additional investment into a reconfiguration of one's own future. It is also important to note the potential for difference in mourning styles between men and women and among various cultures.

Psychosocial, Emotional, and Spiritual Symptoms

Although we frequently attempt to distinguish among psychosocial, emotional, and spiritual issues, the reality is that the range and depth of being human make it nearly impossible to recognize where one aspect of being ends and another begins. It has been suggested to address these areas as a continuum and view the issues that arise in these aspects of our human functioning at end of life as opportunities rather than as problems (McKinnon & Miller, 2002). "For those caring for the terminally ill, psychosocial and spiritual issues that in the past have been seen as problems can, with information and compassion, become opportunities— opportunities that will allow each of us to live fully until we say goodbye" (McKinnon & Miller, 2002, p. 273) (see **Boxes 27-9** and **27-10**).

Some issues that arise must be viewed in a practical light, because addressing them might assist in providing resources for the dying elderly to promote quality of life and dignity.

Psychosocial Issues

When family members are the primary caregivers of the elderly, role changes are very common. Caregivers may resist providing increasing physical care, not wanting to recognize the decline or not wanting to diminish the dignity of the patient. The patient may resist it as well, resenting the need for the increased level of care because it demonstrates yet more limitations and inabilities in level of independence. Caregivers may not comprehend the emotional changes and resistance of their elder, and may become frustrated with the increasing tasks of care and with the emotional burdens of its constancy.

BOX 27-9   Psychosocial and Spiritual Opportunities Near the End of Life

The opportunity to:

- Reframe society's view of dying: Grow on!
- Expand the definition of quality of life.
- Focus on the individual, not the disease.
- Address as a whole physical pain, psychosocial issues, and spiritual concerns
- Move through fear to peace.
- Move through confusion to meaning.
- Move through despair to hope.

- Move from isolation to community.
- Come to terms with the physical body.
- Move from loss to closure.
- Adjust to new roles.
- Get affairs in order.

Data from Kinzbrunner, B. M., Weinreb, N. J., & Policzer, J. S. (2002). *Twenty common problems in end-of-life care*. New York, NY: McGraw-Hill.

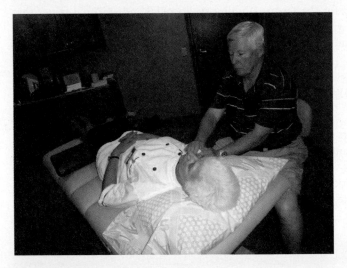

Figure 27-2 Therapeutic touch may be used by trained staff to promote comfort.

It may be helpful for caregivers to view the last year of a person's life as a reversal of the first year of life. This revised perspective helps the caregiver see that the person is not intentionally increasingly helpless or necessarily giving up certain functions. Rather, he or she may be losing abilities in a reverse order of that in which infants gain abilities over the first year of life. These may affect the areas of mobility, activities of daily living, cognition, and personal care needs. As physical ability declines, people begin to withdraw from activities, which may further increase dependence on persons around them and their sense of isolation.

Having sufficient physical care—whether from family, paid caregiver resources, or in assisted living or long-term care facilities—is important for those facing end of life. What constitutes sufficient care may vary with the individual, but it is always an aspect of end-of-life care that will become more important as the person's physical abilities decline. Although some elderly enjoy this increased dependence, very independent individuals often find this increasing caregiver need to be one of the hardest aspects of treatment to accept.

Many patients and families have financial concerns. The concerns are greater, of course, for individuals or families with few resources, or with only some resources (**Figure 27-2**).

Although subsidies for some services are available, many people may not have the ability to access them. The palliative care or hospice team may be helpful in linking the patient and family with appropriate financial resources. Nurses may also want to have basic information available for possible referrals when access to other

BOX 27-11   Special Considerations for Veterans

The We Honor Veterans program is a combined effort of the National Hospice and Palliative Care Association (NHPCO) and the Department of Veterans Affairs (VA) that was launched in September of 2010. This program is designed to recognize and meet the unique needs of dying veterans through education of staff and community, coordinating care with the VA, providing a veteran-to-veteran volunteer, and honoring the veteran for his or her service. A veteran may have special needs depending on many factors, such as:

- Which branch of the military served
- Which war or era served
- If in special forces
- If in combat
- Which theater or geographical area served
- If an officer

- Drafted or enlisted
- Gender

Moral injury (the invisible wounds from war) can also complicate a veteran's end of life. Because these men and women gave so much of themselves for freedom, it is important for healthcare providers to learn about their needs to be able to serve them in the last days or months of their lives. More information can be found at http://www.WeHonorVeterans.org. A Military History Checklist and a Military History Tool Kit are available to assist care providers with this assessment and can be accessed at: http://www.wehonorveterans.org/get-practical-resources/resources-topic/medical-needs and http://www.wehonorveterans.org/get-practical-resources/resources-topic/intakeadmission

team members is not available. There are agencies and individuals available to augment the family's ability to provide care. Most require private pay resources, but some are government sponsored in order to keep people in their homes a bit longer (e.g., Some Medicaid-sponsored hours to provide in-home support are available in some states for those individuals who financially qualify. The Veterans Administration (VA) also has some financial resources for those who qualify (see **Box 27-11**)

Emotional Issues

A person's place in the life cycle affects the person's reaction to end-of-life circumstances. As an elderly person faces death, the individual looks back upon life and reflects upon its experiences. There is an attempt to emotionally integrate all the aspects of one's life, including determination of its meaning and acceptance of its uniqueness (Rando, 1984). It is an unfair exaggeration to imply that all elderly persons are at peace with their coming death. Some are and some are not. Older adults do appear to see death as an important issue, one they often think about and plan for. Caring intervention should continue to facilitate an appropriate death for the aged individual according to the patient's desires, not what the medical personnel deem appropriate.

Anticipatory grief is a process of adjustment during the course of the terminal illness that is faced by the patient as well as by the family and caregivers. It usually begins at the time of diagnosis and can be caused by a variety of adjustments and secondary losses experienced by and required of the individual. These might include loss of control, independence, productivity, security, various abilities, predictability and consistency, future existence, pleasure, ability to complete plans and projects, significant others, meaning, dreams, and hopes for the future (Rando, 1984).

Persons who are facing end of life often encounter feelings of hopelessness. They may find comfort and be helped to adjust to their changing condition by recognizing a changing focus of *hope*. "A patient can hear a terminal diagnosis and still have hopes for the type of life remaining" (Rando, 1984, p. 270). When a person is confronted with the possibility of a life-ending illness, usually the first response is: "I hope it's nothing serious or that it can be easily treated without much disruption in my life." As treatment is not successful and as the illness progresses, one might hope that "my family and I will have the opportunity to get things done . . . have closure . . . see my granddaughter get married."

When getting better or prolonging life is not feasible, one is often confronted with giving up hope altogether. That is how some people feel when they choose hospice or palliative care. That is, in fact, what some physicians imply when they say, "There is nothing more that can be done for you." Hospice and palliative care personnel believe that hope can continue—but the focus of hope moves away from that of getting better. One can hope for the appropriate help and support for themselves and their families through the transitions that end of life brings. They can hope they will be provided with guidance and emotional comfort and their care will be provided with respect for their dignity through the dying process. They can hope that their passing will be comfortable and pain-free. They can hope that their families will receive the appropriate support before and after their death. They can hope to be treated holistically—as an individual with unique needs, wishes, and desires.

Four powerful statements proposed by Ira Byock provide a clear path to emotional wellness throughout a lifetime. They also provide a format for resolving some personal, emotional, and/or spiritual issues at end of life. They are (Byock, 2004, p. 3):

1. Please forgive me.
2. I forgive you.
3. Thank you.
4. I love you

Spiritual or Cultural Issue

Spiritual issues may or may not be related to the person's relationship or lack thereof with an organized religion. Some may find great peace and comfort in a religion and its practices and rituals. Others are just as spiritual, without the link to religious ties and practices, perhaps finding comfort in nature or some other source.

Spiritual and cultural rituals may be important for some people at end of life. Nurses may be in a position to help patients and families obtain access to the rituals that may be important as a person is nearing death. For some religions, this may mean obtaining appropriate clergy for confession, communion, and anointing. For others it may mean a more general ritual for commendation of the dying. In some cultures, certain foods, fasting, handling of the body, and placement in a certain position to facilitate burial may be important (Kirkwood, 1993)

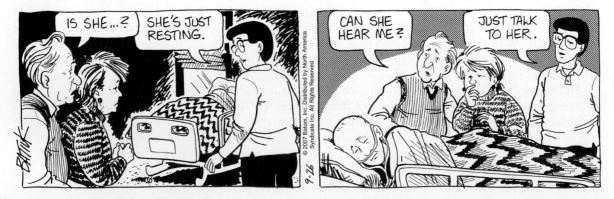

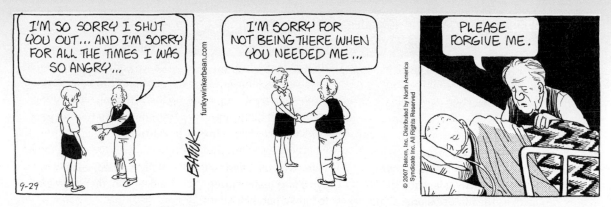

(see **Table 27-3**). As in other aspects of individualized care, it is appropriate to ask the patient and/or family about these preferences.

To formalize this asking, several brief assessments have been developed for use by nurses to incorporate a spiritual component into their nursing plan of care. These are available for detailed review in *Spiritual Care in Nursing Practice* (Mauk & Schmidt, 2004) (see **Box 27-12**). The assessments are easy to incorporate, using acronyms as reminders in obtaining the spiritual history content (see **Boxes 27-13** and **27-14**).

The information obtained by the nurse may be useful for interventions with the patient and family by other members of the care team, regardless of the setting in which care is provided.

Caregiver Issues and Compassion Fatigue

Because providing care for a patient over an extended period of time is common in hospice and palliative care, it is important to recognize issues that may affect a person's ability to provide this care. In hospice care, the Social Work Assessment Tool (SWAT) has been developed to help measure not only the patient's adjustments to aspects of the dying experience, but also those of the caregivers. It encompasses decision making, anxiety about death, environmental preferences, safety, comfort, finances, anticipatory grief, and others. It is designed to show progression in the patient's and caregiver's adjustments over time (NHPCO, 2016).

Nurses are at moderate to high risk for the development of compassion fatigue—a condition that is commonly present when a caregiver continues to provide compassionate care to others in stressful situations without practicing good self-care for himself to herself. Stress, trauma, anxiety, life demands, and excessive empathy (caring more for patient's needs than their own) were key determinants of compassion fatigue risk. Because the risk is apparent, compassion fatigue is preventable and treatable (Abendroth & Flannery, 2006). Awareness is the first step in treatment of compassion fatigue. Authentic, sustainable self-care is possible with education, clarification of personal and professional boundaries, healthy living choices (eating, sleeping, and exercise), stress management, and a healthy support system—living life in balance (Compassion Fatigue Awareness Project, 2012).

Components of Peaceful Dying

It may be possible to plan for a peaceful death, given the knowledge of having a terminal illness. "The key to peaceful dying is achieving the components of peaceful living during the time you have left" (Preston, 2000, p. 161).

TABLE 27-3   Cultural and Religious Practices at End of Life

Religion	During Sickness	Dying and Death	After Dying
Buddhism	Important to die in positive state of mind; organ donation permitted	Help die peacefully by encouraging forgiveness; position on right side, left hand on left thigh, legs stretched out; no special body preparations	Leave body alone as long as possible to avoid disturbing the consciousness during transition from death to new life
Hinduism	Family does daily care; father/oldest son makes health decisions; same-sex caregiver due to modesty	With terminal diagnosis, dying information given to family, not the patient; family decides how much info to share with the patient	Body washed, usually by eldest son, then cremated
Islam	Prayer five times per day; clean area of any body waste, including person and sheets; can use pitcher and basin provided; use clean sheet to cover patient during prayer. Best efforts provided to maintain life; hardship is a test from Allah; can remove life support; natural death will allow person to accept the will of Allah	Body on its side, facing Mecca; friends and loved ones pray for mercy, forgiveness, and blessings of Allah	Person of same gender prepares body for burial; same day as death if possible; cremation forbidden.
Jehovah's Witness	No blood transfusions; organ transplants per individual conscience	Respectful care for dying person and family; respond to their individual needs	Generally follow traditional state mandates for burial or cremation
Judaism	In serious illness, patient is not to be left alone—to be attended by family; doctor's duty to prolong life unless death is imminent and certain; cannot hasten death	Autopsy not permitted unless required by law; organ donation only after person declared dead (not at all by Orthodox)	Cremation forbidden; focus on deceased and funeral; mourning occurs in the home for 7 days after the funeral. Orthodox: extend arms alongside the body, fingers outstretched; tubing, body fluids, sheets/blankets with blood are buried with the body; designated Orthodox Jew should clean the body. Someone stays with body, praying until body enters ground.

TABLE 27-3	Cultural and Religious Practices at End of Life (*continued*)		
Religion	**During Sickness**	**Dying and Death**	**After Dying**
Christianity (general)	Respect and dignity for body; organ donation and autopsy allowed; if treatment is of no benefit or unreasonable burden, may forgo and allow natural death; decision up to patient/family	Open to pastoral care; some have a rite of anointing by a priest; some have service of commendation of the dying	Practices may vary by denomination, but commonly include a gathering with family and friends after the funeral or memorial service.
Orthodox Christianity	Fasting on certain days = no meat, milk, fish, eggs; no eating before communion; can use drugs to reduce pain/suffering; removing life supports done after prayer and discussion with family members, medical professional, and spiritual director; organ donation acceptable	Family encouraged to be at bedside; invite priest; Anointing of the Sick (Holy Unction)	Body buried in ground, w/coffin, grave liner, monument with image of the cross; cremation is not allowed.
Roman Catholicism	If possible, fast 1 hour before receiving Eucharist; moral obligation to use ordinary or proportionate means of preserving life (in judgment of patient)	Sacrament of Anointing of the Sick before surgery, for elderly in weakened condition, by a priest	May be cremated; cremains may be brought to funeral mass.

Data from Toole, M. M. (2006). *Handbook for chaplains: Comfort my people.* New York, NY: Paulist Press. Copyright 2006 by Mary M. Toole/Paulist Press. Retrieved from www.paulistpress.com

Some components are accomplished only by the individual, whereas others may require the assistance of family and medical providers, such as the following (Preston, 2000):

> Instilling good memories
> Uniting with family and medical staff
> Avoiding suffering, with relief of pain and other symptoms
> Maintaining alertness, control, privacy, dignity, and support
> Becoming spiritually ready
> Saying goodbye
> Dying quietly

A *good death* is possible and can be facilitated by the nurse who advocates for and works to ensure that the patients, families, and caregivers are free from avoidable distress and suffering, that the process is in accord with the wishes of the patient and family, and that it is consistent with clinical, cultural, and ethical standards (Dobbins, 2005).

CLINICAL TIP

The nurse's goal should be to help a patient have a "good" death.

BOX 27-12   Suggested Resources

Albom, M. (1997). *Tuesdays with Morrie: An old man, a young man, and life's greatest lesson*. New York, NY: Doubleday.

Association for Death Education and Counseling. (2016). Retrieved from http://www.ADEC.org

Bodtke, S., & Logan, K. (2016). *Hospice and palliative medicine handbook: A clinical guide*. Retrieved from http://www.hpmhandbook.com

Byock, I. (2012). *The best care possible: A physician's quest to transform care through the end of life*. New York, NY: Avery.

Callanan, M., & Kelley, P. (1992). *Final gifts: Understanding the special awareness, needs, and communications of the dying*. New York, NY: Poseidon Press.

Hospice Foundation of America: http://www.hospicefoundation.org

Journal of Hospice and Palliative Nursing: http://www.jhpn.com

National Hospice and Palliative Care Organization: http://www.nhpco.org

Nuland, S. B. (1993). *How we die: Reflections on life's final chapter*. New York, NY: Random House.

Project on Death in America. Open Society Institute: http://www.soros.org/initiatives/pdia

Smith, W. J. (2000). *The culture of death: The assault on medical ethics in America*. San Francisco, CA: Encounter Books.

Toole, M. M. (2006). *Handbook for chaplains: Comfort my people*. New York, NY: Paulist Press.

Webb, M. (1997). *The good death: The new American search to reshape the end of life*. New York, NY: Bantam Books.

Wit. (2001). A movie made for HBO and a Pulitzer Prize–winning play by Margaret Edson featuring a single-minded English professor, who in the face of imminent death learns the power and importance of simple acts of human kindness.

BOX 27-13   HOPE Model

H = Sources of hope, meaning, comfort, strength, peace, love, and connection: What do you hold on to during difficult times?

O = Organized religion: Importance? Helpful and nonhelpful aspects?

P = Personal spirituality and practice: Relationship with God? Most helpful aspects of spiritual practices?

E = Effects on medical care and end-of-life issues: Has illness affected your ability to do the things that usually help you spiritually? Are there specific practices to be aware of in providing care? Can I help access resources helpful to you?

Reproduced with permission from American Academy of Family Physicians. (2001). Spirituality and medical practice: Using the HOPE questions as a practical tool for spiritual assessment. © 2001 American Academy of Family Physicians. All rights reserved.

> **BOX 27-14   FICA Model**
>
> **F** = Faith or beliefs (What gives meaning to life?)
>
> **I** = Importance and influence (Is faith important? How do beliefs influence behavior toward illness?)
>
> **C** = Community (Is the spiritual or religious community supportive? How? Person or people important to you? People you love?)
>
> **A** = Address (How would you like healthcare providers to address these issues in your health care?)
>
> Data from Puchalski, C., & Romer, A. L. (2000). Taking a spiritual history allows clinicians to understand patients more fully. *Journal of Palliative Medicine, 3*(1), 129–131.

Postmortem Care

Pronouncing Death

Procedures for pronouncing the death of a person vary across states and institutions. In some states, nurses may be able to pronounce the death, whereas in others this is not allowed. In in-patient settings, policies differ and the individual institutional policies are followed. In hospice home care, generally a nurse makes a visit, determines the lack of vital signs, and contacts the physician who has already agreed to sign the death certificate because the death has been anticipated. The funeral home or mortuary is contacted for removal of the body.

In pronouncing the death, it is customary to identify the patient and note the following (Berry & Griffie, 2006):

> General appearance of the body
> Lack of reaction to verbal or tactile stimulation
> Lack of pupillary light reflex (pupils fixed and dilated)
> Absent breathing and lung sounds
> Absent carotid and apical pulses (in some situations, listening for an apical pulse for a full minute is advisable)

Physical Care of the Body

Care of the body is an important nursing function. It is not surprising that families often recall the actions of the nurse after the death of their loved one. Careful and gentle handling of the body communicates care and concern on the part of the nurse. The nurse should allow the family to spend time with the body if desired. Rituals and customs should have been identified before the death, to now be incorporated into this care, reflecting the patient and family wishes.

Family members should be allowed to touch the body if they so desire and are comfortable with this action. They may wish to select special clothes for their loved one's transfer to the funeral home. If they choose to remain present through the postmortem care, they should be educated about the potential for some body changes. For example, there may be the sound of air escaping from the lungs when the body is turned (a sighing sound), and stool and urine may be present in a previously continent person, as the rectal and urinary bladder sphincters relax. Nursing care also includes the removal of drains, tubes, intravenous lines, and any other devices. Family members may wish to participate in bathing and dressing the body; some may find comfort in the small details of "a favorite gown and the hair just right" (Berry & Griffie, 2006).

Summary

When death approaches for the elderly patient, the role of the nurse changes along with the patient's changing condition. The role moves from a "fix-it" focus to that of "presence"—the ability to be with the patient and with

---

BOX 27-15 Ten Self-Care Tips for the Nurse Caring for Patients at End of Life

1. Become educated—knowledge is power! Develop expertise in symptom management. It lessens anxiety in working with patients and their families.
2. Maintain professional boundaries and relationships with patients and families.
3. Utilize the other palliative care or hospice team members. Each has a perspective and expertise to add to the case. The nurse does not have to do it all.
4. Develop an interdisciplinary care team in your palliative or end-of-life care setting or facility.
5. Utilize all facility staff/team members in their respective roles.
6. Find and maintain balance in your personal life.
7. Locate and use appropriate support persons for debriefing during and after a difficult case.
8. Allow yourself and all team members to grieve the death of your patient.
9. Include the other members of the team (including CNAs, housekeeping, and other staff who knew the patient) in rituals or memorial activities following the death of your patient.
10. Practice good self-care in your personal and professional life. Eat, sleep, play, laugh, cry (. . . enough!!), . . . and wear comfortable shoes.

BOX 27-16 Web Exploration

Explore the Website for the Hospice Foundation of America at http://www.hospicefoundation.org and compare the contents with those at Ira Byock's Website at http://www.dyingwell.com

---

his or her family. This presence involves the provision of comfort measures, lending a listening ear, providing a peaceful environment, and compassionately educating patient and family about the dying process.

Nurses caring for the dying also need to care for themselves (see **Box 27-15**). The nurse's gratification does not come from curing (see **Box 27-16**), but rather from supporting the patient in a peaceful and dignified "good death."

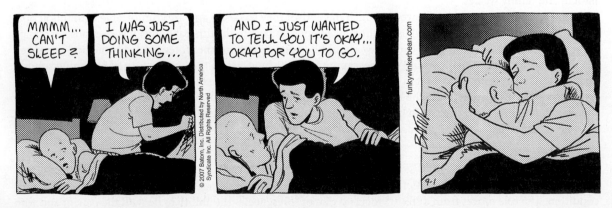

Clinical Reasoning Exercises

1. Visit a funeral home and talk with the funeral home director(s) about their experiences. What are the major components of their job? How do they feel they provide a service to the community?
2. Review your local newspaper and read the obituaries. What are the ages of the persons who have died? Are most of them older or younger?
3. Recall a funeral for a family member that you may have attended in the past. What were the components of the service? How did religious and cultural aspects play a part in the funeral or memorial service? The burial? The grieving and mourning? How did family and friends grieve? How did they remember the loved one?

Personal Reflections

1. This chapter has provided a large amount of information on caring for older adults at end of life. Are there areas of your nursing practice that you need to further develop in order to provide effective care to the dying? List a few of those areas in which you could improve your practice.
2. If an older family member who is close to you was recently given a terminal diagnosis, how would you respond? What questions would you ask of him or her? What actions, if any, would you take?
3. Do you have advance directives or a living will for yourself? Why or why not?
4. Have you ever been with a person when they died? What was that experience like for you?
5. After learning the material in this chapter, do you view any aspects of end of life differently?
6. Have you ever provided postmortem care for a patient? If so, what was the most difficult aspect of that experience?

References

Abendroth, M., & Flannery, J. (2006). Predicting the risk of compassion fatigue: A study of hospice nurses. *Journal of Hospice and Palliative Nursing, 8*(6), 346–356.

Aging with Dignity. (2015). Five wishes: 2015 edition. Retrieved from https://agingwithdignity.org/shop/product-details/five-wishes

Allchin, L. (2006). Caring for the dying: Nursing student perspectives. *Journal of Hospice and Palliative Nursing, 8*(2), 112–115.

Allen, W. (1976). *Without feathers, death* [Play]. Act 1. New York, NY: Ballantine Books.

American Academy of Hospice and Palliative Medicine. (2016). Smartbrief 4/20/16. Retrieved from http://aahpm.org/

Aminoff, B. Z., & Adunsky, A. (2004). Dying dementia patients: Too much suffering, too little palliation. *American Journal of Alzheimer's Disease and Other Dementias, 19*(4), 243–247.

Berry, P., & Griffie, J. (2006). Planning for the actual death. In B. R. Ferrell & N. Coyle (Eds.), *Textbook of palliative nursing* (pp. 561–577). New York, NY: Oxford University Press.

Bodke S., & Ligon, K., (2016). Definitions table. In *Hospice and palliative medicine handbook: A clinical guide* (p. 197). Retrieved from http://www.hpmhandbook.com

Brajtman, S. (2005). Helping the family through the experience of terminal restlessness. *Journal of Hospice and Palliative Nursing, 7*(2), 73–81.

Brennan, C. W., & Mazanec, P. (2011). Dyspnea management across the palliative care continuum. *Journal of Hospice and Palliative Nursing, 13*(3), 130–139.

Byock, I. (2004). *The four things that matter most: A book about living.* New York, NY: Free Press.

Byock, I. (2012). *The best care possible: A physician's quest to transform care through the end of life.* New York, NY: Avery/Penguin.

Centers for Disease Control and Prevention. (2016). Deaths and mortality. Retrieved from https://www.cdc.gov /nchs/fastats/deaths.htm

Center for Ethics in Health Care, Oregon Health & Science University. (2008). Frequently asked questions about physicians orders for life sustaining treatment paradigm. Retrieved from https://www.ohsu.edu/xd /education/continuing-education/center-for-ethics/ethics-outreach/upload/Oregon-Death-with-Dignity -Act-Guidebook.pdf

Centers for Medicare and Medicaid Services. (2012). Hospice payment system. Retrieved from http://www.cms.gov /Outreach-and-Education/Medicare-Learning-Network-MLN/MLNProducts/downloads/hospice_pay_sys_fs.pdf

Centers for Medicare and Medicaid Services. (2016a). Outreach and education. Retrieved from https://www .cms.gov/outreach-and-education/outreach-and-education.htm

Centers for Medicare and Medicaid Services. (2016b). Medicare fee for service payment. Retrieved from https:// www.cms.gov/medicare/medicare-fee-for-service-payment/physicianfeesched/

Compassion Fatigue Awareness Project. (2012). *What is compassion fatigue?* Retrieved from http://www.compassion fatigue.org/pages/compassionfatigue.html

Connor, S. R., Pyenson, B., Fitch, K., Spence, C., & Iwasaki, K. (2007). Comparing hospice and non-hospice patient survival among patients who die within a three-year window. *Journal of Pain and Symptom Management, 33*(3), 238–246.

Derby, S., & O'Mahoney S. (2006). Elderly patients. In B. R. Ferrell & N. Coyle (Eds.), *Textbook of palliative nursing* (pp. 639–640, 646–647). New York, NY: Oxford University Press.

Dobbins, E. H. (2005). Helping your patient to a "good death." *Nursing, 35*(2), 43–45.

Emanuel, L. L., von Gunten, C. F., & Ferris, F. D. (1999). *Trainer's guide, module 2: Communicating bad news. The education for physicians on end-of-life care (EPEC) curriculum.* Princeton, NJ: Robert Wood Johnson Foundation.

Enclara Health Hospice Pharmacy Services. (2011). *Management algorithm pharmacopoeia (MAP) handbook* (3rd ed.). West Deptford, NJ: Enclara Health.

Ferrell, B. R. (1991). Pain in elderly people. *Journal of the American Geriatrics Society, 39*(1), 64–73.

Ferrell, B. R., Grant, M., & Virani, R. (1999). Strengthening nursing education to improve end-of-life care. *Nursing Outlook, 47*(6), 252–256.

Gibson, M., & Schroder, C. (2001). The many faces of pain for older, dying adults. *American Journal of Hospice and Palliative Care, 18*(1), 19–25.

Gidwani, R., Joyce, N., Kinosian, B., Faricy-Anderson, K., Levy, C., Miller, S. C., . . . Mor, V (2016). Gap between recommendations and practice of palliative care and hospice in cancer patients. *Journal of Palliative Medicine.* Retrieved from https://www.ncbi.nlm.nih.gov/pubmed/27228478

Griffie, J., Nelson-Marten, P., & Muchka, S. (2004). Acknowledging the "elephant": Communication in palliative care: Speaking the unspeakable when death is imminent. *American Journal of Nursing, 104*(1), 48–58.

Hillesum, E. (1996). *An interrupted life: The diaries and letters from Westerbork* (p. 155). New York, NY: Henry Holt & Company.

Hogan, C. (2015). Spending in the *last year of life and the impact of hospice on medicare outlays* (p. 36). Washington, D.C.: MedPAC.

Hogan, C., Lunney, J., Gabel, J., & Lynn, J. (2001). Medicare beneficiaries cost of care in the last year of life. *Health Affairs, 20*(4), 188–195.

Hospice and Palliative Nurses Association. (2003). Position paper: Palliative sedation at the end of life. *Journal of Hospice and Palliative Nursing, 5*(4), 235–237.

Hospice and Palliative Nurses Association. (2004a). Pain. *Journal of Hospice and Palliative Nursing, 6*(1), 62–64.

Hospice and Palliative Nurses Association. (2004b). Value of the professional nurse in end-of-life care. *Journal of Hospice and Palliative Nursing, 6*(1), 65–66.

Hospice and Palliative Nurses Association. (2016). HPNA position statement: Artificial nutrition and hydration in advanced illness. Retrieved from https://www.hpna.org/filemaintenance_view.aspx?ID=21

Karnes, B. (2001). *Gone from my sight: The dying experience* (pp. 12–13). Depoe Bay, OR: B. K. Books.

Kinzbrunner, B. M. (2002). Nutritional support and parenteral hydration. In B. M. Kinzbrunner, N. J. Weinreb, & J. S. Policzer (Eds.), *Twenty common problems in end-of-life care* (pp. 313–327). New York, NY: McGraw-Hill.

Kinzbrunner, B. M., Weinreb, N. J., & Policzer, J. S. (2002). *Twenty common problems in end-of-life care.* New York, NY: McGraw-Hill.

Kirkwood, N. A. (1993). *A hospital handbook on multiculturalism and religion: Practical guidelines for health care workers.* Harrisburg, PA: Morehouse.

Kodjak, A. (2016). Arcadia study: Dying in a hospital means more procedures, tests and costs. Retrieved from http://www.npr.org/sections/health-shots/2016/06/15/481992191/dying

Krisman-Scott, M. A. (2003). Origins of hospice in the United States: The care of the dying, 1945–1975. *Journal of Hospice and Palliative Nursing, 5*(4), 205–210.

Kübler-Ross, E., & Kessler, D. (2000). *Life lessons.* New York, NY: Simon and Schuster.

Levi, M. H. (1991). Constipation and diarrhea in cancer patients. *Cancer Bulletin, 43*, 412–422.

Lewis, L. (2001, July). Toward a good death in the nursing home: Pain management and hospice are key. *Caring for the Ages,* 24–27.

Lipman, A. G. (2006). Pharmacotherapy for pain control at end of life. In K. J. Doka (Ed.), *Pain management at the end of life: Bridging the gap between knowledge and practice* (pp. 156–158). Washington, DC: Hospice Foundation of America.

Lowes, R. (2016). Medicare approves payment for end of life counseling. Retrieved from http://www.medscape.com/viewarticle/853541

Mauk, K. L., & Schmidt, N. K. (2004). *Spiritual care in nursing practice.* Philadelphia, PA: Lippincott Williams & Wilkins.

McCaffery, M. (1968). *Nursing practice theories related to cognition, bodily pain, and man-environment interactions.* Los Angeles, CA: University of California at Los Angeles Student Store.

McCaffery, M., & Pasero, C. (1999). *Pain: Clinical manual* (2nd ed.). St. Louis, MO: Mosby.

McKinnis, E. A. (2002). Dyspnea and other respiratory symptoms. In B. M. Kinzbrunner, N. J. Weinreb, & J. S. Policzer (Eds.), *Twenty common problems in end-of-life care* (pp. 147–162). New York, NY: McGraw-Hill.

McKinnon, S. E., & Miller, B. (2002). Psychosocial and spiritual concerns. In B. M. Kinzbrunner, N. J. Weinreb, & J. S. Policzer (Eds.), (2002). *Twenty common problems in end-of-life care* (pp. 257–274). New York, NY: McGraw-Hill.

Mercadante, S., Ferrera, P., Villari, P., & Casuccio, A. (2006). Opioid escalation in patients with cancer pain: The effect of age. *Journal of Pain and Symptom Management, 32*(5), 413–419.

Meyer, C. (2001). Allow natural death: An alternative to DNR? In *Hospice patients alliance.* Retrieved from http://www.hospicepatients.org/and.html

Morrow, A. (2012). What is POLST and do I need one? About.com. Retrieved from http://Dying.about.com/od/ethicsandchoices/f/POLST.htm

National Consensus Project for Quality Palliative Care. (2009). *Clinical practice guidelines for quality palliative care* (2nd ed.). Pittsburgh, PA: Author. Retrieved from www.nationalconsensusproject.org/guideline.pdf

National Hospice and Palliative Care Organization (NHPCO). (2016a). Hospice philosophy statement. Para 1. Retrieved from http://www.nhpco.org/nhpco-0

National Hospice and Palliative Care Organization (NHPCO). (2016b). Public statistics. Retrieved from http://www.nhpco.org/sites/default/files/public/statistics_Research/2015_Facts_Figures.pdf

National Hospice and Palliative Care Organization (NHPCO). (2016c). Social work assessment tool. Retrieved from http://www.nhpco.org/sites/default/files/public/nchpp/SWAT_Information_Booklet.pdf

Perley M. J., & Dahlin, C. (Eds.). (2007). *Core curriculum for the advanced practice hospice and palliative nurse.* Washington, DC: Hospice and Palliative Nurses Association.

Preston, T. A. (2000). *Final victory: Taking charge of the last stages of life, facing death on your own terms.* Roseville, CA: Prima.

Puchalski, C., & Romer, A. L. (2000). Taking a spiritual history allows clinicians to understand patients more fully. *Journal of Palliative Medicine, 3*(1), 129–131.

Quaglietti, S., Blum, L., & Ellis, V. (2004). The role of the adult nurse practitioner in palliative care. *Journal of Hospice and Palliative Nursing, 6*(4), 209–213.

Quint, J. C. (1967). *The nurse and the dying patient.* New York, NY: Macmillan.

Rando, T. A. (1984). *Grief, dying and death: Clinical interventions for caregivers.* Champaign, IL: Research Press.

Rando, T. A. (1993). *Treatment of complicated mourning.* Champaign, IL: Research Press.

Rushton, C. H., Spencer, K. L., & Johanson, W. (2004). Bringing end-of-life care out of the shadows. *Nursing Management, 35*(3), 34–40.

Saunders, C. (1984). On dying well. *Cambridge Review,* 49–52.

Schweitzer, A. (1961). *On the edge of the primeval forest & more from the primeval forest: Experiences and observations of a doctor in equatorial Africa* (p. 62). London, UK: Macmillan.

Sheehan, D. K., & Schirm, V. (2003). End of life care of older adults. *American Journal of Nursing, 103*(11), 48–57.

Storey, P. (1996). *Primer of palliative care* (2nd ed.). Gainesville, FL: American Academy of Hospice and Palliative Medicine.

Temel, J. S., Greer, J. A., Muzikansky, A., Gallagher, E. R., Admane, A., Jackson, V.A., . . . & Lynch, T. J. (2010). Early palliative care for patients with metastatic non-small-cell lung cancer. *New England Journal of Medicine, 363*(30), 733–742.

Toole, M. M. (2006). *Handbook for chaplains: Comfort my people.* New York, NY: Paulist Press.

Towey, J. (2005). *Five wishes: Questions and answers.* Retrieved from http://www.agingwithdignity.org/five-wishes.php

Warden, V., Hurley, A. C., & Volicer, V. (2003). Development in psychometric evaluation of the Pain Assessment in Advanced Dementia (PAINAD) Scale. *Journal of the American Medical Director Association, 4,* 9–15. Developed at New England Geriatric Research Education & Clinical Center, Bedford VAMC, MA.

Weinreb, N. J., Kinzbrunner, B., & Clark, M. (2002). Pain management. In B. M. Kinzbrunner, N. J. Weinreb, & J. S. Policzer (Eds.), *Twenty common problems in end-of-life care* (pp. 91–145). New York, NY: McGraw-Hill.

Wolfelt, A. D. (2001). *Healing a teen's grieving heart: 100 practical ideas.* Ft. Collins, CO: Companion Press.

Wolfelt, A. D. (2012). How to help the grieving. Retrieved from https://www.centerforloss.com/

Wolfelt, A. D. (2016a). Grief. Retrieved from https://www.centerforloss.com/grief/

Wolfelt, A. D. (2016b). The mourner's bill of rights. Retrieved from http://griefwords.com/index.cgi?action=page&page=articles%2Fmourners.html&site_id=5

Wong, D. L, Hockenberry-Eaton, M., Wilson, D., Winkelstein, M. L., & Schwartz, P. (2001). *Wong's essentials of pediatric nursing* (6th ed., p. 1301). St. Louis, MO: Mosby.

Worden, J. W. (1991). *Grief counseling and grief therapy: A handbook for the mental health practitioner.* New York, NY: Springer.

Wright, J. B. (2002). Depression and other common symptoms. In B. M. Kinzbrunner, N. J. Weinreb, & J. S. Policzer (Eds.), *Twenty common problems in end-of-life care* (pp. 221–240). New York, NY: McGraw-Hill.

For a full suite of assignments and additional learning activities, see the access code at the front of your book.

CHAPTER 28

Care Transitions, System Models, and Health Policy in Aging

Carole A. Pepa
Terrie Black
Michelle Camicia

(Competencies 4, 5, 8, 10, 14)

LEARNING OBJECTIVES

At the end of this chapter, the reader will be able to:

> Describe the continuum of care.
> Identify criteria for admission to postacute levels of care.
> Compare the settings available for older adult living.
> Describe the evidence-based care transition models used in different settings.
> Describe models of community-based care management.
> Explain initiatives to increase and ensure quality in healthcare delivery.
> Describe the prospective payment system as it applies to the different levels of care (e.g., home care, acute care, in-patient rehabilitation facilities, long-term care hospitals).
> Compare the U.S. Medicare and Medicaid programs.
> Describe the influence of third-party players on health care.
> Compare the aging policies of Japan, Germany, England, and Canada with those of the United States.
> Discuss the influence of the different stakeholders on health policy formation.
> Explain the role of the gerontological nurse in policy formation and advocacy.

KEY TERMS

Acute in-patient rehabilitation
Adult day services
Advocacy
After discharge care management of
   low-income frail elderly (AD-LIFE)

Agency for Healthcare Research
   and Quality (AHRQ)
Assisted living facilities
Care coordination
Case mix groups

Care transitions intervention

Commission on Accreditation of
Rehabilitation Facilities

Community-based care management
programs

Continuity Assessment Record and
Evaluation (CARE) tool

Copayment

Diagnosis-related groups

Geriatric Resource for Assessment and
Care of Elders

Health information technology

Health policy

Health policy development

Healthy People 2020

In-patient rehabilitation facility

Inpatient Rehabilitation Facility Patient
Assessment Instrument

Institute of Medicine

Joint Commission

Long-term acute care hospitals

Long-term care

Managed care organizations

Medicaid

Medicare

Minimum Data Set

Money Follows the Person

National Quality Forum

National Quality Strategy

Next step in care

Outcome and Assessment Information Set

Patient Protection and Affordable Care Act
of 2010

Postacute care

Potentially avoidable hospitalization

Preferred provider organizations

Preventable hospital readmission

Private insurance

Programs of All-Inclusive Care for the Elderly

Prospective payment system

Public policy

Quality Safety Education for Nurses

Resource utilization groups

Skilled nursing facility

Social policy

Transitional care model (TCM)

Transitional care

Transitional care unit

The healthcare environment evolves as the needs and characteristics of the population change, and new approaches to care delivery become part of the continuum of care. Providers of care, especially gerontological nurses, must be familiar with the needs of older adults and address the challenges faced by them. Services and programs for older adults must be tailored to meet the evolving needs of the aging population. To advocate for the well-being of older adults, care providers must understand different models of care and act to influence *health policy*.

To meet the needs of medically complex issues while decreasing lengths of hospital stays, individuals are moving from acute care hospitals into other *postacute care* (PAC) settings. This has resulted in differing levels of care as well as differing levels of need based on a variety of patient characteristics. The evolving healthcare system requires providers to look beyond the medical model of care and embrace the entire individual's needs in the provision of care. Person-directed care is a philosophy of care that is congruent with current quality goals and favored by patients, advocates, and clinicians alike who seek a transformation of the culture of care from an institution focus to a personal, patient-centered focus.

Continuum of Care

To address quality of care across the continuum, it is critical to be familiar with the different settings of care. With an understanding of these settings, nurses can apply evidence-based practice models to ensure both safe transitions across the care continuum and quality outcomes. Care across the continuum asks that health professionals look critically at the setting of care and anticipate the needs of patients as these settings change.

The determination of the right level of PAC for an individual must be based on the individual's biopsycho-social ecological assessment (Camicia et al., 2014). Factors that must be considered include biological, social, financial resources, environmental, and systems. Biological factors include the individual's medical needs, preinjury or illness level of function, and tolerance of rehabilitation. Social factors include psychological and informal and formal community supports. Other important considerations include financial resources and stressors and the physical environment of the community living setting. Systems factors include the components of care and services, the intensity of service provision (e.g., number of hours of nursing care or therapy), and the structure and process of the program. There is a continuum of rehabilitation care as well. The intensity of services decreases across the continuum from *in-patient rehabilitation facility* (IRF) level of care to the *skilled nursing facility* (SNF) to home health to comprehensive outpatient programs to outpatient programs. To be the most cost and outcome effective, the care setting must be matched to the patients' needs. The nurse coordinates care from the acute setting through the various PAC settings and community to ensure the person's optimal function and participation in the community where he or she lives and plays.

Acute Care Hospital

The acute care hospital is often the point of entry into the healthcare system for older adults. Due in part to the increasing admissions of older adults for hospital care, it is essential that nurses have education specific to the needs of this specialty population. In the acute care setting, the primary focus of nursing care involves caring for acute illnesses, injuries, and exacerbations of chronic diseases such as cardiopulmonary conditions, orthopedic problems, and various cancer treatments. Care of the older adult often begins in the emergency setting and may progress into critical care, general units, or an acute rehabilitation unit or hospital. Regardless of the acute care setting, the optimal goal is to promote recovery and maintain the elder's optimal level of functioning through quality care and the prevention of complications.

Acute In-Patient Rehabilitation

Rehabilitation services begin while in the acute care setting and extend throughout the continuum based on the needs of the older adult. *Acute in-patient rehabilitation* ("acute rehab") is an appropriate option for those who will benefit from an intensive, multidisciplinary approach to care delivery. The typical rehabilitation team consists of nurses, therapists, physicians, and other specialists who work collaboratively with the patient to maximize independence and optimal level of functioning. Additional services such as neuropsychology, speech, and respiratory therapy are also available for patients during their rehabilitation.

> **CLINICAL TIP**
>
> Acute inpatient rehabilitation is most appropriate for those who may benefit from an interprofessional approach to care and are able to tolerate at least 3 hours of therapy per day.

The hours of nursing care and the intensity of therapy in a rehabilitation unit is greater than those services provided in acute or transitional care units and extended care facilities. Each patient admitted to an acute rehabilitation unit receives a minimum of 15 hours per week of combined therapies to fulfill Medicare requirements for admission. Primary conditions necessitating a referral with subsequent admission to an acute rehabilitation facility include conditions such as stroke, head trauma, neurological diseases, amputation, spinal cord injury, major multiple trauma, and orthopedic surgery.

Transitional and Progressive Care Unit

Transitional or progressive care is a broad term that encompasses a variety of skilled nursing services, including subacute, skilled, and some rehabilitative care services. Medically stable patients requiring nursing care beyond the acute illness or injury phase can be managed in a hospital-based *transitional care unit* (TCU) or an SNF on a short-term basis. The terms *transitional care* and *skilled care* are often used interchangeably, but depending on the setting there can be wide variations (Yung, Yeh, & Pressler, 2012). Transitional care bridges the gap for patients with complex or multiple problems who are not stable enough to return to a home setting, but not sick enough to require long-term nursing care. Examples of the conditions included in admission to such a unit are general debility, wound care, gait training, and intravenous therapy.

In a hospital-based TCU setting, patients are transferred to a designated unit from an acute bed to a designated skilled care bed. Hospital-based skilled nursing facilities exist as a distinct part of the hospital and are usually called transitional care units. Skilled care helps patients transition from illness to wellness—from dependence to self-care.

Long-Term Acute Care Hospital

Long-term acute care hospitals (LTACHs) or units furnish extended medical and rehabilitative care to individuals with clinically complex problems, such as multiple acute or chronic conditions, that need hospital-level care for relatively extended periods. The usual length of stay for patients admitted to this type of facility is generally about 25 days.

Although LTACHs are often confused with nursing homes or rehabilitation facilities, there is a significant difference. LTACHs treat patients who might be classified as intensive care patients at short-term hospitals. Some of these facilities are stand-alone hospitals; however, nearly half of all LTACHs are "hospitals within hospitals" because they are hosted by an acute care hospital that leases a floor, wing, or other space to the LTACH (Butcher, 2007).

> ### CLINICAL TIP
> LTACHs provide long-term intensive acute care, such as for patients on a ventilator, often within an acute care hospital setting on a designated floor or wing.

Home Health Care

One of the most sought-out options for older adults requiring observation or nursing care upon discharge from a medical facility may be for home healthcare services. Home health care is designed for those who are homebound due to severity of illness or immobility. For reimbursement of allowable expenses, home health services must be medically necessary, intermittent, and ordered by a healthcare provider.

There has been much growth in the recent past related to the number of home health agencies. This increase is due in part to the desire to be cared for in familiar surroundings by family members and in-home caregivers. Providing care in the home improves the quality of life and increases the likelihood that the person receiving care will remain more active and independent (Kadowaki, Wister, & Chappel, 2015).

Although physical, occupational, and speech therapy may be provided through home care, when nursing care is also ordered, a registered nurse (RN) makes initial contact, completes an in-depth assessment, evaluates the patient, and develops a plan of care to ensure the individual's health condition requires nursing services and qualifies for home health services. If the patient only needs therapy, a RN does not have to make the initial assessment. The majority of home healthcare patients are older adults with a variety of nursing needs, such as wound care, intravenous therapy, management of newly diagnosed diabetes, tube feedings, and skilled assessment for exacerbation of a chronic illness.

Long-Term Care
Nursing Homes

In the United States, the demand for *long-term care* (LTC) is expected to rise exponentially. By the year 2030, 20.3% of the U.S. population will be over 65 years of age, up 13% from 2012. By 2050, it is expected that 21% of those over age 65 years will be 85 years of age or older (Ortman, Velkoff, & Hogan, 2014). In light of these predictions, an older person's likelihood of living in a nursing home (LTC) increases sharply with age. "About 1% of the young elderly (aged 65 to 69 years) currently live in a nursing home or LTC facility. The proportion rises to 3% for ages 75 to 79, 11.2% for ages 85 to 89, 19.8% at ages 90 to 94, 31.0% at ages 95 to 99, and up to 38.2% among centenarians" (Cire, 2011, p. 1).

The LTC industry includes nursing homes, for both custodial and skilled care, assisted living homes, and independent living homes. Initially, the LTC industry was developed to meet the needs of the elderly and infirm in an environment that would embrace efficiency in terms of economies of scale for those requiring care outside the home for long periods of time. Initially, nursing homes were connected to hospitals or physician groups. Medicare and Medicaid provided the funding avenue that allowed nonmedical individuals to open and operate nursing homes as free-standing entities. The LTC industry grew as corporations saw the potential market growth and entered the LTC arena. Eventually, skilled nursing homes offered rehabilitation services when the acute care setting began looking for alternative care environments for those in need of these types of services. These services, while typically less intensive than those offered at an acute rehabilitation hospital, were welcomed by third party payers because they realized cost savings in the acute care settings (Chandra, Dalton, & Holmes, 2013).

Government regulation helped define the care needs of individuals in the nursing home setting, including those individuals at a skilled nursing level. According to the *Medicare Benefits Policy Manual* (MBPM), skilled care requires services provided by a professional. This is contrasted by custodial level care, which is typically provided by unskilled or unlicensed medical personal such as an aide or assistant.

With this differentiation, it became apparent that there was a lower level of care needed to meet the needs of individuals who needed assistance but did not rise to the level of either skilled or custodial care. Assisted living homes were first developed as community-based residential facilities with different levels of care provided. Eventually, the designated title for these homes fell under the umbrella of assisted living. Most individuals living in assisted living pay for these services out of their own pockets because Medicare and Medicaid have not caught up with this level of care in many states. This gap has resulted in individuals without personal funds being admitted to the nursing home setting regardless of their level of care. **Table 28-1** provides a comparison of nursing homes and assisted-living homes in terms of services provided.

Assisted Living Facility

Assisted living facilities (ALFs) provide assistance and monitoring of older residential adults for whom independent living is no longer appropriate but who do not need 24-hour skilled nursing home care. In the United States, ALFs are regulated and licensed at the state level. More than two thirds of the states use the licensure term *assisted living*; other licensure terms include *supportive living facility* (SLF), *residential care home*, and *personal care homes*.

TABLE 28-1 Care Levels in LTC Homes	
Nursing Homes	**Assisted Living Homes**

1. Skilled nursing care of a RN required, such as:
   a. Medication administration
   b. Daily wound care
   c. Assessment
	1. Does not require skilled nursing care services daily

2. Requires assistance with one or more activities of daily living (ADLs) 24 hours/day at the skilled level	2. Supportive care
	   a. Medication management
	   b. Personal care assistance
	   c. Homemaking
	   d. Social activities
	   e. 24-hour supervision

3. Therapy provided if required	3. Health-related services provided on a Limited basis

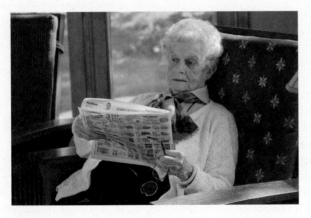

Figure 28-1 Assisted and independent living homes are a growing part of the LTC industry.

Assisted living services vary by facility and recipient need. Independent apartments include handicap-accessible units with grab bars in bathrooms and wall-mounted emergency home response systems. Personal services may include assistance or supervision with activities of daily living (ADLs), medication management, coordination of healthcare-provider services, housekeeping services, financial management, and transportation to medical appointments.

The typical living arrangements for ALFs vary. In general, they replicate the typical apartment settings with various floor plans and sizes to accommodate the needs, finances, and desires of the renter. ALFs generally provide nutritious meals in an aggregate setting, planned activities, common rooms for entertainment, gardens, exercise, and game rooms for the residents, allowing older adults can socialize with others in a safe and protected environment (see **Figures 28-1** and **28-2**).

Adult Day Services

Adult day services (ADSs) provide supervised daily care in a nonresidential facility for the elderly and disabled. ADSs are a growing source of nonresidential LTC, with more than 5,600 adult day care (ADC) centers in the United States (National Adult Day Services Association [NADSA], 2015). In 2012, 273,000 participants were enrolled in ADC centers throughout the United States (U.S. Department of Health and Human Services [USDHHS], 2013).

ADC programs may be sponsored by a variety of organizations, including churches, hospitals, or healthcare systems that includes these facilities. These centers provide socialization, planned outings, nutritional diet-appropriate meals, supervised activity, medication administration, and a safe environment for older adults. Many ADS providers offer 6-, 8-, or 12-hour service options that allow caregivers to continue working or have respite periods. The persons who may benefit from these services are those with chronic health conditions, cognitive impairments, limited mobility or physical disabilities, and safety concerns. Because half all care recipients have some level of dementia, many ADC centers offer dementia care programs and have dementia-trained staff.

The NADSA (2015) reports that most adult day centers are operated on a nonprofit or public basis and the average daily fees across the country are approximately $69. Funding comes from philanthropic or public sources, such as the local agency on aging. Third-party payers (Medicare Part B or health insurance) may cover skilled services or medical therapies. Many services are paid for privately by care recipients and families (NADSA, 2015).

Many older adults prefer to remain in their own homes as they age; however, many persons are faced with the decreased ability to maintain their independence because of age-related physical or cognitive impairments or chronic health conditions. For these individuals, ADS might be an ideal alternative to congregate residential care such as assisted living and nursing homes (Eldercare locator, 2015). ADSs create a partnership among caregivers, families, and professionals in managing the health and well-being of an individual to promote and support aging in place.

There are also opportunities for different levels of independence in community living. **Table 28-2** provides an overview of these alternatives.

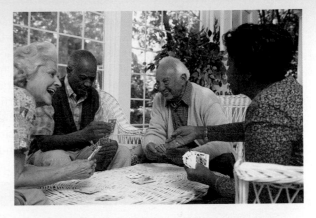

Figure 28-2 Independent and assisted living facilities provide opportunities for safety, comfort, and social networking.
Comstock Images/Alamy Images.

Care Transitions and Care Coordination

Models of *care coordination* were first identified more than a century ago. As demographics shift and the number of older adults increases, the need has increased for models of care that support the older adult in the community. Komisar and Feder (2011) looked at promising models of healthcare delivery that coordinate across a continuum

TABLE 28-2	Stakeholders in Policy Formulation
Patients and consumers	Patients and consumers are those individuals who access health care at any point across the continuum of care due to a healthcare need. The anticipation is that the consumer or patient will receive the care that is needed.
Nurses and providers	Nurses are providers of care. In addition, hospitals, clinics, physicians, home health agencies, hospice, LTC facilities, and any individual or business that provides health care to individuals or groups are considered providers.
Government	The government initiates local, state, and national levels of policy in health care. Locally, city governments are able to develop healthcare policy. Expenditure for health care reached $2.8 trillion by 2008; of this, $1.1 trillion was paid by the government for healthcare services provided. The government provides care to roughly 7.8 million veterans through the Veterans Administration. The government also funds the Indian Health Service, which provides care to about 1.9 million Native Americans across 35 states (Dentzer, 2009).

of care. Key components of successful models included care that is "person-centered"; primary medical care core; an assessment of the older adult's care needs, as well as the needs of the caregiver; coordination of both medical care and LTC needs; a specific focus on transitional needs when moving in or out of a healthcare facility; an ongoing relationship between the care coordinator and the primary care physician (PCP); and an ongoing relationship between the care coordinator and the older adult (Komisar and Feder, 2011).

Care coordination also encourages active patient participation, promotes healthy lifestyle choices, and facilitates better self-management. The focus is on improving continuity of care across settings, promoting the use of effective preventive and community services, increasing accessibility to healthcare providers, and improving communication among the providers and the patient and family (Schraeder & Shelton, 2011).

CLINICAL TIP

Care coordination is often done by gerontological nurses who work with older adults as coaches to help encourage self-care.

Care coordination requires the nurse to work with the older adult as a coach and supporter. The goal of care coordination is to implement evidence-based guidelines for care management and support the older adult in self-management of health. Nurses in this role help the individual focus on personal health and participation goals and support the person through coaching and motivational techniques to reach these goals.

Many new models of care are focused on improving healthcare services for the older adult. The goal of these healthcare services is to provide a continuum of care across the lifespan to promote health and minimize the negative effects of disease and disability in the older adult (**Case study 28-1**). Understanding the use of the different healthcare models and identifying the types of models and services that are appropriate to meet the needs of the older adult at different points in time are essential to providing optimal care.

Components of these models of care include providing care for acute and chronic illness, health promotion, and health maintenance. These healthcare services are provided in a variety of settings and include care coordination during transitions between healthcare settings.

Case Study 28-1

The Borkowskis are a close-knit family of five whose grandfather, Papa B, has been living with them in their home since he was widowed 10 years previously. Papa B is 88 years old and has been recently diagnosed with middle-stage Alzheimer's disease (AD). The family is having increasing difficulty in supervising and providing round-the-clock care for him. Unfortunately, it has gotten to the point at which it is no longer safe for him to be home alone. The adult daughter of Papa B, with whom he resides, works full time, as does her husband. The three children are in school during the day. The family desperately wants to keep Papa B at home, but do not know what resources may be available to them. As their nurse, they come to you for help and guidance.

Questions:

1. What services might the Borkowski family use to help them keep Papa B at home? Do these services seem feasible at this time?
2. As his condition deteriorates further, what services discussed in this chapter might be necessary at various points in time?

Transitional Care Models and Programs

Transitional care focuses on transitions or movements between facilities for the elderly and chronically ill. The goal of transitional care is to provide patients with a seamless transition that does not result in duplication of services or fragmented care. The care coordinator follows the patient through the healthcare system and facilitates open communication and collaboration among all providers. The primary focus is on maintaining continuity of care, enhancing patient and caregiver self-management activities, and preventing complications and hospital readmission.

Transitional care engages with patients while hospitalized and then intensively follows patients after hospital discharge. The role of the nurse in these programs is to assist older adults and their families in ensuring care is continued as planned after an acute care, LTC, or rehabilitation admission.

The role and function of a nurse working in transitional care might include in-hospital assessment, in-home assessments, teaching patients about self-care, managing medications, symptom recognition, scheduling appointments and transportation for follow-up with primary care and specialists, coordination of information with primary care, medication reconciliation, development of a plan of care with the elder and family, and follow-up phone calls.

Often, *transitional care models* emphasize self-care (Coleman, Parry, Chalmers, & Min, 2006), and therefore most of the research originates on cohorts of older adults who are able to manage their care independently or with informal caregiver supports. With very short-term education and coaching by nurses, this level of self-management is greatly improved. Gaps in transitional care interventions for the population of frail older adults include the absence of studies on cognitively impaired adults and medically underserved populations (Golden, Tweary, Dang, & Roos, 2010; Naylor, Aiken, Kurtzman, Olds, & Hirschman, 2011).

The majority of transitional care interventions focus on the transition from acute care hospital to home (BOOST, Care Transitions Program, Transitional Care Model). Other models focus on in-home assessments (GRACE) and additional models focus on LTC (INTERACT). All models focus on the priority of reducing *preventable hospital readmission* and *potentially avoidable hospitalizations*, thus saving money while maintaining quality of life.

Better Outcomes for Older Adults through Safe Transitions

The Better Outcomes for Older Adults through Safe Transitions (BOOST) intervention that includes predischarge and postdischarge interventions to (1) reduce 30-day hospital readmission rates for older adults, (2) improve patient satisfaction, (3) identify high-risk patients to prevent adverse events, (4) improve communication between providers and patients, and (5) better prepare the patient and family for discharge (Society of Hospital Medicine, 2016). BOOST provides tools to support nurses in improving care transitions. One key element of BOOST is the strength of the education and communication tool components. This resource site provides materials to help optimize the discharge process at any institution; it was developed through support from the John A. Hartford Foundation. The program and tools are based on the principles of quality improvement, evidence-based medicine, and personal and institutional experiences. More information is available at http://www.hospitalmedicine.org/BOOST.

Care Transitions Intervention

Developed by Eric Coleman and colleagues at University of Colorado Health Sciences Center, *Care Transitions Intervention* (CTI) is a patient-centered 4-week intervention program designed to improve quality of care and contain costs for patients with complex care needs as they transition across care settings. It is based on four pillars: (1) assistance with self-management of medications, (2) a patient-centered medical record that is kept by the patient, (3) timely follow-up with primary physician or specialist, and (4) a list of signs and symptoms that could indicate worsening of the condition (Coleman et al., 2006).

One of the main features of this model is the use of a Transitions Coach (an advanced practice nurse [APN], RN, social worker, occupational therapist, or other professional or paraprofessional) who follows the patient before and after discharge from the hospital and for follow-up. The coach's role encourages self-management and reinforces important aspects of care, including improved patient–physician communication, offering strategies on how to respond to changes in health or important concerns, and engaging patients in medication reconciliation. Coaches make one home visit after discharge and follow up with phone calls. Outcomes from the use of this model indicate a decrease in hospital readmissions and an increase in patient's self-identified goals regarding symptom management (Coleman et al., 2006). More information and a training program for nurses and others interested in CTI is available at http://www.caretransitions.org/.

Transitional Care Model

The Transitional Care Model (TCM) (Naylor et al., 2011) is a nurse-led model that follows the patient from hospital to home. The nurse acts as the main care manager, who consults with the patient in hospital, at home within 24 hours of discharge, accompanies the patient to postdischarge follow-up visits, and provides weekly home visits and ongoing telephone support for an average of 2 months. The emphasis of TCM is care coordination and continuity of care.

This model includes a patient-centered intervention to improve quality of life, improve patient satisfaction, and reduce readmissions. The TCM was developed to address the needs of elders with complex needs after discharge from the hospital. Key components of this program include (1) continuity of care at hospital discharge, (2) focus on individual and caregiver understanding (including early symptom recognition), (3) management of chronic health issues and prevention of decline, and (4) medication management. Specific research-based nursing protocols were developed to assist the nurse.

Further information on Transitional Care Model training programs can be found at http://www.transitional care.info/.

Community-Based Care Management Programs

To provide choices and informed decision making for older adults, it is imperative that nurses have the knowledge to assist the older adult through improved awareness of community services, availability of services, access points, eligibility for service, and affordability of quality care for older adults (Tang & Pickard, 2008).

Next Step in Care

Next Step in Care provides information and advice to help family caregivers and healthcare providers plan safe and smooth transitions for patients. Next Step in Care's easy-to-use guides help family caregivers and healthcare providers work closely together to plan and implement safe and smooth transitions for chronically or seriously ill patients. More information is available at http://www.nextstepincare.org.

National Transitions of Care Coalition

The National Transitions of Care Coalition provides resources for providers, policymakers, and patients to meet the challenges associated with transitioning patients from one provider to another. These tools are intended to reduce the fragmented service often associated with care transitioning. Through a more collaborative relationship between providers, the transition between providers improves, increasing quality of care and safety for patients, especially older adults. Additional information regarding the National Transitions of Care Coalition can be found by visiting their Website at http://www.ntocc.org/Home.aspx.

Initiative to Reduce Avoidable Hospitalizations

One example of an initiative from the Centers for Medicare and Medicaid Services (CMS) is the Initiative to Reduce Avoidable Hospitalizations. This initiative focused on long-stay nursing facility residents who were enrolled in both Medicare and Medicaid. The goal was to reduce in-patient hospitalizations (CMS, 2016b) Initially funded in 2012, the second phase of this initiative was funded in 2015. For more information about this initiative, review https://innovation.cms.gov/initiatives/rahnfr/

Community-Based Care Transitions

As part of the Patient Protection and Affordable Care Act (PPACA), the Community-Based Care Transitions Program (CCTP) was created to "(a) improve transitions of Medicare beneficiaries from an inpatient hospital setting to another care setting, (b) improve quality of care, (c) reduce readmissions for high risk beneficiaries, and (d) document measurable savings to the Medicare program" (CMS, 2016a, para1). The CMS Website can provide more information about this program at https://innovations.cms.gov/initiatives/CCTP.

Interventions to Reduce Acute Care Transfers

Interventions to Reduce Acute Care Transfers (INTERACT) is a quality improvement program aimed at reducing hospital admissions of nursing home residents; it was initially developed in a project supported by the CMS. Evidence supports that implementing INTERACT interventions has decreased hospitalizations from nursing homes (Ouslander, Bonner, Herndon, & Shutes, 2014; Ouslander et al., 2011). More information about INTERACT interventions can be found at http://interact2.net.

After Discharge Care Management of Low-Income Frail Elderly

An interdisciplinary approach to chronic care management, *After Discharge Care Management of Low-Income Frail Elderly* (AD-LIFE) uses medical and psychosocial care management models to coordinate care of older adults leaving acute care (Wright, Hazelett, Jarjoura, & Allen, 2007). This approach is still under study in a randomized trial (Allen et al., 2011). In their pilot study, the interdisciplinary team (IDT) included an APN, social worker, pharmacist, RN care manager, geriatrician, and other specialists as needed. An initial assessment by the APN prior to the older adult's discharge from acute care was shared with the IDT. The team used evidence-based protocols to generate a care plan. The RN care manager working with the community-based primary care practitioner provided ongoing follow-up care to the older adult (Wright et al., 2007).

Guided Care

Chad Boult, MD, and his colleagues at Johns Hopkins developed the Guided Care model. The team sought to develop a model to improve the health care of older adults with multiple comorbidities by providing comprehensive health care by a nurse–physician team. Guided Care is based in a primary care office and uses RNs trained in Guided Care principles to coordinate cost-effective care (Boyd et al., 2008). The Guided Care nurse curriculum includes training in areas such as transitional care, motivational interviewing, evidence-based guidelines for managing chronic conditions, health insurance coverage, and working with physicians, family caregivers, and community resources (Boult, Karm, & Groves, 2008a, p. 52).

In this model, each patient receives eight services from the Guided Care nurse. These are listed in **Table 28-3**.

The nurse then works with the patient to develop a plan of care that focuses on the patient management of the chronic illness, including medication management, symptom monitoring, and nutritional and activity interventions. This plan of care is central to the care of the individual and used by the nurse in ongoing telephone visits, working with community resources, and, if needed, communicating the older adults' needs during care transition between healthcare facilities.

TABLE 28-3   Services Each Patient Receives from the Guided Care Nurse
1. An in-depth assessment at patient's home
2. Individualized care guide
3. Proactive monitoring with phone contacts
4. Coaching on self-management
5. Referral to a chronic disease self-management course
6. Education of caregivers
7. Coordination of transitions between providers and sites of care
8. Facilitation of access to community resources

Data from Boult, C., Karm, L., & Groves, C. (2008a). Improving chronic care: The "guided care" model. *The Permanente Journal, 12*(1), 50–54. Retrieved from www.ncbi.nlm.nih.gov/pmc/articles /PMC3042340; Boult, C., Reider, L., Frey, K., Leff, B., Boyd, C. M., Wolff, J. L., . . . Scharfstein, D. (2008b). Early effects of "guided care" on the quality of health care for multimorbid older persons: A cluster-randomized controlled trial. *Journals of Gerontology Series A: Biological Sciences & Medical Sciences, 63A* (3), 321–327.

Guided Care is a LTC coordination program. The nurse can visit the home as needed, but manages much of the older adult's needs through routine and episodic phone calls. Nurses working in the Guided Care model are trained in this model and have responsibilities in the clinic environment as well as in the home. Evidence indicates that Guided Care improves quality of care, reduces caregiver strain, improves physician satisfaction, and suggests a reduction in use and cost of expensive services (Boult et al., 2008b, 2011; Boyd et al., 2010).

Geriatric Resource for Assessment and Care of Elders

A model of primary care that focuses on improving the quality of care for low-income seniors by the longitudinal integration of geriatric and primary care services across the continuity of care was developed by Counsell et al. (2007). The *Geriatric Resource for Assessment and Care of Elders* (GRACE) uses a geriatric IDT, including an APN and social worker in collaboration with a PCP and geriatrician. The team develops a plan of care and (with the PCP) modifies the plan if needed. The support team then meets with the patient to review and implement the plan of care. The team conducts an in-home assessment of the older adult and works with a geriatric IDT, using care protocols to evaluate and follow common geriatric conditions.

Comprehensive primary care for these low-income older participants may be provided through a community health center (Boult & Wieland, 2010). The team uses resources such as pharmacy, mental health services, home health care, and other *community-based care management programs* to meet the individual's needs. Ongoing support for the older adult occurs through monthly contacts and a home visit by the APN or social worker after any emergency room visit or hospitalization (Counsell et al., 2007). Nurses working in the GRACE model work as part of the IDT, using care protocols to care for the elderly living in the community.

Programs of All-Inclusive Care for the Elderly

The Balanced Budget Act of 1997 included a state option known as *Programs of All-Inclusive Care for the Elderly* (PACE). PACE provides an alternative to institutional care for persons aged 55 or older who require a nursing-facility level of care. The interdisciplinary PACE team offers and manages all health, medical, and social services and mobilizes other services as needed to provide preventive, rehabilitative, curative, and supportive care. PACE organizations provide these services and care in the home, community, and PACE center. PACE functions within the Medicare and Medicaid programs and becomes the sole provider of services. The PACE program replaces other medical coverage, but individuals can leave the program at any time. In addition to age and level of care requirements, eligibility for PACE includes residence in a service area of a PACE organization and ability to live safely in the community with help from PACE (PACE, 2016).

Risk in Care Transitions

Regardless of which transitions model is applied, transitions in setting of care (hospital, rehabilitation, LTC, home) are considered to be vulnerable exchange points and contribute to the risk of poor health outcomes (Naylor et al., 2011). This risk is higher in older adults who may have several chronic diseases, cognitive dysfunction, sensory impairment, and functional decline that coexist with acute and chronic illnesses. According to the CMS, Medicare patients readmitted to hospitals within 30 days of discharge, added $26 billion a year to healthcare costs (CMS, 2016a). To improve transitions of care and decrease preventable readmissions, resources have been identified and projects have been proposed to discover appropriate interventions across the healthcare continuum. Many of these are listed earlier in this chapter.

CLINICAL TIP

Transitions in settings of care are vulnerable exchange points for older adults. Nurses must pay particular attention during times of care transitions in order to promote quality outcomes for elderly patients.

Key factors that lead to poor outcomes in the transition of care across the continuum include (1) inadequate education to patients and their families about care management, (2) poor communication between patients and care providers, (3) inadequate assessment at point of care, (4) medication discrepancies, (5) lack of follow-up care, (6) health literacy issues, (7) lack of support systems, and (8) cultural barriers.

Effective communication is essential in achieving the goals of remaining functional and stable on return to home. Communication breakdown in information exchange about medications and disease management reflects individual, population, and systematic problems that influence safety. Communication problems within the system of healthcare delivery include both miscommunication and absence of communication about medications and disease management (Arora et al., 2010).

Nursing Responsibility in Transitioning Care

Regardless of nursing care settings, it is a requirement that nurses contribute to the safety and continuity of care for their patients upon discharge to home or transfer to another care setting. Diligence on the part of the discharging nurse and the admission nurse of the receiving facility is essential to ensure care continuity. Safe, timely, and effective transitions across care settings are promoted through optimal collaboration and coordination among the patient, family, and interprofessional team. The nurse participates in the development and evaluation of the transition plan and identifies and communicates any barriers to the plan (Vaughn, 2015).

For interagency transfers, a detailed transfer form must be completed, as well as a verbal report to the accepting facility, prior to discharge or transfer. The basic information that should be included during a transfer is listed in **Box 28-1**.

BOX 28-1   Basic Information to Be Included in a Transfer

- Detailed assessment
- Treatments
- Wounds
- Current medications
- Allergies

- Level of independence
- Recent diagnostic testing
- Primary care practitioner notification upon discharge and admission to the receiving facility

Discharge to a home setting requires detailed discharge instructions for the patient and applicable caregiver. Timely education and planning are essential to ensure that the patient and caregiver are able to appropriately transition care without disruption. To achieve this, the nurse begins planning for discharge at the time of admission. With the ongoing trend for decreased lengths of stay in the acute care facility, time is of the essence. Teaching and understanding of the care needs must be undertaken to determine if additional support services are needed when the patient returns home.

Quality in Health Care

Healthcare systems that collaborate, coordinate care, communicate, and anticipate patients' needs are essential to ensuring quality nursing care that is "safe, effective, patient-centered, timely, efficient, and equitable" (Institute of Medicine [IOM], 2001, p. 6). Regardless of where a patient is on the care continuum, quality is at the forefront of care. Patients are viewed as full partners in healthcare decisions, with trust and transparency being key elements. Patients as consumers are expecting, and even demanding, quality outcomes. This has led to legislation and regulation by the CMS to mandate the reporting of quality indicators by healthcare entities and practitioners to fully disclose to the consumer quality outcomes of care.

Definitions

Quality of health care has been defined by the *Institute of Medicine* (IOM) in several ways. The IOM (see **Box 28-2**) speaking from a standards perspective, called quality "the degree to which health services for individuals and populations increase the likelihood of desired health outcomes and are consistent with current professional knowledge" (IOM, 2001, p. 232). In its landmark report, *Crossing the Quality Chasm*, the IOM (2001) focused on conceptual rather than measureable definitions, defining quality as "safe, effective, patient centered, timely, efficient, and equitable" (p. 6).

Elements of Quality Health Care

Six recommended "Aims for Improvement" from the IOM serve as core elements of quality health care (see **Box 28-3**). A healthcare system that achieves major gains in these six areas would better meet patient needs.

Quality and Safety

Based on the competencies from the IOM to provide a foundation for cultures of safety and quality, the *Quality and Safety Education for Nurses* (QSEN) project redefined the competencies for nursing. The QSEN competencies apply to all areas of nursing and are listed in **Box 28-4**. As evident, the focus of quality and safety has shifted from individual actions to system causes and improvements (Sherwood & Zomorodi, 2014). More information about the competencies can be found at http://www.qsen.org.

Technological Advances

The potential role of technology in quality improvement is expanding. Electronic documentation systems and a broad range of electronic health monitoring equipment applications will be increasingly important to healthcare

BOX 28-2   Institute of Medicine

The IOM provides evidence for informed healthcare decision making to those in both government and the private sector. The IOM is a division of the National Academies of Sciences, Engineering, and Medicine. For more information about the Institute of Medicine and its reports visit https://www.nationalacademies .org/hmd/

BOX 28-3   Institute of Medicine Aims for Improvement

Ideally, a healthcare system should be:

- *Safe:* Avoiding injuries to patients from the care that is intended to help them.
- *Effective:* Providing services based on scientific knowledge to all who could benefit, and refraining from providing services to those not likely to benefit.
- *Patient centered:* Providing care that is respectful of and responsive to individual patient preferences, needs, and values, and ensuring that patient values guide all clinical decisions.

- *Timely:* Reducing waits and sometimes harmful delays for both those who receive and those who give care.
- *Efficient:* Avoiding waste, including waste of equipment, supplies, ideas, and energy.
- *Equitable:* Providing care that does not vary in quality because of personal characteristics such as gender, ethnicity, geographic location, and socioeconomic status

Reproduced from Institute of Medicine. (2001). *Crossing the quality chasm: A new health system for the 21st century* (pp. 5–6). Washington, DC: National Academies Press.

BOX 28-4   QSEN Quality and Safety Competencies for Nursing

- Patient-centered care
- Teamwork and collaboration
- Evidence-based practice (EBP)
- Quality improvement

- Safety
- Informatics

Data from QSEN Institute. (2014). Competencies. Retrieved from http://www.qsen.org

---

outcomes and cost assessments. Provisions in the *Patient Protection and Affordable Care Act of 2010* (PPACA) (also called the Affordable Care Act) focus on *health information technology* (HIT), specifically by increasing quality of data collected, creating new programs that involve HIT, and giving payments to existing entities for the use and improvement of HIT. New operating rules and standards will directly or indirectly control both use and continuing innovation.

National Quality Strategy

The *National Quality Strategy* (NQS) was first published in 2011 and has published yearly updates. It was led by the Agency for Healthcare Research and Quality (AHRQ) on behalf of the Department of Health and Human Services and mandated by the PPACA. The purpose of the NQS is to "set standards and regulations to measure healthcare quality and its impact on public health" (Robert Wood Johnson Foundation [RWJF], 2012, para 3). The NQS established three overall aims (1) make health care more accessible, safe, and patient centered; (2) address environmental, social, and behavioral influences on health and health care; and (3) make care more affordable (RWJF, 2012, para 4). To advance these aims, the NQS focuses on the six priorities listed in Box 28-4. To view more information about the report and annual updates, go to http://www.ahrq.gov/workingforquality. These priorities reflect the recommended aims from the IOM (2001).

The Joint Commission

The vision of the *Joint Commission* is to ensure the safest, highest quality care across all settings. Accreditation through the Joint Commission is voluntary. The Joint Commission uses standards that have been developed with input from government agencies, including the CMS, healthcare professionals, healthcare providers, and research to measure and assess organizational performance. The Joint Commission standards are higher than the standards required by the Centers for Medicare and Medicaid Services Conditions of Participation. Through the rigorous evaluation process developed by the Joint Commission, hospitals that successfully achieve accreditation are recognized internationally for the highest level quality of care. In addition to Accreditation, the Joint Commission also offers Disease Specific Care (DSC) certification. Programs may seek voluntary DSC certification for programs such as Alzheimer's/Memory Care, Stroke Rehabilitation, Comprehensive Stroke Centers, and numerous others as well. Additional information can be obtained by visiting the Joint Commission Website, at http://www.jointcommission.org/

The Commission on Accreditation of Rehabilitation Facilities

The *Commission on Accreditation of Rehabilitation Facilities* (CARF) is another organization that offers voluntary accreditation in a variety of programs and services. The mission of CARF is to promote the quality, value, and optimal outcomes of services through a consultative accreditation process that centers on enhancing the lives of the people served (CARF, 2016). CARF offers certification in Medical Rehabilitation, Aging Services to name a few. For more information, visit http://www.carf.org.

National Quality Forum

The *National Quality Forum* (NQF) is a nonprofit, nonpartisan organization committed to improving the quality of health care in the United States. The NQF sets standards, recommends measures for use in payment and public reporting programs, identifies and accelerates quality improvement priorities, advances electronic measurement, and provides information and instruments to help healthcare decision-makers (National Quality Forum, 2016). More information regarding the National Quality Forum can be obtained by visiting their Website at http://www.qualityforum.org.

Additional agencies and organizations that lead quality improvement efforts in health care are listed in **Box 28-5**.

BOX 28-5 **Agencies and Organizations That Lead Quality Improvement Efforts in Health Care**

Development of Standards

Blue Cross and Blue Shield (BCBS): http://www.bcbs.com

Centers for Medicare and Medicaid Services (CMS): http://www.cms.gov

Institute of Medicine (IOM): http://www.iom.edu

Development of Knowledge and Evidence-Based Best Practices

Agency for Healthcare Research & Quality (AHRQ): http://www.ahrq.gov

American Geriatrics Society (AGS): http://www.americangeriatrics.org

American Medical Association (AMA): http://ama-assn.org

American Nurses Association (ANA): http://www.nursingworld.org

National Patient Safety Foundation (NPSF): http://www.npsf.org

Nursing Alliance for Quality (NAQC): http://naqc.org

Curriculum Content

Hartford Institute for Geriatric Nursing (HIGN): http://www.hartfordign.org

Institute for Healthcare Improvement (IHI): http://www.ihi.org

Awards Programs

American Association of Critical Care Nurses (AACN)

American Nurses Credentialing Center (ANCC)

Beacon Award

Magnet Recognition Program

Quality Indicators
Agency for Healthcare Research and Quality

The *Agency for Healthcare Research and Quality* (AHRQ) produces the National Healthcare Quality Report (NHQR) and the National Healthcare Disparities Report (NHDR). These reports measure trends in effectiveness of care, patient safety, timeliness of care, patient-centeredness, and efficiency of care. The reports present, in chart form, the latest available findings on quality of and access to health care.

The NHQR tracks the healthcare system through quality measures, such as the percentage of heart attack patients who received recommended care when they reached the hospital or the percentage of children who received recommended vaccinations. The NHDR summarizes healthcare quality and access among various racial, ethnic, and income groups and other priority populations, such as residents of rural areas and people with disabilities. These complete reports can be downloaded from the AHRQ Website.

Healthy People 2020

The Healthy People (http://www.healthypeople.gov/2020) agenda provides science-based, 10-year national objectives for improving the health of all Americans. For three decades, Healthy People has established benchmarks and monitored progress over time in order to:

> Encourage collaborations across communities and sectors
> Empower individuals toward making informed health decisions
> Measure the impact of prevention activities

The vision of Healthy People is a society in which all people live long, healthy lives. *Healthy People 2020* strives to:

> Identify nationwide health improvement priorities
> Increase public awareness and understanding of the determinants of health, disease, and disability and the opportunities for progress
> Provide measurable objectives and goals that are applicable at the national, state, and local levels
> Engage multiple sectors to take action to strengthen policies and improve practices that are driven by the best available evidence and knowledge
> Identify critical research, evaluation, and data collection needs

A new goal in Healthy People 2020 involves improving the health and well-being of older adults. Emerging issues for improving the health of older adults include efforts to:

> Coordinate care
> Help older adults manage their own care
> Establish quality measures
> Identify minimum levels of training for people who care for older adults
> Research and analyze appropriate training to equip providers with the tools they need to meet the needs of older adults

In addition to Healthy People 2020, there is a companion document for Rural Healthy People 2020 that specifically targets individuals in rural areas. For more information, go to http://sph.tamhsc.edu/srhrc/rhp2020.html.

Funding Health Care

Quality and health outcomes in a healthcare system are related to funding, among other variables. The U.S. healthcare system is funded through a variety of mechanisms.

Prospective Payment System

The *prospective payment system* (PPS) for acute care hospitals was developed in 1983 to rein in healthcare costs paid by Medicare and Medicaid. This system replaced the fee-for-service system that allowed providers to bill retrospectively for cost of services provided. PPS, on the other hand, is a predetermined, fixed reimbursement based on the classification system of a particular service (CMS, 2015). The following is a brief review of settings affected by PPS:

> *Diagnosis-related groups* (DRGs) are used by acute care hospitals as part of PPS. The DRGs are categories of care based on the diagnosis(es) made for each patient. Each category is weighted according to the average cost of care for Medicare patients with the same diagnosis. Additional payment is provided based on geographic location of the provider and average labor rates (with additional payments in Alaska and Hawaii). Add-on incentives are included for providers treating a high number of low-income patients, if the hospital is a teaching facility, and for unusually costly patient care situations.
> LTC hospitals (LTCHs) also follow a system similar to acute care, but DRGs are weighted to reflect the different resources used by LTCHs. These are referred to as MS-LTC-DRGs. IRFs also have a PPS. The data collection instrument completed upon admission and discharge is known as the *Inpatient Rehabilitation Facility Patient Assessment Instrument* (IRF-PAI). Reimbursement is based upon a patient's Impairment Group Code (such as stroke or hip fracture), the motor score of the IRF-PAI and, in some cases, patient age and the cognitive score from the IRF-PAI. Upon completion of the IRF-PAI, patients are categorized into *Case Mix Groups* (CMGs), which then determine both payment and length of stay for a given case.
> The Balanced Budget Act of 1997 implemented PPS for nursing homes using *resource utilization groups* (RUGs), or categories to determine reimbursement. The RUG scores are based on data collected from resident assessments (MDS 3.0), staffing data, and geographic location. The *Minimum Data Set* (MDS) is an assessment instrument that must be completed for all new admissions to nursing homes. The assessments are also required for changes of condition and as part of quarterly and annual evaluations of every patient (resident) in a nursing home. These evaluations capture the care needed by each patient based on the answers to the questions asked in the MDS. The information provided in the MDS is electronically submitted to the CMS and are used as the basis for RUGs classification for reimbursement.
> The Balanced Budget Act of 1997 implemented PPS for home health agencies, with full implementation in 2000. Payment is based on a 60-day period known as an episode of care. Each 60-day episode is paid separately, with payment determined by Medicare and adjustments made for case mix. There is an additional adjustment if the cost of care provided is exceptionally high due to the needs of the patient. The data collection tool required by home health agencies for reimbursement is the *Outcome and Assessment Information Set* (OASIS).
> Currently, there is an initiative directed by CMS for all PAC settings to utilize the *Continuity Assessment Record and Evaluation (CARE) tool*. The goal is to compare similar items in a uniform manner across the various PAC venues.

The U.S. healthcare system is funded from a variety of sources, including government transfer payments, private insurance, and private funds. Government transfers include funding for Medicare and Medicaid. Additional benefits provided by the government include the services provided by the Veterans Administration and the Indian Health Service.

Medicare

Medicare is Title XVIII of the Social Security Act; it was passed in 1965, after years of trying to provide some kind of universal health insurance. It is an insurance program for those 65 or over who have paid into the Social Security system or railroad fund or are diagnosed with end-stage renal disease. Those collecting Social Security Disability

Insurance (SSDI) are eligible for Medicare after a 24-month waiting period. When Medicare was enacted, nearly one in three elderly were poor and about half of America's elderly did not have hospital insurance (De Lew, 2000).

The four programs of Medicare (Traditional Part A and Part B, Medicare Advantage, and Medicare Part D) are explained in **Table 28-4**. If a physician accepts Medicare assignment, then the physician must accept whatever

TABLE 28-4   Types of Medicare Programs

Program	Coverage	Premium?	Costs
Medicare Part A	Blood, home health services, hospice, inpatient hospital care, SNF care (for transitional care)	No, for those who are eligible for Social Security or Railroad Retirement Benefits. Others can pay a premium to receive Part A.	A deductible applies for each benefit period, but no coinsurance for first 60 days of hospitalization. Coinsurance required after day 60 SNF: No cost for days 1–20 in a benefit period; coinsurance for days 21–100. Home health care: No cost for covered services, but 20% of approved cost for durable medical equipment.
Medicare Part B	Doctor and other healthcare provider services, outpatient care, durable medical equipment, mental health services, some home care services, some screening and preventive services, laboratory services	Yes, automatically deducted from Social Security checks.	For most services, a deductible applies—once the deductible is met, then 20% of Medicare-approved cost.
Medicare Advantage (Medicare Part C)	All covered benefits included in Traditional Medicare Parts A and B, except hospice. May cover additional benefits such as dental, vision, and health and wellness.	Yes	Plans are offered by Medicare-approved private companies and are usually considered managed care programs such as health maintenance organizations or preferred provider organizations. Deductible and coinsurance payments may be different from those required by traditional Medicare Parts A and B.
Medicare Part D (Medicare Prescription Drug Improvement and Modernization Act of 2003)	Multiple plans are offered from which a beneficiary can choose. Plans vary in prescriptions covered, deductible, premium, and *copayment*.	Yes	A coverage gap ("donut hole") exists. Once a certain amount of money is spent during a year, costs increase until the end of the coverage gap is reached.

Data from Centers for Medicare and Medicaid Services. (2015). *Medicare benefit policy manual.* Retrieved from http://www.cms.gov/Regulations-and-Guidance/Guidance/Manuals/Downloads/bp102c08.pdf; Centers for Medicare and Medicaid Services. (2016a). Community-based care transitions program. Retrieved from https://innovations.cms.gov/initiatives/CCTP/

Medicare provides as reimbursement. If the physician does not accept Medicare assignment, then the patient is responsible for any additional cost Medicare does not reimburse the physician. This is a question that all older adults should ask of their physicians prior to a visit.

CLINICAL TIP

Encourage older patients to ask their physician prior to the visit whether or not they accept Medicare assignment. It the physician does not accept Medicare, the patient will have to pay additional costs out of pocket.

Choosing a prescription plan under Medicare Part D is very complex, and plans vary across states. In the booklet *Medicare & You*, plans and options are outlined so beneficiaries can determine which plans to contact for additional information (see **Box 28-6**). Even though this prescription option has saved the elderly money, medication costs can still be very expensive.

Medicaid

Medicaid is Title XIX of the Social Security Act. It is an assistance program that is jointly financed by the state and federal governments, but is administered by the state; therefore, coverage and eligibility differ from state to state. To qualify for Medicaid, an individual must fit into a category of eligibility and meet certain financial and resource standards. Medicaid provides (1) health insurance for low-income families and people with disabilities, (2) nursing facility services for older Americans and persons with disabilities, and (3) Medicare Part B premiums and Medicare Parts A and B deductibles and copayments, as well as some services not covered by Medicare, depending on the benefits that states offer.

Federal funding for Medicaid comes from the general revenues; there is no trust fund set up for Medicaid as there is for Medicare. The state Medicaid office directly pays the doctor, hospital, nursing facility, or other healthcare provider. Not all physicians will accept Medicaid patients because physicians must accept as payment whatever Medicaid reimburses. In some instances, this reimbursement may be less than the cost to provide the service.

The elderly account for a disproportionate share of Medicaid costs. The fact that Medicaid is the primary reimbursement mechanism for LTC explains this phenomenon (Reaves & Musumeci, 2015). In an attempt to decrease high-cost nursing home care, Medicaid instituted a waiver program to facilitate home and community-based care delivery. Many states have instituted programs that support low-income elderly in their homes to prevent or delay nursing home placement. In another attempt to curtail Medicaid spending, many states have initiated a managed care model for Medicaid services.

Although eligibility for Medicaid is different in each state, each state does require an individual and family to use their own resources (spend down) before they can become eligible to receive Medicaid reimbursement for LTC. If the recipient of nursing home care is married, and the spouse is remaining in the couple's home, the spouse is allowed to keep half of the total nonexempt resources jointly owned when the individual entered the nursing home. There are upper as well as lower limits to the amount the spouse can keep. Rules also cover property and other assets given away as gifts, so family members cannot give away resources that could be used to pay for care.

BOX 28-6   Web Link

Browse the free online version of *Medicare & You*, available at https://www.medicare.gov/Pubs /pdf/10050.pdf

The PPACA of 2010 affects Medicaid coverage, because it provides incentives to states to increase home and community-based services. A state's Medicaid program must offer medical assistance for certain basic services to most categorically needy populations. However, states may also receive federal matching funds to provide certain optional services, such as home and community-based care to certain persons with chronic impairments.

Money Follows the Person

The *Money Follows the Person* (MFP) rebalancing demonstration program helps states rebalance their LTC systems by transitioning eligible Medicaid recipients from LTC institutions back to the community. Each state's MFP program is individualized to meet that state's needs and specific goals.

The MFP initiative is based on the premise that many Medicaid beneficiaries residing in LTC facilities would prefer to live in the community and would do so if they had adequate support and services. In addition, the MFP is based on the premise that it would cost less to care for and transition these individuals back into the community than what Medicaid currently spends on their long-term institutionalized care.

The goal of the MFP rebalancing program is to increase the states' ability to serve Medicaid recipients with LTC needs in the community and reduce the use of institutionalized care. Once transitioned into the community, each MFP participant receives home- and community-based service (HCBS) benefits according to their individual needs and services required. The states receive a matching federal fund, Federal Medical Assistance Percentage (FMAP), for each participant they transition into the community. States are required to reinvest these FMAP funds into their LTC systems. This is coined the "rebalancing initiative."

Forty-three states and the District of Columbia have implemented MFP programs. From spring 2008 through December 2010, nearly 12,000 people had transitioned back into the community through MFP programs (Mathematica Policy Research, 2011). The PPAC of 2010 strengthens and further expands the Money Follows the Person program to more states; extends the MFP program through September 30, 2016; and appropriates an additional $2.25 billion over a 4-year period ($450 million for each FY 2012–2016).

Private Insurance

Private health insurance grew from a small service industry to become the second largest third-party payer after the government. Following World War II, government control of pay increases pushed employers to find alternative incentives to attract qualified workers. Benefits provided by employers expanded to include health, dental, vision, disability, and life insurance coverage at no cost to the employee. Over time the cost of doing business has steadily risen, including the cost of healthcare benefits. This has resulted in employers shifting some of the healthcare cost burden to employees in the form of increased premium payments, as well as out-of-pocket payments in the form of copayments and deductibles for healthcare services. There has also been a shift toward wellness, with employees being required to pay copayments based on their level of health. This helps shift the ownership for good or bad health habits onto the employee rather than the employer or the insurance company (Zelman, McCue, & Glick, 2009).

Another element that has developed to control the rising cost of health care are *managed care organizations* (MCOs). Created by insurance companies, MCOs are designed to limit the costs incurred by insurance companies through contracts with providers outlining the cost to the insurance company for services provided to a policy holder. This system of cost control expanded as providers developed relationships with multiple insurance companies in order to be assured of a wide patient base. This relationship proved to control costs, with the beneficiary of these savings being the insurance company.

Preferred Provider Organizations

Preferred provider organizations (PPOs) provide healthcare plans that are comprehensive, providing coverage savings when in-network providers are used. Consumers may also use out-of-network providers at a higher cost.

The payment plan is set up using a system of deductibles and coinsurance payments. In this system, the deductibles are required to be paid first; the coinsurance payments are applied as benefits are used. This system is less expensive than other programs because the consumer pays more up-front costs than in other plans (Cleverley, Song, & Cleverley, 2011).

Health Maintenance Organizations

Health maintenance organizations (HMOs) provide a comprehensive coverage package that coordinates the care providers, with the PCP as gatekeeper. The PCP is responsible for overseeing the care provided to each patient who is part of the HMO, including referrals to specialists and other outpatient services (Cleverley et al., 2011).

Point of Service Plan

The point of service (POS) plan is a combination of the preferred provider organization and the health maintenance organization. A PCP is assigned; however, the patient can be referred to providers both in the network and outside the network, and coverage is available for any provider.

Long-Term-Care Insurance

LTC insurance (LTCI) is offered in the United States as an additional benefit beyond a regular insurance policy. LTC insurance is intended to cover care and services provided that are not covered by regular insurance policies, Medicare, or Medicaid. These policies are obtained by individuals through LTCI providers.

Private Pay

Private pay funds are those funds that come directly from individuals who receive healthcare services. This includes any out-of-pocket expenses incurred by the individual based on their current healthcare coverage. For those individuals who do not have healthcare benefits, the entire cost of the care received is their responsibility unless they qualify for other assistance programs offered through the provider or another agency based on financial status and/or diagnosis.

The Affordable Care Act

The PPACA, signed into law in 2010, was in response to the need for healthcare reform. The intention of the PPACA was to provide affordable health care to enhance quality of life for all Americans. Components of the Act are listed in **Box 28-7.** The primary foci of this Act include quality improvement, cost reduction programs, and increased access to affordable care (USDHHS, 2015).

BOX 28-7   Components of the PPACA

1. Elimination of lifetime limits for health insurance coverage for essential services
2. Elimination of the ability of insurance companies to rescind coverage
3. Free preventive care
4. Development of a prevention and public health fund
5. Increased access to affordable care, including a provision for preexisting conditions
6. Quality improvement and cost reduction programs
7. Increased access to health care in the community or at home, which provides more options for care outside of institutional settings

In 2012, the U.S. Supreme Court upheld provisions of the PPACA as constitutional, including the individual mandate and Medicaid expansion. Since 2015, taxpayers without insurance were penalized.

Global Models of Health Care

The health system in the United States is still evolving. Even with the passage of the PPACA, there is still discussion about how to best provide affordable and acceptable health care across the care continuum to all. Healthcare issues, especially, concern the elderly in the United States. Yet, the aging of the population is a challenge worldwide (Sciegai & Behr, 2010). Comparing models of health care around the world may provide greater insights into how best to meet the challenges the growth in the aging population will create.

Japan

Japan has a universal healthcare system. Insurance is provided through the National Health Insurance, a variety of employer-based health insurance plans, and Health Insurance for the Elderly. Everyone in Japan must enroll in a health insurance plan.

The National Health Insurance covers workers in agriculture, forestry, or fisheries; the self-employed; and those not employed, including students and retirees. Copayments are required for both in-patient and out-patient services and for prescriptions, but there is no deductible (Matsuda, 2015). As with the employer-based insurance plans, premiums are fixed and divided between employers and employees. If there is no employer, the government pays for that portion of the plan. Premiums are automatically deducted from pensions for those who are retired. Catastrophic coverage begins when a set threshold, depending on enrollee age and income, is met (Matsuda, 2015). Japan has one of the largest elderly populations in the world (**Figure 28-3**). In 2014, 26% of the population in Japan was over the age of 65 years (World Bank, 2016). By 2055, the 65 years or older population will comprise 40% of the total population (Oi, 2015).

In 2000, the LTCI program was introduced. The purpose of the LTCI system was to "support the independence and quality of life for frail and impaired elderly persons by providing them with adequate health and welfare services" (Asahara, Momose, & Murashima, 2003, p. 770). Currently, all those age 65 or older are entitled to receive LTC according to their eligibility levels. Eligibility for services under LTCI depends on age and need and is based on a certification process. Once certification is approved, the applicant is placed into one of seven levels of need. A person not eligible for one of the seven levels is classified as independent; this status can be reevaluated in as little as 6 months (Ohwa & Chen, 2012). To fund the program, citizens age 40 and over have to pay premiums. Premiums for those 65 and over are decided by municipalities based on an estimate of expenditures and linked to income (Matsuda, 2015).

The hallmark of Japan's LTCI is that it does not offer monetary benefits; instead, it provides services to help

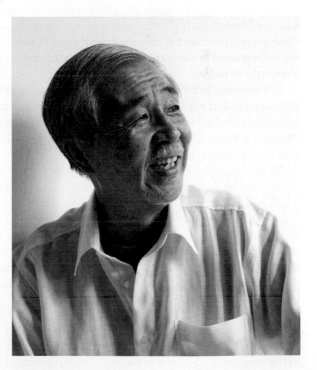

Figure 28-3 Japan has one of the largest elderly populations in the world.
© ICHIRO/Digital Vision/Thinkstock

relieve the stress on caregivers. These include community-based services such as help at home, ADC, respite care, assistive devices, and visiting nurses (Campbell, Ikegami, & Gibdon, 2010). This LTC approach has fostered a change in attitudes in Japan. Traditional Japanese values would neither allow a stranger into the home to provide care nor consider sending the elder out of the home for care (Tamiya et al., 2011). As the community-based services have expanded, they have become more accepted (Tamiya et al., 2011).

Germany

Germany was the first country to establish a national healthcare program. Social insurance in Germany is a mandatory transfer system whereby employees and employers make equal contributions for LTC, social health insurance, pension funds, unemployment, and worker's compensation (Rublee, Spaeth, & Schramm, 2012). The German model of health care is based on the "solidarity principle," which states that "members of society are responsible for providing adequately for another's well-being through collective action" (Geraedts, Heller, & Harrington, 2000, p. 378). The statutory health insurance covers about 86% of the population and provides a wide spectrum of services ranging from preventive care to in-patient and out-patient hospital care. Prescription medications are also covered (Blümell & Busse, 2015). This insurance scheme is operated by over 100 competing sickness funds. Individuals have a choice of sickness funds and may change if not satisfied. The statutory health insurance covers the employee, pensioner, and dependents and is financed through compulsory contributions based on gross earnings. Copayments are required for most services, and, although copayments are required for prescription medications, 5,000 medications are essentially free after adjustments in costs are made.

The remaining population, including civil servants and the self-employed, are covered by private insurance. In addition, those with higher incomes can opt out of the statutory health insurance and choose private insurance. Once private insurance is chosen, the statutory health insurance is no longer an option; therefore, private insurance is regulated by the government so the insured are not faced with large premiums as they age and experience a decrease in income (Busse & Blümell, 2014).

In Germany, individuals have free choice among general practitioners and specialists. There is no formal gatekeeping, and registration with a PCP is not required. However, sickness funds must offer participants the option of enrolling in a family care model. This option offers incentives for complying with gatekeeping rules (Blümell & Busse, 2015). Unlike some other countries' healthcare systems, there is little or no waiting for physician or care access in Germany.

To help meet the needs of the growing older population, LTC coverage is mandated. LTCI is mandatory and is provided by the same public–private mix as the health insurance scheme (Blümell & Busse, 2015). Everyone who has a need can apply for up to 2 years of benefits under LTCI. Applicants are assessed for need and, if need is determined, they are placed in one of three levels of care. Beneficiaries can choose between cash payment or in-kind services. LTCI covers about half of the costs of institutional care (Blümell & Busse, 2015). The goal of the LTCI law was to provide relief from the financial burden of long-term disability and illness. German citizens also can purchase private LTCI in place of the LTCI purchased with statutory health insurance. As the aging population grows, the premiums of private insurance may increase as risk increases, and LTCI premiums may become unaffordable.

Although most aging Germans are still cared for by relatives, the LTCI provides incentives to establish additional home healthcare agencies, short-term institutional care facilities, and assisted living facilities (Geraedts et al., 2000). LTCI also provides cash to family caregivers as well as free training courses; it also makes contributions to the pension fund (Busse & Blümell, 2014). Quality of nursing homes and LTC providers has been monitored since 2009. Costs of the program have remained within the budget, but adjustments may be required in the future as the aging population increases and the younger population decreases.

CLINICAL TIP

The U.S. healthcare system can gain ideas for solutions to common issues by examining how other countries have successfully funded healthcare services.

England

The National Health Service (NHS) in England is a universal system of health care based on clinical need rather than employment status; care is free at point of care. The NHS is divided into two basic sections: primary and secondary care. Primary care is usually the patient's first contact with a healthcare provider. Primary care providers are independent contractors with the NHS and may be general practitioners, dentists, pharmacists, or optometrists (National Health Service [NHS], 2013).

Over 75% of the funding for health care comes from general taxes, with a little over 3% coming from user charges (Harrison, Gregory, Mundle, & Boyle, 2011). Nearly 100% of the population of Great Britain has access to health services. The NHS covers comprehensive care, ranging from preventive services to in-patient and out-patient hospital care. Dental care, some eye care, mental health care, some LTC, and rehabilitation are also covered (Thorlby & Arora, 2015). Private health services are available in England, mostly for over-the-counter medicines, other medical products, and private hospital costs (Thorlby & Arora, 2015).

Wait times, as well as other outcome indicators, have been addressed through several reforms. The latest, passed in 2012, was the Health and Social Care Law. This controversial law created general practitioner managed consortia, abolished the primary care trusts, shifted control from the central government to physicians, emphasized patient-centered care delivery, and provided financial incentives to improve quality (Perlman & Fried, 2012).

LTC, considered social care, has shifted from institutions to community-based care and from public to private sectors. Social care is not provided free as a universal right under the NHS. Charges for residential care are based on income and assets; charges for community-based care, if any, are determined by Councils with Adult Social Services Responsibilities (Boyle, 2011). The 2014 Care Act attempts to limit an individual's risk of catastrophic LTC costs by imposing a gap on expenditures, but needs criteria still apply (Thorlby & Arora, 2015). The NHS provides end-of-life and palliative care in patient homes, hospices, care homes, and hospitals.

In 2014, the Commonwealth Fund compared the healthcare systems of 10 wealthy countries. The NHS Health Service was declared the best system in terms of "efficiency, effective care, safe care, coordinated care, patient-centered care and cost-related problems" (About the NHS in England, 2015, para 4).

Canada

The Canadian healthcare system, known as Medicare, provides universal coverage at no cost at the point-of-care access for physician and hospital services. The Canadian Health Act establishes the standards for medically necessary hospital, diagnostic, and physician services that provincial health plans must follow (Minister of Justice, 2016, p. iii). Each of the 10 provinces is responsible for establishing, maintaining, and evaluating the provision of healthcare services within the province; however, their programs must follow national guidelines of universality, portability, accessibility, and comprehensiveness and be publicly administered (Allin & Rudoler, 2015). Therefore, even though each province has a slightly different coverage plan, a resident could receive covered care in another province if it were necessary. In addition, the services must be based on need, rather than ability to pay.

The healthcare system in Canada is funded primarily through tax monies. Although the federal government provides some money to the provinces, most of the costs are covered by the provinces themselves, which in turn levy taxes to pay for health care. Most physicians are in private practice, and they charge on a fee-for-service basis, though they cannot charge more than the government-established fee schedule. Hospitals are primarily private, not-for-profit institutions. In addition to medical services, most provinces and territories cover the cost of regular vision and dental care for children, seniors, and social assistance recipients. Provinces and territories can also provide services such as prescription drug coverage, long term care, and home care but usually target sub populations, such as seniors, children, and low income adults (Marchildon, 2013). The Canadian Health Act does not guarantee coverage for care provided out of hospital or by providers other than physicians; therefore, LTC services and end-of-life care are not mandated to be insured services (Allin & Rodoler, 2015). While a small number of provinces include hospice palliative care as a core service under their provincial health plans, other provinces may include this care under their provincial home care budgets. These budgets, however, are subject to budget cuts (Canadian Hospice Palliative Care Association [CHPCA], 2014, p.3). Even when health services in residential care facilities are covered, housing and meal costs are generally out-of-pocket unless the patient meets a means test (Allin & Rodoler, 2015). Private insurance may cover long term care and support services. Private insurance in Canada is usually complementary to Medicare and employment-based (Marchildon, 2013).

One criticism of the Canadian system has been the long waiting periods (LaPierre, 2012). Timely access to care is an area of priority for the healthcare system in Canada, and wait times have decreased in targeted areas. All provinces publicly report wait time data, but wait time between referral and visit with specialists is not measured the same consistently (Allin & Rodoler, 2015).

Health Policy

In order to understand the healthcare environment and the changes needed to meet the population needs, an understanding of health policy is needed.

Health policies are decisive actions chosen to respond to an issue in health care. These actions include the actual response to the healthcare issue and the plan to implement the response (Chaffee, Mason, & Leavitt, 2012).

Stakeholders in Policy Formation

Patients/Consumers

Patients and consumers are those individuals who access health care at any point across the continuum of care due to a healthcare need. The anticipation is that the consumer or patient will receive the needed care.

Nurses and Providers

Nurses are providers of care. In addition, hospitals, clinics, physicians, home health agencies, hospice, LTC facilities, and any individual or business that provides health care to individuals or groups are considered providers.

Government

The government initiates local, state, and national levels of policy in health care.

Locally, city governments are able to develop healthcare policy. Expenditure for health care reached $3.3 trillion in 2014; of this, $836 billion was paid by the government for healthcare services provided by Medicare, Medicaid, Children's Health Insurance Program (CHIP), and PPACA subsidies. The government provides care to almost 6 million veterans through the Veterans Administration. The government also funds the Indian Health Service, which provides care to about 1.9 million Native American Indians and Alaska Natives across 35 states (Indian Health Services, n.d.).

Organizations/Nurse Organizations

There are a variety of organizations that have a stake in healthcare policy. These can be at the local, state, or national levels, and each organization develops its own mission, vision, and values based on its core objectives. These objectives are periodically updated to reflect current healthcare issues.

Health Policy Development

Health policy development is dependent on the level of authority of the stakeholders. The government is the primary stakeholder in health policy development. This may include the local, state, or federal government.

The federal government is divided into three branches: the executive, legislative, and judicial branches. The executive branch is led by the President of the United States. The Vice President and the President's cabinet of advisors are also included in the executive branch. The Vice President is elected as the running mate of the president, and the 15 members of the cabinet (see **Box 28-8**) are appointed by the president and affirmed by the Senate.

The DHHS, one of the cabinet departments, provides necessary services to those individuals who need them the most (see **Box 28-9**), including the underserved and vulnerable populations such as the elderly. This department administers Medicare and Medicaid as well as the National Institutes of Health, the Centers for Disease Control and Prevention [CDC], and the Food and Drug Administration (About HHS, 2015). The nurse has the opportunity to advocate for the elderly by understanding the DHHS and what this department is responsible for, especially related to the administration of Medicare and Medicaid. The CMS Website provides additional information relevant to the care and *advocacy* of the elderly at http://www.cms.gov.

The *legislative branch* of the United States government is made up of the Senate and the House of Representatives. For a bill to become law, both the Senate and the House of Representatives must ratify the bill by majority vote. If the President vetoes the bill, the bill can still be passed if the Senate and the House of Representatives override the veto by a two-thirds majority vote (The White House, 2016).

The *judicial branch* of the U.S. government includes the U.S. Supreme Court, U.S. district courts, and 13 U.S. courts of appeal. The district courts oversee federal cases, and the courts of appeal review district court cases. The Supreme Court justices are appointed by the President and affirmed by the Senate. Supreme Court decisions cannot be appealed (The White House, 2016).

BOX 28-8   United States Cabinet

- Department of Agriculture
- Department of Commerce
- Department of Defense
- Department of Education
- Department of Energy
- Department of Health and Human Services
- Department of Homeland Security
- Department of Housing and Urban Development
- Department of the Interior
- Department of Justice
- Department of Labor
- Department of State
- Department of Transportation
- Department of the Treasury
- Department of Veteran Affairs

BOX 28-9   Health Committee Websites to Visit

Committee on Ways and Means (House of Representatives Subcommittee on Health): http://waysandmeans.house.gov

Library of Congress https://www.congress .gov/U.S. Senate Committee on Health, Education,

Labor and Pensions (Senate Subcommittee on Health): http://www.help.senate.goc

To find the Websites for state governmental agencies, go to the Website for your state and search for a health and/or aging committee

BOX 28-10   How a Bill Becomes a Law

1. Bill is written: Anyone can write a bill.
2. Bill is introduced: Only a member of Congress can introduce the bill.
3. Referral to committee: Once introduced, the bill is referred to the appropriate committee for review by a subcommittee. During this review the subcommittee can accept, amend, or reject the bill. Once the bill is approved, the bill is sent to the full committee for review. The full committee can also accept, amend, or reject the bill.
4. If the committee accepts or amends the bill, the bill is then moved forward to the Senate or House.

The majority party determines when and if the bill will be added to the schedule for consideration.

Both the Senate and the House must pass a bill by majority vote before the bill can be sent to the President.

5. The President has several options when presented a bill. The President can sign the bill, and it will be printed in the Statutes at Large. The President can veto the bill, sending it back to Congress for reconsideration. If Congress overrides the veto, the bill will become law and is printed.

Data from The White House. (2016). The legislative branch. Retrieved from https://www.whitehouse.gov/1600/legislative-branch

Lobbying and Lobbyists

Lobbyists are paid individuals who understand the legislative process (see **Box 28-10**) and educate members of the government and their staff on specific needs of an individual or group by preparing and presenting information relevant to those specific needs. Lobbyists may also present this relevant information as part of congressional hearings.

Social Policy

Social policy refers to programs and policies that have an impact on members of a society through the distribution of good and services. The intent of social policy is to improve each individual's access to food, shelter, education, and health care.

Public Policy

Public policy refers to the programs and policies developed by the government in response to the identified needs of the members of the society. The Public Policy Institute of California (http://www.ppic.org/main/about.asp) is an example of an entity designed to improve public policy through research and advocacy. The Commonwealth Fund (http://www.commonwealthfund.org/) provides another example of advocating for public policy in health care through research (**Boxes 28-11** and **28-12**).

Healthcare Policy Related to Aging and Mental Health

The aging population has its own distinctive needs based on a variety of issues related to the aging process, as well as those related to social policy and public policy. Research indicates that mental health is tied to the overall health and well-being of our aging population. According to the CDC (2012), older adults are at greater risk of developing depression and other mental health disorders. To learn more about the role advocacy plays in healthcare policy related to aging and mental health, please visit the following Websites:

> National Coalition on Mental Health and Aging: http://www.ncmha.org/
> National Alzheimer's Project Act: http://aspe.hhs.gov/daltcp/napa/
> World Health Organization: http://www.who.int/mental_health/mhgap/en/

BOX 28-11   Research Highlight

Title: The Effect of a Randomized Trial of Home Telemonitoring on Medical Costs, 30-Day Readmissions, Mortality, and Health-Related Quality of Life in a Cohort of Community-Dwelling Health Failure Patients

Purpose: The purpose of this randomized control trial was to identify the effects of home telemonitoring on medical costs, 30-day hospital readmissions, mortality, and health-related quality of life in heart failure patients living at home.

Methods: From June 2001 through January 2005, 206 participants were recruited from several heart failure services in the Baltimore, Maryland area. At a randomization visit, a heart failure research nurse collected baseline physical data as well as an in-depth history, medication review, Mini-Mental Status Examination (MMSE), Medical Outcomes Short Form (SF-36), and the Minnesota Living with Health Failure Questionnaire (MLHF). All participants received written materials about heart failure and self-management activities. They were randomized into two groups: telemonitored and usual care (control). Daily weights, blood pressure, heart rate, and 15-second heart rhythm strip were sent daily through the monitoring device. If readings were outside individually set parameters, the nurse practitioner with heart failure expertise would contact the participant and make medication adjustments if needed. Participants not contacted in a month because of a red flag were contacted to answer any questions and provide encouragement. All participants were followed until the end of the project on December 31, 2006 or the participant's death, whichever came first. The SF-36, MLHF, and medication review were repeated at 6 months and 1 year. SPSS 18 was used to analyze the data. Of the 206 participants recruited, 3 were eliminated, leaving 101 in the usual care group and 102 in the monitored group. Over the course of the study, 94 participants died.

Findings: Participants were followed for 802 ± 430 days. There were no differences between groups in Medicare payments for in-patient or emergency room visits or lengths of stay. There were no differences in 30-day readmissions or mortality. Although scores for SF-36 and MLHF improved, there was no difference between the groups.

Application to Practice: In an effort to decrease 30-day hospital readmissions, disease management programs have been implemented to assist patients in their transition from hospital to different destinations: community-based care, home care, in-patient rehabilitation, and skilled nursing facilities. In this study, there were no differences between the monitored group and the usual-care group in the study variables. However, in this study, all participants were well managed in their heart failure. All were receiving guideline-based treatment regimens, all were receiving care from a cardiologist, and monitored patients received oversight from a nurse practitioner with heart failure expertise. All participants adhered to their treatment regimens. This study supports the importance of good medical treatment and patient adherence in the treatment of heart failure (p. 520). In addition, the study tends to support the need for a multi-model intervention approach to the treatment of heart failure. The study also supports the need to further study the use of telemonitoring patients after hospital discharge to determine which patients would best benefit from this intervention.

Reproduced from Blum, K., & Gottlieb, S. S. (2014). The effect of a randomized trial of home telemonitoring on medical costs, 30-day readmissions, mortality, and health-related quality of life in a cohort of community dwelling heart failure patients. *Journal of Cardiac Failure*, 20(7), 513–521. Copyright 2014, with permission from Elsevier.

BOX 28-12   Evidence-Based Practice Application

Medicare beneficiaries with chronic illnesses are more likely to be readmitted to the hospital within 30 days after hospital discharge. Research suggests that care transitions management programs can reduce hospital readmissions and increase quality of care of elders. Utilizing evidence about population characteristics, transition care programs, and informatics, a population-based telephone care transition program was created for all Medicare hospitalized patients discharged to self-care. Results of the intervention demonstrated a reduction in hospitalizations of Medicare beneficiaries and cost savings. The author provided a step-by-step description of the process of implementing this evidence-based project.

Data from Hewner, S. (2014). A population-based care transition model for chronically ill elders. *Nursing Economics, 32*(3), 109–116, 141.

Healthcare Policy and Health Disparities

The demographic profile of older Americans provides the foundation for understanding the health disparities that exist. The population of older adults over the age of 65 years continues to climb, with an estimated 55 million individuals by the year 2020. The primary source of income for many individuals over the age of 65 is Social Security. If those same individuals do not have other sources of income, such as savings or pension plans, their median income may not rise above the poverty level. Research indicates that the socioeconomic status of an individual can lead to health disparities. Those with lower incomes tend to have poorer health status than those with higher incomes. An additional issue faced by older adults is the ability to access healthcare services, especially in rural areas of the country where public transportation or other types of transportation services are limited or unavailable. Without access to care, older adults face death and disability due to chronic disease.

The PPACA includes provisions to address several of the healthcare disparities faced by older adults. These provisions include requiring Medicare to pay for preventive care, development of accountable care organizations that will provide coordinated care teams to address the issue of chronic disease management and increased funding for community health centers that will provide care regardless of ability to pay (Alliance for Health Reform, 2012).

Advocacy

Nurses have the capacity to advocate for the uninsured, underinsured, and the impoverished in a variety of ways. As an individual, nurses can meet with government representatives at the local, state, and national levels to advocate. Nurses also can join other nurses to advocate in small groups or in larger groups by joining nurse organizations. Nurse organizations include specialty organizations that are closely aligned to specific clinical specialties, as well as larger organizations that span national or international scopes of involvement. Nurses who are interested in becoming more involved in health policy and advocacy should consider the Nurse in Washington Internship program (NIWI), which is an intensive primer on such topics. For more information, visit http://www.nursing-alliance.org/dnn/Events/NIWI-Nurse-in-Washington-Internship. **Boxes 28-13** and **28-14** give additional resources for nurses in the areas of health policy and advocacy.

Summary

It is imperative that the nurse recognize and institute appropriate patient- and family-specific interventions to decrease the potential risk factors in transitioning across healthcare settings for older adults, as well as utilize various EBP care transition models. Advocacy for the older adult requires that nurses understand their needs

BOX 28-13   Resource List

American Association of Long Term Care Insurance: http://www.aaltci.org

American Nurses Association: http://www.nursingworld.org

American Presidency Project. (2012). *Lyndon B. Johnson. 348-Statement by the President following passage of the Medicare bill by the Senate.* Retrieved from http://www.presidency.ucsb.edu/ws/index.php?pid=27072

Bolin, J. N., Bellamy, G. R., Ferdinand, A. Q., Vuong, A. M., Kash, B. A., Schulze, A., Helduser, J. W. (2015). Rural Healthy People 2020: New decade, same challenges. *Journal of Rural Health, 31*(3), 326–333.

Centers for Medicare and Medicaid Services. Retrieved from http://cms.hhs.gov

Commonwealth Fund. (2016). *The commonwealth fund, a private foundation working toward a high performance health system.* Retrieved from http://www.commonwealthfund.org

Compare nursing homes, hospitals, home healthcare agencies in your area at the Medicare Website: http://www.medicare.gov

Harvard University. (2016). *The Malcolm Weiner center for social policy.* Retrieved from http://www.hks.harvard.edu/centers/wiener

Joint Commission. (2016). Retrieved from http://www.jointcommission.org

Sultz, H. A., & Young, K. M. (2013). *Health care USA: Understanding its organization and delivery* (8th ed.). Burlington, MA: Jones & Bartlett Learning.

U.S. Administration on Aging: http://www.aoa.gov

BOX 28-14   Recommended Readings

Adler-Hilstein, J., Sarma, N., Woskie, L. R., & Jha, A. K. (2014). A comparison of how four countries use health IT to support care for people with chronic conditions. *Health Affairs, 33*(9), 1559–1566.

Ecklund, M. M., & Bloss, J. W. (2015). Progressive mobility as a team effort in transitional care. *Critical Care Nurse, 35*(3), 62–68.

Faith, D., Kilpatrick, K., Reid, K., Carter, N., Bryant-Lukusius, D., Martin-Misener, R., . . . DiCenso, A. (2015). Hospital to community transitional care by nurse practitioners: A systematic review of cost-effectiveness. *International Journal of Nursing Studies, 52*(1), 436–451.

Hung, D., & Leidig, R. C. (2015). Implementing a transitional care program to reduce hospital readmissions among older adults. *Journal of Nursing Care Quality, 30*(2), 121–129.

Nagaya, Y., & Dawson, A. (2014). Community-based care of the elderly in rural Japan: A review of nurse-led interventions and experiences. *Journal of Community Health, 39*(5), 1020–1028.

Shmueli, A., Stam, P., Wasem, J., & Trottmann, M. (2015). Managed care in four managed competition OECD systems. *Health Policy, 119*(7), 860–873.

Vedel, I., & Khanassov, V. (2015). Transitional care for patients with congestive heart failure: A systematic review and meta-analysis. *Annals of Family Medicine, 13*(6), 562–571.

Walker, D. K., Barton-Burke, M., Saria, M. G., Gosselin, T., Ireland, A., Norton, V., & Newton, S. (2015). Everyday advocates: Nursing advocacy is a full time job. *American Journal of Nursing, 115*(8), 66–70.

regardless of the environment in which they live. This chapter presented information regarding the healthcare environment and transitions of care, how health care for older adults is funded, global models of health care, healthcare policy, and healthcare quality for older adults. Gerontological nurses can advocate for older adults by understanding the healthcare environment within which the older adult must navigate.

Clinical Reasoning Exercises

1. In a small group, create a model for healthcare delivery in the year 2040. Identify which features would be present, why these features would be necessary, and how it would be financed. Explain the role of the professional nurse and the advanced practice nurse as well as other healthcare providers.

2. Determine who your elected officials are at the local, state, and national levels. Explore the ways you can contact one elected official regarding a current issue of interest to you. Share this information with another student interested in the same issue.

3. The PPACA was signed into law in 2010. Discuss how this law affects your patient's ability to obtain health care.

4. Providing quality care while maintaining fiscal responsibility is a critical balancing act that must be maintained. Discuss with another student several ways you can provide quality care while helping to control costs.

Personal Reflections

1. Have you ever cared for a patient who was not able to pay for their health care or medications? How did you feel about this situation? Did the care you gave differ from that for a patient who did have healthcare coverage? What can you do to advocate for a patient who is not able to pay for health care or medications?

2. Bed management is an important aspect of health care, both in terms of patient satisfaction and reimbursement. If you had to choose between admitting a private pay patient and a patient receiving Medicaid, which patient would you choose and why? Would your decision criteria change if the payment source was not known?

3. Interview someone who has come from another country. Explore with this person how the elderly were cared for in his or her country. Would that health policy be a viable model in the United States?

References

Allen, K. R., Hazelett, S. E., Jarjoura, D., Wright, K., Forsnight, S. M., Kropp, D. J., . . . Pfister, E. W. (2011). The after discharge care management of low income frail elderly (AD-LIFE) randomized trial: Theoretical framework and study design. *Population Health Management, 14*(3), 137–142.

Alliance for Health Reform. (2012). *Chapter 10: Disparities.* Retrieved form http://www.allhealth.org/sourcebookcontent.asp?CHID=126

Allin, S., & Rudoler, D. (2015). The Canadian health care system, 2014. In E. Mossialos, M. Wenzel, R. Osborn, & C. Anderson (Eds.), *International profiles of health care systems, 2014* (pp. 21–31). New York, NY: The Commonwealth Fund. Retrieved from http://www.commonwealthfund.org/~/media/files/publications/fund-report/2015/jan/1802_mossialos_intl_profiles_2014_v7.pdf

Arora, V. M., Prochaska, M. L., Farnan, J. M., D'Arcy M. J., Schwanz, K. J., Vinci, L. M., . . . Johnson, J. K. (2010). Problems after discharge and understanding of communication with their primary care physicians among hospitalized seniors: A mixed methods study. *Journal of Hospital Medicine, 5*(7), 385–391.

Asahara, K., Momose, Y., & Murashima, S. (2003). Long-term care insurance in Japan. Its frameworks, issues, and roles. *Disease Management & Health Outcomes, 11*, 769–777.

Blum, K., & Gottlieb, S. S. (2014). The effect of a randomized trial of home telemonitoring on medical costs, 30-day readmissions, mortality, and health-related quality of life in a cohort of community dwelling heart failure patients. *Journal of Cardiac Failure, 207*, 513–521.

Blümel, M., & Busse, R. (2015). The German health care system, 2014. In E. Mossialos, M. Wenzel, R. Osborn, & C. Anderson (Eds.), *2014 international profiles of health care systems* (pp. 83–91). New York, NY: The Commonwealth Fund. Retrieved from http://www.commonwealthfund.org/~/media/files/publications /fund-report/2015/jan/1802_mossialos_intl_profiles_2014_v7.pdf

Boult, C., & Wieland, G. D. (2010). Comprehensive primary care for older patients with multiple chronic conditions: "Nobody rushes you through." *Journal of the American Medical Association, 304*(17), 1936–1943.

Boult, C., Karm, L., & Groves, C. (2008a). Improving chronic care: The "guided care" model. *The Permanente Journal, 12*(1), 50–54. Retrieved from http://www.ncbi.nlm.nih.gov/pmc/articles/PMC3042340

Boult, C., Reider, L., Frey, K., Leff, B., Boyd, C. M., Wolff, J. L., . . . Scharfstein, D. (2008b). Early effects of "guided care" on the quality of health care for multimorbid older persons: A cluster-randomized controlled trial. *Journals of Gerontology Series A: Biological Sciences & Medical Sciences, 63A*(3), 321–327.

Boult, C., Reider, L., Leff, B., Frick, K. D., Boyd, C. M., Wolff, J. L., . . . Scharfstein, D. O. (2011). The effect of guided care teams on the use of health services: Results from a cluster-randomized controlled trial. *Archives of Internal Medicine, 171*(5), 460–466.

Boyd, C. M., Reider, L., Frey, K., Scharfstein, D., Leff, B., Wolff, J., . . . Marsteller, J. (2010). The effects of guided care on the perceived quality of health for multi-morbid older persons: 18 month outcomes from a cluster-randomized controlled trial. *Journal of General Internal Medicine, 25*(3), 235–242.

Boyd, C. M., Shadmi, E., Conwell, L. J., Griswold, M., Leff, B., Brager, R., . . . Boult, C. (2008). A pilot test of the effect of guided care on the quality of primary care experiences for multi-morbid older adults. *Journal of General Internal Medicine, 23*(5), 536–542.

Busse, R., & Blümel, M. (2014). Germany: Health system review. *Health Systems in Transition, 16*(2). Copenhagen, Denmark: World Health Organization. Retrieved from http://www.euro.who.int/__data/assets/pdf_file/0008 /255932/HiT-Germany.pdf?ua=1

Boyle, S. (2011). United Kingdom (England) health system review. In A. Maresso (Ed.). *Health Systems in Transition.* Copenhagen, Denmark: World Health Organization. Retrieved from http://www.euro.who.int/__data /assets/pdf_file/0004/135148/e94836.pdf

Butcher, L., (2007, August). Hospitalists and LTACs: For some physicians, it's a perfect fit. *Today's Hospitalist.* Retrieved from http://www.todayshospitalist.com/index.php?b=articles_read&cnt=321

Camicia, M., Black, T., Farrell, J., Waites, K., Wirt, S., & Lutz, B. (2014). The essential role of the rehabilitation nurse in facilitating care transitions. A White paper by the Association of Rehabilitation Nurses. *Rehabilitation Nursing, 39*(1), 3–15.

Campbell, J. C., Ikegami, N., & Gibdon, M. (2010). Lessons from public long-term care insurance in Germany and Japan. *Health Affairs, 29*(1), 87–95.

Canadian Hospice Palliative Care Association. (2014). Fact sheet: Hospice palliative care in Canada. Retrieved from http://www.chpca.net/media/330558/Fact_Sheet_HPC_in_Canada%20Spring%202014%20Final .pdf

Canadian Minister of Health. (2011). *Healthy Canadians: A federal report on comparable health indicators 2010.* Retrieved from http://www.hc-sc.gc.ca/hcs-sss/pubs/system-regime/2010-fed-comp-indicat/index-eng.php

Centers for Disease Control and Prevention. (2012). Depression is not a normal part of growing older. Retrieved from http://www.cdc.gov/aging/mentalhealth/depression.htm

Centers for Medicare and Medicaid Services. (2015). *Medicare benefit policy manual.* Retrieved from http://www .cms.gov/Regulations-and-Guidance/Guidance/Manuals/Downloads/bp102c08.pdf

Centers for Medicare and Medicaid Services. (2016a). Community-based care transitions program. Retrieved from https://innovations.cms.gov/initiatives/CCTP/

Centers for Medicare and Medicaid Services. (2016b). Initiative to reduce avoidable hospitalizations among nursing facility residents. Retrieved from https://innovation.cms.gov/initiatives/rahnfr/

Chaffee, M. W., Mason, D. J., & Leavitt, J. K. (2012). A framework for action in policy and politics. In D. J. Mason, J. K. Leavitt, & M. W. Chaffee (Eds.), *Policy & politics in nursing and health care* (6th ed., pp. 1–11). St. Louis, MO: Saunders.

Chandra, A., Dalton, M. A., & Holmes, J. (2013). Large increases in spending on postacute care in Medicare point to the potential for cost savings in these settings. *Health Affairs, 32*(5), 864–872.

Cire, B. (2011). *NIH-commissioned census bureau report describes oldest Americans—Is 90 the new 85?* National Institutes of Health-National Institute on Aging. Retrieved from http://www.nia.nih.gov/newsroom/2011/11/nih-commissioned-census-bureau-report-describes-oldest-Americans

Cleverley, W. O., Song, P. H., & Cleverley, J. O. (2011). *Essentials of health care finance* (7th ed.). Sudbury, MA: Jones and Bartlett Learning.

Coleman, E. A., Parry, C., Chalmers, S., & Min, S. (2006). The care transitions intervention. *Archives of Internal Medicine, 166*(17), 1822–1828.

Commission on Accreditation of Rehabilitation Facilities. (2016). CARF accreditation focuses on quality, results. Retrieved from http://www.carf.org

Counsell, S. R., Callahan, C. M., Clark, D. O., Tu, W., Buttar, A. B., Stump, T. E., & Ricketts, G. D. (2007). Geriatric care management of low-income seniors: A randomized controlled trial. *Journal of the American Medical Association, 298*(22), 2623–2632.

De Lew, N. (2000). Medicare: 35 years of service. *Health Care Financing Review, 22*(1), 75–103.

Dentzer, S. (2009). Key issues in health reform. Retrieved from http://healthaffairs.org/healthpolicybriefs/brief.php?brief_id=10?view=full

Eldercare locator. (2015). Adult day care. Retrieved from http://www.eldercare.gov/Eldercare.NET/Public/Resources/Factsheets/Adult_Day_care.aspx

Geraedts, M., Heller, G. V., & Harrington, C. A. (2000). Germany's long-term-care insurance: Putting a social insurance model into practice. *The Milbank Quarterly, 78*(3), 375–401.

Golden, A., Tweary, S., Dang, S., & Roos, B. (2010). Care management's challenges and opportunities to reduce the rapid rehospitalization of frail community-dwelling older adults. *The Gerontologist, 50*(4), 451–458.

Harrison, A., Gregory, S., Mundle, C., & Boyle, S. (2011). The English health care system, 2011. In S. Thomson, R. Osborn, D. Squires, & M. J. Reed (Eds.), *International profiles of health care systems, 2011* (pp. 38–44). Publication No. 1562. New York, NY: The Commonwealth Fund. Retrieved from http://www.commonwealthfund.org/Publications/Fund-Reports/2011/Nov/International-Profiles-of-Health-Care-Systems-2011.aspx

Hewner, S. (2014). A population-based care transition model for chronically ill elders. *Nursing Economics, 32*(3), 109–116, 141.

Indian Health Service. (2015). Retrieved from http://www.ihs.gov

Institute of Medicine. (2001). *Crossing the quality chasm: A new health system for the 21st century.* Washington, DC: National Academies Press.

Kadowaki, L., Wister, A. V., & Chappel, N. L. (2015). Influence of home care on life satisfaction, loneliness, and perceived life stress. *Canadian Journal on Aging, 34*(1), 75–84.

Komisar, H. L., & Feder, J. (2011). Transforming care for Medicare beneficiaries with chronic conditions and long-term care needs: Coordinating care across all services. Retrieved from http://www.thescanfoundation.org/sites/default/files/Georgetown_Trnsfrming_Care.pdf

LaPierre, T. A. (2012). Comparing the Canadian and U.S. systems of health care in an era of health care reform. *Journal of Health Care Finance, 38*(4), 1–18.

Marchildon, G. (2013). Canada health system review. *Health Systems in Transition, 15*(1). Retrieved from http://www.euro.who.int/__data/assets/pdf_file/0011/181955/e96759.pdf

Mathematica Policy Research. (2011). *Money follows the person: Expanding options for long term care.* Retrieved from https://www.google.com/webhp?sourceid=chrome-instant&ion=1&espv=2&ie=UTF-8#q=Mathematica+Policy+Research.+(2011).+Money+follows+the+person%3A+Expanding+options+for+long+term+care

Matsuda, R. (2015). The Japanese health care system, 2014. In E. Mossialos, M. Wenzel, R. Osborn, & C. Anderson (Eds.), *International profiles of health care systems, 2014* (pp. 83–91). New York, NY: The Commonwealth Fund. Retrieved from http://www.commonwealthfund.org/~/media/files/publications/fund-report/2015/jan/1802_mossialos_intl_profiles_2014_v7.pdf

Medicare. (2016). Programs of All-Inclusive Care for the Elderly. Retrieved from http://www.medicare.gov/your-medicare-costs/help-paying-costs/pace/pace.html

Minister of Justice. (2016). Canada health act. Retrieved from http://laws-lois.justice.gc.ca/eng/acts/c-6/

National Adult Day Services Association. (2015). About adult day services. Retrieved from http://www.nadsa.org/learn-more/about-adult-day-services/

National Health Service. (2013). Guide to the healthcare system in England. Retrieved from http://www.gov.uk/government/uploads/system/uploads/attachment_data/file/194002/9421-2900878-TSO-NHS_Guide_to_Healthcare_WEB.PDF

National Health Services. (2015). About the NHS. Retrieved from http://www.nhs.uk/NHSEngland/thenhs/about/Pages/overview.aspx

National Quality Forum. (2016). About us. Retrieved from http://www.qualityforum.org

Naylor, M. D., Aiken, L. H., Kurtzman, E. T., Olds, D. M., & Hirschman, K. B. (2011). The importance of transitional care in achieving health reform. *Health Affairs, 30*(4), 746–754.

Ohwa, M., & Chen, L. (2012). Balancing long-term care in Japan. *Journal of Gerontological Social Work, 55*(7), 659–672.

Oi, M. (2015). Who will look after Japan's elderly? Retrieved from http://www.bbc.com/news/world-asia-31901943

Ortman, J. M., Velkoff, V. A., & Hogan, H. (2014). *An aging nation: The older population in the United States: Current Population Reports P25-1140.* Washington, DC: U.S. Census Bureau. Retrieved from http://www.census.gov/prod/2014pubs/p25-1140.pdf

Ouslander, J. G., Bonner, A., Herndon, L., & Shutes, J. (2014). The INTERACT quality improvement program: An overview for medical directors and primary care clinicians in long-term care. *Journal of the American Medical Directors Association, 15*(3), 162–170.

Ouslander, J. G., Lamb, G., Tappen, R., Herndon, L., Diaz, S., Roos, B. A., . . . Bonner, A. (2011). Interventions to reduce hospitalizations from nursing homes: Evaluation of the INTERACT II collaborative quality improvement project. *Journal of the American Geriatrics Society, 59*(4), 745–753.

Perlman, M., & Fried, B. J. (2012). United Kingdom. In B. J. Fried & L.M. Gaydos (Eds.), *World health systems: Challenges & perspectives* (pp. 605–623). Chicago, IL: Health Administration Press.

QSEN Institute. (2014). Competencies. Retrieved from http://www.qsen.org

Reaves, E. L., & Musumeci, M. (2015). Medicaid and long-term services and supports: A primer. Retrieved from http://kff.org/medicaid/report/medicaid-and-long-term-services-and-supports-a-primer/

Robert Wood Johnson Foundation. (2012). What is the national quality strategy? Retrieved from http://www.rwjf.org/en/library/research/2012/01/what-is-the-national-quality-strategy-.html

Rublee, D., Spaeth, B., & Schramm, W. (2012). Germany. In B. J. Fried, & L. M. Gaydos (Eds.), *World health systems: Challenges and perspectives* (pp. 647–661). Chicago, IL: Health Administration Press.

Schraeder, C., & Shelton, P. (2011). *Comprehensive care coordination for chronically ill adults.* West Sussex, UK: Wiley-Blackwell.

Sciegai, M., & Behr, R. A. (2010). Lessons for the United States from countries adapting to the consequences of aging populations. *Technology and Disability, 22,* 83–88.

Sherwood, G., & Zomorodi, M. (2014). A new mindset for quality and safety: The QSEN competencies redefine nurses' role in practice. *Nephrology Nursing Journal, 41*(1), 15–23, 72.

Society of Hospital Medicine. (2016). Project BOOST mentored implementation program. Retrieved from http://www.hospitalmedicine.org/BOOST.

Tamiya, N., Noguchi, H., Nishi, A., Reich, M. R., Ikegami, N., Hashimoto, . . . Kawachi, I. (2011). Population aging and wellbeing: Lessons from Japan's long-term care insurance policy. *Lancet, 378*(9797), 1183–1192.

Tang, F., & Pickard, J. G. (2008). Aging in place or relocation: Perceived awareness of community-based long-term care and services. *Journal of Housing for the Elderly, 22,* 404–422.

The White House. (2016). Retrieved from http://www.whitehouse.gov

Thorlby, R., & Arora, S. (2015). The English health care system, 2014. In E. Mossialos, M. Wenzl, R. Osborn, & C. Anderson (Eds.), *International profiles of health care systems, 2014* (pp. 43–52). New York, NY: The Commonwealth Fund. Retrieved from http://www.commonwealthfund.org/~/media/files/publications /fund-report/2015/jan/1802_mossialos_intl_profiles_2014_v7.pdf

U.S. Department of Health and Human Services. (2013). *Long-term care services in the United States: 2013 overview.* Retrieved from http://www.cdc.gov/nchs/data/nsltcp/long_term_care_services_2013.pdf

U.S. Department of Health and Human Services. (2015). About HHS. Retrieved from www.hhs.gov/about/index .html

U.S. Department of Health and Human Services. (2015). *The Affordable Care Act section by section.* Retrieved from http://www.healthcare.gov/law/timeline/full.html#2010

Vaughn, S., Mauk, K. L., Jacelon, C. S., Larsen, P.D., Rye, J., Wintersgill. W., . . . Dufresne, D. (2015). The competency model for professional rehabilitation nursing. *Rehabilitation Nursing, 41*(1), 33–44.

Wenzl, R., Osborn, R., & Anderson, C. (Eds.), *International profiles of health care systems, 2014* (pp. 43-52). New York, NY: The Commonwealth Fund. Retrieved from http://www.commonwealthfund.org/~/media /files/publications/fund-report/2015/jan/1802_mossialos_intl_profiles_2014_v7.pdf

World Bank. (2016). Population ages 65 and above (%) of total. Retrieved from http://data.worldbank.org/indicator /SP.POP.65UP.TO.ZS

Wright, K., Hazelett, S., Jarjoura, D., & Allen, K. (2007). AD-LIFE Trial: Working to integrate medical and psychosocial care management models. *Home Healthcare Nurse, 25*(5), 308–314.

Yung, M., Yeh, A., & Pressler, S. J. (2012). Heart failure and skilled nursing facilities: Review of the literature. *Journal of Cardiac Failure, 18*(11), 854–871.

Zelman, W. N., McCue, M. J., & Glick, N. D. (2009). *Financial management of health care organizations* (3rd ed.). San Francisco, CA: Jossey-Bass.

For a full suite of assignments and additional learning activities, see the access code at the front of your book.

Glossary

21st-century leadership: Characteristics of leadership needed to transition from an industrial age to a "sociotechnical age," adopting new strategies to meet the changing scene in health care.

Abandonment: Desertion of an older person by an individual who has assumed responsibility for providing care for the older adult or by a person with physical custody.

Abuse: Harm or injury inflicted on another.

Accountability: Being held responsible for acts or omission of an action once a duty, or expected actions and obligations, have been established by the relationship between two parties.

Acculturation: The process by which people from particular ethnic backgrounds have incorporated the cultural attributes (e.g., values, beliefs, language, skills) of the mainstream culture, or a new cultural identity.

Acetylcholine: A neurotransmitter that plays an important role in learning and memory.

Acquired immunity: The branch of the immune system consisting of humoral immunity and cell-mediated immunity.

Actigraphy: The measurement of movement activity data that provides an objective measure of sleep over a 24-hour day, based on algorithms.

Actin: Protein within muscle that, together with myosin, is responsible for muscle contraction.

Active memory: What you are thinking at any given moment.

Activities of daily living: Activities performed in the course of daily life, including bathing, dressing, transferring, walking, eating, and continence.

Acupuncture: Insertion of very thin needles at pathways of meridians in the body to increase the flow of vital energy (qi).

Acute in-patient rehabilitation: Rehabilitation services offered in an acute care hospital or free-standing rehabilitation unit; patients must be able to tolerate 3 hours per day of therapy to be eligible.

Acute pain: Temporary pain, experienced in a time-limited situation, with attainable relief.

Addiction: A primary, chronic, neurobiologic disease, with genetic, psychosocial, and environmental factors influencing its development and manifestation. It is characterized by behaviors that include one or more of the following: impaired control over drug use, compulsive use, continued use despite harm, and craving.

Adjuvant: Any drug that has a primary indication other than pain but has been found to have analgesic qualities.

Adrenal cortex: The outer portion of the adrenal glands.

Adrenal glands: Paired glands located above the kidneys.

Adrenal medulla: The inner portion of the adrenal glands.

Adrenocorticotropic hormone: Pituitary hormone stimulating the release of glucocorticoids and sex hormones from the adrenal cortex.

Adult day care services: In-community, nonresidential group programs designed to meet the needs of older adults with cognitive and/or functional disabilities and provide respite to family caregivers.

Advance directives: Legal documents that record decisions regarding life-saving or life-sustaining care and actions to be taken in a situation in which the patient is no longer able to provide informed consent.

Adverse drug reaction: Unwanted side effect of medication.

Advocacy: The act or process of pleading the case of another.

African Americans: Comprised of those U.S.-born Blacks, foreign-born Blacks, Jamaican, Haitian, Nigerian, Dominican, and Hispanic Blacks

After Discharge Care Management of Low-Income Frail Elderly (AD-LIFE): Interdisciplinary chronic care management program providing medical and social care for low-income older adults in the community.

Ageism: A negative attitude toward aging or older persons.

Agency for Healthcare Research and Quality (AHRQ): An agency of the U.S. Department of Health and Human Services that provides healthcare information, research findings, and data to help health providers, consumers, researchers, insurers, and policymakers to make informed decisions.

Age-related macular degeneration: A condition associated with aging in which the macula of the eye deteriorates, causing loss of central vision.

Aging in place: The idea of providing stability for the older adult by working toward the common goal of either maintaining the current residence or living in a non-healthcare environment.

Agitation: Restlessness that may lead to negative behaviors or aggressive behavior.

Agnosia: Loss of ability to understand auditory, visual, or other sensations.

Agoraphobia: An anxiety disorder in which an individual has attacks of intense fear and anxiety. There is also a fear of being in places where it is difficult to escape or where help might not be available.

Albumin: As a laboratory test, measures amount of protein in body.

Aldosterone: A mineralocorticoid targeting the kidneys and regulating fluid–electrolyte balance.

Allow natural death: Used as an advance directive in some locations instead of a DNR (do not resuscitate) order; promotes a more positive approach to consideration of a person's wishes at end of life.

Alpha-adrenoceptors: Control vessel constriction.

Alveoli: Tiny, spongy air sacs that are the functional units of the lungs and the site of gas exchange.

Alzheimer's disease: A terminal neurological disorder characterized by deterioration of the brain leading to progressive forgetfulness and loss of independence.

American Indian: Many older American Indians prefer the term "Indian" to "Native American," believing that *anyone* born in the United States is a "Native American," and that the term "Indian" reflects the language used in treaties with the federal government. There are at least 558 different federally recognized tribes/nations and 126 tribes/nations applying for recognition in the United States.

Amino acid neurotransmitters: Glutamate is the major excitatory neurotransmitter, and gamma-aminobutyric acid (GABA) is the major inhibitory neurotransmitter.

Andragogy: Related to the teaching of adults.

Andropause: Loss of androgen hormone such as testosterone in aging males.

Anemia: A disease characterized by a deficiency of erythrocytes.

Angina: Chest pain resulting from lack of oxygen to the heart muscle.

Anhedonia: Loss of pleasure and interest in daily activities.

Annoyance: Related to suggestions by friends or family to cut down on drinking.

Anomia: Difficulty naming things.

Anorexia of aging: Age-related decline in food intake.

Anthropometric measures: Important indicators of an older adult's nutritional status; includes items such as body weight, body mass index, triceps skin fold.

Antibodies: Antigen-attacking proteins of the immune system.

Anticholinergic: Medications that block acetylcholine and can cause or worsen confusion.

Antidepressant: A psychiatric medication used to alleviate mood disorders, such as depression, dysthymia, and sometimes anxiety disorders. Most antidepressants work by changing the levels of one or more of the naturally occurring brain chemicals.

Antigen: Any foreign substance invading the body.

Anxiety: A normal human emotion that everyone experiences. It can be expressed as irritability, nervousness, apprehension, or fear.

Anxiolytic: A medication used for the treatment of anxiety when it leads to psychological and physical symptoms.

Aphasia: Impaired ability to communicate.

Apnea: The absence of airflow for 10 seconds or longer at the nose and mouth.

Apolipoprotein E-e4: A protein that carries cholesterol in blood and that appears to play some role in brain function. Variants of this gene are associated with the development of Alzheimer's disease.

Apoptosis: A process of programmed cell death marked by cell shrinkage.

Apraxia: Inability to perform purposeful movements.

Arteries: Carry blood from the heart to the rest of the body or the lungs.

Asian or Pacific Islander: Persons from the continent of Asia, including China, Japan, India, Pakistan, Korea, Vietnam (including Hmong peoples), Laos, Thailand, Philippines, Pacific Islands (Hawaii, Samoa, Tonga), Micronesia (Marianas, Marshalls, Gilbert), or Melanesia (Fiji, Papua New Guinea).

Assault: Threatening to harm.

Assimilation: See Acculturation.

Assisted living facility: In-community, independent living facility for older adults that may provide assistance with certain activities of daily living or medications.

Assistive devices: Any item, piece of equipment, or product system, whether acquired commercially off the shelf, modified, or customized, that is used to increase, maintain, or improve functional capabilities of individuals with disabilities.

Assistive technologies: Technological tools used to access education, employment, recreation, or communication, enabling someone to live as independently as possible.

Atherosclerosis: Hardening and narrowing of the arteries to the heart from plaque buildup in vessel walls.

Atria: The two upper chambers of the heart; they receive blood from the venous system.

Attention: The ability to disengage, reengage, and sustain focus and vigilance.

Attitudes: Values, thoughts, and beliefs held by a person.

Atypical antidepressants: A psychiatric medication used to alleviate mood disorders in the class of antidepressants, but atypical antidepressants affect neurotransmitters, including dopamine, serotonin, and norepinephrine. They work by changing the balance of these chemicals to help brain cells send and receive messages, which usually leads to improved mood.

Augmentative and alternative communication: All forms of communication that enhance or supplement speech and writing, either temporarily or permanently, or that involve the use of personalized methods or devices to aid a person's ability to communicate.

Autoimmunity: The immune system's attack of the body's own cells.

Autonomic nervous system: Part of the peripheral nervous system; contains the sympathetic and parasympathetic pathways.

Autonomy: Referring to self-governance or self-directing freedom; being in charge of one's own being; having moral independence.

Avoidable and unavoidable pressure ulcers: *Avoidable* means that a resident developed a pressure ulcer when the facility did not evaluate the resident's clinical condition and pressure ulcer risk factors; define and implement interventions consistent with the resident's needs, goals, and recognized standards of practice; or monitor and evaluate the impact of the intervention or did not revise the interventions as appropriate to the findings of the evaluation. *Unavoidable* means that a resident developed a pressure ulcer even though the facility had appropriately and comprehensively assessed the resident's clinical condition and risk factors, implemented appropriated interventions, monitored and evaluated the effectiveness of these interventions, and revised them as indicated by the care plan.

Ayurveda: Traditional medical system of India.

B cells: Cells of the immune system that mature in the bone marrow and produce antibodies in response to antigen exposure.

Baby boomers: People born between the years 1946 and 1964, after World War II.

Background noise: Sound other than the voice or sound that is being listened to.

Baroreflex: Reflex stimulated by baroreceptor activity.

Basic multicellular unit: Temporary anatomic structure composed of osteoblasts, osteoclasts, vasculature, nerve supply, and connective tissue; responsible for bone modeling and remodeling.

Battery: The act of touching without permission, as in the case of performing a procedure without consent.

Beers Criteria: A list of potentially inappropriate medications for older adults.

Behavior theory: Comprises four leadership styles, each with unique characteristics.

Beneficence: Doing or producing good.

Benign paroxysmal positional vertigo: One of the more common and treatable causes of dizziness in older adults, resulting from otoconia being displaced in the ear canal.

Benign prostatic hyperplasia: Enlargement of the prostate gland that often occurs with advanced age.

Beta-adrenoceptors: Trigger vessel dilation.

Beta-amyloid plaques: Deposits found in the spaces between nerve cells in the brain that are made of beta-amyloid.

Better Outcomes for Older Adults through Safe Transitions (BOOST) Care Transitions: Transitional care program providing information and tools to help optimize the discharge process.

Bioelectrical impedance analysis: An inexpensive, quick, and noninvasive tool used in clinical practice to estimate fat mass versus lean mass.

Biofeedback: Use of feedback from a machine to control target functions in the body with the mind; eventually the machine feedback is eliminated.

Biological therapies: Targeted therapies that affect the body's immune system and may include interferons, interleukins, monoclonal antibodies, vaccines, and gene therapy.

Biologically based practices: Use of substances found in nature such as botanicals, vitamins, and minerals.

Black American: Individuals of mixed ethnic and cultural heritage. The slave trade resulted in a diaspora (dispersion) from West and Central Africa; this group also includes immigrants from the West Indies, South America, Central America, Haiti, and other Caribbean Islands.

Bladder diary: A daily record of the time and volume of fluid intake, voiding, and incontinence episodes with associated activities.

Bladder training: An intervention that focuses on providing patients with the tools to delay urination and suppress urgency in order to establish more normal voiding intervals.

Body mass index: Used to determine body fat levels, with a BMI less than 18.5 kg/m^2 indicating underweight and increased risk of mortality; a BMI of 18.5 to 24.9 kg/m^2 indicates normal weight, 25 to 29.9 kg/m^2 overweight, and greater than 30 kg/m^2 obesity.

Bone mineral density: Screening test for osteoporosis.

Braden Scale for Pressure Ulcer Risk Assessment: Most widely used tool to assess pressure ulcer risk; a Braden score of 16 or less indicates a high risk of pressure ulcer development in the general population, and a score of 18 or less is indicative of high risk in older adults or persons with darkly pigmented skin.

Breakthrough pain: A transient, moderate to severe pain that increases above the pain addressed by the ongoing analgesics.

Broca's aphasia: Broken speech.

Brown bag assessment: Lay term for when patients bring in all their medications in a brown paper bag and a health professional reviews and assesses them.

Cachexia: Complex metabolic processes associated with an underlying terminal illness (e.g., cancer, end-stage renal disease) and is characterized by loss of muscle mass with or without loss of fat mass.

Calcitonin: A hormone of the thyroid gland that stimulates increased uptake of calcium by bone-forming cells.

Cancer: A malignant or invasive growth or tumor.

Capacity: The ability to make decisions.

Cardiac output: The amount of blood pumped by the heart per minute.

Cardiovascular disease: Includes hypertension, coronary heart disease, congestive heart failure, and stroke.

Care coordination: Often done by gerontological nurses who work with older adults as coaches to help encourage self-care.

Caregiver burden: Emotional and/or physical illness associated with the demands of caring for an ill family member.

Care Transitions Intervention: Transitional care model (Coleman); patient centered to improve quality and contain costs for older adults with complex care needs.

Cartilaginous joints: Joints composed of two bones separated by a layer of cartilage.

Case mix groups: Patient classification system to group patients with similar characteristics.

Cataracts: A clouding of the lens of the eye, its capsule, or both.

Catecholamines: Hormones of the adrenal medulla released in response to sympathetic nervous system activity.

Catheter-associated urinary tract infection: A bladder infection caused by an indwelling urinary catheter.

Causation: Generally determined by a jury and answers the question: Did the defendant's action or failure to act cause, or significantly contribute to, the loss or injury?

Causative factors: Factors that influence pressure ulcer development such as (1) intensity of pressure, (2) duration of pressure, and (3) tissue tolerance, which is the ability of skin and its supporting structures to endure pressure.

CD34$^+$ cells: The primary circulating progenitor stem cells.

Ceiling effect: When the increase in a dose of medication goes beyond a certain point and no longer increases effectiveness but increases risks.

Cell-mediated immunity: The branch of acquired immunity responsible for destroying intracellular antigens.

Centenarian: Someone who is 100 years of age or older.

Center for Science in the Public Interest: An educational and advocacy organization that has a newsletter and has championed many projects for nutrition in various areas

Cerebrovascular accident: Stroke, brain attack.

Certification: A type of credential earned through meeting specific requirements that validate expertise and knowledge in a specialty area.

Cerumen: Ear wax.

Chemical restraint: A medication used to control behavior or restrict the patient's freedom of movement and is not a standard treatment for the patient's medical or psychological condition.

Chemoreceptors: Receptors related to the abilities to smell and taste.

Chemotherapy: A systemic (entire body) therapy that uses chemicals to destroy cancer cells.

Chemotherapy-induced cognitive impairment: Also referred to as "chemo brain"; is a controversial symptom more recently noted in the survivor with cancer, manifesting as weakening or impairment of memory and/or cognitive function associated with cancer treatment, including chemotherapy and hormonal therapy.

Chiropractic practice: Manipulation of the skeletal system by trained practitioners to put the body back in balance.

Cholinergic neurons: Neurons that release the neurotransmitter acetylcholine, which plays a significant role in learning and memory in humans and animals.

Cholinesterase: An enzyme that degrades acetylcholine.

Cholinesterase inhibitor: A medication that inhibits cholinesterase and indirectly increases acetylcholine. Used as a treatment for Alzheimer's disease.

Chronic bronchitis: A type of chronic obstructive pulmonary disease characterized by increased mucus production and scarring of bronchial tubes that obstructs airflow.

Chronic disease: A disease that is ongoing or recurring. Some types of cancer, as well as AIDS, recently have been designated as chronic diseases.

Chronic Disease Self-Management Program: A care model developed by Dr. Kate Lorig, at Stanford University, to facilitate self-management of chronic illnesses.

Chronic obstructive pulmonary disease: A group of diseases related to obstructed airflow in the lungs.

Chronic pain (persistent, nonmalignant): Pain that lasts a month or more beyond the usual expected recovery period or illness or goes on for years.

Chronological aging: The process of physiological change caused only by the passage of time.

Circadian rhythm: Biologically or behaviorally based functions that change systematically over each 24-hour period and can be modified or entrained to cycles of light/dark and sleep/wake.

Circadian rhythm disorders: Sleep disturbance pattern resulting from circadian timing system alterations or from endogenous circadian rhythm and exogenous factor misalignment, affecting sleep timing or duration.

Clonal expansion: A process through which B and T cells of the immune system multiply to produce cellular clones.

Codes of ethics: Codes of moral reasoning used by members of a profession to direct the moral behavior of their work.

Cognition: Group of mental processes including attention, awareness, judgment, memory, perception, and the like.

Cognitive behavioral therapy: A form of psychiatric treatment that focuses on examining the relationships among thoughts, feelings, and behaviors.

Cohort: A group of people with a similar characteristic, such as age or exposure to toxic chemicals, who are studied over time.

Colon: Another term for the large intestine; extends from the small intestine to the rectum.

Combativeness: Aggressive behavior and noncompliance.

Communicating bad news: Module 2 of Education in Palliative and End-of-Life Care (EPEC). This training for medical personnel promotes honest and compassionate discussion about end-of-life care and options for treating life-ending illnesses.

Communication: The giving and receiving of information.

Commission on Accreditation of Rehabilitation of Rehabilitation Facilities: Organization that offers accreditation to a variety of programs and services.

Communication Enhancement Model: Provides direction for effective healthcare provider communication; directs that the younger adult healthcare providers make an individualized assessment of the communication abilities of each older adult and only modify speech as needed to support effective communication with that individual.

Community-based care management programs: A variety of programs based in the community setting that provide choices and informed decision making for older adults

Compensatory scaffolding: A process in which the individual's brain recruits additional neuron connections for maintaining memory and decoding what has been observed.

Compensatory strategies: Focus on providing mechanisms to assist the person with the physical or neurological impairment.

Competence: Having the capacity to function or respond; having requisite or adequate abilities or qualities to perform a task or respond to a situation. Mental competence is evaluated to determine whether a person has adequate capacity to make informed decisions.

Complement system: A collection of proteins of the immune system involved in the destruction of antigens and initiation of the inflammatory response.

Complementary and alternative medicine: Alternative approaches to healing that may include acupuncture, biofeedback, guided therapy, healing touch, herbal and dietary supplements, Reiki, yoga, and the like.

Complementary and alternative therapy: A group of diverse medical and healthcare systems, practices, and products that are not generally considered part of conventional medicine (also called Western or allopathic medicine).

Complexity leadership: Leadership is viewed as an interactive system of dynamic, unpredictable agents that interact with each other in complex feedback networks, which can then produce adaptive outcomes such as knowledge dissemination, learning, innovation, and further adaptation to change.

Conductive hearing loss: Occurs when the cause of hearing loss is located in the outer and/or middle ear.

Confidentiality: Being entrusted with confidences. Maintaining confidentiality is required to protect the right of privacy.

Conflict: Occurs when a choice must be made between two equal options.

Conflict of interest: Conflict that arises from competing loyalties and opportunities. This may include conflicts between the nurse's value system and choices made by the patients, their families, other healthcare team members, the organization, or the insurance company or when incentive systems or other financial gains create conflict between professional integrity and self-interest.

Conflict resolution: Encouraging collaborative decision making to move the team beyond the conflict.

Congestive heart failure: A chronic deficiency in the heart's ability to pump blood to the body.

Constipation: Sluggish bowels that result in hard stool and delay in normal bowel movements.

Continuing care retirement community: A community for the elderly that provides a continuum of care that spans independent living to skilled nursing care in a traditional nursing home setting, all within a single campus setting.

Continuity Assessment Record and Evaluation (Care) Tool: A tool mandated by CMS to compare similar items in a uniform manner across the various PAC venues.

Continuity theory: The view that one's personality (and its influence on behavior) remain somewhat stable over the course of the lifespan.

Continuous bladder irrigation: Used after a transurethral resection of the prostate to flush the bladder.

Contracting: A specific agreement between the nurse and client in which a behavior change is described and a plan for the change is committed to paper.

Copayment: The amount of money one pays to a care provider in addition to what the insurance pays.

Core competencies: The essential skills and knowledge needed to provide high-quality care to older adults.

Core values: Basic beliefs and attitudes of an individual that reflects that individual's thoughts, behaviors, and culture.

Corneal ulcer: Irritation of the cornea that may be caused by stroke, infection, fever, or trauma and often results in scarring.

Coronary artery disease: Also called coronary heart disease or ischemic heart disease; results from atherosclerosis.

Coronary heart disease: Includes myocardial infarction, angina, and other conditions.

Cortical bone: The outer layer of bone; also known as compact bone.

Corticotropin-releasing hormone: Hypothalamic hormone that stimulates release of adrenocorticotropic hormone from the pituitary gland.

Cortisol: The primary glucocorticoid in the human body and a hormone regulating the stress response.

Cultural awareness: Being mindful, attentive, and conscious of similarities and differences among cultural groups.

Cultural congruence: The understanding and application of acceptable beliefs, ideas, and practices that result in an interpersonal, social, and intercultural understanding and acceptance of differences and similarities of all peoples within a worldview.

Cultural humility: The identification of one's own biases and the acknowledgment that those biases must be recognized. Cultural humility acknowledges that it is impossible to be adequately knowledgeable about cultures other than one's own.

Cultural sensitivity: Being aware and sensitive to differences when working with others outside of our own culture.

Culturally competent: awareness of one's personal biases through critical self-reflection and a deliberate understanding of culturally diverse health-related values, beliefs, and behaviors, health disparities in morbidity and mortality, population-specific treatments and skills in working with diverse populations.

Culture: Integrated patterns of human behavior that include the language, thoughts, communications, actions, customs, beliefs, values, and institutions of racial, ethnic, religious, or social groups.

Culture of safety: Safe and appropriate delegation of care.

Cupping: A practice in traditional Chinese medicine in which a cup is placed over intact skin to create a vacuum.

Curative care: Medical care focused on healing and cure of disease.

Curative treatment: Interventions and medications aimed at eradicating disease.

Cut down: Refers to attempts by the client to cut down on drinking.

Cystectomy: Surgical removal of the bladder.

Cytokines: Chemical messengers of the immune, hematopoietic, and other physiological systems.

Damages: Loss or injury.

Daytime sleepiness: An inability to stay awake and alert during the primary episodes of daytime wakefulness.

Declarative memory: Factual information that can be declared and is divided into three types: *episodic* (events), *semantic* (concepts), and *lexical* (word) *memory*.

Deductible: The amount of money one pays to a care provider before the insurance benefits are activated.

Deglutition: Act of chewing.

Dehydroepiandrosterone: An adrenal sex hormone able to convert to a multitude of other hormones, primarily estrogen and testosterone.

Delayed retirement credit: Additional money one can earn in addition to full Social Security benefits if one works past age 65.

Delegation: Process for a nurse to direct another person to perform nursing tasks and activities.

Delirium: Acute confusion caused by physiological illness.

Dementia: A broad term referring to the symptoms associated with a progressive decline in cognitive function to the extent that it interferes with daily life and activities.

Demineralization: A decrease in the amount of minerals or inorganic salts in tissues, as occurs in certain diseases.

Demographic tidal wave: A term that describes the Baby Boomers; a large group about to "crash" into the resources of the United States.

Demyelination: Any disease of the nervous system in which the myelin sheath of neurons is damaged.

Dependence: Physical response to use of opioids, characterized by withdrawal symptoms when the opioid is stopped.

Depression: A mood disorder, common in persons with dementia.

Dermis: The intermediate layer of the skin.

Detrusor: Muscle in the bladder that assists with voiding.

Diabetic retinopathy: Impaired vision due to bleeding in the retina from ruptured vessels.

Diagnosis-related groups: Categories of care based on the diagnosis(es) applied to the patient.

Diaphragm: A sheet of muscle located across the bottom of the chest that aids in respiration through its contraction and relaxation.

Diarrhea: Loose, watery stool.

Diastole: Relaxation of ventricles when filling with blood.

Dietary Approaches to Stop Hypertension (DASH) diet: A diet promoted by the U.S. Department of Health and Human Services that has been proven to be palatable and effective in lowering blood pressure. It is rich in potassium, magnesium, and calcium and low in salt.

Diet history review: A component of nutritional assessment in which the patient reports nutritional intake and behaviors.

Dilemma: Occurs when it appears there are no acceptable choices. To qualify as a dilemma, there must be active engagement in the situation that forces an evaluation of and need for choices. Actions are uncertain because alternatives are equally unattractive.

Direct physical abuse: Mistreatment that involves physical harm such as punching, beating, burning, and sexual abuse; involves the use of physical force to purposefully inflict pain or harm to another.

Disaster: A natural or man-made event that requires resources outside of the local community to respond to the event.

Disaster recovery: The mobilization of resources to assist communities affected by a disaster to return to a state of normality.

Disaster response: Includes the mobilization of manpower and resources to meet the needs of those affected by disaster events, including saving lives, protecting property and the environment, and meeting basic human needs.

Diverticulitis: Inflammation of the intestinal diverticula.

Do not resuscitate: A physician's written order instructing healthcare providers not to attempt cardiopulmonary resuscitation (CPR) in case of cardiac or respiratory arrest.

Dopaminergic system: Releases dopamine, affecting motor control.

Dosha: Energy in the Ayurvedic medical system.

Dry eyes: A lack of usual moisture in the eyes, sometimes associated with older age.

Dual sensory impairment: When one experiences a loss in both vision and hearing.

Due care: The specifics of what is expected of caregivers in their professional role.

Duty: Expected actions and obligations.

Dysarthria: Weakness of the musculature involved in speech.

Dysesthesia: Any impairment of the senses, especially of the sense of touch.

Dyspareunia: Painful intercourse.

Dysphagia: Difficulty in swallowing.

Dysphagia diet: Particular diet that is safe for those with swallowing problems.

Dysthymia: A type of neurotic depression that is a mood disorder consisting of chronic depression, with less severe but longer lasting symptoms than major depressive disorder.

Eden Alternative: In-community, changing the culture of long-term care through ongoing training and continued dedication to creating a life worth living for those living there.

Elastic recoil: A measure of the lungs' ability to expand and contract.

Elder abuse: Mistreatment or harm to older adults via force to a vulnerable elder, whether physical, psychosocial, or financial; a single, or repeated act, or lack of appropriate action, occurring within any relationship in which there is an expectation of trust that causes harm or distress to an older person.

Elderly: Usually described as those persons age 65 or over.

Elder mistreatment: A preferred term to elder abuse; harm to older adults.

Elderspeak: Speech that is overly caring and controlling and less respectful than normal adult-to-adult speech.

Emergency Nurses Association: Professional specialty organization for emergency nurses.

Emergency preparedness: Defined by the U.S. Department of Homeland Security (DHS) as "a continuous cycle of planning, organizing, training, equipping, exercising, evaluating, and taking corrective action in an effort to ensure effective coordination during incident response".

Emergency response system: A device that evaluates self-care and/or physiological parameters and allows a person at high risk (e.g., an older person who lives alone and has a health problem) to get immediate help in the event of an emergency.

Emergency Severity Index (ESI): Red flags that indicate a change in status.

Emotional intelligence: the ability to manage one's emotions

Emotional neglect: when a person receives good or adequate physical care, but is socially isolated

Emphysema: A type of chronic obstructive pulmonary disease that causes irreversible lung damage and results in decreased gas exchange at the alveolar level related to loss of elasticity.

Employee retention: Process and outcome in which a worker remains or is retained at a job.

End of life: Last stages of living; in this context usually caused by a terminal illness.

Environmental and situational factors: The institutional context of communication, including the focus on care tasks, lessened opportunities for communication, and intergenerational communication issues.

Environmental controls: Electronic systems that allow individuals to control lights, heating and cooling, and just about any electrical piece of equipment, such as curtains, garage doors, and gates, from a remote location.

Environmental hazards: Potential hazards in the environment that lead to falls, such as slippery floors, inadequate lighting, loose rugs, unstable furniture, and obstructed walkways.

Epidermis: The thin, outermost layer of the skin.

Epinephrine: A catecholamine of the adrenal medulla that regulates the body's stress response; also known as adrenaline.

Episodic memory: Ability to recall events.

Erectile dysfunction: Impotence; the inability to attain or maintain an erection sufficient for intercourse.

Erythrocytes: Red blood cells.

Esophageal dysphagia: Trouble swallowing that results from motility problems, neuromuscular problems, or obstruction that interferes with the movement of the food bolus through the esophagus into the stomach.

Esophagus: Extends from the pharynx to the stomach.

Established (chronic) incontinence: Incontinence that persists beyond resolution of acute causes or is long-standing.

Ethical principles: Guidelines that evolve from beliefs and values that facilitate decision making and guide practice.

Ethics committee: An interdisciplinary committee that provides insight into ethical issues and makes recommendations, but lacks formal legal authority.

Ethics of care: Ethical principles applied to healthcare situations.

Ethnocentrism: A universal tendency to believe that one's own culture and world view are superior to another's.

Ethnogeriatrics: Health care for elders from diverse ethnic populations.

European Americans: Currently the largest population in the U.S., European Americans include the two major Christian denominations: Catholics and Protestants. Protestant denominations further fracture into, among others, Lutherans (Scandinavian Americans), Presbyterians (German Americans), Methodists (Scottish Americans), and Episcopalians (Anglo Americans). Of note is that these sects are not hard-and-fast rules; many Irish and Italian Americans are not Catholics, but Protestants; likewise many German and Anglo Americans are Catholic.

Evacuation: Removal of persons from their place of residence to a safer location, usually due to a disaster.

Excess disability: More disability or loss of function than can be explained by dementia alone.

Executive function: Higher level function of the cerebral cortex supporting abstraction, planning, sequencing, and decision-making ability.

Exercise: continuous movement that promotes health

Extrinsic aging: Aging due to chronic exposure to external factors such as smoking.

Extrinsic risk factors: Factors that contribute to a fall that are outside of the patient's body, such as a wet, slippery floor; rugs; intravenous access poles; oxygen tubing; or lighting.

Failure to rescue: Neglecting to take action or to recognize a preventable complication.

Fall: Unintentional incident of dropping to the ground or floor, which may or may not result in injury.

Fall injury risk factors: Factors that contribute to a fall injury that are related to a patient's body or health, such as taking warfarin, which increases the risk of bleeding.

Fall risk assessment: Evaluating the individual's risk factors for falling, such as intrinsic factors; extrinsic or environmental factors (in the home setting, e.g., loose rugs); medications that put the patient at risk; and a physical examination, such as strength, balance, and mobility.

Fast-twitch fibers: Muscle fibers that provide short bursts of energy but fatigue easily; used in activities of high intensity and low endurance.

Fatigue: Sense of tiredness.

Fidelity: The state of being faithful and loyal, referring to allegiance to another.

Fiduciary responsibility: An ethical obligation to good stewardship of both the patient's and the organization's funds.

Filipino Americans: Immigrants from the Philippines.

Financial abuse: Mistreatment of an older adult through stealing or misuse of his or her money or property.

Financial exploitation: Using an older person and his or her worldly goods or money for personal gain.

Financial or material exploitation: Illegal or improper use of a person's funds, money, assets.

Five Wishes: An alternative advance directive that gives additional information and explanation about a person's wishes for end-of-life care; not legally recognized in all states.

Follicle-stimulating hormone: Hormone released from the pituitary that stimulates follicle production in females and sperm in males.

Forced expiratory volume: The amount of air that can be forcefully expelled in 1 second.

Foreign-born: Born outside of the United States; not a U.S. citizen at birth.

Fortified foods: Those foods chosen based on their enhancement during processing (with vitamins and minerals) or enhanced with butter or cream during preparation.

Framingham Heart Study: A 50-year, longitudinal study of over 5,000 subjects designed to identify factors that cause and prevent cardiovascular disease.

Free radicals: Molecules with an unpaired electron in the outer shell of electrons that remain unstable until paired with another molecule.

Frequency: Number of vibrations that particles make in a certain period of time.

Functional decline: Decreased ability to independently perform activities of independent living or instrumental activities of daily living, such as dressing, bathing, shopping, and bill paying.

Functional urinary incontinence: The genitourinary tract is functioning, and incontinence is due to immobility or cognitive limitations.

Gallbladder: A small sac located below the liver that stores the bile sent from the liver.

Gastroesophageal reflux disease: When gastric acid and/or stomach contents come up into the esophagus.

Gastrointestinal immunity: Antibodies in the intestine that block antigens and bacteria in addition to neutralizing toxins.

General anxiety disorder: Extreme, excessive, unrealistic worry or nervousness and tension, even if there is minimal cause to provoke the anxiety. GAD is an anxiety disorder that is characterized by excessive, uncontrollable, and often irrational worry about everyday things that is disproportionate to the actual source of worry. In the case of this disorder, symptoms must last at least 6 months. This excessive worry often interferes with daily functioning, with many individuals with GAD typically anticipating disaster and being overly concerned about everyday matters. Individuals often exhibit a variety of physical symptoms, including fatigue, fidgeting, headaches, nausea, numbness in hands and feet, muscle tension, muscle aches, difficulty swallowing, bouts of shortness of breath, difficulty concentrating, trembling, twitching, irritability, agitation, sweating, restlessness, insomnia, hot flashes, and rashes, as well as the inability to fully control the anxiety symptoms.

Genetics: The study of heredity and the transmission of certain genes through generations.

Genomics: The identification of gene sequences in the DNA.

Geriatric assessment interdisciplinary team: An interdisciplinary training model developed in Maryland as an elective for students from various healthcare disciplines.

Geriatric assessment team: An interdisciplinary team of professionals specializing in assessment of the elderly.

Geriatric evaluation and management: Defined in-patient units or services by which the elderly are assessed and treated.

Geriatric interdisciplinary team training: An organized training program for professionals of various disciplines focused on learning about working in teams and the use of teams in gerontology.

Geriatric Resource for Assessment and Care of Elders: In-community model of primary care for low-income seniors.

Geriatric resource nurse: In-hospital, geriatric-trained acute care nurse.

Geriatrics: Medical care of the aged.

Geriatric syndrome: A common health condition in older adults that does not fit into the category of a discrete disease (such as polypharmacy, delirium, anxiety etc. . .) but that can negatively affect health outcomes

Gerocompetencies: A set of standards or competencies to meet in order to provide high-quality care to older adults.

Gerogogy: Related to the teaching of older adults.

Gerontological nursing: A specialty within nursing practice in which the clients, patients, and residents are older persons.

Gerontological rehabilitation nursing: Gerontological nursing care of older persons in which rehabilitation is emphasized; care for those with rehabilitation problems such as stroke, brain injury, neurological disorders, or orthopedic surgeries.

Gerontology: The study of aging or the aging process.

Geropharmacology: A specialty in medications and pharmacy of older adults.

Glasgow Coma Score: Tool used to classify low-level brain injury or coma in three areas: best motor, best verbal, and best eye response.

Glaucoma: A group of degenerative eye diseases in which vision is damaged by high intraocular pressure.

Global aphasia: Both receptive and expressive aphasia.

Glomerular filtration rate: Kidney filtration system for waste and toxins.

Glomeruli: Bundles of capillaries located in the kidneys.

Glucagon: A pancreatic hormone regulating blood glucose levels through stimulation of the release of stored glucose.

Glaucoma: A group of eye conditions that are one of the leading causes of blindness in older adults.

Glucocorticoids: Hormones of the adrenal cortex involved in both metabolic and antiinflammatory functions.

Glucose tolerance: The ability to respond effectively to dramatic rises in blood glucose levels.

GLUT4: An insulin-mediated glucose transporter protein located within cytoplasmic vesicles.

Gonadotropin-releasing hormone (GnRH): Released by the hypothalamus and stimulates the synthesis and release of follicle-stimulating hormone (FSH) and luteinizing hormone (LH).

Gonioscopy: Tool to directly examine the eye.

Good death: Death free from avoidable distress and suffering, according to patient and family wishes, consistent with clinical, cultural, and ethical standards.

Graying of America: Similar to the aging of America, referring to the increase in numbers of older Americans.

Green House: In-community, long-term skilled care model, providing care in small homes through self-managed team of cross-trained direct care workers.

Grief: A natural and normal reaction to a loss of any kind.

Growth hormone: A pituitary hormone that stimulates amino acid uptake and synthesis of proteins.

Guardianship: The appointment of another person to help with decision-making for an incapacitated or incompetent adult.

Guided Care: In-community model of comprehensive primary care provided by physician/nurse teams for older adult patients with complex chronic conditions.

Guided imagery: Use of imagery to elicit responses in the body.

Guilt: Feelings of worry related to an action or behavior.

Hallucinations: False sensory beliefs, such as seeing, hearing, feeling, tasting, or smelling things that others do not.

Hawaiian and other Pacific Islands ("the Pacific Rim" or "Oceania"): From Hawaii and/or Pacific Islands, including Samoa, Tonga, Micronesia, Fiji, Guam, Palau, and Marina, Papua New Guinea and Marshall Islands.

HCHAPS surveys: The first national, standardized, public report of patient's satisfaction with hospital care.

Health behavior change: Attempts to explain the processes underlying the learning of new health behaviors. The two most widely cited theories of behavior change are social cognitive theory and stages of change.

Healthcare environment: The system in which care is provided, made up of multiple, intricate relationships among stakeholders. These relationships are built on needs and ability to meet those needs. The primary relationship is between providers and consumers.

Health contract/calendar: A behavior-changing tool that borrows concepts from a variety of theories. It relies on the self-management capability of a client, after initial assistance is provided by a clinician or health educator. The client is helped to choose an appropriate behavior change goal and to create and implement a plan to accomplish that goal. The statement of the goal and the plan of action are then written into a contract format.

Health disparities: A particular type of health difference that is closely linked with social, economic, and/or environmental disadvantage.

Health–illness continuum: The degree of client wellness that exists at any point in time, ranging from an optimal wellness condition (with available energy at the maximum) to death (which demonstrates total energy depletion).

Health information technology: Decisive action chosen to respond to an issue in health care. This action includes the actual response to the healthcare issue and the plan to implement the response.

Health literacy: The degree to which individuals have the capacity to obtain, process, and understand basic health information and services needed to make appropriate health decisions.

Health policy: Decisive action chosen to respond to an issue in health care. This action includes the actual response to the healthcare issue and the plan to implement the response.

Health policy development: Creation of policy related to the well-being of individuals and/or communities. Policy development depends on the needs of the individuals and communities and the interest and perspective of the stake-holders.

Health promotion: Activities aimed at improving or enhancing health.

Health screening: Population-wide efforts to detect early disease.

Healthy People 2020: Launched in December 2010 to create an ambitious, yet achievable, 10-year agenda for health promotion and disease prevention activities aimed at improving the health of the United States.

Hearing aid: A device that amplifies sound.

Helicobacter pylori: A common bacterial contributor to symptoms of gastritis and peptic ulcers.

Hematopoiesis: The process of blood cell production.

Hemiparesis: Weakness of one side of the body.

Hemiplegia: Paralysis of one side of the body.

Hendrich II Fall Risk Model: A fall risk model with high validity and reliability.

Herpes zoster: The virus that causes chickenpox and shingles.

High-performance work team: A group of high-performing individuals who have brilliance, drive, and the ability to propose solutions to problems.

Hispanic/Latino: Includes the diversity of the subgroups of Mexican American, Cuban American, and Puerto Rican populations within a broader context. The U.S. Bureau of the Census uses the term "Hispanic" as an ethnicity category referring to persons who trace their origin or descent to Mexico, Puerto Rico, Cuba, Central or South America, or Spain, regardless of race. Hispanics/Latinos can trace their ancestry back to the indigenous people of North America as well as to Spanish/European, Asian, and African roots.

Histamine 2 (H2) blockers: Medications used for the treatment of gastroesophageal reflux disease.

Holistic: Viewing, assessing, and treating the whole person; identifying equal value for the individual's status of mind, body, and spirit as a complex, dynamic entity.

Home care: Services provided in the home of a home-bound person; may include skilled nursing, therapy, and home health aides.

Home health care: Care provided in the home for those who are homebound due to severity of illness or immobility.

Homeopathy: Medical system that follows the natural law of "like cures like."

Homeostasis: The ability to maintain balance in the organ systems.

Homeostatic sleep drive or pressure: A building drive or pressure for sleep based on prolonged wakefulness.

Hope: To expect with confidence.

Hormones: Chemical messengers of the endocrine system.

Hospice care: A program to deliver palliative care to individuals in the final stages of a terminal illness; additionally provides personal support and care to the patient, and supports to the patient's family or caregivers while the patient is dying; provides bereavement support after the patient's death.

Hospital Elder Life Program: A program that aides in reducing falls in cognitively impaired older adults (particularly targeting prevention of delirium and functional decline).

Human needs theory: Maslow surmised that a hierarchy of five needs motivates human behavior: physiologic, safety and security, love and belonging, self-esteem, and self-actualization.

Humoral immunity: The branch of acquired immunity mediated by antibodies and responsible for defending the body against extracellular antigens.

Hwalek–Sengstock Elder Abuse Screening Test: A tool to use for screening for elder abuse or mistreatment.

Hyperactive form: Most recognized form of delirium that often manifests with psychomotor agitation and a plethora of psychiatric symptoms, such as confusion, hallucinations, or delusions.

Hypersomnias: A group of sleep disorders with the main symptom of daytime sleepiness unrelated to other causes of sleep disturbance such as circadian rhythm or sleep-related breathing disorders, including narcolepsy; recurrent and idiopathic hypersomnias; hypersomnias due to medical conditions, drugs, or substances; and behaviorally induced insufficient sleep syndrome.

Hypertension: Currently defined as a consistently elevated reading of 140/90 mm Hg.

Hypoactive form: Delirium characterized by a flat affect or apathy; may mimic stupor or coma; often present in otherwise calm and seemingly alert patients.

Hypogeusia: Age-related decline in taste.

Hypophysiotropic: Acting on the pituitary gland.

Hypopnea: A reduced airflow of 10 seconds or longer in duration.

Hypothalamic-pituitary-adrenal (HPA) axis: Regulates glucocorticoid levels in the body and allows the body to respond to stressful conditions.

Iatrogenic harm/iatrogenesis: Doctor- or healthcare-created harm.

Immigrant: An individual who moves into a country or region to settle there.

Immovable joints: Joints composed of collagen fibers that allow only minimal bone shifting; also known as fibrous joints.

Immunocompromise: A change or alteration of the immune system that normally fight off infections and other illnesses.

Immunomodulation: The effects of various chemical mediators, hormones, and drugs on the immune system.

Immunosenescence: Aging of the immune system.

Incompetence: Lacking competence; this is a judgment of the court and limits the person's legal rights.

Incontinence: Involuntary loss of stool or urine.

Independent living: Older adults caring for themselves, but can occur in a wide variety of settings from the home to senior living apartments or continuing care retirement communities.

Indian Health Service: An agency of the Department of Health and Human Services that provides health services to American Indians and Alaskan Natives. It now serves over 1.9 million American Indians and Alaskan Natives in 35 states.

Infection: Invasion of pathogens in a bodily part or tissue.

Inflammatory response: Redness, swelling, and warmth produced in response to infection.

Informed consent: A legally binding and voluntary decision regarding a proposed treatment based on information regarding the risks, benefits, and alternatives to a procedure or treatment.

Inhibin B: Glycoprotein that suppresses follicle-stimulating hormone.

Injury Severity Score: Descriptors of anatomic injury to describe injury severity; helps predict outcomes after injury.

Innate immunity: The branch of the immune system with which a person is born and that is the body's first line of defense against invading antigens.

In-patient rehabilitation facility: Acute 24 hour per day inpatient rehabilitation services in which patients qualify by being able to complete at least 3 hours of therapy per day.

Inpatient Rehabilitation Facility Patient Assessment Instrument: The data collection instrument completed upon admission to and discharge from inpatient rehabilitation facilities.

Insomnia: Repeated difficulty with sleep initiation, duration, consolidation, or quality despite adequate time and opportunity for sleep; it is associated with some form of daytime impairment.

Institute of Medicine: An independent, nonprofit organization that works outside of government to provide unbiased and authoritative advice to decision-makers and the public. The IOM asks and answers the nation's most pressing questions about health and health care.

Instrumental activities of daily living: Activities related to independent living; they include meal preparation, money management, shopping, housework, and using a telephone.

Insulin: A pancreatic hormone regulating blood glucose levels through stimulation of glucose uptake.

Insulin resistance: Resistance to the actions of insulin.

Interdisciplinary collaboration: When a team of professionals from different disciplines collaborates around common goals.

Interdisciplinary group/team: Professional staff and volunteers who focus on physical, emotional, psychological, social, and spiritual aspects of a person in designing and/or implementing holistic care; common in hospice and palliative care and other care settings. A team in which members of various disciplines interact, collaborate, and work together for common goals.

Intergenerational care: In the community, multiple generations receive ongoing services and/or programming at the same site and interact through planned activities.

Integrative health care: Coordinated, integrated, systematic, comprehensive care.

International models of health care: The healthcare delivery systems of countries in the world.

Internet: A vast collection of resources that includes people, information, and multimedia and is best characterized as the biggest labyrinth of computer networks on earth.

Interpretation: The oral conversion of verbal statement(s) said in one language to another language without adding, omitting, or distorting meaning.

Interprofessional team: Many diverse team members working together with common goals toward better patient outcomes.

Intractable pain: Chronic and persistent pain that can be psychogenic and not relieved by ordinary medical, surgical, and nursing measures.

Intradisciplinary team: A team in which members are within a discipline but members may be at different levels of preparation; may also refer to members of various disciplines working with similar patients, but not necessarily with common goals.

Intraocular pressure: The amount of pressure inside the eye; normal is 9 to 21 mm Hg.

Intrinsic risk factors: Factors that contribute to a fall that are related to a patient's physiology or current medical problems; anything the patient carries within his or her body.

Islets of Langerhans: Glandular cells of the pancreas.

Isolation: State of being alone or separated.

Joint Commission: An independent nonprofit organization that accredits healthcare organizations and programs in the United States.

Justice: Conformity to principles of what is right and fair; establishment of rights following rules of equity.

Keratinocytes: Cells of the epidermis that produce the protein keratin.

Ketones: Acetone bodies in the urine indicating inadequate management of diabetes mellitus.

Killer T cells: T cells that directly attack and destroy infected cells within the body; also termed cytotoxic T cells.

Korean War: June 27, 1950 through January 31, 1955.

Kotter's Change Model: A model that helps leaders generate positive feelings among employees toward change. It allows leaders to instill feelings of action in employees' hearts, by helping them envision the problem and identify solutions to the problem.

Lack of opportunities: Fewer opportunities to communicate with peers and loved ones that often comes with advancing age.

Landmarks in gerontological nursing: Key events in the development of the specialty of gerontological nursing.

Langerhans cells: Cells of the epidermis involved in immune response.

Language: The symbol system used by a shared group of people for communication.

Late-onset depression: Depression occurring for the first time in later life (after the age of 60); differs from early-onset (recurrent) depression, which is depression that occurs after the age of 60, but the individual has had a previous bout of depression at an earlier age.

Leaders: Visionaries who create the systems that managers manage and change them in fundamental ways to take advantage of opportunities and to avoid hazards.

Legal nurse consultant: A nurse expert who provides analysis and informed opinion on legal matters related to health care.

Leptin: Clinical predictor of nutritional status in the elderly.

Leukocytes: White blood cells.

Lexical memory: Ability to store words.

Liability: Any legally enforceable obligation.

Life expectancy: How long one can expect to live based on statistical probability; usually calculated at birth and at age 65.

Lifelong learning: Learning that occurs throughout life, motivated by situational and developmental periods.

Life review: An autobiographical effort that can be preserved in print, by tape recording, or on videotape.

Limited English Proficiency: Individuals who do not speak English as their primary language and who have a limited ability to read, speak, write, or understand English.

Lipofuscin: An undegradable material that decreases lysosomal function; age pigment. A brown pigment found in aging cells relating to oxidative mechanisms.

Literacy: Ability to read and understand.

Liver: The largest gland in the body; secretes bile in the small intestine and screens blood from the stomach and intestines for toxins.

Living will: A document that provides information about the types of treatment persons would or would not wish to have if they were unable to speak for themselves.

Longevity: A long life.

Long-term acute care hospitals: Hospitals that furnish extended medical and rehabilitative care to individuals with clinically complex problems, such as multiple acute or chronic conditions, who need hospital-level care for relatively extended periods.

Long-term care: A variety of services to help persons with personal or healthcare needs over a period of time; usually custodial care in a nursing home type facility.

Long-term care facility: Also known as a nursing home; a facility in which care is provided primarily for older adults or any persons who have lost some or all of their ability for self-care due to illness, disability, or advanced dementia.

Long-term memory: Memory that is much more expansive than short-term memory; there is no limit as to how long information can be stored there.

Luteinizing hormone: A hormone released from the pituitary that stimulates ovulation and corpus luteum growth in females; stimulates testosterone production in males.

Macrophage: An immune cell that acts as a scavenger, engulfing foreign substances, dead cells, and other debris through phagocytosis.

Macular degeneration: Loss of central vision, associated with aging; see also ARMD.

Major depression: A mood disorder characterized by an all-encompassing low mood accompanied by low self-esteem and by loss of interest or pleasure in normally enjoyable activities and hobbies.

Malnutrition: The state of being poorly nourished.

Malpractice: Failure to meet the standard of care that results in harm to the patient.

Managed care organizations: Created by insurance companies, MCOs are designed to limit the costs incurred by insurance companies through contracts with providers outlining the cost to the insurance company for services provided to a policy holder.

Maslow: Maslow surmised that a hierarchy of five needs motivates human behavior: physiologic, safety and security, love and belonging, self-esteem, and self-actualization.

Massage therapy: Manipulation of soft tissues in the body by kneading or other techniques.

Mauk model for poststroke recovery: A theoretical model derived using grounded theory methods that suggests a common process for stroke recovery and rehabilitation.

Mechanoreceptors: Receptors related to the ability to touch.

Medicaid: A government program first developed to provide care to the indigent elderly population. It was expanded to include women and children living below the poverty level, as well as individuals with disabilities. Benefits are all-inclusive, requiring the recipients to seek out providers who take patients receiving Medicaid. Medicaid is funded through state and federal governments.

Medical anthropology: A subfield of anthropology that draws upon social, cultural, biological, and linguistic anthropology to better understand factors that influence health and well-being (broadly defined), the experience and distribution of illness, the prevention and treatment of sickness, healing processes, the social relations of therapy management, and the cultural importance and utilization of pluralistic medical systems.

Medical interpreter: A trained staff member who is determined to have native knowledge of the target language and has undergone (typically) 45 hours of medical interpreter training to effectively provide verbal interpretation services in the healthcare field.

Medicare: A government program that pays for healthcare services for individuals over the age of 65, as well as for specific diagnoses to individuals who qualify. Benefits include acute care, outpatient services approved by the primary care physician, and hospice. Medicare also provides recipients with a drug program that includes an additional expense for recipients to be covered.

Medicare prevention: Preventive services covered by Medicare which may include an initial physical examination that includes prevention counseling, annual wellness visits, smoking cessation, comprehensive health programs that include complementary and alternative practices, screening and intensive behavioral therapy for obesity, depression screening, alcohol misuse counseling sessions.

Medication administration record: A strategy used to assess medication compliance; the patient (or family) lists the medications taken daily and tracks days 1 to 31 regarding what was taken at what time of day, including missed doses.

Medication-related problem (MRP): Drug-related problem that often results in negative outcomes and increased cost.

Meditation: A conscious process used to produce the relaxation response.

Mediterranean diet: This near-vegetarian diet is high on unrefined grains, potatoes, fruit, vegetables, fish, wine, and olive oil, and low on meat, cheese, refined sugar or flour, butter, and margarine.

Melanin: A pigment produced by melanocytes and essential to protecting the body against ultraviolet radiation.

Melanocytes: Cells located within the epidermis that produce melanin.

Melatonin: A hormone produced by the pineal gland that is linked to sleep and wake cycles.

Memory care: Units designed for seniors with Alzheimer's or other forms of dementia.

Meniere's syndrome: A common cause of vertigo in the elderly characterized by dizziness and tinnitus.

Menopause: Cessation of menstrual cycles within the aging female.

Mental health: State of mental well-being.

Meridian: Disease is seen as an imbalance between yin and yang; this imbalance impedes the flow of vital energy (*qi* or *chi*) and blood along pathways called meridians.

Metastasis: Spreading of cancer to other organs beyond the primary site.

Mid-upper arm circumference: A predictor of mortality in older adults living in long-term care facilities; the mid-point of the upper arm is measured with a tape measure placed snugly against the skin.

Mind–body medicine: Use of the powers of the mind to alter physical states in the body.

Mineralocorticoids: Hormones of the adrenal cortex involved in the regulation of extracellular mineral concentrations.

Minimum Data Set: Part of the U.S. federally mandated process for clinical assessment of all residents in Medicare- or Medicaid-certified nursing homes.

Minor depression: A mood disorder that does not meet full criteria for major depressive disorder but in which at least two depressive symptoms are present for 2 weeks.

Minority: Subgroup within a population. In social science, it is used to identify a group that suffers subordination and discrimination within a society, usually because of their race, ethnicity, or national origin. The term is used by the federal government to describe protected and/or disadvantaged ethnic or racial populations.

Mitochondria: Parts of a cell that transform organic compounds into energy.

Mixed form: Delirium that presents with both hyperactive and hypoactive features.

Mixed hearing loss: Both conductive and sensorineural hearing loss are present.

Mixed urinary incontinence: The existence of urge and stress urinary incontinence symptoms at the same time.

Model health promotion programs: Programs, often developed with federal funding, that promote the health and wellness of older adults.

Money Follows the Person: Transitional and community care, federal program that transitions eligible Medicaid recipients from nursing homes back to the community with community resources and services.

Monoaminergic system: Release of the neurotransmitters norepinephrine and serotonin.

Moral dilemma: Arises when two or more moral principles apply that support mutually inconsistent actions.

Moral distress: Occurs when someone wants to do the right thing but is limited by the constraints of the organization or society.

Moral injury: (The invisible wounds from war) that can also complicate a veteran's end of life.

Moral principles: Those values, ethics, beliefs, and positions that guide behavior and thought.

Moral sensitivity: Responsiveness to moral principles and morality.

Moral uncertainty: The confusion surrounding situations in which a person is uncertain what the moral problem is or which moral principles or values apply to it.

Morbidity: Related to incidence of illness.

Mortality: Death.

Motor unit: The combination of a single nerve and all the muscle fibers it innervates.

Mourning: The outward demonstration of a person's grief responses to a loss.

Moxibustion: A therapy of traditional Chinese medicine in which moxa floss is used to apply heat to certain points in the body.

Mucositis: Inflammation of the mucosa.

Multidisciplinary team: A team made up of members of various disciplines.

Muscle quality: Strength generated per unit of muscle mass.

Muscle strength: The capacity of muscle to generate force.

Music therapy: Use of music to enhance physical and psychological well-being.

Myelosuppression: The decrease in the production of blood cells.

Myocardial cells: Cells located in the heart; also known as cardiomyocytes.

Myocardial infarction: Heart attack.

Myofascial: Muscle pain.

Myofibril: A contractile filament that comprises skeletal muscle fibers; composed of actin and myosin proteins.

Myosin: Protein within muscle that, together with actin, is responsible for muscle contraction.

Myth: Thought that evidence-informed research notes are false.

Nasogastric tube: A commonly used method of short-term enteral feeding in which a tube is passed through the nares into the stomach as a means to provide nutrition.

National Pressure Ulcer Advisory Panel: An expert group convened to develop a common classification systems for pressure ulcers.

National Quality Forum: A not-for-profit, nonpartisan organization committed to improving the quality of health care in the United States.

National Quality Strategy: The national effort to get stakeholders to work together to achieve better health and healthcare for all Americans. It was mandated by the Patient Protection and Affordable Care Act.

National Transitions of Care Coalition (NTOCC): Transitional care tools and resources for providers, consumers, and caregivers.

Native American: Those original Americans from over 500 tribes within the United States, and nearly half of these 2.4 million people reside in the western part of the country due to forced migration. The two predominant tribes are the Cherokee and the Navajo, each with more than a quarter million people.

Native-born: A citizen at birth.

Naturally occurring retirement community: Living communities specifically for older adults. Most are duplexes, condominiums, apartments, trailers, or single-family homes that are all located in the same neighborhood.

Natural killer (NK) cells: Cells of the immune system that attack and destroy infected cells.

Natural products: A category of complementary health approaches that includes herbs, proteins, probiotics, vitamins, minerals, fatty acids, and whole diets.

Naturopathic medicine: A variety of healing practices that support the body to heal itself.

Nausea and vomiting: Symptoms of gastric upset and expelling gastric contents.

Negligence: is deviation of accepted practice, a wrongful act, or failure to act by a healthcare professional, usually due to lack of knowledge or skill or poor judgment in application of the knowledge and skill.

Nephrons: Located in the kidneys; combination of the Bowman's capsule and renal tubule with the glomerulus.

Nerve cells: Neurons within the nervous system that transmit chemical and electrical signals.

Neurofibrillary tangles: Collections of twisted tau found in the cell bodies of neurons; a symptom of Alzheimer's disease.

Neurogenesis: Formation of new neurons.

Neuropathic: A pathological change in the central or peripheral nervous system.

Neurotransmitters: Substances that carry nerve impulses across nerve synapses, such as norepinephrine.

Next Step in Care: Transitional care; eight easy-to-use guides to help family caregivers and providers plan and implement transitions.

Nociceptive: The process of detection and signaling the presence of a noxious stimulus.

Nocturia: The awakening from sleep to urinate more than once during the night.

Nondeclarative memory: Includes motor skills, cognitive skills, reflex responses, priming, and condition responses.

Non-Hispanic white: Those who are of the white race and are not of Hispanic or Latino origin/ethnicity.

Nonmaleficence: Not committing harm or evil.

Non-rapid eye movement sleep: Refers to stages N1 through N3 of sleep.

Nonrestraint fall prevention interventions: Behavioral interventions in persons with agitation, having family or a sitter stay at bedside of high-risk fallers or those with cognitive impairment or moving a patient closer to the nurse's station.

Nonstochastic theories of aging: Theories stating that a series of genetically programmed events occur to all organisms with aging.

Nonverbal communication: Includes tone of voice and physical behaviors such as body language and eye contact.

Norepinephrine: A catecholamine of the adrenal medulla that regulates the stress response; also known as noradrenaline.

Nurse delegation: The National Council of State Board of Nurses addresses the circumstances under which a licensed nurse delegates a nursing function to an unlicensed person to carry out specific activities.

Nurse manager: Nurse who acts as administrative manager of a unit.

Nurse Manager Leadership Partnership Learning Domain Framework: Describes essential functions of nurse managers and outlines opportunities that may be useful to achieve mastery of these functions. The framework includes three domains: (1) the leader within: creating the leader in yourself; (2) the art of leadership: leading people; and (3) the science of leadership: managing the business.

Nurses Improving Care for the Hospitalized Elderly: In the hospital, tools and processes to educate nursing staff in specialized care of the hospitalized older adults.

Nursing home: A facility that provides daily help for residents with physical or other problems who are unable to live on their own.

Nursing informatics: A blending of computer, information, and nursing science designed to assist in the management and processing of nursing data, information, and knowledge to support the practice of nursing and the delivery of nursing care.

Nutrition: One component in the development and exacerbation of disease related to dietary practices and habits.

Nutrition bull's eye: Goal is for people to consume the nutritious foods that are listed in the center of the bull's-eye. These foods are low in saturated fat, sugar, and sodium, and high in fiber.

Nutrition Screening Initiative: A multidisciplinary effort led by the American Academy of Family Physicians and the American Dietetic Association to promote the integration of nutrition screening and dietary interventions into health care for the elderly.

Obsessive-compulsive disorder: Constant thoughts or fears that cause the individual to perform certain rituals repeatedly or follow certain routines. The disturbing thoughts are obsessive, and the routines or rituals are called compulsions. An example is a person with an unreasonable fear of germs who will not touch another person, washes his or her hands repeatedly, or uses only plastic utensils (never using a utensil that another person has touched to eat).

Obstructive sleep apnea: A breathing disorder in which breathing repeatedly stops and starts during sleep.

Older adult: Person over the age of 65 years.

Oldest old: Someone 85 years of age or older.

Olfaction: The ability to smell.

Oncologic emergency: An urgent, immediate event that results in medical care.

Orientation: A function of memory and involves awareness of the dimensions of person, place, and time.

Oropharyngeal dysphagia: Trouble swallowing usually related to neuromuscular impairments affecting the tongue, pharynx, and upper esophageal sphincter.

Osteoarthritis: Deterioration of joints and vertebrae as a consequence of wear and tear.

Osteoblast: Bone cell responsible for formation of new bone and repair of damaged or broken bone.

Osteoclast: Bone cell responsible for bone resorption.

Osteocyte: Dormant osteoblast embedded in bone matrix.

Osteoporosis: Demineralization of the bones; decreased bone density.

Otoconia: "Stones" in the ear canal that affect balance.

Otosclerosis: Damage to the inner ear of unknown cause that leads to progressive deafness.

Outcome and Assessment Information Set: Data collection instrument required by home health agencies for reimbursement.

Overflow incontinence: Incontinence that occurs because the bladder has not been emptied and has become overdistended.

Pacific Islanders: Persons from the area that consists of three distinct island groups in the Pacific Ocean: Micronesia, Melanesia, and Polynesia.

Pain: An unpleasant sensory and emotional experience associated with actual or potential tissue damage or described in terms of such damage.

Pain scales: Measurement options by which medical personnel can translate a person's self-assessment of pain for appropriate intervention decisions.

Palliative and hospice care team: A team whose focus is comfort and/or end of life care.

Palliative care: Concept of care designed to promote comfort and holistic management of symptoms at any stage of illness or disease.

Pancreas: A gland located below the stomach and above the small intestine; secretes pancreatic fluid that neutralizes stomach acid and breaks down large nutrients.

Panic attack: Feelings of terror that strike suddenly and repeatedly with no warning. Symptoms can include extreme nervousness, increased heart rate, increased blood pressure, sweating, chest pain, palpitations (irregular heartbeats), and a feeling of smothering or choking that may make the person feel like he or she is having a heart attack or "going crazy."

Paranoia: False thoughts that others are conspiring against one's self; unfounded mistrust of others.

Parasomnias: Undesirable physical events or experiences that occur during entry into sleep, within sleep, or during arousals from sleep.

Parathyroid gland: A group of cells located at the back of the thyroid gland that secretes parathyroid hormone.

Parathyroid hormone: A hormone of the parathyroid gland involved in promoting elevation of blood calcium levels.

Parkinson's disease: A neurological disorder characterized by lack of dopamine in the brain secondary to loss of neurons in the basal ganglia.

Partnering communication: Involves a person-centered approach such as the 5Ps, being respectful, and being flexible to accomplish all that is needed for the patient. It allows patients to participate in their own care as well as partnering with them for the care they must provide to the patient.

Pathophysiology: The study of the changes of normal mechanical, physiological, and biochemical functions, either caused by a disease or resulting from an abnormal syndrome.

Patient-centered communication: Consistent and clear communication between patient and clinician in which the patient is at the center.

Patient Protection and Affordable Care Act of 2010: Also known as Obamacare, a comprehensive health reform law signed into law in 2010 in response to the need for healthcare reform. The intention of the Affordable Care Act was to provide affordable health care to enhance quality of life for all Americans.

Patient rights: Rights to which patients are entitled; usually defined or described by the organization charged with providing care or protecting patients.

Pedagogy: Principles of teaching.

Pelvic floor muscle exercises: Muscle exercises, often called Kegel exercises, that strengthen the pelvic floor and are often used for the treatment of urinary incontinence.

Pelvic muscle rehabilitation: An exercise program designed to increase the strength, tone, and control of the pelvic floor muscles to facilitate a person's ability to voluntarily control the flow of urine and suppress urgency.

Percutaneous endoscopic gastrostomy: Invasive insertion of a feeding tube through the anterior abdominal wall to provide a vehicle for nutrition.

Periodic limb movements of sleep: Repetitive, highly stereotyped, limb movements that occur during sleep.

Peripheral artery disease: A problem with blood flow in the arteries due to blockage or narrowing.

Peripheral neuropathy: A disorder of peripheral nerves in which symptoms (most often in the lower extremities) are often described as numbing, tingling, burning, and painful.

Peripheral vascular disease: The most common form of peripheral artery disease.

Personal amplification device: Devices that aid in hearing; can be developed to account for individual hearing loss.

Person-first language: Person-centered communication (such as "the person with diabetes" versus "the diabetic").

Personhood: The status of being a person; being human.

Pet-assisted therapy: Use of animals to decrease stress and increase feelings of well-being.

Phantom limb pain: Pain in an absent or amputated extremity.

Pharmacodynamics: How drugs work in the body and a person's ability to manage medications.

Pharmacogenomics: A genetic, set-at-birth capacity to metabolize medications through numerous different pathways, each one working at a different rate in different people.

Pharmacokinetics: How drugs are absorbed, metabolized, and eliminated.

Pharynx: Connects the oral cavity to the esophagus.

Photoaging: The process of change in skin structure and function resulting only from exposure to ultraviolet radiation.

Physical abuse: The use of physical force to purposefully inflict pain or harm to another. Direct abuse includes assault and aggressive violence such as hitting, kicking, biting, punching, pushing, shoving, burning, restraining, overmedicating, and slapping. Sexual assault and rape are also included in this category

Physical dependence: A state of adaptation that is manifested by a drug class–specific withdrawal syndrome that can be produced by abrupt cessation, rapid dose reduction, decreasing blood level of the drug, and/or administration of an antagonist.

Physical restraint: Any manual method, physical or mechanical device, material, or equipment that immobilizes or reduces the ability of a patient to move his or her arms, legs, body, or head freely.

Physician's Orders for Life-Sustaining Treatment: A document that states what type of care a person wants at the end of life.

Pig in a python: A descriptor of the Baby Boomers, as if they were a large lump inside a snake that is slowly moving along toward the tail; in other words, a bulge in population moving slowly through time.

Pineal gland: A small gland located deep in the brain that secretes melatonin.

Pioneer Network: A nonprofit organization formed in 1997 to advocate for person-directed care in long-term care.

Plaques: Made up of the amyloid beta-peptide shown to be neurotoxic; occur outside of the neuronal cell and consist of gray matter with a protein core surrounded by abnormal neurites.

Plasma cell: An antibody-producing B cell.

Plasticity: The ability to form new neuronal connections onto available existing neurons.

Pluripotent stem cells: Cells possessing the ability to differentiate into cells of any other type.

Polydipsia: Excessive thirst.

Polyphagia: Excessive eating.

Polypharmacy: Concurrent use of multiple medications.

Polysomnography: The monitoring of sleep in detail (as in an overnight sleep study).

Polyuria: Excessive urination.

Postacute care: Care provided after inpatient acute care; may include skilled care, rehabilitation, long-term care.

Posttraumatic stress disorder: A severe anxiety disorder that develops after exposure to any significant traumatic event.

Potentially avoidable hospitalization: Hospitalizations that may not have been necessary if certain acute conditions and exacerbations of chronic illness had been identified and treated successfully in the primary care setting.

Power of attorney: Someone designated to make treatment decisions when a person is unable to express his or her wishes.

Prayer: A conversation with a higher being.

Prealbumin: A hepatic protein that may indicate a more recent change in nutritional status.

Precipitating factors: Those events or conditions that occur during hospitalization to trigger a delirium.

Predisposing factors: Those baseline vulnerabilities that are possessed by the patient prior to hospitalization.

Presbycusis: Age-related hearing loss that generally occurs at higher frequencies first.

Presbyopia: Age-related vision loss of objects at close range; known as farsightedness.

Prescribing cascade: When medication side effects are treated with other medications.

Pressure injury: Formerly known as pressure ulcers, but now encompassing deep tissue injury as well as wounds and other damage from excess pressure.

Pressure redistribution: The ability of a support surface to distribute load over the contact areas of the human body to reduce the overall pressure and avoid areas of focal pressure.

Pressure ulcer: "A pressure ulcer is localized injury to the skin and/or underlying tissue usually over a bony prominence, as a result of pressure, or pressure in combination with shear. A number of contributing or confounding factors are also associated with pressure ulcers; the significance of these factors is yet to be elucidated" (National Pressure Ulcer Advisory Panel [NPUAP] and European Pressure Ulcer Advisory Panel [EPUAP], 2009, p. 7).

Pressure ulcer management: Includes nursing assessment, accurate staging (classification) of the pressure ulcer, and documentation of the onset and assessed stage.

Pressure ulcer risk assessment: Evaluating for risk factors for pressure ulcer development, including advanced age; immobility; malnutrition; incontinence; diminished level of consciousness; impaired sensation; history of pressure ulcers; multiple comorbidities such as diabetes, chronic obstructive pulmonary disease, renal disease, and arterial and vascular disease; medication history; and previous treatment with steroids, radiation, or chemotherapy.

Pressure ulcer staging system: Developed by the NPUAP to provide a common classification for wounds and pressure ulcers.

Preventable hospital readmission: Readmissions that occur within 30 days of hospital discharge possibly related to inadequate quality of care in hospital or lack of appropriate coordination of postdischarge care.

Primary prevention: Activities designed to completely prevent a disease from occurring, such as immunization against pneumonia or influenza.

Private insurance: Coverage by a health plan that is not government provided, but rather provided through an employer or union or purchased by an individual from a private health insurer.

Proactive intervention: Vital energy that cannot be measured.

Programs of All-Inclusive Care for the Elderly: In-community, Medicare and Medicaid program that utilizes an interprofessional team that assesses, plans, implements, and monitors interventions for the older adult.

Proliferative retinopathy: The fourth and most advanced stage of diabetic retinopathy in which abnormal and fragile vessels develop to compensate for blocked blood flow to the retina; this leads to visual disturbances and often blindness.

Prompted voiding: A scheduled intervention aimed at helping the individual recognize and act effectively on the sensation of the need to void.

Prospective payment system: A method of reimbursement used by Medicare based on a predetermined fixed amount. Payment for a specific service is based on a classification system for that service. For example, reimbursement to an acute care hospital would be based on the patient's DRGs.

Prostate-specific antigen: A serum screening test for prostate cancer.

Proton pump inhibitors: Medications used to treat GERD, including include omeprazole, lansoprazole, rabeprazole, pantoprazole, and esomeprazole.

Psychological or emotional abuse: The infliction of anguish, pain, or distress through verbal or nonverbal acts.

Psychological or emotional neglect: Not providing for physical or emotional needs of an elder; may be present when a person receives good or adequate physical care, but is socially isolated.

Public policy: Programs and policies developed by the government in response to the needs of the members of the society that have been identified by the government or another entity.

Qi (chi): The circulating life energy that in Chinese philosophy is thought to be inherent in all things.

Qigong: A traditional Chinese medicine practice that uses physical activity and meditation to encourage the free flow of energy (qi) through the body

Quality of life: An individual's perception about the value and benefits of life.

Quality and Safety Education for Nurses: Competencies for safety and quality for nursing. These are based on the IOM competencies which provide a foundation for a culture of quality and safety.

Radiation therapy: Cancer treatment that uses special equipment to provide a precise dose of radiation to the tumor.

Radical prostatectomy: Surgical removal of the prostate as a treatment for cancer.

Radicular: Pertaining to a nerve root.

Rapid eye movement sleep: Refers to stage R of sleep, which is characterized by rapid eye movements and muscle atonia.

Reactive oxygen species: Short-lived, highly reactive products of mitochondrial oxidative metabolism that destroy proteins, lipids, and nucleic acids.

Reciprocity: Referring to a mutual exchange of privileges, such as the ability to be true to one's self while respecting and supporting the values and views of another.

Reiki: Holistic Japanese technique of stress reduction in which life force energy is transferred to the client through the practitioner's hands.

Relational teaching: Style of instruction having many levels, from a toxic to a powerfully life-sustaining relationship; the latter takes a deep understanding of self on the part of the instructor

Relaxation techniques: A group of complementary health approaches that produce the body's relaxation response. Included are breathing exercises, guided imagery, progressive, muscle relaxation, self-hypnosis.

Religiosity: Refers to believing in a god, organized rituals, and specific dogma, related to a superior being.

REM behavior disorder: A parasomnia characterized by abnormal behaviors emerging during REM sleep that cause injury or sleep disruption.

Replicative senescence: A phenomenon in which cells are able to undergo only a finite number of divisions.

Reproductive axis: Integration of the hypothalamus, pituitary, and gonad to control reproductive hormones.

Resource utilization groups: Categories to determine reimbursement. The RUG scores are based on data collected from resident assessments (MDS 3.0), staffing data, and geographic location.

Respite care: Services that provide a break for caregivers by providing care in the home or a facility.

Respondeat superior: Transfers the liability to the employer, who then becomes the principal from whom the accuser hopes to recover a perceived loss.

Restless legs syndrome: A sensorimotor disorder characterized by a complaint of a strong, nearly irresistible, urge to move the legs.

Restorative strategies: Interventions that address rebuilding skills that are impaired.

Retinal detachment: Situation in which the retina becomes displaced due to trauma or illness and requires immediate medical attention to restore vision.

Revised Trauma Score: A tool to help identify physiological response to injury. An essential process that enables the facility to identify sources of loss, financial risk, and potential for liability.

Sadness: Mood associated with, or characterized by, feelings of loss, despair, helplessness, sorrow, fear, and rage.

Safety promotion: Activities and strategies focusing on increasing safety and preventing injury.

Sanctity of life: The belief that all life is of value and that this value is not based on how functional or effective a person's life is, but rather that all have a right to life.

Sarcomere: Muscle compartments containing actin and myosin.

Sarcopenia: Age-related loss of muscle mass.

Sarcoplasmic reticulum: A portion of the endoplasmic reticulum; membrane network in the cell cytoplasm in striated muscle fibers.

Scatter laser treatment: Treatment for diabetic retinopathy in which a laser burns abnormal vessels away from the retina to reduce further vision loss.

Scaffolding Theory of Aging and Cognition: A process in which the individual's brain recruits additional neuron connections for maintaining memory and decoding what has been observed.

Secondary prevention: Efforts directed toward early detection and management of disease, such as the use of colonoscopy to detect small cancerous polyps.

Selective serotonin reuptake inhibitors: A psychiatric medication used to alleviate mood disorders in the class of antidepressants. SSRIs are called selective because they primarily affect serotonin, not the other neurotransmitters.

Selective serotonin-norepinephrine reuptake inhibitors: A psychiatric medication used to alleviate mood disorders in the class of antidepressants. SNRIs block the reabsorption (reuptake) of the neurotransmitters serotonin and norepinephrine in the brain.

Self-neglect: A behavior in which a person neglects to attend to basic needs, such as personal hygiene (bathing and grooming), appropriate clothing, eating, or neglecting to care for their medical conditions.

Semantic memory: Concept memory.

Senescence: The process of growing old.

Senior citizen: Those age 65 years and older.

Sensorineural hearing loss: Damage that occurs in the inner ear and/or auditory nerve fiber.

Servant leadership: Focus is on the leader meeting the needs of the followers before the needs of the leader or the organization are met.

Sexual abuse: Nonconsensual sexual contact of any kind such as touching, rape, unwanted sexual photography and the like

Sexual intimacy: Closeness experienced through acts related to sex.

Sexuality: The total experience of being a sexual being; more than sexual intercourse.

Short-term memory: Memory that is limited in capacity and information remains for only a few seconds.

Silver tsunami: Term referring to the large wave of older adults reaching older age as Baby Boomers retire.

Skeletal muscle: Muscle under voluntary control; comprises the majority of all muscle mass and is also known as voluntary or striated muscle.

Skilled nursing facility: A facility that provides skilled, professional medical, nursing, and therapy care according to the CMS guidelines and regulations.

Sleep architecture: Refers to the different stages of sleep and their relative amounts within the sleep cycle and to timing of the sleep cycle.

Sleep cycle: The combination of NREM and REM stages of sleep, usually a period of 90 to 110 minutes duration, occurring three to five times per night.

Sleep efficiency: The time spent asleep during the time spent in bed attempting to sleep; calculated as total sleep time $\times$ 100/time in bed and expressed as a percentage.

Sleep fragmentation: Systematic disturbance of the cumulative sleep process by brief periodic arousals, resulting in reduced restoration similar to that found following sleep deprivation.

Sleep quality: Variously defined, but often refers to the subjective perception of feeling rested or restored upon waking.

Sleep-related breathing disorders: Syndromes characterized by disordered respiration during sleep, including central and obstructive sleep apnea syndromes, as well as sleep-related hypoventilation syndromes.

Sleep-wake disorders: Alterations of the sleep-wake cycle, often resulting in lack of quality sleep.

Slow-twitch fibers: Muscle fibers that contract steadily but are not easily fatigued; used in activities of low intensity and high endurance.

Smart homes: Assistive domotics, which is an application of home automation that focuses on enabling older adults or disabled persons to live at their home instead of a healthcare facility.

Social determinants of health: The conditions in which people are born, grow, live, work, and age, including the health system.

Social networks: Social engagements that provide support and socialization.

Social policy: Programs and policies that affect members of a society through how goods and services are distributed among members of that society. The intent of social policy is to improve each individual's access to food, shelter, education, and health care.

Social Security: A federal program that provides financial assistance to the elderly and disabled; federal "old age" pension program.

Somatic: Pertaining to the body wall, in contrast to the viscera.

Sound energy therapy: Use of sound frequencies to facilitate healing.

Speech: Production of sounds used for communication.

Spiritual assessment: An integral part of comprehensive assessment, this is a dynamic record of the client's core values and beliefs based on personal philosophy and meanings.

Spiritual baseline assessment: The initial documentation about the client's values and beliefs based on personal philosophy, understanding, and meaning of life.

Spirituality: The feeling of connectedness with something higher than one's self, whether it be a god, nature, or another being.

Spiritual resources: Internal and external assistance utilized to support efforts toward meeting optimal level of spiritual functioning.

Spiritually centric: Taking the perspective that everyone else shares the same meaning and practice of spirituality as I do, because my spirituality is the only correct one.

Spiritual well-being: Wellness or health of all the inner resources of a person, which is the ultimate concern around which all other values (of the individual) are focused.

Staging: The objective description of the extent of the disease and the determination of whether the person's cancer has spread.

Standards of care: The degree of care that can be expected of a reasonably prudent person of the same profession in a similar situation.

Stakeholders in policy formation: Individuals who influence or are influenced by the creation of a policy.

START criteria: Screening Tool to Alert doctors to the Right Treatment.

Stem cell progenitors: The progeny cells of pluripotent stem cells.

Stereotype: A simplified standardized conception, image, opinion, or belief about a person or group.

Stochastic theories of aging: Theories stating that random events occurring in one's life cause damage that accumulates with aging.

STOPP criteria: Screening Tool of Older People's potentially inappropriate Prescriptions.

STRATIFY scale: Evidence based risk assessment tool (STRATIFY) to predict which elderly inpatients will fall.

Stress incontinence: Leaking of urine occurs during activities that increase abdominal pressure, such as laughing, sneezing, and exercising.

Stroke: An interruption of the blood supply to the brain.

Subcutaneous layer: The innermost layer of the skin.

Substance-induced anxiety disorder: A mood disorder in which a person exhibits anxious symptoms. Symptoms may include irritability, nervousness, apprehension, or fear.

Successful aging: Includes not only maintaining physical, cognitive, and functional abilities, but also maintaining engagement with others through communication.

Suicidal ideation: Thoughts about suicide that may be as detailed as a formulated plan, without the suicidal act itself.

Suicide: The act of intentionally causing one's own death.

SUPPORT study: The Study to Understand Prognoses and Preferences for Outcomes and Risks of Treatment; it revealed deficiencies in care and treatment of the terminally ill in U.S. medical practices.

Suppressor T cells: T cells that suppress the immune response.

Suprachiasmatic nucleus: The primary circadian rhythm pacemaker (in humans).

Survivor: A person living from the time of a cancer diagnosis for the balance of life.

Survivorship: The survivor is in the transition from active treatment to surveillance care.

Symptom management: Focus on promotion of comfort and alleviation of a variety of symptoms.

Symptoms: Characteristics signs of disease or illness.

Synapses: Space between the dendrites on neurons where chemical signals via neurotransmitters are relayed to other neurons.

Synaptogenesis: Generation of new synapses.

Synovial fluid: Fluid secreted by the synovium that allows smooth, easy movement of the bones comprising a synovial joint.

Synovial joint: Joint connecting two bones containing smooth cartilage on their opposing ends.

Synovium: Synovial joint capsule membrane that secretes synovial fluid.

Systole: Contraction of the heart that forces blood into the aorta.

T cells: Cells of the immune system that mature in the thymus and play a critical role in cell-mediated immunity.

Tai Chi: A martial art comprised of slow and flowing movements combined with meditation; improves balance and motion

T-helper cells: T cells that regulate the immune system.

Tangles: Paired helical filaments and a few straight filaments that occur in the neuronal cell body; the main protein associated with neurofibrillary tangles is known as tau.

Task talk: Nurse–patient conversations in healthcare settings in which heavy workloads and staffing shortages contribute to the communication with patients being almost exclusively about care tasks.

Teach-back method: After providing health information, have patients repeat back what information they have received.

Telomerase: An enzyme that regulates chromosomal aging by its action on telomeres.

Telomere: Repeated sequences of DNA that protect the tips of the outermost appendages of the chromosome arms.

Tertiary prevention: Efforts used to manage clinical diseases in order to prevent them from progressing or to avoid complications of the disease, as is done when beta-blockers are used to help remodel the heart in congestive heart failure.

Theory of adult learning: Developed by Malcolm Knowles, applies principles to enhance learning in adults over 18 years old who have completed mandatory public education.

Theory of self-efficacy: The belief that one's actions influence outcomes; self-efficacy and outcomes expectations affect behavior, motivation, thought patterns, and emotions.

Therapeutic (healing) touch: Movement of the practitioner's hands over a patient's body to balance its energy fields.

Thrombocytes: Blood platelets responsible for blood clotting.

Thrombocytopenia: An inadequate number of platelets.

Thyroid: A small, butterfly-shaped gland located in the lower front portion of the neck.

Thyroid-stimulating hormone: A pituitary hormone stimulating the synthesis and release of triiodothyronine and thyroxine.

Thyroxine: A thyroid hormone involved in metabolic and thermal regulation.

Timed Up and Go Test: A simple and reliable test for mobility.

Tinnitus: Ringing in the ears.

Titration: The gradual increase or decrease of medication to reduce or eliminate pain while allowing the body to accommodate the side effects or toxicity.

Tolerance: A state of adaptation in which exposure to a drug induces changes that result in a diminution of one or more of the drug's effects over time.

Tonometer: An instrument used to measure intraocular pressure.

Total lung capacity: The maximum volume to which the lungs can expand during the greatest inspiratory effort.

Total sleep time: The total minutes of sleep, including all stages of NREM plus REM sleep.

t-PA (tissue plasminogen activator): Used to treat acute ischemic stroke.

Trabecular bone: The inner portion of bone; also known as spongy bone.

Traditional Chinese Medicine: The medical system that balances the opposing forces of yin and yang.

Transactional leadership: Style in which leaders seek to engage individuals in the recognition and pursuit of a commonly held goal.

Transcultural: A term used widely in nursing to apply to people of diverse cultures.

Transformational or charismatic leadership: Transformational leaders seeking to attain a collective goal for the organization and stimulating innovative thinking to transform followers' beliefs. They understand the need for change in the organization and clearly communicate the vision to achieve the change.

Transforming Care at the Bedside: In-hospital care model to improve the quality of care for patients discharged from medical and surgical units *within* hospitals, discharged from the hospital to home, or discharged to another healthcare facility.

Transient (acute) urinary incontinence: Incontinence caused by the onset of an acute problem that once successfully treated will result in resolution of the incontinence.

Transient ischemic attack: Stroke symptoms that last from minutes to less than 24 hours with no residual effects.

Transitional care: Care that facilitates the move between healthcare settings with an emphasis on self-care.

Transitional Care Model: Patient-centered care model to improve quality of life, increase patient satisfaction, and reduce hospital readmissions (Naylor).

Transitional care unit: Facilitates the move among healthcare settings with an emphasis on self-care.

Translation: The most accurate, written conversion of a written document from one language into another without adding, omitting, or distorting meaning.

Transurethral resection of the prostate: Surgical intervention for benign prostatic hyperplasia.

Treatment options: The range of interventions available.

Triage: Meaning "to sort" a system of classification of severity of illness, injury, or trauma.

Triceps skin fold: Measured using a skin fold caliper by measuring the mid-point between the acromion process and the olecranon process of the upper arm; reflects fat stores.

Triiodothyronine: A thyroid hormone involved in metabolic and thermal regulation.

Triphasic model of human sexual response: Three phases of sexual response: excitement, plateau, and orgasm.

Tuberculosis: Disease caused by *Mycobacterium tuberculosis*; can affect any body part, but particularly the lungs.

Ureters: Tubes connecting the kidneys to the bladder.

Urethra: Canal that leads from the bladder out of the body.

Urge suppression techniques: Strategies that help control bladder contractions and therefore minimize or resolve urgency.

Urge urinary incontinence: Associated with a strong, abrupt desire to void and the inability to inhibit leakage before reaching the toilet.

Urinary tract infection: Bacterial invasion of the bladder or urinary tract.

Urostomy: Stoma through which urine passes into a receptacle on the outside of the body; used when the bladder has been removed.

U.S. Preventive Services Task Force: A task force convened by the U.S. Public Health Service to systematically review the evidence of effectiveness of clinical preventive services. Its mission is to evaluate the benefits of individual services and to create age-, gender-, and risk-based recommendations about services that should routinely be incorporated into primary medical care.

Values: Beliefs and attitudes that reflect a person's thoughts and culture.

Vasopressin: A pituitary hormone responsible for regulation of blood and osmotic pressure.

Ventilatory rate: The volume of air inspired in a normal breath multiplied by the frequency of breaths per minute; also known as the minute respiratory rate.

Ventricles: The two lower chambers of the heart; the left ventricle expels oxygen-rich blood into the aorta to be delivered to the entire body, excluding the lungs, and the right ventricle expels oxygen-poor blood into pulmonary arteries traveling to the lungs for reoxygenation.

Veracity: To tell the truth.

Verbal communication: Relies on knowledge of a common language as well as the ability to produce words.

Veritable energy field: Energy that can be measured.

Veteran: A person who has served active duty in the armed forces (41.9% of persons over 65 years of age).

Veterans Administration: An agency of the federal government that provides benefits and services to veterans as well as survivors of veterans. The Veterans Administration operates acute care centers, clinics, and long-term care facilities across the United States that provide medical, surgical, and rehabilitation services.

Vicarious liability: A legal relationship between two entities, such as an employer and employee or independent contractor, where liability is shared.

Vietnamese: Immigrants from Vietnam, Laos, Cambodia, and Hmong (the mountainous regions of China, Vietnam, Laos, and Thailand).

Vietnam War: August 5, 1964 (February 28, 1961, for Veterans who served "in country" before August 5, 1964), through May 7, 1975.

Violation of personal rights: Failure to acknowledge and enforce the rights of a competent older adult.

Visceral: Pertaining to a bodily organ.

Vital capacity: The maximum amount of air that can be expelled from the lungs following a maximum inspiration.

Vitrectomy: Evacuation of the vitreous humor to remove blood that has leaked from damaged vessels in diabetic retinopathy.

Wandering: Tendency to walk around that may result in elopement; a common symptom in individuals with cognitive impairment, including delirium and dementia.

Weight loss: A decrease in body weight; can be predictive of mortality in older adults.

Wernicke's aphasia: Difficulty comprehending speech; fluent and rhythmic but lacks meaning.

Whole medical systems: Complete systems of diagnosis and practice.

Working memory: Memory that includes executive functions such as planning, attention, inhibition, encoding, and monitoring.

World War II: December 7, 1941 through December 31, 1946.

World Wide Web: A system of clients (Web browsers or software applications used to locate and display Web pages) and servers that use the Internet for data exchange.

Yang: Half of the principle of opposites; it represents the bright, active, upward, hot, male force in traditional Chinese medicine.

Yin: Half of the principle of opposites; it represents the cold, dark, weak, female force in traditional Chinese medicine.

Index

Note: Page numbers followed by *b*, *f*, or *t* indicate material in boxes, figures, or tables, respectively.